Hospital
Infections

# HOSPITAL INFECTIONS

## Second Edition

EDITED BY

John V. Bennett, M.D.
*Assistant Director for Medical Science, Center for Infectious Diseases, Centers for Disease Control, U.S. Public Health Service, Atlanta*

Philip S. Brachman, M.D.
*Director, Global EIS Program, Centers for Disease Control, U.S. Public Health Service; Clinical Professor of Community Health, Emory University School of Medicine, Atlanta*

Foreword by
Maxwell Finland, M.D.
*Professor Emeritus of Medicine, Harvard Medical School; Hospital Epidemiologist, Boston City Hospital, Boston*

Donald E. Craven, M.D.
*Associate Professor of Medicine, Boston University School of Medicine; Hospital Epidemiologist, Boston City Hospital, Boston*

Foreword by
William A. Altemeier, M.D.[†]
*Formerly Professor and Chairman, Department of Surgery, University of Cincinnati College of Medicine, Cincinnati*
[†]Deceased

LITTLE, BROWN AND COMPANY
BOSTON/TORONTO

Library of Congress Catalog Card No. 85-81300

ISBN 0-316-08990-7

Printed in the United States of America

MV

# CONTENTS

## II.  ENDEMIC AND EPIDEMIC HOSPITAL INFECTIONS

# FOREWORD

In the introduction to their book *The Control of Infections in Hospitals* (1966), LeRiche and co-workers date the beginnings of hospitals, as an expression of charity, to A.D. 325 when the bishops at the Council of Nicaea were instructed to provide a hospital in every cathedral city. For more than half a millennium, hospitals mixed all patients within their wards, including those convalescing from, or still ill with, active and terminal infections. Thus, the prevalent plagues—cholera, smallpox, typhoid fever, and others—were introduced and spread to those not already dying of other causes. In addition, infections of surgical wounds were almost inevitable, and most of them were fatal. In the middle of the nineteenth century, James Simpson reported that the mortality rate following amputations was four times higher in hospitalized patients compared to those who remained at home and was directly proportional to the size of the hospital.

In 1843, Oliver Wendell Holmes, in his classic paper *On the Contagiousness of Childbed Fever,* postulated that puerperal infections were spread physically to parturient women by physicians from infected materials in autopsies they had performed or from infected women they had attended. A few years later, Ignaz P. Semmelweis published his epochal findings on puerperal fever, which showed that women delivered by physicians were infected four times as often as those delivered at home by midwives, and that hospitals without students had better results, except in Paris where midwives did their own autopsies. He effected a marked reduction in maternal mortality through the practice of proper hand washing by attending physicians. In the decades that followed, Joseph Lister, in his historic essay *On the Antiseptic Principle in the Practice of Surgery,* introduced the principles of antisepsis and thereafter the science of bacteriology was created with the studies of Louis Pasteur.

The beginnings of epidemiology were traced by Leslie T. Webster to the Books of Hippocrates in the fifth century B.C. Those works contained observations on different types of sickness and on fluctuations in their prevalence, from which Hippocrates concluded that individuals and populations differ among themselves and undergo changes in resistance to various sicknesses. Webster also mentions the treatise on contagion published by Franciscatus in 1576.

Webster's own studies were focused on the role of susceptibility and immunity of individuals within a population in the origins, spread, course, and termination of epidemics of infection; he used a single strain of organism in closed and controlled populations of experimental animals for his model. Similar studies had been reported earlier by Topley and Greenwood in England as well as by Harold Amos at the Rockefeller Institute, where Webster worked.

The principles derived from experimental epidemiology are clearly applicable to hospital infections. In the experimental model, however, a single virulent strain of organism was used to infect one or more susceptible animals that were then introduced into closed populations of other susceptible animals of the same breed. The organism spread to some of the uninfected susceptible animals, and produced infections from which some died while others survived. Those that survived either cleared their organisms or became carriers, with or without residual infected focuses. New groups of susceptible animals introduced into this residual population had the same fate as the original population, and the infection was perpetuated by continuous introduction of new susceptible individuals.

Needless to say, humans—particularly hospitalized patients—are far more complex with respect to their susceptibility or resistance to infection than are the purebred stocks of laboratory animals used in experimental epidemiology. Also, the hospital is a far more threatening environment than the carefully arranged cages in the animal quarters. Instead of the single strain of infecting organism that is introduced to an animal colony, a variable number of virulent pathogens are brought to the hospital from the community by patients admitted with infections. In addition, inpatients are exposed to the indigenous hospital flora of other infected patients and the hospital staff. The hospitalized patient is more susceptible than a healthy individual because of underlying disease or tissue injury either acquired outside the hospital or inflicted by surgical procedures and instrumentation.

The present volume deals with the many facets of the hospital environment as well as the numerous invasive procedures frequently used in patient management. The large number of chapters and the size of this text attest to the magnitude and complexity of such problems and to the large amount of available information. This material is based on extensive investigations throughout the country, and it is reinforced by the experiences of personnel at the U.S. Public Health Service's Centers for Disease Control (CDC). Furthermore, the effects of the extensive usage of antimicrobial agents in hospitalized patients on the occurrence and character of nosocomial infections are reviewed.

Interest in nosocomial infections has grown at a very rapid rate since the early 1960s, when it was stimulated by the alarming increase in the numbers of serious staphylococcal infections encountered in hospitals throughout the United States and other countries. More recently, serious infections with gram-negative rods have superseded in importance the infections due to staphylococci, except perhaps in newborn nurseries. Of greater concern are the outbreaks of multi-drug resistant staphylococci and gram-negative bacilli. Partly as a result of experiences with such outbreaks, several important conferences and symposia dealing with nosocomial infections and their control were convened in the United States and the United Kingdom. The transactions of those assemblies have been published and contain many important contributions. Other textbooks and monographs dealing with this subject have also been published during this time, in addition to the increased attention being given to infectious disease problems published by national organizations such as the American Public Health Association, American Hospital Association, American Academy of Pediatrics, American College of Surgeons, and the CDC.

Why, then, publish a second edition of this book at this time? First, there is the rapidly changing character and increasing seriousness of the infections being encountered and the increasing difficulty of controlling them. Second, the character of the hospitals and the increasing number and complexity of the services they provide are rapidly changing. The latter have involved organ transplantation, implantation of foreign bodies, and the repair or replacement of defective tissues. Such procedures often involve extensive and intensive use of immunosuppressive agents previously employed for the management of neoplastic or chronic diseases. There has also been a marked increase in the use of invasive devices and hospitalization in intensive care units. In addition, more frequent use of multiple broad-spectrum antimicrobial agents has permitted many patients to survive serious infections.

As a result of the growing interest in infection control and hospital epidemiology, there has been a rapid increase in the numbers of hospital personnel involved in the early recognition of nosocomial infections, as well as an increase in efforts to reduce the enormous amount of illness, disability, mortality, and economic burden they entail. Thus, over the past decade the number of physicians, nurses, hospital administrators, and others who are interested in infectious diseases and hospital epidemiology has risen markedly. Many of these people have joined a new society, the Association for Practitioners in Infection Control (APIC). Furthermore, another new organization, The Society of Hospital Epidemiologists of

America (SHEA), has been formed. There have also been greater emphasis and increasing activity on the part of Infection Control Committees within hospitals. The use of periodic or continuous surveillance of infections is being introduced in more and more hospitals, and many of them are making increasing use of computers to compile, store, retrieve, and analyze information on hospital infections.

At the First International Conference on Nosocomial Infections, Sir Robert Williams concluded,

My main regret, therefore, in reviewing the discussions at the meeting is that we have so little documentation of the good achieved for individual patients. I believe that one of the reasons we have so often failed to persuade our colleagues in hospitals to do the antiseptic things we think they ought to is that we have so rarely provided them with convincing evidence that, if they do, their patients will get better more quickly or survive in significantly greater numbers.

This challenge was reiterated in 1980 by Theodore Eickhoff at the beginning of the Second Annual Conference on Nosocomial Infections. Clearly, we have made inroads into our understanding of nosocomial infections, and the massive Study of the Efficacy of Nosocomial Infection Control (SENIC) has substantiated the importance of infection control programs. However, the challenge issued by Sir Robert Williams and Theodore Eickhoff remains the credo for the next decade. In addition to garnering sound scientific data we have to consider streamlining our policies in accordance with mounting economic limitations. This will require selecting practices that substantially reduce or prevent nosocomial infections.

This volume contains well-documented material in each aspect of infection control and epidemiology. It does more than merely provide a syllabus or systematic guide to the procedures involved in the recognition of infections and in their control; it provides an up-to-date analysis of each problem and basis for current practice.

The editors of this volume are therefore to be commended for undertaking and updating this authoritative source book on hospital infections. It has been and will continue to be a valuable text for reference and guidance to students and practitioners in the fields of infectious diseases and epidemiology and to all physicians caring for hospitalized patients.

*Maxwell Finland*
*Donald E. Craven*

# FOREWORD

My first and welcome responsibility in writing a foreword to the second edition of *Hospital Infections* is to recognize its timeliness and its continuing importance in surgical practice. Although considerable progress has been made in understanding the nature, causes, and control of these infections in the past 20 years, they continue to present many significant problems. Thus, the need for providing solutions to old problems and emerging new ones persists since successful surgery is singularly dependent upon the prevention and control of postoperative and posttrauma wound and other nosocomial infections. For *patients*, the significance of these infections is related to the associated increase in morbidity, pain, and discomfort; the resulting prolongation of hospitalization; the additional medical expense; and the added threat of increased mortality, disability, or possible cosmetic disfigurement, which may affect the patient's job, family, and quality of life. For the *physician*, and particularly the surgeon, the development of a postoperative infection is often of special significance because of its effect on the success of the operation, the occurrence of other associated complications, the added responsibilities from the increased morbidity and the possibility of mortality, a challenge to his professional reputation, and the threat of malpractice liability.

The second edition of *Hospital Infections* will be a valuable addition to other advances which have been made in the field of surgical infections by medicine and surgery. Some of the highlights indicative of other developments include the following:

1. The designation of etiologic factors of wound infections under the categories of *microbial, nonmicrobial,* and *associated* or *predisposing.*

2. The classification of infections in surgical patients, according to patient risk, into *clean elective, clean-contaminated, contaminated,* and *dirty* or *infected.* Although this classification had been developed in a ten-university study of wounds and burns under the auspices of the National Research Council and the Office of the Scientific and Research Development between 1942 and 1946, it was not widely accepted before its use by the five-university collaborative ultraviolet study under the auspices of the National Institutes of Health and the National Research Council, 1960–1963. The general adoption of this classification of infections by risk has been a great step forward in clearing up much of the confusion in collecting and reporting data on the incidence and types of wound infections.

3. The continuing activities of the Subcommittee on Prevention and Control of Infection in Surgical

Patients of the American College of Surgeons which has been productive of four international symposia with the establishment of a current data base (1970–1973) on knowledge on the nature and control of surgical infections, the publication of the *Manual on Prevention and Control of Infection in Surgical Patients* in 1976 and its revised and updated second edition published in October, 1983.

4. During this same period, members of the Centers for Disease Control (CDC) have shown leadership in the development of the *Manual for Isolation Procedures* and the organization and pursuit of an important National Nosocomial Infection Study in approximately 80 hospitals in the United States. In the latter, the progressive collection of data and regular communication to local hospitals have provided much useful information and have emphasized the importance of not only collecting such data, but also of using it to provide valuable feedback with its appropriate distribution. While most of the progress made in statistical analysis of the factors studied were related to the clean-elective classification of wounds, similar valuable information has also been obtained and extended to clean-contaminated wounds.

5. The CDC Study of the Efficacy of Nosocomial Infection Control (SENIC) has not only shown the effectiveness of various measures and activities in reducing the occurrence of nosocomial infections but has also provided some extremely useful descriptive data extending our knowledge of surgical as well as other nosocomial infections.

6. During 1982, CDC initiated the publication of a very valuable series of *Guidelines and Recommendations for the Prevention of Infections and Infection Control in Hospitals.*

Other manifestations of increased interest in the field of hospital infections can be found in the activities of the Committee on Operating Room Environment of the American College of Surgeons, and the organization of the Surgical Infection Society in 1980 for the purpose of establishing and maintaining a critical mass of surgeons and other scientists interested in the prevention and control of infections on an ongoing basis.

Thus, the second edition of *Hospital Infections* comes at an opportune time in our continuing efforts to prevent and control nosocomial infections. It reflects the rapid increase in related knowledge and should bring to a wide spectrum of physicians, nurses, and scientists valuable and useful information.

*William A. Altemeier*

# PREFACE

Nosocomial infections are a major public health problem in hospitals throughout the world. The impact of infections upon the patient, hospital personnel, family, and the community are such that nosocomial infections are an important challenge to those committed to improving the health of all people. Patterns of nosocomial infections continue to evolve, representing changes involving agents, sources, methods of transmission, host risk factors, and the environment. Nonetheless, effective measures for their control and prevention have been identified and publicized, personnel have been trained, consensus guidelines developed, and disease-specific recommendations promoted.

An important investigation, the Study of the Efficacy of Nosocomial Infection Control (SENIC), has shown that with optimal surveillance and control programs, the employment of an infection control nurse for every 250 beds, and the involvement of a trained infection control physician, approximately one-third of selected infections (urinary tract infections [36%], surgical wound infections [48%], pneumonias [7%], and bacteremias [28%]) can be prevented. Most hospitals, recognizing the problems and aware of licensing regulations, have appointed infection control personnel, instituted surveillance programs, and developed procedures for infection control within their institutions. Only about one-fourth of all infections potentially preventable with highly effective programs were being prevented in the mid-1980s, and substantial opportunities to further decrease the number of cases of infection doubtlessly still exist in most hospitals. However, prevention of infections will become increasingly more challenging as a result of the ever-expanding use of new invasive and immunocompromising diagnostic and therapeutic techniques, the aging population, and the increasing prevalence of chronic diseases that predispose to infections.

The increasing concern over nosocomial infections has been demonstrated by the publication of several new medical journals devoted to articles dealing with such infections, the formation of new specialty societies with the purposes of highlighting the problems and initiating discussions of methods of control and prevention, and institution of a number of training courses for persons involved in the control and prevention of nosocomial infections. The revision of the first edition of this book also reflects this increasing concern.

This second edition follows the format of the first edition, with emphasis on the epidemiology of the infections. It is directed to individuals who are responsible for controlling and preventing nosocomial infections. Part I defines the overall problem, focusing on the general concepts of control and prevention, and discusses areas of special concern. Part II includes comprehensive discussions of specific infection problems related to organ systems and procedures. Every chapter has been revised and some have been significantly changed in content and direction. New chapters have been added that encompass statistics, multiply resistant pathogens, molecular biology, dialysis units, and extended-care facilities. Infection surveillance and control recommendations have been extensively revised in accord with data from the SENIC project.

The authors have been selected because of their personal commitment to and involvement in the area of nosocomial infections. They have summarized their own relevant work and the work of others as reported in the scientific literature. We are grateful to them for their dedication in preparing their chapters and their willingness to share their knowledge and expertise with others. We also express our appreciation to the publisher, Little, Brown and Company, and to the many other persons who made multiple contributions to the preparation of this book.

*J. V. B.*
*P. S. B.*

# CONTRIBUTING AUTHORS

Robert C. Aber, M.D.
*Associate Professor, Department of Medicine, Pennsylvania State University College of Medicine; Vice Chairman, Department of Medicine, The Milton S. Hershey Medical Center, Hershey, Pennsylvania*

J. Wesley Alexander, M.D., Sc.D.
*Professor of Surgery, University of Cincinnati College of Medicine; Director, Department of Research, Shriners Burns Institute, Cincinnati*

James R. Allen, M.D., M.P.H.
*Chief, Transfusion and Blood Studies, Center for Infectious Diseases, AIDS Activity, Centers for Disease Control, U.S. Public Health Service, Atlanta*

John V. Bennett, M.D.
*Assistant Director for Medical Science, Center for Infectious Diseases, Centers for Disease Control, U.S. Public Health Service, Atlanta*

Philip S. Brachman, M.D.
*Director, Global EIS Program, Centers for Disease Control, U.S. Public Health Service; Clinical Professor of Community Health, Emory University School of Medicine, Atlanta*

Robert G. Brooks, M.D.
*Assistant Director, Internal Medicine Training Program, Department of Internal Medicine, Orlando Regional Medical Center, Orlando, Florida*

Claire V. Broome, M.D.
*Chief, Respiratory and Special Pathogens Branch, Division of Bacterial Diseases, Center for Infectious Diseases, Centers for Disease Control, U.S. Public Health Service, Atlanta*

John P. Burke, M.D.
*Professor of Medicine, University of Utah College of Medicine; Chief, Infectious Disease Division, LDS Hospital, Salt Lake City*

Marie B. Coyle, Ph.D.
*Associate Professor of Laboratory Medicine, Departments of Microbiology and Immunology, University of Washington School of Medicine; Director, Clinical Microbiology Laboratory, Harborview Medical Center, Seattle*

Peter Cruse, M.B., Ch.B., F.R.C.S. (Ed.), F.R.C.S. (C.), F.A.C.S.
*Professor and Head, Department of Surgery, The University of Calgary; Professor and Head, Department of Surgery, Foothills Hospital, Calgary, Alberta*

**Richard E. Dixon, M.D.**
*Associate Professor of Medicine, Hahnemann University School of Medicine, Philadelphia; Director, Department of Medicine, Helene Fuld Medical Center, Trenton, New Jersey*

**Herbert L. DuPont, M.D.**
*Professor of Medicine and Director, Program in Infectious Diseases and Clinical Microbiology, The University of Texas Medical School at Houston; Attending Physician and Chairman, Infection Control Committee, Hermann Hospital, Houston*

**Theodore C. Eickhoff, M.D.**
*Professor of Medicine, University of Colorado School of Medicine; Director, Department of Internal Medicine, Presbyterian/St. Luke's Medical Center, Denver*

**William F. Enneking, M.D.**
*Distinguished Service Professor, Department of Orthopaedic Surgery, University of Florida College of Medicine, Gainesville*

**Martin S. Favero, Ph.D.**
*Chief, Nosocomial Infections Laboratory Branch, Center for Infectious Diseases, Centers for Disease Control, U.S. Public Health Service, Atlanta*

**Jorge Franco, Ph.D.**
*Visiting Assistant Professor, Department of Microbiology and Immunology, Hahnemann University School of Medicine; Manager of Microbiology and Immunology, Smith Kline Bioscience Laboratories, Philadelphia*

**Eugene J. Gangarosa, M.D.**
*Professor and Director, Master of Public Health Program, Emory University School of Medicine, Atlanta*

**Richard A. Garibaldi, M.D.**
*Associate Professor of Medicine, University of Connecticut School of Medicine; Hospital Epidemiologist, University of Connecticut Health Center, Farmington*

**Julia S. Garner, R.N., M.N.**
*Chief, Prevention Activity, Hospital Infections Program, Center for Infectious Diseases, Centers for Disease Control, U.S. Public Health Service, Atlanta*

**Donald A. Goldmann, M.D.**
*Associate Professor of Pediatrics, Harvard Medical School; Hospital Epidemiologist, Children's Hospital, Boston*

**Robert W. Haley, M.D.**
*Associate Professor, Division of Epidemiology and Preventive Medicine, Department of Internal Medicine, University of Texas Health Science Center at Dallas, Southwestern Medical School; Attending Physician, Internal Medicine Service, Parkland Memorial Hospital, Dallas*

**Walter J. Hierholzer, Jr., M.D.**
*Professor of Medicine and Epidemiology, Yale University School of Medicine; Hospital Epidemiologist, Yale-New Haven Hospital, New Haven*

**Ian Alan Holder, Ph.D.**
*Professor of Research, Surgery, and Microbiology, University of Cincinnati College of Medicine; Director, Department of Microbiology, Shriners Burns Institute, Cincinnati*

**James M. Hughes, M.D.**
*Director, Hospital Infections Program, Center for Infectious Diseases, Centers for Disease Control, U.S. Public Health Service, Atlanta*

**Marguerite M. Jackson, R.N., M.S.**
*Assistant Clinical Professor, Department of Community and Family Medicine, University of California, San Diego, School of Medicine; Coordinator, Infection Control Team, UCSD Medical Center, San Diego*

**Andrew Moss Kaunitz, M.D.**
*Assistant Professor, Department of Obstetrics and Gynecology, University of Florida College of Medicine, Gainesville; Director, Division of Ambulatory Care, Department of Obstetrics and Gynecology, University Hospital, Jacksonville, Florida*

**Karen Rose Koppel Kaunitz, Esq.**
*Assistant Vice President of Legal Affairs, Methodist Hospital Inc., Jacksonville, Florida*

**Harold Laufman, M.D., Ph.D.**
*Professor Emeritus of Surgery, Albert Einstein College of Medicine of Yeshiva University; Attending Surgeon Emeritus and Director, Institute for Surgical Studies, Montefiore Hospital and Medical Center, New York City*

**William J. Ledger, M.D.**
*Given Foundation Professor of Obstetrics and Gynecology, Cornell University Medical College; Obstetrician and Gynecologist-in-Chief, The New York Hospital-Cornell Medical Center, New York City*

**Patricia Lynch, R.N., B.S.N.**
*Clinical Instructor, School of Community Medicine and Public Health, University of Washington; Infection Control Coordinator, St. Cabrini Hospital, Seattle*

**Bruce G. MacMillan, M.D.**
*Shrine Professor of Surgery, University of Cincinnati College of Medicine; Chief of Staff, Shriners Burns Institute, Cincinnati*

**Dennis G. Maki, M.D.**
*Ovid O. Meyer Professor of Medicine and Director, Trauma and Life Support Center, Infectious Disease Section, Department of Medicine, University of Wisconsin Clinical Sciences Center, Madison*

**George F. Mallison, M.P.H., P.E.**
*Consultant, Environmental and Infection Control, Glen Rock, New Jersey*

**Stanley M. Martin, M.S.**
*Chief, Statistical Services Activity, Division of Bacterial Diseases, Center for Infectious Diseases, Centers for Disease Control, U.S. Public Health Service, Atlanta*

**R. Michael Massanari, M.D.**
*Associate Professor of Pathology and Medicine, University of Iowa College of Medicine; Associate Hospital Epidemiologist, University of Iowa Hospitals and Clinics, Iowa City*

**John E. McGowan, Jr., M.D.**
*Professor of Pathology and Laboratory Medicine and Professor of Medicine, Department of Infectious Diseases, Emory University School of Medicine; Director of Clinical Microbiology, Grady Memorial Hospital, Atlanta*

**William Petty, M.D.**
*Professor and Chairman, Department of Orthopaedics, University of Florida College of Medicine; Attending Surgeon and Chairman, Department of Orthopaedics, Shands Hospital, Gainesville*

**Arthur L. Reingold, M.D.**
*Assistant Chief, Respiratory and Special Pathogens Branch, Division of Bacterial Diseases, Center for Infectious Diseases, Centers for Disease Control, U.S. Public Health Service, Atlanta*

**Jack S. Remington, M.D.**
*Professor of Medicine, Division of Infectious Diseases, Stanford University School of Medicine; Chairman, Department of Immunology and Infectious Diseases, Research Institute, Palo Alto Medical Foundation, Palo Alto, California*

**Frank S. Rhame, M.D.**
*Assistant Professor, Departments of Medicine and Laboratory Medicine and Pathology, University of Minnesota Medical School; Hospital Epidemiologist, University of Minnesota Hospitals and Clinics, Minneapolis*

**Bruce S. Ribner, M.D.**
*Associate Professor of Medicine, Program in Infectious Diseases and Clinical Microbiology, University of Texas Medical School at Houston; Attending Physician and Hospital Epidemiologist, Hermann Hospital, Houston*

**Jay P. Sanford, M.D.**
*President and Dean, Uniformed Services University of the Health Sciences, Bethesda, Maryland; Attending Physician, Walter Reed Army Medical Center and National Naval Medical Center, Washington, D.C.*

**Dennis R. Schaberg, M.D.**
*Associate Professor of Medicine, Division of Infectious Diseases, University of Michigan Medical School, Ann Arbor*

**William Schaffner, M.D.**
*Chairman, Department of Preventive Medicine, and Chief, Division of Infectious Disease, Department of Medicine, Vanderbilt University School of Medicine; Hospital Epidemiologist, Vanderbilt University Hospital, Nashville*

**Fritz D. Schoenknecht, M.D.**
*Professor of Laboratory Medicine and Professor of Microbiology and Immunology, University of Washington School of Medicine; Director, Clinical Microbiology Laboratory, University Hospital, Seattle*

**Bryan P. Simmons, M.D.**
*Infectious Diseases Fellow, Emory University School of Medicine, Atlanta*

**Walter E. Stamm, M.D.**
*Associate Professor of Medicine, University of Washington School of Medicine; Head, Infectious Disease Division, Harborview Medical Center, Seattle*

**William M. Valenti, M.D.**
*Associate Professor, Department of Medicine, University of Rochester School of Medicine; Hospital Epidemiologist, Strong Memorial Hospital, Rochester, New York*

**Paul F. Wehrle, M.D.**
*Hastings Professor of Pediatrics, University of California, Los Angeles, UCLA School of Medicine; Director of Pediatrics, Los Angeles County–USC Medical Center, Los Angeles*

**Robert A. Weinstein, M.D.**
*Associate Professor, University of Chicago, Division of the Biological Sciences, Pritzker School of Medicine; Hospital Epidemiologist, Department of Medicine, Michael Reese Hospital and Medical Center, Chicago*

**Walter W. Williams, M.D., M.P.H.**
*Medical Epidemiologist, Surveillance, Investigations, and Research Branch, Division of Immunization, Center for Prevention Services, Centers for Disease Control, U.S. Public Health Service, Atlanta*

# I BASIC CONSIDERATIONS OF HOSPITAL INFECTIONS

## 1 EPIDEMIOLOGY OF NOSOCOMIAL INFECTIONS

Philip S. Brachman

### BASIC CONSIDERATIONS

This chapter is a review of the basic principles of epidemiology as they relate to nosocomial infections. An understanding of the epidemiology of nosocomial infections is necessary for the development and implementation of effective and efficient control and prevention measures. One uses epidemiologic methods to define the factors related to the occurrence of disease, including the relations among the agent, its reservoir and source, the route of transmission, the host, and the environment. Once these relations have been defined for a specific disease, the most appropriate means of control and prevention should become apparent. Without defining each of these relations, control and prevention efforts are, at best, a gamble. Defining the epidemiologic relations introduces science into control and prevention and leads to more effective and economical use of all resources.

#### Definitions

EPIDEMIOLOGY   The term *epidemiology* is derived from the Greek *epi* (on or upon), *demos* (people or population), and *logos* (word or reason). Literally, it means the study of things that happen to people; historically, it has involved the study of epidemics. Epidemiology is the dynamic study of the determinants, occurrence, and distribution of health and disease in a population, which—for nosocomial infections—is the hospital population. Epidemiology defines the relation of disease to the population at risk and in volves the determination, analysis, and interpretation of rates. There are many different rates used by epidemiologists; the most common is the attack rate, which is the number of cases of the disease divided by the population at risk. Calculation of other rates helps define the outbreak, for example, calculation of rates among a selected comparison group to compare with the group in which cases occurred (see Chapter 6).

INFECTION   *Infection* entails the replication of organisms in the tissues of a host; the related development of overt clinical manifestations is known as *disease;* however, if the infection provokes an immune response only, without overt clinical disease, it is referred to as an inapparent or subclinical infection. *Colonization* implies the presence of a microorganism in or on a host with growth and multiplication of the microorganism, but without any overt clinical expression or detected immune reaction at the time it is isolated. *Subclinical* (or *inapparent*) *infection* refers

3

to a relation between the host and microorganism in which the microorganism is present; there is no overt expression of the presence of the microorganism, but there is interaction between the host and microorganism that results in a detectable immune response, such as a serologic reaction. Therefore, special serologic tests may be needed to differentiate colonization from subclinical infection. In the absence of such information, it is customary to employ the term colonization. A *carrier* (or colonized person) is an individual colonized with a specific microorganism and from whom the organism can be recovered (i.e., cultured) but who shows no overt expression of the presence of the microorganism at the time it is isolated; a carrier can have a history of previous disease due to that organism, such as typhoid. The carrier state may be *transient* (or short-term), *intermittent* (or occasional), or *chronic* (long-term, persistent, or permanent). We have found, for example, in culture studies of hospital staff for nasal carriage of *Staphylococcus aureus,* that approximately 15 to 20 percent are noncarriers, 60 to 70 percent are intermittent carriers, and 10 to 15 percent are persistent carriers. Epidemiologically, the important consideration is whether the carrier is the source of the infection for another individual; any carrier who is disseminating or shedding the organism may subsequently infect another person. Also, the carrier may develop disease with the source of the organism being him- or herself (endogenous source).

DISSEMINATION    *Dissemination,* or shedding of microorganisms, refers to the movement of organisms from a person carrying them into the immediate environment. To show this, one cultures samples of air or surfaces and swabs objects onto which microorganisms from the carrier may have been deposited. Shedding studies may be conducted in specially constructed chambers designed to quantitate dissemination. While shedding studies have occasionally been useful to document unusual dissemination, they have not generally been useful in identifying carriers whose dissemination has resulted in infection in other persons. In the hospital setting, dissemination is most efficiently identified by means of surveillance, in which the occurrence of infection among contacts is noted. When infection is shown to result from dissemination of organisms from a person, that person is known as a "dangerous disseminator."

The demonstration by culturing techniques that an individual is carrying a certain organism defines a potential problem, whereas epidemiologic demonstration by surveillance and investigative techniques defines the real problem. In some hospitals, routine culture surveys of all or selected asymptomatic staff may be conducted in an attempt to identify carriers of certain organisms, but such surveys lack practical relevance unless the results are related to specific cases or an outbreak of disease. This practice only identifies those who are culture-positive and does not in itself reliably separate colonized persons into disseminators as distinct from nondisseminators. Usually only a fraction of colonized persons are disseminating; thus the nondisseminators are not associated with the actual spread of infection. If disease transmission has occurred and a human source of infection is suspected, culture surveys in conjunction with epidemiologic investigation to identify the potential source are realistic, and additional laboratory study to confirm the presence of a dangerous disseminator may then be undertaken. Thus culture surveys and microbiologic studies of dissemination in the absence of disease problems are usually inappropriate and wasteful of resources.

In some instances, dissemination from a carrier has been reported to be influenced by the occurrence of an unrelated disease such as a second infection. One report, for example, suggested that infants carrying staphylococci in their nares disseminate staphylococci only after the onset of a viral respiratory infection. Such infants are called "cloud babies" (see Chapter 5). In another instance, a physician disseminated staphylococci from his skin because of a reactivation of chronic dermatitis. Desquamation of his skin led to the transmission of staphylococci to patients with whom he had contact. Dissemination has been reported of tetracycline-resistant *Staphylococcus aureus* from individuals carrying this organism who were treated with tetracycline. Dissemination may be constant or sporadic. If sporadic, it may result from the intermittent occurrence of some precipitating event, such as a second infection, or it may be due to other, unknown factors. The risk of dissemination is generally greater from individuals with disease caused by that organism than from individuals with subclinical infection or who are colonized with the organism.

*Contamination* refers to microorganisms that are transiently present on body surface (such as hands) without tissue invasion or physiologic reaction. Contamination also refers to the presence of microorganisms on or in an inanimate object.

NOSOCOMIAL INFECTIONS    *Nosocomial infections* are infections that develop within a hospital or are produced by microorganisms acquired during hospitalization. Nosocomial infections may involve not only patients, but also anyone else who has contact with a hospital, including members of the staff, volunteers, visitors, workers, salespersons, and delivery personnel. The majority of nosocomial infections become clinically apparent while the patients are still hospitalized; however, the onset of disease can occur after a patient has been discharged. As many as 25 percent of postoperative wound infections, for example, become symptomatic after the patient has been discharged (see Chapter 27). In these cases the patient became colonized or infected while in the hospital, but the incubation period was longer than the patient's hospital stay. This sequence is also seen in some infections of newborns and in most breast abscesses of new mothers. Hepatitis B is an example of a nosocomial disease with a long incubation period; its clinical onset usually occurs long after the patient is discharged from the hospital.

Infections incubating at the time of the patient's admission to the hospital are not nosocomial; they are community-acquired, unless of course they result from a previous hospitalization. Community-acquired infections can serve as a ready source of infection for other patients or personnel and thus must be considered in the total scope of hospital-related infections.

The term *preventable infection* implies that some event related to the infection could have been altered and that such alteration would have prevented the infection from occurring. A medical attendant who does not wash his or her hands between contacts with the urinary collection equipment of two patients, for example, may transmit gram-negative organisms from the first patient to the second, which may result in a urinary tract infection. Hand-washing might have prevented this infection from occurring. The identification of such an event in retrospect, however, is likely to be impossible; at best, the situation is difficult to distinguish from circumstances in which both patients developed infections from their own autogenous flora (e.g., from *Escherichia coli*). It is often impossible to identify the precise mode of acquisition of individual nosocomial infections. More than one mode may contribute to the development of the same infection, and not all modes may be preventable.

A *nonpreventable infection* is one that will occur despite all possible precautions, for example, infection in an immunosuppressed patient due to his or her own flora. It has been estimated that approximately 30 percent of all reported nosocomial infections are preventable. Given ideal circumstances, many infections caused by flora acquired during hospitalization are avoidable by prevention of nosocomial acquisition or avoidance of predisposing procedures in those who have acquired nosocomial strains. Epidemics, especially common-vehicle epidemics, are potentially preventable; however, epidemics account for only a small

number of the nosocomial infections that occur. Prompt investigation and the institution of rational control measures should reduce the number of cases involved in outbreaks. Endemic infections account for the majority of nosocomial infections, and the consistent application of recognized, effective control measures for endemic infections is probably the single most important factor in reducing the overall level of nosocomial infections.

SOURCE: ENDOGENOUS (OR AUTOGENOUS), EXOGENOUS   Organisms that cause nosocomial infections come from either endogenous (autogenous) or exogenous sources. *Endogenous* infections are caused by the patient's own flora; *exogenous* infections result from transmission of organisms from a source other than the patient. Either endogenous organisms are brought into the hospital by a patient (this represents colonization outside the hospital), or the patient becomes colonized after being admitted to the hospital. In either instance, the organisms colonizing the patient may subsequently cause a nosocomial infection. It may not always be possible to determine whether a particular organism isolated from the patient with an infection caused by that organism is exogenous or endogenous, and the term *autogenous* should be used in this situation. Autogenous infection indicates that the infection was derived from the flora of the patient, whether or not the infecting organism became part of the patient's flora subsequent to admission. Information about current disease problems in the community or in hospital contacts may be useful in differentiating the two sources. Microbiologic determinations of the characteristics of the organism—such as phage typing, antibiograms, biochemical reactions, or genetic analysis—may help identify strains of nosocomial origin (see Chapters 7, 11, and 12).

SPECTRUM OF OCCURRENCE OF CASES   To determine whether a nosocomial infection problem exists in a particular hospital, one must relate the current frequency of cases to the past history of the disease in that institution. To characterize a disease's frequency as sporadic, endemic, or epidemic, investigators must know something of the past occurrence of that disease in relation to time, place, and person. *Sporadic* means that cases occur occasionally and irregularly, without any specific pattern. *Endemic* means that the disease occurs with ongoing frequency in a specific geographic area in a finite population and over a defined time period. *Hyperendemic* refers to what appears to be a gradual increase in the occurrence of a disease in a defined area beyond the expected number of cases;

however, it may not be certain whether the disease will occur at epidemic proportions. An *epidemic* is a definite increase in the incidence of a disease above its expected endemic occurrence. *Outbreak* is used interchangeably with epidemic; however, some people use outbreak to mean an increased rate of occurrence, but not at levels as serious as an epidemic (see Chapter 4).

An occasional gas gangrene infection among postoperative patients is an example of a sporadic infection. An endemic nosocomial infection is represented by the regular occurrence of infections—either in a particular site or at different sites—that are due to the same organism, occur at a nearly constant rate, and are generally considered by the hospital staff to be within "expected and acceptable" limits. Surgical wound infections due to a single organism that follow operations classified as "contaminated surgery," for example, could represent the endemic level of postoperative wound infections.

An epidemic classically begins with a sudden increase in the occurrence of disease among susceptible persons who have had contact with a contaminated source, but the onset of disease occurs at an unusually high frequency relative to that expected. On the other hand, an epidemic may also result from prolonged exposure to the source of the organism, with cases occurring sporadically due to sporadic dissemination or distribution of the agent, sporadic contact between the agent and a susceptible host, or sporadic presence of a susceptible host. Cases of salmonellosis, for example, may result from contact with a contaminated food that patients and staff are exposed to over a long period of time, possibly months before it is identified. Only an occasional case of salmonellosis may result from this exposure, but depending on the past history of salmonellosis in the institution, these cases may represent "epidemic" salmonellosis.

A characteristic sharp and abrupt increase in the number of cases may fail to occur with diseases having a long and variable incubation period. Many people may be exposed to hepatitis B at one particular time, for example, but the appearance of the resulting disease may be spread out over several weeks, thereby obscuring the presence of an epidemic (see Chapter 5).

INCIDENCE AND PREVALENCE   Occurrence of infection is quantified by calculating its incidence and prevalence. *Incidence* is the number of new cases in a specific population in a defined time period. To determine the true incidence of a disease, culture or serologic surveys may be necessary. *Prevalence* is the total number of current cases of an infection in a defined population at one point in time (point prevalence) or over a longer period of time (period prevalence). The prevalence rate will include cases of recent onset as well as cases of earlier onset that are still clinically apparent (see Chapter 4).

## EPIDEMIOLOGIC METHODS

There are generally three techniques used in epidemiologic studies—descriptive, analytic, and experimental—all of which may be used in investigating nosocomial infections. Additionally, the principles involved in these methods have application to surveillance; surveillance data are commonly analyzed by the descriptive method, and such analysis may suggest the need for analytic studies to identify certain features of a disease. Furthermore, analysis of surveillance data may lead to the development of experimental studies to deal with a specific disease.

### Descriptive Epidemiology

The basic epidemiologic method, descriptive epidemiology, is used in most investigations. Once the initial problem has been defined, however, additional studies using one of the other two methods can be conducted to develop more information about the epidemic, confirm initial impressions, prove and disprove hypotheses, and evaluate the effectiveness of control measures, prevention measures, or both.

*Descriptive epidemiology* describes the occurrence of disease in terms of time, place, and person; each case of a disease is first characterized by describing these three attributes (see Chapter 5). When data from the individual cases are combined and analyzed, the parameters of the epidemic or disease problem should be characterized.

TIME   There are four time trends to consider: secular, periodic, seasonal, and acute. *Secular* trends are long-term trends in the occurrence of a disease, that is, variations that occur over a period of years. The gradual but steady reduction in the incidence of diphtheria in the United States over the past 50 years, for example, is the secular trend of that disease. The secular trend generally reflects the immunologic, socioeconomic, and nutritional levels of the population from which the secular data have been reported. In diphtheria, the downward trend generally reflects the rising immunity and improved socioeconomic and nutritional levels of the overall population.

*Periodic* trends are temporal interruptions of the secular trend and usually reflect changes in the overall susceptibility to the disease in the population. The upsurge in influenza A activity every two to three years, for instance, reflects the periodic trend of this disease and is generally the result of antigenic drift of the influenza A virus.

*Seasonal* trends are the annual variations in disease incidence that are related in part to seasons. In general, the occurrence of a particular communicable disease increases when the circumstances that influence its transmission are favorable. The seasonal pattern of both community-acquired and nosocomial respiratory disease, for example, involves high incidence in the fall and winter months, when transmission through the air is enhanced because people are together in rooms with closed windows and are breathing unfiltered, recirculating air. Thus they have greater contact with each other and with droplets as well as droplet nuclei. There may also be agent and host factors that influence the seasonal trends. The seasonal trend of foodborne disease involves higher incidence in the summer months when ambient temperatures are elevated and refrigeration may be inadequate. Foods contaminated with non-disease-producing levels of microorganisms may be allowed to incubate, resulting in the attainment of infectious doses.

The fourth type of time variation is the *acute* or epidemic occurrence of a disease with its characteristic upsurge in incidence. The overall shape of the epidemic curve depends on the interaction of many factors: characteristics of the specific agent; its pathogenicity, concentration, and incubation period; the mode and ease of its transmission; host factors, including the susceptibility and concentration of susceptible individuals; and environmental factors, such as temperature, humidity, movement of air, and general housekeeping.

An epidemic can be portrayed by an *epidemic curve,* that is, a graphic representation of the number of cases of the disease plotted against time (see Chapter 5). The time scale will vary according to the incubation or latency period, ranging from minutes, as in an outbreak of disease following exposure to a toxin or a chemical, to months, as in a nosocomial epidemic of hepatitis B. The time scale (abscissa or horizontal scale) should be selected with three facts in mind: (1) the unit time interval should be equal to or less than the average incubation period so that the true nature of the epidemic curve will be apparent (i.e., all the cases will not be bunched together); (2) the scale should be carried out far enough in time to allow all cases to be plotted; and (3) any cases that occurred before the epidemic should be plotted to give a basis for comparison with the epidemic experience.

If the epidemic curve starts with the *index case* (i.e., the first case in the outbreak), the time between the index case and onset of the next case is the *incubation period* if transmission was from the index case directly to the next case, that is, from person to person. The upslope in the curve is determined by the incubation period, the number and concentration of exposed susceptible persons, and the ease of transmission. The height of the peak of the curve is influenced by the total number of cases and the time interval over which they occur. The downslope of the curve is usually more gradual than the upslope; its gradual change reflects cases with longer incubation periods and the decreasing number of susceptible individuals. Cases resulting from *secondary transmission*—that is, resulting from contact with earlier cases in the epidemic— will also be represented on the downslope of the epidemic curve or, occasionally, by a second upswing, which reflects a second, distinct, and usually smaller "wave" of disease following the main outbreak. Consecutive waves of disease may represent ongoing transmission from new focuses or from one focus that is intermittently or periodically infective or from which organisms are periodically disseminated. In a common-vehicle epidemic, the epidemic curve usually rises rather sharply and then gradually falls off. In a contact-spread epidemic (person-to-person), the epidemic curve usually rises gradually, has a flatter peak than the common-vehicle curve, and then falls off.

PLACE The second feature of descriptive epidemiology is place; in an investigation there may be three different places that need to be defined. The first is where the patient is when disease is diagnosed, and the second is where contact occurred between the patient and the agent. If a vehicle of infection is involved, the third place is where the vehicle became infected. To implement the most appropriate control and preventive measures, it is necessary to distinguish between these three geographic areas; certain actions may control additional spread from a specific focus but may not prevent new cases from occurring if the source continues to infect new vehicles. Several examples will help to emphasize the importance of carefully describing place or places involved in disease outbreaks.

In an outbreak of nosocomial salmonellosis, the patients were located on various wards throughout the hospital at the time they developed disease. Individual control measures were directed at each patient in the various wards; however, the place of infection was the radiology department, where barium used for gastrointestinal tract roentgenographic examinations was contaminated with salmonella. Because the barium had been contaminated in the radiology department, preventive measures were directed there.

Another example involves outbreaks of septicemia associated with intravenous fluids. In these instances, it is important to determine whether the fluid became contaminated in the process of manufacture (*intrinsic* contamination) or after the fluid had been bottled (*extrinsic* contamination). Extrinsic contamination can occur during shipment to the hospital, after being brought into the hospital, while being prepared for use, or during actual use.

PERSON    The third major component of descriptive epidemiology is person. Careful evaluation of host factors related to the individual person includes consideration of age, sex, race, immunization status, competence of immune system, and presence of underlying disease that may influence susceptibility (acute or chronic), therapeutic or diagnostic procedures, medications, and nutritional status (see Chapter 5). In essence, any host factor that can influence the development of disease must be considered and described. Those that increase the patient's chance of developing disease are known as risk factors.

Age sometimes influences the occurrence of diseases and also provides a clue regarding the cause of an outbreak. Persons at either end of the age spectrum—the young and the elderly—are generally more susceptible to disease. Such susceptibility may reflect levels of immunity, both active and passive, as well as the level of less specific personal factors of protection against development of disease. Age can also be an important clue to the source of an outbreak of disease. If, in an apparent common-source outbreak, for example, all ages from infancy to old age are involved, then the source of the outbreak must have been available to patients scattered through at least several wards. On the other hand, if all the patients involved in an epidemic are women in the childbearing ages, then in attempting to identify the place of the exposure, the investigation can be narrowed to the obstetric or possibly the gynecologic ward.

Consideration of therapeutic procedures may be of similar importance. If all patients who developed bacteremia due to the same organism have received intravenous-fluid therapy, then a common source of intravenous fluids would be suspected as the cause of the outbreak.

These few examples demonstrate that the description of individual host factors among involved patients may point to important information that may lead to a solution of the epidemic problem.

*Analytic Epidemiology*

The second method of epidemiologic investigation is *analytic epidemiology,* in which the determinants of disease distribution are evaluated in terms of possible causal relations. Two basic methods are used: case-control and cohort studies. In both instances, relations between cause and effect are analyzed: the *case-control* method starts with the effect and searches for the cause: the *cohort* method starts with the cause and evaluates the effect. The case-control and cohort methods have also been referred to as retrospective and prospective studies, respectively; both methods, however, can be either retrospective or prospective. These terms indicate the temporal frame of reference for the collection of specific data: in a *retrospective* study, data are collected after the event has occurred; in a *prospective* study, the data are collected as the event occurs.

CASE-CONTROL STUDY    The case-control method starts with an allocation of persons between a study group (those already affected with the disease) and a comparison-control group or groups (see Chapter 5). Any differences between these groups are then determined. In an outbreak of nosocomial urinary tract infections due to *Proteus rettgeri,* for example, a group of patients with this infection was compared to a group that did not have urinary tract infection due to *P. rettgeri.* It was shown that the infected patients were more likely than the comparison group patients to have had indwelling urinary tract catheters, to have been located in the same area of the hospital, and to have previously received systemic antibiotic therapy. Thus it was concluded that in this epidemic, indwelling urethral catheters, proximity of patients to one another, and previous systemic antibiotic therapy were directly related to the subsequent development of urinary tract infections due to *P. rettgeri.*

The case-control approach has the advantages of being inexpensive, relatively quick, and easily reproducible. It is used most often in acute disease investigations, since the epidemiologist arrives after a problem is recognized and often after the peak of the epidemic has passed. This approach, however, may introduce bias into the selection of the control group since it may be difficult to retrospectively reconstruct the involved and noninvolved populations. In selecting a comparison-control group, bias may be introduced if one is unable to exclude patients who are asymptomatically infected with the causative agent being studied. A lesser problem but a real one is ascertaining in retrospect that a patient actually had disease, rather than was asymptomatically infected or colonized. This latter circumstance presents considerable difficulty in categorizing critically ill patients with manifestations that resemble those of infection but stem from other causes. Fortunately, the search for sources can be pursued by including all culture-positive persons in the case definition, and thus it need not be restricted to those with clinical disease. This approach does, however, jeopardize the search for important host factors related to disease occurrence. Another limitation is the memory of the involved patients for past events, the specification of which may be important to the investigation. Also, the hospital records may lack documentation of events important to the investigation. These limitations derive from the retrospective approach rather than deficiencies in the case-control approach per se. Indeed prospective case-control studies can be implemented, but usually they have little usefulness in outbreak investigations.

COHORT STUDY    In the cohort method, patients exposed to a "cause" are compared with a group not exposed to the cause to see what the effect will be. In the above outbreak of *P. rettgeri* urinary tract infections, for example, the importance of the proximity of patients with catheters—an infectious risk—was prospectively analyzed by scattering certain patients with urethral catheters throughout the hospital. Inhibition of the nosocomial spread of infection was demonstrated by this cohort approach.

The advantage of the cohort study is that it provides a direct estimate of the risk provided by a particular factor for disease occurrence, and this is relatively easy to accomplish when the incubation period is short. Although bias may still be a problem, it is less likely to be introduced in this type of study, which usually is conducted prospectively. The cohort study, however, is usually more difficult, more expensive, and more time-consuming than retrospective studies. For diseases with long incubation periods, the difficulties may be insurmountable. An example of a prospective cohort study is one in which a cohort of patients who received blood transfusions over a specific period of time is followed to see which ones develop hepatitis B. A retrospective cohort study would involve studying a cohort of patients who developed hepatitis to see which ones received blood transfusions within the past six months.

Another technique of analytic epidemiology is a cross-sectional survey, which allows for collection of data over a specific limited period of time. It makes possible an accessing of the relation between two or more factors whose presence can be confirmed at the time of the survey.

### Experimental Epidemiology

The third method of epidemiologic investigation is the *experimental method,* which is a definitive method of proving or disproving a hypothesis. The experimental method assumes that causes are followed by effects and that a deliberate manipulation of the cause is predictably followed by an alteration in the effect that could rarely be explained by chance. The two groups selected for study are similar in all respects except for the presence of the study factor in one group. Either the case-control or the cohort method is used to evaluate the interaction between the cause and the effect.

An example of the experimental method is the evaluation of a new drug as treatment for a disease: a group of patients with the disease is randomly divided into two subgroups that are equal in all respects, except one of the subgroups is treated with the drug and the other subgroup (the control group) is given a placebo. If there is no other variation between the two groups, any difference in the course of the disease may be ascribed to the use of the drug.

The experimental method has less direct use in the investigation of outbreaks of nosocomial disease today than the other two methods. This method, however, does have usefulness in assessing general patient-care practices and in evaluating new methods to control and prevent epidemics as long as the patient is not at any increased health risk. It has less use in therapeutic studies because of the need for informed consent and the need to prevent placing the patient at an unjustified or greater risk in attempting to conduct a specific study.

## CHAIN OF INFECTION
### General Aspects
Infection results from the interaction between an infectious agent and a susceptible host. This interaction—called *transmission*—occurs by means of contact between the agent and the host. Three interrelated factors—the agent, transmission, and the host—represent the *chain of infection.*

The links interrelate in and are affected by the environment; this relation is referred to as the *ecology of infection,* that is, the relation of microorganisms to disease as affected by the factors of their environment. In attempting to control nosocomial infections, an attack on the chain of infection at its weakest link is generally the most effective procedure. With definition of the links in the chain for each nosocomial infection, future trends of the disease should be predictable, and it should be possible to develop effective control and prevention techniques. Defining the chain of infection leads to specific action, in contrast to the incorporation of nonspecific actions in an attempt to control a nosocomial infection problem.

Disease causation is multifactorial; that is, disease results from the interaction of many factors related to the agent, transmission, and host. The development of disease reflects the interaction of these factors as they affect a person. Thus some people exposed to an infectious agent develop disease and others do not. For example, among a group of people exposed to β-hemolytic streptococci, usually only some develop disease; this reflects the variability in the various factors related to the development of disease.

*Agent*

The first link in the chain of infection is the microbial agent, which may be a bacterium, virus, fungus, or parasite. The majority of nosocomial infection problems are caused by bacteria and viruses; fungi occasionally and parasites rarely cause nosocomial infections.

PATHOGENICITY   The measure of the ability of microorganisms to induce disease is referred to as *pathogenicity,* and it may be assessed by disease-colonization ratios. One organism with high pathogenicity is *Yersinia pestis;* it almost always causes clinical disease in a host. An organism with low pathogenicity is α-hemolytic streptococcus; it commonly colonizes in humans but only rarely causes clinical disease. The pathogenicity of an organism is additionally described by characterizing the organism's virulence and invasiveness.

*Virulence* is the measure of the severity of the disease. In epidemiologic studies, virulence is defined more specifically by assessing morbidity and mortality rates and the degree of communicability. The virulence of organisms ranges from slightly to highly virulent. Although some organisms are described as avirulent, it appears that any organism can cause disease under certain circumstances. It may be possible to reduce virulence by a deliberate manipulation of the organism, for example, by repeated subculturing on a specific medium or by exposure to a certain drug or to radiation. Purposeful attempts to develop "avirulent" strains have been related to efforts to develop a microbial strain for vaccination purposes, such as the attenuated poliomyelitis virus used for oral vaccination. Under certain host-factor conditions, however, clinical poliomyelitis can result from oral "vaccination" with the attenuated strain. Some naturally occurring organisms have been considered avirulent or of low virulence; however, under certain conditions—such as high doses, reduced or defective host resistance, or both—disease has resulted from contact with these organisms. For years, *Serratia marcescens,* for example, was considered to be an avirulent organism; because of this and because certain strains produce easily recognizable red pigment, these organisms were used for environmental studies in hospitals. However, as hospitalized patients became more susceptible to developing infections—due to advancing age, presence of chronic diseases, and the effects of new diagnostic and therapeutic measures—nosocomial disease due to *S. marcescens* organisms subsequently became recognized and reported. It became apparent that this organism could cause disease in individuals with compromised defense systems. Thus avirulence is a relative term; whether an organism is "avirulent" depends on host factors such as susceptibility, agent factors such as dose, and other characteristics of the agent that influence the occurrence of disease.

*Invasiveness* describes the ability of microorganisms to invade tissues. Some organisms can penetrate the intact integument, whereas other microorganisms can enter only through a break in the skin or mucous membranes. An example of the former is *Leptospira* and of the latter *Clostridium tetani. Vibrio cholerae* organisms are noninvasive; once in the gastrointestinal tract, they do not invade the endothelium; rather, they elaborate a toxin that reacts with the mucosal tissue and causes diarrhea. *Shigella* organisms are highly invasive and cause a symptomatic response by invading the submucosal tissue.

DOSE   Another important "agent" factor is *dose,* that is, the number of organisms available to cause infection. The *infective dose* of an agent is that quantity of the agent necessary to cause infection. The number of organisms necessary to cause infection varies from organism to organism and from host to host, and it will be influenced by the mode of transmission. The relation of dose to the onset of typhoid fever, for example, was shown in volunteer studies by Hornick [2], who demonstrated that with an inoculum of $10^3$ *Salmonella typhosa,* no clinical disease developed in normal volunteers. However, when the inoculum was increased to $10^7$ salmonellae, there was a 50 percent attack rate among the volunteers, and with an inoculum of $10^9$ organisms, there was a 95 percent attack rate.

SPECIFICITY   Microorganisms may be specific with respect to their range of hosts. St. Louis encephalitis virus, for example, has a broad range of hosts, including many avian species, mammals, and mosquitoes. On the other hand, *Rickettsia prowazekii,* the species that causes typhus, has a very narrow host range, involving body lice and man. *Brucella abortus* is highly communicable in cattle but not in man. Some *Salmonella* species, such as *S. typhimurium,* are common to both animals and humans, but others have a narrow range of specificity; for example, *S. dublin* primarily infects bovines, and *S. typhosa* is known to infect only humans.

OTHER AGENT FACTORS   Other characteristics of the organism, such as the production of enzymes, are directed toward overcoming the defense mechanisms of the host. The streptococci, for example, produce leukocidin, hemolysin, and proteinase, all of which are directed toward overcoming humoral and tissue defense mechanisms of the host. Some agents produce polysaccharide capsules and others, toxins, that may give an advantage to the organism.

Certain antigenic variations within species of microorganisms influence the disease-producing potential of the organism. Of the 83 different pneumococcal serotypes, for instance, 14 cause over 80 percent of human pneumococcal pneumonia infections. Among streptococci, group A organisms are associated with infections of the pharynx, whereas group B organisms are primarily associated with infections of the genitourinary tract.

The antigenic makeup of an organism may change, allowing a new variant to spread through a population because of the lack of host resistance to the new variant. This is seen with influenza A; every two to three years, a modified variant becomes prevalent and spreads throughout the country. This phenomenon is known as *antigenic drift.* More significant changes in influenza A occur every seven to ten years (e.g., Asian strain, 1958-59; Hong Kong strain, 1968-69; Victoria strain, 1975-76); these changes are known as *major antigenic shifts.*

Resistance-transfer plasmids also influence the occurrence of nosocomial disease (see Chapter 12). The transfer of R plasmids from one enteric organism to another has occurred in hospital outbreaks and may account for a change in the antibiotic sensitivity of a strain. The antibiotic sensitivity of "hospital organisms" is also influenced by the use of antibiotics in the hospital (see Chapter 11); more resistant strains are selected as a result of the increased use of a particular antibiotic (or antibiotics) against which specific resistance plasmids are commonly carried by prevalent nosocomial strains. If a common R-plasmid-mediated resistance pattern of *Escherichia coli* in a hospital is ampicillin, tetracycline, and sulfonamide, for example, then the pressures deriving from the use of any one of these drugs will concurrently select for strains with the other two resistances as well. This change in antibiotic sensitivity may make therapy difficult; it can result in an increasing prevalence of the resistant strain, reduce the infecting or colonizing doses of the organism in those receiving drugs to which these strains are resistant, increase the numbers of organisms disseminated from persons colonized with these strains, and subsequently cause a greater frequency of nosocomial infections due to this more resistant strain.

Other organism factors, some plasmid-mediated, include the ability to adhere to intestinal mucosa, resist gastric acid and disinfectants, and produce bacteriocins active against endogenous flora.

RESERVOIR AND SOURCE   All organisms have a reservoir and a source; these may be the same or different, and it is important to distinguish between these potentially different sites if control and/or prevention measures are to be directed at this aspect of the chain of infection. The *reservoir* is the place where the organism maintains its presence, metabolizes, and replicates. Viruses generally survive better in human reservoirs; the reservoir of gram-positive bacteria is usually a human, whereas gram-negative bacteria may have either a human or animal reservoir, (e.g., *Salmonella*) or an inanimate reservoir (e.g., *Pseudomonas* in water). The reservoir may be quite specific: for poliomyelitis virus, for example, the reservoir is always human. On the other hand, *Pseudomonas* species may be found in either an animate or an inanimate reservoir.

The *source* is the place from which the infectious agent passes to the host, either by direct contact or by indirect contact through a vehicle as the means of transmission. Sources also may be animate or inanimate. The reservoir and source may be the same location, or the source may become contaminated from the reservoir. For example, a reservoir for *Pseudomonas* organisms may be the tap water in a hospital; however, the source from which it is transmitted to the patient may be a humidifier that has been filled directly with the contaminated tap water. In a common-source outbreak of measles, the reservoir and source may be the same person.

The source may be mobile or fixed. A susceptible patient may be brought to a fixed source (e.g., a patient who comes to use a contaminated whirlpool bath), or the source may be mobile and brought to the patient (e.g., contaminated food brought from the kitchen to the patient's bedside).

PERIOD OF INFECTIVITY   *Infectivity* refers to the ability of an organism to spread from a source to a host. An infected human may be infective during the incubation period, the clinical disease state, or convalescence. Additionally, an asymptomatic carrier (or colonized person), who does not show evidence of clinical disease, may be infective. An example of a disease that is primarily infectious during the incubation period is hepatitis A: the infected individual is infective during the latter half of the incubation period and during the first several days of clinical disease. In measles, the patient is infective during the prodromal stage to approximately four days after the onset of the rash. In chickenpox, the individual is infective from approximately five days before the skin eruption to not more than six days after the appearance of the eruption. A disease in which the individual is infective primarily during the initial clinical-disease phase is exemplified by influenza, in which the individual is infective for a period of several days after the onset of symptoms. In cases of tuberculosis and typhoid fever, the individual may be infective for essentially the entire pretreatment clinical phase, with infectivity usually significantly decreasing when there is clinical evidence of successful chemotherapy. Examples of diseases that are infectious into the convalescent period are salmonellosis, shigellosis, and diphtheria. In some diseases, such as typhoid fever and hepatitis B, a chronic carrier state may develop in which the individual may be infective for a long time, possibly years, while showing no symptoms of illness. However, the microorganisms that most commonly cause nosocomial infections—such as *E. coli, Klebsiella, Enterobacter,* and *Pseudomonas*—do not demonstrate the same patterns of infectivity or evoke the protective immune responses that typhoid fever and hepatitis B do.

Asymptomatic or subclinical carriers may also be infective for brief periods and continue to be the source of infection for susceptible individuals for long periods. This is seen, for example, in poliomyelitis and hepatitis A. In poliomyelitis, the ratio is approximately 100 carriers to one clinical case, and in hepatitis A, ten to one. In spite of not showing clinical evidence of infection, the person with a subclinical infection may be an active transmitter of infection, and clinical disease may result from such transmission. Dissemination from an asymptomatic carrier may be related to a specific event, such as the occurrence of a second disease process (see previous discussion). However, dissemination may also occur that is unrelated to any definable event. The staphylococcus carrier provides a classic example of the asymptomatic dissemination of infectious organisms; in this case, the site of dissemination may be the anterior nares or, at times, the skin. Similarly, the site of asymptomatic streptococcal carriage may be in the pharynx, perianal area, or vagina.

The source of an infection may be an atypical case of a specific disease whose clinical course has been modified either by therapy, vaccine (as in measles), or prophylaxis (such as the use of immune serum globulin in hepatitis A). Also, the source may be an abortive case of disease in which the typical expression of the disease has been modified by treatment with antibiotics.

Animals may also provide a source of infection, although this is of less concern in the hospital setting.

EXIT   The portal of exit for organisms from humans is usually single, although it may be multiple. It may not always be the obvious portal of exit; in bubonic plague, for example, in which the skin lesions are the most visible concern, exit by the airborne route from unrecognized secondary pneumonia is also of great importance in transmission. In general, the major portals of exit are the respiratory and gastrointestinal tracts as well as the skin and wounds. Blood may also be the portal of exit, as in hepatitis B infections.

*Transmission*

Transmission, the second link in the chain of infection, describes the movement of organisms from the source to the host. Spread may occur through one or more of four different routes: contact, common-vehicle, airborne, or vectorborne. An organism may have a single route of transmission, or it may be transmissible by two or more routes. Tuberculosis, for example, is almost always transmitted by the airborne route; measles is primarily a contact-spread disease but may also be transmitted through the air; salmonellae may be transmitted by contact or by the common-vehicle or airborne route. Thus in defining the route of transmission, although one route may be the obvious one involved in a nosocomial infection problem, another route may also be operative. Knowledge regarding the route of transmission for a specific disease can be very helpful in the investigation of a nosocomial infection problem. Such information can point to the source and may allow control measures to be introduced more rapidly.

CONTACT SPREAD   In contact-spread disease, the victim has contact with the source, and that contact is either direct, indirect, or by droplets. *Direct contact,* of which person-to-person spread is an example, occurs when there is actual physical contact between the source and the victim, such as in the fecal-oral spread of hepatitis A virus. Infections resulting from organisms within the patient may be referred to as *autogenous infections;* that is, the mode of acquisition is autogenous, even though transmission occurred earlier, namely, at the time the host became colonized with the organism. A postoperative cholecystectomy wound infection due to coliform organisms from the patient's own gallbladder, for instance, would represent an autogenous contact infection.

*Indirect-contact* transmission is distinguished from direct-contact transmission by the participation of an intermediate object (usually inanimate) that is passively involved in the transmission of the infectious agent from the source to the victim. The intermediate object may become contaminated from an animate or inanimate source. An example is the transfer to susceptible hosts of enteric organisms on an endoscope that initially became contaminated when brought in contact with an infected patient (the index patient).

*Droplet spread* refers to the brief passage of the infectious agent through the air when the source and the victim are relatively near each other, usually within several feet, such as when there is transmission by talking or sneezing. Droplets are large particles that rapidly settle out on horizontal surfaces; thus they are not transmitted beyond a radius of several feet from the source. Examples of droplet-spread infections include measles and streptococcal pharyngitis.

COMMON-VEHICLE SPREAD   In *common-vehicle* spread infection, a contaminated inanimate vehicle serves as the vector for transmission of the agent to multiple persons. The victims become infected after contact with the common vehicle. This transmission may be active if the organisms replicate while in the vehicle, such as salmonellae in food, or passive if the organisms are passively carried by the vehicle, such as hepatitis A in food. Other types of common vehicles include blood and blood products (hepatitis B), intravenous fluids (gram-negative septicemia), and drugs (salmonellosis), in which units or batches of a product become contaminated from a common source and serve as a common vehicle for multiple infections. Thus multiple vehicles may all become contaminated from a single common source. Even though there are multiple vehicles involved, these infections may be considered to be transmitted by a common vehicle because the epidemiologic principles are the same. It should be noted that "common source" and "common vehicle" are not interchangeable terms. A common source is just that: a source common to multiple vehicles from which the vehicles become infected. A common vehicle, on the other hand, is a vehicle of infection associated with two or more cases of a disease. If only a single infection results, the designation of direct-contact or indirect-contact spread, whichever is appropriate for the circumstances, should be used.

AIRBORNE SPREAD   *Airborne* transmission describes organisms that have a true airborne phase in their route of dissemination, which usually involves a distance of more than several feet between the source and the victim. The organisms are contained within droplet nuclei or dust particles; the former are airborne particles that result from the evaporation of droplets, are 5 $\mu$ or smaller in size, and may remain suspended in air for prolonged periods of time. Dust particles that have settled on surfaces may become resuspended by physical action and may also remain airborne for a prolonged period. Skin squamae may become airborne and provide a mechanism for the airborne transmission of organisms such as staphylococci. Airborne particles may remain suspended for hours or possibly days, depending on environmental factors. Movement may be within a room, or—again depending on environmental factors, especially air currents—transmission may be over a longer distance. The size and density of the airborne particle will also influence the distance it moves.

Airborne spread by means of droplet nuclei is exemplified in the transmission of tuberculosis and, in some instances, staphylococcal infections. The classic experiments of Riley [3] demonstrated the airborne route of infection for tubercle bacilli, in which the source of the organisms was disseminating patients with active, sputum-positive, cavitary disease. Some nosocomial staphylococcal disease has been shown to be transmitted by the airborne route. In one report [4], several postoperative wound infections were said to have resulted from the airborne spread of staphylococci from a staff member who remained at the periphery of the operating room throughout the surgical procedure; the only route for transmission of the organisms was through the air, there being no opportunity in this case for contact or common-vehicle spread.

Organisms may be transmitted in dust, as was seen, for example, in an outbreak of salmonellosis, in which transmission occurred by means of contaminated dust contained in a vacuum cleaner bag; the dust became resuspended each time the vacuum cleaner was used [1].

The airborne route of transmission is more frequently assumed to be the route of an infection than is the case. Creation of an infectious aerosol is more difficult than is usually recognized.

VECTORBORNE SPREAD   Vectorborne-spread nosocomial disease, although unreported in the United States, could occur; it includes external and internal vector transmission. *External vectorborne transmission* refers to the mechanical transfer of microorganisms on the body or appendages of the vector; shigellae and salmonellae are transferred in this way by flies, for example. *Internal vectorborne transmission* includes harborage and biologic transmission. In transmission by harborage, there is no biologic action between the vector and the agent; this is seen with *Yersinia pestis* organisms in the gastrointestinal tract of the flea. *Biologic* transmission occurs when the agent (e.g., a parasite) goes through biologic changes within the vector, as malaria parasites do within the mosquito.

## Host
The third link in the chain of infection is the host or victim. Disease does not always follow the transmission of infectious agents to a host. As previously discussed, various agent factors play a part; similarly, a variety of host factors must also be surmounted before infection occurs and disease develops. Host factors that influence the development of infections are the site of deposition of the agent and the host's defense mechanisms, both specific and nonspecific.

ENTRANCE   Sites of deposition include the skin, mucous membranes, and respiratory, gastrointestinal, and urinary tracts. Organisms such as leptospires can gain entrance through normal skin. Other organisms, such as staphylococci, need a minute breach in the integrity of the skin to gain entrance to the body. There may be mechanical transmission through the normal skin, as with hepatitis B virus on a contaminated needle. Abnormal skin, such as a preexisting wound, may be the site of deposition of organisms such as *Pseudomonas aeruginosa*. Mucous membranes may be the site of entrance, as the conjunctiva is for adenovirus type 8.

Another site of deposition is the respiratory tract. The exact area of deposition will depend on the size of the airborne particle and the aerodynamics at the time of transmission. Generally, particles 5 $\mu$ or larger in diameter will be deposited in the upper respiratory tract, whereas those less than 5 $\mu$ in diameter will be deposited in the lower respiratory tract.

Infectious agents may gain entrance to the body through the intestinal tract by means of ingestion of contaminated foods or liquids, through contaminated supplemental feedings, or through contaminated equipment, such as endoscopes inserted into the intestinal tract. Within the gastrointestinal tract, some organisms cause disease by secreting a toxin that is absorbed through the mucosa (enterotoxigenic *E. coli*), while others invade the wall of the intestinal tract (*Shigella*). Some microorganisms involve primarily the upper part of the gastrointestinal tract (*Staphylococcus*), and others, the lower part of the tract (*Shigella*). The urinary tract may become infected from contaminated foreign objects such as catheters or cystoscopes inserted into the urethra, or by the retrograde movement of organisms on the external surface of a catheter inserted into the bladder.

Organisms may gain entrance into the host via the placenta, as occurs in rubella and toxoplasmosis. Transplantation is another method by which microorganisms enter the host; infection may follow renal transplantation if the donated kidney is infected with cytomegalovirus.

An organism may colonize one site and cause no disease, but the same organism at another site may result in clinical disease. *E. coli,* for example, routinely colonizes the gastrointestinal tract and under normal circumstances does not cause disease; however, the same organism in the urinary tract may very well cause infection. *S. aureus* may colonize the external nares without any evidence of disease, but when the same organism colonizes a fresh surgical wound, a postoperative wound infection may develop.

DEFENSE MECHANISMS: NONSPECIFIC   A host's defense mechanisms may be nonspecific or specific; the quantity and quality of these mechanisms will vary from person to person. Nonspecific defense mechanisms include the skin, mucous membranes, and certain bodily secretions. The skin forms the first barrier against infection; it is a mechanical barrier and contains secretions that have an antibacterial action. Tears, a form of epithelial secretion, have an antibacterial action (due to lysozyme), and they also mechanically remove entrapped organisms. The gastrointestinal tract secretes acid that acts as a barrier against enteric organisms. Other secretions, such as mucus and enzymes, bolster the defense mechanisms. The muscular contractions of the intestinal tract act to move the contents through the tract and thus reduce the available time for organisms to invade the mucosa. Within the nose and upper respiratory tract, the cilia act to remove organisms that impinge on them. The blanket of mucus serves to entrap and remove infectious agents. The lower respiratory tract is protected by secretions and macrophages that ingest microorganisms and carry them to regional lymph nodes.

The local inflammatory response provides another nonspecific host defense mechanism. Other nonspecific protective mechanisms include genetic, hormonal, and nutritional factors, as well as behavioral patterns and personal hygiene. Age, as influenced by these nonspecific factors, is associated with decreased resistance at either end of the spectrum; the very young and the very old frequently are more susceptible to infection. Surgery and the presence of chronic diseases—such as diabetes, blood disorders, certain lymphomas, and collagen diseases—alter host resistance, which again reflects the influence of the above nonspecific factors.

DEFENSE MECHANISMS: SPECIFIC    Specific immunity results from either natural events or artificially induced events. *Natural immunity* results from having had certain diseases—such as rubella and poliomyelitis (type-specific)—and usually persists for the life of the host. Immunity may also develop after inapparent infection, such as in diphtheria or poliomyelitis. With other diseases, there is a latent stage following clinical illness in which immunity is imperfect; the agent will remain in the latent stage until some triggering mechanism initiates disease. Such latency is shown in infection with herpes simplex virus and cytomegalovirus.

*Artificial immunity* can be either active or passive. *Active* artificial immunity follows the use of vaccines. There are attenuated vaccines, such as those used against poliomyelitis, yellow fever, and tuberculosis; killed vaccines, used against such diseases as typhoid fever and pertussis; and toxoids, which are used against diphtheria and tetanus. *Passive* immunity results from the use of immune serum globulin (i.e., serum that contains antibody); this is employed, for example, in prophylaxis against hepatitis A infections. Transplacental antibodies, such as measles antibodies, also provide an example of passive antibody protection. Passive antibody protects the individual from disease, but it neither protects against infection nor prevents subsequent spread of the agent to others. Passive protection is of relatively short duration, usually several months at most.

HOST RESPONSE    The spectrum of the host's response to a microorganism may range from a subclinical (or inapparent) infection to a clinically apparent illness, the extreme being death.

The clinical spectrum of disease varies from mild, to a "typical" course (although a disease may typically be mild), to severe disease and possible death. The degree of host response is determined by both agent and host factors and includes the dose of the infecting organism, its organ specificity, the pathogenicity of the infecting organism, its virulence and invasiveness, and its portal of entry. Host factors include the quantitative and qualitative level of the specific and nonspecific immunologic factors previously discussed.

The same organism infecting different hosts can result in a clinical spectrum of disease that is the same, similar, or different in various individuals. In an epidemic, for example, many cases of what appears to be the epidemic disease may meet the clinical case definition, while other cases that epidemiologically are related to the same outbreak may not meet the same case definition. They may, in fact, be cases of the epidemic disease, but with a different clinical spectrum (as can occasionally be demonstrated by serologic tests). They may also be cases of other diseases occurring concurrently with the epidemic.

*Environment*
The environment significantly influences the multiple factors in the chain of infection. The transmission of the agent from its source to the host occurs in an "environment" that represents the summation of many individual factors; changes in any of these can have an impact on any link in the chain of infection. Some environmental factors are under strict control, such as the air in an operating room, whereas others are not.

At times, too much emphasis is placed on the role of the environment; for example, it is inappropriate to take environmental cultures routinely throughout a hospital (see Part I, Chapters 7 and 14). In other instances, not enough attention is paid to the environment. There needs to be a healthy respect for the environment, with maintenance that does not deliberately promote the transmission of disease-causing agents to hosts, but without excessive control measures that impose unnecessary and ineffective actions on the hospital staff and a consequent loss of efficiency and effectiveness, and a wasting of resources such as personnel time and money. Knowledge of environmental factors and their influence on the chain of infection and an awareness of adverse changes in the environment should be sufficient to alert one to the need to investigate these environmental factors to ascertain their role in a nosocomial infection problem.

Some environmental factors can influence all the links in the chain of infection, while others are more limited in their range of action. Humidity, for example, can influence a multiplicity of factors; it can affect the persistence of an agent at its source, its transmission through the air, and the effectiveness of a host's mucous membranes in resisting infection.

Other environmental factors, however, have a more limited effect on the occurrence of infection; for example, the temperature-pressure relation in a specific autoclave affects sterilization within that autoclave, but it has no direct effect on the host.

Certain environmental factors directly affect the agent. Replication of the agent at its reservoir may depend on certain substances in the environment. The agent's survival is influenced by the temperature, humidity, pH, and radiation at its reservoir or source; its survival is even influenced by such factors during its transmission. There may also be toxic substances in the environment that are lethal for the agent.

The transmission of agents will be affected by environmental factors such as temperature and humidity, as mentioned above. Airborne transmission is influenced by air velocity and the direction of its movement. The stability and concentration of an aerosol are directly related to environmental factors. In winter people tend to be indoors with closed windows and reduced air circulation, and this increases the risk of airborne disease compared with summer, when room air is air-conditioned or diluted with outside air. In outbreaks associated with common-vehicle transmission, the temperature of the environment will influence the level of contamination in the vehicle. The spread of vectorborne disease also reflects favorable conditions in the environment for the survival and movement of the vector.

The host's resistance mechanisms are affected by environmental factors; for example, in an excessively dry atmosphere, mucous membranes become dry and are less able to protect against microbial invasion. Also, the host's behavioral patterns are influenced by temperature.

Only after each link in the chain of infection has been carefully described can the most appropriate methods of control and prevention be determined. There may be similarities among cases of disease in different outbreaks; until all the factors involved in the chain of infection are determined for each outbreak, however, it is not possible to be certain that extrapolation of control and preventive measures from one outbreak will be appropriate to another outbreak.

## REFERENCES

1. Bate, J., and James, U. *Salmonella typhimurium* infection dust-borne in a children's ward. *Lancet* 2:713, 1958.
2. Hornick, R. B., Greisman, S. E., and Woodward, T. E. Typhoid fever: Pathogenesis and immunologic control. *N. Engl. J. Med.* 283:686, 1970.
3. Riley, R. L., et al. Aerial dissemination of pulmonary tuberculosis: A two-year study of contagion in a tuberculosis ward. *Am. J. Hyg.* 70:185, 1959.
4. Waller, C. W., Kuntsin, R. B., and Brubaker, M. M. The incidence of airborne wound infections during operation. *J.A.M.A.* 186:908, 1963.

# 2 PERSONNEL HEALTH SERVICES

Walter W. Williams
Julia S. Garner

Ages ago, Hippocrates exhorted his followers, "First do no harm." Nowhere does this charge seem more relevant today than in hospitals. In the United States, about 5 million persons work in more than 7000 hospitals. These persons may become infected through exposure to infected patients or exposure outside the hospital. In either case they may transmit the infection to patients, other hospital personnel, members of their households, or other community contacts.

Persons who have direct contact with patients, including nurses, medical house staff, clinical faculty, attending physicians, paramedical personnel, and nursing and medical students, are more likely than other hospital personnel to be involved in disease transmission. Nevertheless, other hospital personnel may occasionally have contact with patients that is comparable in quality, intensity, and duration to that of patient-care personnel. Risk to patients and personnel who have only brief, casual contact with each other is generally felt to be low.

In this chapter we outline the infection control objectives of a hospital personnel health service and discuss the epidemiology and control of selected infections transmitted among patient-care personnel and patients. The program we outline does not provide a blueprint for comprehensive health care; rather, it presents a general viewpoint regarding what a hospital personnel health service might do to prevent transmission of infection to and from patient-care personnel. The objectives and control measures presented here reflect recommendations outlined in the Centers for Disease Control Guideline for Infection Control in Hospital Personnel [84], which can be consulted for specific details not covered in this chapter.

## INFECTION CONTROL OBJECTIVES OF A PERSONNEL HEALTH SERVICE

The Centers for Disease Control (CDC) recommends that the infection control objectives of a personnel health service be part of the hospital's general program for infection control [84]. The objectives can include (1) stressing maintenance of sound habits in personal hygiene and individual responsibility in infection control; (2) monitoring and investigating infectious diseases, potentially harmful infectious exposures, and outbreaks of infections among personnel; (3) providing care to personnel for work-related illnesses or exposures; (4) identifying infection risks related to employment and instituting appropriate preventive measures; and (5) containing costs by eliminating unnecessary procedures and preventing infectious disease that results in absenteeism and disability. For these objectives to be met, the support of the administration, medical staff, and other hospital personnel is essential.

Regardless of whether the hospital's personnel health service is devoted mainly to controlling infectious diseases or to providing a comprehensive health program for personnel, the same elements will assist in controlling infection. These elements include placement evaluations, personnel health and safety education, immunization programs, protocols for surveillance and management of job-related illnesses and exposures to infectious diseases, counseling services for personnel regarding infection risks related to employment or special conditions, guidelines for restricting work because of infectious disease, and maintenance of health records. Each of these elements is discussed below.

### Placement Evaluations

When personnel are appointed initially or reassigned to different jobs or areas, a placement evaluation can be used to ensure that persons are not placed in jobs that would pose undue risk of infection to them, other personnel, patients, or visitors. It is important that initial placement evaluations be done when personnel are hired or as soon after as possible. After the placement evaluation, later appraisals can be done as needed for ongoing programs or evaluation of work-related problems.

A health inventory is an important part of the placement evaluation. This inventory can include determining a health worker's immunization status and obtaining a history of any conditions that may predispose the health worker to acquire or transmit infectious diseases, for example, obtaining a history of childhood diseases such as chickenpox and measles, and documenting exposure to or treatment for tuberculosis, hepatitis, dermatologic conditions, chronic draining infections or open wounds, and immunodeficient conditions. The health inventory can be used to determine whether physical examinations or laboratory tests are needed.

Physical examinations may help detect unusual susceptibility to infection or conditions that may increase the likelihood of transmitting disease to patients, and serve as a baseline for determining whether future problems are work-related. There are no data, however, to suggest that routine complete physical examinations are needed for infection control purposes. Neither are there data to suggest that routine laboratory testing (such as complete blood counts, serologic tests for syphilis, urinalysis, or chest roentgenograms) or preemployment screening for enteric or other pathogens are cost-beneficial. In some areas, however, local public health ordinances may still mandate that certain screening procedures be used.

### Personnel Health and Safety Education

Personnel are more likely to comply with a health program if they understand its rationale. Thus education is a central focus of a personnel health program. This includes initial job orientation and ongoing inservice education about the infection control aspects of personnel health and the proper use of the personnel health service. Not all personnel need the same degree of instruction in infection control, and educational programs need to be matched to the needs of employees in different job categories.

The personnel health service has a unique opportunity to initiate health education even before the person's hospital duties are assumed. The preplacement evaluation can be used in part to provide personnel with oral and written guidance about their role in the prevention of nosocomial infections. This is an excellent time to stress that *patient-care personnel can decrease the risk of acquiring or transmitting infection by careful hand-washing after touching a source that is likely to be contaminated and by taking care of patients with transmissible infections according to the published Guideline for Isolation Precautions in Hospitals* [35]. Other helpful suggestions by the health service about using appropriate precautions to avoid illness or on bringing illness promptly to medical attention may also be presented to personnel.

### Immunization Programs

Since hospital personnel are at risk of exposure to and possible transmission of vaccine-preventable diseases, maintaining immunity is an essential part of a hospital's personnel health and infection control program. Optimal use of immunizing agents will safeguard the health of personnel, obviate unnecessary work restrictions, and protect patients from becoming infected by personnel. Therefore, each hospital's staff should formulate a comprehensive policy on immunizing hospital personnel [84].

Immunization recommendations are made by the U.S. Public Health Service Immunization Practices Advisory Committee (ACIP) and are published periodically in the CDC *Morbidity and Mortality Weekly Report*. Indications for use of licensed vaccines are generally the same for hospital personnel as for the general population; however, immunity to some diseases, such as rubella, may be more important for persons who work in hospitals. Decisions about which vaccines to include in immunization programs can be made by considering the (1) risk of exposure to an agent in a given area, (2) nature of employment, and (3) size and kind of institution. Table 2-1 lists immunization recommendations from the Guideline for Infection Control in Hospital Personnel [84] that can be considered by hospitals in formulating policies.

SCREENING FOR SUSCEPTIBILITY TO HEPATITIS B OR RUBELLA   The decision to screen potential vaccine recipients for susceptibility to hepatitis B virus (HBV) is an economic one, since vaccinating HBV carriers or persons already immune does not appear to present a hazard [30,74]. In the United States, the cost-effectiveness of screening is usually determined by the prevalence of previous infection in any targeted group, the cost of screening, and the cost of immunizing personnel [46,56]. Routine serologic tests to ensure that rubella vaccine is given only to those proved susceptible may be very expensive. The ACIP states that rubella immunization of men and of women not known to be pregnant is justifiable without serologic testing [47].

VACCINE ADMINISTRATION   The most efficient use of vaccines with high-risk groups is to immunize personnel before they enter high-risk situations. It is crucial that persons administering immunizing agents be well-informed about indications, storage, dosage, preparation, and contraindications for each of the vaccines, toxoids, and immune globulins they may use. Product information should be available at all times, and a pertinent health history should be obtained from each health worker before an agent is given [84].

### Work Restrictions and Management of Job-related Illnesses and Exposures

Optimal safeguarding of patients and personnel calls for prompt evaluation and administrative action on the basis of signs and symptoms of transmissible infectious diseases or significant exposures of personnel to a transmissible agent. Therefore, a major function of the personnel health service is to arrange for prompt diagnosis and management of job-related illnesses and provide prophylaxis for certain preventable diseases to which personnel may be exposed. Hospitals are advised to have well-defined policies for personnel who have transmissible infections [84]. Such policies should govern personnel responsibility in using the health service and reporting illness, as well as rules for excluding personnel from direct contact with patients and giving clearance after work restriction because of an infectious disease. For any exclusion

policy to be enforceable and effective, all personnel—especially department heads, area supervisors, and head nurses—must know when an illness is to be reported. Those with the authority to relieve personnel of duties also need to be identified. Any policy for work restriction should be designed to encourage personnel to report their illnesses or exposures and not penalize them with loss of wages, benefits, or job status [84].

Table 2-2 lists recommendations from the Guideline for Infection Control in Hospital Personnel [84] for prophylaxis of hospital personnel after important exposures. Table 2-3 summarizes important recommendations and suggested work restrictions listed in this guideline [84] for personnel with selected infectious diseases.

### Health Counseling

All personnel need to know about infection risks related to employment; therefore, a readily available mechanism is needed for personnel to obtain advice about illnesses they may acquire from or transmit to patients [84]. Access to health counseling about transmissible illnesses is especially important for women of childbearing age. Personnel who are pregnant, may be pregnant, or might become pregnant need to know about potential risks to the fetus due to work assignments and about preventive measures that will reduce those risks. Diseases that, if contracted by the mother, are a potential risk to the fetus include cytomegalovirus infection, hepatitis B, and rubella (see Chapter 35).

### Coordinated Planning With Other Departments

The infection control activities of the personnel health service should be coordinated with the infection control program and other hospital departments [84]. This coordination will help ensure adequate surveillance and follow-up of infections in personnel. Moreover during case investigations, outbreaks, and other epidemiologic studies involving hospital personnel, this coordination will promote efficient investigations and prompt implementation of control measures. Such coordination can be accomplished more easily if a representative of the personnel health service is on the Infection Control Committee.

## EPIDEMIOLOGY AND CONTROL OF SELECTED INFECTIONS TRANSMITTED AMONG HOSPITAL PERSONNEL AND PATIENTS

The hazard of nosocomial spread of infection from hospital personnel to patients was recognized during

TABLE 2-1. Recommendations for immunization of hospital personnel

| Disease or agent | Immunization guideline | Other recommendations |
|---|---|---|
| Rubella | All personnel (male or female) considered at increased risk of contact with patients with rubella or likely to have direct contact with pregnant patients should be immune to rubella[a] (Category I) | Before immunizing, serologic screening for rubella need not be done unless the hospital considers it cost-effective or the potential vaccinee requests it (Category II). Persons can be considered susceptible unless they have laboratory evidence of immunity or documented immunization with live virus vaccine on or after their first birthday.<br>Consideration should be given to using rubella vaccine in combination with measles and mumps vaccines (measles-mumps-rubella [MMR] trivalent vaccine) |
| Hepatitis B | Persons at substantial risk of HBV infection who are demonstrated or judged likely to be susceptible should be actively immunized (see text) (Category II) | Before immunizing, serologic screening for hepatitis B need not be done unless the hospital policy considers it cost-effective or the potential vaccinee requests it (Category I)<br>Prophylaxis with an immune globulin (passive immunization) should be used when indicated, such as following needle-stick exposure to blood that is at high-risk of being HB$_s$Ag-positive (Category I). Immune globulins should not be used as a substitute for active immunization (Category I) |
| Measles | All persons susceptible by history or serologic study who are considered at increased risk of contact with patients infected with measles should be protected (Category I) | Most persons born before 1957 have probably been infected naturally and generally need not be considered susceptible. Younger persons can be considered immune only if they have documentation of (1) physician-diagnosed measles, (2) laboratory evidence of measles immunity, or (3) adequate immunization with live measles vaccine on or after the first birthday<br>Consideration should be given to administering measles vaccine in combination with rubella and mumps vaccine (measles-mumps-rubella [MMR] trivalent vaccine) |
| Poliomyelitis | Routine primary immunization for adults in the United States is not recommended. Personnel who may have direct contact with patients who may be excreting polioviruses should complete a primary series. Primary immunization with IPV instead of OPV is recommended for these persons whenever feasible (Category I). (IPV is preferred because the risk of vaccine-associated paralysis following OPV is slightly higher in adults than in children and because personnel may shed | |

TABLE 2-1. (CONTINUED)

| Disease or agent | Immunization guideline | Other recommendations |
|---|---|---|
| | virus after OPV and inadvertently expose susceptible or immunocompromised patients to live virus)<br>In an outbreak, OPV should be provided to anyone who has not been completely immunized or whose immunization status is unknown[b] (Category I) | |
| Influenza | To avoid problems with staffing during the influenza season and to prevent spread of influenza from personnel to patients, efforts should be made to immunize hospital personnel against influenza in the fall of each year (Category II) | |
| Diphtheria, pneumococcal disease, mumps, tetanus | Because hospital personnel are not at substantially higher risk than the general adult population of acquiring these diseases, they should seek these immunizations from their primary care provider, according to the recommendations of the ACIP (Category I) | |
| Pertussis, tuberculosis, cholera, meningococcal disease, plague, rabies, typhoid, typhus, yellow fever | Hospitals should not assume responsibility for routine immunization of hospital personnel against these diseases (Category I) | |

IPV = inactivated polio vaccine; OPV = oral polio vaccine; ACIP = Immunization Practices Advisory Committee; Category I = strongly recommended; Category II = moderately recommended.
[a]Pregnancy is a contraindication. Vaccine should not be given to pregnant women or those who may become pregnant within three months.
[b]Exceptions to this recommendation are discussed in the current ACIP recommendations under the heading *Precautions and Contraindications: Immunodeficiency*. (Immunization Practices Advisory Committee. *Morbid. Mortal. Weekly Rep.* 31:32, 1982.)
Source: Adapted from Williams, W. W. *Infect. Control* 4 (Suppl.):326, 1983. Consult current ACIP recommendations for a detailed discussion of the rationale for each recommendation.

the last century at the time Semmelweis and his contemporaries enunciated the concept of hospital-acquired infection. Patient-care personnel have long since been implicated as reservoirs and vectors of organisms causing nosocomial outbreaks. During the past decade the occupational risks caused by infection transmitted from patients to personnel have received even more attention.

The purpose of this section is to discuss the major hazards of infection transmitted to and from hospital personnel. It should be kept in mind that almost any transmissible infection may occur in the community at large or within the hospital and can affect both personnel and patients; however, only those infectious diseases that are most important to personnel are discussed here. Relevant epidemiology, microbiology, and preventive measures applicable to personnel health are reviewed for each disease.

## ACQUIRED IMMUNODEFICIENCY SYNDROME (AIDS)

At the time of this writing, evidence implicates a newly recognized retrovirus as the cause of AIDS (see Chapter 35). Epidemiologic data suggest that the virus has been transmitted through intimate sexual contact; sharing contaminated needles; transfusion of whole blood, blood cellular components, plasma, or clotting factor concentrates that have not been heat-treated; or from infected mother to child before, at, or shortly after the time of birth. There has been no evidence of transmission by casual contact or airborne spread, nor have there been cases of AIDS in health-care or laboratory personnel that can be definitely ascribed to specific occupational exposures. The distribution of disease and modes of spread appear to be similar to those found in hepatitis B virus infection.

TABLE 2-2. Recommendations for prophylaxis after exposure

| Disease | Recommendations |
| --- | --- |
| General | When prophylactic treatment with drugs, vaccines, or immune globulins is deemed necessary and is offered, personnel should be informed of alternative means of prophylaxis, risk of infection if known if treatment is not accepted, degree of protection provided by the therapy, and potential side effects (Category I) |
| Hepatitis A | Personnel who have had direct fecal-oral exposure to excretions from a patient incubating hepatitis A should be given IG (0.02 ml/kg) (Category I). Prophylaxis with IG for all personnel who take care of patients with hepatitis A (other than as suggested above) should not be given (Category I) |
| Hepatitis B | For prophylaxis after percutaneous (needle-stick) or mucous membrane exposure to blood that might be infective, the recommendations in Table 2-4 should be followed (Category I) |
| Hepatitis non-A, non-B | For needle-stick exposures involving patients known to have hepatitis non-A, non-B, IG (0.06 ml/kg) should be given (Category II) |
| Meningococcal disease | Antimicrobial prophylaxis should be offered immediately to personnel who have had intensive direct contact with an infected patient without using proper precautions. If prophylaxis is deemed necessary, treatment should not await results of antimicrobial sensitivity testing (Category I) |
| Pertussis | Antimicrobial prophylaxis should be offered immediately to personnel who have had intensive contact with an infected patient without using proper precautions (Category II) |
| Rabies | Hospital personnel who either have been bitten by a human with rabies or have scratches, abrasions, open wounds, or mucous membranes contaminated with saliva or other potentially infective material from a human with rabies should receive a full course of antirabies treatment (Category I) |

IG = immune globulin; Category I = strongly recommended; Category II = moderately recommended.
Source: Adapted from Williams, W. W. *Infect. Control* 4 (Suppl.):326, 1983.

Precautions have been advised for persons and specimens from persons considered to be part of the "AIDS spectrum" [17], which includes (1) persons who meet the surveillance definition of AIDS, that is, persons with opportunistic infections not associated with underlying immunosuppressive disease or therapy or Kaposi's sarcoma (patients under 60 years of age); (2) persons with chronic generalized lymphadenopathy, unexplained weight loss, and/or prolonged unexplained fever when the history suggests an epidemiologic risk for AIDS; and (3) other patients whose clinical condition and epidemiologic history are suggestive of AIDS. Any new information on the cause and transmission of AIDS should be considered when precautions are designed or changed.

With present knowledge, it appears prudent for hospital personnel to use precautions in taking care of patients with AIDS similar to those used for patients with hepatitis B virus infection [17,35] (see Chapter 9). It also appears prudent for hospital personnel who have AIDS to use precautions similar to those suggested for known carriers of hepatitis B surface antigen (HBsAg) to minimize their infectious risk to others (see hepatitis discussion following).

Personnel considered to have any of the clinical features described in the AIDS spectrum should be counseled about precautions to minimize their risk of infecting others. Moreover personnel considered to have any of the clinical features described in the AIDS spectrum who have no exudative lesions on the hands should wear gloves for procedures that involve trauma to tissues or direct contact with mucous membranes or nonintact skin. Personnel considered to have any of the clinical features described in the AIDS spectrum and who have exudative lesions on the hands either should wear gloves for all direct patient contact and when handling equipment that will touch mucous membranes or nonintact skin or should abstain from all direct patient contact [84].

Personnel must take special care to avoid accidental wounds from sharp instruments contaminated with potentially infective material and avoid contact of

TABLE 2-3. Summary of important recommendations and work restriction for personnel with selected infectious diseases

| Disease/problem | Relieve from direct patient contact | Partial work restriction | Duration |
|---|---|---|---|
| Conjunctivitis, infectious | Yes | | Until discharge ceases |
| Cytomegalovirus infections | No | | |
| Diarrhea | | | |
|   Acute stage (diarrhea with other symptoms) | Yes | | Until symptoms resolve and infection with *Salmonella* is ruled out |
|   Convalescent stage *Salmonella* (nontyphoidal) | No | Personnel should not take care of high-risk patients | Until stool is free of the infecting organism on two consecutive cultures not less than 24 hours apart |
|   Other enteric pathogens | No | See text | |
| Enteroviral infections | No | Personnel should not take care of infants or newborns | Until symptoms resolve |
| Group A streptococcal disease | Yes | | Until 24 hours after adequate treatment is started |
| Hepatitis A | Yes | | Until 7 days after onset of jaundice |
| Hepatitis B | | | |
|   Acute | No | Personnel should wear gloves for procedures that involve trauma to tissues or contact with mucous membranes or nonintact skin | Until antigenemia resolves |
|   Chronic antigenemia | No | Same as acute illness | Until antigenemia resolves |
| Hepatitis NANB | No | Same as acute hepatitis B | Period of infectivity has not been determined |
| Herpes simplex | | | |
|   Genital | No | | |
|   Hands (herpetic whitlow) | Yes | It is not known whether gloves prevent transmission | Until lesions heal |
|   Orofacial | No | Personnel should not take care of high-risk patients | Until lesions heal |
| Measles | | | |
|   Active | Yes | | Until 7 days after the rash appears |
|   Postexposure (susceptible personnel) | Yes | | From the 5th through 21st day after exposure and/or 7 days after the rash appears |
| Mumps | | | |
|   Active | Yes | | Until 9 days after onset of parotitis |
|   Postexposure | Yes[a] | | From the 12th through 26th day after exposure or until 9 days after onset of parotitis |
| Pertussis | | | |
|   Active | Yes | | From the beginning of the catarrhal stage through the 3rd week after onset of paroxysms or until 7 days after start of effective therapy |
|   Postexposure (asymptomatic personnel) | No | | |

TABLE 2-3. (CONTINUED)

| Disease/problem | Relieve from direct patient contact | Partial work restriction | Duration |
|---|---|---|---|
| Postexposure (symptomatic personnel) | Yes | | Same as active pertussis |
| Rubella | | | |
|   Active | Yes | | Until 5 days after rash appears |
|   Postexposure (susceptible personnel) | Yes | | From the 7th through 21st day after exposure and/or 5 days after rash appears |
| Scabies | Yes | | Until treated |
| *Staphylococcus aureus* (skin lesions) | Yes | | Until lesions resolve |
| Upper respiratory infections (high-risk patients) | Yes | Personnel should not take care of high-risk patients | Until acute symptoms resolve |
| Varicella (chickenpox) | | | |
|   Active | Yes | | Until all lesions dry and crust |
|   Postexposure | Yes | | From the 10th through 21st day after exposure or, if varicella occurs, until all lesions dry and crust |
| Zoster (shingles) | | | |
|   Active | No | Appropriate barrier desirable | Until lesions dry and crust, personnel should not take care of high-risk patients |
|   Postexposure (susceptible personnel) | Yes | | From the 10th through 21st day after exposure or, if varicella occurs, until all lesions dry and crust |

<sup>a</sup>Mumps vaccine may be offered to susceptible personnel. When given after exposure, mumps vaccine may not provide protection; however, if exposure did not result in infection, immunizing exposed personnel should protect against subsequent infection. Neither mumps immune globulin nor immune serum globulin is of established value in postexposure prophylaxis. Transmission of mumps among personnel and patients has not been a major problem in hospitals in the United States, probably due to multiple factors including high levels of natural and vaccine-induced immunity.

Source: Adapted from Williams, W. W. *Infect. Control* 4 (Suppl.):326, 1983.

mucous membranes and open skin lesions with potentially infective materials from AIDS patients. Because of the lack of pertinent information, no particular course of action can be recommended in the event of accidental percutaneous or mucosal exposure to potentially infective material from patients with AIDS. Since patients with AIDS are often in high-risk groups for hepatitis B, a hospital's staff may consider implementing recommendations for exposures to blood suspected of being positive for HBsAg (Table 2-4).

## ACUTE DIARRHEA

Various agents may cause diarrhea in patients and hospital personnel. *Salmonella, Shigella,* and *Campy-* *lobacter* species are among the common bacterial enteric pathogens. Infection with these agents may produce mild symptoms of diarrhea but is often accompanied by other symptoms, such as abdominal cramps, fever, or bloody diarrhea. Diarrheal illness accompanied by such symptoms suggests a bacterial cause. Rotavirus and the 27-nanometer (Norwalk and Norwalk-like) agents are among the chief causes of sporadic and epidemic viral gastroenteritis (see Chapter 35). *Giardia lamblia* and other protozoa are also frequent causes of diarrhea. Any of these agents may be transmitted in hospitals via the hands of infected personnel.

If personnel develop an acute diarrheal illness accompanied by fever, cramps, or bloody stools, they are likely to be excreting potentially infective organisms in high titer in their feces. The specific cause

TABLE 2-4. Summary of postexposure prophylaxis for acute percutaneous (needle-stick) exposures to HBV

| Status of patient's blood | HBsAg testing recommended | Recommended prophylaxis[a] |
|---|---|---|
| HBsAg-positive | No | HBIG (0.06 ml/kg IM or 5 ml immediately plus hepatitis B vaccine series, if indicated, *or* second dose HBIG 1 month after needle-stick (if HBV vaccine not given) |
| HBsAg status unknown | | |
| Source known | | IG (0.06 ml/kg) immediately; *if test positive,* |
|   Blood at *high risk* of being HBsAg positive[b] | Yes[c] | HBIG (0.06 ml/kg IM or 5 ml) immediately plus hepatitis B vaccine series, if indicated, *or* second dose HBIG 1 month after needle-stick (if HBV vaccine not given); *if test negative,* nothing |
|   Blood at *low risk* of being HBsAg-positive[d] | No | Nothing or IG (0.06 ml/kg) |
|   HBsAg status unknown; source unknown | No | Nothing or IG (0.06 ml/kg) |

HBV = hepatitis B virus; HBIG = hepatitis B immune globulin; IG = immune globulin (formerly called immune serum globulin, ISG, or gamma globulin).
[a]Consult current ACIP recommendations (*Morbid. Mortal. Weekly Rep.* 30:423, 1981, and 33:285, 1984) for important details.
[b]*High risk that source is HBsAg-positive* occurs in patients with acute, unconfirmed viral hepatitis; patients institutionalized with Down's syndrome; patients on hemodialysis; persons of Asian origin; homosexual men; and users of illicit intravenous drugs.
[c]If results can be known within 7 days after exposure. Although prophylaxis may be given up to 7 days after exposure, it is most effective when given as soon after exposure as possible, preferably within 24-48 hours. Screening of exposed personnel to determine susceptibility may also be considered, but the decision to screen should not delay the administration of globulin.
[d]*Low risk that the source is HBsAg-positive* occurs in the average hospital patient.
Source: Modified from Williams, W. W. *Infect. Control* 4 (Suppl.):326, 1983.

of acute diarrhea, however, cannot be determined solely on the basis of clinical symptoms; thus appropriate laboratory tests are important. Not allowing these persons to take care of patients pending evaluation will prevent transmission. Evaluation of personnel may usually be limited to an initial culture for bacterial pathogens and stool examination for intestinal protozoa; repeat studies may be indicated if the results of the first tests are negative and the illness persists. Whenever appropriate, specific treatment for documented infection with enteric pathogens is recommended for infected personnel [84].

*Carriage of Enteric Pathogens by Personnel*
Carriage of enteric pathogens may persist after resolution of the acute illness. Once the person has clinically recovered and is having formed stools, however, there should be little hazard to patients, provided normal hygienic practices are observed. Existing data suggest that appropriate antibiotic therapy may eradicate fecal excretion of *Shigella* or *Campylobacter*. If persons take antibiotics, any follow-up cultures are

best taken 48 hours after the last dose. Carriage of *Salmonella* by personnel, however, calls for special precautions regarding contact with high-risk patients. This is because carriage may be prolonged, and the clinical sequelae of acute salmonellosis are often severe in high-risk patients—newborns, the elderly, immunocompromised patients, and the severely ill, such as those in intensive care units (see Chapter 32). Antibiotic therapy may prolong *Salmonella* excretion or lead to emergence of resistant strains and is not generally indicated. Personnel with nontyphoidal *Salmonella* enteric infections should be excluded from direct contact with high-risk patients until stool cultures are *Salmonella*-free on two consecutive specimens collected not less than 24 hours apart. However, personnel infected by enteric pathogens other than *Salmonella* may return to work after symptoms resolve. Before they return to work, these persons need to be individually counseled about the importance of hand-washing [84].

Generally, personal hygiene, particularly hand-washing by personnel before and after all patient contacts, will minimize the risk of acquiring or transmitting enteric pathogens.

## CYTOMEGALOVIRUS

Personnel may be exposed to patients with cytomegalovirus (CMV) infection, but the risk of acquiring CMV infection from patients appears to be small (see Chapter 35). The two principal reservoirs of CMV in hospitals are (1) infants infected with CMV and (2) immunocompromised patients, such as oncology patients and those undergoing kidney or bone marrow transplant. Available data show no evidence of greater risk of CMV transmission to personnel working in dialysis units [78], oncology wards [31], or pediatric areas compared to personnel having no patient contact [1,85]. However, evidence is accumulating to suggest sexual contact as a significant mode of CMV transmission outside the hospital environment [28,49]. Large, well-controlled studies are needed to document the validity of these observations.

The precise mechanism of CMV transmission is unknown; however, infection appears to be acquired only through intimate, direct contact with an excreter of CMV or with contaminated secretions. The virus can be shed in the urine, saliva, respiratory secretions, tears, feces, breast milk, semen, and cervical secretions.

### Screening Programs for CMV Infection
Because infection with CMV during pregnancy may damage the fetus, protecting women of childbearing age from persons who are excreting the virus is of primary concern (see Chapter 29). Most infants infected with CMV are asymptomatic. Screening programs to detect such patients are not practical, however, because the tests are time-consuming, costly, and entail screening all newborns. Mass screening of personnel is not likely to provide useful information because the available complement fixation (CF) tests are not reliable indicators of immunity. These tests lack sensitivity, and the antigen most commonly used for serologic testing (the AD 169 strain) may not cross-react with all other known CMV strains. Furthermore, identifying women as seropositive does not guarantee they cannot transmit infection to the fetus if they become pregnant because congenital infection may result from reactivation of latent infection [2,71] and, theoretically, from exogenous reinfection. In addition, since there are no studies clearly indicating that personnel may be protected by transfer to areas requiring less contact with infants and children [1,85], identifying women as seronegative to institute such

measures may not reduce the number of primary infections.

### Preventing Transmission of CMV
When hygienic practices are used, the risk of acquiring infection through patient contact is low [1]. Therefore, a practical approach to reducing the risk of infection with CMV is to stress careful hand-washing after all patient contacts and avoidance of contact with areas or materials that are potentially infective [35]. Patients infected with CMV can be identified, and this information can be used in counseling pregnant personnel and determining their work assignments.

Personnel who contract illnesses thought to be due to CMV need not be restricted from work [84]. They can reduce the risk of transmission to patients or other personnel by careful hand-washing and preventing their body fluids from contacting other persons.

## HEPATITIS

Viral hepatitis has long been recognized as a nosocomial hazard (see Chapter 35). The agents that most commonly cause viral hepatitis are hepatitis A virus (HAV), hepatitis B virus (HBV), and one or more viruses currently designated non-A, non-B (NANB).

### Hepatitis A
Nosocomial hepatitis A occurs infrequently and is associated with two unusual circumstances: (1) the source of infection is a patient hospitalized for other reasons whose hepatitis is not apparent, and (2) the patient is fecally incontinent. These circumstances may occur in adult and pediatric patients.

Hepatitis A is transmitted primarily by the fecal-oral route. It has not been reported to occur after inadvertent needle sticks. Personnel who have frequent contact with blood, such as those who work in dialysis units, do not show evidence of increased infections with HAV [54]. Hepatitis A, however, has been reported to be transmitted by blood transfusion [67].

Fecal excretion of HAV is greatest during the incubation period of disease before the onset of jaundice. Once disease is clinically obvious, the risk of transmitting infection is decreased. However, some patients admitted to the hospital with hepatitis A may still be shedding virus [16,25] and are potentially infective. Fecal shedding of HAV can continue for up to two to three weeks after onset of dark urine; in most persons, however, viral shedding is complete about seven days after dark urine appears [25]. Anicteric infection may also occur, especially in young children. There is no evidence supporting the existence of a chronic HAV carrier state.

Personnel can help protect themselves and others from infection with HAV by always maintaining good personal hygiene, practicing thorough hand-washing at all times, and taking care of patients known to be infected with HAV according to published recommendations [35]. Personnel who are suspected of being infected with HAV are advised not to take care of patients until seven days after the onset of jaundice, when viral shedding in most persons is complete [84].

### Hepatitis B

Most nosocomial cases of hepatitis B unrelated to the transfusion of blood or blood products occur in hospital personnel rather than patients. Transmission occurs by parenteral or mucosal exposure to HBsAg-positive blood from persons who are carriers or have acute HBV infection. The principal modes of HBV transmission have been discussed elsewhere (see Chapters 17 and 35). Often carriers of HbsAg and persons with acute infections are unrecognized and therefore not known to be infective. The infectivity of blood is best correlated with the presence of hepatitis B "e" antigen (HBeAg); however, any blood that is HBsAg-positive is potentially infective. Presence of HBeAg correlates strongly with the number of infective HBV in the serum.

The principal modes of HBV transmission are given below in order of decreasing efficiency:

1. *Overt parenteral transmission.* Direct percutaneous inoculation by needle or instrument contaminated with serum or plasma (e.g., accidental needle sticks, transfusion of contaminated blood or blood products, and acupuncture)
2. *Inapparent parenteral transmission*
   a. Percutaneous inoculation with infective serum or plasma without overt needle puncture (e.g., contamination of fresh cutaneous scratches, abrasions, burns, or other lesions)
   b. Contamination of mucosal surfaces with infective serum or plasma (e.g., mouth pipetting accidents, accidental eye splash, and other direct contact with mucous membranes of the eyes or mouth, such as hand to mouth or eye when contaminated with infective blood or serum)
   c. Transfer of infective material to skin lesions or mucous membranes via inanimate environmental surfaces (e.g., surfaces of various types of hospital equipment, devices, and rubber gloves)
   d. Contamination of mucosal surfaces with infective secretions other than serum or plasma (e.g., contact involving saliva or semen)

Fecal-oral transmission of HBV does not appear to occur; however, transmission among homosexual men has been described, possibly via contamination from asymptomatic rectal mucosal lesions at sites of sexual contact [61]. Airborne spread of HBV by droplet nuclei does not appear to be epidemiologically important [59,60]. Transmission of HBV in dental operatories, however, by large droplets that may strike mucous membranes or contaminate environmental surfaces has not been ruled out [59].

Within the hospital setting certain work locations and occupational categories have been identified as showing increased risk for hepatitis B infection [29,43,48,51,52,54,58,76]. Generally the highest risk of HBV infection is associated with locations and occupations in which contact with blood from infected patients is frequent. The locations and occupations are as follows:*

| *Work locations* | *Occupational categories* |
|---|---|
| Blood banks | Dentists and dental |
| Clinical laboratories | surgeons |
| Dental clinics | Dialysis technicians |
| Dialysis wards | Laboratory technicians |
| Emergency rooms | Nurses |
| Hematology/oncology wards | Physicians (especially |
| Operating and recovery | surgeons and |
| rooms | pathologists) |
| Pathology laboratories | |

Hospital personnel not physically exposed to blood are at no greater risk than the general population. Patient contact without physical exposure to blood has not been documented to be a risk factor.

To prevent transmission of hepatitis B, hospital personnel must be aware of the modes of transmission and the appropriate precautions in taking care of infected patients or handling their clinical specimens [35]. In general the major emphasis is on applying blood precautions, practicing proper hand-washing, having minimal contact with blood or blood-contaminated excretions, and handling the blood of all patients as potentially infective material [35].

Since droplets from the patient's mouth reach the face of the dentist during certain procedures, dentists should consider protecting their eyes, nose, and mouth from such exposure by using masks and protective eyewear [84]. They can prevent direct contact with infective material in the patient's mouth by routinely wearing gloves during dental procedures.

*Adapted from Maynard, J. E. *Am. J. Med.* 70:440, 1981.

*Acute HBV Infection in Personnel
and HBsAg Carriers*

A carrier is a person who is HBsAg-positive on at
least two occasions at least six months apart. After
acute infection with HBV, the likelihood of developing the carrier state lessens as the person gets older
and depends on the host's immune responsiveness.
Carriers and persons with acute disease have the highest concentrations of HBV in the blood and serous
fluids. The risk of transmission of HBV by HBsAg-
positive health professionals has been examined in
recent reports [3,15,24,38,62,63,70]. Transmission
has been documented in some instances from oral
surgeons, gynecologists performing complex pelvic
surgery, and a general practitioner. HBsAg-positive
personnel with exudative dermatitis on body areas
that may contact patients may also pose a risk to
patients [70].

Among dental practitioners who do not routinely
wear gloves, a greater risk of transmitting infection
appears to be associated more with highly traumatic
dental work, such as tooth extractions and surgery,
than with less traumatic work such as examinations
and restorations. Transmission by surgeons has been
related to type of surgery, in particular major operative procedures, such as laparotomy, hysterectomy,
and major repairs, during which the chance of accidental puncture wounds is presumably greater. In
one instance, transmission by a hospital worker with
a severe exudative dermatitis on both hands appeared
to be related to contamination of indwelling arterial
catheters [70].

The asymptomatic carrier of HBsAg and the person
with an acute case do not appear to endanger susceptible persons except through direct inoculation of
his or her blood or contaminated secretions. Thus
these persons need not be restricted from patient-care
responsibilities unless there is epidemiologic evidence
that the worker is transmitting infection [84].

Personnel who are HBsAg-positive may be able to
reduce or eliminate their risk of infecting patients by
wearing gloves during high-risk procedures in which
their blood or body fluids may contact patients [38,63].
Double-gloving during complex surgery might also
help interrupt transmission [15]. Personnel who have
no exudative lesions on the hands and are acutely
infected with HBV or known to carry HBsAg should
wear gloves for procedures involving trauma to tissues
or direct contact with mucous membranes and nonintact skin. Moreover personnel with exudative lesions on the hands should either wear gloves for all
direct patient contact and when handling equipment
that will touch mucous membranes or nonintact skin
or abstain from all direct patient care [84]. Further-

more, it is crucial to counsel known carriers of HBsAg
about practicing good personal hygiene, preventing
their blood and potentially infective body fluids from
contacting other persons, and refraining from donating blood.

*Hemodialysis Centers*

Infection with HBV has represented a great hazard
to both patients and personnel in hemodialysis centers. If adequate infection control strategies are not
practiced, hepatitis B infection, once introduced, can
become endemic, with patients and environmental
surfaces acting as reservoirs. Placing patients on isolation precautions or segregating patients who are
HBV carriers and assigning seropositive personnel to
take care of these patients has greatly decreased transmission of HBV in this environment. A complete
discussion of the modes of transmission and control
measures for hepatitis B in dialysis centers has been
published [18] and is discussed in Chapter 17 in this
textbook.

*Pregnant Personnel*

Pregnant personnel are at no greater risk of contracting hepatitis than other personnel; however, if a woman
develops hepatitis B during pregnancy and is HBsAg-
positive at the time of delivery, the infant is at high
risk of developing neonatal hepatitis and becoming
an HBsAg carrier [66,79]. Because of this risk, it is
important that pregnant personnel know the dangers
of working in high-risk departments and the precautions that should be used [18]. Female personnel of
childbearing age may also consider immunization with
hepatitis B virus vaccine.

*Hepatitis B Virus (HBV) Vaccine*

An inactivated vaccine of high immunogenicity and
efficacy is commercially available. The application of
the vaccine in acute-care hospitals will depend on the
risk of HBV infection for hospital personnel and the
cost of vaccine.

Present estimates of risk have been based primarily
on studies of the prevalence of hepatitis serum markers in selected groups [29,48,51,52,58,76]. Incidence studies of HBV infection among hospital personnel have been few [21,26,43] and have not included
all groups of hospital personnel and appropriate community controls. Thus data that can be used to analyze the cost-effectiveness of administering vaccine to
hospital personnel are not complete.

Because the risk that hospital personnel will acquire hepatitis B varies among hospitals and among

different occupational groups within hospitals, each hospital should formulate its own specific immunization strategy. In developing these strategies, hospitals can use available published data regarding the risk of infection [21,26,29,43,48,51,52,58,76]. Some institutions may instead choose to screen personnel serologically in various occupational categories or work locations to determine the prevalence of seropositivity in these groups.

The decision to screen potential vaccine recipients for susceptibility to hepatitis B is an economic one; immunizing HBV carriers and persons already immune does not appear to present a hazard [30,74]. In the United States, the cost-effectiveness of screening is usually determined by the prevalence of previous infection in any targeted group, the cost of screening, and the cost of immunizing personnel [46,56].

Although HBV vaccine is intended primarily for preexposure prophylaxis, it has been recommended for postexposure use in persons, such as health-care personnel, who belong to a high-risk group for whom preexposure administration of vaccine is recommended [44]. HBV vaccine in combination with hepatitis B immune globulin (HBIG) provides sustained protective levels of antibody and obviates the need for a second dose of HBIG in such exposures.

HBV vaccine is reported to be safe [20,22,34, 73,75]. The Immunization Practices Advisory Committee has published a discussion of this vaccine and its use [46].

## Non-A, Non-B Hepatitis

The epidemiology of NANB hepatitis in the United States more closely resembles that of hepatitis B than that of hepatitis A. Important aspects of NANB infections are (1) the NANB agent or agents circulate in the blood in acute cases; (2) there appears to be a chronic blood carrier state during which blood may remain infective; and (3) transmission of NANB infection is usually associated with percutaneous needle exposure or other exposure to blood or with inapparent parenteral transmission. Since blood containing HBsAg is not used for transfusions, most posttransfusion hepatitis in the United States is NANB. Thus emphasis on blood precautions, as with hepatitis B, seems the most reasonable current approach to preventing transmission from patients to personnel. For personnel with this illness, precautions suggested for hepatitis B should be adequate to prevent transmission to patients. Techniques are not yet available to detect specific antigens and antibodies or to determine the period of infectivity after acute infection.

## Needle-stick Injuries

Needle-stick injuries account for a large number of work-related accidents reported in hospitals [55]. Most injuries occur on patient-care units when personnel are (1) disposing of used needles, (2) administering parenteral injections or infusion therapy (especially to uncooperative patients), (3) drawing blood, (4) recapping needles after use, (5) handling linens or trash containing uncapped needles, or (6) cleaning up after patient-care procedures in which needles are used. Although other infections have been reported to be transmitted by accidental needle sticks, hepatitis B and probably NANB pose the greatest risks to hospital personnel. In the absence of immunoprophylaxis, the risk of acquiring overt hepatitis B through an accidental puncture wound from a needle used on an HBsAg-positive patient is about 6 percent [68].

The risk of needle-stick injuries can be reduced by discarding used needles in puncture-resistant disposal units without first recapping them or purposely bending or breaking them by hand. Risk of injury may also be reduced by obtaining assistance when administering injections or infusion therapy to uncooperative patients and by using caution when cleaning up after procedures that include the use of needles. Training or instruction of personnel should include discussions of methods to prevent needle-stick injuries. Additionally the incidence of needle-stick injuries may be reduced by providing needle-disposal units throughout the hospital in locations that encourage their immediate use, for example, in nursing stations, patient rooms, laboratories, and utility rooms [57]. When some needle-cutting devices are used, blood may spatter onto environmental surfaces. However, no current data are available from controlled studies examining the effect, if any, of needle-cutting devices on the incidence of needle-stick injuries.

After some needle-stick injuries, immunoprophylaxis for hepatitis B or NANB may be advisable [44,45] (Table 2-4). Immune globulins for protection against viral hepatitis are most effective when given soon after exposure.

## HERPES SIMPLEX VIRUSES

Herpes simplex viruses (HSV) can be transmitted among personnel and patients through direct contact either with primary or recurrent lesions or with secretions (such as saliva, vaginal secretions, and infected amniotic fluid) that can contain the virus when no lesions are obvious (see Chapter 35). Although many sites can become infected, exposed areas of skin are most likely to be involved, particularly when minor cuts, abrasions, or other skin lesions are present.

### Transmission of HSV from Patients to Personnel

Personnel may develop an infection of the fingers (herpetic whitlow or paronychia) from exposure to contaminated oral secretions. Such exposure is a distinct hazard for nurses, anesthesiologists, dentists, respiratory care personnel, and other personnel who may have direct (usually hand) contact with either oral lesions or respiratory secretions from patients. Less frequently, personnel may develop infection of the fingers from exposure to contaminated genital secretions or lesions on skin or mucous membranes. Personnel can protect themselves from such infection by (1) avoiding direct contact with lesions, (2) wearing gloves on both hands or using "no-touch" technique for all contact with oral or vaginal secretions, and (3) thorough hand-washing after patient contact [35].

### Transmission of HSV from Personnel to Patients

Currently there is no evidence that personnel with genital infections pose a high risk to patients if personnel follow good patient-care practices. The risk posed by personnel with orofacial herpes to patients is unknown. Personnel with oral infections, however, can reduce the risk of infecting patients by (1) wearing an appropriate barrier, such as a mask or gauze dressing, to prevent hand contact with the lesion; (2) washing hands well before all patient care; and (3) whenever possible, not taking care of patients at high risk of severe infection, such as neonates, patients with severe malnutrition, severely burned patients, and patients in immunodeficient states, until the lesions are healed. The potential risk of infecting high-risk patients must be weighed against the possibility of compromising patient care by excluding personnel with orofacial herpes.

Personnel with herpetic whitlow may be more likely to transmit infection by contact. Personnel can prevent transmission of HSV to patients by not having direct contact with patients until lesions are healed. Although some have suggested that personnel with herpetic whitlow may have patient contact if they wear gloves [4,37], the adequacy of this method in preventing transmission of infection is unknown.

## MENINGOCOCCAL DISEASE

Nosocomial transmission of *Neisseria meningitidis* to hospital personnel taking care of patients with men-

ingococcemia, meningococcal meningitis, or lower respiratory infections is uncommon. In rare instances transmission to personnel from patients with meningococcemia or meningococcal meningitis has occurred through intensive direct contact with the infected person and direct contact with respiratory secretions without use of proper precautions (see Chapter 34). The most likely mode of spread from a person with infections at these sites is by large droplet secretions. Risk to personnel from casual contact (e.g., as usually occurs with housekeepers and with laboratory contact with clinical specimens) appears to be negligible.

Meningococcal lower respiratory infections, however, may present a greater risk of transmission than meningococcemia or meningitis alone [23,64], especially if the patient has an active, productive cough [23]. Possible airborne transmission (droplet nuclei) to persons who did not have close contact with the infected patient has been suggested [23]; however, droplet spread cannot be excluded.

When taking care of patients with suspected *N. meningitidis* infection at any site, personnel can decrease the risk of infection by using proper precautions [35].

### Prophylaxis After Unprotected Exposure

Antimicrobial prophylaxis can eradicate carriage of *N. meningitidis* and prevent infections in personnel who have unprotected exposure to patients with meningococcal infections. Prophylaxis is indicated for persons who have intensive direct contact with infected patients and who do not use proper precautions [84]. Personnel who have close contact with patients with unrecognized meningococcal lower respiratory infection and therefore do not use proper precautions might also need prophylaxis [23]. Additional studies will be important to define the need for prophylaxis in this situation.

When prophylaxis is deemed necessary, it is important to begin treatment immediately [84]. Often prophylaxis must be started before results of antimicrobial testing are available. Rifampin is now the drug of choice for prophylaxis. Because sulfonamide-resistant meningococci are prevalent, sulfonamides should be used only if the organism has been found to be sulfonamide-sensitive [84].

### Carriage of N. meningitidis by Personnel

Carriage of *N. meningitidis* in the nasopharynx of healthy persons has been recognized for many years, but the prevalence is quite variable. Carriage may be transient, intermittent, or chronic. Surveillance of hospital personnel to determine carriage is useful only during special epidemiologic studies. In nonoutbreak situations, asymptomatic carriers among personnel need not be identified, treated, or removed from patient-care activities [84]. The management of carriers identified during special studies is not within the scope of this chapter.

## PERTUSSIS

Pertussis, caused by *Bordetella pertussis,* is highly communicable. The secondary attack rate is determined primarily by the immune status of those exposed; age may also be a factor. Unless infected persons are treated with an effective antibiotic, the period of communicability extends from the beginning of the catarrhal stage to approximately three weeks after onset of paroxysms.

Nosocomial transmission of pertussis has been reported infrequently. Although infection occurs less commonly in adults and may be limited to mild respiratory illness, personnel with pediatric patient contact may be involved in transmission of pertussis to patients [50,53]. However, the risk of pertussis infection and dissemination is probably not serious enough to warrant routine immunization of hospital personnel with current vaccines. Immunizing persons over age six is not recommended because of the increased frequency of adverse reactions. In addition current vaccines do not confer complete immunity, and protection against pertussis may decrease as the interval between immunization and reexposure increases. Natural immunity appears to be long-lasting, although infection in persons who reportedly had pertussis in the past has been reported [50].

During an outbreak, restricting personnel with cough or upper respiratory tract symptoms from taking care of patients may be important in preventing additional spread [53]. Personnel with symptoms of infection should be restricted from direct patient care from the beginning of the catarrhal stage through the third week after onset of paroxysms or until seven days after the start of effective therapy [84]. Erythromycin prophylaxis of exposed susceptible patients who are infected may abort or attenuate illness if administered in the early, preparoxysmal cough stage of the illness. Prophylaxis of less than 14 days is frequently followed by bacteriologic relapse. Infected contacts may be identified rapidly by the fluorescent antibody (FA) technique; culture techniques identify infection more reliably than FA examination, however, because both false-positive and false-negative

results occur with the FA method. Asymptomatic carriage of pertussis is very unusual; persons with positive cultures generally develop symptoms. Asymptomatic personnel who have had contact with patients presumed to have pertussis can be observed and treated if symptoms develop within the incubation period (up to 21 days).

## SCABIES

Scabies is a disease caused by infestation with the mite *Sarcoptes scabiei.* It is transmitted in hospitals primarily through intimate direct contact with an infested person, even when high levels of personal hygiene are maintained [12,14,36]. Transmission to personnel has occurred during activities such as spongebathing patients or applying body lotions. Transmission between patients may also be possible when patients are ambulatory. Transmission by casual contact, such as holding hands, has been infrequently reported [42]. Transmission via infested bedding, clothes, or other fomites has not been implicated as a major mode of transferring mites [32,36].

Treatment is recommended for persons with active infestation. A single correct application [32,36] of agents used to treat scabies is curative in most cases and appears to eliminate the risk of transmission immediately after the first treatment [12,32,36]. Treatment destroys both eggs and the active forms of the mites; however, ovicidal activity has not been fully substantiated for all available agents. Repeating the treatment seven to ten days after the initial therapy will kill any newly hatched mites. Between treatments the risk of transmission is felt to be negligible.

Using appropriate precautions when taking care of infested patients will decrease the risk of transmission to personnel [35]. If personnel are infested with the mite, transmission can be prevented by excluding them from work until they are treated.

## STAPHYLOCOCCUS AUREUS AND STREPTOCOCCUS, GROUP A AND GROUP B

### Staphylococcus aureus Disease and Carriage
Staphylococcal carriage or infection occurs frequently in humans (see Chapter 31). There are two sources of nosocomial transmission: persons with lesions and asymptomatic carriers. Persons with skin lesions due to *S. aureus* are most likely to disseminate these organisms. Direct contact is the major route of trans-

mission. Even minor disease or entirely inapparent infections in personnel may represent a prime hazard to patients. One way to decrease the possibility of dissemination is not to allow patient-care personnel to work until skin disease caused by this organism is resolved.

The anterior nares is one of the most commonly colonized sites, but carriage of *S. aureus* may occur at other sites, such as any draining or crusted lesion, the nasopharynx and oropharynx, and the skin of the axilla, fingers, and perineum. The epidemiology of methicillin-resistant staphylococci does not appear to be different, except that nasal carriage may be less frequent, and outbreaks tend to occur more frequently in intensive care and burn units (see Chapter 10).

Culture surveys of personnel can detect *S. aureus* carriers but do not indicate whether carriers are likely to disseminate their organisms. Thus a more reasonable approach is to emphasize effective surveillance that permits prompt recognition of staphylococcal disease in personnel and patients. If personnel are linked epidemiologically to an increased number or unusual cluster of cases of staphylococcal disease, these persons should be cultured and, if positive, removed from patient contact until carriage is eradicated [84]. Discussion of treatment regimens, follow-up of implicated personnel, and management of outbreaks is beyond the scope of this chapter (see Chapter 31).

### Group A Streptococcus Carriage

Although strains from all streptococcal serologic groups may occasionally cause infection, strains from groups A and B are the more important pathogens that potentially involve hospital personnel. In nosocomial transmission, the main reservoirs for group A *Streptococcus* appear to be the pharynx, skin, rectum, and female genital tract. Direct contact and large droplets are the major modes of transmitting this organism; however, airborne spread has been suggested [13,72].

Although pharyngeal and skin infections are the most common group A streptococcal infections, outbreaks of surgical wound infections caused by this organism have been more important in hospitals. Sporadic outbreaks have been traced to carriers among personnel. Since group A streptococcal surgical wound infections are infrequent, the occurrence of cases should prompt a search for a carrier. If personnel are linked epidemiologically to the occurrence of disease, they should be cultured, and if positive, removed from patient contact until carriage is eradicated [84]. Routine screening, however, is not recommended. Discussion of treatment regimens, follow-up of impli-

cated personnel, and management of outbreaks is beyond the scope of this chapter (see Chapter 31).

### Group B Streptococcus Carriage

Carriage of group B *Streptococcus* by personnel does not appear to be important in nosocomial transmission. The epidemiology of group B streptococcal infections in neonates suggests that maternal colonization with group B *Streptococcus,* followed by the infant's acquisition during passage through the birth canal, accounts for most cases of disease that have onset soon after birth. Spread of the organism from colonized to uncolonized infants via the hands of personnel, however, may play a role in late-onset neonatal disease. Careful hand-washing by personnel will minimize the risk of spread from colonized to uncolonized infants.

## TUBERCULOSIS

Even though the risk of nosocomial infection with *Mycobacterium tuberculosis* is low, tuberculosis (TB) continues to pose a problem for health-care personnel. In the hospital infection is most likely to occur when a patient has unsuspected pulmonary or laryngeal TB, has bacillus-laden sputum or respiratory secretions, and is coughing or sneezing into air that remains in circulation (see Chapter 26). The best ways to protect others from a patient with TB are to maintain a high index of suspicion for TB and to institute appropriate isolation precautions [35]. The most widely accepted approach to the care of personnel in health-care facilities follows the recommendations for surveillance and control in the general population issued jointly by the American Thoracic Society, the American Lung Association, and CDC [8], and those of the CDC Guidelines for Prevention of TB Transmission in Hospitals [19] and the Guideline for Infection Control in Hospital Personnel [84].

### Screening Programs

A tuberculosis screening and prevention program for personnel is important in protecting personnel and patients [7,27]. It is important that all institutions have a screening program; however, the program should be based on local epidemiologic data because risk of transmission varies widely among different segments of the population and in different locations [84]. It is important to identify hospital personnel with tuberculosis infection without evidence of current (active) disease because preventive treatment with isoniazid may be indicated [8]. Persons with tuberculous infection are those with a significant skin-test reaction, usually defined as 10 mm or more of induration to 5 tuberculin units (TU) of purified protein derivative–standard (PPD-S) administered via the Mantoux technique.

The tuberculin skin test is the method of choice for TB screening. The Mantoux technique (intracutaneous injection of 0.1 ml of PPD-tuberculin containing 5 TU) is preferred for screening persons for TB infection [10] because it is the most accurate test available. A two-step procedure [77] can be used to minimize the likelihood of misinterpreting a boosted reaction as a true conversion due to recent infection [9,77]. In the two-step procedure, an initial tuberculin skin test (Mantoux, 5 TU PPD) is given. If this test result is 0–9 mm of induration, a second test is given at least one week and no more than three weeks after the first. The result of the second test is used as the baseline test in determining treatment and follow-up of these personnel [84]. A skin test result of 10 mm of induration or more is considered to be significant.

The two-step procedure, however, may not always be necessary. Personnel in the second or third decade of life may be less likely to have had remote infection with *M. tuberculosis.* Thus the age of personnel in an institution and the epidemiology of nontuberculous mycobacterial infection in the geographic location may determine the frequency of the booster phenomenon [80]. Depending on these factors, the two-step method may not detect any more reactors than a single test. A pilot study may be useful to assess the frequency of the booster phenomenon in a given hospital and thus the need for the two-step test [80].

Multipuncture skin-test methods deliver an unknown quantity of antigen and may produce both false-positive and false-negative results. When repeated tuberculin testing is required or in postexposure testing, multipuncture methods do not allow precise interpretation of test results and proper counseling.

After the initial TB screening test, policies for repeat testing can be established by considering factors that contribute to the individual's risk of acquiring new infection [7]. These factors include the location and prevalence of untreated TB in the community, in the institution, and among personnel [7]. For personnel considered to be at significant risk, repeat skin tests may be necessary on a routine basis (e.g., every 3–6 months or yearly). If the risk of exposure to TB is small, it is not necessary to repeat skin tests routinely.

During TB screening, it is important to obtain an initial chest roentgenogram on persons with significant skin-test reactions, those whose skin tests convert, or those who have pulmonary symptoms that may be due to TB. There is no need to obtain routine chest films of asymptomatic, tuberculin-negative personnel [84].

After initial chest films of persons with significant reactions, repeated chest x-ray examinations have not been found to be of sufficient clinical value or to be cost-effective in monitoring persons for development of disease [11]. Thus personnel known to have a significant reaction, including those who have completed adequate preventive treatment, do not need repeat chest films unless they have pulmonary symptoms that may be due to TB [6,11].

*Management of Personnel After Exposure*
If personnel are exposed to an infective patient with TB and proper precautions are not used, it is important to skin-test these personnel ten weeks after the exposure. Ten weeks is the upper limit of time required for an infected person to develop hypersensitivity to tuberculin. Unless a recent skin test was given—for example, during the three months before the exposure—a baseline test may be needed as soon as possible after the exposure, to help decide whether a significant reaction at ten weeks represents a recent conversion related to the exposure [84].

Because the size of the skin-test reaction can be so important, the Mantoux technique is preferred for postexposure evaluations. Those already known to have significant reactions need not be skin-tested. Those who have significant reactions on testing need chest roentgenograms to exclude the possibility of tuberculous pulmonary disease. If chest films are normal, these persons can be advised to receive preventive treatment, unless such treatment is contraindicated. If the chest film has abnormalities compatible with pulmonary TB, these personnel need evaluation to rule out the possibility of current disease [84].

*BCG Vaccination*
Many bacille Calmette-Guérin (BCG) vaccines are available today, and they vary in immunogenicity, efficacy, and reactogenicity. Controlled trials of previous vaccines conducted before 1955 showed protection ranging from 0 to 80 percent; however, the efficacy of vaccines currently available in the United States has not been demonstrated directly and can only be inferred. Thus the skin-test reaction after BCG vaccination may be quite variable, and it cannot be distinguished from that due to virulent tuberculous infection. Caution is necessary in attributing a significant skin-test reaction to previous BCG vaccination, especially if the person vaccinated has recently been exposed to infective tuberculosis. A his-

tory of BCG vaccination, then, should not preclude an initial screening test, and it is important to manage a significant reaction in BCG-vaccinated persons as a possible tuberculous infection [84].

Skin testing after BCG vaccination or natural infection with mycobacteria may be associated with adverse reactions, including severe or prolonged ulceration at the test site. Initial use of 1 TU PPD or a partial dose of 5 TU PPD may be useful in avoiding untoward reactions in persons who might be expected to have a severe reaction, such as those with an undocumented history of a large reaction in the past. A full 5 TU dose may be used safely if the initial skin test is negative [84]. The efficacy of this method, however, has not been examined in controlled trials.

Generally in the United States, adequate surveillance and control measures rather than BCG vaccination are recommended to protect hospital personnel and patients.

*Preventive Treatment and Work Restrictions*
Preventive treatment of persons with significant tuberculin reactions may decrease the risk that their subclinical infections will progress to clinical disease. In determining priorities for preventive therapy, the decision-maker must weigh the person's risk of developing current tuberculosis against the risk of isoniazid toxicity, the ease of identifying and supervising those to whom preventive therapy is offered, and the likelihood of the patients' infecting others. About 5 percent of persons who have recently converted will develop current disease in the first one to two years after infection; the risk of developing current disease gradually declines thereafter. Persons for whom preventive treatment is recommended include newly infected persons; significant reactors with abnormal chest roentgenograms and negative bacteriologic findings; persons with special clinical conditions; significant reactors less than 35 years old, even in the absence of additional risk factors; and members of the household of persons with newly discovered TB [8].

Contraindications to treatment include (1) previous isoniazid-associated hepatic injury or other severe adverse reactions (e.g., drug fever, chills, and arthritis) and (2) acute liver disease of any cause. Persons 35 years old or more may need preventive treatment if the potential exists for transmitting disease if it develops [8]. Since the risk of developing current disease is low, work restrictions may not be necessary for otherwise healthy persons who do not accept preventive therapy. However, it is essential that they be instructed to seek evaluation promptly if symptoms develop that may be caused by TB,

especially if they have contact with high-risk patients [84].

Personnel with current pulmonary or laryngeal TB pose a risk to patients and other personnel while they are infective. Stringent requirements regarding work restrictions for hospital personnel are necessary because of this special situation. Objective measures of lack of infectivity are negative cultures and sputum smears that are free of bacilli. The American Thoracic Society recommends that criteria for removing from or returning to work always be tailored to the individual. Moreover they recommend that multiple factors be considered, including those that influence the expulsion of infective particles in the work air space (mainly coughing), the characteristics of potential contacts in the work environment, and the possible consequences if personnel become infected [5].

## VARICELLA-ZOSTER

Varicella-zoster virus (VZV) is the causative agent of varicella (chickenpox) and zoster (shingles). The virus is highly communicable, leading to high attack rates of exanthematous chickenpox among healthy susceptible children. A small proportion of adults have escaped even asymptomatic childhood varicella and remain susceptible. Nosocomial transmission of varicella-zoster infection among personnel and patients is well-recognized (see Chapter 35). While varicella is usually a benign disease of childhood, it can cause severe illness in patients with impaired immunity. Appropriate isolation precautions for hospitalized patients with known or suspected varicella or zoster can reduce the risk of transmission to personnel [35]. It is advisable to allow only personnel who have had varicella or those with serologic evidence of immunity to take care of these patients. It is worth stressing here that no person who may have or may be incubating VZV infection should enter a hospital unnecessarily.

Varicella is transmitted primarily via airborne spread by small-particle aerosols (droplet nuclei) and by contact spread by large particles (droplets). The virus may also be spread by direct contact but is not likely to be spread by inanimate objects, because it is extremely labile. The incubation period for varicella in the normal host ranges from 10 to 21 days.

Even though personnel who are susceptible to varicella may be few, it is useful to identify such persons at the time of the placement evaluation. Most persons with a clearly positive history of previous varicella are probably immune. Many with negative or unknown histories may be immune, but some may also be susceptible [65]. When available, serologic screening may be used to define susceptibility more precisely. In institutions in which varicella is prevalent or there are many high-risk patients, it may be useful to screen personnel who have a negative or equivocal history of varicella for the presence of serum antibodies to VZV to document susceptibility or immunity. This knowledge will help in assigning personnel to areas in which VZV infection is present, avoiding unnecessary work restrictions and disruption of patient services if exposure occurs, and reducing the chance of nosocomial transmission [41]. Sensitive screening techniques exist, for example, fluorescent antibody to membrane antigen (FAMA), immune adherence hemagglutination (IAH), enzyme-linked immunosorbent assay (ELISA), or varicella skin tests, but they may not be readily available. The complement fixation (CF) test is not considered reliable because of the false-negative results obtained.

Zoster appears to result from activation of latent VZV. There is scant evidence to support the view that zoster can be contracted by exposure to persons with varicella or zoster. However, varicella-zoster virus can be transmitted by direct contact with a person with zoster.

If susceptible personnel are exposed to persons with varicella, these personnel are potentially infective during the incubation period (10 to 21 days after exposure). If varicella occurs, transmission is possible until all lesions are dry and crusted. If susceptible personnel are exposed to zoster, varicella may occur; thus these persons may transmit VZV during the incubation period of varicella. After exposure to varicella or zoster, personnel not known to be immune to varicella (by history or serologic study) should be excluded from work beginning on the tenth day after exposure and remain away from work for the maximum incubation period of varicella (21 days). Personnel who have varicella should be excluded from work at least until all lesions have dried and crusted [84].

In addition, because of the possibility of transmission and development of severe illness in high-risk patients, it may be advisable to exclude personnel with zoster from taking care of high-risk patients until all lesions are crusted. Personnel with zoster may not pose a special risk to other patients if the lesions can be covered [84].

## VIRAL RESPIRATORY INFECTIONS

The role of viruses in nosocomial infections has been discussed recently in the literature [69,81,82,83].

The three chief mechanisms of transmission of respiratory viruses are (1) small-particle aerosols (droplet nuclei), (2) large particles (droplets), and (3) inoculation of viruses after direct contact with infective areas or materials. Different respiratory viruses may vary in the way in which they are transmitted (see Chapter 26).

Pediatric patients appear to be at particular risk of complications from nosocomial respiratory tract infections. Infection in the elderly, patients with chronic underlying illness, and immunocompromised patients may also be associated with significant morbidity. Thus it may be prudent to exclude personnel with viral respiratory infections from the care of these high-risk patients [84]. Because large numbers of personnel may have viral respiratory illnesses during the winter, it may not be possible to restrict all such personnel from taking care of patients who are not in high-risk groups. In all instances, careful hand-washing before patient contact is essential in preventing transmission. If hand-washing is done appropriately, gloves and routine use of gowns may have no additional benefit in preventing transmission to patients [39,40]. Masks might be beneficial in preventing transmission by large droplets from personnel to patients on close contact. However, masks probably will not completely protect personnel from patients with respiratory illnesses because large particles and aerosols may still reach the eyes, and self-inoculation from contaminated hands can still occur by touching the eyes.

Because influenza epidemics are unpredictable, hospitals may want to revise their policy regarding influenza immunization each year, taking note of the recommendations from the Immunization Practices Advisory Committee, which are revised annually. Nosocomial spread of influenza might be reduced by immunizing personnel and high-risk patients several weeks or longer before the influenza season. Amantadine may be useful to limit spread to and from patients and unimmunized personnel during an epidemic of influenza A.

## REFERENCES

1. Ahlfors, K., Ivarsson, S.-A., Johnsson, T., and Renmarker, K. Risk of cytomegalovirus infection in nurses and congenital infection in their offspring. *Acta Paediatr. Scand.* 70:819, 1981.
2. Ahlfors, K., Ivarsson, S.-A., Johnsson, T., and Svanberg, L. Primary and secondary maternal cytomegalovirus infections and their relation to

congenital infection. *Acta Paediatr. Scand.* 71:109, 1982.

3. Alter, H. J., Chalmers, T. C., Freeman, B. M., et al. Health-care workers positive for hepatitis B surface antigen: Are their contacts at risk? *N. Engl. J. Med.* 292:454, 1975.

4. American Academy of Pediatrics, Committee on Fetus and Newborn. Perinatal herpes simplex viral infections. *Pediatrics* 66:147, 1980.

5. American Thoracic Society. Guidelines for work for patients with tuberculosis. *Am. Rev. Respir. Dis.* 108:160, 1973.

6. American Thoracic Society, Ad Hoc Committee of the Scientific Assembly on Tuberculosis. Discharge of tuberculosis patients from medical surveillance. *Am. Rev. Respir. Dis.* 113:709, 1976.

7. American Thoracic Society, Ad Hoc Committee of the Scientific Assembly on Tuberculosis. Screening for pulmonary tuberculosis in institutions. *Am. Rev. Respir. Dis.* 115:901, 1977.

8. American Thoracic Society, American Lung Association, and Centers for Disease Control. Preventive therapy of tuberculous infection. *Am. Rev. Respir. Dis.* 110:371, 1974.

9. American Thoracic Society Executive Committee. Diagnostic standards and classification of tuberculosis and other mycobacterial disease (14th ed.). *Am. Rev. Respir. Dis.* 123:343, 1981.

10. American Thoracic Society Executive Committee. The tuberculin skin test. *Am. Rev. Respir. Dis.* 124:356, 1981.

11. Barrett-Connor, E. The periodic chest roentgenogram for the control of tuberculosis in health care personnel. *Am. Rev. Respir. Dis.* 122:153, 1980.

12. Belle, E. A., D'Souza T. J., Zarzour J. Y., et al. Hospital epidemic of scabies: Diagnosis and control. *Can. J. Public Health* 70:133, 1979.

13. Berkelman, R. L., Martin, D., Graham, D. R., et al. Streptococcal wound infections caused by a vaginal carrier. *J.A.M.A.* 247:2680, 1982.

14. Bernstein, B., and Mihan, R. Hospital epidemic of scabies. *J. Pediatr.* 83:1086, 1973.

15. Carl, M., Francis, D. P., Blakey, D. L., and Maynard, J. E. Interruption of hepatitis B transmission by modification of a gynecologist's surgical technique. *Lancet* 1:731, 1982.

16. Carl, M., Kantor, R. J., Webster, H. M., et al. Excretion of hepatitis A virus in the stools of hospitalized patients. *J. Med. Virol.* 9:125, 1982.

17. Centers for Disease Control. Acquired immune deficiency syndrome (AIDS): Precautions for clinical and laboratory staffs. *Morbid. Mortal. Weekly Rep.* 31:577, 1982.

18. Centers for Disease Control. *Control Measures for Hepatitis B in Dialysis Centers.* Atlanta: Department of Health, Education, and Welfare, Public Health Service, Viral Hepatitis Investigations and Control Series, HEW publication no. (CDC) 78-8358, November 1977.

19. Centers for Disease Control. *Guidelines for Prevention of TB Transmission in Hospitals.* Atlanta: U.S. Department of Health and Human Services, HHS publication no. (CDC) 82-8371, 1982.

20. Centers for Disease Control. Hepatitis B virus vaccine safety: Report of an inter-agency group. *Morbid. Mortal. Weekly Rep.* 31:465, 1982.

21. Centers for Disease Control. *Hepatitis Surveillance Report No. 47,* December 1981.

22. Centers for Disease Control. The safety of hepatitis B virus vaccine. *Morbid. Mortal. Weekly Rep.* 32:134, 1983.

23. Cohen, M. S., Steere, A. C., Baltimore, R., et al. Possible nosocomial transmission of group Y *Neisseria meningitidis* among oncology patients. *Ann. Intern. Med.* 91:7, 1979.

24. Communicable Disease Surveillance Centre and the Epidemiological Research Laboratory of the Public Health Laboratory Service, London. Acute hepatitis B associated with gynecological surgery. *Lancet* 1:1, 1980.

25. Coulepis, A. G., Locarnini, S. A., Lehmann, N. I., and Gust, I. D. Detection of hepatitis A virus in the feces of patients with naturally acquired infections. *J. Infect. Dis.* 141:151, 1980.

26. Craig, C. P., Gribble, C., Suarez, K. Risk of hepatitis B among phlebotomists. *Am. J. Infect. Control* 9:11, 1981.

27. Craven, R. B., Wenzel, R. P., and Atuk, N. O. Minimizing tuberculosis risk to hospital personnel and students exposed to unsuspected disease. *Ann. Intern. Med.* 82:628, 1975.

28. Davis, L. E., Stewart, J. A., and Garvin, S. Cytomegalovirus infection: A seroepidemiologic comparison of nuns and women from a venereal disease clinic. *Am. J. Epidemiol.* 102:327, 1975.

29. Dienstag, J. L., and Ryan, D. M. Occupational exposure to hepatitis B virus in hospital personnel: Infection or immunization? *Am. J. Epidemiol.* 115:26, 1982.

30. Dienstag, J. L., Stevens, C. E., Bhan, A. K., and Szmuness, W. Hepatitis B vaccine administered to chronic carriers of hepatitis B surface antigen. *Ann. Intern. Med.* 96:575, 1982.

31. Duvall, C. P., Casazza, A. R., Grimley, P.M., et al. Recovery of cytomegalovirus from adults with neoplastic disease. *Ann. Intern. Med.* 65:531, 1966.

32. Estes, S. A. Diagnosis and management of scabies. *Med. Clin. North Am.* 66:955, 1982.

33. Favero, M. S., Maynard, J. E., Leger, R. T., Graham, D. R., and Dixon, R. E. Guidelines for care of patients hospitalized with viral hepatitis. *Ann. Intern. Med.* 91:872, 1979.

34. Francis, D. P., Hadler, S. C., Thompson, S. E., et al. The prevention of hepatitis B with vaccine: Report of the CDC multi-center efficacy trial among homosexual men. *Ann. Intern. Med.* 97:362, 1982.

35. Garner, S. J., and Simmons, B. P. CDC guideline for isolation precautions in hospitals. *Infect. Control.* 4(Suppl.):245, 1983.

36. Gooch, J. J., Strasius, S. R., Beamer, B., et al. Nosocomial outbreak of scabies. *Arch. Dermatol.* 114:897, 1978.

37. Greaves, W. L., Kaiser, A. B., Alford, R. H., and Schaffner W. The problem of herpetic whitlow among hospital personnel. *Infect. Control* 1:381, 1980.

38. Hadler, S. C., Sorley, D. L., Acree, K. H., et al. An outbreak of hepatitis B in a dental practice. *Ann. Intern. Med.* 95:133, 1981.

39. Hall, C. B., and Douglass, R. G., Jr. Modes of transmission of respiratory syncytial virus. *J. Pediatr.* 99:100, 1981.

40. Hall, C. D., and Douglass, R. G., Jr. Nosocomial respiratory syncytial viral infections: Should gowns and masks be used? *Am. J. Dis. Child* 135:512, 1981.

41. Hayden, G. F., Meyers, J. D., and Dixon, R. E. Nosocomial varicella. II. Suggested guidelines for management. *West. J. Med.* 130:300, 1979.

42. Haydon, J. R., Jr., and Caplan, R. M. Epidemic scabies. *Arch. Dermatol.* 103:168, 1971.

43. Hirschowitz, B. A., Dasher, C. A., Whitt, F. J., and Cole, G. W. Hepatitis B antigen and antibody and tests of liver function: A prospective study of 310 hospital laboratory workers. *Am. J. Clin. Pathol.* 73:63, 1980.

44. Immunization Practices Advisory Committee. Postexposure prophylaxis of hepatitis B. *Morbid. Mortal. Weekly Rep.* 33:285, 1984.

45. Immunization Practices Advisory Committee. Recommendation on immune globulins for protection against viral hepatitis. *Morbid. Mortal. Weekly Rep.* 30:423, 1981.

46. Immunization Practices Advisory Committee. Recommendation on inactivated hepatitis B virus vaccine. *Morbid. Mortal. Weekly Rep.* 31:317, 1982.

47. Immunization Practices Advisory Committee. Recommendation on rubella prevention. *Morbid. Mortal. Weekly Rep.* 30:37, 1981.

48. Janzen, J., Tripatzis, I., Wagner, U., et al. Epidemiology of hepatitis B surface antigen (HB$_s$Ag) and antibody to HB$_s$Ag in hospital personnel. *J. Infect. Dis.* 137:261, 1978.

49. Jordan, M. C., Rousseau, W. E., Noble, G. R., et al. Association of cervical cytomegalovirus with venereal disease. *N. Engl. J. Med.* 288:932, 1973.

50. Kurt, T. L., Yeager, S. A., Guenette, S., and Dunlop S. Spread of pertussis by hospital staff. *J.A.M.A.* 221:264, 1972.

51. Leers, W. D., and Kouroupis, G. M. Prevalence of hepatitis B antibodies in hospital personnel. *Can. Med. Assoc. J.* 113:844, 1975.

52. Levy, B. S., Harris, J. C., Smith, J. L., et al. Hepatitis B in ward and clinical laboratory employees of a general hospital. *Am. J. Epidemiol.* 106:330, 1977.

53. Linnemann, C. C., Jr., Ramundo, N., Perlstein, P. H., Minton, S. D., and Englender, G. S. Use of pertussis vaccine in an epidemic involving hospital staff. *Lancet* 2:540, 1975.

54. Maynard, J. E. Viral Hepatitis as an Occupational Hazard in the Health Care Profession. In G. N. Vyas, S. N. Cohen, and R. Schmid (Eds.), *Viral Hepatitis: A Contemporary Assessment of Epidemiology, Pathogenesis, and Prevention.* Philadelphia: Franklin Institute Press, 1978, p. 321.

55. McCormick, R. D., and Maki, D. G. Epidemiology of needle-stick injuries in hospital personnel. *Am. J. Med.* 70:928, 1981.

56. Mulley, A. G., Silverstein, M. D., and Dienstag, J. L. Indications for use of hepatitis B vaccine, based on cost-effectiveness analysis. *N. Engl. J. Med.* 307:644, 1982.

57. Osterman, C. A. Relationship of new disposal unit to risk of needle puncture injuries. *Hosp. Top.* 53:12, 1975.

58. Pattison, C. P., Maynard, J. E., Berquist, K. R., et al. Epidemiology of hepatitis B in hospital personnel. *Am. J. Epidemiol.* 101:59, 1975.

59. Petersen, N. J., Bond, W. W., and Favero, M. S. Air sampling for hepatitis B surface antigen in a dental operatory. *J. Am. Dent. Assoc.* 99:465, 1979.

60. Petersen, N. J., Bond, W. W., Marshall, J. H., et al. An air sampling technique for hepatitis B surface antigen. *Health Lab. Sci.* 13:233, 1976.

61. Reiner, N. E., Judson, F. N., Bond, W. W., et al. Asymptomatic rectal mucosal lesions and hepatitis B surface antigen at sites of sexual contact in homosexual men with persistent hepatitis B virus infection: Evidence for de facto parenteral transmission. *Ann. Intern. Med.* 96:170, 1982.

62. Reingold, A. L., Kane, M. A., Murphy, B. L., et al. Transmission of hepatitis B by an oral surgeon. *J. Infect. Dis.* 145:262, 1982.

63. Rimland, D., Parkin, W. E., Miller, G. B., and Schrack, W. D. Hepatitis B outbreak traced to an oral surgeon. *N. Engl. J. Med.* 296:953, 1977.

64. Rose, H. D., Lenz, I. E., and Sheth, N. K. Meningococcal pneumonia: A source of nosocomial infection. *Arch. Intern. Med.* 141:575, 1981.

65. Ross, A. H. Modification of chickenpox in family contacts by administration of gamma globulin. *N. Engl. J. Med.* 267:369, 1962.

66. Schweitzer, I. L., Dunn, A. E., Peters, R. L., and Spears, R. L. Viral hepatitis B in neonates and infants. *Am. J. Med.* 55:762, 1973.

67. Seeberg, S., Bandberg, A., Hermodsson, S., et al. Hospital outbreak of hepatitis A secondary to blood exchange in a baby (letter). *Lancet* 1:1155, 1981.

68. Seeff, L. B., Wright, E. C., Zimmerman, H. J., et al. Type B hepatitis after needle-stick exposure: Prevention with hepatitis B immune globulin: Final report of the Veterans Administration Cooperative Study. *Ann. Intern. Med.* 88:285, 1978.

69. Simmons, B. P., and Wong, E. S. CDC guideline for prevention of nosocomial pneumonia. *Infect. Control* 3:327, 1982.

70. Snydman, D. R., Hindman, S. H., Wineland, M. D., et al. Nosocomial viral hepatitis B: A cluster among staff with subsequent transmission to patients. *Ann. Intern. Med.* 85:573, 1976.

71. Stagno, S., Reynolds, D. W., Huang, E.-S., et al. Congenital cytomegalovirus infection: Occurrence in an immune population. *N. Engl. J. Med.* 296:1254, 1977.

72. Stamm, W. E., Feeley, J. C., and Facklam, R. R. Wound infections due to group A *Streptococcus* traced to a vaginal carrier. *J. Infect. Dis.* 138:287, 1978.

73. Szmuness, W., Stevens, C. E., Harley, E. J., et al. Hepatitis B vaccine: Demonstration of efficacy in a controlled clinical trial in a high-risk population in the United States. *N. Engl. J. Med.* 303:833, 1980.

74. Szmuness, W., Stevens, C. E., Oleszko, W. R., and Goodman, A. Passive-active immunization against hepatitis B: Immunogenicity studies in adult Americans. *Lancet* 1:575, 1981.

75. Szmuness, W., Stevens, C. E., Zang, E. A., et al. A controlled clinical trial of the efficacy of the hepatitis B vaccine (Heptavax-B): A final report. *Hepatology* 1:377, 1981.

76. Tabor, E., Gerety, R. J., Mott, M., and Wilbur, J. Prevalence of hepatitis B in a high-risk setting: A serologic study of patients and staff in a pediatric oncology unit. *Pediatrics* 61:711, 1978.

77. Thompson, N. J., Glassroth, J. L., Snider, D. E., and Farer, L. S. The booster phenomenon in serial tuberculin testing. *Am. Rev. Respir. Dis.* 119:587, 1979.

78. Tolkoff-Rubin, N. E., Rubin, R. H., Keller, E. E., et al. Cytomegalovirus infection in dialysis patients and personnel. *Ann. Intern. Med.* 89:625, 1978.

79. Tong, M. J., Thursby, M., Rakela, J., et al. Studies on the maternal-infant transmission of the viruses which cause acute hepatitis. *Gastroenterology* 80:999, 1981.

80. Valenti, W. M., Andrews, B. A., Presley, B. A., and Reifler, C. B. Absence of the booster phenomenon in serial tuberculin skin testing. *Am. Rev. Respir. Dis.* 125:323, 1982.

81. Valenti, W. M., Betts, R. F., Hall, C. B., et al. Nosocomial viral infections. II. Guidelines for prevention and control of respiratory viruses, herpes viruses, and hepatitis viruses. *Infect. Control* 1:165, 1981.

82. Valenti, W. M., Hall, C. B., Douglas, R. G., Jr., et al. Nosocomial viral infections. I. Epidemiology and significance. *Infect. Control* 1:33, 1980.

83. Valenti, W. M., Hruska, J. F., Menegus, M. A., and Freeburn, M. J. Nosocomial viral infections. III. Guidelines for prevention and control of exanthematous viruses, gastroenteritis viruses, picornaviruses, and uncommonly seen viruses. *Infect. Control* 2:38, 1981.

84. Williams, W. W. CDC guideline for infection control in hospital personnel. *Infect. Control* 4 (Suppl.):326, 1983.

85. Yeager, A. S. Longitudinal, serological study of cytomegalovirus infections in nurses and in personnel without patient contact. *J. Clin. Microbiol.* 2:448, 1975.

## 3  INFECTION SURVEILLANCE AND CONTROL PROGRAMS

Robert W. Haley
Julia S. Garner

## HISTORY

Nosocomial infections have been a serious problem ever since sick patients were first congregated in hospitals. The explosiveness of spread of the classic epidemic diseases led to the concept of quarantine, from which evolved modern techniques of isolation. The ubiquitous threat of wound infections following surgery stimulated the stringent aseptic tradition of the operating room, including meticulous aseptic surgical technique, environmental cleanliness, and disinfection and sterilization processes. The observations of Semmelweis and Holmes, later bolstered by the popularization of the germ theory of infectious diseases, established the importance of hand-washing for reducing the spread of infection among patients. The unique observations and management abilities of Florence Nightingale established the modern basis for the design of hospitals and the strategies for patient care that minimize infection risks. And finally, the advent and widespread availability of antimicrobial agents in the 1940s revolutionized the treatment of infectious diseases and promised virtually to eliminate infections as a threat to hospitalized patients. Thus by the postwar period of the late 1940s most of the concepts and tools for preventing nosocomial infections were in the hands of individual physicians and nurses who were to apply them, but no organized group at the hospital level was considered necessary to oversee the activity of infection control.

In the mid-1950s, hospitals in the United States and abroad were struck by a pandemic of staphylococci that were increasingly resistant to available antibiotics and more virulent than previous strains. In response to this widespread problem, hospitals organized Infection Control Committees to develop new strategies for controlling the epidemic and for coordinating the infection control efforts of the diverse groups and departments of the hospital. In addition the Centers for Disease Control (CDC), then called the Communicable Disease Center, designated a new investigations unit, one purpose of which was to assist Infection Control Committees in investigating hospital epidemics. This nationwide effort was summarized and discussed at two national conferences on the control of staphylococcal disease in 1958. The proceedings of the conferences indicated the leading approaches to be stringent disinfection and monitoring of the inanimate environment, detection and treatment of staphylococcal carriers among the hospital staff, more vigorous encouragement of aseptic technique, and the reporting of staphylococcal infections to the Infection Control Committee [33, 34].

By the mid-1960s the pandemic began to subside for reasons that are still unclear. It left in its wake, however, a new awareness of nosocomial infections and committees of hospital personnel interested in controlling the problem. At the same time hospitals were experiencing another strong current of change— the use of increasingly complex technology bequeathed by the World War II technologic "push" and the burgeoning space race. Thus, as staphylococcal epidemics declined, new types of infections were seen involving "opportunistic" pathogens, such as gram-negative rods, fungi, and parasites, infecting an increasing number of highly compromised and immunosuppressed patients undergoing new medical treatments. These developments were described in 1963 at the National Conference on Institutionally Acquired Infections, the name of the conference well illustrating the awareness that a broader problem was emerging. The proceedings of the conference indicated the development of a much wider range of approaches to control of the problem, including the application of epidemiologic methods, the recommendation of organized systems for surveillance of nosocomial infections, and the importance of personnel education [35].

Through the mid- and late 1960s a few hospitals developed organized infection control programs to conduct surveillance, develop control measures, and monitor the control process for the Infection Control Committee, although most hospitals continued to depend on the individual efforts of doctors and nurses. These programs were focused somewhat and encouraged by an infection control manual published and distributed widely by the American Hospital Association's Committee on Infections Within Hospitals [1]. Meanwhile researchers at the CDC were conducting pilot studies in several community hospitals to develop and test technology for conducting more effective surveillance of nosocomial infections [9]. After demonstrating the futility of depending on voluntary reporting of infections by doctors or nurses, these pilot studies first relied on a physician infection control officer to identify infections. Later, borrowing from the British the concept of the "infection control sister" [13], which was being tried in two other U.S. hospitals [32, 36], the CDC researchers thoroughly tested the feasibility of surveillance by trained infection control nurses and found that one full-time-equivalent nurse was needed to perform surveillance and control for approximately every 250 beds [5]. On the basis of these findings, the CDC set up a training course for infection control nurses that held

its first classes in 1968. These developments were summarized and discussed in the First International Conference on Nosocomial Infections held at the CDC in 1970. The proceedings focused on a debate between the proponents of surveillance of infections by infection control nurses and their critics, who considered the approach either infeasible, unnecessary, or too costly [6].

Following the First International Conference, the CDC developed a strong recommendation for the surveillance approach, which was also supported and promoted by the American Hospital Association [2, 31]. Popularized by scientific papers, presentations at scientific meetings and regional and local conferences, practical manuals, training courses, and individual consultations with hospital staffs by medical and nurse epidemiologists from CDC, the approach was adopted in varying degrees by virtually all U.S. hospitals in the early-to-middle 1970s. For example, although Infection Control Committees had emerged earlier, in 1970 few hospitals had infection control nurses, practiced active surveillance of infections, or had formal policies prescribing aseptic practices; by 1976, however, the majority of hospitals had adopted these and had begun reducing their levels of wasteful routine environmental culturing [22]. Since there were virtually no government or private regulations or standards of much force during those years, this revolution in infection control was entirely a voluntary movement by hospitals to address an emerging problem. Noteworthy signs of the vitality of the movement were the demand for the CDC training course for infection control nurses, the huge circulation of the various books and manuals on infection control, and the formation of a professional society for infection control nurses (the Association for Practitioners in Infection Control [APIC] established in 1972). During the 1970s the CDC operated a network of 70 voluntary hospitals, the National Nosocomial Infections Study (NNIS), to maintain nationwide surveillance of the problem [4].

In 1974 the CDC began a nationwide study to evaluate the effectiveness of the approach that had been adopted throughout the country. Termed the SENIC Project (Study on the Efficacy of Nosocomial Infection Control), the multiphased study had two objectives: first, to measure the extent to which these new programs, labeled "infection surveillance and control programs" (ISCPs), had been adopted by U.S. hospitals; and second, to determine whether these programs had reduced nosocomial infection rates in the country and if so to what extent [19]. The study was stimulated by the prediction that future financial pressures on hospitals would cause them to discontinue costly preventive programs of unproven value. If the programs were truly effective, their efficacy should be documented scientifically to perpetuate their support; if not, a demonstration of the lack of efficacy should help to redirect the efforts of the nation's hospitals toward more effective approaches. (See summary of the results of the SENIC evaluation, following.)

During the 10 years (1974–1983) that the SENIC Project was conducted, the infection control movement in U.S. hospitals was going through a maturation phase. In this period over 5000 infection control nurses received training in the CDC training courses, and diverse organizations began sponsoring their own courses for nurses, physicians, and microbiologists; a professional society for physician epidemiologists, the Society of Hospital Epidemiologists of America (SHEA), was formed in 1980; more efficient methods of detecting infections through surveillance were developed; extensive environmental culturing programs virtually disappeared; national conferences on infection control, including the Second International Conference on Nosocomial Infections in 1980, disseminated new information and provided a forum for infection control personnel to exchange experiences; and a host of new risk factors that predispose patients to infection and cause epidemics were identified and studied. Despite much continued debate over the cost-effectiveness of routine infection surveillance, the hospitals that increased the intensity of their surveillance efforts outnumbered those that reduced or discontinued the activity [18].

The early 1980s saw a consolidation of the experiences of the past decade. Of particular importance was the CDC project to record the increasingly complex set of findings and recommendations into a series of guidelines for hospitals. The physician- and nurse-epidemiologists of the CDC Hospital Infections Program had been providing consultation to hospital personnel on diverse technical issues ranging from questions on disinfection techniques to the management of outbreak investigations. By 1980 they were responding to over 10,000 inquiries per year. The philosophy behind the effort to write guidelines was to provide to all U.S. hospitals simultaneously the answers to the most important and frequently recurring questions [14]. In the end the effort produced a valuable checklist of the issues that should be addressed in policies of all hospitals [3]. To make the guidelines most useful, each recommendation was classified according to the strength of its backing by scientific evidence or the consensus of experts. This was to allow hospitals to discriminate between approaches very likely to prevent infections and those

with a good rationale but of untested value. The intent of the process was to provide a body of useful information and to avoid the aura of governmental regulatory pressures.

The mid-1980s promises to provide great opportunities for increasing the effectiveness of infection surveillance and control efforts of hospitals. The publication of the results of the SENIC Project showing the effectiveness of the surveillance and control approach will fortuitously coincide with the initial stages of the new prospective payment system of government financing for hospital care [17, 23]. Using the system of diagnosis-related groups (DRGs), the reimbursement system should create a strong incentive for hospitals to prevent costly nosocomial infections. Thus by 1990 efforts by hospitals could be preventing a much larger proportion of nosocomial infections than before.

## STRATEGIES FOR SURVEILLANCE AND CONTROL

The main lesson derived from the past two decades of research and experience is that preventing nosocomial infections and controlling infection outbreaks in hospitals requires an organized management system staffed by dedicated personnel to influence the behavior of practicing doctors, nurses, and paramedical workers [17]. In this respect the system is similar to an office or department of quality control on the management staff of an industrial corporation. Many nosocomial infections are analogous to product defects resulting from the human errors of workers on the assembly line. Without careful management to ensure quality and without statistical feedback of the product defect rates, quality tends to decline, whereas a system for managing quality usually improves the products. This is the general rationale behind the need for an organized infection surveillance and control program.

The basic model for an effective ISCP is portrayed in Figure 3-1 [19]. The nosocomial infections that are preventable, perhaps between 30 and 50 percent, are primarily caused by problems in *patient-care practices,* such as the use and care of urinary catheters, intravenous and central venous monitoring catheters, and respiratory therapy equipment, as well as handwashing practices and surgical skill. As in most work situations, in the absence of a system for managing these practices, they are generally determined by the *inertia of ward routine,* that is, the apprentice system, in which practices are passed on from generation to generation of doctors and other hospital workers. Since

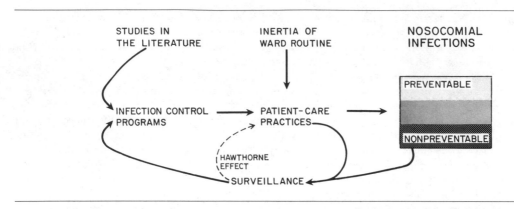

FIG. 3-1. Simplified theoretical model of an infection surveillance and control program. (From Haley, R. W., et al., *Am. J. Epidemiol.* 111:474, 1980, with permission of the journal.)

old practices become strongly ingrained, changing behavior in the hospital environment meets stiff resistance and, if pursued persistently, generates interpersonal conflict. To change old practices to preventive practices requires an infection control program, consisting of an organized intervention system with specific goals for changing behavior. For this program to be successful it must be guided by sound principles and current information; consequently, the infection control personnel must learn correct preventive practices from studying the published literature, including articles in scientific journals, textbooks, and technical manuals, and they must conduct regular surveillance over the occurrence of nosocomial infections and the patient-care practices in their hospital. The information obtained from surveillance not only allows infection control personnel to direct their efforts toward the most serious problems, but also arms them with information with which to obtain the support of hospital workers and provide feedback on the results of preventive changes. Information is power, and the more immediately relevant it is to the individual hospital's situation, the more powerful it is.

A more detailed model of the infection control process is pictured in Figure 3-2 [20]. There are basically two routes for the infection control staff to influence patient-care practices and reduce infection risks: taking direct action to change behavior without having to rely on the voluntary compliance of hospital personnel (the direct approach), and working with hospital personnel through training or other activities to motivate them to practice correct techniques (the indirect approach). Taking the direct approach, for example having the purchasing department switch to a new sterile closed urinary drainage system that cannot be opened, generally requires a less personnel-intensive effort and is more certain to be effective, but unfortunately only a minority of infection risks are susceptible to this approach.

In contrast, the majority of infection risks require changing behavior, a more difficult and less certain endeavor [26–28]. To change behavior successfully requires a complex management process involving the following steps. First, the preventive practice must be correctly defined; all too frequently medical, nursing, or support service departments use written or informal policies that run counter to proven preventive approaches. Given correct policies, the infection control staff must achieve a unity of purpose among the power brokers of the hospital, for example the hospital administrator, nursing service director, chiefs of involved medical departments, or directors of support service departments. A dissenting department head will ensure the failure of any attempt to influence patient care in his or her domain. Achieving unity of purpose requires a skillful and diplomatic approach, involving a realistic effort to balance infection control needs against practical constraints. The importance of peer relations must be recognized by having a knowledgeable infection control physician to deal with the medical staff and an influential nurse as the infection control coordinator to work with the nursing and support service staffs.

With unity of purpose established, training efforts must be designed to provide all relevant personnel with the skills and knowledge required to carry out

FIG. 3-2. Detailed conceptual model of an infection surveillance and control program. Shaded areas represent background/contextual influences. ISCP-infection surveillance and control program. (From Haley, R. W. et al., *Am. J. Epidemiol.* 111:609, 1980, with permission of the journal.)

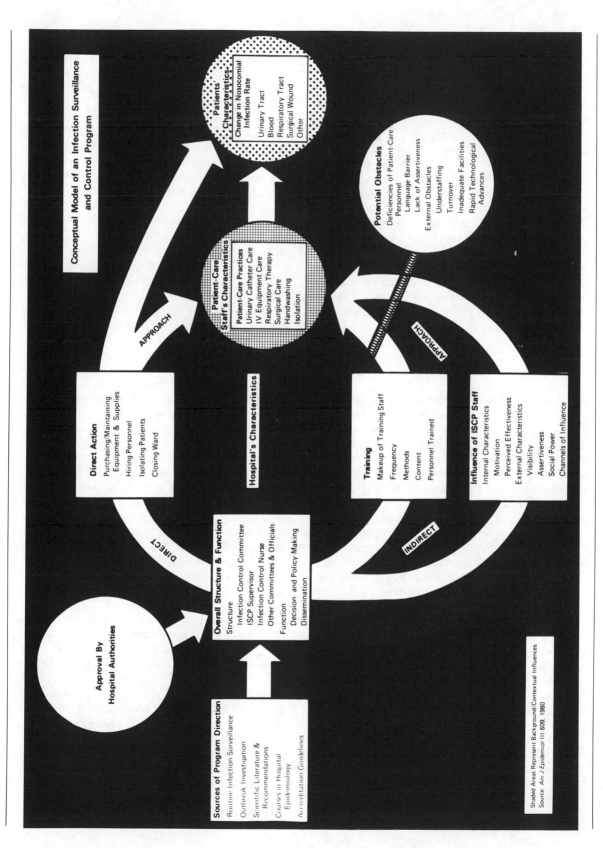

**Conceptual Model of an Infection Surveillance and Control Program**

Patients' Characteristics

Change in Nosocomial Infection Rate
Urinary Tract
Blood
Respiratory Tract
Surgical Wound
Other

Potential Obstacles

Deficiencies of Patient-Care Personnel
Language Barrier
Lack of Assertiveness
External Obstacles
Understaffing
Turnover
Inadequate Facilities
Rapid Technological Advances

Patient-Care Staff's Characteristics

Patient-Care Practices
Urinary Catheter Care
IV Equipment Care
Respiratory Therapy
Surgical Care
Handwashing
Isolation

APPROACH

APPROACH

**Direct Action**

Purchasing/Maintaining Equipment & Supplies
Hiring Personnel
Isolating Patients
Closing Ward

**Hospital's Characteristics**

**Training**

Makeup of Training Staff
Frequency
Methods
Content
Personnel Trained

**Influence of ISCP Staff**

Internal Characteristics
Motivation
Perceived Effectiveness
External Characteristics
Visibility
Assertiveness
Social Power
Channels of Influence

INDIRECT

DIRECT

**Overall Structure & Function**

Structure
Infection Control Committee
ISCP Supervisor
Infection Control Nurse
Other Committees & Officials
Function
Decision- and Policy-Making
Dissemination

**Approval By Hospital Authorities**

**Sources of Program Direction**

Routine Infection Surveillance
Outbreak Investigation
Scientific Literature & Recommendations
Courses in Hospital Epidemiology
Accreditation Guidelines

Shaded Areas Represent Background/Contextual Influences.
Source. *Am J Epidemiol* III:609, 1980.

the new preventive practice according to the agreed on standard. Various motivational techniques can be used to increase compliance; potential obstacles to correct performance, such as understaffing or inadequate hand-washing facilities, must be removed. Once these prerequisite steps are taken, the practice must be monitored to measure compliance, and the results· must be reported to department heads and particularly to first-line workers to reward the desired behaviors and focus attention on breakdowns in performance. With unity of purpose among supervisors and department heads *and* quantitative data on performance, correct practice can be maximized. If any of the steps in the process is neglected or fails, the degree of prevention will be reduced. Since halfway programs are often ineffective, a well-organized system to manage the process of infection control is essential to have a substantial effect in the rapidly changing technologic milieu of the modern hospital.

## PERSONNEL AND ORGANIZATION

### Infection Control Committee

An Infection Control Committee is present in virtually every hospital in the United States and usually functions as the hospital's central decision- and policy-making body [24]. Its decisions are often independent and binding throughout the hospital, but may require review and approval by higher authorities such as the hospital administration. Since its purpose is to be the hospital's advocate for prevention of infections, it is usually placed above the various clinical and support service departments. Most committees are composed of representatives from most of the hospital's departments and meet regularly, usually monthly, to deal with current developments and problems. Its multidisciplinary representation is important for at least three reasons. First, since infection problems and control measures often cross departmental lines, effective decision-making requires regular participation of members from most departments. Second, to carry out the committee's decisions it is often most effective to have committee members exert inside influence in their respective departments to ensure agreement and compliance. Third, the multidepartmental representation of the committee bolsters its authority as an advocate for the hospital that transcends the special interests of any single department. When a committee decision is opposed, as for example by a strong department head, this overall authority can be quite important to ensure that the final compromise position is in the best interests of patient care in all departments.

The activities of the infection control staff members, such as the infection control nurse and the hospital epidemiologist or infection control physician (see section following), are generally performed, at least in principle, at the direction of the Infection Control Committee. In the role of executive staff of the committee, their job is to provide technical information and surveillance data, to draft policies for the committee's use in the final decision-making process, and to carry out or promote many of the prevention and control measures that are adopted.

### Infection Control Physician

Almost all hospitals have a physician acting as the chairperson of the Infection Control Committee [15]. An increasing number of committees, particularly in the larger hospitals and in those affiliated with medical schools, also have a full- or part-time position for a physician with special training in hospital epidemiology functioning as the hospital epidemiologist. The hospital epidemiologist may be the chairperson of the committee or may occupy a separate position as either a technical advisor or a member of the executive staff of the committee. The former seems preferable in smaller hospitals, whereas the latter creates a separation of the epidemiologic and decision-making roles that could strengthen both activities, particularly in the more complex situations present in larger hospitals.

Most of those occupying these positions are practicing physicians, who serve on a part-time basis, often in a two-year committee assignment [15]. In the mid-1970s, 40 percent were pathologists, 18 percent internists (about half of these were infectious disease specialists), 12 percent surgeons, and 20 percent other types of physicians; in 10 percent of U.S. hospitals, the position was held by someone other than a physician, most commonly a microbiologist. By 1983 the tendency was toward increased representation of internists, particularly infectious disease specialists, and a commensurate decrease of nonphysicians and pathologists [unpublished SENIC data]. The average tenure in this position tends to be two to three years and most tend to spend less than four hours per week, although pathologists and infectious disease specialists tend to remain much longer and devote more time. An increasing number of hospitals, particularly those that are large and affiliated with medical schools, are creating full-time positions for hospital epidemiologists, some of whom provide the same service for groups of smaller hospitals in the surrounding locale.

The degree of knowledge and interest of these infection control physicians appears to vary widely. In the mid-1970s only about 60 percent of U.S. hospitals had an infection control physician who indicated special interest in the problem, and by 1983 the percentage had not increased [18]. In both periods only about a third of the physicians had taken a training course in infection control. Without a training course physicians are generally unprepared to manage infection control activities since little if any time has been devoted to the subject in the curricula of medical schools, medical residencies, or even infectious disease fellowships. Consequently the role of the infection control physician appears to be the area of infection control most in need of a focus in the near future.

*Infection Control Nurse*

The infection control nurse (ICN) occupies the key position in the infection surveillance and control program. Without a qualified energetic person in this position, the efforts of the Infection Control Committee will be largely ineffective. This fact has become so apparent that by 1983 virtually 100 percent of U.S. hospitals had established such a position on at least a part-time basis [18].

Of the people holding this position, over 95 percent have been nurses [11]. Their most common job titles are infection control nurse (34 percent of U.S. hospitals), infection control coordinator (18 percent), and nurse epidemiologist (12 percent) [unpublished SENIC data]. The term *infection control practitioner* has been commonly used in published articles but is rarely used in practice (only 5 percent). Additionally, this term may cause confusion with the term *nurse practitioner,* which refers to a group with different skills, training, responsibilities, and legal standing.

In U.S. hospitals, only about one-fourth of the ICNs work on infection control full-time. A much higher percentage (over 70 percent) work full-time in larger hospitals (over 300 beds) in contrast to a much lower percentage (14 percent) in smaller hospitals [11]. In 1976 only about one-half of U.S. hospitals met the recommendation for one full-time-equivalent ICN per 250 hospital beds [11]. Since most hospitals tended to have either one half-time or one full-time ICN position, smaller hospitals were more likely to have met this recommendation than large hospitals, even though some larger hospitals have more than one position. By 1983, however, two-thirds of hospitals had established enough ICN positions to meet the recommendation [18]. In small hospitals in which ICNs work less than full-time on infection control, the appointee often has one or more other titles including director or assistant director of

nursing service, inservice education coordinator, operating room supervisor, utilization review nurse, or more recently, risk management coordinator [11]. In an increasing number of large medical school–affiliated hospitals, infection control is combined with risk management or utilization review in a single department. Although this situation offers advantages in efficient use of personnel and bringing epidemiologic techniques to the risk-management or utilization review activities, it runs the risk of seriously reducing the personnel commitment to infection control if sufficient staff are not provided to cover all of the added responsibilities.

The ICN position is most often located organizationally in the nursing service department, although the ICN usually obtains advice and supervision from the infection control physician, if one is present in the hospital [11]. The majority of ICNs hold a nursing position equivalent to nursing supervisor or higher. Choosing more experienced nurses for the job is important to give the ICN a greater insight into the patient-care practices that are to be influenced and more experience in the clinical milieu, which facilitates the detection of infections for surveillance and increases rapport with clinical nurses and doctors. In contrast to the levels of training of infection control physicians, almost all ICNs have taken at least one training course in infection control; two-thirds of these were trained in the CDC training course, but an increasing number are taking courses offered by local and national APIC organizations, academic institutions, and private firms [11]. In 1983, as an indication of the increased training opportunities available for ICNs, the CDC in cooperation with the Association of Schools of Public Health consulted with a group of infection control training experts and recommended that the CDC reduce or discontinue its direct training efforts and turn these resources toward developing training materials and guidelines for others to use in training [7].

ICNs across the country tend to spend their time in very similar ways. Regardless of the number of hours per week worked or the size of the hospital, they spend on the average about half of their time on surveillance of infections, about a fourth on policy development, and the rest about equally divided among training, consulting, and investigating potential outbreaks [11]. In the early 1970s it appeared that there would be a high turnover rate of nurses in the ICN position; however, by the mid-1970s the turnover rate had fallen significantly below that of hospital nurses in general, suggesting that the earlier trend was a temporary feature of the position's formative period [11].

A particularly interesting controversy of the early 1980s has been the debate over whether the ICN position should continue to be filled by nurses or whether persons with different training should be used. By the mid-1970s only 6 percent of the positions were filled by persons other than nurses, almost all being bachelor's- or master's-level microbiologists, and most of these were employed in larger medical school–affiliated hospitals that already had at least one ICN [10]. Although far outnumbered, these microbiologists tended to be far more active in the national APIC organization and to participate more in authoring papers for the infection control journals. The only study that has compared ICNs with these infection control laboratorians (ICLs) found that the ICNs tended to spend more time teaching hospital personnel about infection control practices, whereas the ICLs spent more time and appeared more proficient in investigating potential outbreaks [10]. In addition ICNs appeared to exert more influence on the clinical nurses; they were reported by nurses to be more visible on the wards, more readily available for discussing clinical questions related to infection control, and less reluctant to speak up to personnel observed disregarding prescribed hand-washing practices. From these findings, it was concluded that ICNs and ICLs offered different skills, all of which appear potentially useful to the infection control effort [10].

Perhaps a prudent employment policy would be the following. In all hospitals a nurse is preferentially considered to ensure the greatest degree of influence in the patient-care setting; however, in hospitals, particularly large ones, in which more than one position is needed, a person with other skills is considered for one of the additional positions to expand the expertise of the program. The increasing number of persons with specific training in epidemiology (e.g., a master's degree in public health or epidemiology) might be particularly useful, followed by microbiologists and even statisticians or computer programmers, depending on the particular needs of the program. A priority for the near future is to determine what combination of qualifications and training is optimal for the person in this vital position. Perhaps nurses should take extended formal training in epidemiology and microbiology, and laboratorians or epidemiologists should undergo training similar to that of at least a licensed practical nurse. Since the ideal has not yet been established, the current trends toward certification testing of infection control personnel should be kept flexible to incorporate new standards as they emerge.

## EFFICACY OF SURVEILLANCE AND CONTROL PROGRAMS

The question of the efficacy of infection surveillance and control programs has been posed almost from the beginning of the movement in the 1960s but has been of increasing interest since the First International Conference in 1970. This debate has centered on several issues, including the efficacy and cost-effectiveness of routine infection surveillance over and above vigorous control measures; the need for ICNs; the best ratio of ICNs to hospital beds; the need for interested and trained infection control physicians; and the effectiveness of reporting surgical wound infection rates to surgeons. Although several studies in individual hospitals have demonstrated dramatic reductions of their nosocomial infection rates following the establishment of various combinations of these characteristics, they have not been influential in settling the efficacy questions because of the lack of simultaneous control observations, the possibility of selective reporting of positive results in the literature, and other methodologic problems [8, 12, 25, 30, 32].

In the early 1970s, CDC investigators designed the protocol for a large historical prospective study, building in numerous design features to avoid or control for the many potential biases that might be encountered. After clearance through internal scientific peer review at the CDC, presentations at scientific meetings, and formal review in government channels, the project was undertaken by the CDC staff with technical assistance from the Department of Biostatistics of the University of North Carolina School of Public Health, the UCLA Institute for Social Science Research, and the National Center for Health Statistics, with financial support from the CDC, the National Institute of Allergy and Infectious Diseases, the Health Care Financing Administration, and the office of the Assistant Secretary for Health, HHS.

After the initial design phase spanning 1974 to 1976, pilot studies were completed to validate the various data collection methods developed specifically for the project [19]. The study was then performed in three phases. First, a questionnaire was mailed to all U.S. hospitals to measure specific surveillance and control characteristics needed to construct indices of these activities and other measures of the ICN, the infection control physician, and the other components under study. After stratifying all acute-care U.S. hospitals with these two indices, 338 hospitals were selected randomly from the strata [19]. The sample provided a representative group of hospitals that had established different levels of surveillance and control efforts, including hospitals that had established no programs at all. Second, each of the 338 sample hospitals was visited by trained CDC interviewers to validate the surveillance and control indices and collect more detailed descriptive information about the programs.

The third phase involved a review by trained CDC medical records analysts of random samples of the medical records of patients admitted in 1970 and in 1975–1976 to the 338 sample hospitals. In each hospital 500 patients were selected randomly from each of the two years, and their records were reviewed to diagnose all nosocomial urinary tract infections, surgical wound infections, pneumonia, and bacteremia from the clinical data found in all parts of the record. These four sites account for over 80 percent of nosocomial infections. From these data on approximately 339,000 patients, the change of the nosocomial infection rates from 1970 (before any of

the hospitals had programs) to 1975–1976 (after the program activities measured in the first two phases had been established) were estimated. In addition measurements were made of other hospital and patient characteristics, changes in which could have confounded the evaluation. Following the data collection phase (1976–1978), the large computerized data base was extensively edited and made ready for analysis (1978–1980), and the statistical analysis of the influence of the programs on the change in infection rates, controlling for changes in other characteristics, was performed (1980–1983).

The results, published in early 1985 [17], are summarized in Table 3-1. In comparison with hospitals that started no program activities, those that established infection surveillance and control programs with a full-time-equivalent ICN per 250 occupied beds, an effectual infection control physician with special interest in infection control, and a program for reporting wound infection rates to surgeons reduced their nosocomial infection rates by approximately 32

TABLE 3-1. Percentage of nosocomial infections prevented by the most effective infection surveillance and control programs

| Type of infection | Components of most effective programs | Percent prevented |
|---|---|---|
| Surgical wound infection (SWI) | An organized hospitalwide program with Intensive surveillance and control Reporting SWI rates to surgeons Plus | 20 |
| | An effectual physician with special interest and knowledge in infection control | 35 |
| Urinary tract infection | An organized hospitalwide program with Intensive surveillance in operation for at least a year An ICN per 250 beds | 38 |
| Nosocomial bacteremia | An organized hospitalwide program with Intensive control alone Plus | 15 |
| | Moderately intensive surveillance in operation for at least a year An ICN per 250 beds An infection control physician or microbiologist | 35 |
| Postoperative pneumonia in surgical patients | An organized hospitalwide program with Intensive surveillance An ICN per 250 beds | 27 |
| Pneumonia in medical patients | An organized hospitalwide program with Intensive surveillance and control | 13 |
| All types of nosocomial infections | An organized hospitalwide program with All of the components listed above | 32 |

percent, a result that was highly statistically significant for all four types of infections studied. Separate analyses for cohorts of high- and low-risk patients showed similar results for each type of infection, although programs to prevent infections among low-risk patients had to be somewhat more intensive than those needed for high-risk patients. The importance of these results was emphasized by the finding that among hospitals that started no programs the nosocomial infection rate was increasing at a rate of 18 percent over five years, presumably reflecting the increasing infection risks accompanying the continual introduction of invasive and immunocompromising medical technology.

Whereas about one-third of nosocomial infections *could* be prevented if all U.S. hospitals had established the programs found to be the most effective, the fact that relatively few hospitals actually had all of the required components meant that in the mid-1970s only 6 percent of nosocomial infections were actually being prevented nationwide [17]. The widespread adoption of the most effective programs might therefore be expected to prevent an additional one-fourth of the infections. A resurvey of a random sample of U.S. hospitals in 1983 found that hospitals had substantially increased the intensity of their surveillance and control activities, but the failure to implement certain specific critical components, such as an adequate staffing ratio for ICNs, training of hospital epidemiologists, or reporting wound infection rates to surgeons, had muted the degree of improvement in prevention to the extent that still only 9 percent of infections were being prevented [18]. It seems likely, however, that the publication of the first controlled studies on the efficacy of the programs from the SENIC Project coincident with the beginning of prospective payment system will stimulate substantial improvements by the mid- or late 1980s.

## COST-BENEFIT ANALYSIS OF SURVEILLANCE AND CONTROL PROGRAMS

In the planning stage of the SENIC Project, a preliminary cost-benefit analysis of infection surveillance and control programs was developed, using equivalent estimates of costs and benefits in 1975 dollars [16, 29]. Based on a nosocomial infection rate just over 5 percent occurring among the over 37 million patient admissions to U.S. general hospitals each year, the number of infections occurring nationwide would exceed 2 million per year. Assuming an average extra charge per infection in 1975 of $600, an empirically

derived figure that is among the lower published estimates [21], the total extra cost would be on the order of 1 billion dollars per year in 1975 dollars. In view of inflation in hospital costs of 14 to 18 percent per year since 1975, that estimate can be expected to have tripled by 1985 (see Chapter 24).

On the other hand, assuming a 1975 salary cost of $12,000 for an ICN, $5000 for consultation by a part-time infection control physician, $2000 for part-time clerical assistance, and $1000 for miscellaneous expenses—the costs necessary to perform surveillance and control for 250 hospital beds—the total cost would be approximately $20,000 per 250 beds. With approximately 898,000 beds among all U.S. hospitals in 1975, the cost of adding an effective program would be approximately 72 million dollars—again in 1975 dollars.

Dividing the cost of the programs by the cost of the infections indicates that only about 6 percent of the costs of infections would have to be prevented to offset exactly the costs of the programs. If the programs are exactly 6 percent effective, an estimated 100,000 nosocomial infections would be prevented nationwide, and the net cost would be close to zero. Given, however, the estimate of 32 percent effectiveness derived from the SENIC Project [17], the nationwide establishment of the most effective programs can be expected to prevent at least 732,000 nosocomial infections at a net savings of approximately 1.3 billion dollars per year in 1985 dollars.

In past years when patients and third-party agencies paid the extra costs of nosocomial infections, it was not entirely clear whether the hospitals' expenditures would actually be offset by preventing infections. Certainly the economic advantage was not realized by hospitals directly. With reimbursement of hospitals by a flat fee determined by a patient's DRG, it appears that the extra costs of most infectious complications of hospitalization will now be borne directly by the hospitals as operating deficits. If this remains so, as reimbursement agencies tighten the DRG-specific reimbursement rates, hospitals will be forced to take all proven money-saving measures to remain financially solvent. Thus the intense financial pressures that are likely to develop should establish the most effective infection surveillance and control programs in all U.S. hospitals.

## REFERENCES

1. American Hospital Association. *Infection Control in the Hospital.* Chicago: AHA, 1968.

2. American Hospital Association. *Infection Control in the Hospital* (Revised ed.). Chicago: AHA, 1970.

3. Centers for Disease Control. *Guidelines for the Prevention and Control of Nosocomial Infections.* Springfield, Va.: National Technical Information Service, U.S. Department of Commerce, 1982.

4. Centers for Disease Control. *National Nosocomial Infections Study Quarterly Reports.* Atlanta: CDC, 1970–1983.

5. Centers for Disease Control. *Outline for Surveillance and Control of Nosocomial Infections.* Atlanta: CDC, 1972 (reprinted September 1973, May 1974, November 1976).

6. Centers for Disease Control. *Proceedings of the First International Conference on Nosocomial Infections,* August 5–8, 1970, Atlanta. Chicago: American Hospital Association, 1970.

7. Centers for Disease Control, Association of Schools of Public Health. *A Report of the Meeting of the CDC/ASPH Working Group on Nosocomial Infection Control Training,* April 12–13, 1983, Atlanta. Atlanta: CDC, 1983.

8. Cruse, P. J. E., and Foord, R. The epidemiology of wound infection: A 10-year prospective study of 62,939 wounds. *Surg. Clin. North Am.* 60:27, 1980.

9. Eickhoff, T. C., Brachman, P. S., Bennett, J. V., and Brown, J. F. Surveillance of nosocomial infections in community hospitals. I. Surveillance methods, effectiveness, and initial results. *J. Infect. Dis.* 120:305, 1969.

10. Emori, T. G., Haley, R. W., Garner, J. S., et al. Comparison of surveillance and control activities of infection control nurses and infection control laboratorians in United States hospitals, 1976–1977. *Am. J. Infect. Control* 10:3, 1982.

11. Emori, T. G., Haley, R. W., and Stanley, R. C. The infection control nurse in U.S. hospitals, 1976–1977: Characteristics of the position and its occupant. *Am. J. Epidemiol.* 111:592, 1980.

12. Fuchs, P. C. *Epidemiology of Hospital-Associated Infections.* Chicago: American Society of Clinical Pathologists, 1979, pp. 74–78.

13. Gardner, A. M. N., Stamp, M., Bowgen, J. A., and Moore, B. The infection control sister. *Lancet* 2:710, 1962.

14. Haley, R. W. CDC guidelines on infection control: Introduction. *Infect. Control* 2:117, 1981.

15. Haley, R. W. The "hospital epidemiologist" in U.S. hospitals, 1976–1977: A description of the head of the infection surveillance and control program. *Infect. Control* 1:21, 1980.

16. Haley, R. W. Preliminary cost-benefit analysis of hospital infection control programs (the SENIC Project). In Dascher, F. (Ed.), *Proven and Unproven Methods in Hospital Infection Control.* New York: Gustav Fischer Verlag, 1978, pp. 93–96.

17. Haley, R. W., Culver, D. H., White, J. W., Morgan, W. M., Emori, T. G., Munn, V. P., and Hooton, T. M. The efficacy of infection surveillance and control programs in preventing nosocomial infections in U.S. hospitals. *Am. J. Epidemiol.* 121:182, 1984.

18. Haley, R. W., Morgan, W. M., Culver, D. H., et al. Hospital infection control: Recent progress and opportunities under prospective payment. *Am. J. Infect. Control* 13:78, 1985.

19. Haley, R. W., Quade, D., Freeman, H. E., et al. Study on the efficacy of nosocomial infection control (SENIC Project): Summary of study design. *Am. J. Epidemiol.* 111:472, 1980.

20. Haley, R. W., Quade, D., Freeman, H. E., et al. Study on the efficacy of nosocomial infection control (SENIC Project): Summary of study design (Appendix A). *Am. J. Epidemiol.* 111:608, 1980.

21. Haley, R. W., Schaberg, D. R., Crossley, K. B., Von Allmen, S. D., and McGowan, J. E., Jr. Extra days and prolongation of stay attributable to nosocomial infections: A prospective interhospital comparison. *Am. J. Med.* 70:51, 1981.

22. Haley, R. W., and Shachtman, R. H. The emergence of infection surveillance and control programs in U.S. hospitals: An assessment, 1976. *Am. J. Epidemiol.* 111:574, 1980.

23. Inglehart, J. K. The new era of prospective payment for hospitals. *N. Engl. J. Med.* 307:1288, 1982.

24. Joint Commission on Accreditation of Hospitals. Infection Control. In *Accreditation Manual for Hospitals.* Chicago: Joint Commission on Accreditation of Hospitals, 1976.

25. Moore, W. L., Jr. Nosocomial infections: An overview. *Am. J. Hosp. Pharm.* 351:832, 1974.

26. Raven, B. H., Freeman, H. E., and Haley, R. W. Social science perspectives in hospital infection control. In Johnson, A. W., Grusky, O., and Raven, B. H. (Eds.), *Contemporary Health Services: Social Science Perspectives.* Boston: Auburn House Publishing Co., 1981, pp. 137–176.

27. Raven, B. H., and Haley, R. W. Social influence in a medical context. In Bickman, L. (Ed.), *Applied Social Psychology Annual,* Vol. I. Beverly Hills, Calif.: Sage, 1980, pp. 255–277.

28. Raven, B. H., and Haley, R. W. Social Influence and Compliance of Hospital Nurses with Infection Control Policies. In Eiser, J. R. (Ed.), *Social*

*Psychology and Behavioral Medicine.* New York: Wiley, 1980, pp. 413–438.

29. Sencer, D. J., and Axnick, N. W. Utilization of cost-benefit analysis in planning prevention programs. *Acta Med. Scand.* 576(Suppl.):123, 1975.

30. Shoji, K. T., Axnick, K., and Rytel, M. W. Infections and antibiotic use in a large municipal hospital, 1970–1972: A prospective analysis of the effectiveness of a continuous surveillance program. *Health Lab. Sci.* 11:283, 1974.

31. Stamm, W. E. Elements of an active, effective infection control program. *Hospitals* 50:60, 1976.

32. Streeter, S., Dunn, H., and Lepper, M. Hospital infection: A necessary risk? *Am. J. Nurs.* 67:526, 1967.

33. U.S. Public Health Service Communicable Diseases Center and the National Academy of Sciences National Research Council. *Proceedings of the National Conference on Hospital-Acquired Staphylococcal Disease,* September 15–17, 1958, Atlanta. Atlanta: CDC, 1958.

34. U.S. Public Health Service Communicable Diseases Center and the National Academy of Sciences National Research Council. *Proceedings of the Conference on Relation of the Environment to Hospital-Acquired Staphylococcal Disease,* December 1–2, 1958, Atlanta. Atlanta: CDC, 1958.

35. University of Michigan School of Public Health, Mayo Foundation Communicable Disease Center. *Proceedings of the National Conference on Institutionally Acquired Infections,* September 4–6, 1963, Minneapolis. Atlanta: CDC; 1963.

36. Wenzel, K. S. The role of the infection control nurse. *Nurs. Clin. North Am.* 5:89, 1970.

# 4 SURVEILLANCE OF NOSOCOMIAL INFECTIONS

Robert W. Haley
Robert C. Aber
John V. Bennett

## DEFINITION OF SURVEILLANCE

Surveillance, when applied to disease, may be defined as the systematic, active, ongoing observation of the occurrence and distribution of disease within a population and of the events or conditions that increase or decrease the risk of such disease occurrence. The term implies that the observational data are regularly analyzed and disseminated to those who need the information to take appropriate actions.

Surveillance of disease should be a continuous process that consists of the following elements: (1) defining the events to be surveyed as concisely and precisely as possible, (2) collecting the relevant data in a systematic way, (3) consolidating or tabulating the data into meaningful arrangements, (4) analyzing and interpreting the data, and (5) disseminating the data and interpretations to those who need to know them.

Some argue that surveillance implies more than the monitoring of infections and that taking appropriate actions based on analysis and interpretation of the data is also entailed in the concept. We prefer to classify the actions taken on the basis of the knowledge gained from surveillance as "infection control efforts" rather than as an integral part of the surveillance activity per se.

## HISTORY

In the six years since the first edition of this book appeared, a great deal of discussion and debate has taken place concerning the desirability of continuing routine surveillance, argued by some to be too personnel-intensive in a milieu of constrained hospital budgets. As this discussion continues, it is useful to know how the modern concepts and techniques of surveillance came about—how we got where we are now. Many of these practices were developed to meet emerging problems, and the basic concept has been found to be effective in reducing infection risks. Knowledge of the historical reasons for these developments may help in improving the efficiency and effectiveness of surveillance without discarding well-conceived approaches that are still effective.

The use of surveillance methods to control nosocomial infections dates back at least to the classic work of Dr. Ignaz Semmelweis in Vienna in the 1840s [22]. Although the Semmelweis story is best remembered as the first demonstration of the importance of person-to-person spread of puerperal sepsis and of the effectiveness of washing hands with an antiseptic solution, an equally important achievement was his rigorous approach to the collection, analysis, and use of surveillance data. In contrast, the concurrent work of Dr. Oliver Wendell Holmes on the same subject in the United States was based primarily on the traditional anecdotal case-study approach of clinical medicine.

Semmelweis' investigation is an amazingly contemporary example of the effective use of surveillance in addressing a widespread infection problem. When he assumed the directorship of the obstetric service at the Vienna Lying-In Hospital in 1847, the apparent risk of maternal mortality had been at high levels for over 20 years—so long that the eminent clinicians of the day considered the risks to be no more than the expected endemic occurrence and that they could not be influenced.

Semmelweis first undertook a retrospective investigation of the problem and set up a prospective surveillance system to monitor the problem and the effects of later control measures. The initial results of his retrospective study of yearly hospital mortality lists showed clearly that the maternal mortality level, which he measured by calculating yearly mortality rates, had indeed increased 10-fold following the introduction in the 1820s of the new anatomic school of pathology, which used the autopsy as its main teaching tool. His second discovery, based on the use of ward-specific mortality rates, was that the risk of death in the ward used for teaching medical students was at least four times higher than that in the ward used for teaching midwifery students. After the septic death of his mentor suggested the presence of a transmissible agent, Semmelweis used the findings from his retrospective surveillance to implicate the practices of the medical students. After observing their daily routines, he surmised correctly that they were transferring the infection from their cadavers to the parturient women and that washing hands with a chlorine solution would prevent transmission. Subsequently his prospective surveillance data confirmed the effectiveness of the control measure in dramatically reducing the maternal mortality rate.

Here the great insights of Semmelweis ended, as often happens to infection control efforts today. Apparently due to his abrasive manner and lack of diplomacy, as well as an inability to organize his statistical data into a concise, convincing report, he failed to win over his clinical colleagues to his discovery. Within two years he was dismissed from the staff of the hospital, and his successor gradually allowed the strict hand-washing measures to decline. In the absence of continuing surveillance, the epidemic promptly resumed and lasted well into the early part of the twentieth century, its severity and means of prevention apparently unappreciated by several more generations of clinicians.

This story well illustrates one of the main impediments to infection control today: that in the absence of careful analysis of epidemiologic data and a diplomatic presentation, clinicians, who are oriented almost entirely toward the treatment of their patients, often fail to appreciate the severity of the problem and sometimes even resist control measures. It also points out the usefulness of surveillance in identifying problems and developing and applying control measures. From a methodologic viewpoint, Semmelweis' efforts encompassed almost all aspects of the modern surveillance approach: retrospective collection of data to confirm the presence of a problem; analysis of the data to localize the risks in time, place, and person; controlled comparisons of high- and low-risk groups to identify risk factors; formulation and application of control measures; and prospective surveillance to monitor the problem, evaluate the control measures, and detect future recurrences. The main shortcoming of his approach was his failure to educate his powerful colleagues diplomatically with a careful report of his findings.

As good a model as Semmelweis' work was, the modern era of nosocomial infection surveillance grew as much out of different currents of the midtwentieth century as from the Semmelweis tradition. The importance of surveillance for disease control in general arose in the United States as a central concept in the effort to control tropical diseases among troops stationed in the Pacific Theater in World War II. At the end of the war, the core of the epidemiologists of the Malaria Control in War Areas Unit were transferred to a civilian facility within the Public Health Service to apply their surveillance and control strategies to the control of malaria in the southern United States. Located in Atlanta near the endemic areas, the unit was first named the Communicable Diseases Center (CDC) and later the Centers for Disease Control (CDC). Since the large volume of reports of malaria indicated the disease to be widespread, a surveillance system was immediately set up to define the problem. But as investigators examined each reported case, they found virtually all of the reports to contain errors in diagnosis. Thus the mere activity of surveillance "eradicated" the malaria epidemic in the United States.

With this and similar successes fresh in memory when the pandemic of staphylococcal infections swept the nation's hospitals in the mid-1950s, the CDC staff members were quick to apply the concepts of surveillance to the problem. When asked to assist in investigating a staphylococcal epidemic in a hospital, those early investigators often met strong resistance from clinicians and hospital administrators convinced that no unusual infection problems were present in their hospital. In instances in which the investigators were able to continue the investigations, the collection and reporting of surveillance data regularly changed those attitudes to strong concern over the documented problems and eagerness to apply control measures. These initial investigations confirmed a nationwide epidemic and led the CDC to sponsor several national conferences to discuss the problem.

As the epidemic subsided in the early 1960s, CDC's Surveillance Unit continued to develop more effective surveillance methods specifically geared to the hospital situation. By 1970, on the basis of pilot studies, the CDC was recommending that surveillance be practiced routinely in all hospitals. By the late 1970s almost all U.S. hospitals had adopted the approach, and surveillance culturing of the inanimate environment, which previously had enjoyed a degree of popularity, had been virtually abandoned (see Chapters 3 and 14). In 1976 the Joint Commission on Accredditation of Hospitals incorporated a detailed surveillance system into its standards for accreditation.

By the early 1980s the pendulum began swinging back in the opposite direction as critics questioned the effectiveness and cost-benefit of routine infection surveillance, although more hospitals still were increasing their surveillance efforts than were decreasing them. There is some indication that the inability of some larger hospitals to establish an adequate number of positions for infection control nurses (one full-time-equivalent per 250 beds) was a major contributor to the disenchantment with routine infection surveillance. As this rethinking gathered momentum, the announcement of the results of the SENIC Project strongly substantiated the necessity of surveillance along with control measures to reduce infection rates [10]. The strong conclusion was that without an organized routine hospitalwide surveillance system, even the most vigorous control policies are unlikely to be fully successful. To the extent that these results are accepted, the continuing discussions of surveillance can be expected to turn away from questioning the value of surveillance to identifying how to perform surveillance most efficiently without reducing its proven effectiveness.

## THE TECHNIQUE OF SURVEILLANCE

### Surveillance by Objectives
Throughout the 1970s a growing concern was that excessive personnel and financial resources were being spent in collecting large amounts of routine surveillance data that were not being used to prevent infections. Although descriptive information from the SENIC Project suggests that this fear was not widely held by infection control personnel in U.S. hospitals, it illustrates the intellectual struggle of the decade over how most efficiently to integrate surveillance into an infection control program to increase its impact. In short, this view expressed the concern that surveillance activities were being routinely practiced without clear objectives.

OUTCOME OBJECTIVES   In setting up a new surveillance system or in revamping an old one, the easiest, although least desirable, approach is to examine the surveillance practices of other local hospitals or those recommended by authoritative experts and begin practicing them on a routine basis. Given the increasing financial constraints on hospital budgets and the often limited size of their infection control staffs, it has become increasingly necessary to plan surveillance efforts with the opposite approach, that is, by proceeding from the statement of clear objectives to the design of a surveillance system to achieve these objectives. Surveillance without objectives has become indefensible.

Of course the ultimate *outcome objective* of surveillance is to reduce the risks of nosocomial infections among hospitalized patients. Thus when evaluating the need for particular surveillance activities, one should ask how the activity can be expected to result in the reduction of infection. Activities not directly justified on this basis should probably be discontinued and the resources redirected to more clearly objective-oriented activities. This approach has been referred to as "surveillance by objectives" [10].

PROCESS OBJECTIVES   Unlike intervention or control activities, the mere act of collecting surveillance data does not usually influence infection risks appreciably, although in some serious epidemic situations a highly visible investigation may change patient-care behaviors and end the problem. Usually, however, to translate surveillance efforts into infection prevention, it is necessary to identify and state intermediate, or process, objectives that if achieved by surveillance will in turn reduce infection risks. Process objectives are often referred to loosely as the "uses of surveillance." These may include such things as documenting baseline rates of endemic infections, identifying epidemics or other infection problems, convincing key clinicians or other hospital personnel of the seriousness of a problem and the need for vigorous control measures, evaluating the effects of control measures, reinforcing preventive patient-care practices, satisfying standards, defending the hospital against malpractice claims and litigation over nosocomial infections, and conducting research.

*Baseline rates.* The most fundamental use of surveillance is the measurement of baseline rates of endemic nosocomial infections. Its prime function is to provide objective quantitative knowledge of the ongoing infection risks in the hospital and to serve as the basis for the other uses of surveillance. It can also lead directly to the prevention of infections. Finding the endemic infection rates higher than anticipated often stimulates a search for unsuspected causes that would not have been made without the impetus of having baseline rates available. In the SENIC interview survey in 1976, surveillance was reported to be used for this purpose in 91 percent of hospitals [6]. This process is aided by analyzing the surveillance data to obtain infection rates that are readily interpretable, such as rates by type of infection, pathogen, service or hospital area, and in some instances, by individual hospital personnel. Approximately three-fourths of hospitals reported performing these types of analyses of their surveillance data [6].

*Identifying epidemics.* The most frequently discussed use of surveillance is for the identification of epidemics. In the SENIC interview survey this use was reported by 81 percent of hospitals [6]. By regularly measuring the infection rates, one can recognize deviations from the baseline rates that sometimes represent epidemics due to a new common source of infection, the introduction of a new virulent pathogen, or increased person-to-person spread from a breakdown in patient-care practices. Although it has been argued that epidemics can often be recognized without the effort required for routine surveillance, the monitoring of baseline rates provides two important advantages. It allows fewer outbreaks to escape notice and more to be detected in an earlier stage, thereby reducing the number of cases that occur. Thus hospitals with organized routine surveillance systems can expect to have fewer nosocomial infections due to epidemics.

Justifying the relatively time-consuming activity of routine surveillance and calculation of baseline rates is a complex management issue. On the one hand when a serious epidemic occurs, particularly when one or more deaths are attributed to it, hospital officials are usually quite anxious to have baseline data with which to confirm quickly the extent of the problem, pinpoint precisely what changes have occurred in the rates, and demonstrate that all appropriate measures are being taken. Historically the usefulness of such data in an epidemic investigation and their perceived value in prevention or earlier recognition of future problems have often been the justification for establishing ongoing surveillance activities. On the other hand, since only a minority of nosocomial infections occur in outbreaks or epidemics, the justification for routine surveillance must include additional uses that contribute to the control of both endemic and epidemic infections.

*Convincing clinicians.* Perhaps the most important use of surveillance—ironically, the one most often overlooked—is to arm the infection control staff with information that will allow them to convince physicians, nurses, and hospital administrators of the need for preventive actions. Typically infection control personnel feel that their most difficult problem is to get hospital personnel to agree when there are serious problems and to adopt the recommended preventive practices.

Sociologic theory on the means by which people or groups are influenced lists six fundamental steps that form the bases of social power: (1) providing information that will influence behavior (information power), (2) presenting oneself as an expert whose advice should be followed (expert power), (3) presenting oneself as a legitimate authority with the right to require compliance (legitimacy power), (4) referring to the acceptable conduct of one's peers to obtain their compliance (referent power), (5) threatening punishments for failure to conform (coercion power), and (6) offering rewards for conformity (reward power). From the SENIC interview survey, it appears that information and expert power were the only bases of social power used by most infection control nurses, Infection Control Committee chairpersons, and hospital epidemiologists [18]. Staff nurses indicated that their practices would be influenced almost exclusively by these two as well. Conversely, referent, legitimacy, coercion, and reward power were perceived as ineffective and were rarely used by infection control personnel.

If this survey is accurate, how does the infection control staff either obtain sufficiently convincing information or become sufficiently recognized as experts to use these two bases of social power fully? A favorite way of achieving both is to become thoroughly familiar with the scientific literature on hospital epidemiology and infection control. Thus when trying to influence a colleague one can quote relevant references to establish expertise and to provide convincing information. This approach, however, is only as effective as the information is relevant to the specific situation. And since most scientific articles are unable to anticipate the many varied circumstances that affect infection risks in different hospitals, relying entirely on the body of scientific publications, although useful to a point, is ultimately a losing strategy.

Maintaining current surveillance data allows the infection control staff to present an accurate, quantitative, and timely picture of most infection problems that might arise. Since the epidemiologic analysis of patients in the aggregate is not part of the clinical training of physicians or nurses, having such information elevates the infection control staff to a unique position of expertise and respect. If the data are analyzed correctly and expeditiously and are presented skillfully, clinicians usually come to rely strongly on them for guidance. A particularly effective example is the practice of regularly reporting individual surgeons' wound infection rates to them on a regular basis to allow them to assess their surgical skill in comparison with their peers. In contrast hospital administrators are accustomed to viewing problems in aggregate statistical terms, and often expect proposals, particularly those for money or extra resources, to be formulated in an organized quantitative manner and supported by relevant evidence. In short, having routine surveillance data gives the infection control staff both the information and the expert position necessary to influence key hospital staff members in critical situations.

*Evaluating control measures.* Once problems have been recognized through surveillance, potential risk factors identified through epidemiologic analysis, and staff members influenced to carry out the control measures, continued surveillance is usually necessary to ensure that the problem comes under control and remains so. One of the unfortunate realities of controlling infections is that even the most rational control measures based on the best information and sound judgment sometimes prove to be ineffective. In the absence of continued formal surveillance, it may take a long time to discover that the expected reduction in infections did not occur. Even worse, clinicians recalling the experiences of their own patients may disagree about the effects or argue that control is unnecessary or futile. Providing continuing evidence of the progress of the control effort at least places the discussions on a factual basis with the total picture in view, and at best points the way to new control strategies that will prove more effective. Even after control measures have been found effective, contin-

uing surveillance can be important. For example, finding a recrudescence of the problem following initial successful control could lead to the identification of a breakdown in the control measures.

*Reinforcing practices.* The most important measure in maintaining a sustained reduction in endemic nosocomial infection rates and in preventing epidemics due to known risk factors is to perpetuate certain critical patient-care practices that reduce infection risks, the so-called preventive patient-care practices (e.g., aseptic urinary catheter care, changing intravenous cannulas, encouraging coughing and deep breathing in postoperative patients, hand-washing). Besides the obvious prerequisites to gaining compliance such as formulating correct policies, obtaining agreement of key authorities, and training personnel, surveillance can contribute substantially to sustained compliance by providing feedback to the staff on their performance. In the SENIC interview survey, the infection control staff in approximately 80 percent of hospitals reported monitoring practices and reporting surveillance results in inservice education [6].

This feedback can entail either process evaluations that report rates of compliance with the policy or outcome evaluations that report the changes in infection rates related to the policy. Process evaluations require continuing surveillance of preventive patient-care practices, whereas outcome evaluations require surveillance of nosocomial infections. In some circumstances it may be most appropriate to report these findings directly to the patient-care personnel (e.g., wound infection rates to surgeons), and in others it might be preferable to report them to the supervisor or chief of service (e.g., a high rate of septicemia in an intensive care unit). For this activity to be most effective, it must be designed to provide relatively immediate positive reinforcement for proper compliance and to identify deficiencies at which corrective action can be directed.

*Satisfying standards.* In the SENIC interview survey, surveillance was used by the largest percentage of hospitals (93 percent) to satisfy the requirements of the Joint Commission on Accreditation of Hospitals (JCAH) [6]. In 1976 the JCAH revised its interpretation of standards dealing with the infection control program, and it currently directs each Infection Control Committee to develop a practical surveillance system for reporting, evaluating, and keeping records of infections among patients and hospital personnel to provide an indication of the endemic level of all nosocomial infections, identify the sources of infections, and discover real or potential epidemics [16]. Satisfying this standard is clearly a legitimate use of surveillance in the practical operation of an infection control program, and it can be used effectively as leverage to obtain approval for adequate program resources and for implementing infection control policies.

*Malpractice claims.* In earlier decades one of the often voiced criticisms of surveillance was that it created a record that could be used against the hospital in litigation of a malpractice claim related to a nosocomial infection. Based on more extensive experience with malpractice claims and litigation, most legal experts now take just the opposite view, primarily for two reasons. First, in most states the records of internal hospital committees, including the Infection Control Committee, are considered privileged and not discoverable in civil court proceedings. Second, the ability to show that the hospital has a vigorous surveillance system for detecting problems that might occur is thought to be among the most important defenses against unwarranted claims (see Chapter 13). In 1976 fewer than 10 percent of hospital administrators considered surveillance data to be more often a hindrance than a help in these situations [6].

*Conducting research.* Apart from its fundamental place in a hospital's infection control effort, surveillance methods have formed the basis for conducting much valuable research in controlling infections in all hospitals. Early studies using surveillance to measure infection risks identified the risk factors on which many of the current infection control policies and recommendations are based. More recently, experiments such as those comparing the safety of different intervals for changing respirator breathing circuits have used routine surveillance methods to evaluate alternative practices. The pooling of surveillance data from many hospitals has formed the basis for CDC's National Nosocomial Infection Study and for a similar statewide network in Virginia. Such systems allow the detection or confirmation of infection problems with nationwide distributions. Even though the accuracy of surveillance systems varies substantially, when consistent definitions and data collection methods have been used this limitation appears to have been of little practical significance in many research efforts.

## Methods of Surveillance

COLLECTING THE DATA *Defining events to be surveyed.* It is of utmost importance in developing a surveillance system to define carefully those events to be surveyed and to apply the accepted definitions systematically in the data-collecting process. In attempting to understand the relation between urinary tract infection and urinary catheterization, for ex-

ample, it is necessary first to define or establish criteria to decide what will be called a "urinary tract infection" and what will be considered "urinary catheterization." Once the event to be surveyed has been defined as concisely and precisely as possible and the criteria for determining its presence or absence have been established, it is imperative that these definitions and criteria be applied systematically and uniformly henceforth. Ideally all members of the population judged at risk for the occurrence of the event would be systematically and continuously assessed for the presence or absence of the properties specified by the criteria that define the event or infection being sought. By 1976 written definitions for nosocomial infections were being used in three-fourths of U.S. hospitals [6].

The Centers for Disease Control has published guidelines for determining the presence and classification of infection [3]. These guidelines are not rigorous definitions of disease but rather serve as practical, operational definitions for most hospitals, regardless of their size or medical sophistication. In constructing the criteria to be used in surveillance, the exact definitions decided on are not as critical as the stipulation that the Infection Control Committee obtain the concurrence of key hospital staff members. Such widespread advance agreement is necessary to avoid having the results of surveillance later disqualified by disagreements over the definitions.

It is also important that consistent criteria be used in determining the service to which a patient belongs. The service to which the patient was assigned at the time of acquisition of the infection should be used. If this determination is not possible, the patient should be assigned to the service on which he or she resided at the time of onset of the infection.

*Role of the infection control nurse.* A number of methods of collecting infection data have been described in the literature. In general the most satisfactory and practical method at present employs a person (or persons), often called the infection control nurse (ICN), whose job description includes collecting and analyzing surveillance data. Details of the qualifications, functions, and responsibilities of the ICN were given previously (see Chapter 3). The ICN is responsible to the Infection Control Committee and should be under the immediate supervision of the committee chairperson or hospital epidemiologist, if the hospital has one. The choice of a nurse to fill this position has been primarily based on professional training and ability to interact with other nursing personnel in the data-collection process, but experience has shown that persons other than nurses can also function well, particularly in the surveillance process. One ICN can conduct surveillance for about 250 acute-care hospital beds and have sufficient time remaining for other infection control duties and responsibilities [3].

*Minimal data to collect.* The precise information collected in conjunction with each infection may vary according to the institution, service, site of infection, or causative agent. Certain essential identifying data, however, can be recommended: the patient's name, age, sex, hospital identification number, ward or location within the hospital, service, and date of admission; the date of onset of the infection; the site of infection; the organism or organisms isolated in culture studies; and the antimicrobial susceptibility pattern of the organisms isolated. Additional information should be collected only if it will be analyzed and used by the hospital. Some institutions may wish to include the primary diagnoses of the infected patients, an assessment of the severity of underlying illnesses, the names of the attending physicians or other staff who attended the patient, whether exposure occurred before the onset of infection to therapies that may predispose to infection (e.g., surgery, antibiotic, steroid, or immunosuppressive therapy; instrumentation), what antimicrobial agents were used to treat the infection, and some assessment of mortality related to the infection. Recording the presence or absence of particular exposure factors may be useful for certain types of infections, for example, urinary catheterization for urinary tract infections; respiratory therapy equipment for respiratory infections; and the use of intravenous, subclavian, or arterial catheters for primary bacteremia.

This information may be recorded on a file card or sheet by the ICN, and it may subsequently be transferred to a computer for analysis if one is available. It is important to update the infection file—whether it be on cards, sheets, or a computer—as new information becomes available.

*Denominators.* Denominator information for calculating rates can usually be obtained from the medical records department. The number of admissions or discharges by ward and service for a specified period of time (usually a month or longer) should be obtained. The number of admissions is theoretically superior to the number of discharges in reflecting the number of patients at risk, since patients who die may not be included in discharges. Practically, however, these differences do not significantly affect the rates of infection, and the choice between them is usually decided on the basis of the ease with which they can be obtained. Also, the census of hospitalized patients at the start of the surveillance interval theoretically needs to be added to the number of ad-

missions to yield the precise number of patients at risk during the surveillance interval, which is usually one month. This correction is customarily ignored, since this census is small in comparison to the total number of admissions to an acute-care hospital over a period of a month or longer. This correction, however, can become highly important when the surveillance intervals are short (e.g., one week or less) or when the average duration of hospital stay is excessively long (e.g., in a chronic-care facility).

Special denominators—such as the number of intensive-care unit admissions or discharges or the number of patients undergoing a surgical procedure—must sometimes be obtained from special log books maintained within the appropriate hospital area. Such denominators as the number of patients receiving indwelling urinary catheters, intravenous catheters, or other predisposing factors by service or hospital location are often more difficult to obtain. Central supply and pharmacy records may be useful; in some hospitals, such data may be retrieved from the computer files of the hospital's business office (see p. 68).

SOURCES OF INFECTION DATA The effective infection control nurse must use a wide variety of sources of infection information, from both within and outside the hospital, to ensure the most complete enumeration of infections. The main methods used for detecting cases of infection and the frequency of use of each among U.S. hospitals in the mid-1970s are shown in Figure 4-1. The active techniques of case-finding, which are used in almost all hospitals, are strongly preferred to the passive techniques. The active techniques not only allow more complete detection of cases but also provide the opportunity for the infection control nurse to visit the patient-care areas regularly, interact with and provide consultation to the medical and nursing staffs, and gain first-hand awareness of the infection problems. The passive techniques, particularly the practice of expecting physicians or staff nurses to fill out infection report forms, have been shown to be extremely inaccurate for the routine detection of infections. Hospitals relying on passive techniques typically find extremely low nosocomial infection rates, but these rates are due to extreme underreporting rather than extraordinary practice.

*The microbiology laboratory.* Of the case-finding methods listed in Figure 4-1, one of the most useful is the periodic (usually daily) review of microbiology laboratory reports. This may be performed each morning before making ward rounds, so that any new or potential infections can be inspected during the rounds. Such review implies an understanding by the

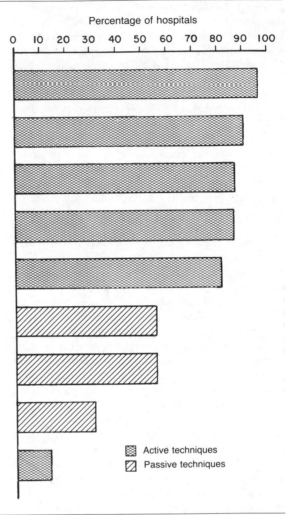

Percentage of hospitals

FIG. 4-1. Active and passive case-finding methods used in surveillance.

ICN of the infectious and epidemiologic potential of various microorganisms; such knowledge might be achieved in a laboratory training period at the time of employment and reinforced by periodic inservice review sessions. It must be stressed that a review of the microbiology laboratory reports alone is not sufficient for the identification of nosocomial infections, because cultures are not obtained for all infections or may be handled incorrectly; some infectious agents (e.g., viruses) will not be identified in many hospital laboratories; and for some types of infections (e.g., surgical wound infections and pneumonia), the identification of a potentially pathogenic organism from a culture specimen does not mean that infection is present; such infections require clinical verification.

*Ward rounds.* Periodic (preferably daily) ward rounds by the ICN should be included as an integral part of an effective surveillance program. The purposes of such rounds are to identify new infections, follow up previously identified infections, and consult with the nursing staff about infection control policies and practices. New infections may be identified outright by physicians or nurses working in the area visited, review of temperature records, follow-up of suspicious microbiology laboratory reports, review of patients having high-risk procedures (such as surgery, urinary tract instrumentation, or indwelling urinary or intravenous catheters), and review of patients in isolation or receiving antimicrobial therapy. Ward visitation also allows direct inspection and documentation of visible infections, which increase the validity of the data collected.

*Other sources.* Additional infection information may
be obtained through a periodic review of x-ray laboratory reports, records of personnel health clinic visits, and autopsy reports. The surveillance of infection
in discharged patients, although often neglected, may
be of particular value in newborn infants and postoperative patients. These patients are often discharged within the incubation period of their characteristic infections. Telephone or mail surveys or
reports from patients' private physicians may be of
assistance in detecting such infections.

The exclusive use of alternative methods of infection data collection, such as the review of postdischarge medical records or the use of infection report
sheets filled out by attending physicians or floor nurses,
is less satisfactory from the standpoint of infection
control. The former method suffers from its ex post
facto nature. Valuable time may be lost between the
onset of the infection and its discovery by this method,
and such delay may result in excessive morbidity or
mortality among patients or hospital personnel. The
latter method has been used in a number of hospitals,
but it suffers from the lack of systematic application
of standard definitions and criteria for detecting infection, as well as from great variation from person
to person in the completeness of reporting infection.

CONSOLIDATING AND TABULATING DATA   Since it is
difficult to recognize potentially important relations
or patterns of infection from the raw data on the file
cards, worksheets, or line-listing forms, it is necessary to consolidate the data in ways that make them
more understandable. This step simply involves
counting and recording the number of infections in
single-variable frequency tables (e.g., number of infections by service, site, or pathogen) and two-way
cross-tabulations (e.g., number of infections by site
on each hospital service, by pathogen on each hospital
service, and by pathogen for each site). A separate
table should be prepared for each of these analyses.
In addition, the antimicrobial susceptibility patterns
should be tallied by pathogen for each site. It is
usually practical to perform the single-variable frequency tables and two-way cross-tabulations by hand,
but three-way (e.g., pathogen-by-site-by-service), four-
way (e.g., susceptibility patterns–by-pathogen-by-
site-by-service), and more complex cross-tabulations
usually require mechanical or computer assistance.

Although beginning infection control personnel
should first master the standard frequency and cross-
tabulation routines mentioned previously, more experienced personnel should begin to try more creative
ways of organizing the infection data. The basic purpose of tabulating the infections is to gain a new

understanding of when, where, and in whom the
infections are occurring. One of the most frequent
mistakes made at this stage is to do the initial tabulations hastily and proceed with calculating rates
without pausing to examine and contemplate the data.
It is often very useful simply to read over the original
listings and initial simple tabulations to let the mind
synthesize the data and suggest additional tabulations, graphs, and listings. For example, finding an
increased rate of bacteremias on the surgery wards
might call for a tabulation of bacteremias for each
surgical subspecialty, or for each surgical ward and
the surgical intensive care unit, and comparisons with
similar rates from previous months or for the same
months the previous year. This process of free-wheel-
ing exploration of the data has no rigid rules; that is
right which works!

CALCULATING RATES  *Definition of rate.*  After the
initial tabulations of the infections are complete, the
infection control staff should have strong suspicions
of where infection problems might be occurring. Since
these hunches are based only on examination of infections (numerator data), additional analysis involving the calculation of *rates* is necessary to develop
stronger evidence. A practical way of doing this is
to write in the "denominator data," obtained in the
data collection stage, below the appropriate numerator figures in the frequency and cross-tables of infections tabulated earlier. From these numerators (indicating the numbers of infections) and their
denominators (indicating the numbers of patients at
risk for the infections), infection rates can be calculated.

A *rate* is an expression of the probability of occurrence of some particular event, and it has the form
$k(x/y)$, where $x$, the numerator, equals the number
of times an event has occurred during a specific time
interval; $y$, the denominator, equals a population from
which those experiencing the event were derived during the same time interval; and $k$ equals a round
number (100, 1000, 10,000, 100,000, and so on),
called a base. The *base* used depends on the magnitude
of $x/y$ and is selected to permit the rate to be expressed
as a convenient whole number. For example, if 5
infections were found among 100 patients in a given
month, the value of $x/y$ would be 0.05 infections per
patient per month; to express the rate as a convenient
whole number, $x/y$ would be multiplied by the base
number 100, giving 5 infections per 100 patients
per month. If 50 infections were found among 10,000
patients in a month, the base number 1000 would
be used to express the rate as 5 infections per 1000
patients per month. It is important to emphasize that

in determining a rate, both the time interval and the population must be specified, and these must apply to both the numerator ($x$) and the denominator ($y$) of the rate expression.

*Types of rates.*    Three specific kinds of rates—prevalence, incidence, and attack rate—are fundamental tools of epidemiology and must be familiar to infection control personnel. *Prevalence* is the number of cases of the disease found to be *active* within a defined population either during a specified period of time (period prevalence) or at a specified point in time (point prevalence); these concepts are discussed in a later section of this chapter. *Incidence* is the number of *new* cases of disease that occur in a defined population during a specified period of time. The *incidence rate* is obtained by dividing the number of new cases by the number of people in the population at risk during the specified time period. In Figure 4-2, which portrays the infection status of ten hospitalized patients, the incidence of infection during either time period A or B, for example, would be three, since three new infections began among the ten patients in each time period. Assuming that period A was one month and period B was three months, the incidence *rates* would be three infections per ten patients at risk (30 percent) per month in period A, and 10 percent per month in period B (i.e., exactly equivalent to 30 percent per three months).

An *attack rate* is a special kind of incidence rate. It is usually expressed as a percentage (i.e., $k = 100$

in the rate expression), and it is used almost exclusively for describing epidemics in which particular populations are exposed for limited periods of time (e.g., common-source outbreaks). Since the duration of the epidemic is reasonably short, the period of time to which the rate refers is not stated explicitly, but assumed. This is what distinguishes an attack rate from an incidence rate, in which the period of time is always stated. For example, if 100 infants in a newborn nursery were exposed to a contaminated lot of infant formula over a three-week period, and if 14 of the infants developed a characteristic illness thought to be caused by the contaminated formula, then the attack rate for those infants exposed to the formula would be 14 percent. Notice that the incidence rate would be 14 cases per 100 infants per three weeks, preferably expressed as 4.67 cases per 100 infants per week.

*Choice of numerator and denominator.*    The fact that multiple infections occasionally occur in individual patients somewhat complicates the calculation of rates. Basically two types of incidence rates can be calculated: the "infection ratio" is the number of *infections*

FIG. 4-2. Infection status of ten hospitalized patients. *Incidence* of infection during time period A or B is three (three new cases were added during each time period); *period prevalence rate* of infection during time period A is 40 percent and during B, 60 percent (four cases and six cases, respectively, occur in each period of time); and *point prevalence rate* of infection at time C is 30 percent (three cases exist at that point in time).

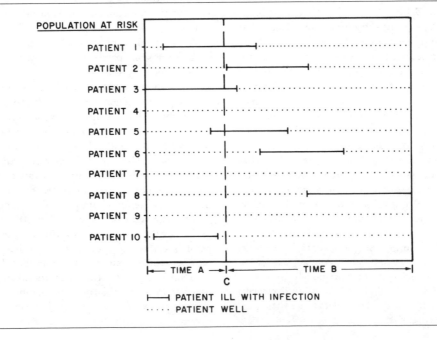

divided by the number of patients at risk during the specified period, and the "infection proportion" is the number of *patients with one or more infections* divided by the number of patients at risk during the time period. Since about 18 percent of patients with nosocomial infections have more than one infection, the infection ratio is usually about 1.27 times larger than the infection proportion [13]. In practice, most investigators have found the infection ratio to be far easier to obtain than, and equally as useful as, the infection proportion, and consequently the commonly used term "infection rate" has come to refer specifically to the infection ratio. In either case, however, when presenting the results it is important to specify which method has been used for calculating the rate.

In determining what type of denominator to use, we have found that for acute-care hospitals infection rates using the number of patients at risk (e.g., the number of admissions or discharges) as the denominator are adequate for most epidemiologic purposes. Another approach, much discussed but little used in hospital epidemiology, is to make the denominator the number of patient-days at risk during the period of surveillance (i.e., the sum of all days spent by all patients in the specified area during the time period covered). Referred to as the "incidence density," it is primarily of use when most patients have long hospitalizations, such as in nursing homes, where the number of admissions or discharges does not closely reflect the number of patients at risk. To get an idea of how the two types of rates compare, rates based on the number of patient-days ($R$) are usually smaller than those based on admissions or discharges ($r$) by a factor approximately equal to the average length of stay of the patients ($k$); that is, $R = k \cdot r$. For example, if the infection rate were found to be 5 infections per 100 admissions per month and the patients' average length of stay was ten days, one would expect to find a rate of approximately 5 infections per 1000 patient-days.

In acute-care hospitals, in which relatively few patients stay in the hospital longer than 10 days, the statistical advantage of using patient-days as the denominator is generally not sufficient to outweigh the disadvantage of its more abstract interpretation. In analyzing surveillance data in which controlling for length of stay might be important, there are more efficient statistical techniques to accomplish this, such as cross-table analysis stratified by categories of length of stay (e.g., the Mantel-Haenzel technique), standardization of rates on length of stay, and multiple linear or logistic regression analysis treating length of stay as a "covariate" [7, 20].

It is especially important that the denominator reflect the appropriate population at risk as precisely as possible. In determining the attack rate of surgical wound infection among patients on the urology service, for example, ideally only those urology patients who actually undergo a surgical procedure that results in a wound capable of being infected would be included in the denominator. Practical difficulties in obtaining such refined denominators, however, often dictate the use of a less precise denominator, such as the total number of admissions or discharges from the urology service during the appropriate period of time.

Calculated rates may be displayed in graphic form to facilitate visual assimilation of the data. Simple, creative, and neatly drawn graphics are particularly effective when presenting important findings to clinicians or administrators to convince them of the existence of a problem and the need for preventive action.

ANALYSIS *Comparing patient groups.* Analysis implies careful examination of the body of tabulated data in an attempt to determine the nature and relations of its component parts. This includes comparison of current infection rates to determine whether significant differences exist among different groups of patients. Suppose, for instance, that both the gynecology and general surgery services have had eight catheter-associated urinary tract infections during a given month; during the same month, however, there were 20 patients who had indwelling catheters discharged from the gynecology service and 100 such patients discharged from the general surgery service. Thus the respective rates for gynecology and general surgery patients were 40 percent and 8 percent. Determination of whether the difference observed between these infection rates is significant (i.e., greater than what we would expect by random or chance occurrence alone if indeed no real difference exists) requires the use of a statistical process known as *significance testing.*

Several tests of significance—such as the chi-square test, Fisher's Exact test for cross-tables, and Student's $t$ test for comparison of sample means—should be familiar to epidemiologists and ICNs (see Chapter 6). Currently available routines for programmable calculators and the many statistical software packages for microcomputers (see p. 68) make even the most sophisticated statistical testing procedures quite accessible to all infection control departments. In the preceding example, the difference between the observed infection rates (40 percent versus 8 percent) is highly significant at $p$ less than 0.001 according to the Fisher's Exact test. This means that a difference as large as or larger than that observed (40 percent versus 8 percent) would be expected to occur by chance alone less than one time in 1000. Thus it is quite likely that there is a real difference between the infection rates on the two services, and additional investigation is indicated to explain why such a difference exists.

*Comparing rates over time.*   Another type of analysis involves the comparison of current infection rates with those established in the past to determine whether significant changes have occurred over time. Tables of the rates for the present month and each of several preceding months can simply be visually inspected, or the rates can be plotted on graph paper to detect changes of potential importance. Potentially important deviations from baseline rates should be subjected to tests of statistical significance (see Chapter 6), and additional investigation undertaken if indicated (see Chapter 5).

An interesting approach to screening large amounts of surveillance data for potential epidemics was developed in the CDC's National Nosocomial Infections Study. Called "computerized epidemic threshold analysis," this technique uses the infection experience for the same month over the past several years as a baseline for predicting the rate to be expected in the present month. To allow for random statistical variation in the rates, an upper boundary, or "threshold," is set, usually at 2 or 3 standard deviations above the predicted rate. Any of the current month's rates that significantly exceed their threshold rates are flagged by the program and recorded on a printout as suspicious rate increases to be investigated further. This routine is repeated automatically for the rates in all the cells of the various rate tables of interest (e.g., tables of rates by service, ward, site, site by pathogen, and so on).

One present disadvantage of this method is the obvious need for rather sophisticated computer equipment and software to accomplish the large number of comparisons required. Another difficulty is deciding how high to set the threshold. This problem arises from the fact that the sensitivity (the proportion of true outbreaks detected) and the specificity (the proportion of random increases that are falsely called outbreaks) of the method are affected in opposite directions by the level of the threshold. If one raises the threshold, the sensitivity decreases and the specificity increases; this causes fewer true outbreaks to be detected but increases the likelihood that any increase flagged by the program represents a true outbreak. Conversely, decreasing the threshold has the opposite effect of allowing the identification of more

true outbreaks but reducing the likelihood that any flagged increase is a true outbreak. Thus to use the program wisely requires careful judgment to set the threshold at just the right level that will pick up the most true outbreaks while minimizing the amount of investigation wasted on purely random fluctuations (see Chapter 5).

*Clusters.*   Screening for clustering of specific patterns of antimicrobial susceptibility of organisms is another potentially valuable analytic tool for detecting outbreaks, especially when it is applied to particular pathogens on specific wards or in particular geographic areas.

INTERPRETATION   Interpretation of the data is considered by many as the final step in analysis; it is simply an intellectual process by which some meaning is ascribed to the tabulated and analyzed body of information. The interpretation may vary from no significant change in the current infection rates to the detection of a possible outbreak in the hospital. Often, however, more information—particularly that obtained through additional investigation directed specifically at problem areas identified by means of the analysis of the surveillance data—will be necessary for final interpretation of the data. Additional uses of other information collected through surveillance, such as the time of onset of infection, are described in Chapters 3 and 5.

REPORTING THE DATA   It is essential that the tabulated data—or at least the analyses and interpretations of the data—get to those people in the hospital who need to know them to take appropriate actions. A monthly report containing the tabulated data and analytic results and their interpretations should routinely be submitted to the Infection Control Committee and maintained on record in the hospital. Of course, weekly or even daily reports may be necessary during epidemics or unusual situations. It is not necessary—in fact, it is often very inefficient—to include a line listing of infections in this report. Also the analysis of a single month of infection data may yield some tables that contain insufficient data to justify inclusion in the report. These tables should be retained and a summary table released whenever sufficient monthly data have accumulated.

Summary reports or graphic representations of the data should also be widely distributed to the professional staff of the hospital. Summary data may be placed on bulletin boards and sent to local or state health departments, other local hospitals, or elsewhere as judged necessary or desirable by the Infection Control Committee to achieve specific objectives.

In the reporting phase, as well as throughout the surveillance process, measures should be taken to ensure the privacy of the information collected on patients and hospital staff members. For example, the infection control nurse should keep all surveillance forms that list patients by name under very tight security, such as a locked filing cabinet or other secure storage method. Reports should not mention patients or staff members by name unless there is a good reason, and if it is necessary, the distribution of the reports should be limited. The Infection Control Committee should establish a policy on privacy of information, prescribing the procedures for handling records or reports that identify patients or staff members (e.g., surgeon-specific wound infection rates or laboratory data implicating an employee as a human disseminator of an epidemic organism).

*Prevalence*

DEFINITION   *Prevalence* measures the number of all current cases of active disease (new and old) within a specified population at risk during a specified period of time, and the *prevalence rate* is the prevalence divided by the number of patients at risk during the period. When the period of time used for the calculation is relatively long, usually a month or longer, the measurement is called *period prevalence.* In Figure 4-2, the period prevalence rate of infection during time period A would be 4/10, or 40 percent, and during time period B, 6/10, or 60 percent. When the period of time used for the calculation is relatively short, such as one day or less, the measurement is called *point prevalence* (i.e., the frequency of all currently active cases of disease, old and new, at a given instant in time). For example, the point prevalence rate of infection at point C in Figure 4-2 would be 3/10, or 30 percent. It should be apparent that the difference between point and period prevalence is arbitrary; an interval that is considered a "point" on one time scale may become a "period" on a different time scale.

THE PREVALENCE SURVEY   The *prevalence survey,* as it is applied to nosocomial infections, consists of a systematic study of a defined population for evidence of infection at a given point in time; such a survey derives the point prevalence rate for the population. Typically after a short period of training to standardize definitions and methods, a team of surveyors visits every patient in the hospital on a single day and detects all active infections from studying the medical record and examining the patient or discussing the case with the clinical staff when necessary. When there are more beds than the survey team can

visit in one day, the prevalence survey is conducted over several days with care to ensure that each bed is visited only once.

If the object is to obtain the prevalence rate of *infections* (the usual procedure), then those infections that have resolved before the day of the visit are not counted, and the point prevalence rate is calculated simply by dividing the number of infections active on the day of the visit by the number of beds visited and multiplying by an appropriate base number (usually 100). If, on the other hand, the object is to obtain the point prevalence rate of *infected patients,* then all patients with currently active or resolved infections contracted during the current hospitalization are counted, and the point prevalence rate is calculated simply by dividing the number of infected patients by the number of beds visited and multiplying by the appropriate base number. To be consistent with the usual way of defining the incidence rate (i.e., the infection ratio), prevalence surveys should be designed to measure the point prevalence rate of infections.

The relative magnitudes of these various measures are complicated but can be deduced from the fundamental relation between prevalence and incidence:

$$\text{Prevalence} \propto \text{incidence} \times \text{duration.}$$

From this general relation it is apparent that prevalence rates (both point and period prevalence) are always higher than the comparable incidence rates, and the longer the duration of the infections the greater the difference will become. As explained in the earlier discussion of the two types of incidence rates, the infection ratio is always higher than the infection proportion measured on the same population as long as some patients develop more than one infection. In contrast, the prevalence rate of infections is always lower than the prevalence rate of infected patients, because the "duration" of an infected patient's stay in the hospital is almost always longer than the "duration" of the active infection. Interestingly, point prevalence and period prevalence rates measured on the same population are usually approximately the same, although due to the larger number of patients studied in a period prevalence survey, estimates of period prevalence are usually more precise than those of point prevalence.

In general the most useful measure to derive from surveillance is the incidence rate because it provides an estimate of the risk of infection, uncluttered by differences in the durations of various infections. The main reason that prevalence rates were used in the past was simply that a point prevalence survey requires much less effort and can be completed much more rapidly than developing incidence rates, which require ongoing, daily surveillance. There are two main disadvantages of point prevalence surveys: first, due to the complex influence of the duration of infections, the prevalence rate overestimates patients' risks of acquiring infection; and second, except in the largest hospitals, the number of patients included in a point prevalence survey (i.e., the number of beds) is usually too small to obtain precise enough estimates of rates to detect important differences (e.g., a difference between the bacteremia rates on medicine and surgery) with statistical significance. Because of these limitations, prevalence surveys are generally useful primarily when a "quick and dirty" estimate is needed and there is insufficient time or resources to obtain a more useful measure of the incidence.

USES OF PREVALENCE SURVEYS *Secular trends.* Repeated prevalence surveys in the same institution have been used to document secular trends in the epidemiology of nosocomial infections. Prevalence studies in large hospitals have demonstrated such changes as shifts in the predominant pathogens associated with nosocomial infections and in the patterns of antimicrobial use for hospitalized patients [17]. However, limitations in the numbers of patients studied and variations in types of prevalence rates determined in the various surveys have complicated the interpretation of these results. In general, incidence rates derived from ongoing surveillance, although more time-consuming, are much better suited for detecting and examining secular trends.

*Estimating surveillance accuracy.* Prevalence surveys have been used to determine the completeness of ascertainment of a hospital's ongoing surveillance system. Typically a survey team, using the same standard definitions used for routine surveillance by the ICN, visits all patients in the hospital to detect all active infections. By comparing the infections identified by the survey team during the prevalence survey with those detected by the routine surveillance system, and under the assumption that the survey team correctly detected all active infections, an estimate is derived of the percentage of true infections detected by the routine surveillance system. Although this percentage approximates the sensitivity of routine surveillance (i.e., the probability that the routine surveillance system will detect a true infection), the statistic has been referred to as an "efficiency factor," since the difficulty of determining reliably whether infections are active at the time of the prevalence survey introduces some error into the assessment [2]. Since the efficiency factor approximates the sensitivity, it can be used to correct the monthly routine

estimates of the incidence rates for the degree of underascertainment. Past experience indicates that approximately 60 percent efficiency is usual and that 80 percent or greater is often possible.

One of the weaknesses of this application in past studies has been the failure to estimate the specificity of routine surveillance in addition to its sensitivity (efficiency). Specificity is the probability of correctly classifying a patient as uninfected when he or she in fact develops no infection, and it reflects how often the ICN records an infection when one was not really present. Unfortunately, the specificity of ICNs in estimating incidence rates in routine surveillance has not been thoroughly studied [15, 24]. The process of correcting incidence rates with the efficiency factor assumes that specificity is a perfect 1.0. Corrections for lower levels of specificity would give lower estimates of the incidence rates.

*Estimating incidence from prevalence.* Modified prevalence surveys can be used to derive a crude approximation of the incidence rates that would have been obtained from continuous surveillance [23]. Surveys are performed at regular intervals (e.g., weekly) that must be considerably less than the average duration of stay of infected patients. Only infections that began since the preceding survey are tabulated. The denominator of the rates should probably include the number of admissions during the interval plus the census at the start of the period. Obviously the shorter the interval between prevalence surveys, the more closely the final estimate approximates the true incidence rate. Some loss in completeness, accuracy, and timeliness in detecting infections—as compared to the results of surveillance studies—must be weighed against the potential benefit from a smaller time commitment to case-finding.

Alternatively, various formulas have been derived to allow the estimation of incidence rates from data collected in a single prevalence survey [8, 19]. These techniques were of particular interest in the early 1970s when prevalence surveys were being used more commonly. Since incidence rates are currently being obtained by ongoing surveillance in most U.S. hospitals, however, these statistical conversion techniques have not been widely applied.

*Other uses.* Perhaps the best uses of prevalence studies are to make valuable estimates of antimicrobial usage patterns, evaluate the adherence to proper isolation practices, monitor practices related to high-risk procedures such as intravenous and urinary catheterization, and so on [17, 21]. Prevalence surveys have also been useful for increasing the awareness of nosocomial infection problems in hospitals without surveillance programs. Indeed, the results of such surveys have often been important in a hospital staff's decision to institute a more extensive ongoing surveillance system.

### Targeted Surveillance

A recent trend in the development of the concept of surveillance has been to find creative ways of targeting surveillance more directly toward potential infection problems. The purpose of these efforts is to obtain the greatest preventive impact from the effort invested in surveillance. As such, these ideas indicate a greater awareness of the need to direct surveillance efforts toward specific preventive objectives. Although these new approaches were generally motivated by the need to reduce the amount of personnel time devoted to surveillance in hospitals with inadequately staffed programs, the ideas, if proved as effective as routine continuous hospitalwide surveillance, might greatly increase the efficiency of surveillance in all hospitals.

UNIT-DIRECTED SURVEILLANCE   In some large hospitals faced with insufficient numbers of ICNs to maintain comprehensive surveillance over all of the beds, one approach has been to direct the available personnel time to the surveillance of infections in areas with the highest infection risks, such as intensive care units or oncology units [24]. These units tend to contain the patients that are most susceptible to infection, that is, the patients most likely to have suppressed immunologic systems, to be undergoing invasive diagnostic and therapeutic procedures, and to be receiving intensive nursing and medical care with the attendant risk of person-to-person spread of infection. Focusing scarce resources on a few relatively small units has the advantages of greatly simplifying the surveillance effort and of preventing infections in the patients with the highest risks and greatest likelihood of suffering severe and life-threatening infections. Despite the inordinately high infection risks in these units, a relatively small percentage of patients are treated in them, and therefore only a minority of all nosocomial infections occur there. Thus limiting surveillance to such small units sacrifices potential prevention of the majority of infections occurring among general patients.

ROTATING SURVEILLANCE   Another approach is to rotate the surveillance efforts around the hospital in an effort to identify and eliminate infection risks in discrete departments or areas in a sequential manner. Typically in a large hospital with an insufficient number of ICNs, the infection control staff divide the hospital into convenient geographic areas to be sur-

veyed for a month each in sequential fashion. Throughout the month the ICN performs careful, continuous surveillance of all nosocomial infections occurring among the patients or personnel of the area and of all patient-care practices related to infection risks. At the end of the month the surveillance data are tabulated, analyzed, and discussed by the Infection Control Committee. From the discussion a final report is written to present the findings, point out the problems, and make recommendations for corrective actions. The report is then given to the appropriate medical, nursing, and other department heads of the area surveyed. After an appropriate time for study, the infection control staff meet with the department heads to achieve a concensus on the corrective actions to take. These actions are then written officially into procedure manuals, presented to and discussed with the patient-care personnel involved, and carried out under the supervision of the regular medical and nursing management staff. Usually within a year or so this area is resurveyed in a similar fashion according to a rotating schedule, and the degree of adherence to and effectiveness of the recommendations are assessed while simultaneously searching for new problems to correct.

This approach avoids the main disadvantage of the unit-directed approach by sequentially covering all areas, but it sacrifices the ability to detect problems that emerge in the large areas not under surveillance at a given time. Its main attraction lies in the fact that at least once a year every area of the hospital is subjected to a detailed infection control evaluation directed specifically at the objective of eliminating or reducing identified infection risks. When coupled with a commitment to investigating outbreaks or other problems that come to attention in areas not under scrutiny at the time and other regular control measures, this method appears to offer some advantages over the unit-directed approach when resources are limited.

PRIORITY-DIRECTED SURVEILLANCE   A third alternative attempts to assign the levels of surveillance effort to various infection problems on the basis of priority levels to which they are assigned [10]. Instead of basing effort on geographic areas, as the previous two alternatives do, the priority-directed approach focuses on the types of infections to be prevented and assigns levels of effort commensurate with the relative seriousness of the problems.

The first prerequisite of this approach is to establish the relative seriousness of the different types of infections to form the basis of the priority rankings. Several possible parameters for setting these priorities are compared in Table 4-1, based on additional analysis of data collected in three hospitals in the SENIC pilot studies [14]. In the past the main parameter used for assessing this has been simply the relative frequency of the different types of infections, since these figures have been familiar for many years. If this measure were used, urinary tract infections would be given the highest priority, followed by surgical wound infections and pneumonia, with primary bacteremia receiving a lower priority just ahead of a large number of relatively rare infections such as hepatitis and tuberculosis.

An alternative parameter that appears to be a better measure of the relative seriousness of the various types of infections is the total of extra hospital costs attributable to each of the infections. This measure reflects both the relative frequency of the infections and the relative degree of morbidity expressed by the costs of the extra days and extra ancillary services necessary to treat the infections. By this criterion surgical wound infections would constitute the most serious problem, followed by pneumonia, with urinary tract infection and bacteremia in remote third and fourth places (Table 4-1). Basing time commitments on these priorities, one would concentrate about one-half of available surveillance time on surgical wound infections, one-third on pneumonia, relatively small amounts of carefully planned time on urinary tract infections and bacteremia, and only occasional effort on the less common infections. These relative levels of effort might be used to the best advantage by the following plan that uses the surveillance methods likely to produce the greatest amounts of prevention within the times available.

*Surgical wound infections.* With half of the time available for surgical wound infections, all patients undergoing operations would be enrolled in a surveillance registry at the time of the operation, and information on several key risk factors (e.g., wound classification, type and duration of operation, and number of underlying diagnoses) would be recorded at that time. All these patients would be visited regularly during hospitalization by the ICN to detect all surgical wound infections. If the time constraint permitted, the ICN would also follow up all or a subset of the patients for infections occurring after discharge.

Each month the tabulation process would involve three steps, ideally accomplished with the aid of a computer (see p. 68). First, each patient would be assigned to an intrinsic infection risk category, using either the familiar surgical wound classes [1] or a multivariate risk factor scale [12]. Second, the surgical wound infection rate would be calculated for each surgeon's patients within *each* category of the infection risk classification—not just for patients with clean wounds or in low-risk categories. Third, two reports would be compiled, one displaying each surgeon's category-specific monthly rates over time (e.g., over a year or two), and a second comparing the category-specific rates of each surgeon with those of his or her colleagues and for the service overall. And finally, the reports would be discussed at the infection control meeting and given to the chief of the surgical service to distribute among and discuss with the practicing surgeons. With this plan, the one-half of surveillance time devoted to surgical wound infections would be directed toward the surveillance effort shown to be the most effective in reducing the problem [5, 11].

*Pneumonia.* With only about one-third of the available time assigned to the surveillance of pneumonia, a plan more narrowly targeted toward specific prevention objectives must be used. The first consideration is to separate the generically different problems of pneumonia among surgical and medical patients. The vast majority of preventable cases of pneumonia among surgical patients are postoperative

TABLE 4-1. Comparison of the relative frequency of the major types of nosocomial infections and alternative measures of their relative importance

| | Percent of all nosocomial infections | Total extra days[a] | (%) | Total extra charges[a] | (%) | Percent preventable[b] |
|---|---|---|---|---|---|---|
| Surgical wound infection | 24 | 889 | 57 | 102,286 | 42 | 35 |
| Pneumonia | 10 | 370 | 24 | 95,229 | 39 | 22 |
| Urinary tract infection | 42 | 175 | 11 | 32,081 | 13 | 33 |
| Bacteremia | 5 | 59 | 4 | 7,478 | 3 | 35 |
| Other | 19 | 69 | 4 | 8,680 | 3 | 32 |
| All sites | 100 | 1,562 | 100 | 245,754 | 100 | 32 |

[a]From SENIC pilot studies [13]; charges are in 1975 dollars.
[b]From SENIC analysis of efficacy [11].

pulmonary infections representing progression of the usual atelectasis syndrome most commonly following operations of the upper abdomen. In contrast, most preventable pneumonias among adult medical patients are hypostatic infections related to the failure to turn patients with diminished levels of consciousness frequently enough. On pediatric and newborn services, the most serious preventable pneumonias follow person-to-person spread of nosocomial infections with viruses such as respiratory syncytial virus (RSV) (see Chapter 35).

Since all surgical patients are routinely followed closely for wound infections, postoperative pneumonias can be detected with little additional effort. Analysis of these rates within appropriate risk categories can be performed for each nursing unit or for the patients of each surgeon. Reports of these analyses should then be discussed just as the wound infection rates are (see preceding section).

For medical patients, a unit-directed approach should be used. The ICN should identify nursing units or intensive care units in which patients with strokes, drug overdoses, and high risk of hypostatic pneumonia are congregated. In these areas patients at high risk may be followed regularly to detect all cases of pneumonia, and the pneumonia rates among these patients should be regularly reported to the head nurse and charge nurses of the specified nursing units; concurrently there should be continuing inservice education regarding the importance of frequently turning patients to prevent pneumonia.

The ICN should regularly visit units caring for infants or children at high risk of serious pneumonia from RSV and similar agents to monitor informally the frequency of upper respiratory infections among patients and employees. When the frequency of these infections appears to have risen, virologic studies should be done immediately to detect the presence of virulent viruses. When they are found, the staff members should be warned of the imminent danger and instructed in meticulous contact precautions for infected patients and employees [9].

*Bacteremia.* With little time assigned for the surveillance of bacteremias, the object of the limited effort must be to detect clusters of nosocomial bacteremia that may be related to correctable errors in patient management, such as habitual contamination of venous or arterial catheters, failure to change the site of intravenous catheters frequently enough, or improper sterilization of arterial pressure monitoring devices. Since collecting sufficient data to calculate routinely the specific bacteremia infection rates for all the possible risk factors would be far too time-consuming, the ICN should conduct only "numer-

ator surveillance." This involves investigating briefly all cases of bacteremia reported by the microbiology laboratory each day. The object of this brief daily activity is to recognize common factors that might tie the cases together, such as a single unusual organism, spatial clustering, or a relation with some diagnostic or therapeutic device. Only when a suspicious cluster or relation is found would a more detailed investigation involving the calculation of rates be undertaken. Since these problems are likely to occur infrequently, little time will be spent on this problem, but the time spent will be directed to maximize the chance of detecting a problem.

*Urinary tract infections.* The modest surveillance efforts allowable here should be directed toward identifying areas in which patient-care personnel are not managing urinary catheters or other urinary instrumentations properly. The most efficient way of achieving this goal is to perform part-time rotating surveillance on different wards or nursing units to measure catheter-associated urinary tract infection rates (stratified or adjusted by categories of the duration of catheterization) and to assess the indications for inserting and discontinuing catheters and the techniques of aseptically caring for them. By periodically reporting comparisons of urinary tract infection rates of different units, practices can be improved in the units found to have problems. Alternatively, the infection control staff can relax other surveillance activities for one month each year to devote full time to hospitalwide surveillance of urinary tract infections and catheter-care practices. This amount of effort would be commensurate with the magnitude of the problem and would reinforce preventive efforts at least on a yearly basis.

*Other infections.* Virtually no time should be spent routinely performing formal surveillance of other infections. Instead the ICN should depend on other hospital departments to recognize the rare outbreaks of unusual infections. For example, the employee health service should maintain surveillance to recognize problems of tuberculosis transmission to employees; the director of the newborn nursery should be counted on to recognize and notify the ICN of clusters of staphylococcal pyoderma; and someone in the microbiology laboratory should be alert to clusters of unusual pathogens. Again the level of effort is commensurate with the magnitude of the problems, but the efforts are likely to detect problems if they occur.

### The Role of Computers in Surveillance

Few technologies have offered as much promise to infection control, yet produced as little tangible benefit, as the digital computer. This is ironic since much of the drudgery and time expenditure of surveillance is consumed in keeping lists of patients, counting and recording denominators, and repeating standard infection rate tabulations month after month—jobs that would seem maximally suited for computerization. In most hospitals, however, the past experience was that if you put your data into a computer you could never get it back out.

The reasons for this disappointment are actually rather simple. Computers were designed fundamentally for business and accounting purposes rather than for scientific uses, and until recently the only computers available to the infection control staff were large mainframe machines owned by and operated solely for the hospital's business office. Given that infection control personnel generally have been inexperienced in the use of computers, it is not surprising that they have been unable to redirect a machine poorly designed for their needs in the first place.

MAINFRAME COMPUTERS   Recently, however, two developments have greatly changed the prospects for computer use in surveillance. First, hospitals have increasingly adopted integrated data base management systems for efficiently organizing most information on all hospitalized patients on their mainframe computers. Although administrative efficiency, not infection control, was the objective for these systems, they offer a dramatic opportunity to the infection control staff, particularly in large hospitals, for greatly reducing the work of surveillance. With the demographic, business, pharmacy, laboratory, and other records of all patients residing in one, or a system of, computerized files, only two things are needed to generate surveillance reports directly from the mainframe: first, a mechanism for entering information on nosocomial infections obtained through surveillance into a file in the data base management system; and second, a software package for merging infection information into the patient data base by patient identification numbers, making the required tabulations and rate calculations, and constructing the various tables and figures for printed reports.

Although several such systems are commercially available for hospitals' mainframe computers, the initial investment is usually high, and operating costs may be prohibitive if the infection control program is charged for computer time and programming. To find out whether such a system is available for the computer at a particular hospital, the marketing representative of the company that manufactured the hospital's business computer should be consulted with the assistance of the hospital's data processing manager.

MICROCOMPUTERS   The second development is the more recent introduction of the personal microcomputer at prices that have suddenly put potentially powerful computers literally on the desks of the infection control staff. Initially, the usefulness of microcomputers was severely limited by the unavailability of software designed to accomplish the unique tasks required in infection control, but recently, commercial software products have made the microcomputer a potentially very useful tool for infection surveillance and control activity. In view of the large reductions in length of hospital stay and operating expenses that have been shown to be possible by the SENIC Project [11], hospital administrators are likely to be increasingly willing to invest in microcomputers and software for infection control.

*Functions of microcomputer software.*   The best software packages for infection control serve three important functions: learning aid, planning guide, and "workhorse" for performing surveillance. To serve as a learning aid, a good software package must be designed by infection control experts who structure the computer functions and the user's manual to teach the surveillance approaches that have been proven effective. In this way, software products become a powerful vehicle for increasing the sophistication of infection control staff members in all types of hospitals.

To serve as a planning guide, the software package must have the versatility to create special surveillance files and user-defined codes that allow the infection control staff to design new surveillance systems aimed at achieving specific prevention objectives. The user's manual should include sections that guide the infection control staff through the process of planning a new surveillance system and possess the versatility to support most foreseeable surveillance functions. The infection control staff should be particularly skeptical of packages that are oriented mainly toward microbiologic information or have objectives that are too broad (e.g., infection control plus risk management, quality assurance and employee health) unless their usefulness and efficiency for infection control per se are demonstrated.

To serve as a "workhorse" for surveillance the software system must be designed to handle the required data quickly while minimizing the time required to enter data, edit the files, and produce reports. To run efficiently, it should be programmed in an efficient language (e.g., assembly language or the C language), and the choice of data items to be collected and processed should be limited to those essential for preventing infections, with only a few non-specific fields that can be defined by the user for special purposes. For data entry efficiency, it should have a menu-driven format with appropriate help screens, and the data entry fields should fit on as few screens as possible to reduce time-consuming page turning. All fields, except perhaps a "comments" field, should have structured codes with internal edit checks to prevent entry of invalid responses. Since open-ended (non-coded) responses cannot be analyzed easily, such data is rarely used and only reduces efficiency of storage and processing. Codes should be user-designed wherever possible. The package should allow the creation of separate files for special surveillance projects such as surgical wound, intensive care unit, or procedure surveillance, and ideally infections entered into any special file should be automatically added to an infection master file to facilitate overall hospital analysis if needed. Efficient file structures should be provided for entering, storing, and retrieving large "denominator files" (e.g., a record for each surgical operation) and later adding infection information to those cases in which infections occurred (e.g., wound infection data). It should be possible to enter only "numerator data" (e.g., infections) and supply numerical denominators in the analysis stage. An effective report generator should be able to select records based on a string of search criteria, sort the resulting file, and print line-listings of cases, two- and three-way cross-tabulations and selected rates for virtually all variables in the data base. It should also have the ability to display graphics, including "epidemic curves," line graphs, and bar charts, on the computer screen as well as in printed form, and the ability to output data files to other computers or statistical packages.

Developing the type of compact and highly efficient software systems needed for routine use in community hospitals is made difficult by the need to limit the amount of information collected in order to maximize efficiency of computer usage and staff time. To limit the amount of information appropriately, a software designer must make difficult judgmental decisions about what is the minimum of information essential for effective infection control. The designer must be ruthless about excluding extra data fields that might have research or other appeal but have only marginal or no actual infection control impact. Since this requires astute epidemiologic insight into the priorities and functioning of infection control programs rather than statistical or computer programming judgment, slower progress and fewer good products can be anticipated in this class of soft-

ware packages. As a result, great care must be taken in choosing an infection surveillance software package.

SELECTING THE BEST SOFTWARE PACKAGE    As discussed in the earlier sections on Surveillance by Objectives and Priority-Directed Surveillance, the most important decisions that must be made before selecting a software system are the objectives to be achieved by the surveillance activity. In view of the substantial differences among the packages currently available for testing, it is apparent that a system selected before objectives are written and agreed upon may not meet the owner's needs when put into use. For example, if the objectives of surveillance include research, the best software package might be one of the general-purpose data base management packages that allow complete flexibility but require far greater computer skills and more time. On the other hand, if the objectives are limited to controlling and preventing infections, one of the software packages designed specifically for infection control would probably be the best choice. Furthermore, a significant change in the infection control program's objectives may require the acquisition of a new software package.

A particularly important consideration is the size of the surveillance task. This is determined by the number of patients on whom surveillance data is to be stored, which is in turn a function of the size of the hospital, the number of patients included, and the size of any special surveillance projects undertaken. Before purchasing a software package, the infection control staff should estimate the number of records to be collected per year and should study the capacities of both the hardware and the software packages available. Hospitals with small surveillance tasks can generally get along reasonably well with a dual-drive microcomputer system and any of the available software packages that do not require more extensive hardware (e.g., a "hard" disc or large amounts of internal memory). Hospitals with large surveillance tasks (e.g., large or university-affiliated hospitals) may need more expensive hardware including "hard" discs (e.g., ten megabytes or larger), larger internal memory size (e.g., possibly in the megabyte range), and perhaps more rapid microprocessors.

STARTING A COMPUTERIZED SURVEILLANCE SYSTEM    Perhaps the greatest impediment to the effective use of microcomputers in infection control is the lack of computer literacy among adults. Microcomputers and powerful software systems have often been purchased and placed in the infection control office only to sit idle because of growing disillusionment with computers. This is frequently due to the inability of the staff to master the basic workings of the computer rather than deficiencies in the hardware or software. To avoid this common pitfall, the infection control staff should either take a computer literacy course at a local school or computer store or find a friend or colleague who could act as a personal advisor in beginning computer skills. After mastering the basics, one should allow at least a month to read the infection control software manual thoroughly, become familiar with its functions, and design the surveillance system, including the types of surveillance studies to be performed, the user-defined variables and codes, and the types of reports that will be needed. All of this planning should be based on the objectives to be accomplished and should be approved by the infection control committee before the system is put into operation. The microcomputer, if introduced in this carefully planned manner, can indeed become the fundamental tool for infection surveillance in the hospital.

# REFERENCES

1. Altemeir, W. A., Burke, J. F., Pruitt, B. A., et al. (Eds.). *Manual on the Control of Infection in Surgical Patients.* Philadelphia: Lippincott, 1976, pp. 29–30.
2. Bennett, J. V., Scheckler, W. E., Maki, D. G., and Brachman, P. S. Current National Patterns: United States. In Brachman, P. S., and Eickhoff, T. C. (Eds.), *Proceedings of the International Conference on Nosocomial Infections.* Chicago: American Hospital Association, 1971.
3. Center for Disease Control. *Outline for Surveillance and Control of Nosocomial Infections.* Atlanta: CDC, 1972.
4. Centers for Disease Control. *Guidelines for the Prevention and Control of Nosocomial Infections.* Springfield, Va.: National Technical Information Service. U.S. Department of Commerce, 1982.
5. Cruse, P. J. E., and Foord, R. The epidemiology of wound infection: A 10-year prospective study of 62,939 wounds. *Surg. Clin. North Am.* 60:27, 1980.
6. Emori, T. G., Haley, R. W., and Garner, J. S. Techniques and uses of nosocomial infection surveillance in U.S. hospitals, 1976–77. *Am. J. Med.* 70:933, 1981.
7. Fleiss, J. L. *Statistical Methods for Rates and Proportions.* New York: Wiley, 1973.
8. Freeman, J., and McGowan, J. E., Jr. Day-specific incidence of nosocomial infection estimated from a prevalence survey. *Am. J. Epidemiol.* 114:888, 1981.
9. Garner, J. S., and Simmons, B. P. (Eds.). CDC guideline for isolation precautions in hospitals. *Infect. Control* 4:245, 1983.
10. Haley, R. W. Surveillance by objectives: A priority-directed approach to the surveillance of nosocomial infection. *Am. J. Infect. Control.* 13:78, 1985.
11. Haley, R. W., Culver, D. H., White, J. W., Morgan, W. M., and Emori, T. G. The efficacy of infection surveillance and control programs in preventing nosocomial infections in U.S. hospitals. *Am. J. Epidemiol.* 121:182, 1984.
12. Haley, R. W., Culver, D. H., White, J. W., Morgan, W. M., and Emori, T. G. Identifying patients at high risk of surgical wound infection: A simple multivariate index of patient susceptibility and wound contamination. *Am. J. Epidemiol.* 121:206, 1984.
13. Haley, R. W., Hooton, T. M., Culver, D. H., et al. Nosocomial infections in U.S. hospitals, 1975–76: Estimated nationwide frequency by selected characteristics of patients. *Am. J. Med.* 70:947, 1981.
14. Haley, R. W., Schaberg, D. R., Crossley, K. B., Von Allmen, S. D., and McGowan, J. E., Jr. Extra days and prolongation of stay attributable to nosocomial infections: A prospective interhospital comparison. *Am. J. Med.* 70:51, 1981.
15. Haley, R. W., Schaberg, D. R., McClish, D. K., et al. The accuracy of retrospective chart review in measuring nosocomial infection rates: Results of validation studies in pilot hospitals. *Am. J. Epidemiol.* 111:534, 1980.
16. Joint Commission on Accreditation of Hospitals. Infection Control. In *Accreditation Manual for Hospitals.* Chicago: Joint Commission on Accreditation of Hospitals, 1976.
17. McGowan, J. E., and Finland, M. Infection and usage of antibiotics at Boston City Hospital: Changes in prevalence during the decade 1964–1973. *J. Infect. Dis.* 129:421, 1974.
18. Raven, B. H., and Haley, R. W. Social influence and compliance of hospital nurses with infection control policies. In Eiser, J. R. (Ed.), *Social Psychology and Behavioral Medicine.* New York: Wiley, 1982.

19. Rhame, F. S., and Sudderth, W. D. Incidence and prevalence as used in the analysis of the occurrence of nosocomial infections. *Am. J. Epidemiol.* 113:1, 1981.

20. Rothman, K. J., and Boice, J. D., Jr. *Epidemiologic Analysis with a Programmable Calculator.* Boston: Epidemiology Resources, 1982.

21. Scheckler, W. E., Garner, J. S., Kaiser, A. B., and Bennett, J. V. Prevalence of infections and antibiotic usage in eight community hospitals. In Brachman, P. S., and Eickhoff, T. C. (Eds.), *Proceedings of the International Conference on Nosocomial Infections.* Chicago: American Hospital Association, 1971.

22. Semmelweis, I. P. The etiology, the concept and the prophylaxis of childbed fever. Leipzig: C. A. Hartleben, 1861 (reprinted in translation by F. P. Murphy, *Med. Classics* 5:334).

23. Wenzel, R. P., Osterman, C. A., Hunting, K. J., and Gwaltney, J. M., Jr. Hospital-acquired infections. I. Surveillance in a university hospital. *Am. J. Epidemiol.* 103:251, 1976.

24. Wenzel, R. P., Thompson, R. L., Landry, S. M., et al. Hospital-acquired infections in intensive care unit patients: An overview with emphasis on epidemics. *Infect. Control* 4:371, 1983.

# 5 INVESTIGATION OF ENDEMIC AND EPIDEMIC NOSOCOMIAL INFECTIONS

Richard E. Dixon

Although effective infection control programs reduce the incidence of nosocomial infections, these infections continue to be a problem even in hospitals with very effective programs. Some nosocomial infections are unavoidable using techniques now available, but many can be prevented, and a hospital's infection control program should be designed to identify preventable infections, determine why they occur, and reduce the probability of their occurrence.

This chapter provides guidelines that hospital infection control personnel can use to determine when epidemiologic investigations should be initiated and introduces techniques that can be used in those investigations.

## CRITERIA FOR INITIATING INVESTIGATIONS

An epidemiologic investigation may be useful whenever a hospital has a potential nosocomial infection problem, such as when the incidence of infections is excessively high. Because no hospital can—or should—investigate every nosocomial infection that occurs, infection control programs should focus efforts on preventable infections, rather than waste time and money evaluating issues that cannot be affected by changes in hospital practices. Frequently, however, neither clinical nor epidemiologic findings indicate whether specific infections are preventable; therefore, the hospital epidemiologist must establish additional criteria to identify the kinds of infections to investigate.

In many instances, definitive criteria do not exist to identify problems that require evaluation, and hospitals are so variable that it is unlikely that absolute criteria can be established. As a result, the decision to investigate a potential problem depends ultimately on the judgment of the hospital epidemiologist, who must decide whether a problem exists but may not have definitive criteria on which to make that decision. The epidemiologist must recognize that it is usually possible to find some reasonable explanation to discount the possibility of a problem. Reasons commonly advanced to argue that a *potential* problem is not a *real* problem and therefore does not need evaluation include the following: the hospital has recently been treating more susceptible patients than in the past, surveillance has been especially vigorous, or infecting strains do not all share the same characteristics. Infection control programs should guard against accepting these explanations too readily. The

73

epidemiologist should generally assume that a potential problem is both real and important until evidence is collected to indicate otherwise, since the goal of the infection control program is to prevent infections, not explain them away.

The following information may be useful to epidemiologists when setting priorities for investigations.

### Epidemic Infections

Infections that occur as part of an epidemic are traditionally considered to be among the most preventable of all infections, and any cluster of infections that appears to be epidemic should be evaluated. On occasion, however, it may be difficult to decide, before an assessment has been conducted, whether a cluster of infections actually represents an epidemic. By definition, a classic epidemic is marked by an unusual, statistically significant increase in the incidence of a particular disease; it usually occurs during a brief interval, involves a specific patient population with defined susceptibility factors, and is caused by a single microbial strain.

This classic definition is useful for identifying some problems, but it fails to characterize all nosocomial and community-acquired infection epidemics. For example, the epidemiologist may not know whether an apparent increase in infection incidence indicates the presence of an epidemic or merely reflects an appropriate fluctuation associated with variations in the host susceptibility characteristics of hospitalized patients. Nor can the epidemiologist rely on the criterion that a single disease and unique microorganism are seen in a typical epidemic, since nosocomial infection epidemics often involve several diseases or multiple pathogens, such as occurs when an especially virulent strain causes infection at multiple sites or when a breakdown in routine patient-care practices allows the spread of several different microorganisms. Finally, the epidemiologist should not always expect to see an abrupt rise in the incidence of infections since the rates of infection may have been excessive for prolonged periods without recognition. Thus, although recognized epidemics almost always require an assessment, the epidemiologist will also need to consider investigating other infections that do not fulfill classic epidemic criteria.

### Endemic Infections

Sporadic (endemic) infections represent the bulk of preventable nosocomial infections, and their control should be a primary objective of ongoing infection control activities. Comparisons of infection rates in similar hospitals show variations that cannot be explained by differences in epidemic experiences, patient characteristics, kinds of treatment provided, or other hospital characteristics. Some of these differences in infection rates can be explained by the existence of more effective infection control programs in some hospitals than in others. Therefore, the hospital epidemiologist should also consider endemic infections worthy of epidemiologic investigation if the local rates of infection appear to be higher than they should be.

INFECTION RATE IS GREATER THAN ACCEPTED THRESHOLD  Few published criteria define acceptable epidemic or endemic infection rate thresholds in hospitals. One such criterion has been offered by the American Public Health Association, which stated that "The occurrence of two or more concurrent cases of staphyloccocal disease related to a nursery or a maternity ward is presumptive evidence of an epidemic and warrants investigation" [1].

Recently, increasing numbers of epidemiologic studies have described infection rates for certain defined patient populations, such as patients undergoing specific surgical procedures or exposed to particular medical devices or treatments. Although such reports often fail to control for degree of host susceptibility or other factors that may influence infection risk, they may provide useful benchmarks against which the epidemiologist may compare local endemic infection rates.

As hospitals begin to characterize patients by diagnosis related groupings (DRGs) for reimbursement, additional data may become available that will control, at least in part, for variations in the extent of underlying illnesses and thereby allow more meaningful comparisons than have previously been possible.

RECOGNIZED PROBLEM IN OTHER HOSPITALS  Hospitals generally have similar practices and use similar therapeutic approaches, so the recognition of an infection control problem in another hospital should prompt an evaluation of local practices. For example, infection control programs began to recognize epidemics of bacteremia associated with use of arterial pressure monitoring devices as they became widely used in intensive care units, and within a brief period a variety of problems and infection control measures were reported in the literature. These reports stimulated other hospitals to evaluate their use of these devices, and similar problems were found on occasion.

The infection control staff are not obligated to

institute every infection control measure suggested in the literature, however, for some may not be appropriate for widespread application. The epidemiologist may wish to conduct an epidemiologic study to determine whether new procedures are needed, in light of local infection experiences.

SIGNIFICANT INCREASE IN INFECTION RATE   The need to conduct ongoing, total hospital surveillance for nosocomial infections remains controversial, and many excellent infection control programs have instituted limited or targeted surveillance (see Chapter 4).

FIG. 5-1. Upper limits of expected number of infections for selected endemic infection rates. For each endemic infection rate (0.001, 0.005, 0.01, 0.02), the upper limit of numbers of infections that would be expected to occur is plotted against the number of patients at risk of infection. In ≤ 5 percent of instances, a larger number of infections might be expected to occur by chance alone. The formula used to calculate the plots is

$$p_x = \frac{e^{-N\lambda}\,(N\lambda)^x}{x!}$$

where $e$ = base of natural log, $x$ = number of observed infections, $N$ = number of subjects available, $\lambda$ = baseline level of occurrence, and $p$ = probability of occurrence. The probabilities ($p$) were summed until the cumulative probability reached or exceeded 0.95. (The author gratefully acknowledges the assistance of Stanley M. Martin, M.S., Centers for Disease Control, in constructing this figure.)

Nonetheless, systematic and rigorously applied surveillance remains a powerful technique for recognizing subtle but important changes in a hospital's infection experience. Such surveillance may be unnecessary to identify explosive or very large problems leading to clinically serious disease, but more subtle problems, such as gradual increases in infection rates, outbreaks caused by several pathogens, and serious problems occurring in small patient populations (such as surgical wound infections associated with a single surgeon or procedure) may be difficult to identify without systematic data collection.

Many hospital infection control programs do not have ready access to sophisticated statistical analyses of their infection surveillance data. Even without formal statistical analyses, however, an infection control program can establish its own thresholds for evaluating potential problems. For example, a 2- to 2.5-fold increase in the infection rate of any site, pathogen, or site-pathogen combination would almost always justify an evaluation. For infections with a high baseline incidence, a smaller rise in infection rate would call for investigation.

Figure 5-1 provides a statistical guideline that might be used to establish general thresholds for concern. The number of infections is plotted against the population at risk. A family of curves for a range of baseline infection rates, ranging from 1 per thousand to 20 per thousand, indicates the upper 95 percent limit of the expected number of infections for each

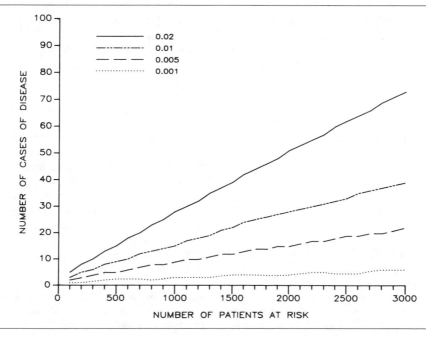

baseline rate. For example, if the expected baseline incidence of an infection is believed to be 5 cases per thousand and if 1000 patients have been at risk of acquiring that infection, we would expect to observe fewer than 10 cases of infection 95 percent of the time. If a larger number is seen, an investigation might profitably be instituted.

Although Figure 5-1 may be useful as a guideline, it must be used cautiously. It cannot be used arbitrarily as a criterion for deciding when to evaluate a potential problem since fewer than the threshold number of cases may represent an important problem on occasion and, in approximately 5 percent of instances, a larger number may be due to chance alone.

SELECTED HIGH-PRIORITY INFECTIONS  Certain nosocomial infections are either so uncommon or sufficiently important that their occurrence almost invariably suggests a potential problem without regard to the size of the hospital or the characteristics of the host population. In modern U.S. hospitals, for example, group A streptococcal infections occur rarely, and the occurrence of two or more nosocomial infections with this pathogen within a brief period of time usually suggests an infection control problem.

Multiply-drug-resistant microorganisms, once established in a hospital, complicate patient management and have been notoriously difficult to eradicate. Many hospitals consider the isolation of a new antimicrobial-resistant strain to require investigation and control, even if the strain does not produce disease. The identification of multiple isolations of a new nosocomial strain may similarly call for an epidemiologic assessment, even if the strain does not obviously cause patient illness, since this may also be an indication that a new mechanism of transmission or a new reservoir has become established.

Although every hospital epidemiologist would undoubtedly identify different high-priority infections, selected site-pathogen combinations that frequently suggested infection control problems during CDC investigations are listed in Table 5-1.

## PRINCIPLES OF EPIDEMIOLOGIC INVESTIGATIONS

For an infection to occur, a sufficient number of pathogenic microorganisms (the agent) must be present; an individual (the host) must be susceptible to infection; and a means for the agent to have appropriate contact with the host (mode of transmission) must be present. An infection may be prevented by altering any one of these factors. The goal of an epidemiologic investigation is to determine which of these factors may be most easily altered to prevent disease.

When a potential problem is first recognized, many factors may seem important. There may be, for example, many potential reservoirs, numerous possible host susceptibility factors, and various modes of transmission that might be responsible for disease acquisition. Which of these is actually related to the occurrence of disease is unknown, and it is therefore difficult to know how to control the problem. An investigation is designed to discover which factors are relevant so that control efforts can be efficiently instituted and concern about irrelevant factors discarded.

In the classic, formal investigation, identification of important factors is accomplished by comparing the characteristics of affected persons (the case population) with those of a similar group of unaffected persons (the control population). The major differences between the case and control populations are assumed to play a role in determining the occurrence of disease.

As discussed in the next section, on occasion effective control measures may be confidently designed without a formal investigation. In these settings, control measures can generally be taken because formal investigations have previously identified the important variables and have demonstrated effective control measures.

Epidemiologic investigations use the same basic study-design and analytic principles as are used in other kinds of biomedical research. Several principles must be emphasized, however.

First, an investigation may show association but be unable to prove causation. For example, the risk of nosocomial pneumonia may be demonstrated to be strongly associated with recent thoracic or abdominal surgery. This does not prove that the surgery causes pneumonia; it merely indicates that something about the surgery—or the patients who typically undergo that kind of surgery—increases the risk of pneumonia. In some instances, however, the epidemiologic associations are sufficiently strong to allow a conclusion to be drawn about causation. A very strong association between exposure to a particular intravenous medication and primary bacteremia implies that the medication may be contaminated, especially if no other strong association is demonstrable. If the weight of epidemiologic evidence finds very strong associations and if those associations are biologically plausible as causal factors, the epidemiologist should be able to draw strong conclusions about causes of

TABLE 5-1. Investigation of infections

| Pathogens | Systemic and blood | Surg. wound | CNS | Respiratory | UTI | Skin | Gastroenteritis |
|---|---|---|---|---|---|---|---|
| **Bacteria** | | | | | | | |
| *Acinetobacter* | | | * | | | | |
| *Citrobacter* | * | | * | | | | |
| *Clostridium perfringens* | | * | | | | | |
| *Corynebacterium diphtheria* | * | | | * | | * | |
| *Enterobacter* | * | | * | | | | |
| *Escherichia coli* | | | * | | | | |
| *Klebsiella* | | | * | | | | |
| *Legionella* | | | | * | | | |
| *Listeria monocytogenes* | * | | * | | | | |
| *Neisseria meningitidis* | * | | * | * | | | |
| *Pseudomonas aeruginosa* | | * | * | | | | |
| *Pseudomonas cepacia* | * | * | * | * | * | | |
| *Salmonella* | * | * | * | | * | | * |
| *Serratia* | * | | | | | | |
| *Shigella* | | * | | | | | * |
| *Staphylococcus aureus* | | | * | | | | |
| *Staphylococcus epidermidis* | | | * | | | | |
| *Streptococcus*, group A | * | * | * | | | * | |
| *Streptococcus*, group B | * | | * | | | | |
| **Other microorganisms and diseases** | | | | | | | |
| *Aspergillus* | * | * | | * | | | |
| Herpes simplex | * | * | | | | | |
| *Pneumocystis* | | | | * | | | |
| Varicella-zoster | * | | | | | * | |

CNS = central nervous system; UTI = urinary tract infection.
Note: The combinations of microorganisms and sites of infection shown with an asterisk are unusual or serious in most U.S. hospitals, without regard to hospital size or type. The occurrence of two or more cases of nosocomial *Disease* in a 30-day period generally deserves an evaluation. Isolation of *Corynebacterium diphtheriae* deserves assessment, even if not associated with disease.

illness, and these conclusions can reasonably become the basis for institution of control measures.

Second, the epidemiologist should not expect to find that every case patient is exposed to the factor that is implicated as causing disease. Even in epidemics, in which specific factors are often proved responsible for disease, one occasionally identifies case patients who fulfill the criteria for being part of the outbreak but have no demonstrable association with the presumed causal factor. It must be remembered that even in epidemic situations, endemic disease continues to occur and that these patients may be difficult to separate from the epidemic cases on clinical or epidemiologic grounds. This is illustrated in the epidemiologic studies showing the relation be-

tween cigarette smoking and the development of lung cancer. Not everyone who smokes will acquire cancer, and some persons acquire lung cancer without exposure to cigarette smoking. Nonetheless, the associations between smoking and development of cancer are exceedingly strong and, moreover, the possibility that smoking causes lung cancer is biologically plausible. Therefore, most observers have concluded that a direct, causal link exists, and efforts to encourage less smoking have been widely adopted.

Third, the epidemiologist uses clinical data somewhat differently from the clinician. If a nursing mother has a breast abscess, for example, her physician would prefer microbiologic proof before making the diagnosis of staphylococcal infection. In contrast, if the same patient's records are reviewed by an epidemiologist during the investigation of a nursery staphylococcal outbreak and if the woman's infant had staphylococcal disease, the epidemiologist should assume that she, too, had a staphylococcal infection, whether a culture was obtained or not.

## PROTOCOL FOR EPIDEMIOLOGIC INVESTIGATIONS IN THE HOSPITAL

Some investigations of nosocomial infection problems are quite complex, requiring that investigators be skilled in epidemiology and statistics, that resources be available for sophisticated analyses of complex data, or that specialized laboratory facilities be readily available. Most epidemiologic investigations of nosocomial infections do not require special resources, however, and every hospital's infection control staff should be able to perform at least the initial phases of most investigations.

Each epidemiologic study is different, and there is no simple, standardized approach to conducting an investigation. Not only is each epidemiologist likely to approach a problem differently, but the relative importance and sequence of steps will necessarily differ according to the nature of the problem. Nonetheless, there are general approaches to epidemiologic investigation that have proved practical and effective when employed by CDC epidemiologists in investigating nosocomial infection problems, and these steps are summarized in this section.

Figure 5-2 illustrates a decision pathway to help determine whether a formal, classic, case-control investigation (a "major" investigation) is required or whether a more limited study (a "basic" investigation) will suffice. The basic investigation is adequate to solve most nosocomial infection problems and should be within the capabilities of most infection control programs. The major investigation is required for unique, very serious, or complex problems, and such investigations may require outside assistance in many institutions. The initial steps are similar for both kinds of investigations, however.

### Initial Evaluation
As illustrated in Figure 5-2, an initial investigation should be instituted whenever the hospital's established threshold of concern, as described above, is surpassed.

CONDUCT PRELIMINARY CASE REVIEW  The epidemiologist first reviews the clinical and epidemiologic characteristics of affected patients. At this stage, the epidemiologist may choose to study a convenient sample of patients—the purpose of the review is to establish the nature and seriousness of the potential problem in general terms, not to characterize it completely. This patient sample may include persons present in the hospital, those identified by routine surveillance, or those whose medical records are conveniently available.

It is important to remember, however, that study subjects who are selected because they are readily available (i.e., a sample of convenience) may not accurately reflect the characteristics of other affected patients and may introduce bias into the investigation that can be quite misleading. For example, neonatal staphylococcal infection has an incubation period of about seven days. As a result, staphylococcal disease in full-term infants often begins after hospital discharge, and disease with onset during hospitalization occurs more often in hospitalized infants with prolonged stay. Therefore, although a nursery staphylococcal problem may initially seem to be limited to premature infants or those born by cesarean section, thorough case-finding may identify a large number of term infants also affected. The epidemiologist who relies solely on a sample of convenience, in this example, hospitalized infants, may fail to recognize the full scope of a problem. More systematic case finding is generally required at later stages for all but the simplest outbreaks.

EVALUATE CLINICAL SEVERITY  During the initial clinical and epidemiologic review, the epidemiologist should determine whether disease is present. The absence of actual disease does not indicate the absence of an infection control problem, however, and the epidemiologist often needs to continue an investigation even in such circumstances.

Approximately 11 percent of formal nosocomial epidemiologic investigations conducted by CDC investigators between 1956 and 1979 were determined to be pseudoepidemics, generally caused by surveillance artifacts or laboratory errors [2]. Although pseudoepidemics may not be associated with patient illness, they are nonetheless important to identify since they may affect the quality of patient care. Errors in processing or interpreting laboratory specimens should be identified since they may lead to faulty clinical diagnoses or inappropriate patient treatment. Faulty surveillance should be corrected so that actual infections are not missed and infection control information is reliable.

On occasion microbial colonization without disease may reflect an important problem, such as when a colonizing strain is resistant to multiple antimicrobial

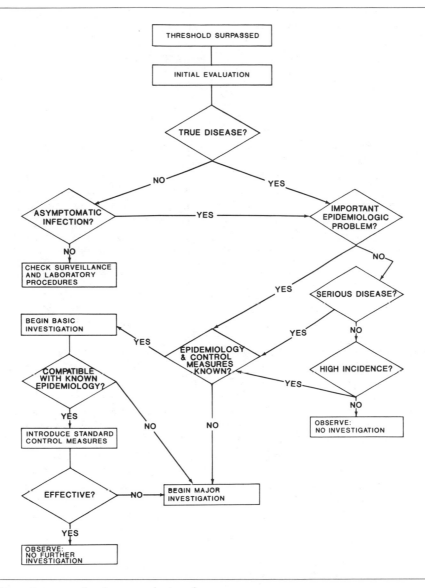

FIG. 5-2. Decision pathway to select between a basic and major epidemiologic investigation.

agents and may serve as a source for subsequent transmission. In other instances, an epidemic of colonization may indicate a breakdown in basic infection control techniques that allows the colonizing strain to spread from patient to patient. In a setting such as this, more virulent strains might also be easily spread, so an investigation into the mechanism of transmission may be useful.

The epidemiologist may choose not to investigate a problem that involves few patients, causes inconsequential disease, or does not seem likely to result from a fundamental breakdown of routine infection control practices. In such circumstances, implementation of empirical control measures or continued monitoring of the problem using surveillance may be all that is necessary. Serious disease or infections affecting large numbers of persons will usually call for an active investigation.

If, on the other hand, serious clinical disease occurs, infections occur at high frequency, or a potentially serious infection control problem is identified, either a basic or major investigation is indicated.

If the epidemiologist's initial assessment suggests that the hospital's problem is similar to ones that have previously occurred and that effective infection prevention and control measures are well known, it is reasonable to begin a basic investigation. A major investigation should be begun at this point if the problem seems to be unusual and control measures are not readily apparent.

As is illustrated in Figure 5-2, a basic investigation may be begun during which the epidemiologist may decide that a formal case-control evaluation is required. Additional evaluation during the basic investigation may show that the problem is actually unique or that the control measures that initially seemed reasonable are inappropriate. Later, those standard control measures that have been implemented may not be effective in solving the problem. In each circumstance, a major investigation should be begun.

*The Basic Investigation*
The basic epidemiologic investigation is a useful and efficient technique for evaluating simple, uncomplicated, and generally nonserious infection problems. It allows the hospital to implement reasonable control measures that have been previously developed, evaluated, and found to be effective. The majority of common problems in hospitals can be managed by this approach.

The basic investigation is especially useful when the clinical and epidemiologic characteristics of case patients are similar to those described elsewhere and when prevention and control measures have been documented to be effective.

In the basic investigation, unlike the major investigation, prevention and control techniques that are likely to be effective are applied empirically. Furthermore, epidemiologic techniques are not used to demonstrate differences between case and control patients. As a result, the basic investigation is unlikely to provide scientific evidence about the cause of the problem being investigated and should not be used if the problem requires continuing scientific study or if the investigator wishes to publish the result of the investigation.

COLLECT CRITICAL DATA AND SPECIMENS   Early in the investigation, the epidemiologist needs to ensure that critical data, specimens, and observations that may be needed during the subsequent phases of the investigation are preserved. Samples of microbial strains believed to be implicated in the problem (epidemic strains) should be saved by the microbiology laboratory. Hospital practices prevailing during the period should be documented since widespread changes in practices often occur once an investigation is be-

gun, and it may not be possible to reconstruct the procedures later in the investigation. Any commercially supplied medications, devices, or materials that may be associated with the problem should be placed in quarantine and saved for public health authorities such as those of the Food and Drug Administration (FDA); all too frequently, such materials are discarded or returned to the manufacturer during the early phases of investigations, making them unavailable for subsequent independent testing if they are implicated in causing disease. Selected specimens of materials likely to be relevant should be collected for testing since such materials are often cleaned or discarded early in investigations. Although it is quite uneconomical and generally unrewarding to initiate widespread, indiscriminate culturing of specimens from patients, personnel, or the inanimate environment, the epidemiologist must judiciously select for sampling those sources that are highly suspect on the basis of past experiences.

INSTITUTE EMPIRICAL CONTROL MEASURES   The epidemiologist should institute control measures based on previous experiences with similar problems and that are appropriate to the problem as defined in the patient-case review. It is sometimes impossible to implement any reasonable control measure until an epidemiologic investigation has identified the cause of the problem, and in such instances a major investigation is warranted. In other instances the problem may have many potential causes, and it is impractical to institute control measures for each; here too a major investigation is useful. For most problems, however, a large body of experience exists to guide the epidemiologist in selecting the appropriate prevention and control measures and to assist in deciding their priorities.

IDENTIFY AFFECTED PATIENTS   The epidemiologist initiates a systematic attempt to identify as many affected patients as possible, recognizing, as discussed earlier, that readily available case patients may not represent the actual affected population.

Formulation of a "tentative case definition" will help guide the search for potential patients with disease. The case definition is simply the epidemiologist's best description of the probable characteristics of case patients. It often includes descriptions of the host group affected and a definition of the kind of disease that occurs; at the point, it must be based on the findings of the preliminary review. For example, the case definition in a nursery staphylococcal outbreak might simply be: An infant, born in the past three months, with (1) skin lesions characteristic of staphylococcal pustulosis and/or (2) a positive culture for *Staphylococcus aureus* from any site.

At this early phase in the investigation, the case definition should be broad since the full scope of the outbreak cannot be known with certainty. An overly broad case definition may lead to a review of patients who are not part of the problem, but they can be subsequently excluded from analysis. An excessively restrictive case definition tends to exclude patients from being evaluated, and the failure to study such patients may seriously jeopardize the investigation.

Case-finding methods are determined by the problem being investigated, but in the majority of epidemiologic investigations in hospitals, a reasonably complete listing of probable case patients can be readily obtained by reviewing surveillance and microbiology records.

Carefully collected surveillance data are a prime resource, but case-finding should not be limited to these data since surveillance typically fails to identify all nosocomial infections even when excellent surveillance methods are employed. Surveillance is especially likely to miss patients with mild or asymptomatic infection or those who have onset of clinical disease after discharge.

Microbiology records should generally be reviewed as a matter of course to identify other potentially affected individuals. The investigator should seek not only to identify patients with infection at the site or with the microorganism that prompted the investigation, but also to review similar strains and potentially related sites of infection to ensure that the problem is not more widespread than originally thought. On occasion patients who have had negative results on laboratory studies may need to be evaluated, for they too may be part of the outbreak.

In certain outbreaks specialized case-finding techniques are required. A carefully designed questionnaire or telephone survey of selected physicians or recently discharged patients may be useful if a characteristic clinical syndrome, unlikely to be identified by hospital surveillance or culturing, is being investigated. If onset of disease may occur after hospital discharge, inquiries to other hospitals, community physicians, and local health departments may be particularly helpful. Clinical examination, culture surveys, skin tests, or serologic surveys may also be useful in some instances.

REVIEW CHARACTERISTICS OF REPRESENTATIVE CASE PATIENTS  The epidemiologist next reviews a sufficient number of case patients to define the clinical and epidemiologic characteristics of the potential problem. In this review the epidemiologist is particularly interested in identifying common host or exposure features of case patients.

When possible, all potentially affected patients should be reviewed. In very large outbreaks (e.g., involving more than 50 patients), it is appropriate to study a sample of patient cases.

Various techniques are available to select samples of patients for review. Whatever scheme is used, the epidemiologist must take care that the sampling process selects a group for study that is *representative* of the total population. In general, randomized sampling is least likely to introduce bias and therefore should be used unless there are strong arguments for using an alternative technique. Systematic sampling can be used in hospital studies if the investigator can be assured that the systematic sampling interval does not correspond to patterns within the hospital that might bias case selection. Samples of convenience—the selection of patients who are readily available—should generally be avoided.

Basic patient identifying information should be recorded that will allow subsequent retrieval of clinical records, and selected clinical and epidemiologic data should be abstracted. The data to be abstracted fall into several categories that are considered epidemiologically in terms of time, place, and person (see also Chapter 1).

*Time.*  The time course of an infection problem provides valuable epidemiologic information. An *epidemic curve*—a graph showing the number of cases of disease according to the time of onset—should be plotted. This curve allows ready comparison of an epidemic period with a preepidemic, or baseline, period, and in addition may allow identification of temporal clusters of cases of disease. The characteristics of the epidemic curve often suggest how disease is spread. An abrupt increase in the number of cases suggests a single exposure to a point source of contamination, as is shown in Figure 5-3A. A more protracted course may be compatible with person-to-person spread (Fig. 5-3B). Mixed modes of transmission may be implied by curves such as that shown in Figure 5-3C, and, as in Figure 5-3D, the epidemic curve is occasionally consistent with several distinct modes of spread.

When the epidemic curve is drawn, the time-scale intervals should be shorter than the presumed incubation period of the disease since person-to-person spread may appear to be common-source spread if longer intervals are used (Fig. 5-4).

Similar plots showing dates of exposure to potential sources of disease, rather than dates of clinical onset, may be especially useful when the disease has a long or variable incubation period. Such plots may

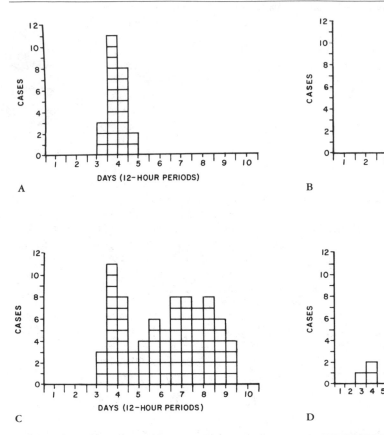

FIG. 5-3. Epidemic curves depicting commonly observed temporal characteristics of outbreaks in hospitals. *A*. A common-source outbreak of disease with an incubation period of 18 to 36 hours. Disease occurrence reaches its peak rapidly. *B*. Person-to-person transmission of a disease with a similar incubation period. The first case of disease (index case) is followed by increasing numbers of cases as the disease spreads. *C*. Mixed common-source and person-to-person transmission of the same disease. The initial peak represents those patients exposed to the contaminated common source, and the later, broader peak represents secondary spread of the disease. *D*. Intermittent exposure to a common source is represented by an indeterminate pattern. This pattern is also consistent with that of a common-source outbreak of disease with a variable incubation period, that of spread from asymptomatic carriers, or that of spread from infected persons who have prolonged carriage. This pattern may also be seen when many persons have asymptomatic infection and only few have clinically apparent disease.

suggest common exposures that are not apparent in curves showing the dates of disease onset.

*Place.* Geographic clustering should also be evaluated. Pictorial representation in the form of *spot maps* is useful—each case of disease is located by its geographic point of onset or acquisition. This simple technique often makes prominent otherwise inapparent clustering and may also suggest the mode of spread. Clustering in a single ward implies a common source or person-to-person spread. Hospital airflow patterns may explain the spatial clustering of disease, as is shown in Figure 5-5 [3]; this spot map shows the distribution of cases of smallpox in a German hospital (see also Chapter 35). The index case (patient 1) had no direct or indirect contact with any of the other cases (secondary and tertiary cases). All secondary and tertiary cases, however, occurred in rooms that received air that flowed from the room of the index case.

A disease scattered at random throughout the hospital is compatible with an autogenous source, widespread distribution of a contaminated common source, or an extensive breakdown in patient-care practices.

Not only should the place of primary residence of patients be considered, but their exposures to other hospital areas should also be evaluated. Surgical wound

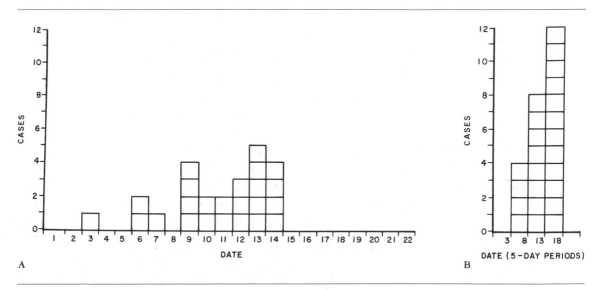

A

B

FIG. 5-4. Effects of the time scale on the appearance of the epidemic curve. The epidemic curves represent the same outbreak caused by a pathogen with a two-day incubation period. A. The curve can correctly suggest person-to-person spread if the time scale has intervals slightly shorter than the incubation period. B. When long intervals are used, the curve incorrectly suggests a common-source exposure.

FIG. 5-5. Spot map showing location of patients with nosocomial smallpox and relation to airflow patterns in a hospital in Meschede, Germany. Patient 1 was the index case. Shaded areas show flow of air from the room of patient 1 to other areas of the hospital. (From Center for Disease Control. Follow-up smallpox—Federal Republic of Germany. *Morbid. Mortal. Weekly Rep.* 19:234, 1970. Adapted from World Health Organization, Smallpox surveillance. *Weekly Epidemiol. Rec.* 45:249, 1970.)

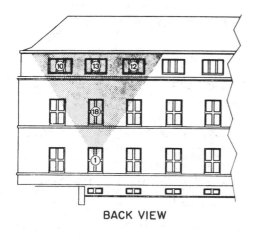

BACK VIEW

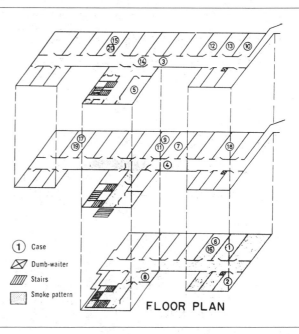

FLOOR PLAN

① Case
⊠ Dumb-waiter
/// Stairs
▨ Smoke pattern

infections, for example, may be specifically associated with a particular operating room.

Time and place descriptions can be combined to reconstruct the dynamic spread of infection through the hospital. Here again, graphic or pictorial representation may be useful. Geographic exposures may be added to a standard epidemic curve, or sequential spot maps may be constructed to trace the spread of disease.

*Person.* A thorough description of the case population is the most important part of this phase of the investigation. The goals of this description are to define the specific underlying host characteristics that predispose to infection and to evaluate all exposures that may alter susceptibility or provide an opportunity for contact with the infecting agent. Here a deliberate, exhaustive search for common features shared by the cases of infection is crucial. Patient host factors that may influence susceptibility to disease should be recorded such as age, sex, nutritional status, types of underlying diseases, history of active or passive immunization, and the receipt of antimicrobial or immunosuppressive medications. For some diseases, specific host factors are important. Patients with gastric achlorhydria are especially susceptible to shigellosis and other enteric diseases, for example.

Exposure factors should also be recorded, both animate and inanimate. Contacts with people should be considered, even when disease is usually considered to be acquired from autogenous sources. The source for gram-negative microorganisms such as *Escherichia coli,* for example, is usually thought to be autogenous carriage or exogenous acquisition from the inanimate environment. These infections may, however, be transmitted from person-to-person; frequently, such spread occurs by way of patient-care personnel.

Therapeutic measures may alter intrinsic host susceptibility or provide the opportunity for contact with the infecting pathogen. Antimicrobial therapy should generally be considered since it may predispose to colonization or disease if the infecting strain is resistant or it may prevent disease if the strain is susceptible. Specific treatments may provide a portal of entry for the infecting microorganism: urinary catheterization, for example, provides a direct route by which bacteria may enter the bladder, and intravenous cannulas provide direct access to the vascular system. Knowledge of such exposures may point to the source of the infecting strain.

METHODS TO OBTAIN AND PROCESS DATA   The case review may be aided by careful design of the data-collection forms. It should be remembered that the goal of the investigation is to characterize selected aspects of the entire affected population, not every detail about each individual case. Thus simple descriptive characteristics (e.g., age, sex, nature of underlying diseases) and notations as to the presence or absence of selected exposures (e.g., geographic areas, personnel, medications, procedures) are all that are generally required.

A simple line-listing form is usually the most efficient way to record these data (Fig. 5-6). Each patient is listed on the form, and the appropriate characteristics checked off or otherwise summarized.

If many patients must be evaluated or numerous host and exposure factors analyzed, data-processing techniques may aid in the analysis of data. Mini- or microcomputers and sophisticated data-base management and statistical software programs are widely available in hospitals, and infection control personnel may elect to develop skills in their use. Unless extensive data are collected and the investigators are familiar with computerized data-processing techniques (or have readily available support from others who can assist with the design of computer-based analytic programs), however, computerization of the investigation is likely to entail more work and require more time than manual tabulation.

FIG. 5-6. Portion of a typical line-listing form used to tabulate data during an epidemiologic investigation. The items to be tabulated are determined by the nature of the problem under investigation.

| CASE NO. | PATIENT I.D. NO. | DATES | | | AGE | SEX | SERVICE | WARD | SITE INFCT | DATE ONSET | ANTIMICROBIAL RESISTANCE (X) | | | | | | | | | | | | | IV | URINE CATH |
| --- | --- | --- | --- | --- | --- | --- | --- | --- | --- | --- | --- | --- | --- | --- | --- | --- | --- | --- | --- | --- | --- | --- | --- | --- | --- |
| | | Adm | Disch | Death | | | | | | | 1 | 2 | 3 | 4 | 5 | 6 | 7 | 8 | 9 | 10 | 11 | 12 | | | |
| 1 | 42266 | 4/27 | 6/1 | | 46 | M | Surg | 4B | Blood | 5/16 | X | X | | X | X | X | | X | X | I | X | X | 5/15-5/28 | 4/27-6/1 |
| 2 | 05819 | 5/17 | | 5/24 | 32 | F | OB | 6A | Blood | 5/18 | X | X | | X | X | X | | X | X | I | X | X | 5/18-5/19 | |
| 3 | 38776 | 5/8 | | 5/18 | 76 | M | Med | 2B | Blood | 5/18 | X | X | | X | X | X | | X | X | X | X | X | 5/8-5/18 | 5/12-5/18 |
| | | | | | | | | | | | | | | | | | | | | | | | | | |
| | | | | | | | | | | | | | | | | | | | | | | | | | |

REFINE THE CASE DEFINITION    After the patient-case review has been completed, the epidemiologist should be able to define the general nature of the problem. This is usually done by refining the preliminary case definition developed at the beginning of the investigation. The case definition should now describe the essential features of affected patients: are the illnesses nosocomial or community-acquired; what particular patient populations are affected; what are the clinical sites of infection; what microorganisms are involved; during what period of time does the problem occur?

As a rule, the full extent of the problem is seldom recognized early in the investigation. Patients initially considered to be cases may now need to be discarded from the study population, and additional patients may need to be added to the study group as the investigation proceeds and the epidemiologist develops a better understanding of the characteristics of the problem.

Although the epidemiologist may reasonably decide to take expedient shortcuts in many phases of the epidemiologic investigation, great care should be taken at this stage to establish an accurate case definition since this definition guides all subsequent phases of the investigation. If this case definition is inaccurate, the conclusions drawn from the investigation are likely to be faulty, and control measures may not be accurately identified.

An overly restrictive case definition will exclude true case patients and make it more difficult to show statistically significant differences between case and control patients. An inappropriately inclusive case definition will dilute true case patients with those who are not a part of the problem and may obscure associations with disease. In general it is best to be overly inclusive during the early stages of the investigation but as restrictive as possible at this stage. If it is impossible to determine whether or not some patients should be included as case patients, the epidemiologist may label them as "possible" or "probable" cases and conduct analyses with those patients both included and excluded from the analysis group.

RECONSIDER WHETHER MAJOR INVESTIGATION IS NEEDED    After collecting epidemiologic and clinical data from case patients, the epidemiologist should decide whether the characteristics of the problem are similar to those described in other institutions and whether reasonable control measures have already been established elsewhere. If the problem is not unique, empirical control measures should be implemented. If, on the other hand, the characteristics of the cases are not consistent with what is known about similar problems, a major investigation should be initiated.

INSTITUTE APPROPRIATE CONTROL MEASURES    Steps to prevent or control disease are often taken immediately—even before the investigation is begun—especially when the problem is serious. If such control measures have not been introduced, the epidemiologist should consider whether any are likely to be effective on the basis of what has been learned from the patient case review. Numerous control measures are frequently available for use, varying in cost, complexity, and efficacy.

A decision about the kinds of control measures to implement should be based on the urgency of control. Major, disruptive, or costly control measures may not be indicated if the clinical and epidemiologic problems are not serious. If effective control measures have not been established or established measures appear to be inappropriate to the epidemiologic situation, the epidemiologist may elect to initiate a major investigation.

MONITOR EFFECTIVENESS OF CONTROL MEASURES    The institution of control measures may be followed by an apparent resolution of the problem. It must be recognized that the control measures may have had no actual effect and that a temporary reduction in disease occurrence may be fortuitous. The infection control program must continue to monitor the problem, therefore, to ensure that it does not recur. Although standard surveillance techniques occasionally are adequate to monitor a problem, specific techniques are frequently necessary, including careful follow-up of high-risk patients, ongoing surveillance of patient-care techniques, or selective culturing of patients or their environment. Ultimately control measures should be judged successful only if an acceptable rate of patient infection is maintained.

If control measures reduce the incidence of disease to acceptable levels for an appropriate period of time, no additional investigation is required, but if the control measures are ineffective or the problem recurs while those control measures are in effect, a major epidemiologic investigation should be instituted immediately.

*The Major Epidemiologic Investigation*
The major investigation—a more rigorous scientific evaluation than the basic investigation, typically involving careful comparisons of case and control populations—should be conducted when a problem is unusual, complex, or of substantial scientific importance, or when the basic investigation has been unsuccessful.

Many of the studies conducted in the early portion of the basic investigation are also done in the major

TABLE 5-2. Steps in initial, basic,
and major epidemiologic investigations

Initial investigation
    Conduct preliminary case review
    Evaluate severity of problem
    Select basic or major investigation
Basic investigation
    Collect critical data and specimens
    Institute control measures
    Identify affected patients
    Review case characteristics (time, place, person)
    Refine case definition
    Reconsider major investigation
    Institute control measures
    Monitor effectiveness control measures
    Reconsider major investigation
Major investigation
    Collect critical data and specimens
    Consider institution of control measures
    Identify affected patients
    Review case characteristics (time, place, person)
    Refine case definition
    Determine if consultation needed
    Formulate tentative hypotheses
    Test hypotheses
    Institute control measures
    Evaluate control measures

investigation, but, as noted in Table 5-2, the strategies diverge after the epidemiologist has reviewed the clinical and epidemiologic characteristics of case patients. Rather than institute empirical control measures, as in the basic investigation, the epidemiologist attempts to identify the causes of the problem through a series of case-control studies and analyses.

If a major investigation is undertaken after a basic investigation has failed to solve a problem, the steps already conducted need not be repeated. However, the investigator should reevaluate the methods used in the basic investigation to be certain that shortcuts were not taken that might impair the validity of the more rigorous evaluation. In particular the epidemiologist should review the adequacy of previous attempts to (1) develop a case definition, (2) identify all infected patients, and (3) characterize the case patients clinically and epidemiologically.

REFINE CASE DEFINITION    If a preliminary basic investigation has failed to identify the problem, the preliminary case definition may have been faulty. Commonly the initial, working case definition is too restrictive and has thereby failed to identify major segments of the affected population. When beginning a formal investigation, the initial case definition should

be reconsidered and broadened if necessary. The revised case definition will continue to be refined as the investigation progresses, and patients can be removed from the case group if the subsequent investigation indicates they are not part of the problem.

REFINE CASE-FINDING TECHNIQUES    During a basic investigation the epidemiologist often takes expedient shortcuts, such as identifying and reviewing only a sample of affected patients. On beginning a major investigation, aggressive steps should be taken to identify *all* potential cases. It is especially important that a broad case definition be used for case-finding so that few cases of infection will be missed. Case-finding should extend sufficiently into previous time periods to identify when the first cases of disease occurred, since the most recently occurring cases may have different epidemiologic characteristics from those of cases occurring earlier.

REVIEW CASES OF DISEASE    In all but the largest outbreaks, the epidemiologist conducting a major investigation should attempt to review all identified cases of disease. In very large outbreaks, this may be impractical, but special care must then be taken to ensure that the sample of patients reviewed is representative. Again random sampling techniques are preferred, and patients should be selected for review from the complete potential case listing. On occasion stratified random sampling can compensate for small numbers of patients in important risk groups.

It is useful to reevaluate the case records of all affected patients, even if they have been previously evaluated during an earlier, more limited assessment. For those patients, as well as for new patients not previously studied, a thorough tabulation of epidemiologic characteristics (time, place, and person) is necessary. The epidemiologist should not only look for factors that have been documented as important in previous investigations but also be prepared to identify previously unrecognized associations.

If a major investigation is undertaken from the start, the steps listed in Table 5-2 and described for the basic investigation should be completed.

DETERMINE WHETHER CONSULTATION IS REQUIRED
Early in the major investigation, the epidemiologist should consider whether outside assistance is likely to be necessary; the investigation may require a substantial investment of time as well as sophisticated laboratory or statistical support. Many state and local health departments are able to advise hospitals regarding epidemiologic investigations and often can assist in arranging epidemiologic and laboratory sup-

port when indicated. Universities with an academic and research interest in nosocomial infections as well as private consulting epidemiologists provide additional sources for assistance. State health departments may request direct assistance from the CDC if needed, and the CDC also provides advice to hospital personnel about strategies that can be used in investigations.

When contamination of a commercially supplied medication or device is suspected, public health authorities should be notified immediately. In particular, the FDA and CDC should be notified; other hospitals may also be affected, and these federal agencies are responsible for evaluation and control of such problems.

FORMULATE TENTATIVE HYPOTHESES  After completing the review of the clinical and exposure data available for affected patients, the epidemiologist prepares a profile of cases, which is a summary of host factors and exposures of patient cases developed by tabulating the presence or absence of the time, place, and person characteristics previously described. In this profile the epidemiologist seeks to identify common features among the cases, the assumption being that at least one of these common features will account for the susceptibility to infection.

The list of common features may be short or long. On rare occasions one feature is so prominent among cases that only a single explanation for the infection problem need reasonably be considered. More often a large list is developed, and there are numerous reasonable hypotheses that may be advanced to explain the problem. The following hypothetical example illustrates the process of hypothesis formulation:

An investigation of epidemic *Proteus rettgeri* urinary tract infection (UTI) shows that all patients infected with the epidemic strain were hospitalized on a single ward, and each had indwelling urinary catheterization before the onset of infection. The epidemic strain neither had been isolated elsewhere in the hospital nor had caused disease other than UTI.

From the case review, the problem appears uniquely to affect patients on a single ward who have been catheterized. These two associations suggest a number of hypotheses, some of which follow. The geographic clustering may have several explanations: it may result from practices in obtaining culture specimens that are unique to the affected ward, a common source such as a medication or an infected staff member may be present on the ward, or ward patients themselves who are already infected may provide a

source for the epidemic strain. The association with urinary catheterization also suggests several hypotheses. The catheter may be related because it leads to a breach in bladder defenses. Alternatively, the catheter or some agent associated with catheter insertion may be contaminated with the epidemic strain. The catheter may be a proxy for the true risk factor, urinary irrigation, which is not routinely recorded in the patient record. Finally, if every patient on the ward is catheterized, catheterization may be quite unrelated to the risk of disease.

No factor can be excluded as unimportant simply because it is not present in each patient defined as a case. Rarely are all host and exposure factors identified with certainty, and furthermore, sporadic cases of disease—those that are, in fact, unrelated to the problem being investigated—may occur during an outbreak; these cases may be difficult to distinguish from the outbreak cases.

TEST THE HYPOTHESES  A valid hypothesis should explain not only why some patients acquire disease, but also why other patients do not. Most of the explanations in the example provided above are reasonable to explain UTI due to *Proteus* organisms, but if information is obtained only about the infected patients, the absence of disease in other patients remains an enigma. The crucial next step of the major investigation allows refinement of the hypotheses so that fortuitous associations can be discarded and causal factors more clearly delineated.

Three basic techniques are commonly used to refine hypotheses: case-control, cohort, and prospective intervention studies.

*Case-control study.*  Retrospectively conducted case-control evaluation is the most effective technique for investigating most hospital epidemics, and it is also often useful for investigating hyperendemic problems (see Chapter 1). In such a study, a group of uninfected patients (the *control group*) is compared with infected patients (the *case group*), and differences in susceptibility and exposure factors are examined. If a proper control group is selected, statistically significant differences between groups are likely to identify the cause of the problem. The value of the case-control study is illustrated in the following example, which, although simplified, is based on an actual investigation.

Over a four-month period, 50 patients on a urology service had UTI due to *Pseudomonas cepacia*. A review of the charts of the patient cases showed that 48 (96 percent) had urinary tract irrigation before infection. No other factor was seen so often: previous cystoscopy was performed in 45 (90 percent), no single physician treated more than 20 percent of infected patients, and only 62 percent could be documented to have had contact with another known case.

From the case data, urinary tract irrigation appeared to be strongly implicated. To test this hypothesis, a control population composed of 84 uninfected urology patients hospitalized in the same period was evaluated. In this control population, it was found that irrigation was indeed common; uninfected control patients had irrigation almost as often as did cases (Table 5-3). Only 24 of the 84 control patients, however, had previous cystoscopy. This suggested that the cystoscopy procedure may have been more important. Even this association, however, did not prove that cystoscopy was responsible for the outbreak. Why did some cystoscopy patients develop infection, while others did not?

Uninfected cystoscopy patients were used as a second control group, and comparison of the data pointed up yet another significant association: there was a marked difference between the groups of physicians who treated the cases and controls (Table 5-4). In this analysis, treatment by one group of urologists (group A) was associated with only two cases of infection, but these physicians treated 12 of the uninfected control patients. In contrast, infection occurred in 43 of 55 cystoscopy patients treated by the other group (group B) of urologists. Additional investigation revealed that the group having fewer cases disinfected cystoscopy instruments with glutaraldehyde, whereas the group with the higher attack rate preferred the use of an aqueous quaternary ammonium disinfectant. On culture, the quaternary ammonium disinfectant yielded the epidemic strain of *P. cepacia*.

This hypothetical example, based on an actual outbreak, illustrates that several control groups are often required to identify the susceptibility and exposure factors responsible for an outbreak of disease. It is also apparent that the epidemiologist selects each control group to test one or more specific hypotheses. A basic strategy for selecting control groups in a stepwise manner can now be described.

First, the epidemiologist should identify important host factors that influence susceptibility to infection. How, for example, do cases differ from other hospitalized patients in terms of age, sex, underlying disease, immune status, and antimicrobial therapy. Often it is not necessary to select a formal control group to evaluate some of these factors. If disease occurs only in neonates, it is not necessary to use a formal control group of the general hospital population to show that age is an important factor. It may be necessary, however, to compare gestational age,

TABLE 5-3. *Pseudomonas cepacia* urinary tract infection outbreak: exposures of cases and controls

| Patient category | Cases (%) | Controls (%) |
|---|---|---|
| Total patients | 50 | 84 |
| Exposed to urinary irrigation | 48 (96) | 80 (95) |
| Exposed to cystoscopy | 45 (90) | 24 (29) |

TABLE 5-4. *Pseudomonas cepacia* urinary tract infection outbreak: exposures to two physician groups, cystoscopy cases versus cystoscopy controls

| Patient category | Cystoscopy cases | Cystoscopy controls | Total exposed | Infection rates (%) |
|---|---|---|---|---|
| Total patients | 45 | 24 | 69 | — |
| Exposed to group A | 2 | 12 | 14 | 14 |
| Exposed to group B | 43 | 12 | 55 | 78 |

birth weight, or Apgar score of infected and uninfected infants.

Since susceptibility alone is not sufficient to explain infection (appropriate exposure to a pathogen is also required), one must next evaluate exposure factors. As with the case review, time, place, and person characteristics should be studied. In this phase of the investigation, susceptibility factors can be controlled by using patients in the control group with similar susceptibility factors; for example, if patients with disease are significantly older than control patients, subsequent control populations should be selected to contain an age distribution comparable to that found for cases. As another example, if patients with gastroenteritis due to *Salmonella* have a significantly higher occurrence of peptic ulcer disease, subsequent control groups should be selected to include a comparable proportion of patients with ulcer.

If all cases have a single susceptibility factor, all controls should have that factor. More commonly, several susceptibility factors occur in varying proportions and with varying degrees of statistical significance when case populations are compared with controls. To deal with this problem, the control populations should be stratified to ensure comparability. Age is one such susceptibility variable that is amenable to stratification. Table 5-5 shows the distribution of ages for hypothetical case and control populations. Although the patients with cases of disease

TABLE 5-5. Percentage distribution of patient ages: cases
of disease compared with random control population

| Age range (years) | Cases (%) | Controls (%) |
|---|---|---|
| Birrh–9 | 0 | 7 |
| 10–19 | 0 | 4 |
| 20–29 | 0 | 12 |
| 30–39 | 2 | 9 |
| 40–49 | 22 | 18 |
| 50–59 | 26 | 21 |
| 60–69 | 28 | 18 |
| 70–79 | 18 | 8 |
| 80 and over | 4 | 3 |

are significantly older than the patients in the control
population, young patients also have disease. To control for age adequately, subsequent control populations should be stratified to ensure that they have a
similar age distribution to the case group.

If an outbreak occurs during a discrete period, two
control populations are possible. First, uninfected patients hospitalized before or after the outbreak may
be compared with those with disease to identify significantly different exposures to people, procedures,
or other factors. Next, uninfected patients hospitalized during the epidemic period may be studied to
test whether these differences are important; that is,
if the differences remain, such exposures may be important.

Exposure to various hospital locations can be similarly examined. If hemodialysis patients with hepatitis B had a significantly higher exposure to a single
dialysis station than dialysis patients without hepatitis who were treated during the same period, the
dialysis station is implicated as potentially important.

Finally, exposures to personnel, other patients,
procedures, and medications should be evaluated. Using a control population that is similar to the case
group in terms of disease susceptibility and time and
place characteristics, the exposure to the infecting
pathogen should be found to occur significantly more
frequently among cases than controls.

This progressive use of multiple control populations, controlling at each step for previously identified significant factors, may seem tedious and ar-
duous. This description of the process, however,
overemphasizes the number of separate steps required. The steps listed separately can often be combined, for it is usually possible to evaluate several
time, place, and person exposures at the same time
by using the same carefully selected control group.
It must be recognized, however, that the process

described above should not be ignored lest the chance
of bias, with the resulting risk of deriving a faulty
conclusion, be introduced.

On rare occasions no difference in host susceptibility can be established on comparison of cases and
controls. This occurs most frequently when the infecting agent is quite virulent or when the portal of
infection is such that, on exposure, every patient
develops disease. Similarly, the case-control evaluation may fail to demonstrate significant differences
in exposures between infected and uninfected patients. Most commonly this occurs when there is
widespread or unrecognized infection in the control
population, when the disease results from endogenous
colonization present at the time of admission, or when
case records do not document the truly significant
exposure. Each of these possibilities must be evaluated with the prospective techniques described below.

Hospitalization itself can have a profound effect on
host susceptibility, and this can complicate the interpretation of case-control studies. As an illustration,
patients with lymphoma may have similar susceptibilities to infection at time of admission to the hospital. After treatment is initiated, however, their
susceptibilities are altered. If infected and uninfected
lymphoma patients are compared for host factors apparent at the time of their admission, no major differences in susceptibility may be apparent. To obtain
a clearer definition of susceptibility factors, it may
be necessary to compare these factors after a period
of hospitalization. In this example, the epidemiologist might calculate the average interval between the
time of admission and that of the onset of disease in
case patients and then compare the host characteristics of cases and controls at that point.

*Methods for selection of control groups.*   Before selecting the members of a control group, the epidemiologist must decide the number of control patients
required and the specific technique for determining
which uninfected patients will be selected.

The number of control patients required to show
differences between case and control patients depends
on a number of factors, including the relative frequencies with which the factor to be compared occurs
in each population and the statistical certainty required by the investigator in showing differences or
no differences. Statistical techniques are available for
estimating the size of control groups, but it is often
unnecessary to calculate the control group size precisely. If the factor to be compared occurs either very
frequently or very infrequently in patients with disease, one control patient for each case patient is usually sufficient; on the other hand, if the factor occurs
in approximately half of the case patients, several

control patients for each case are usually necessary. Almost always, at least one control patient for each case patient should be chosen.

Next, the epidemiologist must select a method to choose control patients. Individual control patients may be selected by including all in the pool of appropriate uninfected patients (a universal sample) or by taking a portion of that pool according to a sampling scheme.

When small populations are studied, all available controls may be required. If the potential pool of control patients is large, this universal sampling method is inefficient, since more control patients than are necessary will be evaluated. In such circumstances, matched, random, or stratified random-sampling schemes may be used.

A *matched sample* may be used when there are only a few general factors that must be controlled, such as age or date of hospitalization. With the matching procedure, each case patient is matched with one or more uninfected control patients according to specified matching characteristics. It is relatively easy to find an appropriate match when a single factor needs to be controlled. As the number of factors increases or the matching factors become quite specific (e.g., the type and duration of surgical procedure), matching becomes more difficult. Even if successful, large numbers of records of potential control patients must be reviewed and discarded to obtain each successful match.

A *random sample* does not require the tedious selection process used in developing a matched sample. Instead, the epidemiologist relies on the powerful effect of chance to ensure that a representative, nonbiased population is selected. Various randomization schemes are available, but the use of a random number table is probably simplest for the hospital epidemiologist. To use a random number table for selecting 20 patients from a pool of 200 potential controls, for example, each potential control is given a number between 001 and 200. The first 20 three-digit numbers found in the table that fall within the range 001 to 200 identify the patients to be selected. Other techniques have been used, such as using patient record numbers, selecting control patients admitted just before or after case patients, or selecting every *n*th patient (e.g., every fifth bacteremia case or every seventh admission). These systematic sampling methods may lead to nonrandom selection, however; for example, patients are neither admitted nor operated on randomly, few elective surgical patients are admitted on Saturdays, and more difficult surgical procedures are usually scheduled early in the day.

The random selection of control patients is most useful when one does not need to control for specific factors within the pool of patients available as controls. If there are no age, sex, or other susceptibility factors identified as important in an outbreak of wound infection following cardiac surgery, for example, one can quickly obtain an appropriate control group by randomly selecting uninfected patients who had cardiac surgery in the appropriate period.

How can a control population be selected if it is necessary to control for numerous factors such as age, sex, and type of operation? As noted, matching on these factors would be quite tedious, and furthermore, one might have difficulty finding control patients who match appropriately each case patient with regard to each factor. For this problem, a *stratified random sample* can be used. It is almost as convenient to select as a true random sample, and it allows almost the same degree of control over important variables as does the matching strategy. To draw a stratified random sample, the potential pool of control patients is divided into groups that correspond to the factors that must be controlled. Then, from each group, a separate random sample is chosen. To illustrate, consider the need to control for the type of operation when 50 percent of case patients had cholecystectomy, 30 percent had herniorrhaphy, and 20 percent had chest surgery. Potential control patients would be divided into groups according to the type of surgery. The epidemiologist would then select, with a separate random pick, half of the controls from the cholecystectomy group, 30 percent from the herniorrhaphy group, and the remainder from the chest-surgery group.

*Analysis of case-control data.*   The frequencies of various susceptibility and exposure factors among cases and controls are tabulated. All differences between the two groups are considered potentially important. When possible, statistical techniques should be used to calculate the probabilities that the observed differences could have occurred by chance. Statistically significant differences are highly suggestive, but of course the presence or absence of statistical significance does not prove or disprove causation.

The case-control study may not provide the solution for a problem. Under such circumstances, other epidemiologic techniques—such as a cohort study or a prospective intervention study—may be employed.

*Cohort study.*   A cohort study may be conducted prospectively or retrospectively (see Chapter 1). For the investigation of nosocomial infection problems, a retrospective cohort study is seldom useful, since case-control techniques are generally more powerful.

If, however, a case-control review fails to solve a problem because the data available retrospectively are inadequate or, as noted in the next section, it is necessary to confirm the results of the case-control study, then a defined high-risk population (the cohort) may be identified and followed prospectively. Necessary clinical and laboratory observations can then be made. After a period of time, differences in susceptibility or host factors among ill and well patients may become apparent that will identify the source of the infection problem.

Rarely is a cohort study conducted independently of a restrospective case-control study. Usually, the case-control study is used to narrow the list of hypotheses and to identify the high-risk populations that are studied prospectively.

*Prospective intervention study.* The prospective trial (an experimental epidemiologic study), like the cohort study, is rarely used primarily in studying nosocomial infection problems (see Chapter 1). It also usually grows out of the findings of a retrospective case-control study. Here, a hypothesis is tested experimentally by intervening with specific measures to correct a presumed infection problem and measuring the impact of that intervention on infection rates. When feasible, such trials should be controlled; that is, the intervention should be applied to one segment of the population at risk but not to a comparable group of control patients. Only by comparing disease risk in the treated group versus the control group can one reliably interpret the results of such a trial.

Illustrations of the ways that uncontrolled trials have been misleading are legion and fall into several broad groups. First, disease occurrence may decline independently of the intervention; without a control group, the drop in infection rate may inappropriately be attributed to a beneficial effect of the intervention. Of course, it is also possible that the treatment regimen may be harmful; again, the use of an untreated control group allows documentation of this effect. It is also possible that an intervention may be beneficial but fail to alter the observed disease risk in the treated population. This might occur if the benefit were offset by some new event that independently increased the disease risk. When a control group is used for comparison, disease risk would also increase more in the untreated population, therby indicating benefit in the treated group. Of course, there are situations in which a controlled trial is difficult to justify; this occurs, for example, when the disease under study is very serious and when the intervention measures are highly likely to be useful. Even in these circumstances, however, a controlled trial should be strongly considered for the reasons outlined.

*Microbiologic study.* It is a common mistake, when an infection problem is first investigated, to obtain large numbers of microbiologic cultures. As noted earlier, some carefully selected culture specimens may be obtained from persons or the inanimate environment if they will not be available later because of the institution of control measures. It must be stressed, however, that such surveys should supplement the epidemiologic investigation, not direct it. Furthermore, the cultures should be obtained only from sites that are likely to be epidemiologically relevant.

Beginning epidemiologists at CDC are cautioned, only partly in jest, that if the epidemiologic and laboratory data disagree, they should disregard the laboratory data. This advice may seem radical, especially to those who consider laboratory data to be "hard" and real and who view statistical and epidemiologic data as "soft" and speculative. The above advice, however, is valuable for several reasons.

First, the isolation of a microorganism by itself rarely explains the occurrence of a disease. The hospital is not a sterile environment, and viable, pathogenic microorganisms may be isolated from most hospital locations. As one example, large numbers of personnel are often colonized by the epidemic strain during a staphylococcal outbreak. However, these personnel are often, like the affected patients, victims of the outbreak rather than its causes. Similar arguments can be made about isolation of microorganisms from sink drains, floors, air, or whatever. Unless there is an epidemiologic link between the source of the isolate and the occurrence of patient disease, the mere isolation of a microorganism, even of an epidemic strain, may mean little.

Second, the failure to isolate a microorganism from a presumed source or reservoir does not vindicate that site. The culture determinations may be negative because they were improperly collected or processed, because adequate technologic procedures were not available for primary isolation, or because too few specimen samples were obtained. This last possibility is dramatically illustrated by the outbreaks of disease caused by contaminated, commercially supplied intravenous medications. In several of these outbreaks contamination had occurred in a very small proportion of individual units (approximately one in 5000 to 10,000 units in some outbreaks), and many negative culture specimens were processed before the first positive result was obtained. If the epidemiologic data had not strongly implicated intrinsic contamination of such fluids, extensive culturing could not have been justified and would not have been undertaken. With direction provided by the epidemiologic findings, however, examinations continued until positive results were obtained.

As another example, several outbreaks of group-A streptococcal surgical wound infections have been traced to medical personnel who had negative pharyngeal culture specimens for group-A streptococci. Because of the epidemiologic association of the disease with these persons, extensive examinations were conducted, and asymptomatic anal carriage of the epidemic strain was documented. The initial failure to isolate a strain does not discredit the epidemiologic findings; instead, it requires that both the epidemiologic and microbiologic techniques be reevaluated.

INSTITUTE AND EVALUATE CONTROL MEASURES As soon as the explanation for a nosocomial infection problem is found, control measures should be vigorously applied. These control measures may be used to confirm the validity of that explanation. The effectiveness of such control measures should be evaluated by continued surveillance for disease and, if necessary, by prospective study.

EVALUATE OTHER HOSPITAL PRACTICES A thorough epidemiologic investigation of a nosocomial infection problem often leads to improved infection control practices not only in the areas where the problem occurred but also throughout the hospital. An outbreak of disease might be considered to be an experiment of nature; that is, the factors that permit epidemic infections to occur are often responsible for endemic infections as well. Investigations of UTIs caused by multiply-drug-resistant Enterobacteriaceae, for example, have documented that many of these infections are transmitted by way of personnel from infected, catheterized patients to neighboring patients who are also catheterized. It is highly likely that infections with other microorganisms are also transmitted by this mechanism, but the mode is more difficult to recognize if common pathogens are involved. Thus measures to control the spread of an epidemic strain may also be expected to control the spread of other strains. The epidemiologist should therefore review practices and procedures throughout the hospital when an epidemiologic study is completed and should institute reasonable control or preventive measures throughout the institution. Hospital personnel should be informed about the investigation and its results.

*Responsibilities for Dissemination of Information*
Hospitals are an integral part of larger communities, and their personnel and patients come from and return to that community. Infection problems in the community influence the hospital, and, conversely, infection problems within the hospital may be spread to the community by patients or personnel. Because of this intimate association between the community and the hospital, the institution's infection control personnel must cooperate with local public health authorities by reporting and assisting in the investigation of problems.

Each hospital is also a part of the larger community of other hospitals. Patients may be transferred from one institution to another and carry their infections with them. Accordingly, frank and frequent exchanges of information between hospitals are important. Although each hospital has its unique practices and policies, a problem in one institution may also be a problem in other hospitals that have the same practices. Thus the results of epidemiologic investigations should be disseminated widely. Finally, hospitals may be affected by outbreaks caused by a contaminated common vehicle that is commercially available to other institutions. When problems with such products are discovered, the hospital epidemiologist has the responsibility to notify promptly not only the manufacturer or distributor of the product, but also the appropriate public health authorities. Local and state health authorities, the FDA, and the CDC cooperate closely in monitoring and attempting to control the contamination of such products, and if such a problem is suspected, these agencies should be notified immediately.

*Administrative Aspects*
An epidemiologic investigation requires vigorous action by hospital personnel. Because of this, each hospital should have an administrative structure that will allow uninhibited investigation of infection problems. The requirements are several.

First, the hospital must have access to someone trained and interested in hospital epidemiology. Often responsibilities for infection control are delegated to an infection control team composed of one or more infection control nurses and a physician hospital epidemiologist (see Chapter 2). This team should be given adequate resources to conduct investigations. Their continuing education should be supported. Sufficient time should be set aside in advance and adequate financial backing must be available to support investigations. The infection control team should have the administrative authority to conduct efficient and wide-range investigations and should specifically have the authority to evaluate patients, take appropriate culture specimens from patients and personnel, and consult with outside experts. That administrative authority must also provide a mechanism that allows the team to make emergency decisions when an infection problem threatens the health and safety of patients and personnel.

Most important, the infection control effort must have adequate support from other departments in the hospital. The microbiology laboratory must maintain the ability to process the specimens required for an epidemiologic investigation, and laboratory personnel should be able to serve as expert consultants in selecting the appropriate microbiologic and serologic techniques required in these investigations (see Chapter 7). The hospital's engineering and housekeeping departments must be ready to provide consultation regarding environmental control. Nursing services must work with the infection control program in conducting epidemiologic studies as well as in applying control measures. Finally, the infection control program must have the wholehearted support and assistance of the medical staff. If the infection control effort takes place without the interest or support of other personnel in the hospital, little can be accomplished.

## REFERENCES

1. Benenson, A. S. (Ed.). *Control of Communicable Diseases in Man* (14th ed.). New York: American Public Health Association, 1985, p. 363.
2. Stamm, W. E., Weinstein, R. A., and Dixon, R. E. Comparison of Endemic and Epidemic Nosocomial Infections. In Dixon, R. E., (Ed.), *Nosocomial Infections*. New York: Yorke Medical Books, 1975, pp. 9–13.
3. Center for Disease Control. Follow-up smallpox—Federal Republic of Germany. *Morbid. Mortal. Weekly Rep.* 19:234, 1970. (Adapted from World Health Organization. Smallpox surveillance. *Weekly Epidemiol. Rec.* 45:249, 1970.)

# 6 STATISTICAL CONSIDERATIONS FOR ANALYSIS OF NOSOCOMIAL INFECTION DATA

Stanley M. Martin

Data that have been collected in a study of nosocomial infections must be reduced from observations on every included patient to summary statistics describing particular groups of patients. While culture results or other information about one or two patients can be important in understanding the cause of infection, information from more patients is needed to determine which of several potentially important factors contributed to the infection. A transition from clinical diagnosis of illness in a single patient to understanding illness in populations of patients must underlie the study of nosocomial infections; the physician's diagnosis of illness in single patients must change to the statistical "diagnosis" of illness in the population of patients.

This chapter describes some basic statistical considerations for understanding nosocomial infection data from the collection phase through the interpretation. Several study-design considerations are presented as reminders of necessary precursors of a good study. Among these, control group selection by either an independent or matched procedure influences which statistical test should be used in the analysis. Emphasis is placed on data collection procedures because of the need for careful definition of data to be collected and as much standardization of the collection process as possible. Finally, a scheme for choosing appropriate significance tests is presented.

## DATA COLLECTION

In many epidemiologic studies the failure of investigators to reach conclusions frequently is attributable to the collection of data with little or no previous planning of the objectives of the study, what data should be collected to achieve the objectives, what populations should be studied, the best locations in the hospital to find the data, who will record the data, and what period should be covered. In the investigation of possible outbreaks of a particular infection type, the investigator should also consider whether it is necessary to extend the scope of investigation beyond the inpatient population of the hospital to the outpatient department, beyond the primary hospital of interest to other hospitals of a similar type or in the same location, or beyond hospitals to the community.

Studies of nosocomial infections previously have involved the collection of data from personal interviews, patient examinations, patient chart reviews, laboratory records, personnel health clinic records, or autopsy data. These sources of data, singly or in combination with one another, continue to provide reliable information for many hospitals. However, the proliferation of computing equipment in the management of patient-related data in hospitals is offering a source of more easily obtainable data for investigating nosocomial infections. The investigator of nosocomial infections should learn about the administrative processes within the hospital that can generate useful "machine-readable" patient records. For example, admissions office personnel may enter demographic data and admitting diagnoses on all patients via a computer terminal or keypunched record. Other hospital locations such as the pharmacy and various laboratories may generate additional records that arrive in the central computer area for the same patients. Medical procedures, operations, diagnoses, and costs may be entered into the computer system from still other sources, possibly for billing purposes; discharge diagnoses and other information may be added as well see Chapter 4).

Although these records are potentially a valuable resource in hospitals having well-planned computer systems, it is doubtful that most physicians and nursing personnel are aware of the availability and completeness of these computer records. These can be available with relatively little work beyond determining from administrative personnel, the accounting office, laboratories, and pharmacy what data are part of the hospital computer system, and from the computer center how to gain access to the needed data. Preliminary inquiries of this kind can offer the potential for larger and better controlled studies because of less cost and time in the data collection phase.

## CONTROL GROUPS

Little information about the association of any factor that may predispose a patient to infection can be gained by studying only a group of patients who have been exposed to the factor. Similarly, studying cases only is descriptive but may not lead to assessment of risks associated with a factor. For example, an attempt to study the association of excisional surgical wound infections caused by *Staphylococcus aureus* with operations by a particular surgeon will be of limited benefit unless a suitable comparison group is also studied. The surgeon performing the operation may be only one of several factors that can potentially influence the risk of incisional infections. Therefore, a suitable control group should include patients receiving the same operation from another surgeon or patients receiving the operation from any of the entire surgical staff performing operations in the hospital other than the suspect surgeon. The control group should include patients expected to be like the infected group with respect to all known possible risk factors except for the surgeon performing the operation. Differences in infection rates between the control group and the group receiving the operation from the suspect surgeon could then be associated with this surgeon.

Studies of this kind can be successfully controlled within a hospital because both exposed and nonexposed patients are present. However, the study of association of infection with the use of a particular, possibly contaminated, product or apparatus may require a multihospital study or an "intervention" study within a single hospital. It would be impossible to study the association of pneumonia with cleaning techniques of respiratory therapy equipment within a single hospital if the hospital's policy dictates one particular cleaning technique for all such apparatus. This is because no control group would be available, unless for purposes of the study the policy could be changed for at least a portion of the equipment. Intervention in the hospital policy regarding the cleaning of respiratory therapy equipment would allow the investigator to design a study to compare pneumonia rates between a group of patients using respiratory therapy equipment cleaned in the usual way and a group of patients using the same type of equipment during the same period but cleaned by a different technique. Of course intervention studies of this kind should be preceded by careful attention to ethical concerns for the welfare of the patient.

Even though patients can be stratified into groups according to exposure or nonexposure to the factor under consideration, comparability of the patients included in each group must be ensured. The underlying risks of patients for acquiring the infection under study can differ drastically even without considering exposure to a single factor. For example, patients with a particular diagnosis may be immunosuppressed and more susceptible to infection. Other factors such as catheterization, exposure to respiratory therapy equipment, prophylactic or therapeutic antibiotics, and intravenous fluids can predispose patients to a greater risk of infection. A well-designed study will attempt to balance the patients in the control and study groups with respect to such known factors that can alter the patients' risk to infection. This may require that control patients be matched to the study patients on these factors. The objective, whether control patients are selected by an independent selection process or matched to the study patients, is to remove the effect of underlying factors that might mask or exaggerate the effect of a particular factor under study.

Multihospital studies require more than a single "study" hospital and a single "control" hospital. Generally it is not reasonable to expect many of the same potentially important, but not necessarily obvious, factors to emerge in any two hospitals. Studies involving more than one hospital must include adequate numbers of hospitals in both the study group and the control group. Factors such as number of beds, hospital policies, ratio of staff to patients, patient characteristics, numbers of discharges, and hospital type must be considered in selecting suitable study and control groups of hospitals. The scope of this chapter is limited to studies within a single hospital to avoid lengthy discussions of the sampling problems and other statistical problems accompanying multihospital studies.

## SUMMARY STATISTICS

When confronted with pages of written observations on infected and noninfected patients, little can be learned about the association between infection and a factor under study until an appropriate summary statistic is found to describe a "typical" value of the factor for the whole group. For example, the proportion of patients who became infected shortly after urinary catheterization can be compared with the proportion of a similar group of patients who were not catheterized and became infected. The proportion summarizes the infection experience in each of the two groups, catheterized and noncatheterized patients. It relates the number of infected patients to the total number at risk of becoming infected in the two groups. The "at risk" population usually includes all patients exposed to a factor or combination of factors. It can include all patients admitted or discharged (e.g., "exposed" to the hospital or a particular service) during a particular period, only patients with a particular diagnosis, or only patients who received a particular procedure or drug.

The actual number of patients "at risk" may be the best available denominator; however, some investigators can measure the "at risk" portion of the summary statistic in terms of the actual duration that each patient was potentially exposed to risk. This can be the number of days hospitalized, number of hours with inserted catheter, or other time of exposure. If the numerator represents the number of patients with a particular infection, the investigator should subtract from the "at risk" period in the denominator the total time patients were exposed after they were in-

fected, since exposure while a patient is infected contributes no additional risk. However, this additional exposure should be included in the denominator, if the numerator represents the number of episodes for infections for each patient.

The numerator of the summary statistic also can be formed in different ways. A single patient may experience more than one infection episode due to the same organism. In this case one must decide whether these patients have had a recurrence of infection from the initial organism or a reinfection with the same organism. If multiple infections occur, the summary statistic can be a count of the total number of infections relative to the total number of patients for whom the numerator was counted. This statistic would be the average number of infections per patient. Decisions about the association of a particular factor with infection can usually be made using the number of infected patients for the numerator and the number of patients at risk (or patient-time exposure) for the denominator.

## STUDY DESIGN

Proportions or other summary statistics are obtained to decide whether hospitalized patients exposed to the factor under consideration are at higher risk of infection than patients who are not exposed to the factor. A significance test is used to determine the probability that a difference as large as the observed difference between the two proportions could have occurred by chance. A small probability of chance occurrence of a difference as large as the observed difference leads the observer to conclude that patients exposed to the factor are likely to be at higher risk of infection. The question then becomes, "How small should the probability be so that a conclusion associating infection with the factor is correct?" In fact there are two probabilities of primary concern in significance testing [12]; these are stated below as questions for the investigator of nosocomial infections:

*Type 1.* Given that there actually is *no difference* between the proportion of patients infected among thoses exposed to the factor and the proportion of patients infected among those not exposed to the factor, what is the probability that the particular samples of patients observed in this study would indicate a *difference* by chance?

*Type 2.* Given that there actually is a *difference* between the proportion of patients infected among those exposed to the factor and the proportion of patients infected among those not exposed to the factor, what is the probability that the particular samples of patients observed in this study would indicate *no difference* by chance?

These two probabilities of error form the basis for decisions from significance tests and are determined by the investigator in the planning stage of the study. A summary of the major steps leading to significance testing for the difference between proportions is presented below. All these should be considered in planning studies of nosocomial infections.

### State Hypothesis to be Tested and Alternative Hypothesis

As an example, the hypothesis that there is no difference between the proportions versus the hypothesis that there is a difference between the proportions can be written as

$H_0: P_E = P_{NE}$

$AH: P_E \neq P_{NE}$ ,

where $P_E$ and $P_{NE}$ are the proportions infected in the exposed and nonexposed groups, respectively. $H_0$, the "null" hypothesis, states that the proportion infected in the exposed group is the same as the proportion infected in the nonexposed group. AH, the alternative hypothesis, states that the proportion infected in the exposed group is not the same as the proportion infected in the nonexposed group. Because the alternative hypothesis does not state the direction of the difference (and would be favored whether $P_E$ were significantly greater than or significantly less than $P_{NE}$), significance tests used to test these hypotheses must consider differences in both directions. These are called 2-tailed tests and are generally useful when the investigator does not know before the data are collected whether to expect exposure to the factor to increase or diminish the patients' risk of infection. When the investigator has reason to believe that exposure to the factor would increase (or decrease) the patients' risk of infection, a 1-tailed test should be used. The hypotheses may be stated as

$H_0: P_E \leq P_{NE}$

$AH: P_E > P_{NE}$

In this case the null hypothesis, $H_0$, states that $P_E$ is less than or equal to $P_{NE}$, while the alternative hypothesis, AH, states that $P_E$ is greater than $P_{NE}$. This is a directional difference because the investigator expects exposure to increase the patient's risk of infection, if a difference exists at all. Considering

the purpose of studies of infection outbreaks within the hospital, one must conclude that 1-tailed tests of significance are generally appropriate.

### State Desired Probability Levels for Type-1 and Type-2 Errors

These probabilities are not based on statistical computations but on the investigator's willingness to chance an error of either kind. Stating the type-2 error indirectly states another probability that is also important in determining how likely the study is to succeed. This probability, defined by

$p = (1 - \text{type-2 error})$,

is called the power of the test. $p$ is the probability that, if a difference actually exists (i.e., that the alternative hypothesis is true), the significance test will reject the null hypothesis in favor of the alternative hypothesis. The power of the test is used in initial planning of the study to ensure an adequate study size to achieve the objectives.

### Determine Study Design to Achieve Desired Objective

A primary consideration in study design is that of deciding whether the study and control groups should be selected independently or whether patients selected for the control group should be matched on certain variables to patients in the study group. That is, for each study patient one or more control patients could be selected to match the study patient on factors determined ahead of time. Many studies of nosocomial infections have required that patients be matched on factors such as age, sex, underlying diagnoses, and predisposing therapeutic factors for validity. In outbreak investigations, it may not be possible to know the specific factors that should be studied; therefore, the study population may consist of all patients who were infected and the control population may include patients who were like the infected patients but were not infected. The proportion exposed to particular factors would then be determined from samples of each of these two populations. Whether patients are matched or unmatched, most studies of nosocomial infection outbreaks involve comparisons of these proportions. The single direction hypotheses would be written as

$H_0: P_I \leq P_{NI}$

$AH: P_I > P_{NI}$ ,

where $P_I$ and $P_{NI}$ are the proportions exposed to the factor under study in the infected and noninfected groups of patients, respectively. Study design must include consideration of study size. This should be based on the requirements to test certain hypotheses or estimate certain parameters and to achieve predetermined error probability levels. Sometimes the size of the study is limited by the time or resources available. In this case it should be understood that a low power or large type-2 error may be associated with the study because inadequate sample sizes are involved, and a decision must be made about the value of doing the study under these circumstances. Approaches to determining sample size requirements for testing the difference between two proportions often involve approximation formulas that can be programmed relatively easily [16].

## Plan Data Collection Procedures and Train Data Collectors

A main consideration in planning the study is the choice of personnel to collect the data. Deciding whether a patient is infected requires a level of medical knowledge that may be beyond that of a secretary or clerical person. Regardless of who the data collectors are, they must be given standard procedures for deciding about each data item such as the case definition. Some verification of the data collection process should be planned to avoid problems such as drifting away from established procedures, misunderstanding procedures, inability to follow procedures, and random errors. Too often inadequate attention is given to quality of data collection because data checking and editing require extra "trouble" for the investigator. Often it is tempting to assume good data quality when the data are collected as computer records. When this happens, the study can become a victim of poor or misleading data instead of contributing valuable information for control of nosocomial infections. Decisions about data handling must be planned in advance to avoid delays. If computer records are involved, coordination with a programmer or other computer personnel is necessary before the study begins.

## Collect Data and Begin Data Processing

One early consideration in study design is the data collection instrument. Designing the form with the intention to use present computer technology requires knowledge of computer input mechanisms and coding schemes that can be used. A common tendency is to ask for too much data on a form, but a well-planned study will pare down the questionnaire to include the important questions only. Simplicity for understanding, recording data, and tabulating is the key to a successful data collection document. Data

processing may involve no more than hand tabulation, but it can involve detailed computer programs for sophisticated analyses. Realizing beforehand that substantial time of nursing staff or other personnel may be required in both the collection and processing phases, and planning for this, can avoid overburdening these people at what may be an inopportune time.

## Perform Analysis and Report Results

A common error of an investigator heading a study is to spend unlimited effort collecting data, but to allow only a very short time for the analysis. However, analyses must take into account all the design considerations, hypotheses to be tested, and level of measurement of the data. Enough analysis time should be allocated to understand thoroughly what the data say. Simply summarizing findings with "$p$ values" is usually an indication that the data have not been thoroughly analyzed. Studies planned to meet some types of objectives can begin with examination of the stated hypotheses, followed by determination of other features of the data that support the conclusions. However, the analysis of data from nosocomial infection outbreaks can require a different approach. Usually there is not a single hypothesis to be tested, and the study objective for infection outbreak data is to determine which factors increase the patients' risk of infection. One approach is to test several factors, looking for an association of any factor with infection. When this procedure is used and the seemingly important factors tested, attention must be given to the effect of multiple significance testing on the overall type-1 error. One way to compensate for several significance tests is to set the type-1 error probability for each test low enough to yield a specified type-1 error over all tests. For example, if it is desired to perform $k$ tests with an overall type-1 error of $\alpha$, then the type-1 error for each test could be set approximately to

$$A = \frac{\alpha}{k}$$

where $A$ is the approximate significance level for each year [11].

## SIGNIFICANCE TESTING

Before presenting directions for choosing a significance test for a particular study, it is necessary to mention briefly two statistical terms. Significance tests can be separated into two categories—*parametric* and *nonparametric*. Use of parametric statistics requires assumptions about the parent population from which the study samples were drawn. For example, observations of urine output volume on a sample of infected patients could be assumed to have come from a population of urine output volumes that were normally distributed around a mean, $\mu$, and variance, $\sigma^2$. Because the assumption is made that these values are normally distributed, the significance testing procedure involves a parametric test. On the other hand, if one is not willing to make assumptions about the parameters of the parent distribution, one may choose a nonparametric test.

The parametric test is usually preferred as long as it is reasonable to make the assumptions for it, because there is an associated gain in power. Although the loss of power accompanying the use of a nonparametric test can be substantial, some of the nonparametric tests actually offer power comparable to parametric tests. When both parametric and nonparametric tests are presented in this chapter, the power of the nonparametric test is reasonably close to that of the corresponding parametric test; the tests mentioned here are commonly used in the analysis of nosocomial infection data.

The decision of which of the many statistical tests to use requires, in addition to thought about the hypotheses and study design, consideration of the level of measurement of the observations. For the sake of simplicity, the discussion in this chapter of level of measurement will be limited to two classifications, *attributes* and *measurements*. Usually data collected on nosocomial infections involve answers to questions such as

Was the patient infected or not infected?
Was the patient exposed or not exposed?
Was the change in a measurement positive or negative?

Attribute responses—yes or no, plus or minus, zero or one—simply give the direction of differences, while measurement data—height, weight, blood sugar level—give the direction and magnitude of the differences. The scheme shown in Figure 6-1 for selecting an appropriate test takes into account the issues mentioned above and should help the investigator choose a significance test by making three simple choices [8]. This scheme uses a partial list of tests and is not intended to limit broader choices that are available [15].

Two sets of data will be used to illustrate the test procedures listed in Figure 6-1. First, assuming that the samples were selected independently, the tests listed for independent samples will be illustrated.

Next the tests listed for matched samples will be illustrated, using the assumption that the same samples were selected with control (noninfected) patients matched to study (infected) patients.

*Example 1—Attribute data.* Suppose 100 patients on the general medicine service acquired *Escherichia coli* urinary tract infections during a six-month period. A sample of 30 of these patients is randomly selected to determine whether the infection is associated with urinary catheterization. A control group of 30 noninfected patients is selected from among all other patients on the general medicine service during the same six-month period. The status of patients in each group with respect to catheterization is presented in Table 6-1.

*Example 2—Measurement data.* Suppose times from admission to onset of *E. coli* urinary tract infection for the 30 infected patients and times from admission to discharge of the 30 noninfected patients from example 1 are observed to determine whether infection occurred at about the time the patients who were infected would have been discharged if they had not been infected. The time in hours observed for each patient is given in Table 6-2.

The examples will be used first to illustrate the tests employed when the samples of infected and noninfected persons are independently selected. Since studies of nosocomial infection outbreaks usually involve 1-tailed tests, the tests illustrated here, except for the chi-square tests, will be 1-tailed.

The observations from example 1 can be summarized into a 2 × 2 table to determine if there is an association of catheters with infection. A high proportion (22/30) of infected patients and a low proportion (5/30) of noninfected patients were catheterized (Table 6-3). The purpose of the significance test of these data is to determine whether the proportion catheterized was significantly larger among infected patients ($P_I$) than among noninfected patients ($P_{NI}$). The single-direction hypotheses can be stated as

$H_0: P_I \leq P_{NI}$

$AH: P_I > P_{NI}$

### Fisher's Exact Test

Fisher's Exact test [4] computes the probability of occurrence of the observed arrangement of the data in Table 6-3 plus the probability of occurrence of all other arrangements more divergent than the observed data in the direction of the alternative hypothesis, subject to the condition that all marginal totals of

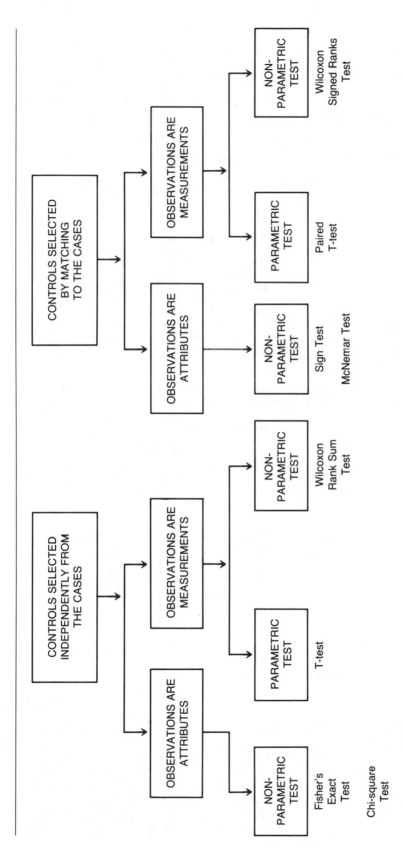

FIG. 6-1. Scheme for selecting an appropriate significance test. (From Martin, S. M. Choosing the Correct Statistical Tests. In R. P. Wenzel (Ed.), *Handbook of Hospital Acquired Infections.* Boca Raton, Fla.: CRC Press, 1981.)

TABLE 6-1. Catheterization status of patients on general medicine service (example 1)

| Infected patients | | | | | | Noninfected patients | | | | | |
|---|---|---|---|---|---|---|---|---|---|---|---|
| Pt. no. | Cath. | No cath. | Pt. no. | Cath. | No cath. | Pt. no. | Cath. | No cath. | Pt. no. | Cath. | No cath. |
| 1. | X | | 16. | X | | 1. | | X | 16. | | X |
| 2. | X | | 17. | X | | 2. | | X | 17. | | X |
| 3. | X | | 18. | X | | 3. | | X | 18. | | X |
| 4. | | X | 19. | X | | 4. | X | | 19. | | X |
| 5. | X | | 20. | X | | 5. | | X | 20. | X | |
| 6. | | X | 21. | X | | 6. | | X | 21. | | X |
| 7. | | X | 22. | X | | 7. | | X | 22. | | X |
| 8. | | X | 23. | | X | 8. | | X | 23. | | X |
| 9. | X | | 24. | X | | 9. | | X | 24. | | X |
| 10. | X | | 25. | | X | 10. | | X | 25. | X | |
| 11. | X | | 26. | X | | 11. | | X | 26. | | X |
| 12. | | X | 27. | X | | 12. | X | | 27. | | X |
| 13. | X | | 28. | X | | 13. | | X | 28. | | X |
| 14. | | X | 29. | X | | 14. | | X | 29. | | X |
| 15. | X | | 30. | X | | 15. | X | | 30. | | X |

Pt. no. = patient number; Cath. = catheterization.

TABLE 6-2. Intervals of exposure to the hospital for infected and noninfected patients (example 2)

| Time in hours from admission to onset of infection (infected patients) | | | | Time in hours from admission to discharge (noninfected patients) | | | |
|---|---|---|---|---|---|---|---|
| Pt. no. | Hrs. | Pt. no. | Hrs. | Pt. no. | Hrs. | Pt. no. | Hrs. |
| 1. | 216 | 16. | 234 | 1. | 253 | 16. | 242 |
| 2. | 187 | 17. | 205 | 2. | 82 | 17. | 233 |
| 3. | 88 | 18. | 136 | 3. | 125 | 18. | 133 |
| 4. | 280 | 19. | 253 | 4. | 138 | 19. | 342 |
| 5. | 310 | 20. | 165 | 5. | 137 | 20. | 102 |
| 6. | 239 | 21. | 340 | 6. | 116 | 21. | 93 |
| 7. | 344 | 22. | 325 | 7. | 232 | 22. | 82 |
| 8. | 315 | 23. | 178 | 8. | 327 | 23. | 248 |
| 9. | 280 | 24. | 153 | 9. | 171 | 24. | 113 |
| 10. | 293 | 25. | 355 | 10. | 338 | 25. | 294 |
| 11. | 200 | 26. | 338 | 11. | 335 | 26. | 304 |
| 12. | 229 | 27. | 77 | 12. | 109 | 27. | 211 |
| 13. | 208 | 28. | 335 | 13. | 126 | 28. | 104 |
| 14. | 233 | 29. | 261 | 14. | 182 | 29. | 261 |
| 15. | 190 | 30. | 93 | 15. | 247 | 30. | 269 |

Pt. no. = patient number.

the tables remain fixed. The formula for computing the test probability for each derived table can be stated in terms of the cell values given in Table 6-4. The probability of the observed arrangement for each table is computed by

$$p_k = \frac{(a + b)! \, (c + d)! \, (a + c)! \, (b + d)!}{a! \, b! \, c! \, d! \, n!},$$

where $p_{k=0}$ is the probability computed for the observed table, $p_{k=1}$ is the probability computed for the next most divergent table, and so on, until the probabilities for all such tables are computed. The next most divergent tables can be generated easily by successively adding 1 to the "$a$" and "$d$" cells while subtracting 1 from the "$b$" and "$c$" cells, when the data are arranged as shown in Table 6-4. Note that

TABLE 6-3. Catheterization status of infected and noninfected patients (example 1)

|  | Infected | Noninfected | Total |
|---|---|---|---|
| Catheter | 22 | 5 | 27 |
| No catheter | 8 | 25 | 33 |
| Total | 30 | 30 | 60 |

TABLE 6-4. General table for summarizing the association of a factor with infection

|  | Infected | Noninfected | Total |
|---|---|---|---|
| Catheter | $a$ | $b$ | $a + b$ |
| No Catheter | $c$ | $d$ | $c + d$ |
| Total | $a + c$ | $b + d$ | $n$ |

this procedure leaves the marginal totals unchanged, a requirement for this test. The probability is computed for each successive table and the final probability is determined by summing these.

$$p_0 = \frac{27! \; 33! \; 30! \; 30!}{22! \; 5! \; 8! \; 25! \; 60!} = .0000094776297$$

$$p_1 = \frac{27! \; 33! \; 30! \; 30!}{23! \; 4! \; 7! \; 26! \; 60!} = .0000006339551$$

$$p_2 = \frac{27! \; 33! \; 30! \; 30!}{24! \; 3! \; 6! \; 27! \; 60!} = .0000000273931$$

$$p_3 = \frac{27! \; 33! \; 30! \; 30!}{25! \; 2! \; 5! \; 28! \; 60!} = .0000000007044$$

$$p_4 = \frac{27! \; 33! \; 30! \; 30!}{26! \; 1! \; 4! \; 29! \; 60!} = .0000000000093$$

$$p_5 = \frac{27! \; 33! \; 30! \; 30!}{27! \; 0! \; 3! \; 30! \; 60!} = .0000000000013$$

$$p_{Tot} = .00001014$$

Because the total probability ($p_{Tot} = .00001014$) is small (less than .05), the conclusion is that there is an increased risk of infection among catheterized patients in this hospital.

It is important to note that the 2-tailed probability for testing the hypotheses,

$H_0: P_I = P_{NI}$

$AH: P_I \neq P_{NI}$,

can be computed by repeating the computations for the opposite direction, determining the appropriate tables for the other tail of the test. This is accomplished by determining the probabilities for tables for which the proportion of catheterized patients is lower in the infected group than in the noninfected group subject to the condition that the marginal totals remain fixed (i.e., the total numbers of infected and noninfected patients is kept constant). Then the second tail of the test is computed by summing the probabilities for all tables in the second direction that have probabilities less than or equal to the probability for the observed table. The probability for the 2-tailed test would then be found by summing the probabilities for each of the 2 tails. When the number of infected patients sampled, $n_I$, is equal to the number of noninfected patients sampled, $n_{NI}$, simply doubling the probability for 1 tail will produce the 2-tailed probability [9].

*Chi-Square for Independent Samples*
Computations for the Fisher's Exact test are tedious without the assistance of a programmable calculator or computer. Chi-square is a suitable approximation when the expected cell frequencies of the 2 × 2 table are sufficiently large. Some authors [16] have recommended that the approximation is inadequate if the total sample size, $n = n_I + n_{NI}$, is less than 20 or if the total sample size is between 20 and 40 with one or more expected cell frequencies as small as 5. Chi-square is a test of independence of the factor and infection, or equivalently, a test of the hypotheses,

$H_0: P_I = P_{NI}$

$AH: P_I \neq P_{NI}$

A simple computational formula makes this test easy to compute:

$$\chi^2 = \frac{(n) \times \left( |ad - bc| - \frac{n_I + n_{NI}}{2} \right)^2}{(a + b)(c + d)(a + c)(b + d)}$$

$$= \frac{(60) \times \left( |22 \times 25 - 8 \times 5| - \frac{60}{2} \right)^2}{27 \times 33 \times 30 \times 30}$$

$$= \frac{13824000}{801900}$$

$$= 17.239$$

This value is greater than the tabulated value of the chi-square distribution (readily available in standard statistical tables) corresponding to a significance level (type-1 error) of 0.05 ($\chi^2 = 3.84$). Therefore, the test leads to the conclusion that $P_I = P_{NI}$, or that infection is not independent of catheterization.

## t-test

Here example 2 will be used to illustrate two tests for measurement data. The assumption that time intervals were sampled from a normal distribution of time intervals permits use of the $t$-test. This is a parametric test of the difference between two means from independent samples. The hypotheses can be written as follows:

$H_0$: $\mu_I \leq \mu_{NI}$

AH: $\mu_I > \mu_{NI}$,

where $\mu_I$ and $\mu_{NI}$ are the means of time intervals for the infected and noninfected populations, respectively, from which the samples were drawn. The definitions of symbols used in the formula for the $t$-test are given below and are more completely discussed elsewhere [17].

$x_{I_i}$ = one time interval measured for the $i^{th}$ selected infected patient.
$x_{NI_i}$ = one time interval measured for the $i^{th}$ selected noninfected patient.
$n_I$ = number of infected patients selected.
$n_{NI}$ = number of noninfected patients selected.

The mean interval from the sample of infected patients is calculated as

$$\bar{x}_I = \frac{\sum_{i=1}^{n_I} x_{I_i}}{n_I}$$

The mean interval from the sample of noninfected patients is calculated as

$$\bar{x}_{NI} = \frac{\sum_{i=1}^{n_{NI}} x_{NI_i}}{n_{NI}}$$

The variance estimate from the sample of infected patients is calculated as

$$s_I^2 = \frac{\sum_{i=1}^{n_I} (x_{I_i} - \bar{x}_I)^2}{n_I - 1} = \frac{\sum_{i=1}^{n_I} x_{I_i}^2 - \dfrac{\left(\sum_{i=1}^{n_I} x_{I_i}\right)^2}{n_I}}{n_I - 1}$$

The variance estimate from the sample of noninfected patients is calculated as

$$s_{NI}^2 = \frac{\sum_{i=1}^{n_{NI}} (x_{NI_i} - \bar{x}_{NI})^2}{n_{NI} - 1} = \frac{\sum_{i=1}^{n_{NI}} x_{NI_i}^2 - \dfrac{\left(\sum_{i=1}^{n_{NI}} x_{NI_i}\right)^2}{n_{NI}}}{n_{NI} - 1}$$

The variance of the difference between sample means is calculated as

$$s_{(\bar{x}_I - \bar{x}_{NI})}^2 = \frac{(n_I - 1) s_I^2 + (n_{NI} - 1) s_{NI}^2}{(n_I + n_{NI} - 2)} \times \left(\frac{1}{n_I} + \frac{1}{n_{NI}}\right)$$

The $t$-statistic is calculated as

$$t = \frac{\bar{x}_I - \bar{x}_{NI}}{s_{(\bar{x}_I - \bar{x}_{NI})}}$$

These values for the data of example 2 (Table 6-2) are given below:

$$\bar{x}_I = \frac{7060}{30} = 235.33$$

$$\bar{x}_{NI} = \frac{5949}{30} = 198.30$$

$$s_I^2 = \frac{1846916 - \dfrac{7060^2}{30}}{30 - 1} = 6395.2644$$

$$s_{NI}^2 = \frac{1398207 - \dfrac{5949^2}{30}}{30 - 1} = 7535.1828$$

$$s_{(\bar{x}_I - \bar{x}_{NI})}^2 = \frac{(29)(6395.2644) + (29)(7535.1828)}{58}$$
$$\times \left(\frac{1}{30} + \frac{1}{30}\right)$$

$$= 464.3482$$

$$t = \frac{235.33 - 198.30}{21.5487} = 1.718$$

A comparison of this computed value of $t$ with tabulated values of the $t$ distribution ($n_I + n_{NI} - 2$ degrees of freedom) reveals that the probability of a chance occurrence of the observed data is less than .05, the value often used as a criterion for judging significance. Therefore, the null hypothesis is rejected, and the mean time from admission to onset of infection in the infected group is considered significantly greater than the mean time from admission to discharge in the noninfected group.

If, on the other hand, the investigator decides it is unreasonable to assume that the samples were drawn from normally distributed populations, a nonparametric test can be chosen to test the difference between the means. In the following section, the data from example 2 are used without the normality assumption to demonstrate a nonparametric test for comparing two sample means, again assuming that the samples were independently selected.

*Wilcoxon Rank Sum Test*
This test procedure begins by ranking the individual observations of numbers of hours from 1 to $n$ ($n = n_I + n_{NI}$), with the least number of hours receiving a rank of 1. The ranks are assigned without regard to which sample the observations are from. When the original values are tied, equal ranks are assigned as the average of the ranks that would have been assigned to the tied observations if they had not been tied. One of several ties in the example occurred between the time intervals for infected patient number 19 and noninfected patient number 1 (Tables 6-2 and 6-5). Each of these was assigned a rank of 39.5, the average of the next two ranks that would have been assigned if they had not been tied. The ranking

(Table 6-5) begins with the assignment of rank 1 to infected patient number 27 and ends with the assignment of rank 60 to infected patient number 25.

After the ranking is completed, the ranks are separated into two groups corresponding to the original samples (Table 6-5). The sum of ranks for the sample having the fewer number of observations is obtained. Since in this example the number of observations is the same for both the infected and noninfected groups, the sum of ranks of either of these can be used.

The sum of ranks for the infected and noninfected groups are 1070 and 812, respectively. Referring to the tables for the Wilcoxon Rank Sum test [18,19] for a 1-tailed probability at $p = .05$, the upper boundary is 1027. Since the sum of ranks for this example is greater than 1027, the investigator would conclude that the average time from admission to onset for infected patients is significantly longer than the time from admission to discharge of noninfected patients.

In the design of a study of nosocomial infections, it is usually necessary to match the controls (noninfected patients) to the infected patients. It is difficult to interpret conclusions about the association of factors with nosocomial infection when controls and study groups are selected independently. If the groups are independent, as in the previous examples, no infor-

TABLE 6-5. Intervals and ranks for infected and noninfected patients (example 2)

| Ranks and time in hours from admission to onset of infection (infected patients) | | | | | | Ranks and time in hours from admission to discharge (noninfected patients) | | | | | |
|---|---|---|---|---|---|---|---|---|---|---|---|
| Pt. no. | Hrs. | Rank | Pt. no. | Hrs. | Rank | Pt. no. | Hrs. | Rank | Pt. no. | Hrs. | Rank |
| 1. | 216 | 29 | 16. | 234 | 34 | 1. | 253 | 39.5 | 16. | 242 | 36 |
| 2. | 187 | 23 | 17. | 205 | 26 | 2. | 82 | 2.5 | 17. | 233 | 32.5 |
| 3. | 88 | 4 | 18. | 136 | 15 | 3. | 125 | 12 | 18. | 133 | 14 |
| 4. | 280 | 44.5 | 19. | 253 | 39.5 | 4. | 138 | 19 | 19. | 342 | 58 |
| 5. | 310 | 49 | 20. | 165 | 19 | 5. | 137 | 16 | 20. | 102 | 7 |
| 6. | 239 | 35 | 21. | 340 | 57 | 6. | 116 | 11 | 21. | 93 | 5.5 |
| 7. | 344 | 59 | 22. | 325 | 51 | 7. | 232 | 31 | 22. | 82 | 2.5 |
| 8. | 315 | 50 | 23. | 178 | 21 | 8. | 327 | 52 | 23. | 248 | 38 |
| 9. | 280 | 44.5 | 24. | 153 | 18 | 9. | 171 | 20 | 24. | 113 | 10 |
| 10. | 293 | 46 | 25. | 355 | 60 | 10. | 338 | 55.5 | 25. | 294 | 47 |
| 11. | 200 | 25 | 26. | 338 | 55.5 | 11. | 335 | 53.5 | 26. | 304 | 48 |
| 12. | 229 | 30 | 27. | 77 | 1 | 12. | 109 | 9 | 27. | 211 | 28 |
| 13. | 208 | 27 | 28. | 335 | 53.5 | 13. | 126 | 13 | 28. | 104 | 8 |
| 14. | 233 | 32.5 | 29. | 261 | 41.5 | 14. | 182 | 22 | 29. | 261 | 41.5 |
| 15. | 190 | 24 | 30. | 93 | 55.5 | 15. | 247 | 37 | 30. | 269 | 43 |

Pt. no. = patient number.

mation is available to allow the investigator to determine whether infected patients really had onset of infection at about the same time as noninfected patients were being discharged. If the noninfected patients generally were admitted with more serious underlying illness than the infected patients, their length of stay in the hospital could have been prolonged on the average longer than their length of stay had they been admitted with illnesses comparable to those of the infected patients. The time from admission to onset of infection could have appeared from the data to be about the same as the interval from admission to discharge of noninfected patients, yet in truth could have exceeded the admission-to-discharge interval. In this case the investigator could overlook an important feature of the observations under study, that is, that infections were occurring after prolonged stay beyond the usual length of stay for patients with underlying illnesses like those of the infected group. Matching the noninfected patients to the infected patients on such important variables can avoid this problem.

If we discard the assumption that the samples from examples 1 and 2 were independent and assume that patients in the noninfected group were matched to patients in the infected group on day of admission, underlying diagnosis, age, and sex, then a new group of tests can be introduced (Fig. 6-1). Although these examples illustrate the situation for one-to-one matching of controls to cases only, testing procedures are available for situations in which a variable number of controls is matched to cases [13].

First, two tests for attribute data from matched samples are illustrated using example 1. The data from example 1 must be summarized and tested differently if the patients are matched [2]; the arrangements of Tables 6-3 and 6-4 are for the unmatched situation. Infected–noninfected pairs rather than individual patients are counted in the 2 × 2 table for matched studies (Table 6-6).

There were 20 pairs in which the infected patient

was catheterized while the matched, noninfected patient was not catheterized. Only three pairs occurred with infected patients not catheterized while their noninfected matches were catheterized. The two cells (Table 6-7) that count the number of pairs having both patients catheterized or neither of the patients catheterized (two and five pairs, respectively) contribute no information about whether infected or noninfected patients were catheterized more often. Therefore, these two cells are not used in the significance tests for attributes. Only the cells counting discordant pairs add information about the association of infection and catheterization. The effective sample size for this example, therefore, is 23 pairs.

*Sign Test*
The sign test takes into account only the direction of differences between members of each pair and has a relatively low power. If there were no difference in the frequency of catheterization among infected and noninfected patients, there would be as many pairs in which the infected patient was catheterized and the matched, noninfected patient not catheterized as there were pairs with the infected patient not catheterized and the matched, noninfected patient catheterized. For this example of 23 untied pairs it is expected that, if no difference in the frequency of catheterization exists between infected and noninfected patients, there should be 11.5 pairs with a catheterized, infected patient and a noncatheterized, noninfected patient, and 11.5 pairs with a noncatheterized, infected patient and a catheterized, noninfected patient. The probability of observing a given number of pairs or fewer having a noncatheterized, infected patient and a catheterized, noninfected patient is given by the sum of binomial probabilities:

$$p_{\text{Tot}} = \sum_{x=0}^{c} \frac{n!}{x! \, (n - x)!} \, (.5)^x \, (1 - .5)^{n-x} \, ,$$

where $n$ is the number of untied pairs [12], and $c$ is

TABLE 6-6. General table for summarizing the association of a factor with infection-matched data

| | | Infected | | |
| | | Catheter | No Catheter | Total |
|---|---|---|---|---|
| Noninfected | Catheter | $a$ | $b$ | $a + b$ |
| | No Catheter | $c$ | $d$ | $c + d$ |
| | Total | $a + c$ | $b + d$ | $n$ |

TABLE 6-7. Pairs of patients by catheterization status (example 1)

| | | Infected | | |
| | | Catheter | No Catheter | Total |
|---|---|---|---|---|
| Noninfected | Catheter | 2 | 3 | 5 |
| | No Catheter | 20 | 5 | 25 |
| | Total | 22 | 8 | 30 |

the smaller of the two cells (b and c) in Table 6-6. The formula sums the probabilities of obtaining 0, 1, . . ., $c$ noncatheterized, infected patients paired with a catheterized, noninfected patient, when half the total untied pairs, 11.5, are expected to be in this cell. The probabilities for example 1 are:

$$p_x = \frac{23!}{x! \, (23 - x)!} (.5)^x (1 - .5)^{23 - x}$$

$$p_0 = \frac{23!}{0! \, (23 - 0)!} (.5)^x (1 - .5)^{23 - 0}$$

$$= 1.19209290 \times 10^{-7}$$

$$p_1 = \frac{23!}{1! \, (23 - 1)!} (.5)^x (1 - .5)^{23 - 1}$$

$$= 2.74181366 \times 10^{-6}$$

$$p_2 = \frac{23!}{2! \, (23 - 2)!} (.5)^x (1 - .5)^{23 - 2}$$

$$= 3.01599503 \times 10^{-5}$$

$$p_3 = \frac{23!}{3! \, (23 - 3)!} (.5)^x (1 - .5)^{23 - 3}$$

$$= \frac{2.11119652 \times 10^{-4}}{}$$

$$p_{Tot} = 2.44140625 \times 10^{-4}$$

This low probability leads to a rejection of the null hypothesis:

$$H_0: P_I \leq P_{NI}$$

in favor of the alternative hypothesis:

$$AH: P_I > P_{NI}$$

The conclusion is that catheterized patients were at higher risk of infection.

## McNemar Test

The McNemar test [10] is a chi-square test that uses pairs of patients rather than individuals; therefore, it differs from the ordinary chi-square test presented earlier. As in the sign test, the McNemar test uses only those pairs with untied observations for the infected and noninfected patients. The formula presented below and the previous formula for chi-square for independent observations both include a correction for continuity. Many elementary statistics textbooks present discussions of appropriate use of the continuity correction [16, 17].

$$\chi^2 = \frac{(|b - c| - 1)^2}{b + c}$$

$$= \frac{(|3 - 20| - 1)^2}{23}$$

$$= \frac{(|-17| - 1)^2}{23}$$

$$= \frac{16^2}{23}$$

$$= 11.13$$

Again this is a 2-tailed test for an association between infection and catheterization in either direction (i.e., more risk associated with catheterization or less risk associated with catheterization). Although computed from matched samples, the value of chi-square from the McNemar test should be compared to the same tabulated values of the chi-square distribution that were used for the chi-square test computed from independent samples. The inference about the populations from which the samples from example 1 were drawn, if they were matched, would be that catheterization is associated with infection, since the probability associated with a chi-square of 11.13 is only .00085.

Next, tests for measurement data from matched samples are presented, using example 2 and assuming that the noninfected patients were selected by matching to the infected patients. These tests use the differences between observations for members of the pairs instead of the two observations separately. The hypotheses to be tested are

$$H_0: \mu_I \leq \mu_{NI}$$

$$AH: \mu_I > \mu_{NI}$$

The hypothesis that the mean of the intervals from admission to onset of infection for infected patients is less than or equal to the mean of the intervals from admission to discharge for noninfected patients is tested against the alternative hypothesis that the mean interval from admission to onset of infection for the infected patients exceeds the mean interval from admission to discharge of noninfected patients. The investigator wishes to decide whether the risk of infection is increased because hospital stay is longer than it would have been if the patients had not acquired infections, or whether the length of stay for infected patients is increased because of infection. If the mean time from admission to onset of infection is about the same as the mean time from admission to discharge of noninfected patients, the investigator could conclude that prolonged stay in the hospital is not the underlying cause of infection. Additional study such as examining the distribution of intervals from onset of infection to discharge would then be necessary to understand to what extent infections actually increased the length of stay. The assumption that the sample observations were selected from a population of normally distributed time intervals must be made for the parametric test presented next.

### Paired t-test

The paired *t*-test uses the statistical theorem that the distribution of differences between two normally distributed, random variables (the sample time intervals) is also normal. Once these differences (Table 6-8) between the time intervals of the two members of each pair are determined, the *t*-test can be used to decide if the mean difference is greater than zero. The formula for this *t*-test is

$$t = \frac{\bar{d}}{s_{\bar{d}}}$$

where $d_i$ is the difference between time intervals for the members of the $i^{th}$ pair,

$$\text{where } \bar{d} = \frac{\sum\limits_{i=1}^{n} d_i}{n} = \frac{1111}{30} = 37.0333$$

$$\text{and } s^2 = \frac{\sum\limits_{i=1}^{n} (d_i - \bar{d})^2}{n(n-1)} = \frac{\sum\limits_{i=1}^{n} d_i^2 - \frac{\left(\sum\limits_{i=1}^{n} d_i\right)^2}{n}}{n(n-1)}$$

$$= \frac{397253 - \frac{(1111)^2}{30}}{30(30-1)}$$

$$= 409.3206$$

are the mean and standard error of the mean of differences in the time intervals, and where $n$ is the number of pairs. Then

$$t = \frac{37.0333}{20.2317} = 1.83$$

is greater than 1.699, the tabulated value of $t$ with $n - 1 = 29$ degrees of freedom corresponding to a 1-tailed probability of .05. The null hypothesis that the interval from admission to onset of infection is less than or equal to the interval from admission to

discharge of noninfected patients is rejected in favor of the alternative hypothesis, that $\mu_I > \mu_{NI}$. These data would support the hypothesis that infections occurred after a prolonged stay in the hospital rather than that prolonged stay resulted from infection.

### Wilcoxon Signed Ranks Test

If the assumption of normality is not acceptable, the hypothesis can be tested from the matched data using a nonparametric test. The Wilcoxon Signed Ranks test [19] is easy to apply in this case. The results of each step in the test procedure are given in Table 6-9. First the differences are determined (column 4) for all pairs without considering the sign of the difference. Then these unsigned differences are ranked from lowest to highest (column 5), with the smallest difference receiving rank 1 (pair number 18). Differences of 0 (e.g., pair number 29) are omitted from the test procedure. Tied differences are assigned the average value of the ranks that would have been assigned if the differences had not been tied (e.g., pair number 1 and pair number 3). Finally, the signs of differences are assigned to the ranks (column 6) and the sums of absolute values of positive and negative ranks are obtained separately. The value of the smaller of the two sums is compared to the critical value [18] for a 1-tailed test at the .05 level. This value, 140, is exceeded by the sum of negative ranks in this example, supporting the hypothesis that the mean interval from admission to onset was greater than the mean interval from admission to discharge of the noninfected patients.

### DISCUSSION

Several principles of study design and a potentially new source of data in hospitals have been presented to remind those responsible for studying nosocomial infections of ways to improve their studies and potentially gain access to computer records for selecting study and control patients. Some simple testing procedures and a scheme for deciding when each is appropriate have been presented. The investigator must be careful to avoid oversimplification of the problems associated with data on nosocomial infections. The use of a simple significance test without understanding the underlying assumptions, without considering the study design, and without giving attention to possible confounding variables can lead to meaningless interpretation of the data. The significance tests presented in this chapter are in no way intended as a complete list of available tests. They were chosen as commonly used examples that are available in each

TABLE 6-8. Summary of differences for the paired *t*-test (example 2)

| Pair no. | Infected patient | Noninfected patient | Difference | Pair no. | Infected patient | Noninfected patient | Difference |
|---|---|---|---|---|---|---|---|
| 1. | 216 | 253 | − 37 | 16. | 234 | 242 | − 8 |
| 2. | 187 | 82 | 105 | 17. | 205 | 233 | − 28 |
| 3. | 88 | 125 | − 37 | 18. | 136 | 133 | 3 |
| 4. | 280 | 138 | 142 | 19. | 253 | 342 | − 89 |
| 5. | 310 | 137 | 173 | 20. | 165 | 102 | 63 |
| 6. | 239 | 116 | 123 | 21. | 340 | 93 | 247 |
| 7. | 344 | 232 | 112 | 22. | 325 | 82 | 243 |
| 8. | 315 | 327 | − 12 | 23. | 178 | 248 | − 70 |
| 9. | 280 | 171 | 109 | 24. | 153 | 113 | 40 |
| 10. | 293 | 338 | − 45 | 25. | 355 | 294 | 61 |
| 11. | 200 | 335 | − 135 | 26. | 338 | 304 | 34 |
| 12. | 229 | 109 | 120 | 27. | 77 | 211 | − 134 |
| 13. | 208 | 126 | 82 | 28. | 335 | 104 | 231 |
| 14. | 233 | 182 | 51 | 29. | 261 | 261 | 0 |
| 15. | 190 | 247 | − 57 | 30. | 93 | 269 | − 176 |

TABLE 6-9. Summary of the ranking procedure for Wilcoxon signed ranks test (example 2)

| Pair no. | Infected patient | Noninfected patient | Difference (unsigned) | Rank (unsigned) | Rank (signed)* |
|---|---|---|---|---|---|
| 1. | 216 | 253 | 37 | 6.5 | − 6.5 |
| 2. | 187 | 82 | 105 | 17 | 17 |
| 3. | 88 | 125 | 37 | 6.5 | − 6.5 |
| 4. | 280 | 138 | 142 | 24 | 24 |
| 5. | 310 | 137 | 173 | 25 | 25 |
| 6. | 239 | 116 | 123 | 21 | 21 |
| 7. | 344 | 232 | 112 | 19 | 19 |
| 8. | 315 | 327 | 12 | 3 | − 3 |
| 9. | 280 | 171 | 109 | 18 | 18 |
| 10. | 293 | 338 | 45 | 9 | − 9 |
| 11. | 200 | 335 | 135 | 23 | − 23 |
| 12. | 229 | 109 | 120 | 20 | 20 |
| 13. | 208 | 126 | 82 | 15 | 15 |
| 14. | 233 | 182 | 51 | 10 | 10 |
| 15. | 190 | 247 | 57 | 11 | − 11 |
| 16. | 234 | 242 | 8 | 2 | − 2 |
| 17. | 205 | 233 | 28 | 4 | − 4 |
| 18. | 136 | 133 | 3 | 1 | 1 |
| 19. | 253 | 342 | 89 | 16 | − 16 |
| 20. | 165 | 102 | 63 | 13 | 13 |
| 21. | 340 | 93 | 247 | 29 | 29 |
| 22. | 325 | 82 | 243 | 28 | 28 |
| 23. | 178 | 248 | 70 | 14 | − 14 |
| 24. | 153 | 113 | 40 | 8 | 8 |
| 25. | 355 | 294 | 61 | 12 | 12 |
| 26. | 338 | 304 | 34 | 5 | 5 |
| 27. | 77 | 211 | 134 | 22 | − 22 |
| 28. | 335 | 104 | 231 | 27 | 27 |
| 29. | 261 | 261 | 0 | Omit | Omit |
| 30. | 93 | 269 | 176 | 26 | − 26 |

*Sum of positive ranks = 292; sum of negative ranks = 143

of the situations presented. The objective has been to show the readers, presumably hospital personnel, how the approach to analyzing nosocomial infection data is affected by assumptions, study design, and level of measurement of data. There is no intention to limit analyses to a single factor in any study. Although the scope of this chapter is limited to the single factor (univariate) case, help for analyses of multiple factors (multivariate) can be found in the references cited.

The selection scheme (Fig. 6-1) is intended to assist with correct application of common test procedures, but even the correct choice of test for a single variable (univariate test) may not produce an accurate conclusion about the association of the factor and infection. There are two reasons for this. First, conclusions from hypothesis testing are based on error probabilities that the investigator sets before the data are collected.

Second, the investigator must understand the complete data set, possibly including interrelations among several factors. For the data of example 1, inquiring into the possible increased risk of infection caused by catheterization would include examination of underlying illnesses and other factors that might be considered confounding factors. A factor that may itself be associated with exposure to the factor under study and with the risk to infection should be considered as a potential confounding factor. One might ask whether the catheterized patients were infected as a result of catheterization or whether their infections occurred as a result of serious underlying illness that not only predisposed the patients to infection but also required that the patients be catheterized. Questions like these can sometimes be answered on the basis of a scan of cross-tabulations of the data. Some of these possible confounding variables can be handled in the study design by matching [3]. However, multivariate statistical tools are also available to help in understanding the effects of several variables at the same time.

One of these methods is the Mantel-Haenszel procedure [7], which tests the hypothesis of association of a single variable with infection while keeping a second variable fixed. This allows the second variable to be tested in the presence of the first variable.

Another method for examining more than one variable and even joint effects of variables involves regression techniques. During the past decade multiple linear logistic regression techniques have been applied to a variety of situations, including matched study designs [1,5,14]. These procedures permit the investigator to develop models including potentially important variables and interaction terms for determining possible joint effects of variables. This is a particularly helpful development for the study of nosocomial infection outbreaks when the causative factors are unknown, because one can explore the data for associations of several potential factors with infection. However, the computations are beyond those that can be done practically with a small calculator. Computer programs that require access to a large computer have been published for this procedure [6].

The study of nosocomial infections can be simplified as previously suggested by taking advantage of data that may be routinely collected in machine-readable form. Rarely do such data contain judgments of infected or noninfected status of patients; therefore, many data items such as culture results, pharmaceuticals, or other indicators must be used to signal that a particular record may be for an infected patient. Usually the infection control practitioner, the hospital epidemiologist, or the Infection Control Committee must solicit the hospital computer center to make provision for entry of the infection status and data about the infection. Of course this requires active infection surveillance or comprehensive record review by the infection control practitioner. The return in simplified selection of study and control groups from computer files and the potential for computer-assisted analysis can in many instances easily offset the cost of additional data collection efforts to obtain machine-readable records.

## REFERENCES

1. Breslow, N. E., and Day, N. E. *Statistical Methods in Cancer Research, Vol. 1. The Analysis of Case-Control Studies* (International Agency for Research on Cancer, Scientific Publications, No. 32). Lyon, France: International Agency for Research on Cancer, 1980, pp. 192–279.
2. Cochran, W. G. The comparison of percentages in matched samples. *Biometrika* 37:256, 1971.
3. Cornfield, J., and Haenszel, W. Some aspects of retrospective studies. *J. Chronic Dis.* 11:523, 1960.
4. Fisher, R. A. *Statistical Methods for Research Workers*. Darien, Conn.: Hafner, 1970, pp. 96–97.
5. Gail, M. H., Lubin, J. H., and Rubenstein, L. V. Likelihood calculations for matched case-control studies and survival studies with tied death times. *Biometrika* 68:703, 1981.
6. Lubin, J. H. A computer program for the analysis of matched case-control studies. *Computers and Biomedical Research* 14:138, 1981.
7. Mantel, N., and Haenszel, W. Statistical aspects of the analysis of data from retrospective studies of disease. *J. Natl. Cancer Inst.* 22:719, 1959.

8. Martin, S. M. Choosing the Correct Statistical Tests. In Wenzel, R. P. (Ed.), *Handbook of Hospital-Acquired Infections*. Boca Raton, Fla.: CRC Press, 1981.

9. Maxwell, A. E. *Analysing Qualitative Data*. London: Methuen, 1971, p. 23.

10. McNemar, Q. *Psychological Statistics*. New York: Wiley, 1955.

11. Miller, R. B., Jr., *Simultaneous Statistical Inferences* (2nd ed.). New York: Springer-Verlag, 1981, p. 67.

12. Ostle, B. *Statistics in Research*. Ames, Iowa: Iowa State University Press, 1954.

13. Pike, M. C., and Morrow, R. H. Statistical analysis of patient-control studies in epidemiology, factor under investigation an all-or-none variable. *Br. J. Prev. Soc. Med.* 24:42, 1970.

14. Schlesselman, J. J. *Case-Control Studies*. New York: Oxford University Press, 1982, pp. 227–280.

15. Siegel, S. *Nonparametric Statistics for the Behavioral Sciences*. New York: McGraw-Hill, 1956.

16. Snedecor, G. W., and Cochran, W. G. *Statistical Methods*. Ames, Iowa: Iowa State University Press, 1968.

17. Steel, G. D., and Torrie, J. H. *Principles and Procedures of Statistics*. New York: McGraw-Hill, 1960.

18. Wilcoxon, F., Katti, S. K., and Wilcox, R. A. *Critical Values and Probability Levels for the Wilcoxon Rank Sum Test and the Wilcoxon Signed Rank Test*. Pearl River, N.Y.: American Cyanamid Co. and Florida State University, 1963.

19. Wilcoxon, F., and Wilcox, R. A. *Some Rapid Approximate Statistical Procedures*. Pearl River, N.Y.: American Cyanamid Co., 1964.

# 7 THE ROLE OF THE LABORATORY IN CONTROL OF NOSOCOMIAL INFECTION

John E. McGowan, Jr.
Robert A. Weinstein
George F. Mallison

Nosocomial infections continue to present a major problem in hospitals today. Because of the importance of this subject, each hospital laboratory has the responsibility of supporting activities related to surveillance, control, and prevention of nosocomial infections, even though resources often are strained by the usual patient-care workload. Each laboratory can make major contributions toward infection control, as long as the persons responsible for infection control efforts and those in charge of the clinical microbiology laboratory cooperate closely to attack this problem. Often the same persons have both of these responsibilities [42].

Laboratory personnel attempt to minimize the occurrence of nosocomial infection in the following seven ways: (1) participation in activities of the hospital Infection Control Committee; (2) accurate identification of responsible organisms; (3) careful attention to antibiotic susceptibility testing; (4) timely reporting of laboratory data and participation in surveillance of nosocomial infection; (5) provision of additional studies, when necessary, to establish similarity or difference of organisms; (6) provision, on occasion, of microbiologic studies of the hospital environment; and (7) training of infection control personnel.

## PARTICIPATION IN INFECTION CONTROL COMMITTEE

### Relationship to Infection Control Committee

A clinically oriented member of the laboratory staff can contribute significantly by serving on the Infection Control Committee. Such participation is essential in contributing to a harmonious relationship among clinical, infection control, and microbiology personnel.

In the typical hospital, the majority of members of the Infection Control Committee do not have a background in microbiology. Thus it is of great importance for the representative of the laboratory to provide the microbiologic expertise that is critical to many decisions of the group. This knowledge may be required for the assessment of the significance of culture data, for determining the validity of laboratory techniques used to identify cases of nosocomial infection, and in the design and implementation of investigations and survey projects.

The diagnostic microbiology laboratory is engaged primarily in the evaluation of cultures related to infection. Because these are crucial data for successful infection control, the laboratory activities should be closely coordinated with the Infection Control Committee. For example, the adequacy of the basic techniques for primary isolation, speciation, and antimicrobial susceptibility testing should be discussed by the microbiologists and the Infection Control Committee. Laboratory resources often are stretched by patient-care requirements, especially in smaller hospitals [13]. Support for infection control activities must be given with discretion. For example, use of laboratory resources to assess colonization or to sample personnel and the environment for bacterial or other organisms should never be permitted when the epidemiologic indications are unclear.

Major changes are occurring currently in reimbursement methods for hospitals in the United States [48]. In view of these changes, there seems to be an added service that the laboratory microbiologist can provide to the Infection Control Committee. As prospective reimbursement takes effect, there will be new and intensive attempts to evaluate the validity and usefulness of hospital programs such as infection control [68]. Techniques for assessment are the bread and butter activity of clinical microbiology personnel, who have to make similar cost-benefit judgments for laboratory equipment, instruments, and procedures almost daily [14,34]. The insights and methods used for such laboratory activities should be helpful to the infection control team and the Infection Control Committee members as they review the benefit of their activities and attempt to improve the productivity of the program.

*Budgetary Considerations*
Costs for laboratory procedures that are not related directly to care of patients (e.g., bacteriologic sampling of personnel and the environment) should be borne by a budget separate from that of the laboratory. To facilitate all the microbiologic activities necessitated by an outbreak, the laboratory (or the hospital epidemiologist, or the Infection Control Committee, depending on the organizational structure of the hospital) should have a contingency fund to enable personnel, materials, and space to be temporarily assigned to epidemic aid support. An investigation of an outbreak should not be financed by charging individual patients for cultures taken during the study.

## ACCURATE IDENTIFICATION OF ORGANISMS INVOLVED IN NOSOCOMIAL INFECTION

Infection control personnel search constantly for evidence that a common organism has spread from pa-

tient to patient or from employee to patient. Thus information permitting the successful tracing of organism movements within the hospital may be of value to the hospital infection control team, whether the positive cultures represent episodes of infection or indicate colonization of the patient [1]. While some clinical features of illness provide information about etiology, the main sources for this determination usually are the data provided by the clinical laboratory. Thus the ability of the laboratory staff to isolate and identify responsible microorganisms is crucial to infection control [36].

*Collection and Transport of Specimens*
Specimen collection, transport, and handling must be of sufficiently high quality to provide valid data. Specimens that are not collected or transported properly may give inaccurate results, even when handled as well as possible once they reach the laboratory. In turn these inaccurate results may lead to improper clinical decisions by physicians, unnecessary labor by laboratory personnel, and unnecessary patient charges. The laboratory must monitor specimen handling continually and work closely with the wards and clinics to make sure that the possibility of contaminated specimens is minimized. This is a necessity to ensure that laboratory information presented to the hospital epidemiologist reports organisms actually associated with the patient's site of culture rather than contaminants.

Certain laboratory findings suggest specific handling errors [106]. For example, a frequent failure to isolate organisms from deep wounds or abscesses of patients who are not on antibiotics, or inability to recover pathogens seen on Gram stain in cases of presumed anaerobic infections, suggests inadequate anaerobic transport media, delay or inappropriate refrigeration of specimens in transit, or use of inadequate techniques for isolating anaerobes. The frequent recovery of three or more different organisms in clean-voided "midstream" urine specimens suggests unsatisfactory technique in collecting specimens, a delay in transporting specimens to the laboratory, or a delay in culturing the specimens. The finding of negative mycobacterial cultures from a high percentage of patients with positive smears for acid-fast bacilli suggests unsatisfactory sputum collection or handling, errors in staining, or errors in culture techniques [107].

Specimen collection and handling should be assessed regularly to detect and correct such problems; the frequency with which probable contaminants are isolated from clinical specimens can be a measure of the quality of specimen collection in a specific hospital area. For example, determining frequency of urine specimens with characteristics that suggest specimen contamination permits wards with high rates to be singled out for evaluation and, if necessary, for inservice education programs instituted by laboratory or infection control personnel. In addition, identifying persons who draw blood cultures that frequently contain diphtheroids, coagulase-negative staphylococci, or other probable skin contaminants may permit reinstruction of these personnel in aseptic technique. Periodic review of the relative incidence of false-positive smears for acid-fast bacilli may highlight problems in sputum collection and processing [107].

Some hospitals use laboratory slips with space to record both the time the specimen was collected and the time the laboratory received it so that transport time can be monitored periodically or continuously and the culturing of old specimens avoided [106].

*Initial Evaluation of Specimens*

Assessment of specimens at the time they are received in the laboratory is one of the best ways to evaluate their suitabililty. For example, microscopic review of Gram stain of sputum specimens remains the best way to determine whether or not these specimens are contaminated [109]; specimens identified as inadequate are not processed further and do not confuse either clinician or epidemiologist. Sputum specimens containing fewer polymorphonuclear leukocytes than squamous epithelial cells are likely to be oropharyngeal material [9,109]. Such specimens should not be processed further, and a new specimen should be requested unless the clinician provides notice of special circumstances (e.g. immunosuppression) that might make it worthwhile to proceed with culture.

Culture or smear results for other types of specimens may also suggest contamination at the time of collection. Scoring systems for use in determining acceptable wound, vaginal, cervical, and other specimens also have been described [6,7]. Application of such criteria will ensure that the information generated from the specimens that are processed completely will more likely correlate with true infecting organisms and will reduce unnecessary laboratory costs. Repeat specimen collection should be requested for these inadequate specimens, and additional processing of organisms isolated from such specimens (e.g., speciation, susceptibility testing) should be limited. The culture report should alert the clinician about the questionable value of the specimen so that results will be used cautiously, if at all, for guidance in diagnosis and therapy.

For specimens from sputum and wounds, reporting of the morphologic characteristics of bacteria seen on Gram stain may be misleading if no statement is made regarding the presence or absence of white blood cells. Both sites may be extensively contaminated with skin, oropharyngeal, or intestinal bacterial flora. When organisms are found only in the presence of abundant squamous epithelial cells, it is unlikely that they are the causative agents, and reports of such mixed flora without qualification about the accompanying cells may lead the clinician falsely to assume mixed flora as the cause of the infection. Substantial effort will be conserved and superior information ultimately provided if repeat collection is requested for such specimens.

Microscopy at the time of specimen submission can help other aspects of microbiologic diagnosis. For example, examination on Gram stain for morphology can identify organisms that might be epidemiologically important but not reflected by culture. Thus presence of a mixed flora on Gram stain of a sputum specimen, when coupled with an aerobic culture yielding only *Hemophilus influenzae*, may indicate possible mixed aerobic-anaerobic infection rather than pneumonia due to *Hemophilus*. Because infection-control implications of these two causes may differ, evaluations of this type by the laboratory can be important. Similarly, nonculture methods for identifying the presence of rotavirus (e.g., demonstration by electron microscopy or immunologic assays) have helped us learn more about this organism as a cause of infection in older patients [24].

Anaerobic culture of specimens should be limited to (1) those that show leukocytes on Gram stain, (2) those with no evidence of contaminating squamous cells and organisms suggestive of anaerobic species, or (3) specimens from patients whose unusual circumstances suggest a need for anaerobic culture. This limitation results in reporting of isolates that have a much higher probability of association with infection. The application of sensitive techniques for culturing and identifying anaerobes [30] to specimens containing endogenous flora is costly and productive of misleading information. It has been estimated that the cost of processing wound and cervical cultures would increase 107 percent if direct anaerobic culturing were done for all specimens [8]. Large numbers of anaerobic organisms are present in the normal flora of skin, oral cavity, and genital and gastrointestinal tracts. Thus swabs from superficial portions of skin or mucous membrane lesions, specimens of expectorated sputum, and any materials contaminated with feces should be considered inappropriate for anaerobic culture [30]. Submission for anaerobic culture of such specimens or of specimens from sites that are rarely infected by anaerobes (e.g., urine) suggests the need for inservice education of hospital personnel.

Isolation of *Candida* from a series of specimens or the demonstration of abundant pseudohyphae usually is required before serious consideration is given to the organism's pathogenicity. Yeasts frequently are isolated from respiratory tract secretions and other clinical specimens, but most represent colonization and are not causing infection. Microbiologists should store cultures of yeasts that are isolated in pure culture, or from several consecutive specimens, for two or three days and append a comment to the report requesting the physician to consult the laboratory if complete identification is indicated. Few such requests are received in the usual hospital, which substantially reduces unnecessary work.

Efforts such as those outlined will substantially reduce errors in diagnosis and use of unnecessary antimicrobial therapy. Such an approach will also improve the specificity of infection surveillance data, which otherwise might include isolates of questionable etiologic significance.

## Identification of Isolates

Once a specimen has been received in the laboratory, it must be processed in a way that will maximize the likelihood of recovering older agents as well as the many newer agents causing hospital cross-infection.

Often it is difficult to determine the causative agents in nosocomial infection. Thus etiologic diagnosis cannot be made with certainty in many cases. The majority of cases today for which the cause is known involve gram-negative aerobic bacilli [12]. Most frequent among these gram-negative rods are *Klebsiella*, *Enterobacter*, *Pseudomonas*, *Serratia*, *Proteus*, and *Escherichia coli* (in approximately that order). In recent years, organisms such as *Acinetobacter*, *Flavobacterium*, and *Pseudomonas* species other than *Pseudomonas aeruginosa* have become increasingly prominent [36].

Anaerobic bacterial organisms (usually found in mixed aerobic-anaerobic infections), viral agents (e.g., rotavirus), and fungi and parasites such as *Pneumocystis* and *Toxoplasma* have been identified as important causes of nosocomial infection [12]. New bacterial agents such as the now numerous species of *Legionella* have been implicated in both epidemic and endemic nosocomial disease [31]. This expansion of the list of possible microbial pathogens for hospitalized patients has made it more difficult for both microbiologist and clinician to deal effectively with hospital infection. Effective handling of such problems requires the laboratory staff to keep up with the steadily un-

folding panorama of organisms important in cross-infection and to implement and maintain culture and other techniques that will bring these to light.

## Need for Complete Identification

The degree to which organism identification routinely is carried can be important to nosocomial infection control efforts. Infection control personnel constantly are searching for evidence that a common organism has spread from patient to patient [37]. The ability to detect such an event is enhanced by identification of the organism at least to the level of species. Reporting of "biotyping" information (pattern of response to biochemical testing) can be of value in differentiating organisms that are frequently encountered, but the need for this identification on a routine basis has not been established [36,37,42].

When organisms are to be identified completely, it is important that standard criteria and nomenclature be consistently applied. Otherwise, attack rates for nosocomial infections with various species may identify false problems (e.g., because of previously unreported species or strains) or fail to identify true problems. Furthermore, such surveillance data may not be comparable to data developed in other institutions or in cooperative surveillance programs.

Even more important, incomplete or incorrect identification of organisms may obscure real problems and make retrospective epidemiologic investigation impossible. For example, a report of "*Klebsiella-Enterobacter* group" (formerly "*Klebsiella-Aerobacter* group") fails to distinguish between two organisms (*Klebsiella* and *Enterobacter*) that have different epidemiologic patterns of infection within the hospital [91]. Similarly, identifying an isolate as *Pseudomonas cepacia*, an organism frequently associated with illness or pseudoepidemics caused by contaminated water or other solutions [65], provides more useful epidemiologic information than identifying the organism only as "*Pseudomonas* species," in which the strain is lumped with a group of organisms that may not have as characteristic a hospital reservoir.

Because of these considerations, it seems reasonable to ask the laboratory personnel to identify to the species level all isolates from blood and other normally sterile body fluids [7,8,106]. Laboratories should maintain the capability to identify gram-negative aerobic bacilli to the genus level with at least 95 percent accuracy, and such identification should be a routine part of laboratory procedure. The laboratory should also have the capability of identifying these organisms to the species level when special or recurring problems in a given institution make such information useful for dealing with nosocomial infection problems.

Many hospitals find it advantageous to employ commercial, multiple test media for biochemical testing that provide this degree of characterization [66]. Acceptable methods for microbiologic identification procedures are described in detail elsewhere [58]; additional assistance in identifying unusual isolates beyond the stated expertise of an individual laboratory is available from state and national reference laboratories.

Sometimes it is the pattern of susceptibility to antimicrobials that discriminates epidemiologically significant organisms from other apparently similar hospital organisms. For example, many U. S. hospitals currently encounter nosocomial infections due to *Staphylococcus aureus* strains resistant to methicillin [100]. Such organisms can be the subject of infection control activities only if the laboratory maintains effective and efficient means for their identification.

### Need for Accuracy and Consistency

Many spurious outbreaks have been traced to inaccurate or inconsistent microbiologic procedures. An "outbreak" of *S. aureus* infection, for example, may be caused by delayed reading of coagulase tests, resulting in misidentification of coagulase-negative organisms as coagulase-positive. Similarly, the renaming of organisms that results from better knowledge of organism relationships can cause confusion. For example, the renaming as *Acinetobacter calcoaceticus* var. *anitratus* of the organism formerly called *Herrellea vaginicola* gave false alarm to institutions not used to seeing or dealing with what appeared to be a new intruder.

### Introduction of New Procedures

The laboratory must also consider whether additional laboratory techniques can make testing results more relevant. For example, cultures of intravenous catheter tips may become positive because of contamination at the time of catheter removal or from the intravascular device becoming infected. The semiquantitative method for culture of intravenous catheters [62] has been shown to be useful in distinguishing between these possibilities (see Chapter 36). Similar claims of usefulness have been made for cultures of burn wounds (see Chapter 30) and surgical wounds [22] (see Chapter 27). These special techniques generate useful information for the clinician in planning therapy, as they indicate the likelihood that sepsis arose from the source at hand. In addition, such information is quite helpful to the infection

control officer's assessment of whether nosocomial infection is present.

### Role in Epidemic Investigation

Outbreaks of nosocomial infection must be dealt with as rapidly as possible [12]. This means that the laboratory may face exceptional demands for service at the beginning of, and throughout, an epidemic period [37]. Advance preparation for such situations makes response easier in the time of need. The laboratory personnel should prepare contingency plans for the types of outbreaks that have occurred most frequently in the past in the hospital so that they are ready to deal with these exceptional requests in a smooth fashion.

Investigation of an outbreak of nosocomial infection may require isolation and identification of isolates in specimens not only from patients but also from personnel who might be colonized with the outbreak strain and from environmental objects that might be similarly contaminated [37,95]. Such activity may require the laboratory staff to process and evaluate large numbers of cultures, and special techniques may be necessary to accomplish such projects. For example reliable detection of *Salmonella* carriage, rather than infection with this organism, requires enhancement of growth by use of selective media [36]. The laboratory staff and the infection control team can process this work efficiently by making careful assessment of the sites to be cultured and determining which culture media and techniques will be employed.

In the absence of an outbreak, routine culture of hospital patients and personnel has little place in the usual hospital infection control program [69,95,106]. Culture of various animate and inanimate sites on a routine basis has been advocated in the past, but data now suggest that high cost outweighs any clinical or epidemiologic benefits [56].

### Quality Control

Just as an effective clinical microbiology laboratory is essential to an effective infection control program, adequate quality control is essential to the practice of good clinical microbiology [9]. Such a quality program begins with a comprehensive procedure manual that establishes standards for performance, including definition of acceptable and unacceptable quality of specimens and specimen containers, permissible delay between collection and receipt of the specimen in the laboratory, and times during which specimens are accepted for processing. The action to be taken by workers when specimens are not in accord with these standards also must be defined. These standards should be communicated to clinicians and nurses as well as to laboratory personnel.

The procedure manual also should cover administrative aspects of laboratory operation related to infection control and employee safety [86]. Minimum standards for identification of isolates should be provided, including a listing of the equipment and reagents to be monitored and the measures to be made to ensure reproducible and accurate performance. The periodic evaluation of skills of all workers, including evening, night, and weekend workers, should be included in the program.

Participating in proficiency testing programs helps the laboratory maintain competence, particularly if proficiency test specimens are submitted to the laboratory in a blind fashion and are handled by routine procedures. If problems develop with such evaluation, the identity of the problem specimens should be made known, and the personnel challenged to deal with the specimen in as careful a fashion as possible, to ensure that the laboratory actually has within its capability the correct handling and identification of the organisms.

In addition to such outcome-oriented projects, periodic review of selected laboratory materials, media, and other equipment should be performed. On occasion, erroneous microbiologic results related to the inadvertent use of contaminated or faulty materials may occur. For example, nonviable contaminants were found in specimen tubes in commercial lumbar puncture trays; these resulted in the assumption that an outbreak was occurring of nosocomial meningitis when the contaminants were seen on Gram stains of cerebrospinal fluid [105]. Such "pseudooutbreaks" [60] must be considered when laboratory culture or stain results do not correlate with clinical or epidemiologic findings.

Hospital-supported continuing education is essential for quality work in the microbiology laboratory. It is especially important for personnel in smaller hospital laboratories to stay abreast of technologic advances and trends in nosocomial infection occurrence and diagnosis [13]. Fortunately a number of organizations, including the American Society for Microbiology, the Association for Practitioners in Infection Control, and the American Society of Clinical Pathology, provide frequent programs on nosocomial infection topics.

## ANTIBIOTIC SUSCEPTIBILITY TESTING

A standardized method of antimicrobial susceptibility testing subject to quality-control evaluation is essential in any clinical microbiology laboratory and is equally critical to infection control studies. On occasion the epidemiologist will suspect that a group of nosocomial infections with organisms of the same species have a common origin. To investigate whether strains in this "cluster" [90] are common or different, the usual practice is to examine results of biochemical tests and the pattern of susceptibility to antimicrobial agents. Often these results will answer the question of relationships. Occasionally additional tests are needed; these are described in a later section of this chapter.

The Kirby-Bauer single-disc-diffusion method or an equivalent test system is used in many laboratories for routine testing of antimicrobial susceptibility of bacteria [51]. However, many laboratories are now routinely performing a more quantitative evaluation of sensitivity, using broth-dilution or agar-dilution test methods [51]. In addition, tube dilution or other methods of establishing minimum inhibitory concentration or susceptibility to "gate" concentrations of antibiotic must be used for testing organisms that have not been standardized for testing by a disc method. The latter include a number of anaerobic bacteria, fungi, and yeasts. Other sources may be consulted for detailed discussion of the performance and quality control of these procedures [50,53,58].

Some microorganisms can be additionally differentiated by indicating the relative degree to which susceptibility or resistance to antimicrobials is present [37]. This can be done by noting the absolute value of zone size in agar-diffusion testing or by providing assessment of minimum inhibitory concentration or minimum bactericidal concentration [51]. Situations in which this more quantitative information would be useful should be delineated jointly by the laboratory and infection control team.

### Selection of Strains for Testing

Application of susceptibility tests to bacteria that are doubtfully related to infection must be avoided, and specific guidelines for the selection of isolates for susceptibility determination should be established by the laboratory. For example, the request for testing of susceptibility should be carefully evaluated when the organisms isolated are endogenous flora present at sites in which they are not normally pathogens. Similarly, the testing of organisms from mixed culture should be avoided in most cases because of the unclear role of the various isolates [9]. Direct testing of urine and spinal fluid is not essential in most cases. Direct testing of susceptibility of isolates from blood culture can be useful as long as the results are confirmed by standardized techniques [84]. Potential pathogens with well-established susceptiblity to antimicrobials should not be tested routinely; this group currently includes *Streptococcus pyogenes* and *Streptococcus pneumoniae*, but isolates of the latter from spinal fluid probably should be tested for penicillin susceptibility, in view of the relatively resistant strains being reported in many parts of the United States and other countries [52].

Modified methods are required for the testing of *Neisseria* species and for *Hemophilus influenzae*. *Neisseria meningitidis* does not routinely need to be tested, as strains of this organism have remained uniformly susceptible to penicillin G [75]. In contrast, *H. influenzae* must routinely be tested for presence of β-lactamases, because such enzymes have now become prevalent in both community-acquired and nosocomial strains of this organism. Penicillin resistance that is caused by β-lactamase-producing strains of *Neisseria gonorrhoeae* are being reported from a smattering of areas of the United States, but routine testing of isolates for β-lactamase is recommended only for organisms recovered from blood and other normally sterile body fluids [75]. Patients who fail to respond to adequate doses of penicillin for gonorrhea may be treated with other drugs instead of waiting for laboratory testing for β-lactamase production.

Methicillin-resistant strains of *S. aureus* have been reported from a variety of hospitals in the United States and elsewhere [100]. Strains have been associated predominantly with nosocomial infection, but some community reservoirs are described as well [89]. Laboratories must include testing methods that will rapidly and accurately detect the presence of such resistant strains; methods required vary from those routinely employed, and involve extensive quality-control evaluation to ensure precision [50].

*Selection of Drugs for Routine and Special Testing*
The introduction of Food and Drug Administration (FDA) controls on the certification of discs for use in the Kirby-Bauer agar-diffusion testing method substantially reduced the unnecessary and wasteful testing of related antimicrobials. These guidelines state that, in general, only one drug of a particular class of antibiotics need be tested, since the results will pertain to all members of that class. Continuation of these recommendations for "class disks" by the National Coordinating Committee on Laboratory Standards (NCCLS) has permitted laboratories to cope with the ever-increasing number of newly introduced antimicrobials with similar activity and indications [75].

The selection of drugs for routine testing should be undertaken by the laboratory after consultation with the Infection Control Committee; the chosen agents should reflect both common usage practices of physicians in the hospital and the spectrum of pathogens that are frequently encountered. Occasionally testing of susceptibility to certain drugs will be performed for epidemiologic purposes; results of such testing may be omitted from routine clinical reporting. Similarly, certain antimicrobials for which the hospital wishes to control usage may be tested but not reported routinely, or tested only after consultation [57].

Different groups of antimicrobials often are used for gram-negative and gram-positive aerobic organisms. Drugs included in each panel should be periodically evaluated and updated. The epidemiologic value of susceptibility patterns may be enhanced by inclusion of certain antibiotics that are not in routine clinical use. Such additional information can also provide valuable taxonomic and quality-control information [36], but these benefits must be weighed against the extra time and cost required for testing and recording of the additional studies.

*Quality Control*
Consistent and accurate identification of organisms over time is necessary for susceptibility data to be useful for clinical and epidemiologic purposes. In addition, errors in performance of susceptibility tests may result in information that is misleading about diagnosis and/or therapy. To minimize this possibility, most antibiotic discs should be stored at 4°C to 8°C (39°F to 46°F) and discs containing synthetic penicillins and cephalosporins require storage at $-20$°C ($-4$°F). Desiccant must be provided, and dispensers should be protected from frequent movement between refrigeration temperature and warm humid room air. Every batch of medium used for testing, whether for agar diffusion or dilution systems of testing, should have pH tested and adjusted to standard values. Cultures of control strains of *S. aureus* ATCC 25923, *P. aeruginosa* ATCC 27853, and *E. coli* ATCC 25922 should be tested to ensure that zone diameters fall within the range of acceptability established by the FDA and listed on the disc package insert, or (for dilution methods) fall within the boundaries of acceptable ranges defined by the NCCLS [10,75]. Susceptibility tests depend on correct incubation temperatures; these should be checked routinely during the week. When results of these quality-control tests exceed acceptable limits, reports on clinical isolates can be withheld until satisfactory control results are obtained. The reproducibility of susceptibility tests can also be assessed by participation in quality-control programs of groups like the College of American

Pathologists or the Centers for Disease Control, which periodically distribute unknown specimens for evaluation. Such testing programs focus on clinically and epidemiologically important strains; correct identification assures the laboratory and infection control personnel that the laboratory applies proper techniques and skills. The reader is referred to more detailed presentations of these quality-control considerations [9].

## TIMELY REPORTING OF LABORATORY DATA AND PARTICIPATION IN SURVEILLANCE OF NOSOCOMIAL INFECTION

To deal with individual problems of nosocomial infection in the hospital as they arise, control measures must be taken as quickly as possible and must be based on accurate assessment of the problem and its causes [12,37]. Without rapid identification and reporting of the organisms involved, control measures cannot be efficiently designed and implemented.

### Surveillance
Laboratory records are an important tool for surveillance of infections [39]. More than 80 percent of infections defined by other criteria as nosocomial may be identified by review of positive cultures from the microbiology laboratory [32]. Thus data gathered by infection control personnel during laboratory visits form an important base to which additional surveillance data from clinical rounds must be added. Both sources must be used to obtain an accurate estimate of the true rate of occurrence of nosocomial infection in a given hospital (see Chapter 4).

For both endemic and epidemic nosocomial infection, microbiologic and immunologic reports may be the starting point for additional epidemiologic investigations. These investigations often require information about attributes of the patient, the personnel involved in care, or the diagnostic and therapeutic procedures provided to the patient. Obtaining these nonlaboratory data usually is easier when the patient is still present in the hospital or at least is fresh in the minds of hospital personnel. Prompt reporting of pertinent laboratory results facilitates information retrieval of this type.

Computer programs have been developed to identify clusters of infections with the same organism and susceptibilities that occur at the same time in the same patient-care area (ward or service). Such programs have permitted identification of outbreaks; whether they provide such information in rapid enough fashion to permit use of control measures remains open to question.

The laboratory can indicate only which organisms were present in culture. The epidemiologist must supplement this information with clinical data to determine whether organisms found in culture indicate infection or colonization. If colonization is present, the identification of organisms in the culture may be of little help to the clinician. To the epidemiologist, however, both the organisms involved in episodes of exogenous colonization and those of infection are of interest. Either may be evidence of spread of organisms from one site to another, indicating an area in which control measures may halt transmission. Data used for this purpose must be accurate, which emphasizes the role of continuing quality-control studies in the laboratory.

### Reporting of Results
To facilitate the surveillance of nosocomial infections and of all infections requiring isolation or notification of public health authorities, a copy of positive culture results should be provided to the infection control personnel. Physicians and nurses sometimes are lax about notifying public health authorities of reportable diseases. Isolation of such organisms will be reported to health authorities more efficiently if the responsibility for reporting is delegated to the infection control nurse or some other person designated by the Infection Control Committee (see Chapter 8).

Prompt reporting by telephone to both clinicians and infection control personnel is essential when presumptive identification is made of isolates of nosocomial significance; this is the only way to ensure proper treatment of the patient and the application of proper control measures [49]. Occasions for reporting include incidents such as the presumptive identification of certain agents in meningitis, isolation of salmonellae or shigellae from stool specimens, positive smears and cultures of tuberculosis bacilli from any patient or employee, and isolation of S. aureus from any culture taken of an employee or from lesions of a newborn.

Laboratory studies may provide early warning of the emergence within a hospital of highly infectious microorganisms, multiple-drug-resistant organisms, and clusters of unusual infections. In some hospitals laboratory workers may be the first to detect these and other trends of infection. When findings suggest a possible outbreak, notification requires quicker action than a "final report," because useful epidemiologic investigations triggered by the first preliminary data from the laboratory often are profitable. The major elements needed in an "early warning" are the interest and expertise of the laboratory worker in calling results to the attention of infection control colleagues. This may be done by telephone or page, if urgent; if not, a mention during the daily visit of the infection control staff usually suffices.

Such reporting facilitates the efforts of the infection control personnel. At the same time, "early warning" must not be requested for so many situations that this becomes an unreasonable burden for the laboratory personnel.

*Laboratory Records*
In addition to instituting control measures, infection control workers often need to analyze laboratory data from various periods to try to detect "patterns" of infection [37]. To assist in this effort, it is helpful if the laboratory can provide an "archival" summary of organisms on a periodic basis. Data of particular usefulness here might include compiled listings of organisms by culture site, date, patient, and ward; a summary of susceptibility testing results for various species of organisms for given time periods might also be of help. Guidelines for selection and a reporting format have been developed [36,104]. The specific laboratory data that can aid epidemiologic analyses vary from hospital to hospital; the information to be included and the frequency with which such summaries are made should be determined by the people providing and working with the data in each hospital.

Laboratory records should be retained in such a way that they facilitate such retrospective epidemiologic investigations and quality-control activities. The source of each specimen, date of collection, patient identification, hospital number, hospital service, ward, and organisms identified in the final report should be recorded. Records also should be kept of results of antimicrobial sensitivity tests and of any special biochemical or typing reactions.

All cultures should be recorded so that results are readily available by date, type of specimen, and pathogens isolated. Culture data on inpatients and outpatients should be maintained separately. Computer storage and retrieval of all results is optimal; noncomputerized rapid retrieval and sorting systems may also be useful [92]. These records can be maintained in simple, inexpensive, and epidemiologically useful fashion by bound log books, which are kept chronologically for each major type of specimen (e.g., blood, wound, skin, cerebrospinal fluid, urine, stool, sputum). Sole reliance on a filing system of loose lab slips is not desirable because specific data are difficult to retrieve and easily lost.

The permanent records of the microbiology laboratory should include dates and other details of any major changes in culturing techniques or laboratory procedures. Dates of changes in the criteria for identification and taxonomic designations applied to isolates should be recorded as well.

*Retention Period for Records*
No analysis of previous data can be made if the records are not available. To this end, it is incumbent on the laboratory staff to maintain the microbiologic records in some accessible format (e.g., final report sheets, disc or tape storage) for a reasonable period. The length of time such records can be maintained depends on hospital size, work volume of the laboratory, and available storage facilities, as well as on infection control needs. Thus storage time should be determined by laboratory personnel after consultation with the hospital infection control staff.

*Summary Reports for Clinical Use*
Development of profiles for susceptibility of frequently tested pathogens to drugs commonly in use can be of considerable assistance in guiding therapy for sepsis of unclear cause and other infections. Testing other organisms (e.g., slow-growing bacteria or organisms requiring special test procedures) may be performed at intervals to develop a profile of their susceptibility. As long as susceptibility patterns can be presumed to remain stable, such testing may be a useful substitute for testing each isolate at the time of recovery.

In liaison with the Infection Control Committee, the laboratory should provide at regular intervals a summary of susceptibility patterns, and make it available to the clinicians on the staff. Tabulations that may be of particular use include frequency of susceptibility to individual drugs by site of infection (which may provide guidance to the clinician for empirical therapy of infection before the causative organism has been identified) and tabulation of frequency of susceptibility to individual antimicrobials by pathogen (which may be used to direct therapy after an organism has been identified but before susceptibility tests have been completed). The Infection Control Committee, a medical staff committee, or both, may wish to receive such data to guide their review of antibiotic use [57].

A listing of the relative costs of the currently employed antimicrobials may be developed with cooperation of the pharmacy; inclusion of this information with susceptibility summaries may enhance incentive to reduce costs of antimicrobial usage [57].

## ADDITIONAL STUDIES TO ESTABLISH SIMILARITY OR DIFFERENCE OF ORGANISMS

On occasion the epidemiologist will suspect that a group of nosocomial infections with organisms of the same species have a common origin. To investigate whether strains in this "cluster" [90] are common or different, the usual practice is to examine results of biochemical tests and pattern of susceptibility to antimicrobial agents. However, for organisms commonly encountered in the hospital (e.g., *S. aureus* or *Klebsiella*), the general pattern of these results may be similar on the basis of chance alone. Conversely, for other organisms (e.g. *P. aeruginosa*), the variation in these characteristics from strain to strain is so small that the tests provide little information about similarity or difference of tested strains [1]. Testing of additional antimicrobials not ordinarily included, or of susceptibility to other antibacterial substances (e.g., silver) may differentiate strains in some cases. In situations in which no differences can be shown for the above tests, examination of additional organism characteristics (markers) can be of great assistance [1,37,106].

Although hospital laboratory personnel may not have the facilities to perform specialized typing procedures, they should know which organisms can be typed and which cannot, and where specific proce-

dures can be performed. When epidemiologically important isolates require special typing, it may be necessary to forward them to local or state reference laboratories. Potentially pathogenic materials should be packaged for air transport in conformance with federal regulations [86].

### Typing of Isolates

Selected typing systems of special value in investigating nosocomial infection problems are summarized in Tables 7-1 through 7-3. Many are beyond the capabilities of the usual clinical laboratory, but a number can be conducted when circumstances dictate.

A number of organisms involved in nosocomial infection have been differentiated successfully by antimicrobial susceptibility testing (Table 7-1). This technique was discussed earlier in this chapter. Test antimicrobials not usually employed for routine clinical use can be of assistance here. As noted earlier, a quantitative assessment of the relative degree to which susceptibility or resistance to antimicrobials is present may help make this differentiation [37]. Susceptibility to heavy metals (resistotyping) also has proved of value in selected instances (see preceding section).

*Biotyping* is the use of certain characteristic biochemical reactions to identify subgroups of bacteria. Typing schemes using this method have been devised for a variety of bacterial organisms, both anaerobes and aerobes, and found to be useful in infection control investigations (Table 7-1). These schemes often are used in conjunction with pattern analysis of an-

TABLE 7-1. Typing systems for selected organisms causing nosocomial infection

| Organism | Antimicrobials or heavy metals | Biotyping | Phage susceptibility |
|---|---|---|---|
| *Escherichia coli* | 23*, 27 | 23, 33 | 64 |
| *Enterobacter* | 61 | 76 | |
| *Klebsiella* | 37, 90 | 37, 85 | 85 |
| *Proteus* | 4 | 4, 47 | 46 |
| *Pseudomonas aeruginosa* | 90 | | 59 |
| *Serratia marcescens* | 90 | 81 | 81 |
| *Salmonella* | 72 | | 35, 55 |
| *Shigella* | 26 | | 54 |
| *Yersinia* | 5 | 5, 83 | 5 |
| *Staphylococcus aureus* | 16 | 36 | 97 |
| *Staphylococcus epidermidis* | 17 | 17 | 17, 43 |
| *Listeria* | | | 99 |
| Diphtheroids | 74 | 74 | |
| *Clostridium difficile* | 110 | | 93 |
| *Hemophilus influenzae* | 103 | 103 | |

*Numbers refer to references using the indicated typing scheme for the indicated organism.

timicrobial susceptibility testing to attempt discrimination of isolates. Biotyping has been proposed as a convenient method for discrimination of strains of *Staphylococcus epidermidis*; the clinical and epidemiologic value of such testing has been proved in a few situations [17], but the method probably should be reserved for special circumstances rather than routinely employed.

Susceptibility to bacteriophages (phage typing) is a characteristic used for typing a number of organisms of nosocomial importance (Table 7-1). The technique is especially handy for grouping strains of *S. aureus*. This procedure usually is available only in reference laboratories, and plasmid transfer of phage characteristics apparently can occur, but the procedure continues to be of value in relating isolates obtained from patients, personnel, and the environment under epidemic conditions [71]. It often has been desirable to determine the bacteriophage types of *S. aureus* isolates obtained just before an outbreak for comparison with the pattern of the epidemic strain. Although routine typing of all strains is not cost-effective, some laboratories store isolates for later typing should it prove desirable. Isolates may be conveniently and inexpensively stored by placing a small amount of growth on a blank paper disc that is placed in a 2-ml glass screw-cap vial containing a few granules of silica gel. If the vial is kept tightly closed,

isolates may be held up to six months; they can then be easily retrieved by placing the disc in broth.

*Serotyping* is a major technique used for typing of many gram-negative aerobic bacilli, especially *Klebsiella pneumoniae* isolates (Table 7-2). Serotyping is probably the single most valuable technique for typing *P. aeruginosa*. The technique can be of great help for other organisms shown in the table as well, in both outbreak situations and research investigations [1]. However, the cost of routine serotyping of isolates in the absence of an outbreak has not been justified by demonstration of benefit to patient diagnosis or therapy. See Chapter 32 for a discussion of the value of serotyping of "enteropathogenic" strains of *E. coli*.

Many bacteria produce products that can inhibit the growth of other organisms. Production of such "bacteriocins" by an epidemic strain, or susceptibility of the organism in question to those produced by other bacteria, can be used as a typing tool for a number of organisms (Table 7-2). The method requires careful use of controls, and widespread agreement on standards for reagents and interpretation is unusual. Bacteriophage typing and pyocine typing often permit additional subdivision of *P. aeruginosa* strains of the same serotype; for maximum usefulness, all three procedures probably should be performed [21].

TABLE 7-2. Additional typing systems for selected organisms causing nosocomial infection

| Organism | Serotyping | Bacteriocin production or susceptibility |
|---|---|---|
| *Escherichia coli* | 23* | 45 |
| *Enterobacter* | | 101 |
| *Klebsiella* | 77, 85 | 11 |
| *Proteus* | 4, 79 | 4, 94 |
| *Morganella* | | 79 |
| *Providencia* | 78, 80 | |
| *Pseudomonas aeruginosa* | 21, 28 | 21 |
| *Pseudomonas cepacia* | 44 | |
| *Serratia* | 81 | 81 |
| *Salmonella* | 25 | |
| *Shigella* | 25 | 73 |
| *Yersinia* | 5, 83 | |
| *Campylobacter jejuni* | 88 | |
| *Staphylococcus aureus* | 18 | |
| *Staphylococcus epidermidis* | 18 | |
| *Listeria* | 98 | |
| *Streptococcus* | 41 | |
| *Hemophilus* | 103 | |
| *Legionella* | 108 | |
| *Clostridium difficile* | | 93 |

*Numbers refer to references using the indicated typing scheme for the indicated organism.

TABLE 7-3. Miscellaneous typing methods for organisms causing nosocomial infection

| Typing system | Organism studied | Reference |
| --- | --- | --- |
| Plasmid profile or nucleic acid homology | Multiple organisms | See Chapter 12 |
| Analysis of enzyme production | *Staphylococcus aureus* | 71 |
| Analysis of marker proteins | *Staphylococcus aureus* | 19 |
| Dienes reaction | *Proteus mirabilis* | 46 |
| Serum opacity | Streptococci | 67 |
| Lipopolysaccharide immunotyping | *Pseudomonas aeruginosa* | 21 |
| Colony morphology | Diphtheroids | 74 |
| RNA electrophoresis | Rotavirus | 87 |
| Killer system analysis | *Candida albicans* | 82 |
| Cytotoxicity assay | *Clostridum difficile* | 110 |

A number of other systems for typing have been proposed for organisms important in cross-infection (Table 7-3). The use of plasmid analysis or nucleic acid homology in nosocomial infection studies is discussed elsewhere (see Chapter 12). Production of enzymes or marker proteins has been employed on occasion. One method of typing of swarming strains of *Proteus mirabilis* is known as Dienes' typing, and can readily be performed by hospital laboratories. A line of demarcation develops at the swarming junction when unrelated strains simultaneously are inoculated on the same agar plate, but it does not appear when the same strains are inoculated concurrently. Other examples shown in Table 7-3 have been used in a small number of reports and their relative usefulness is not yet determined.

*Storage of Strains*
For supplemental tests to be performed, such as those described in the preceding section, the organisms must be available. Thus a related duty of the clinical laboratory staff is to retain strains that may relate to nosocomial infection for a given period while it is determined whether additional testing is needed. In cooperation with infection control personnel, the laboratory staff should subculture and save epidemiologically important isolates, whether such isolates are from outbreaks or from single cases of unusual or potentially epidemic diseases. A system for reviewing and periodically discarding these isolates also must be established. How long a storage period is required for this purpose will vary from hospital to hospital, and should be agreed on between epidemiologist and clinical laboratory supervisor [36,70,104,106]. The technique used to ensure the viability of the organisms (e.g., freezing, lyophilization) should be determined by the laboratory staff after considering the equipment and personnel that are available for this task.

## OCCASIONAL MICROBIOLOGIC STUDIES OF HOSPITAL PERSONNEL OR ENVIRONMENT

In some situations nosocomial infection may result from environmental or personnel sources. In evaluating such episodes, the infection control staff may ask the laboratory staff to process specimens from employees, environmental sources, or hospital equipment (e.g., respiratory therapy machines) as part of the investigation [37,69]. It should be emphasized, however, that such environmental culturing should focus on investigation of documented infections in patients. Environmental studies are not recommended as a major practice in the usual situation. This aspect of a control program recently has been reviewed in detail [69,95,106]; it is worth noting that when such culturing is necessary, its costs should be considered part of the hospitals' infection control program, and charges for the cultures should not be billed to the patients involved in the outbreak [36].

A few procedures of this type should be done routinely (Table 7-4). Others are elective, performed in association with episodes of patient illness or as part of an educational program. A third group is specifically not recommended. Each will be dealt with in turn.

*Routine Environmental Sampling*
In the absence of an epidemic, sampling should be minimal; microbiology and infection control personnel should be firm in not conducting indiscriminate routine microbiologic sampling and testing (see Chapter 14). However, routine checks on the adequacy of sterilizer function, culture of certain blood components, culture of infant formula and some other products [69] prepared in the hospital, and periodic checks on the effectiveness of disinfection of certain equip-

TABLE 7-4. Microbiologic studies of
hospital personnel and the hospital environment

I. Recommended for routine performance
  A. Monitoring of sterilization
    1. Steam sterilizers
    2. Ethylene oxide sterilizers
    3. Dry-heat sterilizers
  B. Sampling of infant formula prepared in the
    hospital and other specific high-risk hospital-
    prepared products
  C. Monitoring of blood components prepared in
    open systems
  D. Monitoring of dialysis fluid (if required by
    regulatory agencies)
  E. "Spot" sampling of certain disinfected equipment
    (occasionally)
II. Elective environmental monitoring
  A. Surveys to investigate a specific problem of
    patient infection
  B. Surveys for educational purposes
III. Procedures not recommended
  A. Routine culture surveys of patients or hospital
    personnel
  B. Routine culture of commercial products labeled as
    sterile
  C. Routine testing of antiseptics and disinfectants
  D. Random culture of blood units
  E. Routine monitoring of disinfection process for
    respiratory therapy equipment

ment that directly contacts tissues other than skin
may help prevent infections from these sources.

MONITORING OF STERILIZATION    All steam and ethylene oxide gas sterilizers should be checked at least
once each week with a suitable live-spore preparation
[95]; ethylene oxide gas sterilizers also should be
checked with each load of items that will come into
contact with blood or other tissues. In addition, each
load in either type of sterilizer should be monitored
with a spore test if it contains implantable objects.
These implantable objects should not be used until
the spore test is reported out as negative, usually at
48 hours of incubation. Guidelines from the Centers
for Disease Control additionally recommend that
dry-heat sterilizers be monitored at least once each
month [95].

All sterilizers should be equipped with time-tem-
perature recorders to provide evidence of adequate
exposure for each load. However, evidence that a
sterilizing temperature has been held for an adequate
time does not prove that sterilization took place; the
temperature is measured at the outlet valve and does
not reflect whether adequate sterilization occurred

within dense volumes of fluid or large, dense, fabric-
wrapped packs. The use of chemical monitors (e.g.,
test tapes or heat-sensitive color indicators) within
the autoclave is recommended for the outside of each
package sterilized [95]. This provides an indication
that a sterilizing temperature may have been reached,
although such monitors do not show whether there
was an adequate duration of exposure. Thus additional monitoring systems are required, which ordinarily involve the laboratory—biologic monitoring
with spore strips generally has been accepted as the
most effective way to determine successful sterilization (see Chapter 14).

Microorganisms chosen for spore strip tests are more
resistant to sterilization than are most naturally occurring pathogens. The test organisms are provided
in relatively high concentrations to ensure a margin
of safety. The spores may be provided either in impregnated filter-paper strips or in solution in glass
ampules. For steam sterilization the thermophile *Bacillus stearothermophilus* is used, and for ethylene oxide
and dry-heat sterilizers *B. subtilis* (strain *globigii*, variety *niger*) is employed. Both species frequently are
incorporated simultaneously in the test strips, and
these can be used to test for adequate sterilization
with either procedure.

Most spore strip preparations are packaged in envelopes that contain one or two test strips and a
control strip. The test strips are packaged in separate
envelopes, and are removed and sterilized at the time
other material is processed. Subsequently, the test
strips and control strip are cultured by placing the
strips in a tube of tryptic-digest casein-soy (TS) broth
that is incubated at 37°C (99°F) for spores used to
control gas sterilization, and 56°C (133°F) for those
used to monitor steam sterilization. It is not necessary
to culture a positive control strip for each test; if
strips are obtained from a single lot, only 10 percent
of the positive control strips need be tested.

Spore solutions are prepared in sealed glass ampules
for testing the adequacy of sterilization of fluids. These
ampules should be incubated at 56°C (133°F) in a
water bath. If there is no change in the indicator by
seven days, the test is reported as negative. Alternatively the fluid may be inoculated with a test culture, which may be subcultured after autoclaving.

Other types of spore preparations are commercially
available and require different handling. In each case,
the manufacturer's directions should be followed
closely.

Test strips or spore solutions should always be
placed in the center of the specimen to be tested,
never on an open shelf in the autoclave. The center
of a pack located near the bottom front exhaust valve

will be exposed for the least adequate duration and temperature of sterilization and thus provides the best location for a test measurement. Testing of sterilization of fluids is accomplished by placing an ampule containing a spore solution in the largest vessel.

Use of ampules containing spore solutions is not appropriate for checking sterilization of microbiologic culture media, because these media do not require the duration of exposure that is required for sterilization of material known to contain large populations of bacteria. In fact heating of bacteriologic culture media to a temperature sufficient to ensure sterilization of a test strip or spore ampule will result in damage to the medium through overheating.

The likelihood of cross-contamination can be reduced by minimizing the handling of the strip after sterilization. Test strips can be removed from their envelopes and placed in sterile glass tubes before sterilization. The tube then is sterilized with the screw-cap removed or with other closures permeable to steam in place. After sterilization the tube is sent to the laboratory, where the nutrient broth is added.

The handling of spore strips in the laboratory requires considerable care to prevent secondary contamination. The transfer should be made in a laminar-flow cabinet if available, using sterile forceps and scissors. The forceps and scissors are common sources of contamination, which may be insufficiently sterilized by flaming or wiping with alcohol. Alcohol may contain viable spores that might not be killed by flaming, and flaming may be insufficient to heat instruments to a temperature that will destroy viable spores. Care should be taken not to cross-contaminate the sterilized spore strips with the control strips.

Condensation on the cover of a 56°C (133°F) water bath may cause contamination of the caps and closures of tubes. A heating block may be used to avoid this, or the bath may be left uncovered; the latter will make it necessary to provide a reservoir to maintain the water level, as the evaporation rate is high at this temperature. Uninoculated culture media should be incubated at 35°C (95°F) or at 56°C (133°F) to ensure that contamination will not yield false-positive reports.

Gram staining and subculturing should be performed to detect secondary contamination of test cultures. If organisms other than gram-positive bacilli are observed, the test should be repeated and reported as "possible laboratory contamination, test being repeated."

Whenever positive results are obtained, the sterilizers should be checked immediately for proper use and function [95]. Careful examination must be made of thermometer and pressure-gauge readings, and re-

cent time and temperature records must be reviewed. If any deficiency is observed or if the repeat sterility test still results in growth, engineering personnel and experts in autoclave maintenance and function should be consulted promptly. Objects other than those used for implants do not need to be recalled at this point unless defects are discovered in the sterilizer or its use; if spore tests remain positive after proper use of the sterilizer is documented, the machine should be removed from service until the defects are corrected [95].

SAMPLING OF INFANT FORMULA AND OTHER PRODUCTS PREPARED IN THE HOSPITAL Infant formula prepared in the hospital kitchen should be monitored on a weekly basis [95]. A guideline for interpretation of culture suggests that fewer than 25 organisms per milliliter be present and that no virulent bacteria, such as *Salmonella* or *Shigella*, be present [95]. The guideline is an arbitrary one, however, and should be a matter of local preference.

Other products prepared in hospitals that have been demonstrated to have a potential for causing nosocomial infection also should be monitored. At one hospital these consisted of hyperalimentation fluid prepared in the hospital and breast milk collected for group use [69]. Whether any products fit into this category and the frequency of monitoring for any identified, should be determined by the individual hospital.

CULTURE OF BLOOD COMPONENTS The American Association of Blood Banks does not recommend random culturing of units of blood to ensure sterility. However, "periodic" culturing of products prepared in an "open" system is advocated [2]. An open system is one in which the transfer container "is not integrally attached to the blood container" [102]. Ten-milliliter samples of the component should be cultured both aerobically and anaerobically for ten days. Incubation at both 18°C to 20°C (64°F to 68°F) and at 35°C to 37°C (95°F to 99°F) is advised [3].

CULTURE OF DIALYSIS FLUID The water used for preparation of dialysis fluid should be tested by colony count at least once per month, according to one set of regulatory requirements [95]. The fluid should contain less than 200 viable organisms per milliliter. Defined methods for such testing vary from one regulatory body to the next; in general, they follow Centers for Disease Control (CDC) guidelines [29].

PERIODIC SAMPLING OF DISINFECTED EQUIPMENT Any article that makes direct contact with the vascular system or tissue other than unbroken skin should be sterile. Whenever possible, steam or gas sterilization should be applied. If chemical disinfection or pasteurization rather than sterilization is used on equipment such as cystoscopes and other endoscopes or anesthesia equipment, some authorities recommend (and some require) that periodic microbiologic sampling be done to ensure the absence of pathogens after processing.

The frequency of sampling of such disinfected devices depends on the results of intermittent sampling, any evidence that nosocomial infection is associated with their use, and an assessment by the Infection Control Committee of the adequacy of standards for control of contamination of such equipment. There is little agreement on which items of this type should be tested, or how often. If such a monitoring program is begun, it may be possible to cut back on the frequency of culturing after a period of time in which cultures are negative, as long as no changes are made in equipment and techniques used [69].

Sampling of unused sterile disposable parts is not necessary, but the parts must not be reused. Samples of reusable equipment should be taken after the product has been disinfected and made ready for use on patients.

### Elective Environmental Monitoring

A wide variety of items and substances can be responsible for cross-infection. Thus environmental surveys may be useful during investigation of specific problems within a hospital and should be instituted in response to, and specifically address, epidemiologic findings [69]. Elective culturing programs may also be instituted in association with educational efforts.

SUPPORT FOR INVESTIGATION OF SPECIFIC PROBLEMS A detailed description of suitable culture techniques for every possible vehicle of cross-infection is beyond the practical scope of this chapter. Methods for sampling sites relevant to infections caused by specific pathogens are described in the appropriate chapters of Part II of this text. The infection control worker and laboratorian must be familiar with general aspects of culture procedures discussed in the following sections, but they should not obtain or process such cultures unless surveillance of infections in patients specifically implicates these items as potential sources of nosocomial infection.

Because standard methods for the microbiologic evaluation of such culture procedures do not exist or are of doubtful validity, considerable expense may be incurred in the production of information that is worthless or misleading. Thus requests for such cultures should be approached with caution, and the infection control staff should be clear regarding how the culture results will affect patient care or epidemiologic control measures before undertaking such tasks [69].

*Culture of blood products after transfusion reaction.* If a transfusion reaction occurs, the possibility of bacterial contamination should be considered [2]. After immediate disconnection of the administered unit, sterile shields should be placed over the exposed ends of needles or tubing to prevent subsequent contamination. A 5-ml sample should be removed aseptically from the administration tubing in the laboratory and processed according to the method recommended by the American Association of Blood Banks (described above) [3]. It is desirable as well to collect blood culture specimens at this time by venipuncture from the patient.

*Cultures of parenteral fluids and intravascular therapy equipment.* The investigation of bacteremia associated with parenteral therapy may require investigation of the needle or catheter, portions of the administration set, the fluid being administered, and portions of the cap or closure provided with the fluid [61] (see Chapter 36). Blood culture specimens should be collected simultaneously from the patient. It is especially important to keep careful track of lot numbers, which should be recorded on the patient's chart as well as on all subsequent laboratory records.

Needles and catheters must be submitted separately from the hubs and other portions of the administration set that may have been exposed to superficial contamination. If portions of the administration set are suspected, these must be received properly capped to exclude spurious contamination. The bottle and administration set should remain connected and be placed in a plastic bag to minimize contamination during delivery to the laboratory.

Catheters and needles may be cultured by a swab-rinse technique (as described in the following section), but the semiquantitative culture methods described in Chapter 36 are preferable. Culture methods for intravenous fluid in containers or collected from administration lines are described in Chapter 36 as well. Careful aseptic technique is critical.

*Methods for culturing tubes and containers.* Cultures of external surfaces or internal cavities (e.g., tubes and containers) may be conducted by a swab-rinse technique [10, 106]. Brain-heart infusion broth (BHIB) supplemented with 0.5% beef extract is used. The broth should contain 0.07% lecithin and 0.5% polysorbate 80 as neutralizers whenever the cultured objects are likely to contain residual disinfectants. A cotton applicator swab is immersed in this broth in a screw-cap tube, wrung out, and used to swab the surface to be sampled. The swab is returned to the tube after sampling; the portion of the stick handled by the operator should be broken off.

Containers and the lumens of tubular structures may be sampled by a rinse technique, which is a better and more convenient sampling method than the swab method for such equipment. The rinse technique involves introducing a suitable quantity of BHIB into the lumen of tubular structures (40 to 50 ml for respiratory therapy tubing) and manually tilting the object to produce a rinsing action. Up to 50 agitations are desirable. Following this, a sample of the broth is placed in a screw-cap tube. Bottles and containers such as nebulizer reservoirs may be sampled by adding 10 to 15 ml of rinse broth, inserting a sterile stopper if required, and shaking vigorously for about 30 seconds.

The broth then is decanted or pipetted into a sterile container and sample tubes thoroughly agitated to ensure a homogeneous suspension. Plate counts are made by preparing a series of tenfold solutions in tubes of TS broth using 1 ml of the test sample for the first dilution. From each tube of the dilution series, 0.5 ml are pipetted onto the surface of a TS agar plate, which is supplemented with 5% sheep or rabbit blood. The plate is rocked until the inoculum is thoroughly distributed and then allowed to dry at 35°C (95°F). The plates are then inverted and incubated for 24 hours, after which colony counts are made if colonies appear to be coalescing or spreading; otherwise, counts are made after 48 hours of incubation.

For specific identification of isolates, the original broth sample should be subcultured at 4 hours and 24 hours after removal of the 1 ml that was used for the dilution count. To perform each subculture, 0.5 ml are pipetted onto the surfaces of TS blood agar, MacConkey agar, and cetrimide agar plates. They are rocked to distribute the inoculum and allowed to dry before incubation at 35°C (95°F). At 24 hours, those same media are inoculated from the original BHIB rinse sample that was incubated at 35°C (95°F). If growth seems apparent on the basis of turbidity, a loopful should be subcultured to provide isolated colonies. At least two colonies of each morphologic colony type should be picked for identification.

*Sampling of respiratory therapy equipment.* In situations of high endemic or epidemic levels of occurrence of nosocomial respiratory infections, sampling of respiratory therapy apparatus may be of value [96]. Methods listed above for culturing tubes or containers may be employed. A direct-dilution method of sampling has been reported by one group of investigators

to be satisfactory for detection of organisms in the range of $10^1$ to $10^6$ CFU/ml [63].

*Methods for sampling of air.* Air sampling may be performed with either settling plates or more sophisticated equipment [38]. Airborne spread of nosocomial bacterial or viral infection is known to occur [40] but is probably uncommon; air sampling should be required infrequently.

Particles suspended in hospital air vary greatly in size and in number of microorganisms they contain. The average diameter of airborne microbial particles in ward air is about 13 $\mu$, but 7 percent are less than 4 $\mu$ in size and 30 percent are greater than 18 $\mu$. Particles with a mean size of 13 $\mu$ settle at a rate of approximately one foot per minute. Since the surface of a standard 100-mm Petri dish represents an area of about 1/15 square foot, and assuming that the air in the study area contains particles of average size, an open Petri dish in still air will sample microbial particles from about 1 cubic foot of air during 15 minutes of exposure [106]. Brain-heart infusion (BHI) or trypticase-soy agar (TSA) are recommended media for such sampling [106].

Although this is an inexpensive way to evaluate airborne microbial contamination, quantitative results may correlate poorly with those obtained with mechanical, volumetric air samplers because of variation in particle size and unknown influences of air turbulence. Under low humidity conditions, droplet nuclei of about 3 $\mu$ can remain suspended indefinitely and can be collected only with high-velocity, volumetric air samplers.

The total number of airborne microbial "particles" will not be measured precisely by observing growth after impaction on an agar plate, as an airborne microbial particle may contain more than one viable cell. Air sampling techniques in which volumetric samples are taken by bubbling air through collection fluid will break up airborne particulate matter and better reflect the total number of organisms than will air samplers that impinge contaminated particles on agar.

A slit sampler, such as the one produced by New Brunswick Scientific, Inc. (New Brunswick, N.J.) is suitable for most microbial air sampling applications [106]. BHI or TSA media should be used in the sampling plates. A staged sampler [38,106] should be needed only when there is some reason to determine the size distribution of the particles. This should be an extremely infrequent event in most U.S. hospitals. Efficient vacuum sources must be used for both samplers, and the rate of flow of air must be properly calibrated to ensure accurate results.

*Culture of floors and other surfaces.* Methods for

sampling of floors and other surfaces have been described in detail [10,22,106]. One method in common use is an adaptation of the swab technique previously described. In this case, a 2 × 2 inch square hole is cut from the center of a sheet of heavy paper, which subsequently is sterilized and wrapped. The culture is collected by placing the paper on the surface to be sampled. The swab is rubbed slowly in close, parallel streaks across the exposed area. This procedure is repeated after moving the swab in a direction perpendicular to the first streaks.

Such surfaces also may be sampled conveniently by use of Rodac plates [10], which are designed to permit direct contact of agar with flat surfaces. Such plates should be filled with 16.5 ml of TS agar containing 0.07% lecithin and 0.5% polysorbate 80 as neutralizers of disinfectant. The number of plates to use depends on the size of the surface being sampled and the level of statistical confidence required. Both the plates and the surface to be sampled should be dry at the time the sample is collected. Plates are pressed firmly against the surface, avoiding a rotary or sliding motion. Colonies are counted after incubation at 35°C to 37°C (95°F to 99°F) for 48 hours. The use of various types of automatic or semiautomatic colony counters will save time in counting large numbers of plates.

Standards for acceptable levels of contamination of floors and bedside tables as sampled by the Rodac plate technique have been suggested by a committee of the American Public Health Association [20]. There is no evidence, however, that any particular level of contamination is directly correlated with an increased risk of infection, and such standards probably are useful only in assessing the adequacy of housecleaning procedures.

*Sampling methods for water and ice.*  Water that meets U.S. Public Health Service standards for drinking water frequently contains up to one million or more microorganisms per milliliter, and some of these organisms are potential pathogens. Ice also can contain organisms that can pose a threat of infection, especially in patients with compromised host defenses. However, correlation of levels of microorganisms with occurrence of patient illness has been found only infrequently.

Samples of water or melted ice can be cultured by passing large quantities through a $0.45$-$\mu$ (or $0.22$-$\mu$) Millipore filter and culturing the filter in broth or directly on agar. More than four colonies/100 ml is considered abnormal by this test [10].

Maximum sensitivity is achieved when the previously described 24-hour BHIB dilution method is used. By this technique substantial numbers of bacteria may be isolated, but there is no evidence that this finding by itself indicates a hazard to the consumer. The finding of a most probable number of 2.2 or more colonies by this test is considered abnormal [10].

*Developing selective media for surveys.*  To reduce the workload in the laboratory and to expedite the processing of specimens, selective survey media should be used whenever possible for culturing specimens during outbreak investigations. Susceptibility data on known or suspected epidemic strains may be used to identify an appropriate selective medium for use in surveys of the animate and inanimate environment of the hospital. Once the implicated organism is isolated and tested on appropriate media containing one or more antibiotics to which it is resistant, the media can be used to exclude numerous bacteria unrelated to the outbreak. This may accelerate the detection of contaminated equipment or infected patients. Pretesting of the media is essential because of possible synergy or antagonism between the added antimicrobials or between these drugs and the media; such interactions could cause inhibition of growth of the epidemic strain or failure to inhibit growth of nonimplicated organisms.

Other selective media also may be useful. For example, cetrimide medium may be helpful in selectively isolating *P. aeruginosa* from contaminated material or mixed cultures. Similarly, tetrathionate broth is an excellent medium for selective preenrichment of *Salmonella* cultures. Mueller-Hinton agar containing sorbitol, a pH indicator, and antibiotics (vancomycin, colistin, and nystatin) provides selective differentiation of *Serratia* species. Many epidemic strains of *S. aureus* are resistant to mercuric chloride, and the incorporation of small amounts of this compound in TSA can be helpful in inhibiting nonepidemic strains of *S. aureus*, *S. epidermidis*, and most gram-negative organisms except *Pseudomonas*. Recently, methicillin-resistant strains of *S. aureus* have become a problem in some U.S. hospitals; agar containing small concentrations of methicillin have been of use in investigating hospital problems due to these strains [100]. The resistance of epidemic microorganisms to other heavy metals, dyes, disinfectants, and other antimicrobial substances also may be used to identify and construct selective media for surveys.

SURVEYS FOR EDUCATIONAL PURPOSES  Sampling techniques that are not directly related to epidemiologic surveys may prove useful in educational programs; visible evidence of contamination of hands, clothing, equipment, and surfaces may serve to teach the need for effective aseptic technique and sanitation.

*Sampling that is Not Recommended*

ROUTINE CULTURE SURVEYS OF PATIENTS AND PER-
SONNEL   Routine culturing of patients or hospital
personnel is not recommended (see Chapter 2). Surveys may be useful during investigation of specific
problems within a hospital, and should be instituted
in response to, and specifically address, epidemiologic
findings.

ROUTINE CULTURE OF COMMERCIAL PRODUCTS   Although commercial patient-care items that are labeled
"sterile" (e.g., intravascular catheters and fluids) occasionally have been contaminated with viable organisms that can cause patient disease, routine sampling of these items is not recommended, because
the low frequency of contamination makes it difficult
(because of the large number of specimens that would
have to be taken) and expensive to perform adequate
sterility testing.

ROUTINE TESTING OF ANTISEPTICS AND DISINFEC-
TANTS   In-use testing of antiseptics and disinfectants
should not be a routine procedure for hospital microbiology laboratories [95]. If contamination of
commercial products sold as sterile is suspected, infection control personnel should be notified and the
nearest office of the U.S. Food and Drug Administration contacted immediately [106]. State regulations may require immediate notification of state health
authorities as well.

RANDOM CULTURE OF BLOOD UNITS   The American
Association of Blood Banks does not recommend random culture of blood units to ensure sterility [2].

ROUTINE MONITORING OF DISINFECTION PROCESS FOR
RESPIRATORY THERAPY EQUIPMENT   Guidelines from
the Centers for Disease Control recommend that "in
the absence of an epidemic or high endemic rate of
nosocomial pulmonary infections, the disinfection
process for respiratory therapy equipment should not
be monitored by cultures; that is, routine sampling
should not be done" [96]. Disinfection of respiratory
therapy and anesthesia equipment is discussed additionally in Chapter 26.

Routine sampling of respiratory therapy equipment while it is being used by a patient is not recommended [96].

## TEACHING MICROBIOLOGIC ASPECTS OF NOSOCOMIAL INFECTION TO INFECTION CONTROL PERSONNEL

The persons responsible for infection control usually
are not trained in clinical laboratory procedures. Since
the key to success in infection control efforts is communication, it is necessary that all involved speak
the same language. For this purpose, training of epidemiology personnel in the language of the clinical
laboratory microbiologist is important. The training
of many infection control personnel in microbiology
is inadequate or out-of-date [36,106]. The goal of
such teaching is not necessarily to make the infection
control staff accomplished laboratory workers, but
rather to familiarize them with the procedures and
practices of the laboratory, the microorganisms involved in nosocomial infection, the validity of test
procedures used in identifying these pathogens, and
the strengths and weaknesses of the resulting data.

Similarly, it is important for the microbiologist to
learn some of the concepts of the epidemiologist,
since few laboratory directors or technologists have
adequate grounding in epidemiology [42]. Especially
important are exposure to techniques used for measuring frequency of infection and the concept of colonization versus infection.

Such joint efforts permit ready communication between the two groups of colleagues. Teaching of this
type can be done in a formal fashion but is also
effective when included as part of the day-to-day informal contacts between the infection control staff
and laboratory personnel.

## REFERENCES

1. Aber, R. C., and Mackel, D. C., Epidemiologic
   typing of nosocomial microorganisms. *Am. J.
   Med.* 70:899, 1981.
2. American Association of Blood Banks. *Technical
   Manual of the American Association of Blood Banks*
   (8th ed.). Washington, D.C.: A.A.B.B., 1981,
   Chapter 24.
3. American Association of Blood Banks. *Technical
   Methods and Procedures* (6th ed.). Washington,
   D.C.: A.A.B.B., 1974.
4. Anderson, R. L., and Engley, F. B., Jr. Typing
   methods for *Proteus rettgeri*: Comparison of biotype, antibiograms, serotype, and bacteriocin
   production. *J. Clin. Microbiol.* 8:715, 1978.
5. Baker, P. M., and Farmer, J. J., III. New bacteriophage typing system for *Yersinia enterocolitica, Yersinia kristensenii, Yersinia frederiksenii,* and
   *Yersinia intermedia*: Correlation with serotyping,
   biotyping, and antibiotic susceptibility. *J. Clin.
   Microbiol.* 15:491, 1982.
6. Balows, A., Dehaan, R. M., Dowell, V. R., and
   Guze, L. B. (Eds.). *Anaerobic Bacteria.* Springfield, Ill.: Thomas, 1974.

7. Bartlett, R. C. A plea for clinical relevance in medical microbiology. *Am. J. Clin. Pathol.* 61:867, 1974.

8. Bartlett, R. C. Control of cost and medical relevance in clinical microbiology. *Am. J. Clin. Pathol.* 64:518, 1975.

9. Bartlett, R. C. *Medical Microbiology: Quality, Cost, and Clinical Relevance.* New York: Wiley Interscience, 1974.

10. Bartlett, R. C., Groschell, D. H. M., Mackel, D. C., Mallison, G. F., and Spaulding, E. H. Control of Hospital-Associated Infections. In Lennette, E. H., Spaulding E. H., and Truant, J. P. (Eds.), *Manual of Clinical Microbiology* (2d ed.). Washington, D.C.: American Society for Microbiology, 1974, Chapter 91.

11. Bauernfeind, A., Petermuller, C., and Schneider, R. Bacteriocins as tools in analysis of nosocomial *Klebsiella pneumoniae* infections. *J. Clin. Microbiol.* 14:15, 1981.

12. Brachman, P. S. Nosocomial infection control: An overview. *Rev. Infect. Dis.* 3:640, 1981.

13. Britt, M. R. Infectious diseases in small hospitals: Prevalence of infections and adequacy of microbiology. *Ann. Intern. Med.* 89:757, 1978.

14. Broughton, P. M. G., and Woodford, F. P. Benefits of costing in the clinical laboratory. *J. Clin. Pathol.* 36:1028, 1983.

15. Casewell, M. W., and Talsania, H. G. Multiple antibiotic resistance and capsular types of gentamicin-resistant *Klebsiella aerogenes. J. Antimicrob. Chemother.* 7:237, 1981.

16. Center for Disease Control. The Role of the Microbiology Laboratory in Surveillance and Control of Nosocomial Infections. National Nosocomial Infections Study Report, Annual Summary, 1974. Atlanta: CDC, issued March, 1977, pp. 27–34.

17. Christensen, G. D., Parisi, J. T., Bisno, A. L., Simpson, W. A., and Beachey, E. H. Characterization of clinically significant strains of coagulase-negative staphylococci. *J. Clin. Microbiol.* 18:258, 1983.

18. Cohen, J. O. Serotyping of Staphylococci. In Cohen, J. O. (Ed.), *The Staphylococci.* New York: Wiley Interscience, 1972.

19. Cohen, M. L., Graves, L. M., Hayes, P. S., et. al. Toxic shock syndrome: Modification and comparison of methods for detecting marker proteins in *Staphylococcus aureus. J. Clin. Microbiol.* 18:372, 1983.

20. Committee on Microbial Contamination of Surfaces, Laboratory Section, American Public Health Association. A comparative microbiological evaluation of floor-cleaning procedures in hospital patient rooms. *Health Lab. Sci.* 7:3, 1970.

21. Conroy, J. V., Baltch, A. L., Smith, R. P., et al. Bacteremia due to *Pseudomonas aeruginosa*: Use of a combined typing system in an eight-year study. *J. Infect. Dis.* 148:603, 1983.

22. Craythorn, J. M., Barbour, A. G., Matsen, J. M., Britt, M. R., and Garibaldi, R. A. Membrane filter contact technique for bacteriological sampling of moist surfaces. *J. Clin. Microbiol.* 12:250, 1980.

23. Crichton, P. B., and Old, D. C. Differentiation of strains of *Escherichia coli*: Multiple typing approach. *J. Clin. Microbiol.* 11:635, 1980.

24. Echeverria, P., Blacklow, N. R., Cukor, G. G., Vibulbandhitkit, S., Changchawalit, S., and Boonthai, P. Rotavirus as a cause of severe gastroenteritis in adults. *J. Clin. Microbiol.* 18:663, 1983.

25. Edwards, P. R., and Ewing, W. H. *Identification of Enterobacteriaceae.* Minneapolis: Burgess Publishing, 1972.

26. Elek, S. D., Davies, J. R., and Miles, R. Resistotyping of *Shigella sonnei. J. Med. Microbiol.* 6:329, 1973.

27. Elek, S. D., and Higney, L. Resistogram typing: A new epidemiological tool. Application to *Escherichia coli. J. Med. Microbiol.* 3:103, 1970.

28. Farmer, J. J., III, Weinstein, R. A., Zierdt, C. H., and Brokopp, C. D. Hospital outbreaks caused by *Pseudomonas aeruginosa*: Importance of serogroup 011. *J. Clin. Microbiol.* 16:266, 1982.

29. Favero, M. S., and Peterson, M. J. Microbiologic guidelines for hemodialysis systems. *Dialysis and Transplantation* 6:34, 1977.

30. Finegold, S. M. Pathogenic anaerobes. *Arch. Intern. Med.* 142:1988, 1982.

31. Fraser, D. W. Bacteria newly recognized as nosocomial pathogens. *Am. J. Med.* 70:432, 1981.

32. Freeman, J., and McGowan, J. E., Jr. Methodologic issues in hospital epidemiology. I. Rates, case-finding, and interpretation. *Rev. Infect. Dis.* 3:658, 1981.

33. Gargan, R., Brumfitt, W., and Hamilton-Miller, J. M. T. A concise biotyping system for differentiating strains of *Escherichia coli. J. Clin. Pathol.* 35:1366, 1982.

34. Gavan, T. C. The laboratory microbiologist in clinical medicine. *Ann. Intern. Med.* 89:789, 1978.

35. Gershman, M. Single phage-typing set for differentiating salmonellae. *J. Clin. Microbiol.* 5:302, 1977.

36. Goldmann, D. A. Laboratory procedures for infection control. In Lennette, E. H., Balows, A.,

Hausler, W. J., Jr., and Truant, J. P. (Eds.), *Manual of Clinical Microbiology* (3d ed.). Washington, D.C.: American Society for Microbiology, 1980, Chapter 94, pp. 939–951.

37. Goldmann, D. A., and Macone, A. B. A microbiologic approach to the investigation of bacterial nosocomial infection outbreaks. *Infect. Control* 1:391, 1980.

38. Groschel, D. H. Air sampling in hospitals. *Ann. N.Y. Acad. Sci.* 353:230, 1980.

39. Gross, P. A., Beaugard, A., and Van Antwerpen, C. Surveillance for nosocomial infections: Can the sources of data be reduced? *Infect. Control* 1:233, 1980.

40. Gundermann, K. D. Spread of microorganisms by air-conditioning systems—especially in hospitals. *Ann. N.Y. Acad. Sci.* 353:209, 1980.

41. Hahn, G., and Nyberg, I. Identification of streptococcal groups A,B,C, and G by slide co-agglutination of antibody-sensitized protein A–containing staphylococci. *J. Clin. Microbiol.* 4:99, 1976.

42. Haley, R. W. The "hospital epidemiologist" in U.S. hospitals, 1976–1977: A description of the head of the infection surveillance and control program. *Infect. Control* 1:21, 1980.

43. Heczko, P. B., Pulverer, J. G., Kasprowicz, A., et al. Evaluation of a new bacteriophage set for typing of *Staphylococcus epidermidis* strains. *J. Clin. Microbiol.* 5:573, 1977.

44. Heidt, A., Monteil, H., and Richard, C. O and H serotyping of *Pseudomonas cepacia. J. Clin. Microbiol.* 18:738, 1983.

45. Hettiaratchy, I. G. T., Cooke, E. M., and Shooter, R. A. Colicine production as an epidemiologic marker of *Escherichia coli. J. Med. Microbiol.* 6:1, 1973.

46. Hickman, F. W., and Farmer, J. J., III. Differentiation of *Proteus mirabilis* by bacteriophage typing and the Dienes reaction. *J. Clin. Microbiol.* 3:350, 1976.

47. Huang, C. T. Multi-test media for rapid identification of *Proteus* species with notes on biochemical reactions of strains isolated from urine and pus. *J. Clin. Pathol.* 19:438, 1966.

48. Iglehart, J. K. Health policy report: The new era of prospective payment for hospitals. *N. Engl. J. Med.* 307:1288, 1982.

49. Isenberg, H. D. Microbiology and the Ailing Patient. In Lorian, V. (Ed.), *Significance of Medical Microbiology In the Care of Patients*, (2d ed.), Baltimore: Williams & Wilkins, 1982.

50. Ishida, K., Guze, P. A., Kalmanson, G. M., Albrandt, K., and Guze, L. B. Variables in demonstrating methicillin tolerance in *Staphylococcus aureus* strains. *J. Clin. Microbiol.* 21:688, 1982.

51. Jones, R. N. The Antimicrobial Susceptibility Test: Rapid and Overnight, Agar and Broth, Automated and Conventional, Interpretation and Trend Analysis. In Lorian, V. (Ed.), *Significance of Medical Microbiology in the Care of Patients* (2d ed.). Baltimore: Williams & Wilkins, 1982.

52. Jones, R. N., Edson, D. C., and the CAP Microbiology Resource Committee. The ability of participant laboratories to detect penicillin-resistant pneumococci. *Am. J. Clin. Pathol.* 78(Suppl.):659, 1982.

53. Jones, R. N., Edson, D. C., and the CAP Microbiology Resource Committee. Interlaboratory performance of disk agar diffusion and dilution antimicrobial susceptibility tests, 1979–1981. *Am. J. Clin. Pathol.* 78(Suppl.):651, 1982.

54. Kallings, L. O., Lindberg, A. A., and Sjoberg, L. Phage typing of *Shigella sonnei. Arch. Immunol. Ther. Exp.* (Warsz.) 16:280, 1968.

55. Katsatiya, S., Caprioli, T., and Champoux, S. Bacteriophage typing scheme for *Salmonella infantis. J. Clin. Microbiol.* 10:637, 1978.

56. Kramer, B. S., Pizzo, P. A., Robichaud, K. J., Witebsky, F., and Wesley, R. Role of serial microbiologic surveillance and clinical evaluation in the management of cancer patients with fever and granulocytopenia. *Am. J. Med.* 72:561, 1982.

57. Kunin, C. M. Evaluation of antibiotic usage: A comprehensive look at alternative approaches. *Rev. Infect. Dis.* 3:745, 1981.

58. Lennette, E. H., Balows, A., Hausler, W. J., Jr., and Truant, J. P. (Eds.). *Manual of Clinical Microbiology* (3d ed.). Washington, D.C.: American Society for Microbiology, 1980.

59. Lindberg, R. B., and Latta, R. L. Phage typing of *Pseudomonas aeruginosa*: Clinical and epidemiologic considerations. *J. Infect. Dis.* 130(Suppl.):33, 1974.

60. Maki, D. G. Through the glass darkly: Nosocomial pseudoepidemics and pseudobacteremias. *Arch. Intern. Med.* 140:26, 1980.

61. Maki, D. G., Rhame, F. S., Mackel, D. C., et al. Nationwide epidemic of septicemia caused by contaminated intravenous products. I. Epidemiologic and clinical features. *Am. J. Med.* 60:471, 1976.

62. Maki, D. G., Weise, C. E., and Sarrafin, H. W. A semi-quantitative culture method for identifying intravenous catheter–related infection. *N. Engl. J. Med.* 296:1305, 1977.

63. Malecka-Griggs, B. and Reinhardt, D. J. Direct dilution sampling, quantitation, and microbial

assessment of open-system ventilation circuits in intensive care. *J. Clin. Microbiol.* 17:870, 1983.

64. Marsik, F. J., and Parisi, J. T. Bacteriophage types and O antigen groups of *Escherichia coli* from urine. *Appl. Microbiol.* 22:26, 1971.

65. Martone, W. J., Osterman, C. A., Fisher, K. A., and Wenzel, R. P. *Pseudomonas cepacia*: Implications and control of epidemic nosocomial colonization. *Rev. Infect. Dis.* 3:708, 1981.

66. Marymont, J. H., III, Marymont J. H., Jr., and Gavan, T. L. Performance of *Enterobacteriaceae* identification systems: An analysis of College of American Pathologists survey data. *Am. J. Clin. Pathol.* 70(Suppl.):539, 1978.

67. Maxted, W. R., and Widdowson, J. P. The Protein Antigens of Group A Streptococci. In Wannamaker, L. W., and Matsen, S. M. (Eds.), *Streptococci and Streptococcal Diseases.* New York: Academic, 1972.

68. McGowan, J. E., Jr., Cost and benefit: A critical issue for hospital infection control. Fifth annual National Foundation for Infectious Diseases lecture *Am. J. Infect. Control* 10:100, 1982.

69. McGowan, J. E., Jr. Environmental factors in nosocomial infection: A selective focus. *Rev. Infect. Dis.* 3:760, 1981.

70. McGowan, J. E., Jr., and Boring, J. R., III. Nosocomial respiratory infection: The essential role of the laboratory in control efforts. *Clinics Lab. Med.* 2:415, 1982.

71. McGowan, J. E., Jr., Terry, P. M., Huang, T. S. R., Houk, C. L., and Davies, J. Nosocomial infections with gentamicin-resistant *Staphylococcus aureus*: Plasmid analysis as an epidemiologic tool. *J. Infect. Dis.* 140:864, 1979.

72. McHugh, G. L., Moellering, R. C., Hopkins, C. C., et al. *Salmonella typhimurium* resistant to silver nitrate, chloramphenicol, and ampicillin. *Lancet* 1:235, 1975.

73. Morris, G. K., and Wells, J. G. Colicin typing of *Shigella sonnei. Appl. Microbiol.* 27:312, 1974.

74. Murray, B. E., Karchmer, A. W., and Moellering, R. C., Jr. Diphtheroid prosthetic valve endocarditis: A study of clinical features and infecting organisms. *Am. J. Med.* 69:838, 1980.

75. National Committee for Clinical Laboratory Standards. *Performance Standards for Antimicrobial Disk Susceptibility Tests*, vol. 4, no. 16. Villanova, Pa.: NCCLS, 1984.

76. Old, D. C. Biotyping of *Enterobacter cloacae. J. Clin. Pathol.* 35:875, 1982.

77. Onokodi, J. K., and Wauters, G. Capsular typing of *Klebsiella* by coagglutination and latex agglutination. *J. Clin. Microbiol.* 13:609, 1981.

78. Penner, J. L., and Hennessy, J. N. Application of O-serotyping in a study of *Providencia rettgeri (Proteus rettgeri)* isolated from human and nonhuman sources. *J. Clin. Microbiol.* 10:834, 1979.

79. Penner, J. L., and Hennessy, J. N. O-antigen grouping of *Morganella morganii (Proteus morganii)* by slide agglutination. *J. Clin. Microbiol.* 10:8, 1979.

80. Penner, J. L. Hinton, N. A., Duncan, I. B. R., Hennessy, J. N., and Whiteley, G. R. O-serotyping of *Providencia stuartii* isolates collected from twelve hospitals. *J. Clin. Microbiol.* 9:11, 1979.

81. Pitt, T. L. State of the art: Typing of *Serratia marcescens. J. Hosp. Infect.* 3:9, 1982.

82. Polonelli, L., Archibusacci, C., Sestito, M., and Morace, G. Killer system: A simple method for differentiating *Candida albicans* strains. *J. Clin. Microbiol.* 17:774, 1983.

83. Ratnam, S., Mercer, E., Picco, B., Parsons, S., and Butler, R. A nosocomial outbreak of diarrheal disease due to *Yersinia enterocolitica*, serotype O:5, biotype 1. *J. Infect. Dis.* 145:242, 1982.

84. Reller, L. B., Murray, P. R., and MacLowry, J. D. *Cumitech 1A—Blood Cultures II.* Washington, D.C.: American Society for Microbiology, 1982, pp 1–11.

85. Rennie, R. P., Nord, C. E., Sjoberg, L., and Duncan, I. B. R. Comparison of bacteriophage typing, serotyping, and biotyping as aids in epidemiological surveillance of *Klebsiella* infections. *J. Clin. Microbiol.* 8:638, 1978.

86. Richardson, J. H., and Barkley, W. E. (Eds.). *Biosafety In Microbiological and Biomedical Laboratories.* Washington, D.C.: U.S. Government Printing Office Publication 1983-646-010/8285, 1983.

87. Rodriguez, W. J., Kim, H. W., Brandt, C. D., Gardner, M. K., and Parrott, R. H. Use of electrophoresis of RNA from human rotavirus to establish the identity of strains involved in outbreaks in a tertiary care nursery. *J. Infect. Dis.* 148:34, 1983.

88. Rogol, M., Sechter, I., Braunstein, I., and Gerichter, C. B. Extended scheme for serotyping *Campylobacter jejuni. J. Clin. Microbiol.* 18:283, 1983.

89. Saravolatz, L. D., Pohlod, D. J., and Arking, L. M. Community-acquired methicillin-resistant *Staphylococcus aureus* infections: A new source for nosocomial outbreaks. *Ann. Intern. Med.* 97:325, 1982.

90. Schaberg, D. R., Haley, R. W., Highsmith, A. K., Anderson, R. L., and McGowan, J. E., Jr. Nosocomial bacteriuria: A prospective study of

case clustering and antimicrobial resistance. *Ann. Intern. Med.* 93:420, 1979.

91. Schaberg, D. R., Weinstein, R. A., and Stamm, W. E. Epidemics of nosocomial urinary tract infection caused by multiply resistant gram-negative bacilli: Epidemiology and control. *J. Infect. Dis.* 133:363, 1976.

92. Schneierson, S. S., and Amsterdam, D. A manual punch card system for recording, filing, and analyzing antibiotic sensitivity test results. *Am. J. Clin. Pathol.* 47:818, 1967.

93. Sell, T. L., Schaberg, D. R., and Fekety, F. R. Bacteriophage and bacteriocin typing scheme for *Clostridium difficile. J. Clin. Microbiol.* 17:1148, 1983.

94. Senior, B. W., Typing of *Proteus* strains by proticine production and sensitivity. *J. Med. Microbiol.* 10:7, 1977.

95. Simmons, B. P. Centers for Disease Control guidelines for hospital environmental control: Microbiologic surveillance of the environment and of personnel in the hospital. *Infect. Control* 2:145, 1981.

96. Simmons, B. P., and Wong, E. S. Guideline for prevention of nosocomial pneumonia, *Infect. Control* 3:327, 1982.

97. Smith, P. B. Bacteriophage Typing of *Staphylococcus Aureus.* In Cohen J. O. (Ed.), *The Staphylococci.* New York: Wiley Interscience, 1972.

98. Stamm, A. M., Dismukes, W. E., Simmons, B. P., et al. Listeriosis in renal transplant recipients: Report of an outbreak and review of 102 cases. *Rev. Infect. Dis.* 4:665, 1982.

99. Taylor, A. G., McLauchlin, J., Green, H. T., et al. Hospital cross-infection with *Listeria monocytogenes* confirmed by phage-typing. *Lancet* 2:1106, 1981.

100. Thompson, R. L., Cabezudo, I., and Wenzel, R. P. Epidemiology of nosocomial infections caused by methicillin-resistant *Staphylococcus aureus. Ann. Intern Med.* 97:309, 1982.

101. Traub, W. H., Spohr, M., and Blech, R. Bacteriocin typing of clinical isolates of *Enterobacter cloacae. J. Clin. Microbiol.* 16:885, 1982.

102. U.S. Food and Drug Administration. *Code of Federal Regulations—Food and Drugs.* Title 21, Parts 600 to 799, revised as of April 1, 1983. Washington, D.C., U.S. Government Printing Office, p. 116.

103. Wallace, R. W., Jr., Musher, D. M., Septimus, E. J., et al. *Haemophilus influenzae* infections in adults: Characterization of strains by serotypes, biotypes, and beta-lactamase production. *J. Infect. Dis.* 144:101, 1981.

104. Washington, J. A. Utilization of microbiologic data. *Hum. Pathol.* 6:267, 1975.

105. Weinstein, R. A., Bauer, F. W., Hoffman, R. D., Tyler, P. G., Anderson R. L., and Stamm, W. E. Factitious meningitis. *J.A.M.A.* 233:878, 1975.

106. Weinstein, R. A., and Mallison, G. F. The role of the microbiology laboratory in surveillance and control of nosocomial infections. *Am. J. Clin. Pathol.* 69:130, 1978.

107. Weinstein, R. A., Stamm, W. E., and Anderson, R. L. Early detection of false-positive acid-fast smears. *Lancet* 2:174, 1975.

108. Wilkinson, H. W., Reingold, A. L., Brake, B. J., et. al. Reactivity of serum from patients with suspected legionellosis against 29 antigens of Legionellaceae and *Legionella*-like organisms by indirect immunofluorescence assay. *J. Infect. Dis.* 147:23, 1983.

109. Wong, L. K., Barry, A. L., and Horgan, S. M.: Comparison of six different criteria for judging the acceptability of sputum specimens. *J. Clin. Microbiol.* 16:627, 1982.

110. Wust, J., Sullivan, N. M., Hardegger, U., and Wilkins, T. D. Investigation of an outbreak of antibiotic-associated colitis by various typing methods. *J. Clin. Microbiol.* 16:1096, 1982.

# 8 THE RELATIONSHIP BETWEEN THE HOSPITAL AND THE COMMUNITY

William Schaffner

The hospital is the place in the community where most people both begin and end their lives. It is the most visible health-care institution in the community. In addition to providing inpatient services, many hospitals also contribute to ambulatory health care through their emergency and outpatient departments. The hospital also is a major employer, an educational resource for both medical professionals and the public, and often a focus of community pride and civic volunteer activity. This complex institution has an understandably complex relationship with the community of which it is a part.

We now are aware that the hospital is a *part* of the community and that infectious events in either one may influence the character of infections in the other. This has not always been true. Before World War II and for a short period thereafter, hospital-acquired infections were recognized as an occasional problem, but usually they were thought to be caused by microorganisms that originated in the community.

During the decade of the 1950s, hospitals around the world were struck by the well-known nosocomial epidemic of *Staphylococcus aureus* infections. Thus attention shifted to the hospital as a special environment, *separate* from the community. No matter what was "going around" in the community, staphylococcal infections were prevalent within the hospital. These dire circumstances stimulated intensive laboratory, clinical, and epidemiologic investigation and resulted in the discipline of hospital epidemiology.

The nature of nosocomial infections, however, did not remain constant. As the staphylococcal problem receded during the 1960s and other nosocomial infections were recognized, it became clear that infections that occurred within the hospital had consequences for the surrounding populace. The proverbial street was found to run both ways. Microorganisms acquired in the community continued to pose problems of spread within hospitals, but some infections acquired in the hospital only appeared after the patient was discharged and were now capable of spreading from former patients to community contacts. As these circumstances became known, hospitals began to fear the adverse publicity and lawsuits that could result from nosocomial infections, and patients expressed concern about their admission to institutions that were no longer perceived as completely benign.

## SPREAD OF COMMUNITY-ACQUIRED INFECTIONS IN THE HOSPITAL

Several recent reports remind us that certain community-acquired infections continue to be capable of spread to patients and staff in the hospital. The decline in the new case rate of tuberculosis in the community has had several effects that paradoxically, may have increased the occupational hazard of acquiring tuberculosis infection among hospital personnel. First, most special tuberculosis hospitals have been closed, thereby requiring that general hospitals undertake the care of patients with active tuberculosis. Second, hospital workers are now more apt to be susceptible (tuberculin-negative) and thus at risk of acquiring infection when exposed to tubercle bacilli. Third, the diagnosis of subtle forms of reactivation tuberculosis among the elderly may be delayed, resulting in the close exposure of personnel. Contemporary technology may amplify the hazard, as demonstrated in the report of one patient with unrecognized pulmonary tuberculosis infecting 23 health workers (physicians, medical students, nurses, aides, ward secretary, kitchen worker, and an x-ray technician), some via an unbalanced air-conditioning system [4].

Pertussis is a preventable childhood disease that is not often recognized in adults. It was with some surprise that workers at the University of Colorado Medical Center discovered two small outbreaks of pertussis that originated among children in the community, spread to house officers and nurses, and spread additionally to children in the outpatient department and other adults [8]. Note that the disease originated in the community, was transmitted to medical personnel who, in turn, infected other community contacts.

*Salmonella* infections are notorious for their ability to spread within hospitals (see Chapter 32). A few years ago, a pediatric ward of a midwestern hospital experienced a prolonged outbreak of salmonellosis that was initiated when a child with *Salmonella* gastroenteritis was admitted. Transmission was accomplished by contact spread, most likely by the hands of medical attendants. It is of special interest that the epidemic extended beyond the hospital to a foundling home and to another hospital when infected patients or their community contacts were admitted to those secondary facilities.

Viral infections also may be introduced into hospitals. This occurs regularly during the influenza season and can produce life-threatening pneumonia among patients with preexisting pulmonary disease [2] (see Chapter 35). Epidemic keratoconjunctivitis due to adenovirus type 8 is another classic example; the hands of ophthalmologists, their tonometers, or solutions transfer the virus inoculum [14] (see Chapter 35).

The ease with which chickenpox can spread on pediatric wards makes it an especially vexing problem [7,9] (see Chapter 35). Children who are incubating the infection may be admitted, such as for elective surgery, and move freely about the ward, exposing numerous patients and staff. Nosocomial chickenpox presents a serious threat to immunocompromised children, who constitute a growing proportion of the hospitalized pediatric population.

The transmission of rubella in the hospital to susceptible patients and hospital workers has been demonstrated on numerous occasions (see Chapter 35). This risk is of sufficient concern that many hospitals have incorporated rubella immunization into their employee health programs.

## SPREAD OF HOSPITAL-ACQUIRED INFECTIONS TO THE COMMUNITY

The spread of hospital-acquired infections to community contacts is a phenomenon generally unappreciated by hospital workers, perhaps because once the patient is "out of sight" he or she is also "out of mind." Practicing obstetricians and pediatricians, however, have long been aware that staphylococcal mastitis in nursing mothers occurs after the patient has been discharged from the hospital. The infant becomes colonized with staphylococci while in the newborn nursery and then transmits the organism to his mother at home.

An examination of the antibiotic susceptibilities of staphylococcal strains provides a clear example of how the microflora of hospitals can influence that of the community. For over two decades physicians have had to cope with "hospital staphylococci," which are almost uniformly resistant to penicillin. Infections acquired outside the hospital were thought to be caused by staphylococci that had remained penicillin-sensitive. But the hospital is not a cloistered environment, and most "street strains" of staphylococci now also are resistant to penicillin (68 percent and 84 percent in two populations studied) [11]. It took a little time, but those "hospital" strains have finally made it around town.

The epidemiology of *S. aureus* has just been given a new twist in Detroit [12]. In that city, persons who are intravenous drug users often take a little black-market oral cephalosporin along with their illicit drugs to prevent infections. Unfortunately, staphylococcal endocarditis still occurs, but now the pathogens often are cephalosporin-resistant and methicillin-resistant. When patients with these community-acquired infections are admitted to the hospital, such newly resistant strains can spread to other patients—a reversal of conventional staphylococcal epidemiology.

It also recently has been established that R-factor-carrying enteric organisms can spread from patients to their community contacts [3]. Infants carrying R-factor containing enteric organisms were followed after their discharge from an intensive care nursery. After 12 months almost half of the infants continued to carry these multiresistant organisms, and one-third of their family members also had acquired R-factor-positive strains in their fecal flora. No family members of a control group of infants were colonized with such bacilli. It would seem that some patients become reservoirs of hospital-derived R-factor containing bacteria for considerable periods after their return to the community [10].

One would have thought that an epidemic of nosocomial sepsis due to contaminated intravenous fluid bottles would be a "pure" hospital problem. Not so. A man was admitted to the hospital with an episode of bacteremia and hypotension that was related to such an outbreak [5]. He was maintained on *home* hemodialysis and had a supply of the implicated fluid in his home, which was used for priming the dialysis apparatus. In a sense his home had become an extension of the hospital.

Renal dialysis has provided us with yet another example of how a hosptial pathogen can spread to family contacts. A few years ago hepatitis B became endemic in some dialysis centers. A patient in such a setting had a severe hemorrhage at home because his arterial shunt dislodged. Some three months later, five of nine persons who were present at the time of the hemorrhage developed hepatitis. Hepatitis B was implicated, an example of the nonparenteral spread of this viral agent [6]. Today the rigorous application of control measures in the dialysis unit and the use of hepatitis B vaccine by the family members of patients who are HBsAg carriers have markedly curtailed this risk. Clearly, however, nosocomial infections have public health implications for the community.

## RELATIONSHIP OF THE HOSPITAL WITH HEALTH AUTHORITIES

Hospitals are developing increasingly complex relationships with health authorities at all governmental levels. The requirements of various regulatory agencies that affect hosptial construction, professional standards review, working conditions for employees, and laboratory licensing have a peripheral impact on the problem of nosocomial infection. To explore these is beyond the scope of this chapter, in which we confine ourselves to more traditional concerns.

The hospital looks to health authorities for assistance in three infection control areas: consultation on the establishment of a useful program, training of personnel to carry out the program, and assistance in the investigation of epidemics.

The ability of different health jurisdictions to respond to these needs varies enormously with the resources and personnel available. Health departments and hospitals have largely gone their separate ways in our society—the first concerned with public health and the second with diagnostics and therapeutics. Therefore, the infection control affairs of the hospital often are not thought to be a major concern of the health department. Even when such an interest is acknowledged, implementation may be difficult for several reasons. Health departments have traditional responsiblities of impressive diversity and often must work within the constraints of tight budgets. Furthermore, the doctors and nurses in the health department may not be comfortable in the highly technologic milieu of the contemporary hospital. Small wonder, then, that local health authorities have been hesitant to open the Pandora's box of nosocomial infection. Hospitals, in turn, value their independence and frequently are wary of close associations with governmental agencies.

Appropriate laboratory support is essential to the investigation of all but the simplest hospital outbreaks. Most health department laboratories are reference laboratories, although they may process clinical specimens in such circumscribed areas as *Salmonella*, *Shigella*, and gonococcal bacteriology. The techniques required to perform primary isolation of hospital pathogens from diverse clinical specimens, environmental sampling, and antimicrobial susceptibility testing usually are not in the public health laboratory worker's repertoire. Even more arcane procedures such as those related to gram-negative bacilli (e.g., serotyping and defining plasmid-mediated antimicrobial resistance mechanisms) are becoming increasingly important in delineating nosocomial outbreaks. Laboratory consultation for investigating outbreaks of nosocomial infections sometimes can be obtained from investigators at university medical centers or from the Centers for Disease Control.

Among state health departments, those in Virginia, New Jersey, Iowa, California, Utah, and Tennessee have led in establishing programs for the control of nosocomial infections. Their program content varies, but most have sponsored training courses that emphasize the basic epidemiologic and laboratory aspects of infection control. These courses usually are presented in collaboration with infectious disease faculty at local medical centers. Some state health departments now also employ infection control practitioners who are able to provide advice to individual hospitals about their infection control problems. The Intermountain Regional Medical Program has demonstrated that such a cooperative arrangement is feasible [1]. With the University of Utah Hospital at its hub, consultation in nosocomial infection problems was provided to small hospitals in five states by a physician, nurse-epidemiologist, and microbiology laboratory consultant. Unfortunately, this demonstration project ceased when its grant support ended, emphasizing the need for stable financing of any such program.

A recent example has demonstrated that imaginative local health department officials can provide dynamic leadership in circumstances that combine aspects of nosocomial infection control and community public health. Physicians in New York were the first to recognize patients with features of what since has become known as the acquired immunodeficiency syndrome (AIDS). In addition to their many other contributions to the investigation of this new disease entity, health officials in New York offered a unique service. The Department of Health provided a monthly forum in which the many investigators in the city could share their new information about the clinical and laboratory features of AIDS. The forum met with immediate success and became a vital communications link among the investigators and with the health department. As Sencer has stated vividly, "Here, the health department has acted . . . as skeleton, with the muscle coming from the community" [13]. This example can serve as a model for the synergistic collaboration that can result when health departments and hospitals join their resources for a common purpose.

As the problem of nosocomial infections became increasingly recognized, federal health officials provided important leadership. The Hospital Infections Unit at the Centers for Disease Control (CDC) was established for this purpose. That program remains the most helpful of any governmental program and provides assistance to local hospitals and health departments in developing guidelines for effective programs, by offering training courses for personnel, and assisting in the investigation of epidemics.

As problems with contaminated products have received wider recognition, the relation of hospital infection control programs to another governmental agency, the Food and Drug Administration (FDA), has developed. Hospitals are not the traditional "clients" of the FDA, and appropriate lines of communication are evolving slowly. Indeed, in the past the close relation between hospitals and industry may have hampered the recognition of problems. Hospital pharmacists, for example, are more likely to contact a manufacturer's representative when a question of contaminated intravenous fluid arises than they are to contact either the FDA or the CDC. Anecdotal reports also suggest that some local FDA field representatives are not familiar with hospital-related problems and thus have not been able to offer prompt and incisive assistance. There is the additional difficulty of delineating the area of the FDA's responsibility vis-à-vis that of the CDC. Clearly the CDC has the best perspective regarding the entire hospital infection arena and is the repository of the major epidemiologic expertise needed to delineate and solve problems. The FDA, on the other hand, has regulatory authority over industry and the responsiblity for recalling products suspected of being contaminated. It is expected that the evolution of the relation between these agencies will result in a lesser risk of nosocomial misadventure for our hospitalized patients.

## REPORTING OF COMMUNICABLE DISEASES

Prevention and control of communicable disease is a traditional primary duty of health departments. However, patients with illnesses that may be a threat to the health of the community are attended by scattered individual practitioners. Therefore, it has been recognized that a system of prompt and accurate notification of the occurrence of certain communicable diseases was a requisite to their control. In 1883 the state of Michigan adopted legislation establishing a system of communicable disease reporting, and all other states have since followed suit. These laws have been determined by the courts on numerous occasions not to violate the special nature of the doctor-patient relationship.

The reporting system is pluralist; both physicians and hospitals have an independent obligation to notify the public health authorities if patients with certain illnesses are admitted to their care. Concerns over possible duplication of reports should not deter reporting; health departments have the responsibility for ascertaining the best final case tally.

It is important that hospitals develop a system of disease notification for several reasons. First, by reporting promptly, hospitals can be of assistance to the public health authorities in the control of communicable disease in their own communities. Second, by educating the staff physicians and employees of this responsibility, the hospital becomes an advocate of good preventive medical practice. Third, the hospital's unique role enables it to be a major contributor to the state and national morbidity data collection mechanism, which determines funding priorities for research and control activities. And last, as medicine's capacity to prevent disease increases, there will be a consequent increasing need for precise information on disease occurrence. Subsequent to the widespread use of polio vaccine, for example, there remains a continuing need to evaluate carefully all cases of poliomyelitis-like illness. A documented case may alert authorities to a population of unimmunized children or a problem with the vaccine itself. Unreported, the incident will go uninvestigated. Similarly, as new diseases such as legionnaires' disease, toxic shock syndrome, and AIDS are recognized, they are added to the roster of diseases that are reportable to the health department.

The list of diseases designated as reportable in Tennessee, indicated in Table 8-1, is representative of those found in most states. Although the list appears extensive, most reporting by hospitals involves just a few diseases: hepatitis, viral meningitis, encephalitis, meningococcal infections, salmonellosis, shigellosis, and the venereal diseases, gonorrhea and syphilis. It is the responsiblity of the hospital epidemiologist to establish a valid reporting mechanism. We have designed the following mechanism after consultation with our local and state authorities.

Reporting is weekly, by standard morbidity report card, which is sent to the local health department. Most reports are generated by positive cultures in the bacteriology laboratory, but the nurse-epidemiologist and infectious disease faculty add reports on such diseases as hepatitis and viral meningitis that would not be reflected in the laboratory culture reports. The reports include the name, age, sex, race, and address of the patient. In addition, the bacteriology laboratory routinely sends subcultures of all *Salmonella, Shigella*, and meningococcal isolates to the state reference laboratory for confirmation and serogrouping.

Reporting of venereal diseases is managed in a somewhat different manner. Regarding syphilis, all serologic results positive in a dilution of 1:16 or greater are reported immediately by telephone to the VD investigator in the local health department. All other positive serologic results are reported on each Friday with complete patient identification, including the name of the patient's physician. All isolates

TABLE 8-1. Reportable diseases in Tennessee

*Reportable by name, address, race, sex, and age of the patient*

| | |
|---|---|
| Acquired immunodeficiency syndrome | Plague |
| Botulism | Poliomyelitis |
| Brucellosis | Psittacosis |
| Campylobacteriosis | Rabies, human |
| Cholera | Reye's syndrome |
| Congenital rubella syndrome | Rocky Mountain spotted fever |
| Diphtheria | Rubella |
| Encephalitis | Salmonellosis |
|   Arthropod-borne |   Typhoid fever |
|   Other infectious |   Other |
| Giardiasis, acute | Shigellosis |
| Gonorrhea | Syphilis |
| Legionellosis | Tetanus |
| Leprosy | Toxic shock syndrome |
| Leptospirosis | Trichinosis |
| Lyme disease | Tuberculosis, all forms |
| Malaria | |
| Measles | Tularemia |
| Meningitis | Typhus |
|   Meningococcal | |
|   Other bacterial | |

*Disease outbreaks*

Foodborne
Waterborne
Related to industrial substances

*Reportable by number of cases*

Chickenpox
Influenza
Meningitis, aseptic

of *Neisseria gonorrhoeae* from patients less than ten years of age are reported immediately by telephone, others are reported on Friday. Only patients with positive cultures, not simply positive Gram stains, are reported.

In addition, the occurrence of any illness that may have public health implications is reported. For example, cases of suspected food poisoning seen in the emergency room are promptly reported by telephone so that the authorities can make an investigation. During the winter months we participate in a special surveillance program for influenza organized by the state health department.

Hospitals may employ other methods of notification. Institutions that require admission diagnoses can prepare a daily list of patients admitted with suspected hepatitis, meningitis, and so on. Other institutions rely on final discharge diagnoses for reporting. The former method is less accurate but is of value to local health departments that give a high priority to investigation of communicable diseases. The latter method is more precise, but one loses the advantage of timeliness. The method that best suits local needs can be chosen. Some states have now included among their requirements for hospital licensure demonstrated evidence that the hospital has an approved and functioning communicable disease reporting mechanism.

## BROADER INFLUENCE OF THE HOSPITAL EPIDEMIOLOGIST

As a person in the medical community with a heightened interest in preventive ,medicine, the hospital epidemiologist is occasionally in a position to influence decisions in areas beyond those relating just to nosocomial infections. Indeed, one of my first goals when I assumed this position at the Vanderbilt University Hospital in 1969 was to convince the hospital administration to discontinue the sale of cigarettes in the hospital. As has been the case in other institutions, this was accomplished without any complaints from personnel, patients, or visitors. Unfortunately, I was unable to persuade the administration to post signs near the vending machines explaining the policy, thereby losing an opportunity for public health education.

The Joint Commission on Accreditation of Hospitals now requires that hospitals institute regular reviews of antibiotic usage; the hospital epidemiologist often is involved in these activities.

Another area in which the epidemiologist can be of assistance is in the immediate management of community contacts of patients with certain infections. A 26-year-old married father of two children, for example, is admitted with meningococcal meningitis. Whose responsibility is it to provide antibiotic prophylaxis to his wife and children: the attending internist, the pediatrician, or the local health officer? I believe there can be no absolute rule, but the hospital epidemiologist can act as an ombudsman, providing assurance that this essential preventive medical service is not overlooked.

It is paradoxical that hospitals, society's most visible health care institutions, have lagged in providing preventive medical services for their employees. Hospital epidemiologists have the opportunity to persuade hospitals to provide screening programs for hypertension and other coronary risk factors, tuberculosis, and cervical and breast cancer, as well as to provide comprehensive immunization programs and even family planning services. If these were combined with an educational effort, hospitals, long admired for their sophisticated care of sick patients, could make a more comprehensive contribution to medicine's highest goal—the prevention of disease.

## REFERENCES

1. Britt, M. R., Burke, J. P., Nordquist, A. G., Wilfert, J. N., and Smith, C. B. Infection control in small hospitals: Prevalence surveys in 18 institutions. *J.A.M.A.* 236:1700, 1976.
2. Burk, R. F., Schaffner, W., and Koenig, M. G. Severe influenza virus pneumonia in the pandemic of 1968–1969. *Arch. Intern. Med.* 127:1122, 1971.
3. Damato, J. J., Eitzman, D. V., and Baer, H. Persistence and dissemination in the community of R-factors of nosocomial origin. *J. Infect. Dis.* 129:205, 1974.
4. Ehrenkranz, N. J., and Kicklighter, J. L. Tuberculosis outbreak in a general hospital: Evidence for airborne spread of infection. *Ann. Intern. Med.* 77:377, 1972.
5. Felts, S. K., Schaffner, W., Melly, M. A., and Koenig, M. G. Sepsis caused by contaminated intravenous fluids: Epidemiologic, clinical, and laboratory investigation of an outbreak in one hospital. *Ann. Intern. Med.* 77:881, 1972.
6. Garibaldi, R. A., Hatch, F. E., Bisno, A. L., Hatch, M. H., and Gregg, M. B. Nonparenteral serum hepatitis: Report of an outbreak. *J.A.M.A.* 220:963, 1972.
7. Gustafson, T. L., Lavely, G. B., Brawner, E. R., Hutcheson, R. H., Wright, P. F., and Schaffner, W. An outbreak of airborne nosocomial varicella. *Pediatrics* 70:550, 1982.
8. Kurt, T. L., Yeager, A. S., Guenette, S., and Dunlop, S. Spread of pertussis by hospital staff. *J.A.M.A.* 221:264, 1972.
9. Leclair, J. M., Zaia, J. A., Levin, M. J., Congdon, R. G., and Goldmann, D. A. Airborne transmission of chickenpox in a hospital. *N. Engl. J. Med.* 302:450, 1980.
10. McKee, K. T., Cotton, R. B., Stratton, C. W., Lavely, G. B., Wright, P. F., Shenai, J. P., Evans, M. E., Melly, M. A., Farmer, J. J., Karzon, D. T., and Schaffner, W. Nursery epidemic due to multiply resistant *Klebsiella pneumoniae*: Epidemiologic setting and impact on perinatal health care delivery. *Infect. Cont.* 3:150, 1982.

11. Ross, S., Rodriguez, W., Controni, G., and Khan, W. Staphylococcal susceptibility to penicillin G: The changing pattern among community strains. *J.A.M.A.* 229:1075, 1974.

12. Saravolatz, L. D., Pohlod, D. J., and Arking, L. M. Community-acquired methicillin-resistant *Staphylococcus aureus* infections: A new source for nosocomial outbreaks. *Ann. Intern. Med.* 97:325, 1982.

13. Sencer, D. J. Major urban health departments: The ideal and the real. *Health Affairs* 2:88, 1983.

14. Wegman, D. H., Guinee, V. F., and Millian, S. J. Epidemic keratoconjunctivitis. *Am. J. Public Health* 60:1230, 1970.

# 9  ISOLATION PRECAUTIONS

Julia S. Garner
Bryan P. Simmons

## HISTORICAL REVIEW

Isolation precautions were used in hospitals in the United States even before recommendations for such precautions were published. "Fever hospitals" were opened in the 1700s, primarily during epidemics such as yellow fever, to prevent infection transmission. These were usually closed after the epidemics disappeared or waned [3].

Published recommendations for isolation of patients with communicable diseases appeared in the United States as early as 1877, when a hospital handbook recommended placing patients with communicable diseases in isolation huts [14]. Although patients with communicable diseases were segregated, problems with cross-infection soon resulted; infected patients were not separated from each other according to their disease, and few, if any, aseptic procedures were practiced. As early as 1889, communicable disease hospitals gradually began to combat the problems of cross-infection by setting aside a floor or ward for housing patients with similar communicable diseases [7] and by putting into practice aseptic procedures recommended in nursing textbooks published from 1890 to 1900 [14].

In 1910 isolation practices in the United States were altered by the introduction of the cubicle system for isolating individual patients [7]. With the cubicle system, patients in multiple-bed wards were managed for the first time as if they were in a room by themselves; hospital personnel used separate gowns, washed their hands with antiseptic solutions after patient contact, and disinfected objects contaminated by the patient. The nursing procedures used with the cubicle system were designed to prevent transmission of pathogenic organisms to other patients and personnel; these procedures became known as "barrier nursing."

In the 1950s the general contagious disease hospitals and wards gradually began to close, and patients with communicable diseases were provided care in the general hospital setting. In the mid-1960s, tuberculosis hospitals also began to close, partially because general hospital or outpatient treatment became preferred for patients with tuberculosis. Thus by the late 1960s patients needing isolation precautions were housed in the general hospital on the ward to which they were admitted, either in a specially designed, single-patient isolation room or in a regular single or multiple-patient room.

To assist general hospitals with patients needing isolation precautions, the Centers for Disease Control (CDC) published *Isolation Techniques for Use in Hos-*

*pitals* in 1970 and revised it in 1975 [4]. This publication was a detailed manual of isolation procedures that could be applied in small community hospitals with limited resources as well as in large metropolitan university-associated medical centers. The manual suggested that hospitals use isolation categories determined almost entirely by the epidemiologic features of the disease, primarily the routes of disease transmission, while at the same time considering appropriate agent and host factors. Certain isolation techniques, felt to be the minimum necessary to prevent transmission of *all* diseases in the category, were indicated for each isolation category. Because all diseases in a category did not have exactly the same epidemiology and some required fewer precautions than others, more precautions were suggested for some diseases than were necessary to prevent disease transmission. This disadvantage of "over-isolation" for some diseases was offset by the convenience of having a small number of categories, all easily understood by most hospital personnel. By the mid-1970s, 93 percent of U.S. hospitals had adopted this approach for isolation precautions [12].

By 1980 hospitals were beginning to experience endemic and epidemic nosocomial infection problems, some due to multiple resistant microorganisms and some due to newly recognized syndromes, which required different isolation precautions from those specified by an existing category of isolation. Moreover, the need was voiced for precautions directed more specifically at nosocomial infections in special-care units, rather than directed at the intrahospital spread of classic contagious diseases acquired in the community [17]. Furthermore, new facts about the epidemiology of some diseases made it appropriate for the CDC to consider revising the isolation manual.

Between 1981 and 1983, CDC Hospital Infections Program personnel held discussions with infectious disease specialists representing medicine, pediatrics, and surgery; hospital epidemiologists; and infection control nurses to get advice on revising the isolation manual. The revision was completed in 1983 and entitled *Guideline for Isolation Precautions in Hospitals* [11]. The recommendations have been modified substantially to reflect current knowledge; for example, new categories for contact and tuberculosis isolation have been added, and the category of protective isolation has been deleted. Protective isolation is no longer recommended because it does not appear to be any more effective than strong emphasis on hand-washing when caring for immunologically compromised patients [16]. In addition, the precautions indicated for other categories have been substantially

modified, and many infections have been assigned to new categories. For example, pneumonia caused by *Staphylococcus aureus* or group-A streptococcus, formerly requiring strict isolation, is included in the new contact isolation category.

The most important change in the new guideline, however, is the increased emphasis on decision-making. Unlike the initial isolation manual, which encouraged few decisions on the part of users, the new guideline encourages decision-making at several levels [8]. First, the guideline offers hospital Infection Control Committees an opportunity to choose between two alternative systems: category-specific or disease-specific isolation precautions. Second, the guideline encourages the physician or nurse who places a patient on isolation precautions to make decisions about the individual precautions to be taken, for example, whether the patient's age, mental status, or condition indicates that a private room is needed to prevent sharing of contaminated articles. Third, the guideline generally allows patient-care personnel taking care of patients on isolation precautions to decide whether they need to wear masks, gowns, or gloves based on the likelihood of exposure to infective material. Such decisions are necessary to isolate the disease but not the patient and to reduce the costs associated with unnecessary isolation precautions.

## DEFINITION OF ISOLATION PRECAUTIONS

We are using the words *isolation precautions* in their broadest sense, that is, as steps to prevent the spread of an infectious agent from an infected or colonized person to another person. In this context, isolation precautions should be thought of as on a continuum ranging from the most to the least demanding. They include private rooms or roommate selection, masks, gowns, gloves, special emphasis on hand-washing, and special handling of contaminated articles; these precautions may be critical to prevent spread of some diseases, but all are not necessary for other diseases. The reasons for these differences involve primarily differences in the epidemiology of infection transmission. We do not attempt to define the epidemiology for individual infections because such information is available in many standard references [2,5,6,15]. However, we do discuss the uses of the most important isolation precautions mentioned previously.

Hand-washing is the single most important isolation precaution. Hand-washing is recommended after touching infective material and after taking care of any infected patient or patient colonized by multiply resistant bacteria. If done properly, hand-washing generally removes organisms acquired from infected patients. Use of antimicrobial-containing products for hand-washing is not necessary when caring for infected patients, but these agents may provide an extra margin of safety.

Private rooms are useful as an isolation precaution because they separate patients and lessen the chance of infection transmission by any route. Most patients infected by organisms that can be transmitted by air should be placed in a private room. However, patients infected by organisms spread by direct contact do not need a private room unless the organism frequently causes serious disease if transmitted or the infected patient has poor hygienic habits. We define a patient with poor hygienic habits as a patient who does not wash hands after touching infective material (feces, purulent drainage, or secretions), contaminates the environment, or shares contaminated articles. Such patients may include children, patients who have altered mental status, and those with infective blood who are likely to bleed profusely and cause environmental contamination. Even when a private room is indicated, patients infected or colonized by the same organism can share a room; this sharing (cohorting) may be necessary during epidemics when private rooms may not be readily available (see Chapter 35).

Sometimes a private room with special ventilation is indicated as an isolation precaution because the organism is spread by air and subsequently frequently causes severe infections. Special ventilation is characterized by (1) negative air pressure in the room in relation to the anteroom or hall, (2) a minimum of six air changes per hour, and (3) special handling of ventilation air from the room, either by discharging it outdoors where it will be well diluted or subjecting it to high-efficiency filtration before circulating it to other rooms (see Chapter 14).

Even when a private room is not indicated as an isolation precaution, special emphasis is placed on choosing the room and roommate for an infected patient. Generally it is recommended that infected patients not share a room with a patient who is likely to become infected or for whom consequences of infection are likely to be serious. Such patients include those who are immunocompromised or who are about to undergo extensive surgery with insertion of prosthetic devices.

Use of masks is an isolation precaution intended to prevent transmission of infectious agents through the air. Masks protect the wearer from inhaling (1) large-particle aerosols (droplets) that are transmitted by close contact and generally travel only short distances (up to about three feet) and (2) small-particle aerosols (droplet nuclei) that remain suspended in the air and thus may travel longer distances. Masks generally lose some efficiency when they are wet or after being worn for prolonged periods.

Gowns are indicated as an isolation precaution when soiling of clothes with infective material is likely, because such soiling can potentially transmit infection to personnel or patients. When gowns are indicated, they should be worn only once and discarded rather than saved for reuse.

Gloves are used for several reasons. First, gloves reduce the possibility that personnel will become infected with organisms from infected patients; for example, gloves may prevent personnel from developing herpetic whitlow after touching oral secretions contaminated by herpes simplex virus. Gloves also reduce the likelihood that personnel will transmit microbial flora from their hands to patients, either their own endogenous flora or that transiently acquired from infected patients or the environment. However, gloves are not the only means to prevent transmission of transiently acquired organisms; good hand-washing eliminates these organisms and interrupts transmission without use of gloves. However, gloves are often recommended as an isolation precaution, because personnel frequently do not wash hands when they should [1].

Isolation precautions often include special handling of used articles because such articles may need to be enclosed in an impervious bag before they are removed from the room or cubicle. Such bagging is intended to prevent inadvertent exposures of personnel to articles contaminated with infective material and prevent contamination of the environment. Most articles do not need to be bagged unless they are contaminated (or likely to be contaminated) with infective material. One bag is probably adequate if the bag is impervious and sturdy (not easily penetrated) and if the article can be placed in the bag without contaminating the outside of the bag; otherwise, double bagging should be used.

Disposable or reusable patient-care equipment can be used for patients on isolation precautions. Using disposable equipment reduces the possibility that equipment will serve as a fomite, but such equipment must be disposed of safely and adequately. Disposable equipment that is contaminated (or likely to be contaminated) with infective material such as blood, body fluids, or wound secretions, should be bagged, labeled, and disposed of according to hospital policy for disposal of infective waste. Local regulations may call for incineration or disposal in an authorized sanitary landfill. Ideally reusable patient-care equipment should be returned to a central processing area for decontamination and reprocessing by trained personnel. When contaminated with infective material, it should be bagged and labeled before being removed from the patient's room or cubicle and remain bagged until decontaminated.

Ideally soiled linen from patients on isolation precautions should be handled as little as possible and should be put in a laundry bag in the patient's room or cubicle (see Chapter 15). The bag should be labeled so that whoever receives the linen knows to take special precautions.

Disposable or reusable dishes can be used for patients on isolation precautions. No special precautions are necessary for dishes unless they are visibly contaminated with infective material, for example, with blood, drainage, or secretions. Disposable dishes contaminated with infective material can be handled as disposable patient-care equipment. Reusable dishes visibly contaminated with infective material should be bagged and labeled before being returned to the food service department. Food service personnel who handle these dishes should wash their hands before handling clean dishes or food (see Chapter 16). The combination of water temperature and dishwasher detergents used in hospital dishwashers is sufficient to decontaminate dishes; therefore, sending dishes from patients on isolation precautions to central service for decontamination-sterilization before sending them to the food service department for washing is neither necessary nor indicated.

Routine and terminal cleaning is indicated for the room or cubicle of patients on isolation precautions. For routine daily cleaning, the same procedures that are used in other hospital rooms can be used for patients on isolation precautions (see Chapter 14). For such cleaning, housekeeping personnel should use the same precautions that patient-care personnel use to protect themselves. When isolation precautions have been discontinued, the room or cubicle should be cleaned. Used disposable items should be discarded, and reusable patient-care equipment should be sent for central processing. Furniture and floors should be cleaned with disinfectant-detergent. Washing of walls, blinds, and curtains is not indicated unless they are visibly soiled. Disinfectant fogging is not recommended, and airing the room is not necessary.

Other isolation precautions may be necessary with certain infections but are too specific to be discussed in detail in this chapter. The *Guideline for Isolation Precautions in Hospitals* can be consulted for specific details not covered in this chapter. The entire guideline has been published or reprinted in two infection control journals [10,11]. It is also available for purchase from two governmental agencies.*

## ALTERNATIVE SYSTEMS FOR ISOLATION PRECAUTIONS

The CDC now recommends that hospitals use one of two different systems for isolation precautions: disease-specific or category-specific. Category-specific isolation precautions are derived by grouping diseases for which similar isolation precautions are indicated into a category of isolation. This system has been recommended by the CDC since 1970. In the second, and new, system of isolation precautions recommended by the CDC, disease-specific isolation precautions, each infectious disease is considered individually so that only those precautions (e.g., private room, masks, gowns, and gloves) indicated to interrupt transmission of that disease are recommended. The two systems are compared in Table 9-1.

In deciding between the two alternative systems, hospital staff should consider the relative advantages and disadvantages of each approach. Most important, the category-specific system is a simpler system requiring personnel to learn only a few established routines for applying isolation precautions. Because many different diseases are grouped into seven categories, however, unnecessary precautions will be applied to some diseases and overisolation may occur. Alternatively, the disease-specific system ensures that the isolation precautions applied are the only ones required to interrupt transmission of the infection. Since the set of precautions is individualized to each disease, this system requires more initial training and inservice education and a much higher level of attention from patient-care personnel to be applied correctly in all cases. Although use of disease-specific isolation precautions should result in less overisolation, it also could result in more mistakes in applying precautions. Both isolation systems were designed to be used with a card that is displayed near the patient and that contains the appropriate specifications for isolation precautions. Such a card alerts personnel and visitors that special precautions are necessary. With disease-specific isolation precautions, we recommend

*Superintendent of Documents, U.S. Government Printing Office, Washington, D.C. 20402, Supt. Docs. Stock #017-023-00148-5. National Technical Information Service, U.S. Department of Commerce, 5285 Port Royal Road, Springfield, VA 22161. NTIS Order No. PB 84-923401.

TABLE 9-1. Comparison of category-specific and disease-specific isolation precautions

|  | Category-specific | Disease-specific |
| --- | --- | --- |
| Isolation precautions | Seven categories, each with a different set of precautions | Individualized for each disease |
| Instruction card for door or cubicle | Separate, preprinted, color-coded card for each category | One all-purpose black and white card to be individualized for each patient |
| Advantages | Simpler system; less diagnostic information needed to assign precautions | Minimizes unnecessary precautions; may reduce cost of placing patient on isolation precautions |
|  | Less decision-making needed to assign precautions | May encourage compliance, especially by physicians |
| Disadvantages | Unnecessary precautions taken for some diseases | Requires more skill and responsibility to assign precautions |
|  | May increase cost of isolation | Requires more diagnostic information about disease to assign precautions |

using one black and white instruction card on which the need for specific precautions can be shown by checking appropriate items and filling in blanks. When isolation categories are used, we recommend using standard, preprinted, color-coded category-specific instruction cards.

*Category-Specific Isolation Precautions*

Seven isolation categories are recommended for category-specific isolation precautions: strict isolation, contact isolation, respiratory isolation, tuberculosis isolation, enteric precautions, drainage-secretion precautions, and blood–body fluid precautions. An isolation category ending with the term *isolation* is used in general when a private room is indicated; a category ending with the term *precautions* is used when a private room is optional or not indicated. The purpose and specifications of each isolation category are listed below.

1. *Strict isolation* is an isolation category designed to prevent transmission of highly contagious or virulent infections that may be spread by both air and contact.

    Strict isolation is indicated for patients with pharyngeal diphtheria, Lassa fever or other viral hemorrhagic fevers, pneumonic plague, smallpox, varicella (chickenpox), and zoster that occurs in an immunocompromised host or is disseminated. Patients with smallpox or a viral hemorrhagic fever should be placed in a private room with special ventilation.

    a. Private room is indicated; door should be kept closed. Patients infected by the same organism may share a room.

    b. Masks are indicated for all persons entering the room.

    c. Gowns are indicated for all persons entering the room.

    d. Gloves are indicated for all persons entering the room.

    e. Hands must be washed after touching the patient or potentially contaminated articles and before taking care of another patient.

    f. Articles contaminated with infective material should be discarded or bagged and labeled before being sent for decontamination and reprocessing.

2. *Contact isolation* is designed to prevent transmission of highly transmissible or epidemiologically important infections (or colonization) that do not warrant strict isolation. All diseases or conditions included in this category are spread primarily by direct contact.

    Contact isolation is indicated for (1) pediatric patients with acute respiratory infections, pharyngitis, or pneumonia, (2) newborns with gonococcal conjunctivitis, herpes simplex infection, or staphylococcal skin infections, (3) any patient with group-A streptococcal endometritis, pneumonia, or skin infection, and (4) any patient with cutaneous diphtheria, disseminated herpes simplex infection, infection or colonization by epidemiologically significant multiply resistant bacteria, staphylococcal pneumonia or major skin infections, pediculosis, scabies, rabies, rubella, or vaccinia. Regardless of the pathogens involved, contact isolation is indicated for patients with major skin infections that are draining and cannot be covered adequately with dressings.

a. Private room is indicated. Patients infected by the same organism may share a room. During outbreaks of respiratory diseases, infants and young children with the same respiratory clinical syndrome may share a room.

b. Masks are indicated for those who come close to the patient.

c. Gowns are indicated if soiling is likely.

d. Gloves are indicated for touching infective material.

e. Hands must be washed after touching the patient or potentially contaminated articles and before taking care of another patient.

f. Articles contaminated with infective material should be discarded or bagged and labeled before being sent for decontamination and reprocessing.

3. *Respiratory isolation* is designed primarily to prevent transmission of infectious diseases over short distances through the air (droplet transmission). Direct or indirect contact transmission occurs with some infections in this category but is infrequent.

Respiratory isolation is indicated for patients with the following diseases: erythema infectiosum; measles; *Hemophilus influenzae* epiglottitis, meningitis, or pneumonia in children; serious meningococcal disease (pneumonia, meningitis, sepsis); mumps; and pertussis (whooping cough).

a. Private room is indicated. Patients infected with the same organism may share a room.

b. Masks are indicated for those who come close to the patient.

c. Gowns are not indicated.

d. Gloves are not indicated.

e. Hands must be washed after touching the patient or potentially contaminated articles and before taking care of another patient.

f. Articles contaminated with infective material should be discarded or bagged and labeled before being sent for decontamination and reprocessing.

4. *Tuberculosis isolation* is designed for patients with pulmonary tuberculosis who have a positive sputum smear or a chest x-ray that strongly suggests current (active) tuberculosis. Laryngeal tuberculosis is also included in this isolation category. This category of isolation can be referred to as AFB (for acid-fast bacilli) to protect the patient's privacy.

a. Private room with special ventilation is indicated; door should be kept closed. Patients with active tuberculosis may share a room.

b. Masks are indicated only if the patient is coughing and does not reliably cover mouth.

c. Gowns are indicated only if needed to prevent gross contamination of clothing.

d. Gloves are not indicated.

e. Hands must be washed after touching the patient or potentially contaminated articles and before taking care of another patient.

f. Articles are rarely involved in transmission of tuberculosis. However, articles should be thoroughly cleaned, disinfected, or discarded.

5. *Enteric precautions* are designed to prevent infections that are transmitted by direct or indirect contact with feces.

Enteric precautions are indicated for patients with the following diseases: infectious diarrhea or gastroenteritis caused by amebae, *Vibrio cholerae* and other *Vibrio* species, *Campylobacter*, *Cryptosporidium*, *Dientamoeba*, *Escherichia coli*, *Giardia*, *Salmonella*, *Shigella*, *Yersinia enterocolitica*, and viruses; enteroviral infections, (e.g., pleurodynia, viral meningitis, and poliomyelitis); enterocolitis caused by *Clostridium difficile* or *Staphylococcus aureus*; necrotizing enterocolitis of newborns; and hepatitis A.

a. Private room is indicated if patient hygiene is poor. A patient with poor hygiene is one who cannot or will not wash hands after touching infective material, contaminates the environment with infective material, or shares contaminated articles with other patients.

b. Masks are not indicated.

c. Gowns are indicated if soiling is likely.

d. Gloves are indicated for touching infective material.

e. Hands must be washed after touching the patient or potentially contaminated articles and before taking care of another patient.

f. Articles contaminated with infective material should be discarded or bagged and labeled before being sent for decontamination and reprocessing.

6. *Drainage-secretion* precautions are designed to prevent infections transmitted by direct or indirect contact with purulent material or with drainage from an infected body site.

Infectious diseases included in this category are those resulting in production of infective purulent material, drainage, or secretions, unless the disease is included in another isolation category requiring more rigorous precautions.

a. Private room is not indicated.

b. Masks are not indicated.

c. Gowns are indicated if soiling is likely.

d. Gloves are indicated for touching infective material.

e. Hands must be washed after touching the patient or potentially contaminated articles and before taking care of another patient.

f. Articles contaminated with infective material should be discarded or bagged and labeled before being sent for decontamination and reprocessing.

7. *Blood—body fluid precautions* are designed to prevent infections that are transmitted by direct or indirect contact with infective blood or body fluids. For some diseases included in this category, such as malaria, only blood is infective; for other diseases, such as hepatitis B (including antigen carriers), blood and body fluids (e.g., saliva, semen, peritoneal fluid) are infective.

Infectious diseases included in this category are those resulting in infective blood or body fluids, unless the disease is included in another isolation category requiring more rigorous precautions. Blood—body fluid precautions are indicated for patients with the following diseases: acquired immunodeficiency syndrome (AIDS), arthropod-borne viral fevers, babesiosis, Creutzfeldt-Jakob disease, hepatitis B and non-A, non-B hepatitis, leptospirosis, malaria, rat bite fever, relapsing fever, and syphilis (primary and secondary).

a. Private room is indicated if patient hygiene is poor or if uncontrolled bleeding is likely to cause environmental contamination.

b. Masks are not indicated.

c. Gowns are indicated if soiling of clothing with blood or body fluids is likely.

d. Gloves are indicated for touching blood or body fluids.

e. Hands must be washed immediately if they are potentially contaminated with blood or body fluids and before taking care of another patient.

f. Articles contaminated with blood or body fluids should be discarded or bagged and labeled before being sent for decontamination and reprocessing.

g. Care should be taken to avoid needle-stick injuries. Used needles should not be recapped, purposely bent, or broken by hand; they should be placed in a prominently labeled, punctureresistant container designated specifically for such disposal.

h. Blood spills should be cleaned up promptly with a solution of 5.25% sodium hypochlorite diluted 1:10 with water.

*Disease-Specific Isolation Precautions*
Most of the common infectious agents and diseases that are likely to be found in U.S. hospitals have specific isolation precautions that are indicated to prevent their transmission. Because more than 160 different diseases, syndromes, or conditions have specific isolation precautions, space does not permit a complete listing in this chapter. They are, however, listed in the CDC *Guideline for Isolation Precautions in Hospitals* [10,11] along with other pertinent comments about disease-specific isolation precautions, such as the length of time to apply isolation precautions. For some diseases, such as group-A streptococcal infections, isolation precautions are indicated only for 24 hours after start of effective therapy. Other diseases may require isolation precautions until the patient is culture-negative or clinically improved.

## MODIFICATION OF ISOLATION PRECAUTIONS IN INTENSIVE CARE UNITS

Many intensive care units pose special problems for applying isolation precautions; hence some modifications may be necessary that will not compromise patient care or increase the risk of infection to other patients and personnel. The isolation precaution that will most often have to be modified is the use of a private room. Ideally a private room should be available, but many intensive care units do not have them. When a private room is not available, and if airborne transmission is *not* likely, a cubicle can be used or an "isolation area" designated by partitions and tape on the floor. Instruction cards can be posted to inform personnel and visitors about other isolation precautions that are necessary, such as wearing gowns and gloves (see Chapter 18).

One isolation precaution that should not be modified in intensive care units is frequent and appropriate hand-washing, since patients clustered nearby are often unusually susceptible to infection. Hands should be washed between caring for patients and may need to be washed several times during the care of a patient. Frequent inservice training and close supervision to ensure adequate application of isolation precautions is especially important in intensive care units.

## RESPONSIBILITIES FOR CARRYING OUT ISOLATION PRECAUTIONS

The hospital is responsible for ensuring that patients are placed on appropriate isolation precautions. Each hospital should designate clearly, as a matter of policy, the personnel responsible for placing a patient on isolation precautions and the personnel who have the ultimate authority to make decisions regarding isolation precautions when conflicts arise. Such authority may be delegated to the chairperson of the Infection Control Committee, the hospital epidemiologist, or other infection control personnel. In many hospitals the nurse in charge is given the authority to place a patient on isolation precautions, particularly if the patient's physician is not available. In 1977, the last year for which national data are available, approximately 44 percent of critical care nurses and 40 percent of noncritical care nurses could place a patient on isolation precautions without consulting the attending physician [9]. In a recent report from a university hospital, most isolation precautions were initiated as a nursing rather than medical decision based on clinical rather than laboratory data [13].

Regardless of who initiates isolation precautions, all personnel—physicians, nurses, technicians, students, and others—are responsible for complying with isolation precautions and for tactfully pointing out observed infractions to the attention of offenders. Physicians should observe the proper isolation precautions at all times, teaching by example. The responsibilities of hospital personnel for carrying out isolation precautions cannot be effectively dictated but must arise from a personal sense of responsibility.

Patients and visitors also are responsible for complying with isolation precautions. The appropriate measures should be explained to the patient and visitors by physicians and nurses. An important general patient responsibility is hand-washing after touching infective material and potentially contaminated articles.

Infection control personnel are responsible for advising the Infection Control Committee and other policymakers in the hospital about revising or modifying isolation policies to fit most appropriately the unique needs of their hospital. Patient population, staffing patterns, and design and construction features greatly influence the isolation policies and procedures that can realistically be practiced in a hospital. Hospitals are encouraged to modify or supplement the recommendations presented in this chapter to meet their own needs. Nevertheless, when modifications are made it is essential that the risk to patients and personnel of acquiring nosocomial infections be minimized.

Finally, infection control personnel should keep up-to-date concerning new knowledge of the epidemiology of infectious diseases that may necessitate changes in isolation policies and procedures in their hospital.

## REFERENCES

1. Albert, R. K., and Condie, F. Hand-washing patterns in medical intensive care units. *N. Eng. J. Med.* 304;1465, 1981.
2. American Academy of Pediatrics. *Report of the Committee on Infectious Diseases* (19th ed.). (Klein, J. O. [Ed.]) Evanston, Ill.: American Academy of Pediatrics, 1982.
3. Bordley, J. *Two Centuries of American Medicine, 1776–1976.* Philadelphia: Saunders, 1976.
4. Centers for Disease Control. *Isolation Techniques for Use in Hospitals* (2nd ed.). Washington: U.S. Government Printing Office, DHEW, Publ. No. (CDC) 76-8314, 1975.
5. Evans, A. S. (Ed.). *Viral Infections of Humans: Epidemiology and Control* (3d ed.). New York: Plenum, 1982.
6. Evans, A. S., and Feldman, H. H. (Eds.). *Bacterial Infection of Humans: Epidemiology and Control* (1st ed.). New York: Plenum, 1982.
7. Gage, N. D., Landon, J. F., and Sider, M. T. *Communicable Disease.* Philadelphia: Davis, 1959.
8. Garner, J. S. Comments on CDC guideline for isolation precautions in hospitals, 1984. *Am. J. Infect. Control* 12:163, 1984.
9. Garner, J. S. Isolation techniques in critical care units. *Crit. Care Q.* 3:29, 1980.
10. Garner, J. S., and Simmons, B. P. CDC guideline for isolation precautions in hospitals. *Am. J. Infect. Control* 12:103, 1984.
11. Garner, J. S., and Simmons, B. P. CDC guideline for isolation precautions in hospitals. *Infect. Control* 4:245, 1983.
12. Haley, R. W., and Shachtman, R. H. The emergence of infection surveillance and control programs in U.S. hospitals: An assessment, 1976. *Am. J. Epidemiol.* 111:574, 1980.
13. Larson, E. Compliance with isolation technique. *Am. J. Infect. Control* 11:221, 1983.
14. Lynch, T. I *Communicable Disease Nursing.* St. Louis: Mosby, 1949.
15. Mandel, G. L., Douglas R. G., and Bennett J. E. (Eds.). *Principles and Practices of Infectious Diseases.* New York: Wiley, 1979.
16. Nauseef, W. M., and Maki, D. G. A study of the value of simple protective isolation in patients with granulocytopenia. *N. Engl. J. Med.* 304:448, 1981.
17. Schaffner, W. Infection control: Old myths and new realities. *Infect. Control* 1:330, 1980.

# 10 MULTIPLY RESISTANT STRAINS: EPIDEMIOLOGY AND CONTROL

Robert A. Weinstein

Our antimicrobial pharmacopeia and the organisms that colonize and infect our patients are in a continual competition. At times the lag between introduction of a new antibiotic and increasing prevalence of resistant bacteria (and fungi and viruses) has been quite long; for example, ampicillin was in use for many years before the widespread emergence of resistant *Hemophilus influenzae*. At other times resistance has occurred even before the clinical use of a specific antibiotic; for example, sulfonamide and aminoglycoside resistance can be found in gram-negative bacilli isolated long before our use of these compounds. Such disparities have led to a controversy over whether antibiotic use and abuse or other host and environmental factors are most responsible for the increasing prevalence of antibiotic-resistant microorganisms in the community and in hospitals [59] (see Chapter 11). Nevertheless, it appears to be conventional wisdom that our antibiotic choices seldom remain more than a very few drugs ahead of the resistant strains.

Since the 1960s reports of antibiotic-resistant bacteria in hospitals have appeared with increasing frequency. For example, before 1965 no hospital outbreaks involving multiply resistant gram-negative bacilli were investigated by the Centers for Disease Control. During 1965–75, however, 11 of 15 nosocomial epidemics of Enterobacteriaceae studied involved multiply resistant strains [93]. Among gram-positive bacteria, resistance of *Staphylococcus aureus* to penicillins became epidemic in the early 1960s and ultimately has come to be considered the norm. Since the late 1960s outbreaks of methicillin-resistant *S. aureus* have been reported, first from Europe and more recently from the United States [36] (see Chapter 11). Bacterial resistance has become a fact of hospital life and is so common that it often goes unnoted until it is either extreme or epidemic. In this chapter we review the epidemiology of drug-resistant strains in hospitals and discuss prevention and control strategies.

## DEFINITION, MECHANISMS, AND GENETICS OF MULTIPLE RESISTANCE

Although there is no standard definition for multiple resistance in bacteria, one definition commonly used is resistance to two or more unrelated antibiotics to which the bacteria are "normally considered susceptible" [59,99].

Alternatively, resistance to certain key or first-line drugs may be used as a marker for problems, such as aminoglycoside (gentamicin, tobramycin, amikacin, or netilmicin) resistance in gram-negative bacilli. Indeed our level of concern often depends on the nature and availability of other agents. Thus penicillin-resistant staphylococci were accepted relatively passively once methicillin became available. However, the therapeutic alternative for methicillin-resistant strains, vancomycin, is a relatively toxic agent, which has heightened our concern about "resistant staph."

The most common mechanisms of resistance include production by bacteria of antibiotic-inactivating enzymes, such as penicillinases or aminoglycoside-modifying enzymes; changes in cell wall permeability or uptake of antibiotics; alteration in target sites, such as ribosomes; changes in susceptible metabolic pathways; or changes in cell wall binding sites that prevent antibiotic attachment (see Chapter 12).

Resistance may be mediated by either the bacterial chromosome or extrachromosomal DNA (plasmids) [23] (see Chapters 11 and 12). Chromosomal resistance occurs by spontaneous mutation and darwinian selection of organisms resistant to single (or closely related) agents. In contrast bacteria may acquire resistance rapidly by the accrual of resistance plasmids (R factors), which often encode multiple resistances to unrelated drugs. Plasmids may spread across species lines and even between genera. An example of extensive spread is the presence of the same plasmid-mediated TEM-1 $\beta$-lactamase—an enzyme that confers resistance to ampicillin—in a variety of gram-negative bacteria, including Enterobacteriaceae, gonococci, and H. influenzae.

At the molecular level portions of plasmids, called transposons, may hitchhike from one plasmid to another or between plasmid and bacterial chromosome. Transposons carrying genes for resistance may align with other elements, such as those encoding virulence or colonization factors, creating R factors with an awesome "one-two punch."

## PATHOGENS AND INCIDENCE

The problem of resistance occurs in the community and hospital for both gram-positive and gram-negative bacteria. For example, resistance at the community level has affected Salmonella, Shigella, and Escherichia coli; Neisseria gonorrhoea and H. influenzae; and most recently, Streptococcus pneumoniae. In hospitals resistance has appeared in a variety of gram-negative bacilli as well as in common skin flora such as coagulase-negative staphylococci and corynebacteria. Although the specific "problem bugs" vary from hospital to hospital and depend on the interaction of a number of factors to be described, there are some general correlations between hospital settings and resistant flora (Table 10-1).

One of the greatest concerns in recent years has been the emergence of aminoglycoside resistance in nosocomial Enterobacteriaceae and Pseudomonas. In individual hospitals the prevalence of aminoglycoside-resistant gram-negative bacilli varies considerably, usually being greatest in large hospitals and teaching institutions [16,68,75]. Data from the National Nosocomial Infection Study (NNIS) show that during 1975–82, 52 percent of the 340,000 nosocomial infections reported by approximately 80 participating hospitals were caused by gram-negative bacilli; 5 percent of Enterobacteriaceae were resistant to gentamicin and/or tobramycin, compared to 14 percent of Pseudomonas species [41]. The percentage of Pseudomonas aeruginosa resistant to gentamicin increased from 6.6 percent in 1975 to 13.1 percent in 1979 [2]. Among Enterobacteriaceae, resistance was most frequent in Serratia marcescens (33 percent) and Providencia (32 percent), and in isolates from burn infections (24 percent) and primary bacteremias (9 percent).

In the past resistance of gram-negative bacilli to ampicillin, cephalosporins, and related antimicrobials did not receive great attention, possibly because of the availability of other drugs or because of limited

TABLE 10-1. Resistance problems 1980s

| Setting | Bacteria | Key resistances |
|---|---|---|
| General hospitals | Enterobacteriaceae | Aminoglycosides, newer cephalosporins |
| | Pseudomonas aeruginosa | Aminoglycosides, antipseudomonal penicillins |
| | Staphylococcus aureus | Methicillin, multiple |
| | Streptococcus pneumoniae | Penicillin, multiple |
| Oncology units | Enterobacteriaceae | Trimethoprim |
| | JK diphtheroids | Multiple |
| | Staphylococcus epidermidis | Multiple |
| Geriatric units | Proteus, Providencia, Morganella | Aminoglycosides |

resistance. In one hospital study of the TEM enzyme, the most common plasmidborne β-lactamase in gram-negative bacilli—nurses and hospitalized patients had a greater prevalence of positive strains (20 percent and 15 percent, respectively) than healthy controls (10 percent) [15].

Recently the availability of the "second-generation" cephalosporins, such as cefamandole, cefoxitin, and cefuroxime, and "third-generation" agents, such as cefotaxime, moxalactam, and cefoperazone, has called more attention to this issue. For instance, *Enterobacter* species were initially considered susceptible to cefamandole but frequently developed resistance during therapy (70,82). In Europe, where the second- and third-generation drugs have been available for several years, cefamandole and cefotaxime resistance among *Enterobacter* is widespread. In preliminary analysis of the 1982 NNIS data, resistance of *Pseudomonas* species to cefotaxime and moxalactam appears common, 49 percent and 33 percent, respectively. For Enterobacteriaceae, resistance to cefotaxime and moxalactam, 7 percent and 3 percent, respectively, increased significantly over the 12-month period [42]. The extent to which the regional differences and increases in resistance correlate with the use of these agents needs to be assessed.

FIG. 10-1. Percentage of *Staphylococcus aureus* infections resistant to methicillin as found in the National Nosocomial Infection Study (NNIS). Comparison of 4 NNIS hospitals affiliated with medical schools and having over 600 beds with 59 other NNIS hospitals. * = data for 6 months only. (Reproduced with permission from Haley, R. W., et al. *Ann. Intern. Med.* 97:297, 1982.)

The prevalence of enteric bacilli resistant to trimethoprim (TMP) and TMP-sulfonamide combinations has been variable [33,39]. For example, TMP has been in use in Finland since 1973; in 1980–81, from 8.6 to 38.3 percent of nosocomial urinary isolates (*Pseudomonas* excluded) were resistant, depending on the hospital studied [43]. When TMP-sulfamethoxazole has been used in a variety of settings for prophylaxis, prevalence of resistant strains has varied from 0 to 100 percent.

For gram-positive bacteria, methicillin resistance in *S. aureus* and the increasing occurrence of disease caused by multiply resistant coagulase-negative staphylococci have been of concern. In 63 NNIS hospitals during 1974–81, the percentage of *S. aureus* infections resistant to methicillin rose from a low of 2.4 percent (1975) to a high of 5 percent (1981) [36]. This increase was due entirely to only four large teaching institutions in which the percentages rose from 0 to 5 percent to 15 to 50 percent (Figure 10-1).

In NNIS hospitals, gentamicin resistance in *S. aureus* increased from 1 to 13 percent during 1975–79, while resistance in coagulase-negative staphylococci increased from 2 to 24 percent [2]. The incidence of infection due to all coagulase-negative staphylococci in leukemia patients increased at one large cancer center from 2 per 1000 days of hospitalization in 1974 to 15 per 1000 days in 1979 [98]. Methicillin resistance occurred in 40 percent of 87 strains tested. Multiply resistant coagulase-negative strains have also caused symptomatic bacteremia in 3 percent of newborns in a large referral intensive care unit (ICU) [4]

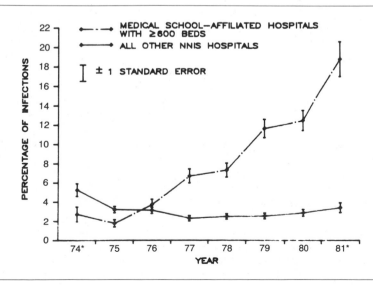

and in increasing numbers of adult patients in some hospitals [12].

## CLASSIFICATION AND DIAGNOSTIC CRITERIA

Determining whether resistant bacteria are hospital-acquired is often problematic since patients may be colonized asymptomatically when they enter the hospital. For example, in our experience [26,101] and others' [10], 15 to 25 percent of patients colonized or infected with aminoglycoside-resistant gram-negative bacilli have brought these strains into the hospital. Moreover, the incubation period for many infections caused by resistant bacteria is not clearly delineated.

In addition to the difficulties in defining hospital acquisition, there is often the question of whether the patient is colonized or has clinical disease due to the resistant strain. Criteria for making this differentiation are discussed in the chapters on site-specific infections; however, we consider colonization an important epidemiologic problem since is increases the reservoir of resistant bacteria and is often a precursor to clinical disease [87].

From a microbiologic standpoint, defining resistance may have pitfalls (see Chapter 7). In testing by disc diffusion, as a general example, antibiotic-containing discs may be outdated or inadequately tamped onto the agar surface, the bacterial inoculum may be too heavy or too light, the depth or pH of the agar may be incorrect, or the wrong drugs may even be used. Some gram-negative bacilli, such as *Flavobacterium,* are intrinsically resistant to the usual gram-negative panel of antibiotics, and unless the appropriate drugs are tested, such bacteria may appear untreatable. Problems in testing specific "drug-bug" combinations are cited in the section Specific Organisms.

## SOURCES OF RESISTANT STRAINS

The source of most resistant strains in hospitals appears to be patients who are colonized or infected [87,99]. Because the normal pharyngeal and intestinal flora of hospitalized patients may be displaced by multiply resistant enteric bacteria and *P. aeruginosa* (urine, perineum, and wounds may be similarly affected [30]), there are often many colonized patients for each patient with recognized infection—the "iceberg effect." This shift in flora often occurs within a very few days of admission (Fig. 10-2) and affects

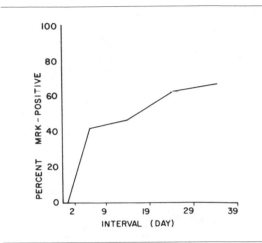

FIG. 10-2. Percentage of 138 patients positive for multiply resistant *Klebsiella* (MRK) on rectal culture, by interval from admission. (Reproduced with permission from Selden, R., et al. *Ann. Intern. Med.* 74:657, 1971.)

the older, generally sicker or more debilitated patients. The importance of various risk factors (e.g., specific exposures vs. more "hands on" care in general) and the pathophysiology of this shift (e.g., possible changes in membrane receptors or ligands, antibiotic suppression of normal flora) are not well delineated [20].

Personnel occasionally have been documented to disseminate resistant gram-positive strains, such as methicillin-resistant *S. aureus* [14] and possibly even coagulase-negative staphylococci. However, personnel carriage of resistant gram-negative bacilli (other than transient hand carriage described in the following section) appears to be very unusual. Exceptions include outbreaks reportedly traced to carriers of *Acinetobacter, Citrobacter,* and *Proteus. Acinetobacter,* one of the few gram-negative bacilli that may be among normal skin flora, was noted in one outbreak to recur periodically despite disinfection of the apparent environmental reservoirs. The outbreak was ultimately traced to the colonized hands of a respiratory therapy technician who had dermatitis and apparently contaminated respiratory therapy equipment while assembling it [8]. There have also been two clusters of *Citrobacter* infections of the central nervous system in neonates, possibly related to hand carriage by nurses [31,71], and an outbreak of *Proteus* infections in newborns traced to a nurse who was a chronic carrier [7].

Foodborne contamination with multiply resistant gram-negative bacilli has been cited in several investigations [50,89] and has been incriminated particularly in oncology units. Despite the potential importance of these observations, however, the overall role of food in introducing resistant strains into the hospital remains unclear.

Environmental sources and reservoirs of resistant strains have been a recurrent problem, especially when patient-care equipment, such as urine-measuring devices, become contaminated with enteric bacilli or *Pseudomonas* [56,99]. Extensive outbreaks of urinary tract infections (and respiratory tract, perineal, and/or intestinal colonization) may result when such contaminated equipment is shared by many patients.

Finally, there has been perennial concern about contamination of many areas of the inanimate environment with which patients do not have direct contact, such as flowerpots [102] and sink traps [22,49,72]. Despite heavy contamination, however, these sites have not been implicated epidemiologically in the spread of bacteria in hospitals.

## MODES OF TRANSMISSION

The most important way that resistant bacteria are spread in the hospital is from an infected patient to

a susceptible patient via transient carriage on hands of personnel. Such spread contributes to the "iceberg" of colonized patients and greatly increases the source and reservoir of resistant strains in the hospital (Fig. 10-3). Most of the evidence incriminating hands of personnel is circumstantial [1,47,81]. However, the weight of experience, dating back to the successful introduction of hand-washing as a control measure by Semmelweis, strongly supports this concept. Indices of "hands on" exposure to personnel, used in a few studies to quantitate patients' risk, have provided an additional measure.

Common-source spread of resistant strains has been noted primarily in outbreak settings. The attention of the medical community (and journal editors) is often attracted to such epidemics because of striking features, such as large numbers of patients infected with very resistant bacteria, unusual breaks in techniques or protocols, or contaminated commercial products. Perhaps more common than such "extravaganzas" are the ongoing episodes of limited cross-infection due to contamination of shared patient-care equipment, such as measuring containers and other environmental reservoirs, which probably account for a significant portion of seemingly "endemic" infections [101].

Airborne spread of resistant bacteria has been documented rarely. For methicillin-resistant *S. aureus,*

FIG. 10-3. The dynamics of nosocomial resistance: "resistance iceberg." (Reproduced with permission from Weinstein, R. A., and Kabins, S. A. *Am. J. Med.* 70:449, 1981.)

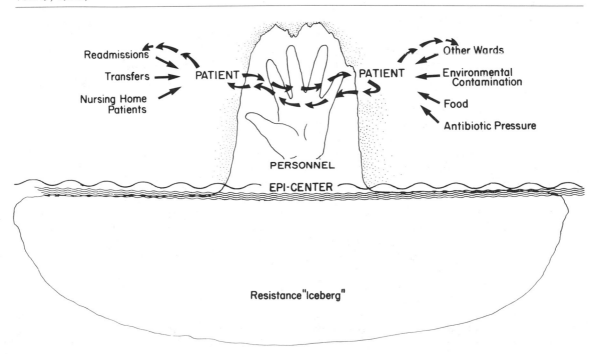

the most recent experience suggests that such spread is not a significant problem. For gram-negative bacilli, there was concern in one hospital that contamination in a 16-story chute-hydropulping waste disposal system led to airborne dispersal and transmission of *Pseudomonas* and enteric bacilli [34]. Waste pulp in the chute had $10^8$ cfu/g; air samples from hallways connecting the chute and nursing units had greater than 150 cfu/ft$^3$ of air. After closing the chute, air counts fell by over 75 percent and the incidence of nosocomial gram-negative bacteremias fell by over 65 percent.

Various insect vectors, such as flies and cockroaches, are probably unimportant in the transmission of resistant bacteria in U.S. hospitals.

## PREDISPOSING FACTORS

### Patients
A number of host factors have been associated with acquisition of antibiotic-resistant bacteria (Table 10-2). Our epidemiologic understanding of these factors has remained somewhat limited because most work has focused on epidemic and few on endemic situations [24,45,75,101], most studies have been retrospective and therefore limited in ability to gather complete host profiles, some studies have not included control groups, and relatively few of the studies have used multivariate analyses to control for relatedness of host factors [11,32]. Indeed many of the factors are undoubtedly "linked" and are serving as indirect markers of frequency of patient-staff contact (i.e., risk of indirect contact spread by hands of personnel).

The outbreaks listed in Table 10-2 include experience with both gram-negative bacilli and gram-positive bacteria. The host factors for both types of epidemics have been generally similar except that gram-negative bacilli involve the urinary tract and associated factors more often, such as indwelling bladder catheters, while gram-positive bacteria affect the skin and related factors somewhat more, such as duration of intravenous catheterization.

Of the many factors, the role of antibiotics has been the most controversial [59] (see Chapters 3 and 12), and several issues warrant emphasis. Many studies document the emergence of aminoglycoside-resistant strains after use of topical aminoglycoside ointments [32], related to nonabsorbable aminoglycosides in enteral regimens for suppression of gut bacteria in oncology patients [26,33], or after parenteral aminoglycoside therapy [3,24,33,54, 57–60,67,76,90]. In some studies resistant strains

TABLE 10-2. Examples of host factors associated with epidemic antimicrobial resistance in selected case-control studies

| Factor | Reference |
|---|---|
| Antimicrobial drugs | |
| Prophylaxis | 32,76,98 |
| Therapy | 6,11,14,27,31,32,35,48, 65,83–85,87,88,92, 95,100,104 |
| Apgar score | 32 |
| Duration of hospital or ICU stay | 8,11,12,27,32,83,87, 104 |
| Decreased WBC | 92 |
| Elderly age | 14,32 |
| Endotracheal intubation (or tracheostomy) | 8,32,66,104 |
| Exchange transfusions | 32 |
| Gastrointestinal colonization | 11,87 |
| Gavage feeding | 31 |
| Genitourinary instrumentation | 85 |
| Hyperalimentation | 12,32 |
| Intravenous therapy | 32 |
| Low birth weight | 32 |
| Mucocutaneous defects | 92 |
| Nasogastric suction | 87 |
| Proximity to other patients | 11,53 |
| Race | 31 |
| Respiratory therapy | 11,87 |
| Severity of underlying disease | 14,100 |
| Sex | 92 |
| Surgery (or number of operations) | 11,14,95 |
| Urinary catheter | |
| Condom | 62 |
| Indwelling | 16,27,76,84,85,104 |
| Urinary irrigation | 85 |

ICU = intensive care unit; WBC = white blood count.

have occurred more frequently in wound and sputum isolates, suggesting emergence of resistance at sites more likely to have poor penetration, and thus subinhibitory levels, of aminoglycosides [101]. The emergence of resistant isolates has also been correlated with inadequate doses of aminoglycosides [24,57,60,101].

There has been some controversy surrounding the relation between amikacin use and resistance [3,60,63,74,103]. Some hospitals have used amikacin extensively without noting any increase in resistance [63]. However, the incidence depends to some extent on how prevalent the various amikacin-inactivating enzymes are in the particular hospital, as well as on the adequacy of dosing. Regardless, cross-resistance to multiple aminoglycosides, including amikacin, occurs in up to 60 percent of gram-negative bacilli resistant to gentamicin or tobramycin [3,40,57,58,86,103].

The use of trimethoprim has been associated with the emergence of trimethoprim-resistant strains in a variety of settings, including treatment of urinary tract infections, prophylaxis of traveler's diarrhea, and gut sterilization in oncology patients. Of particular concern, this resistance is often carried on transferable R factors that confer resistance to multiple antimicrobials, emphasizing the way one agent may effect resistance to many others. In one study 96 percent of 165 TMP-resistant *E. coli* were resistant to at least four drugs, and 25 percent were resistant to seven; TMP resistance was transferable in 40 of 100 strains tested [65].

Regarding gram-positive bacteria, studies in the 1960s suggested that patients were at greater risk of being colonized with *S. aureus* after antibiotic treatment [6]. Recently, methicillin-resistant staphylococci have been found in hospitalized drug addicts who had self-prescribed oral cephalosporins, emphasizing the potential impact of antibiotic use in the community on hospital flora [83].

*Epidemics*
The events leading to any nosocomial epidemic are probably multifactorial. In most outbreaks of multiply drug-resistant bacteria, precipitating events have not been well elucidated. Factors that could increase person-to-person spread include poor aseptic practices, as in crowded units or when the nurse-to-patient ratio becomes too low. Spread from the environment is facilitated by poor housekeeping practices that lead to reservoirs of resistant organisms within the hospital, as when infected urine is allowed to remain in urine measuring or testing devices. Excessive use of antibiotics may increase the selective pressure for resistant strains [59].

Certain fortuitous events may precipitate outbreaks, such as contamination of a commercial product, admission of a patient who is a heavy shedder of multiply resistant bacteria [26], or acquisition of resistance by a bacterial species that is adept at colonization or unusually resistant to disinfection. Also, advances in medical technology, such as transplantation, dialysis, and new prosthetic devices, always create additional epidemic risks.

Particular areas within the hospital, especially intensive care units (see Chapter 18) and burn (see Chapter 30), neurosurgical, and urology units, are prone to outbreaks. These areas house acutely ill patients who are subjected to many invasive procedures

and often exposed to multiple antibiotics under circumstances in which asepsis may be trampled in the rush of crisis care. We have found that multiply resistant bacteria may breed in such units, which we call "epi-centers" (Fig. 10-3) [99]. As colonized patients are transferred to other areas of the hospital, they may leave a trail of resistance.

## PLASMID AND TRANSPOSON OUTBREAKS

Most reported outbreaks have been due to epidemic spread of single strains. In the past few years, however, several "plasmid outbreaks" have been described in which a resistance plasmid has caused either simultaneous or sequential resistance to occur in epidemic fashion in different species or genera (Table 10-3) [18,44,55,78–80,97]. We are also recognizing that transposition of plasmid segments (or other spatial rearrangements of genetic material) may lead to "transposon outbreaks" involving whole families of related resistance plasmids [78].

The epidemiology of most plasmid outbreaks, specifically the reservoirs for the resistance plasmids, time and place of transfer of plasmids, and pressures involved, has been largely speculative [25,59,77]. Transfer can occur in the gut, on skin, in urine, and in the environment (e.g., in urine containers) and may be facilitated by antimicrobial therapy [77]. Moreover, relatively avirulent bacterial strains may serve as reservoirs for resistance. For example, gentamicin resistance in *Staphylococcus epidermidis* or *S. aureus* may be mediated by identical plasmids that can pass between these two species in vitro and on human skin [43].

Plasmid outbreaks may be difficult to detect but should be sought through surveillance for the occurrence of multiple species or genera with identical or very similar multiple drug (or even just key drug) resistance patterns. If available, similar gel electrophoretic patterns of plasmid DNA could facilitate detection (see Chapter 12). Once recognized, plasmid epidemics are at present controlled much like single-strain outbreaks (see section following). In the future, technologic refinements may facilitate more extensive epidemiologic investigation of plasmid and transposon resistance and allow more specific control measures.

*Other Multiple Strain Outbreaks*
Occasionally common sources may become contaminated with several bacterial species, leading to outbreaks of otherwise unrelated strains. For example, one multiple strain outbreak of orthopedic wound

TABLE 10-3. Examples of plasmid outbreaks

| Setting (ref.) | Bacteria (no.) | Predominant infections | Appearance of resistance (duration) | Plasmidborne resistances |
|---|---|---|---|---|
| Neonatal ICU [55] | *Klebsiella* Serotype 30 (21) Serotype 19 (6) | NS | Sequential (9 mo, 5 mo) | Gm, kn, am, cf, cb, |
| Hospitalwide [97] | *Serratia* [71] *Klebsiella Citrobacter Proteus* } (68) *Enterobacter Providencia* | UTI | Simultaneous (3 yr) | Gm, tb, kn, am, cf, cb, st, su |
| Burn unit [18] | *Klebsiella Enterobacter* } (NS) Three other genera | Burn | Simultaneous (11 mo) | Tb, kn, ne, |
| Hospitalwide [80] | *Klebsiella* [69] *Escherichia coli* } (16) *Enterobacter Proteus* | UTI, wd, resp | Index case admitted with epidemic strain; remainder ~ simultaneous (2 yr) | Gm, tb, kn, am, cf, cb, ch, su |

ICU = intensitve care unit; NS = not stated; UTI = urinary tract infection; wd = wound infection; resp = respiratory infection; gm = gentamicin; tb = tobramycin; kn = kanamycin; am = ampicillin; cf = cephalothin; cb = carbenicillin; st = streptomycin; ch = chloramphenicol; su = sulfonamide; ne = neomycin.

infections was traced to a common bucket used to mix cast material. The bucket was not routinely disinfected and contained a variety of contaminants that probably were inoculated into wounds during application of casts. Such outbreaks may go unrecognized unless one strain predominates or the strains or epidemiologic circumstances are very unusual.

## CONTROL

### Control of Epidemic Resistance

Control of resistant bacteria has usually focused on epidemics (Table 10-4) and traditionally has involved efforts to strengthen aseptic practices while an epidemiologic analysis of cases (and controls) is quickly undertaken to exclude common-source exposures [99] (see Chapter 5). Empirical attempts to decrease transmission usually have also included isolating or cohorting infected or colonized patients. Identifying the colonized patients (Fig. 10-3) often requires culture surveys, which may be facilitated by the use of selective media (see Chapter 7). In some outbreaks susceptible patients, such as those with indwelling urinary catheters, have been physically separated to decrease the likelihood that personnel would passively carry pathogens from one patient or drainage bag to the next [53]. In drastic situations, units have been closed to new admissions.

TABLE 10-4. Traditional control measures for epidemic resistance

Identify reservoirs
   Colonized and infected patients
   Environmental contamination
Halt transmission
   Improve hand-washing and asepsis
   Isolate colonized and infected patients
   Eliminate any common source; disinfect environment
   Separate susceptible patients
   Close unit to new admissions if necessary
Modify host risk
   Discontinue compromising factors (Table 10-2) when
     possible
   Control antibiotic use (rotate, restrict, or cease)

In some instances, antibiotic controls may help restrict the spread of resistant bacteria [59,67]. First, in high-density units such as ICUs, restricting antibiotic use may be important [24,25,33,59,67,76]. In rare situations, antibiotic use has been totally and successfully suspended [73]. Second, antibiotic restrictions may decrease selective pressures in some "plasmid outbreaks." Chemicals that "cure" bacterial plasmids in vitro are currently too toxic for use in humans. Safer agents such as nalidixic acid, which may prevent transfer of plasmids [28], have yet to be used for this purpose in clinical situations. Third, more careful dosing with aminoglycosides may decrease the chance that subinhibitory levels will select resistant subpopulations (due to spontaneous chromosomal mutations), particularly in sites that have large bacterial populations, such as wounds or the respiratory tract. Finally, the control of antibiotics that select for sensitive precursors of resistant organisms (e.g., cephalosporins selecting for *Pseudomonas*) may be necessary.

*Experimental Approaches to Epidemic Control*
Table 10-5 lists several methods that have been tried. Topical and nonabsorbable antimicrobials have been used for prophylaxis in several settings, including epidemics of resistant bacteria. For example, polymyxin spray was used experimentally in one ICU to forestall pharyngeal colonization and pneumonia with *Pseudomonas* (see Chapter 26). In limited studies this approach appeared to work, but when applied in the ICU in a continuous fashion, the consequence was a compensatory increase in pneumonias caused by polymyxin-resistant bacilli [22].

In the 1960s attempts were made to use "avirulent" staphylococci to reduce colonization with epidemic strains. This form of bacterial interference has been reexplored recently. In one study, pharyngeal implantation of $\alpha$-hemolytic streptococci successfully displaced resistant enteric organisms in infants in a neonatal ICU [91]. In an outbreak, this approach was used with other measures to control successfully colonization of neonates by amikacin-resistant *Serratia* and *Klebsiella* [13]. However, this work needs to be confirmed and studies extended to adults before any conclusions can be made about its general applicability.

Another control measure from the past that is being reinvestigated is disinfection of urinary catheter drainage bags. Earlier use of this method, with formalin in drainage bottles, ended when closed systems were widely adopted. Unfortunately, closed drainage cannot prevent contamination of collection bags indefinitely; in as many as 30 percent of patients with

TABLE 10-5. Experimental approaches for controlling resistance

Prevention of acquisition by use of topical antimicrobials
   Respiratory spray
   Oral nonabsorbables
   Environmental
Bacterial interference
Treatment of colonized patients
   Topical and/or systemic antimicrobials
Immune enhancement

initially sterile urine, contamination of the bag may precede bladder infection [62]. In a recent study, disinfection of drainage bags with hydrogen peroxide forestalled urinary infections in a small number of patients with acute spinal injury [51]. Organisms may still ascend from the perineum around the catheter, however, and in a controlled study in a large teaching hospital, bag decontamination did not appear to reduce infection rates [96]. Nevertheless, bag disinfection may reduce reservoirs of contaminated urine in the hospital environment [62] and warrants additional controlled study.

Attempts to decontaminate relatively remote environmental reservoirs of resistant bacteria, such as sink traps, have been innovative [52]. However, based on the failure of such efforts to decrease infection rates [22], and on the lack of any epidemiologic link between sink traps and patients [49,72], these extraordinary measures do not appear routinely warranted.

Finally, in drastic situations systemic antibiotics have at times been administered to patients who are only colonized with multiply resistant bacteria (e.g., multiply resistant pneumococci) [48].

*Control of Endemic Resistance*
A variety of epidemic control measures may be applied to endemic situations. For example, we have used "antibiotic resistance precautions" (Fig. 10-4) for all patients who are colonized or infected with resistant gram-negative bacilli [99]. In our experience, such barrier-type precautions have markedly decreased the incidence of aminoglycoside-resistant *E. coli*, *Klebsiella*, and *Enterobacter*, and probably have limited the extent of recurrent miniepidemics of resistant *Serratia* (Fig. 10-5) [101]. In sharp contrast, the incidence of aminoglycoside-resistant *Pseudomonas* infections appears to a greater extent to have paralleled antibiotic use rather than to have been affected appreciably by barrier-type precautions. In fact, we have frequently found that in individual patients *P. aeruginosa* became resistant in the face of aminoglycoside therapy [101].

An update of our experience has confirmed these findings [26]. However, we have found that as barrier-type precautions diminished the incidence of plasmid-mediated resistance in Enterobacteriaceae, the remaining resistant isolates followed a pattern like that of *Pseudomonas*, with broad cross-resistant strains emerging after antibiotic therapy. It is unlikely that the incidence of such strains will be reduced additionally by barrier-type precautions alone.

Based on our studies, we suggest a multifaceted approach to control of endemic aminoglycoside-

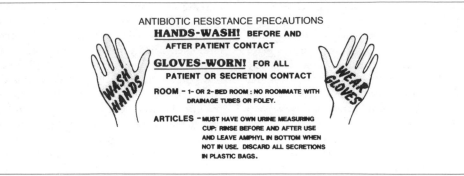

resistant gram-negative bacilli in large acute-care hospitals [99]:

1. Antibiotic-resistance precautions (Fig. 10-4) should be used for all patients who are colonized or infected with aminoglycoside-resistant Enterobacteriaceae. These precautions should be extended to any patient who is a persistent shedder of other multiply resistant bacteria, especially if the patient has draining wounds, receives repeated courses of antibiotics, or requires intensive nursing care.
2. Such precautions should be used while appropriate cultures are being processed from patients who are admitted (or readmitted) with a history of colonization or infection with resistant organisms.
3. Patients transferred from nursing homes or other hospitals should be evaluated for carriage of resistant bacteria [26,35,101]. Certain patients, such as those who are incontinent, have recently received antibiotics, have indwelling urinary cath-

FIG. 10-4. Placard stating barrier-type antibiotic resistance precautions to be placed on door to patient's room and above bed; stickers with similar precautions may be affixed to urinary drainage bag or other items to alert personnel that patient is colonized or infected with resistant bacteria.

eters, or come from large nursing homes or hospitals, may warrant precautions while appropriate cultures are processed.
4. Appropriate aminoglycoside usage and dosage should be ensured to decrease selection of spontaneous mutations among *P. aeruginosa,* and to a lesser extent, among Enterobacteriaceae.

FIG. 10-5. Gentamicin use and gram-negative bacilli resistant to gentamicin at Michael Reese Medical Center, 1970–77. Data are plotted as the monthly average, and averages for the first seven and last five months of 1974 are plotted separately to demonstrate the effect of barrier precautions, which began in August 1974. EKES = *Escherichia coli, Klebsiella, Enterobacter,* and *Serratia.* (Reproduced with permission from Weinstein, R. A., et al. *J. Infect. Dis.* 141:338, 1980.)

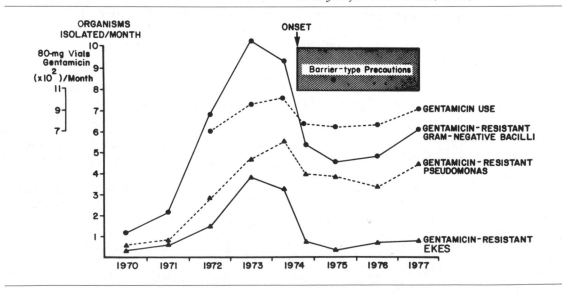

5. Surveillance of patients and clinical laboratory results should be maintained to detect miniepidemics (two or more patients with similarly resistant organisms) so that cross-infection or significant environmental reservoirs can be identified and controlled.

6. When patients who are colonized or infected with resistant bacteria are transferred to another hospital or nursing home, the receiving institution should be notified of the isolation status.

7. Compromising factors (Table 10-2) in high-risk patients should be eliminated whenever possible. In certain specialty units, such as ICUs, control of antibiotic usage as discussed previously may also help to control endemic resistance. However, several factors may limit the efficacy of this measure. First, use of one antibiotic may lead to cross-resistance to others, as seen with aminoglycoside cross-resistance as well as with plasmid colinkage of resistance. Next, sequential acquisition of bacterial resistance when antibiotics are rotated has been well described [69]. Finally, if and when controls are lifted, resistant organisms that have remained in low numbers colonizing patients may reemerge [67].

*Threshold for Investigation and Control*
In certain situations, ongoing control measures are appropriate. First, some organisms always warrant prompt attention because of key resistances. Such bacteria include methicillin-resistant *S. aureus,* high-level penicillin-resistant *S. pneumoniae,* and carbenicillin-aminoglycoside-resistant *P. aeruginosa.* Second, in units such as ICUs, which may serve as epi-centers, aggressive containment of multiply resistant strains can be justified. Third, certain types of patients warrant antibiotic resistance precautions. These include patients who are colonized with multiply resistant strains at several sites and whose severity of illness requires frequent physical attention by physicians, nurses, respiratory therapists and so forth, and thus higher risk for spread of resistant bacteria to other patients.

In other situations, the individual hospital must rely on local surveillance and experience to help set formal or intuitive epidemic thresholds for instituting aggressive containment measures and epidemiologic investigations. The thresholds will probably differ for each hospital and for specific multiply resistant strains. For example, with *Serratia* a low threshold may trigger an investigation because of the iceberg effect often seen in patients with urinary catheters or on respirators. In some hospitals, ongoing laboratory studies, such as serotyping or biotyping, may be used to help

evaluate possible single-strain outbreaks [21] (see Chapter 7). "Plasmid outbreaks" and multiple-strain outbreaks may be more difficult to identify even with ongoing surveillance, and the mere suspicion of clustering of similarly resistant Enterobacteriaceae may warrant an investigation. Finally, if clusters of resistant organisms occur in the face of barrier precautions, our experience suggests that a chronically colonized patient or an environmental source should be sought vigorously [26].

## SPECIFIC ORGANISMS

*Enterobacteriaceae*
Antibiotic-resistant Enterobacteriaceae are common in hospitals, especially aminoglycoside-resistant *Klebsiella, Serratia, Enterbacter,* and *E. coli* [101]. Drug-resistant *Proteus, Providencia,* and *Morganella* are also very common, particularly in geriatric wards and in patients transferred from nursing homes [26,101]. The clinical aspects of infections caused by Enterobacteriaceae are described in chapters on urinary tract infection (see Chapter 25), pneumonia (see Chapter 26), wound infection (see Chapter 27), and bacteremia (see Chapters 36 and 38). Microbiologic diagnosis of these infections usually poses no problem for the modern laboratory, particularly with the availability of newer diagnostic kits (see Chapter 7).

Predisposing factors for, and the epidemiology of, resistant Enterobacteriaceae have differed somewhat from genus to genus (Table 10-6) [85]. Some organisms, such as *Klebsiella,* may be more viable on human skin and thus may have a greater potential for person-to-person spread on the hands of hospital personnel [39]. *Serratia* commonly causes asymptomatic colonization of urinary tract and respiratory tract, and chronically colonized patients are often a source for large numbers of cross-infections [26,84]. There have also been several outbreaks described in which environmental contamination with *Serratia,* notably of graduated cylinders and ventilators, led to epidemics of urinary tract infection, peritonitis, or pneumonia [26]. *Enterobacter* strains often become resistant to second- and third-generation cephalosporins during therapy [70,82], which may explain in part why *Enterobacter* species are a relatively common cause of mediastinitis after open-heart surgery despite cephalosporin prophylaxis [70].

As noted earlier, in some hospitals 15 to 25 percent of all aminoglycoside-resistant Enterobacteriaceae are cultured from patients at the time of admission. Patients with chronic respiratory or urinary tract infections, those who have frequent admissions, and pa-

TABLE 10-6. Epidemiologic patterns in outbreaks of
urinary tract infection by multiply resistant organisms

| Factor | Organism[a] | | |
|---|---|---|---|
| | Klebsiella pneumoniae | Serratia marcescens | Proteus rettgeri |
| Reservoir | | | |
|    Symptomatic GU infection | + + + + | ± | + + |
|    Asymptomatic GU infection | + + | + + + + | + + + |
|    Gastrointestinal colonization | + + | 0 | 0 |
| Mode of transmission | Hands[b] | Hands | Hands |
| Spatial clustering of cases prominent | + + | + + + + | + + + + |
| Risk factors | | | |
|    Urinary catheterization | Yes | Yes | Yes |
|    Broad-spectrum antimicrobial exposure | Yes | Yes | Yes |
|    Urinary catheter irrigation | Yes | No | No |
|    GU instrumentation | No | No | Yes |

GU = genitourinary.
[a]Scale: 0 (no contribution) to + + + + (maximal contribution).
[b]Contact spread on hands of personnel.
Adapted from Schaberg, D. R., et al. *J. Infect. Dis.* 133:363, 1976.

tients transferred from nursing homes or other hospitals are particularly likely to bring resistant strains into the hospital [26,101]. In several instances, such patients have been the index cases in outbreaks [10,17,31] (see Chapter 23).

Since drug-resistant Enterobacteriaceae appear to spread largely from patient to patient on the hands of hospital personnel (Table 10-7), and since colonized or infected patients are usually the major reservoir in the hospital, it has generally been possible to contain resistant Enterobacteriaceae using the precautions described previously [26,99].

### Pseudomonas Aeruginosa

*P. aeruginosa* has intrinsic resistance to most available antibiotics, leaving aminoglycosides, antipseudomonal penicillins, and possibly, newer cephalosporins as treatment options for systemic infection. *Pseudomonas* is ubiquitous in the hospital, frequently colonizing patients (even before admission) and contam-

TABLE 10-7. Epidemiology of endemic aminoglycoside resistance in nosocomial gram-negative bacilli

| Factor | Relative contribution (%) |
|---|---|
| Cross-infection | 30–40 |
| Antibiotic pressures | 20–25 |
| "Community"-acquisition | 20–25 |
| Other (environment, food, personnel, air, unknown) | 20 |

inating water and various foods, particularly salads and fresh vegetables [50,89]. Laboratory identification is not difficult, although aminoglycoside susceptibility testing was confounded until the recognition that the divalent cation content of media needs to be carefully controlled.

There has been considerable controversy over whether aminoglycoside-resistant gram-negative bacilli are less virulent than sensitive strains. In a number of studies using a variety of measures of virulence, such as chills, fever, elevated white count, pyuria, and other local findings of infection, there have been no differences detected [61,76]. In a few studies, however, particularly in oncology patients, aminoglycoside-resistant *Pseudomonas* strains have been less prone to cause bacteremia than sensitive strains [33,46].

Several studies have shown that aminoglycoside-resistant *Pseudomonas* may emerge from sensitive populations of the same serotype during treatment [3,24,101]. In fact, some institutions have found that despite isolating patients with antibiotic-resistant *P. aeruginosa*, the incidence of colonization with these strains has continued to increase [26,50,66,101], in part paralleling the increasing use of aminoglycoside antibiotics.

In epidemic situations, *P. aeruginosa* has been noted to spread from contaminated common sources to persons as well as from person to person [16,21,56]. Such transmission may be more amenable to the control measures outlined previously. However, control of endemic *P. aeruginosa* infections is problematic and may well require more innovative strategies that interfere with the ability of *Pseudomonas* to colonize or invade.

### Staphylococcus Aureus

Resistance of *S. aureus* to methicillin (aminoglycosides, and/or clindamycin) has been reported with increasing frequency in the United States over the past few years [14,36,83,88].

Microbiologic diagnosis is facilitated when the potential causes of false-negative tests for methicillin resistance are recognized. These include use of cloxacillin or dicloxacillin discs, incubation above 35°C (95°F), use of certain automated methods, determination of minimum inhibitory concentrations by standard broth microdilution, and failure to notice small colonies or light growth inside an apparent zone of inhibition [36]. Methicillin-resistant *S. aureus* may be erroneously reported when colonies from mixed cultures of resistant coagulase-negative and sensitive *S. aureus* are not picked carefully. Enterococcal colonies, if picked from blood agar, can give false-positive catalase tests and the impression that the enterococci, which can give positive coagulase tests, are methicillin-resistant *S. aureus*.

The epidemiology of drug-resistant isolates of *S. aureus* appears to be similar to that of susceptible strains (see Chapter 31). Particular reservoirs for methicillin-resistant staphylococci include IV drug addicts, burn-unit patients, nursing-home patients with multiple decubitus ulcers, and hospital personnel with dermatitis. In Detroit methicillin-resistant *S. aureus* arose as a major community problem in drug addicts who frequently self-prescribed antibiotics to forestall or treat infections related to the illicit use of contaminated needles. When these addicts were admitted to hospitals, waves of nosocomial methicillin-resistant infections followed [83].

Once drug-resistant staphylococci have become entrenched in the hospital, eradication is difficult. Control has required accurate laboratory identification, prospective surveillance for colonized and infected patients (including in some hospitals periodic culture surveys of high-risk patients), identification of previously colonized patients at readmission, appropriate isolation of all identified patients, search for environmental and personnel sources, and aggressive antibiotic therapy of infected patients (vancomycin with or without rifampin) [14,36,95].

### Coagulase-Negative Staphylococci

Coagulase-negative staphylococci, formerly thought to be an avirulent part of our normal flora, have become a problem pathogen in patients with implanted prosthetic joints (see Chapter 29), heart valves (see Chapter 28), or neurosurgical shunts (see Chapter 34); in patients with intravascular catheters [4], particularly long-duration central lines [12] such as Hickman catheters (see Chapter 36); and in immunosuppressed patients, particularly those who have received broad-spectrum antibiotics to treat or prevent infection with gram-negative bacilli.

Using gentamicin resistance as a marker, we found that resistant coagulase-negative staphylococci are relatively uncommon in healthy nonhospitalized persons but are rapidly acquired in the hospital, related either to previous antibiotic exposure or ubiquitous environmental contamination [100]. The resistance was plasmid-mediated and could be transferred in vitro or on skin to *S. aureus* [43]. In one study most nosocomial isolates of gentamicin-resistant *S. aureus* appeared to result from in vivo plasmid spread rather than from person-to-person transfer of resistant strains [100].

Since drug-resistant coagulase-negative staphylococci often become part of the patient's normal flora and are so ubiquitous [5,100], control is difficult. In patients with indwelling intravascular catheters or patients undergoing implantation of foreign bodies, preventing infections with coagulase-negative staphylococci at present depends on strict attention to asepsis, and in some situations, antibiotic prophylaxis.

### Penicillin-Resistant Pneumococci

Although multiply resistant *S. pneumoniae* infections have not been a significant nosocomial problem in the United States, they reached epidemic proportions on crowded pediatric wards in South African hospitals in 1977–78 [48]. During that time 48 patients, almost all under three years of age, had positive blood or cerebrospinal fluid cultures, representing 8.5 percent of all pneumococcal isolates from these two sites. In addition, over 300 carriers of resistant pneumococci were found. Successful control measures included restriction of unnecessary antibiotic use (since antibiotic exposure increased the risk of colonization), susceptibility testing of all pneumococci, nasopharyngeal culture surveys, respiratory isolation of all infected and colonized patients, and aggressive use of antimicrobials to eradicate carriage.

### JK Diphtheroids

The JK strain of *Corynebacterium,* often susceptible only to vancomycin, has been noted in the past few years to be an increasingly common pathogen in immunocompromised oncology patients, mostly causing bacteremia or wound infections at bone marrow aspiration and IV catheter sites [29,37,92]. JK diphtheroids appear commonly to colonize the skin of hospitalized patients [29,92], but interestingly are found more often in men and postmenopausal women, suggesting a possible relation between colonization and sebum content of skin. Because of extensive skin colonization, control of endemic infections with JK diphtheroids, like control of coagulase-negative staphylococci, may depend in large part on good aseptic technique. In addition, at least one outbreak of JK diphtheroids has been described in which evidence suggested possible person-to-person spread and a role for careful hand-washing in preventing infections.

### Other Resistant Organisms

High-level resistance of enterococci to aminoglycosides including streptococci, gentamicin, and amikacin is well described but has not been a particularly frequent problem in nosocomial infections. More recently, transmissible penicillin resistance and β-lactamase activity have been demonstrated in a clinical isolate of enterococci [64]. The future impact of such strains on susceptibility of enterococci and other streptococci, in both the hospital and the community, remains an open question.

Clindamycin resistance in the *Bacteroides fragilis* group has been a sporadic, relatively unusual problem that is plasmid-mediated and has occurred in 0 to 10 percent of strains in various medical centers [94]. One author recently described an outbreak of clindamycin-resistant *B. fragilis* on a surgical ward in which 7 (13 percent) of 52 strains were affected [19]; 85 percent of involved patients had received clindamycin or erythromycin before recovery of the resistant strain. Although the epidemiology of this outbreak is not entirely clear, preliminary evidence did not suggest intrahospital transmission.

Resistance of fungi to amphotericin B, 5-flucytosine, and other available antifungal agents has been described. Little is known about the epidemiology, impact, or potential for control of these strains in hospitals. However, as the number of broad spectrum antibacterial agents available in hospitals increases, we may see more overgrowth by fungal organisms, and a new chapter in nosocomial drug resistance may unfold. Similarly, the increasing availability of antiviral agents such as vidarabine and acyclovir presents the potential problem of acquired drug resistance in herpes and other viruses.

## FUTURE CHALLENGES

The ingenious ways in which microorganisms learn to evade our antimicrobial pharmacopeia will no doubt continue to astound, confound, and perplex us. As the pressures of our antimicrobial armamentarium increase, and as our patients are subjected to more invasive procedures and immunosuppressive regimens, we can look forward to greater resistance and more problems with the traditionally avirulent normal flora.

Unfortunately, our control of resistant strains has advanced little since the singular contribution of Semmelweis. Moreover, we still have trouble encouraging and motivating personnel to follow the most basic concepts in asepsis. This issue needs continued attention and study.

At the same time, we need to use advances in microbiologic techniques to obtain a better understanding of the epidemiology of nosocomial resistance, not only in single-strain outbreaks but also in the endemic setting and in plasmid and even transposon outbreaks. As we increase our understanding of bacterial [9] and host factors that control colonization with normal flora and lead to overgrowth of resistant bacteria, new approaches may emerge for preventing colonization with nosocomial pathogens, blocking adherence of unwanted resistant strains, or halting progression from colonization to infection.

In the meantime, I believe the key is not to delay in applying the strategies available to us and not to apply measures in too piecemeal a fashion lest control always lag behind resistance. The growing interchange of resistant bacteria among nursing homes, community hospitals, tertiary care centers, and high-risk outpatient populations emphasizes the need for concerted control efforts.

## REFERENCES

1. Adams, B. G., and Marrie, T. J. Hand carriage of aerobic gram-negative rods may not be transient. *J. Hyg. (Camb.)* 89:33, 1982.
2. Allen, J. R., Hightower, A. W., Martin, S. M., and Dixon, R. E. Secular trends in nosocomial infections: 1970–1979. *Am. J. Med.* 70:389, 1981.
3. Amirak, I. D., Williams, R. J., Noone, P., and Wills, M. R. Amikacin resistance developing in patient with *Pseudomonas aeruginosa* bronchopneumonia. *Lancet* 1:537, 1977.
4. Baumgart, S., Hall, S. E., Campos, J. M., and Polin, R. A. Sepsis with coagulase-negative staphylococci in critically ill newborns. *Am. J. Dis. Child.* 137:461, 1983.
5. Bentley, D. W., Hahn, J. J., and Lepper, M.

H. Transmission of chloramphenicol-resistant *Staphylococcus epidermidis:* Epidemiologic and laboratory studies. *J. Infect. Dis.* 122:365, 1970.

6. Berntsen, C. A., and McDermott, W. Increased transmissibility of staphylococci to patients receiving an antimicrobial drug. *N. Engl. J. Med.* 262:637, 1960.

7. Burke, J. P., Ingall, D., Klein, J. O., Gezon, H. M., and Finland, M. *Proteus mirabilis* infections in a hospital nursery traced to a human carrier. *N. Engl. J. Med.* 284:115,1971.

8. Buxton, A. E., Anderson, R. L., Werdegar, D., and Atlas, E. Nosocomial respiratory tract infection and colonization with *Acinetobacter calcoaceticus:* Epidemiologic characteristics. *Am. J. Med.* 65:507, 1978.

9. Casewell, M. S. The Different Characteristics of Antibiotic-Resistant and Sensitive Bacteria. In Stuart-Harris, C. H., and Harris, D. M., *The Control of Antibiotic-Resistant Bacteria.* London: Academic, 1982, p. 77.

10. Casewell, M. W., Dalton, M. T. Webster, M., and Phillips, I. Gentamicin-resistant *Klebsiella aerogenes* in a urological ward. *Lancet* 2:444, 1977.

11. Chow, A. W., Taylor, P. R., Yoshikawa, T. T., and Guze, L. B. A nosocomial outbreak of infections due to multiply resistant *Proteus mirabilis:* Role of intestinal colonization as a major reservoir. *J. Infect. Dis.* 139:621, 1979.

12. Christensen, G. D., Bisno, A. L., Parisi, J. T., McLaughlin, B., Hester, M. G., and Luther, R. W. Nosocomial septicemia due to multiply antibiotic-resistant *Staphylococcus epidermidis. Ann. Intern. Med.* 96:1, 1982.

13. Cook, L. N., Davis, R. S., Stover, B. H. Outbreak of amikacin-resistant Enterobacteriaceae in an intensive care nursery. *Pediatrics* 65:264, 1980.

14. Craven, D. E., Reed, C., Kollisch, N., DeMaria, A., Lichtenberg, D., Shen, K., and McCabe, W. R. A large outbreak of infections caused by a strain of *Staphylococcus aureus* resistant to oxacillin and aminoglycosides. *Am. J. Med.* 71:53, 1981.

15. Dubois, J., Pechere J. C., and Letarte, R. Factors affecting the increase of R plasmids during hospitalization. *Curr. Microbiol.* 5:219, 1981.

16. Duncan, I. B. R., Rennie, R. P., and Duncan, N. H. A long-term study of gentamicin-resistant *Pseudomonas aeruginosa* in a general hospital. *J. Antimicrob. Chemother.* 7:147, 1981.

17. Edwards, L. D., Cross, A., Levin, S., and Landau, W. Outbreak of a nosocomial infection with a strain of *Proteus rettgeri* resistant to many antibicrobials. *Am. J. Clin. Pathol.* 61:41, 1974.

18. Elwell, L. P., Inamine, J. M., and Minshew, B. H. Common plasmid specifying tobramycin resistance found in two enteric bacteria isolated from burn patients. *Antimicrob. Agents Chemother.* 13:312, 1978.

19. England, A. C., III, Bond, E. J., Livingston, H., and Nelson, K. E. Epidemiology of clindamycin-resistant *Bacteroides fragilis. Programs and Abstracts of the Annual Meeting of the American Society for Microbiology,* March 7–12, 1982, Atlanta, Ga., p. 87, abstract L27.

20. Fainstein, V., Rodriguez, V., Turck, M., Hermann, G., Rosenbaum, B., and Bodey, G. P. Patterns of oropharyngeal and fecal flora in patients with acute leukemia. *J. Infect. Dis.* 144:10, 1981.

21. Farmer, J. J., Weinstein, R. A., Zierdt, C. H., and Brokopp, C. D. Hospital outbreaks caused by *Pseudomonas aeruginosa:* Importance of serogroup 011. *J. Clin. Microbiol.* 16:266, 1982.

22. Feeley, T. W., duMoulin, G. C., Hedley-Whyte, J., Bushnell, L. S., Gilbert, J. P., and Feingold, D. S. Aerosol polymyxin and pneumonia in seriously ill patients. *N. Engl. J. Med.* 293:471, 1975.

23. Foster, T. J. Plasmid-determined resistance to antimicrobial drugs and toxic metal ions in bacteria. *Microbiol. Rev.* 47:361, 1983.

24. Gaman, W., Cates, C., Snelling, C. F. T., Lank, B., and Ronald, A. R., Emergence of gentamicin- and carbenicillin-resistant *Pseudomonas aeruginosa* in a hospital environment. *Antimicrob. Agents Chemother.* 9:474, 1976.

25. Gardner, P., and Smith, D. H. Studies on the epidemiology of resistance (R) factors. I. Analysis of *Klebsiella* isolates in a general hospital. II. A prospective study of R-factor transfer in the host. *Ann. Intern Med.* 71:1, 1969.

26. Gaynes, R. P., Weinstein, R. A., Smith, J., Carman, M., and Kabins, S. A. Control of aminoglycoside resistance by barrier precautions. *Infect. Control* 4:221, 1983.

27. Gerding, D. N., Buxton, A. E., Hughes, R. A., Cleary, P. P., Arbaczawski, J., and Stamm, W. E. Nosocomial multiply resistant *Klebsiella pneumoniae:* Epidemiology of an outbreak of apparent index case origin. *Antimicrob. Agents Chemother.* 15:608, 1979.

28. Gill, S., and Iyer, V. N. Nalidixic acid inhibits the conjugal transfer of conjugative N incompatibility group plasmids. *Can J. Microbiol.* 28:256, 1982.

29. Gill, V. J., Manning, C., Lamson, M., Woltering, P., and Pizzo, P. A. Antibiotic-resistant

group JK bacteria in hospitals. *J. Clin. Microbiol.* 13:472, 1981.

30. Gilmore, D. S., Schick, D. G., and Montgomerie, J. Z. *Pseudomonas aeruginosa* and *Klebsiella pneumoniae* on the perinea of males with spinal cord injuries. *J. Clin. Microbiol.* 16:865, 1982.

31. Graham, D. R., Anderson, R. L., Ariel, F. E., Ehrenkranz, N. J., Rowe, B., Boer, H. R., and Dixon, R. E. Epidemic nosocomial meningitis due to *Citrobacter diversus* in neonates. *J. Infect. Dis.* 144:203, 1981.

32. Graham, D. R., Correa-Villasenor, A., Anderson, R. L., Vollman, J. H., and Baine, W. B. Epidemic neonatal gentamicin-methicillin-resistant *Staphylococcus aureus* infection associated with nonspecific topical use of gentamicin. *J. Pediatr.* 97:972, 1980.

33. Greene, W. H., Moody, M., Schimpff, S., Young, V. M., and Wiernik, P. H. *Pseudomonas aeruginosa* resistant to carbenicillin and gentamicin. *Ann. Intern. Med.* 79:684, 1973.

34. Grieble, H. G., Bird, T. J., Nidea, H. M., and Miller, C. A. Chute-hydropulping waste disposal system: A reservoir of enteric bacilli and *Pseudomonas* in a modern hospital. *J. Infect. Dis.* 130:602, 1974.

35. Gruneberg, R. N., Bendall, M. J. Hospital outbreak of trimethoprim resistance in pathogenic coliform bacteria. *Br. Med. J.* 2:7, 1979.

36. Haley, R. W., Hightower, A. W., Khabbaz, R. F., Thornsberry, C., Martone, W. J., Allen J. R., and Hughes, J. M. The emergence of methicillin-resistant *Staphylococcus aureus* infections in United States hospitals. *Ann. Intern. Med.* 97:297, 1982.

37. Hande, K. R., Witebsky, F. G., Brown, M. S., Schulman, C. B., Anderson, S. E., Levine, A. S., MacLowry, J. D. and Chabner, B. A. Sepsis with a new species of *Corynebacterium*. *Ann. Intern. Med.* 85:423, 1976.

38. Hart, C. A., and Gibson, M. F. Comparative epidemiology of gentamicin-resistant enterobacteria: Persistence of carriage and infection. *J. Clin. Pathol.* 35:452, 1982.

39. Hart, C. A., Gibson, M. F., and Buckles, A. M. Variation in skin and environmental survival of hospital gentamicin-resistant enterobacteria. *J. Hyg. (Camb.)* 87:277, 1981.

40. Houang, E. T., and Greenwood, D. Aminoglycoside cross-resistance patterns of gentamicin-resistant bacteria. *J. Clin. Pathol.* 30:738, 1977.

41. Hughes, J., Jarvis, W., Munn, V., Culver, D., Thornsberry, C., and Haley, R. Nosocomial aminoglycoside-resistant gram-negative bacillary in-

fections in the United States, 1975–1982. *Programs and Abstracts of the 23rd Interscience Conference on Antimicrobial Agents and Chemotherapy,* October 24–26, 1983, Las Vegas, Nev., p. 248, abstract 893.

42. Hughes, J., Jarvis, W., Munn, V., Culver, D., Thornsberry, C., and Haley, R. Resistance of nosocomial gram-negative bacilli to cefotaxime and moxalactam in the United States, 1982. *Programs and Abstracts of the 23rd Interscience Conference on Antimicrobial Agents and Chemotherapy,* October 24–26, 1983, Las Vegas, Nev., p. 162, abstract 427.

43. Huovinen, P., Mantyjarvi, R., and Toivanen, P. Trimethoprim resistance in hospitals. *Br. Med. J.* 284:782, 1982.

43a. Jaffe, H. W., Sweeney, H. M., Nathan C., Weinstein, R. A., Kabins, S. A., and Cohen, S. Identity and interspecific transfer of gentamicin-resistant plasmids in *Staphylococcus aureus* and *Staphylococcus epidermidis*. *J. Infect. Dis.* 141:738, 1980.

44. John, J. F., McKee, K. T., Twitty, J. A., and Schaffner, W. Molecular epidemiology of sequential nursery epidemics caused by multiresistant *Klebsiella pneumoniae*. *J. Pediatr.* 102:825, 1983.

45. Kauffman, C. A., Ramundo, N. C., Williams, S. G., Dey, R., Phair, J. P., and Watanakunakorn, C. Surveillance of gentamicin-resistant gram-negative bacilli in a general hospital. *Antimicrob. Agents Chemother.* 13:918, 1978.

46. Keys, T. F., and Washington, J. A. Gentamicin-resistant *Pseudomonas aeruginosa:* Mayo Clinic experience, 1970–1976, *Mayo. Clin. Proc.* 52:797, 1977.

47. Knittle, M. A., Eitzman, D. V., and Baer, H. Role of hand contamination of personnel in the epidemiology of gram-negative nosocomial infections. *J. Pediatr.* 86:433, 1975.

48. Koornhof, H. J., Jacobs, M. R., Ward, J. I, Appelbaum, P. C., and Hallet, F. A. Therapy and control of Antibiotic-Resistant Pneumococcal Disease. *Microbiology 1979*, p. 286. Washington D.C.: American Society for Microbiology, 1979.

49. Levin, M., Olson, B., Nathan, C. Kabins, S. A., and Weinstein, R. A. Pseudomonas in ICU sinks: Relation to patients. *J. Clin. Pathol.* 37:424, 1984.

50. Lowbury, E. J. L., Thom, B. T., Lilly, H. A., Rabb, J. R., and Whittall, K. Sources of infection with *Pseudomonas aeruginosa* in patients with tracheostomy. *J. Med. Microbiol.* 3:39, 1970.

51. Maizels, M., and Schaeffer, A. J. Decreased incidence of bacteriuria associated with periodic instillations of hydrogen peroxide into the urethral catheter drainage bag. *J. Urol.* 123:841, 1980.

52. Makela, P., Ojajarvi, J., and Salminen, E. Decontaminating waste-trap. *Lancet* 1:1216, 1972.

53. Maki, D. G., Hennekens, C. G., Phillips, C. W., Shaw, W. V., and Bennett, J. V. Nosocomial urinary tract infection with *Serratia marcescens:* An epidemiologic study. *J. Infect. Dis.* 128:579, 1973.

54. Maliwan, N., Grieble, H. G., and Bird, T. J. Hospital *Pseudomonas aeruginosa:* Surveillance of resistance to gentamicin and transfer of aminoglycoside R factor. *Antimicrob. Agents Chemother.* 8:415, 1975.

55. Markowitz, S. M., Veazey, J. M., Macrina, F. L., Mayhall, C. G., and Lamb, V. A. Sequential outbreaks of infection due to *Klebsiella pneumoniae* in a neonatal intensive care unit: Implication of a conjugative R plasmid. *J. Infect. Dis.* 142:106, 1980.

56. Marrie, T. J., Major, H., Gurwith, M., Ronald, A. R., Harding. G. K., Forrest, G., and Forsythe, W. Prolonged outbreak of nosocomial urinary tract infection with a single strain of *Pseudomonas aeruginosa. Can. Med. Assoc. J.* 119:593, 1978.

57. Mathias, R. G., Ronald, A. R., Gurwith, M. J., McCullough, D. W., Stiver, H. G., Berger, J., Cates, C. Y., Fox, L. M., and Lank, B. A. Clinical evaluation of amikacin in treatment of infections due to gram-negative aerobic bacilli. *J. Infect. Dis.* 134:S394, 1976.

58. Mawer, S. L., and Greenwood, D. Aminoglycoside resistance emerging during therapy. *Lancet* 1:749, 1977.

59. McGowan, J E. Antimicrobial resistance in hospital organisms and its relation to antibiotic use. *Rev. Infect. Dis.* 5:1033, 1983.

60. Meyer, R. D. Patterns and mechanisms of emergence of resistance to amikacin. *J. Infect. Dis.* 136:449, 1977.

61. Meyer, R. D., Lewis, R. P., Halter, J., and White, M. Gentamicin-resistant *Pseudomonas aeruginosa* and *Serratia marcescens* in a general hospital. *Lancet* 1:580, 1976.

62. Montgomerie, J. Z., and Morrow, J. W. *Pseudomonas* colonization in patients with spinal cord injury. *Am. J. Epidemiol.* 108:328, 1978.

63. Moody, M. M., deJongh, C. A., Schimpff, S. C., and Tilman, G. L. Long-term amikacin use: Effects on aminoglycoside susceptibility patterns of gram-negative bacilli. *J.A.M.A.* 248:1199, 1982.

64. Murray, B. E., and Mederski-Samaroj, B. Transferable beta-lactamase: A new mechanism for in vitro penicillin resistance in *Streptococcus faecalis. J. Clin. Invest.* 72:1168, 1983.

65. Murray, B. E., Rensimer, E. R., and DuPont, H. L. Emergence of high-level trimethoprim resistance in fecal *Escherichia coli* during oral administration of trimethoprim or trimethoprim-sulfamethoxazole. *N. Engl. J. Med.* 306:130, 1982.

66. Noone, M. R., Pitt, T. L., Bedder, M., Hewlett, A. M., and Rogers, K. B. *Pseudomonas aeruginosa* colonisation in an intensive therapy unit: Role of cross-infection and host factors. *Br. Med. J.* 286:341, 1983.

67. Noriega, E. R., Leibowitz, R. E., Richmond, A. S., Rubinstein, E., Schaefler, S., Simberkoff, M. S., and Rahal, J. J. Nosocomial infection caused by gentamicin-resistant, streptomycin-sensitive *Klebsiella. J. Infect. Dis.* 131:S45, 1975.

68. O'Brien, T. F., Acar, J. F., Medeiros, A. A., Norton, R. A., Goldstein, F., and Kent, R. L. International comparison of prevalence of resistance to antibiotics. *J.A.M.A.* 239:1518, 1978.

69. O'Callaghan, R. J., Rousset, K. M., Harkess, N. K., Murray, M. L., Lewis, A. C., and Williams, W. L. Analysis of increasing antibiotic resistance of *Klebsiella pneumoniae* relative to changes in chemotherapy. *J. Infect. Dis.* 138:293, 1978.

70. Olson, B., Weinstein, R. A., Nathan, C., and Kabins S. A. Broad-spectrum beta-lactum resistance in *Enterobacter:* Emergence during treatment and mechanisms of resistance. *J. Antimicrob. Chemother.* 11:299, 1983.

71. Parry, M. F., Hutchinson, J. H., Brown, N. A., Wu, C. H., and Estreller, L. Gram-negative sepsis in neonates: A nursery outbreak due to hand carriage of *Citrobacter diversus. Pediatrics* 65:1105, 1980.

72. Perryman, F. A., and Flournoy, D. J. Prevalence of gentamicin- and amikacin-resistant bacteria in sink drains. *J. Clin. Microbiol.* 12:79, 1980.

73. Price, D. J. E., and Sleigh, J. D. Control of infection due to *Klebsiella aerogenes* in a neurosurgical unit by withdrawal of all antibiotics. *Lancet* 2:1213, 1970.

74. Price, K. E., Kresel, P. A., Farchione, L. A., Siskin, S. B., and Karpow, S. A. Epidemiological studies of aminoglycoside resistance in the U.S.A. *J. Antimicrob. Chemother.* 8:89, 1981.

75. Rennie, R. P., and Duncan, I. B. R. Emergence of gentamicin-resistant *Klebsiella* in a general hospital. *Antimicrob. Agents Chemother.* 11:179, 1977.

76. Roberts, N. J., and Douglas, R. G. Gentamicin use and *Pseudomonas* and *Serratia* resistance: Effect of a surgical prophylaxis regimen. *Antimicrob. Agents Chemother.* 13:214, 1978.

77. Roe, E. Jones, R. J., and Lowbury, E. J. L. Transfer of antibiotic resistance between *Pseudomonas aeruginosa, Escherichia coli,* and other gram-negative bacilli in burns. *Lancet* 1:149, 1971.

78. Rubens, C. E., Farrar, W. E., McGee, Z. A., and Schaffner, W. Evolution of a plasmid-mediating resistance to multiple antimicrobial agents during a prolonged epidemic of nosocomial infections. *J. Infect. Dis.* 143:170, 1981.

79. Rubens, C. E., McNeill, W. F., and Farrar, W. E. Evolution of multiple-antibiotic-resistance plasmids mediated by transposable plasmid deoxyribonucleic acid sequences. *J. Bacteriol.* 140:713, 1979.

80. Sadowski, P. L., Peterson, B. C., Gerding, D. N., and Cleary, P. P. Physical characterization of ten R plasmids obtained from an outbreak of nosocomial *Klebsiella pneumoniae* infections. *Antimicrob. Agents Chemother.* 15:616, 1979.

81. Salzman, T. C., Clark, J. J, and Klemm, L. Hand contamination of personnel as a mechanism of cross-infection in nosocomial infections with antibiotic-resistant *Escherichia coli* and *Klebsiella aerobacter. Antimicrob. Agents Chemother.* 1967:97, 1968.

82. Sanders, C. C., Moellering, R. C., Martin, R. R., Perkins, R. L., Strike, D. G., Gootz, T. D., and Sanders, W. E. Resistance to cefamandole: A collaborative study of emerging clinical problems. *J. Infect. Dis.* 145:118, 1982.

83. Saravolatz, L. D., Markowitz, N., Arking, L., Pohlod, D., and Fisher, E. Methicillin-resistant *Staphylococcus aureus.* Epidemiologic observations during a community-acquired outbreak. *Ann Intern. Med.* 96:11, 1982.

84. Schaberg, D. R., Alford, R. H., Anderson, R., Farmer, J. J., Melly, M. A., and Schaffner, W. An outbreak of nosocomial infection due to multiply resistant *Serratia marcescens:* Evidence of interhospital spread. *J. Infect. Dis.* 134:181, 1976.

85. Schaberg, D. R., Weinstein, R. A., and Stamm, W. E. Epidemics of nosocomial urinary tract infection caused by multiply resistant gram-negative bacilli: Epidemiology and control. *J. Infect. Dis.* 133:363, 1976.

86. Seal, D. V., and Strangeways, J. E. M. Aminoglycoside resistance due to mutation. *Lancet* I:856, 1977.

87. Selden, R., Lee, S., Wang, W. L. L., Bennett, J. V., and Eickhoff, T. C. Nosocomial *Klebsiella* infections: Intestinal colonization as a reservoir. *Ann. Intern. Med.* 74:657, 1971.

88. Semel, J. D., Trenholme, G. M., and Levin, S. Gentamicin- and clindamycin-resistant *Staphylococcus aureus. Am. J. Med. Sciences* 280:4, 1980.

89. Shooter, R. A. Bowel colonization of hospital patients by *Pseudomonas aeruginosa* and *Escherichia coli. Proc. R. Soc. Med.* 64:27, 1971.

90. Shulman, J. A., Terry, P. M., and Hough, C. E. Colonization with gentamicin-resistant *Pseudomonas aeruginosa,* pyocine type 5, in a burn unit. *J. Infect. Dis.* 124:S18, 1971.

91. Sprunt, K., Leidy, G., Redman, W. Abnormal colonization of neonates in an ICU: Conversion to normal colonization by pharyngeal implantation of alpha-hemolytic *Streptococcus* strain 215. *Pediatr. Res.* 14:308, 1980.

92. Stamm, W. E., Tompkins. L. S., Wagner, K. F., Counts, G. W., Thomas, E. D., and Meyers, J. D. Infection due to *Corynebacterium* species in marrow transplant patients. *Ann. Intern. Med.* 91:167, 1979.

93. Stamm, W. E., Weinstein, R. A., and Dixon, R. E. Comparison of endemic and epidemic nosocomial infections. *Am. J. Med.* 70:393, 1981.

94. Tally, F. P., Cuchural, G. J., Jacobus, N. V., Gorbach, S. L., Aldridge, K. E., Cleary, T. J., Finegold, S. M., Hill, G. B., Iannini, P. B., McCloskey, R. V., O'Keefe, J. P., and Pierson, C. L. Susceptibility of the *Bacteroides fragilis* group in the United States in 1981. *Antimicrob. Agents Chemother.* 23:536, 1983.

95. Thompson, R. L., Cabezudo, I., and Wenzel, R. P. Epidemiology of nosocomial infections caused by methicillin-resistant *Staphylococcus aureus. Ann. Intern. Med.* 97:309, 1982.

96. Thompson, R. L., Haley, C. E., Groschel, D. M., Gillenwater, J. Y., Kaiser, D. L., and Wenzel, R. P. Effect of periodic instillation of hydrogen peroxide ($H_2O_2$) into urinary drainage systems in the prevention of catheter-associated bacteriuria (CAB). *Programs and Abstracts of the 22nd Interscience Conference on Antimicrobial Agents and Chemotherapy,* October 4–6, 1982. Miami Beach, Fla., p. 201, abstract 769.

97. Tompkins, L. S., Plorde, J. J., and Falkow, S. Molecular analysis of R-factors from multiresistant nosocomial isolates. *J. Infect. Dis.* 141:625, 1980.

98. Wade, J. C., Schimpff, S. C., Newman, K. A., and Wiernik, P. H. *Staphylococcus epidermidis:* An increasing cause of infection in patients with granulocytopenia. *Ann. Intern. Med.* 97:503, 1982.

99. Weinstein, R. A., and Kabins, S. A. Strategies

for prevention and control of multiple drug-resistant nosocomial infection. *Am. J. Med.* 70:449, 1981.

100. Weinstein, R. A., Kabins, S. A., Nathan, C., Sweeney, H. M., Jaffe, H. W., and Cohen, S. Gentamicin-resistant staphylococci as hospital flora: Epidemiology and resistance plasmids. *J. Infect. Dis.* 145:374, 1982.

101. Weinstein, R. A., Nathan, C., Gruensfelder, R., and Kabins, S. A. Endemic aminoglycoside resistance in gram-negative bacilli: Epidemiology and mechanisms. *J. Infect. Dis.* 141:338, 1980.

102. Wenzel, R. P., Veazey, J. M., and Townsend, T. R. Role of the Inanimate Environment in Hospital-Acquired Infections. In Cundy, K. R., and Ball, W. (Eds.), *Infection Control in Health Care Facilities: Microbiological Surveillance*. Baltimore, University Park Press, 1977, p. 71.

103. Wormser, G. P., Tatz, J., and Donath, J. Endemic resistance to amikacin among hospital isolates of gram-negative bacilli: Implications for therapy. *Infect. Control* 4:93, 1983.

104. Yu, V. L., Oakes, C. A., Axnick, K. J., and Merigan, T. C. Patient factors contributing to the emergence of gentamicin-resistant *Serratia marcescens*. *Am. J. Med.* 66:468, 1979.

# 11 ANTIBIOTICS AND NOSOCOMIAL INFECTIONS

Theodore C. Eickhoff

The era of chemotherapy for infectious disease is now over 40 years old—40 years marked by the continuous development and introduction of new and potent antimicrobial agents. The contemporary clinician has at his or her disposal a broad array of potent antibiotic agents of proven efficacy and sometimes significant toxicity.

During these 40 years significant changes have occurred in the character of nosocomial infections. The available data strongly suggest that 40 years ago nosocomial infection was generally synonymous with gram-positive coccal infection, most notably with β-hemolytic streptococci and staphylococci. During the 1950s staphylococci—particularly those resistant to the antimicrobial drugs in common use, such as penicillin G, tetracycline, erythromycin, chloramphenicol, and streptomycin—emerged to cause epidemic infection in hospitals. For reasons that are not understood, staphylococci subsided in importance as the major cause of nosocomial infection in the early 1960s, only to be replaced in importance by enteric gram-negative bacilli, enterococci, and fungi [24].

It is tempting to relate the changing character of nosocomial infections, as briefly sketched, to the sequential introduction of new antimicrobial agents and to impute a cause-and-effect relation. No one can seriously doubt that antimicrobial drugs have had a profound effect in shaping the character of nosocomial infections, but such an explanation is greatly oversimplified and fails to take into account the enormous changes in the technology of medicine and patterns of health-care delivery that have also taken place in the past 40 years. In this chapter we explore more fully the way in which antimicrobial drugs are used in hospitals and consider the effects of such drug use on both the host and the microorganism.

## ANTIBIOTIC USE IN HOSPITALS

Data on the overall patterns of antibiotic use within hospitals have appeared in the literature for only two decades. The general thrust of such data indicates that from 25 to 35 percent of hospitalized patients receive systemic antibiotics at any given time [12,54]. Furthermore, sequentially obtained data suggest that there is a trend toward increasing, rather than decreasing, antibiotic use within hospitals.

A series of four prevalence surveys carried out at the Boston City Hospital during January or February of the years 1964, 1967, 1970, and 1973 provides interesting comparative data [63]. In 1964 26 percent of patients in that hospital were receiving at least one systemic antibacterial agent; in 1967 the figure was 27 percent; in 1970 it was 34 percent; and in 1973, 36 percent. In the 1973 survey, 76 percent of patients receiving antibiotics were considered to have an active infection at the time.

Scheckler and Bennett [100] reported on antibiotic use in seven community hospitals scattered throughout the United States; they employed a survey technique comparable to that used in the Boston City Hospital surveys. Twenty-four such prevalence studies carried out between November 1967 and June 1969 indicated that over 30 percent of patients were receiving one or more systemic antibiotics but that only 38 percent of patients receiving antibiotics surveyed in 1969 had recorded evidence of infection. Comparable results were reported by Roberts and Visconti [86] in a single hospital.

Kunin and coworkers [55] reported a study of antibiotic use carried out in 1969 at the University of Virginia Hospital. During a three-month period, all antibiotic therapy given to patients on the medical and surgical services was reviewed by the infectious disease resident and staff, and the use of antibiotics in any given patient was judged by the group to be appropriate or inappropriate. During the survey period, 27 percent of patients admitted to the medical service and 29 percent of patients admitted to the surgical service were given antibiotics. Among patients on the surgical service, 58 percent of the antibiotic therapy given was for prophylaxis, whereas on the medical service, only 6 percent of antibiotic therapy was for prophylaxis.

Inappropriate therapy included instances in which a different drug was thought to be preferable, the dose was considered inappropriate, or the administration of any antimicrobial therapy or prophylaxis was considered unjustified. In the reviewers' judgment, 52 percent of all antimicrobial therapy was inappropriate. On the medical service, 42 percent of all antimicrobial drug use was judged inappropriate, while 62 percent of all antibiotic therapy was considered inappropriate on the surgical service.

A survey carried out in 1979, part of a series of prevalence surveys of infections and antibiotic use at the Latter Day Saints Hospital in Salt Lake City, revealed that the use of systemic antimicrobial agents had increased to 37 percent of all hospitalized surveyed patients, compared to 23 percent of patients found in a comparable survey carried out in 1971 [112]. These investigators found that the increase in antibiotic use could be attributed mainly to increased use of cephalosporin antibiotics for surgical prophy-

laxis. Their definition of "appropriate" use was somewhat less stringent than that of Kunin [55], and overall, 31 percent of antibiotic use was judged to be inappropriate.

Such massive use of antibacterial drugs in hospitals, whether appropriate or inappropriate, has profound effects on both the hosts who receive these drugs, and the bacteria exposed to them. In addition to the ecologic consequences of this massive use of antibiotics, to be discussed in subsequent sections, Kunin [54] has clearly identified the economic consequences, and pointed out the enormous pressures brought to bear by the pharmaceutical industry in the direction of increased antibiotic use. In 1980 $1.55 billion worth of antiinfective drugs were shipped, accounting for approximately 18 percent of all ethical drug products. Markup and administration costs probably doubled that figure to $3 billion. In 1984 the figure is estimated to have reached $5 billion.

## ANTIBIOTICS AND DRUG RESISTANCE OF BACTERIA IN HOSPITALS

Current problems of resistance of bacteria to antimicrobial drugs become more understandable if we recall that in Paul Ehrlich's laboratory, trypanosomes became resistant to the drug $p$-rosaniline after repeated exposures [69]. Similarly, it was shown that pneumococci could develop "resistance" to hydrocupreine derivatives following repeated exposure [25]. In the mid-1940s, shortly after the introduction of penicillin G, it was recognized that certain strains of staphylococci elaborated a potent inactivator of penicillin and that penicillin G had no therapeutic activity in patients with infections caused by such staphylococci. This recognition surely came as a major disappointment but not as a total surprise. In the 40 years that have elapsed since that time, it has become abundantly clear that the major nosocomial pathogens are by and large those organisms that either are naturally resistant to clinically useful antimicrobial drugs or possess the ability to acquire resistance. The best known examples are the staphylococci and aerobic gram-negative bacilli, which together regularly account for the majority of nosocomial infections. No major class of bacterial pathogens has thus far failed to demonstrate an ability to develop resistance to one or more commonly used antimicrobial agents [23].

Selective pressures favoring drug-resistant bacteria conferred by antibiotic therapy may indeed be principally focused in the institutional setting, but they extend widely into the community as well. The increasing prevalence of ampicillin-resistant *Hemophilus influenzae,* the increasing frequency of β-lactamase-producing gonococci, and the emergence of penicillin-insensitive pneumococci are recent examples. In the words of Finland, "little by little, we are experiencing the erosion of the strongest bulwarks against serious bacterial infection" [23].

### Drug Resistance of Staphylococci

ORIGIN The origin of staphylococcal resistance to penicillin G is likely to remain shrouded in mystery. It is clear, however, that penicillinase-producing staphylococci existed before the introduction of penicillin into clinical use. Eight of thirteen strains of *Staphylococcus aureus* isolated from food-poisoning outbreaks before 1940, for example, were found to be resistant to penicillin G through the usual mechanism of penicillinase production [77]. Smith and Marples [107] reported the fascinating observation that penicillin was produced by a dermatophyte responsible for ringworm lesions in New Zealand hedgehogs and that penicillinase-producing strains of *S. aureus* could be recovered from those lesions. Indeed, since penicillin is produced in nature by *Penicillium* species, it should not be a great surprise that certain microorganisms have evolved means of inactivating this compound; our recognition of this phenomenon in clinical medicine represents a relatively late event on the scale of biologic time.

TRENDS Resistance to penicillin G by *S. aureus* appeared rapidly after the introduction of that drug, and by 1949 40 percent of pathogenic strains of *S. aureus* isolated at the Boston City Hospital were resistant to penicillin G [25]. By the early 1950s, 75 percent of pathogenic strains of *S. aureus* from that hospital were resistant to penicillin G. Increasing proportions of staphylococci that are resistant to streptomycin, tetracyclines, and erythromycin were noted in succession within the first few years after each drug was introduced. By 1958 the 80/81 phage type had become predominant in many U. S. hospitals, and at the Boston City Hospital all these strains were resistant to penicillin; in addition, more than 80 percent were resistant to streptomycin, approximately 50 percent to tetracycline, and 10 percent to erythromycin. Of all pathogenic strains of staphylococci isolated from patients who had been in the hospital more than seven days and who had received any antibiotics, nearly all were resistant to penicillin, almost 90 percent were resistant to streptomycin, 80 percent were resistant to tetracycline, and almost 50 percent to erythromycin. In contrast, among strains obtained from outpatients or from patients at the time of their admission to the hospital, about 75 percent were resistant to penicillin, one-third were resistant to streptomycin, 20 percent were resistant to tetracycline, and less than 10 percent were resistant to erythromycin.

By the late 1960s, although the proportion of multiply drug-resistant strains of staphylococci decreased somewhat, there was little overall change in the frequency of penicillin resistance among strains isolated from inpatients. There was, however, an increase in the frequency of penicillin resistance among strains isolated from outpatients; outpatient strains were almost as likely to be resistant to penicillin G as those isolated from inpatients [25].

MECHANISMS OF RESISTANCE In most clinical settings, significant resistance to penicillin G in *S. aureus* is due to the presence of an extrachromosomal element of DNA—a plasmid—that confers on the bacterial cell the ability to produce a β-lactamase enzyme that hydrolyzes and thus inactivates penicillin G (see Chapter 12) [92,93]. The evidence that staphylococcal β-lactamase is the major mechanism of resistance to penicillin G is derived primarily from two readily demonstrable facts: first, small inocula of penicillinase-producing staphylococci are almost as susceptible to penicillin G as are penicillinase-negative strains; and second, penicillinase-negative segregants of penicillinase-producing staphylococci are just as susceptible as strains that apparently never possessed the ability to produce penicillinase.

Plasmid-linked resistance has similarly been demonstrated for tetracycline, chloramphenicol, erythromycin, and the aminoglycosides, as well as certain metallic ions (see Chapter 12). Of major clinical and epidemiologic significance is the fact that such plasmid-linked resistance may be transferable to fully sensitive staphylococci by the mechanism of transduction. Given the selection pressure of antimicrobial therapy present in a hospital setting and the ability of resistant staphylococci, under certain circumstances, to transfer plasmid-linked resistances to sensitive staphylococci via the mechanism of transduction, the scene was set for the emergence in hospitals of staphylococci that are resistant to penicillin G as well as to a variety of other drugs. That this indeed occurred is supported by the observation of Wallmark and Finland [120], of a direct relation between the proportion of drug-resistant strains recovered and the type of previous antibiotic therapy of the patients from whom those strains were recovered. Thus the increased prevalence of resistant strains of *S. aureus* was, at least in part, a direct result of the reduction or elimination of susceptible strains by antibiotic therapy, which permitted resistant strains not only to survive but to multiply and spread.

The mechanism of staphylococcal resistance to drugs other than the penicillins and cephalosporins is less well studied, but in many instances the mechanism of resistance is known [56,72,92]. Tetracycline resistance appears to be a result of altered membrane permeability characteristics within the staphylococcal cell membrane. Chloramphenicol resistance is mediated by the production of the enzyme, chloramphenicol acetyltransferase. Resistance to erythromycin is mediated by modification of the attachment site at the level of the staphylococcal ribosome, which apparently prevents attachment of the drug. Resistance to aminoglycosides is mediated by one or more enzymes catalyzing either phosphorylation, acetylation, or adenylation of the drug.

METHICILLIN RESISTANCE   Naturally occurring methicillin-resistant staphylococci were first reported in Great Britain in 1961 [45] within a very short time after the introduction of the drug. Since that time, there have been numerous reports of the isolation of such organisms, particularly from European sources but from within the United States as well [56,79]. Within a decade of the recognition of methicillin resistance in staphylococci, its epidemiologic and clinical importance was well established in Europe. In 1969 5 percent of all staphylococcal isolates from eight hospitals in London were methicillin-resistant [76]. During the period 1967–70, approximately 40 percent of nosocomial bacteremic strains isolated in Denmark were resistant to methicillin [44].

Kayser and Mak [51] in Zurich, Switzerland, reported that in some hospitals up to 50 percent of staphylococcal disease was caused by methicillin-resistant organisms and that infection caused by methicillin-resistant staphylococci was almost universally nosocomially acquired. Curiously, however, Kayser subsequently reported a spontaneous decline in the frequency of methicillin-resistant staphylococci in the Zurich area, from a high of 28 percent in 1969 to an astonishing 3 percent in 1975 [50]. This spontaneous decline in the prevalence of methicillin-resistant staphylococci did not seem to result from a change in the usage patterns of penicillinase-resistant β-lactam antibiotics, and a conclusive explanation of this regression could not be identified.

The experience in the United States stands in some contrast to that in Europe. Although isolated outbreaks have occurred such as that described by Barrett and colleagues [3] at the Boston City Hospital, methicillin resistance was but a minor problem in the United States during the 1960s and early 1970s. In 1970 it was found in 1 percent or fewer strains in this country [37]. Since 1975, however, there has been a progressive and alarming increase in the frequency of methicillin-resistant staphylococci in U.S. hospitals. Numerous outbreaks have been reported in the United States, particularly within the past five years, occurring most frequently in large tertiary care referral hospitals with medical school affiliation [9,15,18,20,53,59,66,78,103,109,114,115,119].

For example, Haley and his colleagues [37] found that among 63 hospitals participating in the National Nosocomial Infection Survey, the four medical school–affiliated hospitals with over 600 beds reported a frequency of methicillin-resistant staphylococci that increased from 2 percent in 1975 to 18 percent in 1981. The frequency of methicillin-resistant staphylococci in 59 other hospitals participating in the survey remained relatively constant at about 4 percent. Haley and colleagues also suggested that the increase of methicillin-resistant staphylococci in large teaching hospitals was due not only to the large number of patients at high risk of infection and the existence of special care units such as burn units and oncology units, but also to the interhospital spread of the organism by frequent transfer of house staff and by infected patients. Perhaps of greatest concern is the potential for spread of methicillin-resistant staphylococci into the community. As reported by Saravolatz and colleagues [95,96], the proportion of community-acquired methicillin-resistant staphylococcal infections in the Detroit area rose from 3 percent to 38 percent in a single 18-month period in 1980–81. Thus it appears that the United States is encountering an increase in methicillin-resistant staphylococci similar to the one experienced by Great Britain and Europe, albeit some 15 years later.

The mechanism of staphylococcal resistance to methicillin is of some interest because of the abundant evidence that methicillin resistance is not mediated by the production of a β-lactamase enzyme [56,92,93]. The evidence that methicillin resistance in S. aureus is not β-lactamase-mediated is as follows: (1) methicillin-resistant strains produce no more β-lactamase than do most methicillin-susceptible strains; (2) the β-lactamase from methicillin-resistant strains is not different functionally or immunologically from that produced by methicillin-susceptible strains; (3) β-lactamase-negative segregants of methicillin-resistant strains are still methicillin-resistant; and (4) methicillin is not inactivated during incubation with methicillin-resistant strains.

A number of unique properties are common to virtually all methicillin-resistant strains of S. aureus. These include heterogeneous resistance to methicillin and all other penicillins and cephalosporins (whether the strain produces penicillinase or not), high-level resistance to streptomycin, and resistance to tetracyclines and sulfonamides [56,92,93].

The precise nature of methicillin resistance is as yet uncertain, but the evidence suggests that the surface of the bacterial cell and possibly the cell wall structure are slightly different in resistant versus susceptible cells [56,92,93]. Evidence in support of such a difference includes the following: (1) methicillin-resistant cells grow more slowly than do methicillin-susceptible cells; (2) their cell size is larger; (3) they are usually resistant to many other antibiotics; (4) methicillin resistance is more easily detected at lower temperatures or at higher salt concentrations than under usual laboratory conditions; and (5) methicillin-resistant staphylococci are more resistant to lysis by lysostaphin than are methicillin-susceptible organisms.

The fact that methicillin resistance is best expressed at temperatures less than 37°C (99°F) has led Parker and Hewitt [76] to suggest that selection of methicillin-resistant staphylococci may occur in the relatively cooler environment of the skin or anterior nares. The first detection of such strains preceded the introduction of methicillin, and the prevalence of methicillin resistance does not correlate well with the relative clinical use of methicillin or other penicillinase-resistant penicillins. Thus these investigators have suggested that other penicillins, such as penicillin V or ampicillin, might exert selective pressure in favor of methicillin-resistant strains.

PENICILLIN "TOLERANCE" In 1977 Sabath and coworkers [94] described another type of penicillin resistance of *S. aureus,* known as penicillin "tolerance." Such tolerant strains are inhibited by customary concentrations of penicillins, including antistaphylococcal penicillins, but are not killed except by very high concentrations of such drugs. Thus the hallmark of tolerance is a wide discrepancy between the minimal inhibitory and minimal bactericidal concentrations, usually defined as a 32-fold difference or greater. The mechanism of tolerance appears to be decreased autolytic enzyme activity. In Sabath's original report, 44 percent of bacteremic strains studied demonstrated such tolerance. Many strains also showed cross-tolerance with cephalosporins and vancomycin.

The seven years that have elapsed since the first description of penicillin tolerance have not fully clarified either the frequency of the phenomenon of tolerance or the clinical significance, if any, of penicillin tolerance. Results of studies of the frequency of tolerant strains seem to be highly method-dependent

[34,49,82]. Using a method that permitted study of every *S. aureus* organism in each blood culture, rather than merely one or two colonies, Bradley and associates [10,11] reported that every positive blood culture could be shown to contain some tolerant organisms. They suggested that all strains of *S. aureus* could be shown to contain tolerant organisms if large enough numbers of the population were studied. It is not known whether patients infected with strains containing relatively more tolerant subpopulations respond differently to antibiotic therapy than those infected with relatively fewer tolerant subpopulations.

Clinical data are contradictory, with some investigators reporting a higher mortality or longer duration of bacteremia in patients infected with tolerant strains versus those infected with nontolerant strains; other investigators detected no difference in mortality [34,49,82].

In summary three basic forms of staphylococcal resistance to β-lactam drugs have been described [93]:

1. *Enzyme (β-lactamase) mediated* resistance is exceedingly common, results in very high minimum inhibitory concentrations (MICs) and minimum bactericidal concentrations (MBCs), is highly stable, and is of major clinical importance. It is seen in virtually all phage-types of staphylococci.
2. *Intrinsic resistance,* not due to drug inactivation, is chromosomally mediated, is clinically important in methicillin-resistant staphylococci, and usually affects only a very small percentage of cells in a culture. Methicillin-resistant staphylococci are similarly resistant to all other antistaphylococcal β-lactam drugs. This resistance is quite stable and of major clinical importance.
3. *Penicillin tolerance* is characterized by a normal MIC, but an MBC that is at least 32 times and sometimes over 100 times higher than the MIC. This may be a property common to all staphylococci if one tests enough cells of a culture. The mechanism is not drug inactivation but rather deficiency in autolytic enzyme activity necessary for bacteriolysis. The clinical significance of tolerance is uncertain.

### Drug Resistance of Gram-Negative Bacilli

TRENDS The historical development of drug resistance among gram-negative bacilli is perhaps less distinctly characterized than that of staphylococci, but the problems are no less real. The most comprehensive early studies were carried out at the Boston City Hospital, as reviewed by Finland [25]. It is apparent that there has been a progressive decrease in susceptibility to commonly used antimicrobial drugs among strains of *Escherichia coli,* the *Klebsiella-Entero-bacter* group, *Serratia,* and *Proteus,* as well as *Pseudomonas.* In 1935 these organisms accounted for 12 percent of cases and 8 percent of deaths among all bacteremic infections at the Boston City Hospital, but by 1965 they accounted for fully half of all bacteremic infections and 57 percent of deaths from bacteremic infection [24].

The most striking illustration of the development of resistance in enterobacteria occurred in a setting of community-acquired rather than nosocomial infection. This was the extraordinarily rapid development of multiple drug resistance in strains of *Shigella* in Japan. The first multiply drug-resistant strain, isolated in 1955, was resistant to the sulfonamides, streptomycin, tetracycline, and chloramphenicol. In subsequent years the frequency of isolation of *Shigella* strains with identical or additional drug resistances increased; by 1967 almost 50 percent of strains were multiply drug resistant [68].

ORIGIN AND MECHANISM    The identification of multiple drug resistance among strains of *Shigella* in Japan, as outlined, prompted subsequent investigations both in Japan and elsewhere to define the genetic mechanisms involved. Just as many common drug resistances among staphylococci are plasmid-linked, so too the majority of acquired drug resistances among aerobic gram-negative bacilli result from resistance (R) factors present on plasmids, that is, microbial extrachromosomal DNA [17,18]. In the case of aminoglycosides, the major form of acquired resistance is due to R-plasmid-mediated production of enzymes, which inactivate aminoglycosides by acetylation, phosphorylation, or adenylation (see Chapter 12). At least 12 distinct classes of aminoglycoside-modifying enzymes have been described, which vary according to the site of attack on the aminoglycoside and the kind of enzymatic inactivation carried out [17,18,72]. It is worth pointing out that β-lactamase inactivation of all β-lactam drugs is due, finally, to enzymatic hydrolysis of the β-lactam ring; in contrast, aminoglycosides are subject to several different kinds of enzymatic modification and possess numerous sites of attack.

R plasmids, which encode for enzymes that inactivate aminoglycosides, have been found in a wide variety of bacterial genera [1,7,16,17,22,29,38, 41,43,58,71,75,97,124]. Some resistance determinants are self-transmissible, that is, conjugative; other R determinants are on small plasmids that lack the genetic elements necessary for transfer and are referred to as nonconjugative plasmids. In recent years it has become apparent that some R determinants are transposable; these "transposons" are discrete DNA sequences that are capable of movement from one plasmid to another or from chromosome to plasmid or the reverse. If a transposon that mediated, for example, gentamicin resistance, were to become transposed from a nonconjugative to a conjugative plasmid, it would facilitate transfer of that R factor by conjugation from cell to cell within individual genera, among other genera within the Enterobacteriaceae, and sometimes to related gram-negative bacilli outside the Enterbacteriaceae.

In addition to coding for production of aminoglycoside-inactivating enzymes, R factors may also encode for the production of one or more β-lactamase enzymes, and in addition, enzymes that catalyze the inactivation of chloramphenicol, trimethoprim, and several other less frequently used antibiotics [17,72]. In many usually drug-resistant species, such as *Pseudomonas,* the production of drug-inactivating enzymes is chromosomally mediated rather than contained on plasmids.

β-lactamases produced by gram-negative bacilli have been of intense interest in recent years, as β-lactamase-mediated inactivation of penicillins and cephalosporins has been found in enteric gram-negative bacilli, *Pseudomonas, Bacteroides, Neisseria,* and *Hemophilus.* In addition the usefulness of second- and third-generation cephalosporins is related to their ability to resist hydrolysis by these β-lactamases [72]. Six major categories of penicillinases or cephalosporinases are produced by gram-negative bacilli, classified on the basis of their substrate affinity, whether chromosomally or plasmid-mediated, and whether inducible or constitutive.

R factors are often linked, and therefore multiple resistance determinants may be transferred simultaneously. Thus the administration of a single antibiotic may select multiply drug-resistant organisms because of the linkage of multiple-resistance determinants on a single R factor. Thus within a nosocomial setting, a prevalent R factor may be sustained by the use of any drug encompassed in its resistance package. Switching usage patterns from one drug to another, when prevalent R factors mediate resistance to both, may not be attended by a reduction in the frequency of multiply drug-resistant strains. Conversely, any drug in the resistance "package" can exert selective pressure not only for organisms resistant to itself, but also for organisms resistant to any drugs that are linked on the same resistance package.

Investigation of a large outbreak of *Serratia marcescens* at Vanderbilt University was particularly instructive in providing some understanding of the spread of R-factor-mediated resistance in the hospital setting [91,99]. An initial outbreak of gentamicin-resistant *S. marcescens* occurred; this was quickly followed by a major outbreak of infections due to gentamicin-resistant *Klebsiella pneumoniae*, with an identical drug susceptibility pattern. Some years after the outbreak, it became clear that the gentamicin resistance determinant in the initial *Serratia* outbreak was present on a nonconjugative plasmid. The gentamicin resistance determinant subsequently became transposed to a co-resident conjugative plasmid, followed thereafter by intergeneric spread to *K. pneumoniae*, resulting in the second major outbreak.

R-factor transfer probably occurs most commonly in the gastrointestinal tract or on the skin [43,59,65,118]. Resistance transfer among skin bacteria can develop very rapidly, particularly under the selective pressure of topical antimicrobial therapy. In the gastrointestinal tract, resistance transfer may also be facilitated by systemic antibiotics or by residual unabsorbed oral drugs [118]. It may also occur, however, in the absence of any antimicrobial selective pressure. Although R-factor transfer may occur in other body fluids such as urine [98], the urinary tract seems to be of lesser importance as a reservoir for resistant bacteria than is the gastrointestinal tract and skin.

Many investigators have attempted to define the epidemiologic significance of the relative roles played by R-factor transfer in humans, as contrasted to the environmental selection pressure created by antibiotic therapy, with resulting colonization of patients by resistant organisms. Gardner and Smith [29], in studying a nosocomial outbreak due to multiply drug-resistant *Klebsiella*, concluded that colonization of patients with resistant organisms under the selective pressure of antibiotic therapy was of greater epidemiologic significance than R-factor transfer in the gastrointestinal tract. There have been numerous demonstrations of the fact that R-factor transfer can and does occur, and it is clear that both mechanisms operate in the hospital setting, probably closely interrelated [1,17,80,106]. It does appear likely that the development and maintenance of a drug-resistant population of enteric bacteria in the hospital setting is due largely to the selective pressure of antibiotic therapy, whereas linked multiple drug resistance and spread of R determinants to other genera is clearly due to resistance transfer.

ORIGIN OF R FACTORS   As is true of penicillin resistance in staphylococci, available evidence suggests that R factors were present, although far less prevalent, in the preantibiotic era [19,30]. Thus stool cultures from aboriginal populations unexposed to antibiotics were found to contain, in small numbers, strains of *E. coli* with R-factor-mediated resistance to antibiotics. This suggests that a small reservoir of R factors was present to take advantage of the advent of antibiotics, and that R factors were not formed more recently, de novo, after antibiotics came into common use. Recognizing, however, that the R factors present in a linked package may confer resistance not only to a single antibiotic, but also to related and even unrelated antibiotics, it is clear that bacteria containing such R factors possess a survival advantage in any hospital environment in which antibiotics are widely used.

Another major mechanism of aminoglycoside resistance, found among gram-negative bacilli, is restriction of transport of the drug into the bacterial cell [17,18]. It is particularly important in *Pseudomonas aeruginosa*. There is evidence that this type of resistance is increasing, particularly with the currently clinically useful aminoglycosides—gentamicin, tobramycin, amikacin, and netilmicin. This type of "permeability" resistance is relatively easily identified since it results in generalized cross-resistance to each of the aminoglycosides; the levels of resistance tend to be low, and the resistant cells tend to be metabolically impaired and to grow somewhat more slowly than nonresistant organisms. The aminoglycoside resistance spectrum itself, however, as determined by disc-susceptibility testing, is not a reliable means of distinguishing permeability resistance from R-factor-mediated resistance.

*Virulence of Antibiotic-Resistant Bacteria*
The occurrence of nosocomial infection due to multiply drug-resistant organisms is governed by a number of factors including not only antibiotic selection pressure, the nature of the resistance determinant, whether conjugative or nonconjugative plasmid, or transposon, but also possible linkage with other antibiotic resistances and genetic determinants governing adhesion and pathogenicity [17]. Evidence is conflicting regarding altered virulence—whether enhanced or diminished—of drug-resistant bacteria, in contrast to that of drug-susceptible organisms. There may prove to be no single answer to such a question, the answer rather being dependent on the particular bacterial species involved, the specific genetic determinants present, and what these genetic determinants contribute to the metabolic activities of the cell and the specific antigens located on the bacterial cell surface.

Although it is generally true that serious infection, such as bacteremic infection, caused by drug-resistant bacteria results in higher mortality rates than would be true of comparably serious infections caused by drug-susceptible bacteria, it is not at all clear whether the increased mortality is a reflection of increased virulence, diminished effectiveness of antibiotic therapy, or both. Jessen and colleagues [44], for example, who studied the occurrence of methicillin-resistant staphylococci and staphylococcal bacteremia in Denmark, showed that the combined effects of lysogenicity, transduction, and selection not only influenced the phage-type and antibiotic resistance of staphylococci, but also involved properties more directly connected with pathogenicity, such as lipase production, which is thought to facilitate the development of abscesses and to affect adversely the prognosis in bacteremia. The authors could not determine, however, whether the poorer prognosis was due to the shortcomings of antibiotic therapy or to correlated bacterial properties that enhanced virulence.

Taken in totality, the available evidence does not permit a conclusion that drug-resistant bacteria of any given species are more or less virulent than their drug-susceptible relatives.

*Parallels in Antibiotic Use and Antibiotic Resistance*
Evidence from a number of studies suggests that the proportion of bacteria resistant to a given antibiotic may increase as use of the drug increases, or conversely, may decrease if there is decreased use or cessation of use of the drug. Examples of such studies are shown in Tables 11-1 and 11-2.

Lepper and coworkers [57] found that after five months of intensive use of erythromycin for the treatment of all susceptible infections, three-quarters of strains were highly resistant to that drug. When all erythromycin therapy was discontinued and penicillin and tetracycline therapy resumed, the proportion of

erythromycin-resistant strains decreased, whereas the proportion of penicillin-resistant strains, which had declined while erythromycin was exclusively used, rose again rapidly. Similar results were found for tetracycline, to which resistance had increased sharply while it was used for susceptible infections and subsequently declined as its use decreased. Gibson and Thompson [32] described a similar phenomenon with staphylococci from burn wounds that had become highly resistant to tetracycline while that drug was used. When chloramphenicol was substituted for tetracycline, the proportion of chloramphenicol-resistant staphylococci rose sharply during the succeeding six months, while the proportion of tetracycline-resistant staphylococci fell. When chloramphenicol therapy was discontinued, the proportion of chloramphenicol-resistant strains dropped sharply. Bauer and colleagues [6] reported an entirely comparable experience and demonstrated a correlation between the extent of resistance and use of antibiotics. In an extensive study of staphylococci and staphylococcal infection in Great Britain, Barber and her colleagues [2] documented not only a decline in the incidence of staphylococcal infection per patient when a number of anti-cross-infection measures and a controlled antibiotic policy were put into effect, but also a sharp reversal of penicillin and tetracycline resistance of isolates toward increased susceptibility.

Prevailing drug resistance of gram-negative bacilli is also susceptible to alteration by restriction or cessation of use of a given drug. When kanamycin was replaced by gentamicin in an effort to control an outbreak of nosocomial infections caused by kanamycin-resistant enteric organisms, kanamycin-resistant organisms were virtually eliminated from the nursery within a month, which suggested that the selective pressure provided by the extensive use of

TABLE 11-1. Studies demonstrating a temporal relationship between increased use of antimicrobial agents and increased prevalence of resistant hospital organisms

| Year | Reference | Setting for use of antimicrobials | Organisms | Antimicrobials |
|------|-----------|-----------------------------------|-----------|----------------|
| 1953 | 57 | General | *Staphylococcus aureus* | Erythromycin |
|      |    |         | *S. aureus* | Penicillin |
|      |    |         | *S. aureus* | Chlortetracycline |
| 1956 | 32 | Burn ward | *S. aureus* | Chloramphenicol |
|      |    |           | *S. aureus* | Chlortetracycline |
| 1967 | 90 | Surgical prophylaxis | *S. aureus* | Neomycin cream |
| 1971 | 105 | Burn ward | *Pseudomonas aeruginosa* | Gentamicin |
| 1978 | 87 | Surgical prophylaxis | *P. aeruginosa* | Gentamicin |
|      |    |                      | *Serratia* | Gentamicin |
| 1979 | 129 | Postoperative | *Serratia* | Gentamicin |

Adapted from McGowan, J. E., Jr. *Rev. Infect. Dis.* 5:1033, 1983.

TABLE 11-2. Studies demonstrating a temporal relationship between
decreased use of antimicrobial agents and decreased prevalence of organisms

| Year | Reference | Setting for use of antimicrobials | Organisms | Antimicrobials |
|------|-----------|-----------------------------------|-----------|----------------|
| 1953 | 52 | General | *Staphylococcus* | Chloramphenicol |
| 1954 | 57 | General | *S. aureus* | Erythromycin |
| 1956 | 32 | Burn ward | *S. aureus* | Chlortetracycline |
|      |    |           | *S. aureus* | Chloramphenicol |
| 1960 | 2 | General | *S. aureus* | Penicillin |
| 1960 | 6 |         | *S. aureus* | Tetracycline |
| 1966 | 26 | Pediatric ward | *S. aureus* | Erythromycin |
| 1967 | 90 | Surgical prophylaxis | *S. aureus* | Neomycin cream |
| 1970 | 13 | General | *Escherichia coli* | Streptomycin |
|      |    |         | *Klebsiella, Enterobacter* | Streptomycin |
| 1970 | 81 | Neurosurgical unit | *Klebsiella* | "All" |
| 1970 | 84 | General | *S. aureus* | Erythromycin |
|      |    |         | *S. aureus* | Novobiocin |
| 1971 | 105 | Burn wound | *Pseudomonas aeruginosa* | Gentamicin |
| 1972 | 61 | Burn ward | "Enterobacteriaceae" | Carbenicillin |
|      |    |           | *P. aeruginosa* | Carbenicillin |
| 1973 | 27 | Nursery | "Enterobacteria" | Kanamycin |
| 1974 | 108 | Urology ward | "Gram-negative bacilli" | Five agents |
| 1975 | 40 | Nursery | *E. coli* | Kanamycin |
| 1978 | 75 | Surgical prophylaxis | *P. aeruginosa* | Gentamicin |
|      |    |           | *Serratia* | Gentamicin |

Adapted from McGowan, J. E., Jr. *Rev. Infect. Dis.* 5:1033, 1983.

kanamycin was a major factor in causing and propagating the outbreak. As gentamicin was increasingly used, a significant increase in gentamicin resistance of the infants' intestinal flora occurred [27].

Sogaard and colleagues [108], in studying antibiotic-resistant gram-negative bacilli in a urologic ward in Denmark, found a progressive decrease in the incidence of antibiotic resistance among enteric bacteria over a nine-year period that was coincident with a decreasing use of antibiotics in response to a restrictive antibiotic-use policy. In addition the number of more resistant organisms, such as *P. aeruginosa, Proteus, Providencia, Klebsiella,* and *Enterobacter,* declined during the period of study. Bulger and co-workers [13], in surveying resistance among strains of *E. coli* and *Klebsiella-Enterobacter* over a ten-year period, observed a decline in the frequency of resistance to antibiotics; they attributed their findings in part to conservative and selective use of antibiotics and in part to the development of an overall hospital infection control program.

Working in the Birmingham Accident Hospital Burn Unit, Lowbury and associates [61] studied the emergence of strains of *P. aeruginosa* and Enterobacteriaceae that carried an R factor conferring resistance to tetracycline, kanamycin, carbenicillin, ampicillin,

and cephaloridine. These strains emerged under the selective pressure of carbenicillin therapy, which was widely used on the burn unit. After the discontinuation of all use of carbenicillin and restriction on the use of tetracycline, kanamycin, ampicillin, and cephaloridine, strains of *P. aeruginosa* and Enterobacteriaceae carrying this linked multiply drug-resistant pattern disappeared. Price and Sleigh [81] reported an unusually dramatic experience in attempting to control an epidemic of *Klebsiella* infection in a neurosurgical unit; the epidemic was not curtailed by radical measures for the prevention of cross-infection, and the epidemic strain disappeared only when the use of all antibiotics, both prophylactic and therapeutic, was discontinued in the unit.

Based on data such as that reviewed previously, many individuals have felt that a policy of restricting the use of the newest and most broadly active antibiotics would minimize the development of resistance to those drugs and hence prolong their useful life span. In the case of aminoglycosides, however, the situation is somewhat more complicated, owing to the varying substrate specificities of the inactivating enzymes [17,18]. For example, the enzyme 3-acetyltransferase (AAC-3) will inactivate gentamicin and tobramycin, but not amikacin; the enzyme $6^1$-acetyltransferase (AAC-6[1]) will inactivate tobramycin and amikacin, but inactivates gentamicin relatively poorly.

Studies in the United States of the development of amikacin resistance in environments in which amikacin was widely used have suggested, with a few exceptions, that amikacin resistance has not developed significantly [8,14,70,128] and furthermore has resulted in a decrease in gentamicin resistance.

Davies [17] has pointed out that this finding makes sense, inasmuch as organisms that produce the most common gentamicin-inactivating enzymes in the United States would be eliminated by amikacin. Thus depending on the prevalence of specific resistance determinants and the specific enzyme produced, gentamicin use might select out a population of organisms resistant not only to gentamicin, but to tobramycin as well. In Japan, where 6[1]-acetyltransferase-mediated resistance is far more prevalent than in the United States, the use of tobramycin would select a population of organisms resistant not only to itself, but to amikacin as well. Optimal aminoglycoside use, therefore, should be determined not only by prevailing resistance patterns, but also by applying knowledge of the specific enzymes that are prevalent and their pattern of aminoglycoside inactivation.

In an excellent review, McGowan [65] has summarized seven types of evidence linking antimicrobial use in the hospital and antimicrobial resistance in hospital bacteria:

1. Antimicrobial resistance is more prevalent among bacteria causing infection in the nosocomial setting than among bacteria causing community-acquired infection. Although exceptions exist, they have been relatively few, and most of the data support the generalization.
2. In outbreak situations in the nosocomial setting, patients infected with resistant outbreak strains are more likely to have received previous antibiotic therapy than are patients colonized or infected with susceptible strains of the same species. This has been particularly illustrated in recent outbreaks of methicillin-resistant *S. aureus*.
3. Changes in antimicrobial use may lead to parallel changes in the prevalence of resistance to that antibiotic.
4. Areas of most intense antibiotic use within the hospital generally also have had the highest prevalence of antibiotic-resistant bacteria. These are also generally the areas of the hospital in which the most highly susceptible patients are encountered, and include intensive care units, burn units, oncology units, and other special care units.

5. Increased duration of exposure to antibiotics in the hospital generally increases the likelihood of colonization of infection with resistant organisms. This factor may, however, also simply act as a marker for more highly susceptible hosts.
6. The higher the dose of antibiotic given, the greater the likelihood of superinfection or colonization with resistant organisms. Evidence in support of this contention is not well controlled and is most convincing in the case of respiratory tract infection.
7. Finally, the notion of a cause-effect relation seems to fit the existing data, in biologic terms. That is, antibiotic therapy produces marked effects on the host's endogenous flora and exerts selective pressure in favor of resistant organisms. As emphasized by McGowan [65], however, antibiotic therapy appears to act primarily by selecting a drug-resistant causative organism, rather than by increasing the frequency of nosocomial infection.

Drug-resistant organisms—whether mutants, transductants containing plasmids, or conjugants containing R factors—selected by the pressure of antibiotic drugs are probably at a disadvantage, however slight, in the absence of the selective pressure. R determinants must represent an energy "load" for the host bacterium. If this were not so, "wild" bacteria in the community would likely be drug-resistant or would at least be a mixture of sensitive and resistant cells. Although R-factor-containing bacteria acquired in the hospital persist for a time in the community free of the selection pressure of antibiotics, they do decay in the absence of the selective pressure. Only 50 percent of infants who acquired enteric organisms containing R-factor-mediated resistance to kanamycin, for example, still had the original organisms present after one year [16].

## ANTIBIOTICS AND HOST SUSCEPTIBILITY

Antibiotics may affect host susceptibility to infection by either a direct effect on host defense mechanisms or an indirect effect resulting from alteration of the metabolic and immunologic state of the host. Antibiotics additionally exert a profound influence on the nature of host microflora, and although this selection effect may not directly influence host susceptibility to infection, as previously noted, it very directly influences the nature of the organisms that colonize and subsequently infect hospitalized patients.

*Direct Effect of Antibiotics*
*on Host Defense Mechanisms*

The most obvious and dramatic examples of a direct effect of antibiotics on the host defense mechanisms are the instances of granulocytopenia or bone-marrow aplasia occasionally encountered with the use of several antibiotics, notably chloramphenicol and the sulfonamides. Adverse reactions to penicillins, cephalosporins, sulfonamides, and less frequently, other antibiotics may take the form of a severe dermatitis, including exfoliation; such direct immunologic injury to the skin may, of course, enhance host susceptibility to infection. These adverse effects of antibiotic therapy are well known and profoundly influence host susceptibility to infection.

Direct effects of individual antibiotics on the components of host defense, that is, polymorphonuclear leukocyte function, immunoglobulin synthesis and function, and cell-mediated immune mechanisms, have not been systematically studied. There is, however, a gradually increasing body of data from which a few conclusions may be drawn [62,67,116].

With regard to function of polymorphonuclear leukocytes, neither $\beta$-lactam nor aminoglycoside drugs appear to have any deleterious effects on leukocyte function, although there is evidence that tetracycline hydrochloride, chlortetracycline, and doxycycline may inhibit leukocyte chemotaxis and impair phagocytosis. In addition, several sulfonamide drugs, including sulfadiazine, sulfathiazole, and sulfisoxazole, may inhibit leukocyte microbicidal activity. In the case of the tetracyclines, these effects may be seen in clinically attainable concentrations; whether they are of clinical significance has not been established.

Chloramphenicol, in clinically attainable concentrations, can be shown to diminish the antibody response to antigenic stimulation, but this effect has not been shown to be of general clinical significance. Rifampin can be shown in vitro to inhibit antibody production, but the effects of rifampin on antibody response in humans are variable.

Modulation of the host immune response to an infectious agent by specific chemotherapy—such as occurs in the treatment of rickettsial infections with chloramphenicol or tetracycline, penicillin treatment of group-A streptococcal infections, or ampicillin treatment of *H. influenzae* type-B infections—may over long periods of time alter the susceptibility of a population to a particular infectious agent, but this phenomenon probably is of little if any significance in the context of nosocomial infection.

Neither the $\beta$-lactam or aminoglycoside antibiotics are known to have any significant effect on host cell-mediated immune mechanisms. Rifampin, the tetracyclines, and trimethoprim have been shown to suppress lymphocyte blastogenesis at concentrations that might be encountered during clinical use. Several other antibiotics, including clindamycin, erythromycin, and nitrofurantoin, can similarly impair lymphocyte blastogenesis, but only at concentrations rarely achieved during clinical use. Rifampin can also be shown to suppress delayed cutaneous hypersensitivity to purified protein derivative of tuberculin (PPD) in patients with tuberculosis who are receiving the drug. This effect of rifampin, however, has not been shown to alter host susceptibility to infection in patients being treated for tuberculosis, nor to be associated with a poor therapeutic result.

Thus there is little evidence that antibiotic therapy has a major, direct effect on host defense mechanisms, except in instances of adverse drug reactions precipitating severe dermatitis, bone-marrow depression, or other such events.

*Indirect Effect of Antibiotics due to*
*Alteration of Host Metabolic State*

Many antibiotics cause direct toxic or immunologically mediated injury to target organs regulating the metabolic activity of the host, particularly the liver, kidneys, gastrointestinal tract, and lungs. The resulting dysfunction of these organs may alter host susceptibility to infection. These indirect effects of antibiotics can in most instances be minimized or avoided altogether by the rational and careful use of potentially toxic drugs.

KIDNEYS Interstitial nephritis has been associated with a number of drugs, notably the penicillins, including the penicillinase-resistant penicillins. Direct toxic injury to renal tubular epithelium is caused by many drugs, notably cephaloridine, all of the aminoglycosides, the polymyxins, and amphotericin B. Also, glomerulonephritis has been noted shortly after rifampin therapy in persons with previous exposure to the drug. Renal failure and its resulting metabolic consequences have a direct suppressive effect on host defense mechanisms. Clearly, the therapeutic modalities used in the management of renal failure also represent added infection risk factors.

LIVER Minor alterations of hepatic function are found frequently in the course of antibiotic therapy, but in the vast majority of instances such alterations cannot be shown to influence host susceptibility to infection. Intrahepatic cholestasis, such as may occur during therapy with the sodium lauryl sulfate ester of erythromycin, similarly does not appear to represent a major threat to host defense mechanisms. Overwhelming hepatic injury has been associated with both tetracycline and isoniazid therapy, but the unquestionably reduced host resistance to infection is of lesser importance than the more immediate metabolic threat to the host.

COLON  Necrotizing enterocolitis has been recognized as a complication of therapy with many antibiotic drugs, notably penicillins, cephalosporins, and clindamycin. Unlike staphylococcal necrotizing enterocolitis associated with tetracycline therapy, frequently seen during the 1950s and 1960s, most necrotizing enterocolitis seen at present is due to an enterotoxin produced by *Clostridium difficile* [4,5,85]. This adverse effect appears to be related to the alteration of host gastrointestinal tract flora caused by the administered antibiotic.

LUNGS  Immunologically mediated injury to the lungs is an occasional consequence of antibiotic therapy, particularly with penicillins and nitrofurans. It is likely that host susceptibility to infection is only mildly enhanced by such injury.

*Influence of Antibiotic Therapy on Host Microflora*
Virtually all antibiotics in therapeutic doses produce marked changes in the microflora of the skin, upper respiratory tract, gastrointestinal tract, and genital tract—indeed, any site in the host normally colonized by bacteria. Antibiotic-resistant organisms, if present or acquired, are selected out and multiply freely to replace the susceptible organisms inhibited by antibiotic therapy. In the majority of patients, these changes in host microflora are of no demonstrable consequence. As is well recognized, however, the antibiotic-resistant microflora may, on occasion, result in serious or fatal infection. It is through this mechanism that antibiotic therapy appears to exert its major influence on nosocomial infection, that is, by determining the character, rather than the frequency, of nosocomial infections.

Historically, the clearest example of alteration of host microflora that led directly to overgrowth and subsequent infection by antibiotic-resistant bacteria was staphylcoccal enterocolitis associated with or following tetracycline therapy. This appeared to be a direct result of antibiotic therapy, which suppressed the normal gastrointestinal tract flora and permitted rapid and uninhibited overgrowth of drug-resistant staphylococci. In the necrotizing enterocolitis encountered in recent years, the toxin-producing strains of *C. difficile* may not necessarily demonstrate in vitro

resistance to the precipitating antibiotic, but presumably the antibiotic suppresses the more sensitive gastrointestinal tract flora, allowing the less susceptible clostridia to multiply and/or produce enterotoxin [4,5,85].

Colonization of the gastrointestinal tract by multiply drug-resistant gram-negative bacilli, presumably under the influence of antibiotic therapy, has been repeatedly demonstrated [39,89,101,102,118]. In a study at the Denver Veterans Administration Hospital, Selden and associates [102] found that gastrointestinal tract colonization by multiply drug-resistant *Klebsiella* acquired in the hospital was an important intermediary step in the subsequent development of disease caused by that organism. In recent years, evidence has been presented suggesting that hospital food may frequently be contaminated by multiply drug-resistant gram-negative bacilli and that this may be an important source of nosocomial colonization in patients whose normal gastrointestinal tract flora is suppressed by antibiotic therapy. The sources of multiply drug-resistant gram-negative bacilli in hospital food, including, for example, fresh garden salads, has not been clarified.

It has become apparent that some kinds of antibiotics, particularly those active against many components of the anaerobic flora of the gastrointestinal tract, are more likely to be associated with colonization by multiply drug-resistant organisms than are antibiotics less broadly active against the anaerobic flora of the gastrointestinal tract [118]. This has led to the concept of "colonization resistance," suggesting that an intact colonic anaerobic flora is of major importance in preventing colonization by new aerobic gram-negative bacilli.

In a thorough study of bacterial colonization and suprainfection of the respiratory tract, Tillotson and Finland [117] showed that colonization and suprainfection were quite common following high doses of penicillin and aminoglycosides or of broad-spectrum antibiotics alone. They did not, however, find a higher rate of colonization or infection by gram-negative bacilli following treatment with various semisynthetic penicillins, nor did ampicillin therapy appear to confer any additional risk beyond that observed with penicillin G. Louria and Brayton [60] found that the risk of suprainfection following penicillin treatment of pneumonia was related, at least in part, to unnecessarily high doses of penicillin.

It is important to appreciate that antibiotic therapy is by no means the only factor influencing colonization and suprainfection. Johanson and associates [46,47] were among the first to point out the importance of the severity of the underlying disease, independent of antibiotic therapy, in pharyngeal colonization by gram-negative bacilli. Rose and Babcock [88], studying colonization with gram-negative bacilli of patients in an intensive care unit, observed that colonization in surgical patients appeared to be related more strongly to the presence of indwelling tubes and the consequent colonization of multiple sites in the same patient than to the use of antimicrobial drugs. In medical patients, however, colonization appeared to be related primarily to antibiotic therapy. Tenney and associates at the Denver Veterans Administration Hospital [113], who also studied pharyngeal colonization in a medical intensive care unit, found that no single risk factor for gramnegative rod colonization, such as antibiotic therapy, was associated with more than two-thirds of colonized patients and that most risk factors were present in less than one-third. The risk factors studied included, in addition to antibiotic therapy, the severity of the underlying illness, presence of acidosis, steroid therapy, mechanically assisted ventilation, tracheal intubation, nasogastric suction, and others.

Johanson and colleagues [46,47] suggested that the oropharynx is episodically or continually exposed to gram-negative bacilli and *S. aureus,* perhaps in small numbers, and that patients vary in their ability to clear them. Pharyngeal colonization may occur only in patients (1) whose pharyngeal clearance mechanisms are compromised by underlying disease, metabolic state, mechanically assisted respiration, or foreign bodies; (2) who are exposed to large inocula of gram-negative bacilli, for example, by contaminated nebulizers; or (3) in whom gram-negative bacilli are permitted to multiply more rapidly than they can be cleared, such as when antibiotic therapy suppresses normal flora. The risk of disease occurring after colonization has been established is more likely to be related to the state of host pulmonary defense mechanisms and to the virulence of the specific colonizing species than to the use of antibiotic therapy or other risk factors per se.

Sprunt and colleagues [110,111] have suggested that $\alpha$-hemolytic streptococci inhibit the growth of gram-negative bacilli in vitro, and they have furthermore noted the disappearance of inhibitory $\alpha$-hemolytic streptococci from the oropharynx in patients colonized with gram-negative bacilli. Thus bacterial interference, with $\alpha$-hemolytic streptococci acting as the inhibitory species, may be one mechanism for maintaining the normal flora of the upper respiratory tract. If these or other inhibitors are eliminated or depressed by antibiotic therapy, other drugresistant bacteria may be able to multiply to reach detectable levels. This may represent the analogue of

"colonization resistance" within the gastrointestinal tract, and may occur in other areas of the body as well, such as the skin.

In summary, there is abundant evidence that antibiotic therapy is a major determinant of alterations in host microflora and colonization of the host by drug-resistant organisms. There is also evidence, however, indicating that antibiotic therapy is by no means the only determinant involved, and that antibiotic therapy may be only one of a number of risk factors commonly encountered by hospitalized patients that facilitate colonization and often subsequent disease by drug-resistant organisms, including both staphylococci and gram-negative bacilli.

## GENERAL CONCLUSIONS

The interrelation of antibiotic therapy, intrinsic or acquired resistance to antibiotics in bacteria, and nosocomial infection in the hospitalized host represent an extraordinarily complex equation. Considering the large numbers of other risk factors that affect patients in hospitals, it is perhaps not surprising that data simply do not exist that would permit satisfactory and valid conclusions concerning the exact role of antibiotic use in determining either the magnitude or the frequency of hospital infection. As in many areas, there are differences of opinion. In 1970 Williams stated:

I have not referred so far to the factors so often cited as responsible for much of the trouble in hospital infection—abuse of antibiotics—because it seems important to appreciate that the secular changes that we have seen have not been wholly, or even mainly, due to alterations in the use of antibiotics or to the development of staphylococci more resistant to antibiotics [126].

In the same year, Finland wrote:

The major factor presumed to be responsible for the changing ecology of the serious bacterial infections, and for the marked increase in their occurrence, at least at Boston City Hospital, is the selective pressure of the antibiotics so widely and intensively used in therapy, and especially for prophylaxis. Both the large number of drugs and the large doses of each used in the individual patients within the hospital are elements of this selective pressure [24].

This disagreement cannot be resolved in quantitative terms. The use of antimicrobial agents tends to promote the emergence of organisms with intrinsic or acquired resistance to those agents and predisposes patients to colonization by such organisms. With increasing use of instrumentation, immunosuppressive drugs, and other technologic accompaniments of contemporary medical practice, resistant organisms may emerge to cause infection. Infection resulting from multiply drug-resistant bacteria, whether staphylococci or gram-negative bacilli, is notoriously more difficult to treat than infection by drug-susceptible pathogens, and the results of therapy in such compromised hosts are clearly less satisfactory.

Wolff and Bennett have stated the issues very succinctly:

The enhanced risks of acquiring gram-negative rod infections consequent to the proper use of antibiotics for legitimate therapeutic and prophylactic purposes clearly seem outweighed by the anticipated benefits. Such risks represent undesirable but nonetheless acceptable concomitants of medical progress. Use of antibiotics for uncertain or improper indications, however, poses an unacceptable risk [127].

## EVALUATION OF ANTIBIOTIC USE: APPROACHES TO IMPROVEMENT

That antimicrobial agents are both widely misused and widely overused is now established beyond reasonable doubt. From 20 to 35 percent of patients in U.S. hospitals receive antimicrobial agents during the course of their hospitalization, and this accounts for approximately one-third of hospital drug costs. In one study, no evidence of infection was found in as many as 70 percent of patients who received antimicrobial therapy [100]. Kunin has estimated that as many as 50 percent of hospitalized adults who received antibiotic therapy either (1) do not require antibiotic therapy for their medical condition, (2) do not receive the most effective and least expensive drug, or (3) do not receive the lowest dose and duration of therapy that is considered effective [55]. Furthermore, approximately 70 percent of antibiotics used in hospitals are in two highly expensive drug categories—cephalosporins and aminoglycosides [54].

It is important, however, as emphasized by Kunin [54], to place the problem of antibiotic use into broader perspective, rather than to consider it as an isolated example of inappropriate use of drugs. Included in the causation of the problem, and therefore to be considered in resolution of the problem, must be consideration of the ways in which appropriate use of drugs is taught in medical school, how house staff and practicing physicians receive information and advice about new drugs, the nature of the relationship between the pharmaceutical industry and the medical profession, the steadily increasing reliance of the medical profession on drug and laboratory technology in general, and the lack, until very recently, of any significant constraints operating to control the escalating cost of health care.

Viewed in such a context, antibiotic abuse is simply another reflection of what has become known as the "technological imperative," and is quite comparable to well-known problems such as the overuse of psychoactive drugs or excessive use of laboratory testing. There is, however, one major difference between other such problems and antibiotic abuse that is all too often ignored or forgotten—that is, the biologic consequences, or ecologic "fallout," of antibiotic therapy. As previously discussed in this chapter, the widespread use of antimicrobial agents in the hospital setting frequently leads to selection of organisms resistant to those antimicrobial agents and thus creates and maintains a population of drug-resistant nosocomial pathogens in the hospital environment. Physicians have been reluctant to recognize that a decision to use an antimicrobial agent in a given patient has ecologic consequences that extend well beyond the patient at hand.

There are, of course, several different categories of misuse or abuse of antibiotics. For example, antibiotics are widely misused in prophylaxis. A study by the Inter-Society Committee on Antimicrobial Drug Usage organized by the American College of Physicians [104], showed that over 25 percent of the total of antibiotics used in 20 Pennsylvania hospitals was apparently given for surgical prophylaxis and that almost 80 percent of such prophylactic use was accounted for by administration of antibiotic prophylaxis beyond the 24- to 48-hour postoperative period when prophylaxis can be anticipated to be effective. There was in fact a strong correlation between duration of hospital stay and duration of "prophylactic" therapy.

Antibiotics are often used as a diagnostic procedure; frequently, antibiotics are given as an empirical test for patients with fever or other presumed evidence of infection; if the patient "responds" to antibiotic therapy, then infection is presumed to have been the cause. There are, unquestionably, legitimate indications for such use of antibiotics, but most such use—the "take this antibiotic and let's see if your symptoms go away" approach—is clearly inappropriate.

Antibiotics are often used to treat a disease that does not respond to antibiotics. Contributing to abuse in this area are simple physician ignorance [73] and the common use of antibiotics to treat viral respiratory tract infections on the grounds that it is not likely to harm the patient and might prevent subsequent bacterial infection.

There are mistakes in the use of antibiotics, such as incorrect dosage, incorrect route of administration, inappropriate duration of therapy, or inappropriate choice of drug. In addition, physicians frequently fail to look for or recognize adverse reactions; toxic effects are relatively frequent and particularly prominent in aminoglycoside therapy.

The preferential use of newer and more expensive antibiotics, particularly recently introduced cephalosporin drugs, in clinical situations in which older and less expensive drugs have proved effective represents another recently apparent category of misuse. Kunin [54] has referred to many of the antimicrobial agents introduced during the past decade as "drugs of fear," suggesting fear on the part of the physician of not giving the best drug for a presumed infection. The use of second- or third-generation cephalosporins for therapy or surgical prophylaxis in situations in which first-generation cephalosporins have been shown to be effective is a clear example of misuse of "drugs of fear."

Increased recognition of the problem of antibiotic abuse has led to recommendations from advisory bodies, and more recently, demands from the Joint Commission on Accreditation of Hospitals (JCAH), that individual hospitals review their own use of antimicrobial agents. Unfortunately, the mandate to audit preceded the development of techniques demonstrated to be effective in performing such an evaluation, and was issued in the absence of any convincing evidence that self-examination on such a massive scale would beneficially affect the problem.

Nevertheless, a variety of techniques have been employed for carrying out surveillance or monitoring antibiotic use within hospitals. These have been summarized by Kunin [54], as shown in Table 11-3:

1. Gross utilization data based on pharmacy records is relatively inexpensive and may be used to track the costs and trends in use of specific drugs. Such information cannot readily be used for interhospital comparisons unless adjusted for case mix and number of patient days in the hospital. Its major use may be to identify specific problems requiring more detailed investigation.
2. Survey of use on individual services is feasible only if pharmacy records can identify use by specific nursing units or patients assigned to individual services. It is a slight improvement over gross utilization data inasmuch as potential problem areas can be pinpointed more closely.

TABLE 11-3. Methods of surveillance of antimicrobial use in hospitals

1. Gross utilization data based on pharmacy records
2. Survey of use on individual services
3. Survey of routine orders for prophylaxis in surgery
4. Survey of antibiotic therapy for specific infectious diseases
5. Individual case review by independent experts
6. Audits of specific clinical problems based on national criteria

Adapted from Kunin, C. M. *Rev. Infect. Dis.* 3:745, 1981.

3. Survey of routine orders for prophylaxis in surgery is somewhat more labor-intensive and requires individual chart review of all cases for specific operations being surveyed. It does permit interhospital comparison and provides specific data on the practices of individual surgeons; thus such information can be used for educational feedback to the surgical service.
4. Survey of antibiotic orders for specific infectious diseases must, of course, be based on the clinical condition being treated, such as community-acquired pneumonia, hospital-acquired pneumonia, or urinary tract infection. The patterns of practice of individual physicians can be identified and compared. Such information is useful for educational feedback.
5. Individual case review by independent experts is expensive and labor-intensive. It can be useful only if the standards for review are clearly articulated and agreed on by the physicians under review, whether a subspecialty group or an entire service. Lacking that, the findings are less likely to be accepted by the physicians whose antibiotic use is being reviewed.
6. Audits for specific clinical problems based on national criteria represent the most labor-intensive and least documented approach to modifying antibiotic use. Since antibiotic audit is now mandated by the Joint Commission on Accreditation of Hospitals, it may be assumed that hospital and medical staff will expend many hours carrying out this mandate. It is highly desirable, therefore, that this obligation be approached in a way that is likely to be effective educationally and that might have a significant impact on antibiotic use, rather than simply as a pro forma requirement that must be met.

The following suggestions are offered to help maximize the potential benefit of antibiotic audit:

1. Focus should be on several specific clinical issues rather than making an attempt to audit all antimicrobial use. Questions should be constructed quite specifically, remembering that the primary reason for antibiotic audit is to improve medical care and reduce its cost. The purpose is not to introduce conflict into the medical staff, nor to identify one or more physicians as being "guilty" of antibiotic abuse.

2. Concentration should be on areas of therapy or prophylaxis in which generally accepted national standards exist. Such national standards should be developed by, explained to, and agreed on by that segment of the medical staff involved in a given area of audit. The standards should be agreed on by all concerned as representing appropriate standards of therapy or prophylaxis. Reasonable and nationally acceptable standards of therapy exist or could be developed for a number of medical conditions such as pneumonia, intraabdominal infections, septicemia, endocarditis, and osteomyelitis; in many areas of antibiotic therapy, however, controversy exists; often there are legitimate differences of opinion as to the best approach to therapy. It is important that such areas be avoided as subjects for audit and that efforts be concentrated on areas for which acceptable and reasonable standards exist.

3. Audits of the prophylactic use of antibiotics in surgery have been emphasized, since this area has been identified as a major contributor to antibiotic cost and misuse. Procedures for which prophylaxis is currently recommended include prosthetic valve and open heart procedures; coronary artery bypass surgery; insertion of prosthetic joints; colonic surgery; biliary tract surgery in a patient over 70 years of age or with acute cholecystitis, obstructive jaundice, or choledocholithiasis; vaginal hysterectomy; cesarean section; and urologic surgery on bacteriuric patients. It is important to emphasize the appropriate preoperative timing of surgical prophylaxis and that prophylaxis should be terminated within 24 hours after surgery is completed.

4. Antibiotic audit should be by peer review, rather than review by hospital administration, infection control personnel, or pharmacy personnel. Thus it should be a medical staff responsibility, as specified by the JCAH, with standards defined and agreed on by infectious disease consultants within the staff and the medical staff being audited. Infection control personnel and pharmacy personnel may be extraordinarily helpful in the conduct of

the audit but should not have a dominant role in identifying the standards to be met. Broader acceptance of the results of an audit will follow if it is seen as a medical staff review rather than an administration review.

5. Few if any of the standards to be developed should be so rigid as to prohibit exception. Few absolute standards exist; variation from agreed on standards should appropriately prompt additional review but should not be automatically construed as indicating error. Reviewers must allow for the variety of clinical circumstances that might dictate some degree of variation from generally accepted standards.

6. Finally, if problems are identified in a given area of audit, the audit should be used to bring about change. This requires feedback of the information derived to that segment of the medical staff being audited, together with recommendations to improve use. Whether improvement results can be evaluated only by ongoing or repeat audit.

## CONTROL OF ANTIMICROBIAL AGENTS IN HOSPITALS

A number of additional approaches to controlling the use of antimicrobial agents in hospitals have been described. These have been summarized by Kunin, and are outlined in Table 11-4.

Educational programs on the appropriate use of antimicrobial agents have long been a principal approach to minimizing antibiotic abuse. This method has been of particular interest since the dramatic demonstration by Neu and Howrey [72] of major deficiencies in physician knowledge of antibiotic use. On the other hand, evidence that educational programs have been useful in creating change in antibiotic use have been conflicting at best [31,33,42,48,74,130]. In fact several recent reports have suggested that educational programs have little, if any, effect on antimicrobial use in hospitals. Educational programs of other institutions, however, have made a significant impact in the hospital setting, suggesting that continuing, focused, and scientifically supported recommendations do have an effect, especially if supplemented by the feedback of audits of antibiotic use within a specific hospital setting.

Kunin [54] believes strongly that some control of the nature and frequency of contact between pharmaceutical representatives and medical staff physicians is important. Precise guidelines cannot be easily established, but some attention should be given to

TABLE 11-4. Methods for control
of antimicrobial use in hospitals

1. Educational programs on use of antimicrobial agents
   a. Staff conferences
   b. Lectures by outside authorities
   c. Audiovisual programs
   d. Consultations with clinical pharmacists
   e. Hospital-Pharmacy Committee "newsletters"
   f. Independent sources of information (*Medical Letter, AMA Drug Evaluations*)
2. Control of contact between pharmaceutical representatives and staff physicians
   a. Registration in the pharmacy
   b. Visits to staff physicians by appointment only
   c. Policy concerning entry of salespersons to patient-care areas
   d. Restricted time and place of displays
   e. Policy on free samples, fittings
   f. Policy on sponsoring speakers, distribution
3. Hospital formulary
   a. Restriction of formulary to minimal number of agents needed for most effective therapy
   b. Elimination of duplicative agents
   c. Rules for selection of least expensive, most effective agent from a given class of agents
   d. Requirement for generic terminology for all orders and labels
4. Sensitivity tests from the diagnostic microbiology laboratory
   a. Appropriate selection of antibiotic sensitivity tests for organism and site of infection
   b. Use of generic class discs
   c. Restriction of reports on "specialized" agents unless specifically requested or indicated
   d. Use of generic terminology on laboratory report forms
5. Automatic "stop" orders for specific high-cost agents
6. Written justification for high-cost agents in cases in which alternative, equally effective, less expensive, or less toxic agents may be used (e.g., oral cephalosporins, new parenteral aminoglycosides and cephalosporins, lincosamides, chloramphenicol)
7. Required consultation with infectious disease service after administration of first three doses of specific high-cost agents (e.g., aminoglycosides, parenteral cephalosporins, carbenicillin-ticarcillin, lincosamides)
8. Required approval from infectious disease consultants for release of specific agents that may alter ecology of hospital flora (e.g., amikacin, carbenicillin-ticarcillin)
9. Establishment of guidelines and audits of antimicrobial use that permit the hospital staff to set standards of use based on local needs and judgments, guided by independent criteria. Audit is based on voluntary compliance with standards but requires a well-structured channel for authoritative feedback

Adapted from Kunin, C. M. *Rev. Infect. Dis.* 3:745, 1981.

the points listed in Table 11-4. Potential conflicts of interest of speakers sponsored by the pharmaceutical industry should be clearly identified, and it behooves such speakers to discuss their sponsor's product in the perspective of other comparable, and possibly less expensive, products.

The Pharmacy and Therapeutics Committee in a hospital should play a major role in keeping to a minimum the number of agents needed for optimum therapy and in publicizing guidelines for medical staff to select the least expensive effective agent from a drug class such as cephalosporins [130].

The potential role of the diagnostic microbiology laboratory in influencing antibiotic use is often overlooked (see Chapter 7). Use of generic terminology and restriction on the reporting of sensitivity tests with new and costly drugs unless specifically requested or indicated are critically important considerations. Pharmaceutical representatives know only too well that one important way to increase use of their newest product is for the hospital microbiology susceptibility report to contain a specific listing for that drug.

A number of administrative restraints, minor and major, have been effectively used in some hospital settings to modulate antibiotic use, especially the use of new and costly antibiotics [42,64,74,83]. These range from automatic "stop" orders for specific costly drugs, especially if used for surgical prophylaxis, to the requirement for approval from infectious disease consultants for the use of new and costly drugs. The interposition of such administrative restraints must be carefully individualized to the specific hospital setting [54]. For example, the requirement for infectious disease consultation has worked effectively in some academic centers with full-time infectious disease staff and fellows. In community hospital settings, on the other hand, infectious disease consultants on the medical staff have generally rejected the role of "policeman" or "czar" of antibiotic therapy. More broadly applicable is the requirement for written justification, either in the chart or on the order sheet, for costly agents such as new aminoglycosides or cephalosporins, or the requirement for consultation after 24 or 48 hours of use of such agents.

Present problems of antibiotic abuse developed during an era in which there was no restraint on the cost of hospital care other than physician judgment. Costs incurred were simply passed on to patients or their insurance carriers. A major change in the way in which hospitals are reimbursed in the United States is in progress with the advent of non-cost-based, prospective reimbursement, which is based on diagnosis.

The effects of this change will be even more dramatic if and when physician reimbursement and hospital reimbursement are provided by insurance carriers in the form of a single lump-sum payment. It is clearly premature to attempt to assess the impact of these dramatic changes; such an analysis must await a subsequent edition of this volume. Initial informal reports of very limited use of third-generation cephalosporins in hospitals in which their use has not been formally restricted provides some grounds for optimism. There is reason to hope that, given the financial constraints of prospective, fixed-price reimbursement, antibiotic use patterns will change significantly in the direction of more judicious restraint.

# REFERENCES

1. Anderson, F. M., Datta, N., and Shaw, E. J. R factors in hospital infection. *Br. Med. J.* 2:82, 1972.
2. Barber, M., Dutton, A. A. C., Beard, M. A., Elmes, P. C., and Williams, R. Reversal of antibiotic resistance in hospital staphylococcal infection. *Br. Med. J.* 1:11, 1960.
3. Barrett, F. F., McGehee, R. F., and Finland, M. Methicillin-resistant *Staphylococcus aureus* at Boston City Hospital: Bacteriologic and epidemiologic observations. *N. Engl. J. Med.* 279:441, 1968.
4. Bartlett, J. G., Chang, T. W., Gurwith, M., Gorbach, S. L., and Onderdonk, A. B. Antibiotic-associated pseudomembranous colitis due to toxin-producing clostridia. *N. Engl. J. Med.* 298:531, 1978.
5. Bartlett, J. G., Onderdonk, A. B., and Cisneros, R. L. Clindamycin-associated colitis in hamsters due to a toxin-producing clostridial species. *J. Infect. Dis.* 136:701, 1977.
6. Bauer, A. W., Perry, D. M., and Kirby, W. M. M. Drug usage and antibiotic susceptibility of staphylococci. *J.A.M.A.* 173:475, 1960.
7. Benveniste, R., and Davies, J. Mechanisms of antibiotic resistance in bacteria. *Annu. Rev. Biochem.* 42:471, 1973.
8. Betts, R. F., Valenti, W. M., Chapman, S. W., Chonmaitree, T., Mowrer, G., Pincus, P., Messner, M., and Robertson, R. Five-year surveillance of aminoglycoside usage in a university hospital. *Ann. Intern. Med.* 100:219, 1984.
9. Boyce, J. M., White, R. L., and Spruill, E. Y. Impact of methicillin-resistant *Staphylococcus aureus* on the incidence of nosocomial staphylococcal infections. *J. Infect. Dis.* 148:763, 1983.
10. Bradley, H. E., Weldy, P. L., and Hodes, D. S. Tolerance in *Staphylococcus aureus*. *Lancet,* 1:150, 1979.
11. Bradley, H. E., Wetmur, J. G., and Hodes, D. S. Tolerance in *Staphylococcus aureus*. Evidence for bacteriophage role. *J. Infect. Dis.* 141:233, 1980.
12. Buckwold, F. J., and Ronald, A. R. Antimicrobial misuse: Effects and suggestions for control. *J. Antimicrob. Chemother.* 5:129, 1979.
13. Bulger, R. J., Larson, E., and Sherris, J. C. Decreased incidence of resistance to antimicrobial agents among *Escherichia coli* and *Klebsiella-Enterobacter*: Observations in a university hospital over a 10-year period. *Ann. Intern. Med.* 72:65, 1970.
14. Cross, A. S., Opal, S., and Kopecko, D. J. Progressive increase in antibiotic resistance of gram-negative bacterial isolates: Walter Reed Hospital, 1976 to 1980. Specific analysis of gentamicin, tobramycin, and amikacin resistance. *Arch. Intern. Med.* 143:2075, 1983.
15. Crossley, K., Landesman, B., and Saske, D. An outbreak of infections caused by strains of *Staphylococcus aureus* resistant to methicillin and aminoglycosides. II. Epidemiologic studies. *J. Infect. Dis.* 139:280, 1979.
16. Damato, J. J., Eitzman, D. V., and Baer, H. Persistence and dissemination in the community of R factors of nosocomial origin. *J. Infect. Dis.* 129:205, 1974.
17. Davies, J. E. Resistance to aminoglycosides: Mechanisms and frequency. *Rev. Infect. Dis.* 5:S261, 1983.
18. Davies, J. E., and Courvalin, P. Mechanisms of resistance to aminoglycosides. *Am. J. Med.* 62:868, 1977.
19. Davis, C. E., and Anandan, J. The evolution of R factor: A study of a "preantibiotic" community in Borneo. *N. Engl. J. Med.* 282:117, 1970.
20. Dunkle, L. M., Naqvi, S. H., McCallum, R., and Lofgren, J. P. Eradication of epidemic methicillin-gentamicin-resistant *Staphylococcus aureus* in an intensive care nursery. *Am. J. Med.* 70:455, 1981.
21. Eickhoff, T. C., and Young, L. S. Gaps in therapy for infectious diseases: Conference summary. *J. Infect. Dis.* 145:407, 1982.
22. Farrar, W. E., Jr. Molecular analysis of plasmids in epidemiologic investigation. *J. Infect. Dis.* 148:1, 1983.
23. Finland, M. And the walls come tumbling down. More antibiotic resistance, and now the pneumococcus. *N. Engl. J. Med.* 299:770, 1978.

24. Finland, M. Changing ecology of bacterial infections as related to antibacterial therapy. *J. Infect. Dis.* 122:419, 1970.

25. Finland, M. Changing patterns of susceptibility of common bacterial pathogens to antimicrobial agents. *Ann. Intern. Med.* 76:1009, 1972.

26. Forfar, J. O., Keay, A. J., Maccabe, A. F., Gould, J. C., and Bain, A. D. Liberal use of antibiotics and its effect in neonatal staphylococcal infection, with particular reference to erythromycin. *Lancet* 2:295, 1966.

27. Franco, J. A., Eitzman, D. V., and Baer, J. Antibiotic usage and microbial resistance in an intensive care nursery. *Am. J. Dis. Child.* 126:318, 1973.

28. Gardner, P., Bennett, J. V., Burke, J. P., McGowan, J. E., Jr., and Wenzel, R. P. Nosocomial management of resistant gram-negative bacilli (editorial). *J. Infect. Dis.* 141:415, 1980.

29. Gardner, P., and Smith, D. H. Studies on the epidemiology of resistance (R) factors. I. Analysis of *Klebsiella* isolates in a general hospital. II. A prospective study of R-factor transfer in the host. *Ann. Intern. Med.* 71:1, 1969.

30. Gardner, P., Smith, D. H., Beer, H., and Moellering, R. C., Jr. Recovery of resistance (R) factors from a drug-free community. *Lancet* 2:774, 1969.

31. Geddes, A. M., and Gully, P. R. Antibiotic use in hospital. *Lancet* 2:532, 1981.

32. Gibson, C. D., Jr., and Thompson, W. C., Jr. The response of burn wound staphylococci to alternating programs of antibiotic therapy. *Antibiot. Annu.* 1955–56:32, 1956.

33. Gilbert, D. N., and Jackson, J. Effect of an education program on the proper use of gentamicin in a community hospital (abstract). *Clin. Res.* 24:112A, 1976.

34. Goessens, W. H. F., Fontijne, P., van Raffe, M., and Michel, M. F. Tolerance percentage as a criterion for the detection of tolerant *Staphylococcus aureus* strains. *Antimicrob. Agents Chemother.* 25:575, 1984.

35. Greene, W. H., Moody, M., Schimpff, S., Young, V. M., and Wiernik, P. H. *Pseudomonas aeruginosa* resistant to carbenicillin and gentamicin. *Ann. Intern. Med.* 79:684, 1973.

36. Guiney, G. G., Jr. Promiscuous transfer of drug resistance in gram-negative bacteria. *J. Infect. Dis.* 149:320, 1984.

37. Haley, R. W., Hightower, A. W., Khabbaz, R. F., Thornsberry, C., Martone, W. J., Allen, J. R., and Hughes, J. M. The emergence of methicillin-resistant *Staphylococcus aureus* infections in United States hospitals: Possible role of the housestaff-patient transfer circuit. *Ann. Intern. Med.* 97:297, 1982.

38. Hart, C. A. Nosocomial gentamicin and multiply resistant enterobacteria at one hospital. Factors associated with carriage. *J. Hosp. Infect.* 3:165, 1982.

39. Houang, E. T., Caswell, M. W., Simms, P. A., and Horton, R. A. Hospital-acquired faecal klebsiellae as source of multiple resistance in the community. *Lancet* 1:148, 1980.

40. Howard, J. B., and McCracken, G. H., Jr. Reappraisal of kanamycin usage in neonates. *J. Pediatr.* 86:949, 1975.

41. Hughes, V. M., Datta, N., and Faiers, M. C. Interhospital spread of a multiply resistant klebsiella. *Br. Med. J.* 282:696, 1981.

42. Jackson, G. G. Antibiotic policies, practices, and pressures. *J. Antimicrob. Chemother.* 5:1, 1979.

43. Jaffe, H. W., Sweeney, H. M., Nathan, C., Weinstein, R. A., Kabins, S. A., and Cohen, S. Identity and interspecies transfer of gentamicin-resistance plasmids in *Staphylococcus aureus* and *Staphylococcus epidermidis*. *J. Infect. Dis.* 141:738, 1980.

44. Jessen, O., Rosendal, K., Bulow, P., Faber V., and Eriksen, K. R. Changing staphylococci and staphylococcal infections. *N. Engl. J. Med.* 281:627, 1969.

45. Jevons, M. P. "Celbenin"-resistant staphylococci. *Br. Med. J.* 2:124, 1961.

46. Johanson, W. G., Jr., Pierce, A. K., and Sanford, J. P. Changing pharyngeal bacterial flora of hospitalized patients: Emergence of gram-negative bacilli. *N. Engl. J. Med.* 281:1137, 1969.

47. Johanson, W. G., Jr., Pierce, A. K., Sanford, J. P., and Thomas, G. D. Nosocomial respiratory infections with gram-negative bacilli: The significance of colonization of the respiratory tract. *Ann. Intern. Med.* 77:701, 1972.

48. Jones, S. R., Barks, J., Bratton, T., McRee, E., Pannell, J., Yanchick, V. A., Browne, R., and Smith, J. W. The effect of an educational program upon hospital antibiotic use. *Am. J. Med. Sci.* 273:79, 1977.

49. Kaye, D. The clinical significance of tolerance of *Staphylococcus aureus*. *Ann. Intern. Med.* 93:924, 1980.

50. Kayser, F. H. Methicillin-resistant staphylococci, 1965–75. *Lancet* 2:650, 1975.

51. Kayser, F. H., and Mak, T. M. Methicillin-resistant staphylococci. *Am. J. Med. Sci.* 264:197, 1972.

52. Kirby, W. M. M., and Ahern, J. J. Changing

pattern of resistance of staphylococci to anti-biotics. *Antibiot. Chemother.* 3:831, 1953.

53. Klimek, J. J., Marsik, F. J., Bartlett, R. C., Weir, B., Shea, R., and Quintilani, R. Clinical, epidemiologic, and bacteriologic observations of an outbreak of methicillin-resistant *Staphylococcus aureus* at a large community hospital. *Am. J. Med.* 61:340, 1976.

54. Kunin, C. M. Evaluation of antibiotic usage: A comprehensive look at alternative approaches. *Rev. Infect. Dis.* 3:745, 1981.

55. Kunin, C. M., Tupasi, T., and Craig, W. A. Use of antibiotics: A brief exposition of the problem and some tentative solutions. *Ann. Intern. Med.* 79:555, 1973.

56. Lacey, R. W. Antibiotic resistance plasmids of *Staphylococcus aureus* and their clinical importance. *Bacteriol. Rev.* 39:1, 1975.

57. Lepper, M. H., Moulton, B., Dowling, H. F., Jackson, G. G., and Kopman, S. Epidemiology of erythromycin-resistant staphylococci in a hospital population: Effect on therapeutic activity of erythromycin. *Antibiot. Annu.* 1953–54:308, 1954.

58. Levy, S. B. Microbial resistance to antibiotics: An evolving and persistent problem. *Lancet* 2:83, 1982.

59. Locksley, R. M., Cohen, M. L., Quinn, T. C., Tompkins, L. S., Coyle, M. B., Kirihara, J. M., and Counts, G. W. Multiply antibiotic-resistant *Staphylococcus aureus:* Introduction, transmission, and evolution of nosocomial infection. *Ann. Intern. Med.* 97:317, 1982.

60. Louria, D. B., and Brayton, R. G. The efficacy of penicillin regimens: With observations on the frequency of superinfection. *J.A.M.A.* 186:987, 1963.

61. Lowbury, E. J. L., Babb, J. R., and Roe, E. Clearance from a hospital of gram-negative bacilli that transfer carbenicillin resistance to *Pseudomonas aeruginosa. Lancet* 2:941, 1972.

62. Mandell, L. A. Effects of antimicrobial and antineoplastic drugs on the phagocytic and microbicidal function of the polymorphonuclear leukocyte. *Rev. Infect. Dis.* 4:683, 1982.

63. McGowan, J. E., Jr., and Finland, M. Infection and antibiotic usage at Boston City Hospital: Changes in prevalence during the decade 1964–1973. *J. Infect. Dis.* 129:421, 1974.

64. McGowan, J. E., Jr., and Finland, M. Usage of antibiotics in a general hospital: Effect of requiring justification. *J. Infect. Dis.* 130:165, 1974.

65. McGowan, J. E., Jr. Antimicrobial resistance in hospital organisms and its relation to antibiotic

use. *Rev. Infect. Dis.* 5:1033, 1983.

66. McGowan, J. E., Jr., Terry, P. M., Huang, T.-S. R., Houk, C. L., and Davies, J. Nosocomial infections with gentamicin-resistant *Staphylococcus aureus:* Plasmid analysis as an epidemiologic tool. *J. Infect. Dis.* 140:864, 1979.

67. Milatovic, D. Antibiotics and phagocytosis. *Eur. J. Clin. Microbiol.* 2:414, 1983.

68. Mitsuhashi, S. Review: The R factors. *J. Infect. Dis.* 119:89, 1969.

69. Mitsuhashi, S. (Ed.). *Transferable Drug Resistance Factor R.* Baltimore: University Park Press, 1971.

70. Moody, M. M., de Jongh, C. A., Schimpff, S. C., and Tillman, G. L. Long-term amikacin use: Effects on aminoglycoside susceptibility patterns of gram-negative bacilli. *J.A.M.A.* 248:1199, 1982.

71. Murray, B. E., Moellering, R. C., Jr. In-vivo acquisition of two different types of aminoglycoside resistance by a single strain of *Klebsiella pneumoniae* causing severe infection. *Ann. Intern. Med.* 96:176, 1982.

72. Neu, H. C. Changing mechanisms of bacterial resistance. *Am. J. Med.* 77(1B):11, 1984.

73. Neu, H. C., and Howrey, S. P. Testing the physician's knowledge of antibiotic use: Self-assessment and learning via videotape. *N. Engl. J. Med.* 293:1291, 1975.

74. Noone, P., and Shafi, M. S. Controlling infection in a district general hospital. *J. Clin. Pathol.* 26:140, 1973.

75. Palmer, D. L. Epidemiology of antibiotic resistance. *J. Med.* 11:255, 1980.

76. Parker, M. T., and Hewitt, J. H. Methicillin resistance in *Staphylococcus aureus. Lancet* 1:800, 1970.

77. Parker, M. T., and Lapage, S. P. Penicillinase production by *Staphylococcus aureus* strains from outbreaks of food poisoning. *J. Clin. Pathol.* 10:313, 1957.

78. Peacock, J. E., Jr., Marsik, F. J., and Wentzel, R. P. Methicillin-resistant *Staphylococcus aureus:* Introduction and spread within a hospital. *Ann. Intern. Med.* 93:526, 1980.

79. Plorde, J. J., and Sherris, J. C. Staphylococcal resistance to antibiotics: Origin, measurement, and epidemiology. *Ann. N.Y. Acad. Sci.* 236:413, 1974.

80. Pollack, M., Charache, P., Nieman, R. E., Jett, M. P., Reinhardt, J. A., and Hardy, P. H., Jr. Factors influencing colonization and antibiotic-resistance patterns of gram-negative bacteria in hospital patients. *Lancet* 2:668, 1972.

81. Price, D. J. E., and Sleigh, J. D. Control of

infection due to *Klebsiella aerogenes* in a neuro-surgical unit by withdrawal of all antibiotics. *Lancet* 2:1213, 1970.

82. Rajashekaraiah, K. R., Rice, T., Rao, V. S., Marsh, D., Ramakrishna, B., and Kallick, C. A. Clinical significance of tolerant strains of *Staphylococcus aureus* in patients with endocarditis, *Ann. Intern. Med.* 93:796, 1980.

83. Recco, R. A., Gladstone, J. L., Friedman, S. A., and Gerken, E. H. Antibiotic control in a municipal hospital. *J.A.M.A.* 241:2283, 1979.

84. Ridley, M., Barrie, D., Lynn, R., and Stead, K. C. Antibiotic-resistant *Staphylococcus aureus* and hospital antibiotic policies. *Lancet* 1:230, 1970.

85. Rifkin, G. D., Fekety, F. R., and Silva, J. Antibiotic-induced colitis: Implication of a toxin neutralized by *Clostridium sordellii* antitoxin. *Lancet* 2:1103, 1977.

86. Roberts, A. W., and Visconti, J. A. The rational and irrational use of systemic antimicrobial drugs. *Am. J. Hosp. Pharm.* 29:1054, 1972.

87. Roberts, N. J., Jr., and Douglas, R. G., Jr. Gentamicin use and *Pseudomonas* and *Serratia* resistance: Effect of a surgical prophylaxis regimen. *Antimicrob. Agents Chemother.* 13:214, 1978.

88. Rose, H. D., and Babcock, J. B. Colonization of intensive care unit patients with gram-negative bacilli. *Am. J. Epidemiol.* 101:495, 1975.

89. Rose, H. D., and Schreier, J. The effect of hospitalization and antibiotic therapy on the gram-negative fecal flora. *Am. J. Med. Sci.* 255:228, 1968.

90. Rountree, P. M., Beard, M. A., Loewenthal, J., May, J., and Renwick, S. B. Staphylococcal sepsis in a new surgical ward. *Br. Med. J.* 1:132, 1967.

91. Rubens, C. E., Farrar, W. E., Jr., McGee, Z. A., and Schaffner, W. Evolution of a plasmid-mediating resistance of multiple antimicrobial agents during a prolonged epidemic of nosocomial infections. *J. Infect. Dis.* 143:170, 1981.

92. Sabath, L. D. Antimicrobial Resistance: Mechanism of Resistance of Gram-Positive Cocci. In Brachman, P. S., and Eickhoff, T. C. (Eds.), *Proceedings of the International Conference on Nosocomial Infections*. Chicago: American Hospital Association, 1971, pp. 70–75.

93. Sabath, L. D. Mechanisms of resistance to beta-lactam antibiotics in strains of *Staphylococcus aureus*. *Ann. Intern. Med.* 97:339, 1982.

94. Sabath, L. D., Wheeler, N., Laverdiere, M., Blazevic, D., and Wilkinson, B. J. A new type of penicillin resistance of *Staphylococcus aureus*. *Lancet* 1:443, 1977.

95. Saravolatz, L. D., Markowitz, N., Arking, L., Pohlod, D., and Fisher, E. Methicillin-resistant *Staphylococcus aureus*. Epidemiologic observations during a community-acquired outbreak. *Ann. Intern. Med.* 96:11, 1982.

96. Saravolatz, L. D., Pohlod, D. J., and Arking, L. M. Community-acquired methicillin-resistant *Staphylococcus aureus* infections: A new source for nosocomial outbreaks. *Ann. Intern. Med.* 97:325, 1982.

97. Schaberg, D. R., Clewell, D. B., and Glatzer, L. Conjugative transfer of R plasmids from *Streptococcus faecalis* to *Staphylococcus aureus*. *Antimicrob. Agents Chemother.* 22:204, 1982.

98. Schaberg, D. R., Haley, R. W., Highsmith, A. K., Anderson, R. L., and McGowan, J. E., Jr. Nosocomial bacteriuria: A prospective study of case clustering and antimicrobial resistance. *Ann. Intern. Med.* 93:420, 1980.

99. Schaberg, D. R., Rubens, C. E., Alford, R. H., Farrar, W. E., Schaffner, W., and McGee, Z. A. Evolution of antimicrobial resistance and nosocomial infection: Lessons from the Vanderbilt experience. *Am. J. Med.* 70:445, 1981.

100. Scheckler, W. E., and Bennett, J. V. Antibiotic usage in seven community hospitals. *J.A.M.A.* 213:264, 1970.

101. Schimpff, S. C., Young, V. M., Greene, W. H., Vermeulen, G. D., Moody, M. R., and Wiernik, P. H. Origin of infection in acute nonlymphocytic leukemia: Significance of hospital acquisition of pathogens. *Ann. Intern. Med.* 77:707, 1972.

102. Selden, R., Lee, S., Wang, W. L. L., Bennett, J. V., and Eickhoff, T. C. Nosocomial *Klebsiella* infections: Intestinal colonization as a reservoir. *Ann. Intern. Med.* 74:657, 1971.

103. Shanson, D. C. Antibiotic-resistant *Staphylococcus aureus*. *J. Hosp. Infect.* 2:11, 1981.

104. Shapiro, M., Townsend, T. R., Rosner, B., and Kass, E. H. Use of antimicrobial drugs in general hospitals: Patterns of prophylaxis. *N. Engl. J. Med.* 301:351, 1979.

105. Shulman, J. A., Terry, P. M., and Hough, C. E. Colonization with gentamicin-resistant *Pseudomonas aeruginosa*, pyocine type 5, in a burn unit. *J. Infect. Dis.* 124:S18, 1971.

106. Smith, D. H. Mechanisms of Resistance of Gram-Negative Bacilli. In Brachman, P. S., and Eickhoff, T. C. (Eds.), *Proceedings of the International Conference on Nosocomial Infections*. Chicago: American Hospital Association, 1971, pp. 61–69.

107. Smith, J. M. B., and Marples, M. J. A natural

reservoir of penicillin-resistant strains of *Staphylococcus aureus*. *Nature* 201:844, 1964.

108. Sogaard, H., Zimmermann-Nielson, C., and Siboni, K. Antibiotic-resistant gram-negative bacilli in a urological ward for male patients during a nine-year period. Relationship to antibiotic consumption. *J. Infect. Dis.* 130:646, 1974.

109. Speller, D. C. E., Raghunath, D., Stephens, M., Viant, A. C., Reeves, D. S., Wilkinson, P. J., Broughall, J. M., and Holt, H. A. Epidemic infection by a gentamicin-resistant *Staphylococcus aureus* in three hospitals. *Lancet* 1:464, 1976.

110. Sprunt, K., Leidy, G. A., and Redman, W. Prevention of bacterial overgrowth. *J. Infect. Dis.* 123:1, 1971.

111. Sprunt, K., and Redman, W. Evidence suggesting importance of role of interbacterial inhibition in maintaining balance of normal flora. *Ann. Intern. Med.* 68:579, 1968.

112. Stevens, G. P., Jacobson, J. A., and Burke J. P. Changing patterns of hospital infections and antibiotic use: Prevalence surveys in a community hospital. *Arch. Intern. Med.* 141:587, 1981.

113. Tenney, J. H., Hopkins, J. A., LaForce, F. M., and Wang, W.-L. L. Pneumonia and pharyngeal colonization in a medical intensive care unit: Implications for prevention. Submitted for publication.

114. Thompson, R. L., Cabezudo, I., and Wenzel, R. P. Epidemiology of nosocomial infections caused by methicillin-resistant *Staphylococcus aureus*. *Ann. Intern. Med.* 97:309, 1982.

115. Thompson, R. L., and Wenzel, R. P. International recognition of methicillin-resistant strains of *Staphylococcus aureus* (editorial). *Ann. Intern. Med.* 97:925, 1982.

116. Thong, Y. H. Immunomodulation by antimicrobial drugs. *Med. Hypotheses* 8:361, 1982.

117. Tillotson, J. R., and Finland, M. Bacterial colonization and clinical superinfection of the respiratory tract complicating antibiotic treatment of pneumonia. *J. Infect. Dis.* 119:597, 1969.

118. Van der Waaj, D. Colonization resistance of the digestive tract: Clinical consequences and implications. *J. Antimicrob. Chemother.* 10:263, 1982.

119. Vogel, L., Nathan, C., Sweeney, H. M., Kabins, S. A., and Cohen, S. Infections due to gentamicin-resistant *Staphylococcus aureus* strain in a nursery for neonatal infants. *Antimicrob. Agents Chemother.* 13:466, 1978.

120. Wallmark, G., and Finland, M. Phage types and antibiotic susceptibility of pathogenic staphylococci: Results at Boston City Hospital 1959–1960 and comparison of strains of previous years. *J.A.M.A.* 175:886, 1961.

121. Washington, J. A., II. Microbial resistance to β-lactam antibiotics (editorial). *Mayo Clin. Proc.* 57:781, 1982.

122. Weinstein, R. A., and Kabins, S. A. Strategies for prevention and control of multiple drug-resistant nosocomial infections. *Am. J. Med.* 70:449, 1981.

123. Weinstein, R. A., Kabins, S. A., Nathan, C., Sweeney, H. M., Jaffe, H. W., and Cohen, S. Gentamicin-resistant staphylococci as hospital flora: Epidemiology and resistance plasmids. *J. Infect. Dis.* 145:374, 1982.

124. Weinstein, R. A., Nathan, C., Gruensfelder, R., and Kabins, S. A. Endemic aminoglycoside resistance in gram-negative bacilli: Epidemiology and mechanisms. *J. Infect. Dis.* 141:338, 1980.

125. Wenzel, R. P., Osterman, C. A., Donowitz, L. G., Hoyt, J. W., Sande, M. A., Martone, W. J., Peacock, J. E., Jr., Levine, J. I., and Miller, G. B., Jr. Identification of procedure-related nosocomial infections in high-risk patients. *Rev. Infect. Dis.* 3:701, 1981.

126. Williams, R. E. O. Changing Perspectives in Hospital Infection. In Brachman, P. S., and Eickhoff, T. C. (Eds.), *Proceedings of the International Conference on Nosocomial Infections*. Chicago: American Hospital Association, 1971, pp. 1–10.

127. Wolff, S. M., and Bennett, J. V. Gram-negative-rod bacteremia (editorial). *N. Engl. J. Med.* 291:733, 1974.

128. Wormser, G. P., Tatz, J., and Donath, J. Endemic resistance to amikacin among hospital isolates of gram-negative bacilli: Implications for therapy. *Infect. Control* 4:93, 1983.

129. Yu, V. L., Oakes, C. A., Axnick, K. J., and Merigan, T. C. Patient factors contributing to the emergence of gentamicin-resistant *Serratia marcescens*. *Am. J. Med.* 66:468, 1979.

130. Zeman, B. T., Pike, M., and Samet C. The antibiotic utilization committee: An effective tool in the implementation of drug utilization review that monitors the medical justification and cost of antibiotics. *Hospitals* 48:73, 1973.

## 12  R PLASMIDS AND THEIR MOLECULAR BIOLOGY

Dennis R. Schaberg

The development of effective antimicrobial agents has been a significant advance in the treatment of infectious diseases. Based on the idea that mutation would be the primary mechanism for resistance, the development of resistance to antimicrobials was not anticipated as a serious problem. As each new antimicrobial has been introduced, however, bacterial pathogens resistant to that drug have been encountered. The experience with nosocomial *Staphylococcus aureus* infections, summarized by Eickhoff in Chapter 11, is one example of this phenomenon.

The unexpected explanation for much of the resistance encountered was found in the recognition of plasmids, which could be transferred from one bacterial cell to another, carrying genes coding for antimicrobial resistance. These *R plasmids* were first recognized in gram-negative organisms in the enteric pathogen *Shigella,* but since have been found in virtually all clinically important nosocomial pathogens [10].

The hospital presents an environment in which circumstances conspire to accelerate the evolution of antimicrobial resistance. The most frequently encountered nosocomial pathogens—the aerobic gram-negative bacilli, staphylococci, and streptococci—all have the ability to acquire resistance rapidly. Intensive use of antimicrobials exerts extensive selection pressure favoring those organisms that have acquired resistance. In addition, therapy with antimicrobials alters normal flora, which appears to be an important contributor to R-plasmid transfer in vivo in the human GI tract. Transfer also can be readily observed in aqueous reservoirs peculiar to the hospital environment, such as urinary catheter collection bags. Compromised patients receiving antimicrobials who are hospitalized for prolonged periods of time provide an animate reservoir for resistant organisms once selected. In addition, antimicrobials find their way into the general inanimate environment, also contributing to the selective advantage obtained by R-plasmid-containing organisms.

### GENERAL PROPERTIES OF PLASMIDS

Plasmids are self-replicating extrachromosomal genetic elements of bacteria (see Chapter 11). The genetic information necessary for metabolism and growth of the bacterial cell is on the bacterial chromosome. Because this is usually unaltered by plasmid acquisition, plasmids can be acquired or lost without affecting basic cellular function. However, plasmids carry additional genes that often assist the bacterial cell in surviving or competing in adverse environments. This is in contrast to mutation, which results in structural changes in cellular function and metabolism.

Plasmids are isolated from bacterial cells as circular or supercoiled DNA molecules of a mass ranging from 0.5 to 300 $\times$ $10^6$ daltons. The mass of the average bacterial chromosome is approximately $2 \times 10^9$ daltons. The coding capacity of such plasmids can be substantial, with larger plasmids carrying sufficient DNA to code for hundreds of new proteins, if all the plasmid DNA is expressed. For many plasmids known functions can be ascribed, including of course antimicrobial resistance and sometimes virulence factors such as mucosal attachment properties or the ability to scavenge iron from the host. For some plasmids, no phenotypic properties are known. Plasmids with no detectable phenotype are common in many nosocomial isolates and are termed *cryptic plasmids*.

Plasmids are often classified into two general categories based on transmissibility: conjugative and nonconjugative. A plasmid is *conjugative* if it is self-transmissible from one bacterial cell to another. The classic example of a conjugative plasmid is the sex factor F. When a bacterial cell contains this conjugative plasmid, a proteinaceous appendage called a sex pilus is found on the outside of the cell; this together with other plasmid-mediated proteins provides for cell-to-cell transmission of the plasmid DNA. The genes of a conjugative plasmid are usually found in functional clusters, with part of the genes encoding for transfer functions and part devoted to replication; the function of the remaining DNA is often unknown or is concerned with other identifiable functions such as antibiotic resistance.

*Nonconjugative* plasmids are not self-transmissible and do not encode for transfer-specific proteins or a sex pilus. They are usually smaller in mass than conjugative plasmids. Nonconjugative plasmids can be transferred from cell to cell by a process called *mobilization,* in which a co-resident nonconjugative plasmid takes advantage of the transfer of a coexisting conjugative one. In addition, nonconjugative and conjugative plasmids may also be transmitted by bacterial virus vectors called *bacteriophages,* a process termed *transduction.* In this process plasmid DNA instead of phage DNA is packaged within the viral protein coat, and on infection of a suitable recipient cell, the plasmid DNA is released and begins replication within the new host.

Since transduction requires that the plasmid DNA be packaged within the protein coat of a bacteriophage, the amount of plasmid DNA that can be transduced is limited to about the size of the phage genome. This process operates much more efficiently for the smaller nonconjugative plasmids and appears to be an important mechanism of plasmid exchange in *S. aureus.* In gram-negative bacilli and streptococci, on the other hand, conjugation and mobilization seem to be the most common means of transfer. Recently conjugative transfer of resistance has been described in *S. aureus,* and it may be an important mechanism of gene exchange in more recent nosocomial staphylococcal isolates [12,15].

Direct uptake of both conjugative and nonconjugative plasmid DNA by a recipient cell can also occur— a process termed *transformation.* To induce transformation in the laboratory, bacteria are usually treated with calcium chloride to render them able to take up the plasmid DNA—a state referred to as *competence.* The ability to render *Escherichia coli* competent was important in the development of recombinant-DNA technology, since fragments of DNA to be "cloned" are usually inserted into nonconjugative plasmids, which are then transformed into *E. coli* for expression of the cloned DNA. The amount of DNA that can be picked up by a recipient cell is limited, and it is unlikely that transformation plays a significant role in plasmid transfer in the hospital.

In addition to transferability, another important feature of plasmids is *compatibility*. Compatibility refers to the ability of two plasmids to coexist within the same bacterial cell. If two plasmids cannot coexist, they are said to be of the same compatibility class. Compatibility classifications have been applied to plasmids isolated from the various enteric gram-negative bacilli as well as from *Pseudomonas aeruginosa* and to plasmids from *S. aureus.* Compatibility testing has proved useful in several epidemiologic investigations [5]. For example, when R plasmids encoding for chloramphenicol resistance were isolated from both *Salmonella typhi* and *Shigella dysenteriae* in Mexico, many investigators thought that these were closely related R plasmids. Since these R plasmids could coexist in the same cell and were of differing compatibility classes, they were not closely related. Plasmids that are not compatible generally share many genes in common, especially those required for replication.

Transmissibility and compatibility are properties of an entire plasmid. Our understanding of the evolution and diversity of bacterial plasmids has been expanded by the discovery of the process of transposition, whereby plasmid subunits can disperse separately from the entire plasmid. The rapidity with which antimicrobial resistance has been encountered in some organisms is in part related to this process.

A transposition sequence is a well-defined genetic segment, usually of constant size, that can move as an intact unit from one replicating DNA unit to another. These sequences can "jump" from plasmid to plasmid, plasmid to bacteriophage, plasmid to chromosome, or the reverse. Transposition elements specifying resistance, or *transposons,* have been described for most of the widely used antimicrobial agents, including the newer aminoglycosides [11]. In theory any plasmid could gain these elements; it would only be necessary for the DNA containing the transposon to coexist in a cell long enough for transposition to occur.

## MECHANISMS OF RESISTANCE

The resistance genes carried by R plasmids code for the synthesis of new proteins. These proteins frequently provide the bacterial cell with new enzymatic capabilities allowing for resistance. This is in contrast to mutations resulting in resistance, which often alter subcellular structures. These changes in essential cellular components, although resulting in antimicrobial resistance, are also often a disadvantage to the bacterial cell because the function of the component of the cell that is affected is compromised. R plasmids provide an advantage since essential bacterial cell functions are uncompromised. The known modes of R-plasmid-coded resistance have several mechanisms and involve proteins that either enzymatically inactivate the antibiotic, alter the target sites for the antibiotic, block the transport of the antibiotic into the bacterial cell, or bypass the metabolic steps inhibited by the antibiotic.

Plasmid-mediated resistance to ampicillin is an example of enzymatic inactivation. The penicillins and cephalosporins are β-lactam antibiotics, which are important as components of modern antimicrobial therapy. Resistance to these agents stems most often from β-lactamases, enzymes that hydrolyze the β-lactam ring and detoxify the drugs. The β-lactamase can be chromosome- or plasmid-mediated.

An example of plasmid-mediated alteration of an antibiotic-sensitive target is erythromycin resistance in gram-positive bacteria, typically staphylococci and streptococci. In this instance the 23 S RNA of the 50 S ribosome unit is methylated by a plasmid-mediated enzyme. Methylation of specific adenine residues on the RNA prevents binding of the erythro-

mycin and lincomycin classes of antimicrobials, and bacteria containing this plasmid gene exhibit high-level resistance.

A common example of blocking antimicrobial uptake is resistance to aminoglycoside antibiotics. R-plasmid-mediated resistance to aminoglycosides does not show large inoculum effects and the active antibiotic does not disappear from the culture medium after the plasmid-containing organisms are grown. This is true although the mechanism of resistance is due to the presence of plasmid-coded aminoglycoside-modifying enzymes [7].

These enzymes are at the inner membrane of bacterial cells, and the modified aminoglycoside blocks transport of the antibiotic into the cell. The phenotypic expression of aminoglycoside resistance will depend on the site at which the enzyme acts and on whether that site is present or available for enzymatic inactivation on a given aminoglycoside.

Bypass of inhibited metabolism is exemplified by the resistance to sulfonamides and trimethoprim. This is based on a plasmid-coded enzyme that substitutes for a chromosomal enzyme normally inhibited by these drugs. Sulfonamides work through competitive inhibition of the enzyme dihydropteroate synthetase. The plasmid-coded enzyme is smaller, more heat-sensitive, and requires 1000 times as much sulfonamide to inhibit it as does the chromosomal enzyme [27]. Similarly some strains resistant to high levels of trimethoprim, an agent that inhibits dihydrofolate reductase, contain a plasmid-mediated gene coding for a new trimethoprim-resistant dihydrofolate reductase. In each of these instances the plasmids provide a mechanism whereby products vital to the bacterial cell can be synthesized and the inhibiting effect of the drug is bypassed.

## MOLECULAR ANALYSIS OF RESISTANCE

Simplified techniques for isolating and characterizing bacterial plasmids have been developed in recent years [2,8,14,17]. Application of this technology to clinical situations involving antimicrobial resistance has improved our understanding of the evolution of resistance within hospitals. We are aware now that the development of resistance operates at three levels of genetic organization. The first level is dissemination within the hospital of an R-plasmid-containing strain. The next level occurs with plasmid spread, in which an R plasmid is moved from strain to strain or from one species to another. The third level involves transposition of individual resistance determinants from one plasmid to another or from chromosome to plasmid. The latter process may be one way that R plasmids gradually accumulate multiple resistances.

Numerous examples of epidemics due to resistant microorganisms have been reported. A common feature of most of the outbreaks is the emergence of a strain able to resist the action of agents preferred for treating serious infections in hospitalized patients. Most commonly for the gram-negative pathogens, the antimicrobials concerned are newer aminoglycosides, such as gentamicin and tobramycin, or β-lactams, such as carbenicillin and ticarcillin. One such outbreak occurred in Nashville, Tennessee, where resistance to gentamicin was uncommon before 1973. Isolates of *Serratia marcescens* with high-level resistance to gentamicin were first discovered in that year and over the next two years caused a large number of infections. These isolates were of an identical phage-type and serotype and thus represented clonal dissemination of a single strain [25]. Similar hospital outbreaks involving *Klebsiella pneumoniae, P. aeruginosa,* and other gram-negative bacilli have been described.

When strain dissemination is suspected, various techniques can be applied to determine the probable identical nature of strains. The easiest and most available are those used in the routine evaluation of the isolates in the clinical laboratory. Species identification, biotype, and antimicrobial susceptibility pattern all provide useful clues to strain identity. More information is often necessary, however, because many common nosocomial pathogens provide little variability in biotype or susceptibility pattern. This makes accurate determination of the sameness of isolates difficult using the readily available data; additional laboratory study of the strains becomes necessary.

Additional typing information is obtained from referral centers and is usually dependent on the species to be examined [1]. Serotyping, phage-typing, bacteriocin production, and bacteriocin susceptibility can be useful, depending on the organism (see Chapter 7). An additional procedure that has provided information useful for typing isolates is analysis of the total plasmid content of bacterial cells by agarose gel electrophoresis (AGE) [23]. Recent technical advances now allow such analyses to be completed within one day of isolation of an organism in pure culture [2,8,14]. The information generated by AGE is especially important in organisms such as *Citrobacter* species, *Enterobacter,* nonaeruginosa *Pseudomonas* species, and *Staphylococcus epidermidis,* when other typing systems are not available. The presence of cryptic plasmids along with R plasmids in nosocomial isolates often provides a characteristic electrophoretic pattern useful to "fingerprint" a strain. When an outbreak is suspected or an infection problem occurs, such as serial *S. epidermidis* infections in cardiac surgery, in which knowledge of the sameness of multiple isolates would assist in evaluation, AGE can provide useful information rapidly. It also provides information about plasmid content should plasmid spread be suspected. Most large referral hospitals should be able to establish this technique. Smaller institutions can seek assistance from most university centers, especially those involved in recombinant DNA research, where these techniques are applied virtually every day.

Intergeneric R-plasmid exchange can and has contributed to problems encountered with resistant pathogens in a number of hospitals (Table 12-1). Common features of all these reports has been their occurrence in large referral hospitals, involvement of special care units, and simultaneous acquisition by the recipient of the "epidemic" R plasmid of resistance to multiple antimicrobials.

To find out whether there has been possible plasmid spread, comparison of patterns of resistance is coupled with observation of the ability of the natural isolates to transfer similar resistances into reference host strains [3]. *E. coli* strain K-12, onto which resistance to selected antimicrobials such as nalidixic acid or streptomycin has been introduced by mutation, is often chosen to serve as recipient. Similar laboratory strains for use as recipients in *Pseudomonas* transfers also have been developed. The potential donor and recipient are grown in mixed culture, and through use of selective media the ability of the resistance to be transferred can be documented. Strains transferring resistances can then be analyzed by AGE, along with their transconjugants, for total plasmid content. This technique allows the visualization of plasmids and an approximation of their molecular mass. Bacterial lysates are prepared, placed in slots of an agarose slab gel, and separated by electrophoresis. After staining with ethidium bromide, which binds to DNA by inserting between bases, the plasmids can be visualized as discrete bands using ultraviolet light. Photography using special filters provides a permanent record of the gel. R plasmids from a single hospital carrying identical resistances and of similar molecular mass suggest R-plasmid exchange has occurred.

Plasmids encoding similar resistances and of approximately the same size can be additionally explored for identity by endonuclease restriction analysis. Purified plasmid DNA is obtained by ethidium bromide–cesium chloride density centrifugation [19]. The plasmids are then subjected to digestion with

TABLE 12-1. Studies demonstrating intergeneric R-plasmid transfer within the hospital

| Investigator | Geographic location | Species involved | Clinical setting | Molecular mass (md) | Resistances conferred by plasmid |
|---|---|---|---|---|---|
| Thomas, et al. [25] Rubens, et al. [20] | Nashville | *Klebsiella pneumoniae* *Pseudomonas aeruginosa* *Serratia marcescens* | Hospitalwide | 105 | Gm, tm, km, sm, su, tc, cb, ap, cm |
| Elwell, et al. [9] | Dallas | *Klebsiella pneumoniae* *Enterobacter cloacae* | Burn unit | 60 | Tm, km, sm, ap, cb |
| Schaberg, et al. [24] | Dallas | *Klebsiella pneumoniae* *Enterobacter cloacae* | Neonatal intensive care | 80 | Gm, tm, km, cm, ap, cb |
| Tompkins, et al. [26] | Seattle | *Serratia marcescens* *Klebsiella pneumoniae* *Enterobacter aerogenes* *Citrobacter freundii* *Klebsiella oxytoca* *Providencia rettgeri* | Hospitalwide | 45 | Gm, tm, km, ap, cb, cf, sm, su |
| Gerding, et al. [13] Sadowski, et al. [22] | Minneapolis | *Klebsiella pneumoniae* *Escherichia coli* *Enterobacter cloacae* *Morganella morganii* | ICU and hospitalwide | 58 | Gm, tm, km, ap, cb, cf, cm, su |
| O'Brien, et al. [18] | Unknown | *Klebsiella pneumoniae* *Enterobacter aerogenes* *Serratia marcescens* *Escherichia coli* *Citrobacter freundii* *Morganella morganii* | ICU and hospitalwide | 56.5 | Gm, tm, su, cm, ap, cb |
| Knight, et al. [15] | London | *Klebsiella pneumoniae* *Escherichia coli* *Citrobacter freundii* *Enterobacter cloacae* | Hospitalwide | 110 | Gm, tm, km, sm, su, tc, cb, ap, cm |

Antimicrobial abbreviations: gentamicin (gm), tobramycin (tm), kanamycin (km), streptomycin (sm), ampicillin (ap), carbenicillin (cb), cephalothin (cf), chloramphenicol (cm), tetracycline (tc), sulfonamide (su).

endonuclease restriction enzymes, which generates a characteristic DNA fragment pattern depending on the plasmid and particular enzyme used (Fig. 12-1). There are a large number of enzymes available, and each one recognizes discrete nucleotide sequences on a plasmid. Demonstration of identical-sized plasmids encoding for identical resistances with identical restriction-endonuclease fragment patterns is strong evidence that two plasmids are identical. If they come from multiple genera in the same hospital it provides support that intergeneric R-plasmid exchange within the hospital environment is happening. How important R-plasmid exchange is in the overall picture of resistance remains uncertain, but this mechanism does operate in special care areas of large hospitals where selective pressure of therapy is greatest.

Just where antimicrobial resistance genes have originated from and how multiple determinants for antimicrobial resistance accumulate on a given R plasmid is not clear. The movement of resistance genes from plasmid to plasmid or from chromosome to plasmid via transposition may play a role in the "building" of R plasmids. Several studies have shown that this process has worked in the hospital environment [6,20,21]. In the studies by Rubens and co-workers, a gentamicin-resistance determinant originally present on a small nonconjugative plasmid was transposed onto a larger, self-transferable plasmid. Once on the conjugative element, the resistance was efficiently transferred among genera within the hospital. This process provided a mechanism to stack new resistance determinants on a preexisting plasmid and appears to be one way that R-plasmid development can take place. Unfortunately, the techniques for studying transposition remain cumbersome and available only in research laboratories.

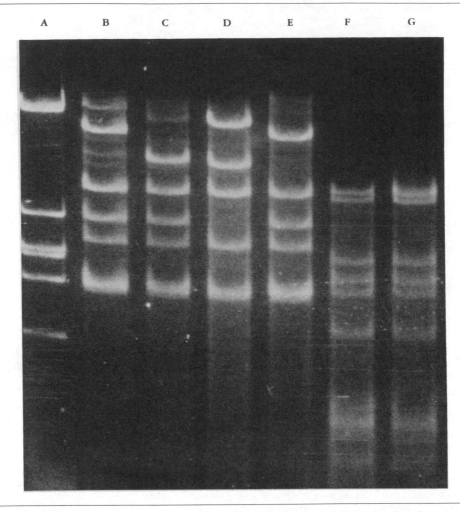

FIG. 12-1. Agarose gel electrophoresis of restriction endonuclease–digested plasmid DNA. Lane A contains bacteriophage lambda DNA digested with EcoR1. Lanes B through E contain gentamicin R plasmids of similar size on screening and thought to be identical. Lanes B and E did give identical patterns as confirmed by digestion with enzyme HindIII shown in F and G. The plasmids in lanes C and D gave different enzyme digestion patterns.

## APPROACH TO CONTROL

In theory one approach to control is to prevent the exchange of R plasmids and interrupt the transposition process in the development of R plasmids. Unfortunately, no agents are available that allow us to do so selectively and efficiently. Rather, we are forced to contend as best we can with the first level of organization, resistant strains, and await modalities to attack the R plasmids specifically.

Adding to the problem is the fact that as many as 10 to 12 resistances may be present on a single R plasmid. The linkage of these resistance determinants makes it possible for therapy with a single antimicrobial to select for resistance to various unrelated antibiotics. Rotation of antibiotics and restricting certain ones may not be as effective as hoped in decreasing resistance. Use of a totally different anti-

microbial, if the plasmid encodes for resistance to both, will continue to select for persistence of the resistant strains.

Measures have been developed that can be successful in controlling dissemination of resistant strains and are based on an understanding of the epidemiology of each circumstance. Strategies of use to many hospitals are summarized by Weinstein in Chapter 38. As we acquire a more clear understanding of the factors in R-plasmid exchange, we hope to be able to intervene in the fundamental processes involved in the evolution of R plasmids and prevent the development of multiply resistant strains.

## REFERENCES

1. Aber, R. C., and Mackel, D. C. Epidemiologic typing of nosocomial microorganisms. *Am. J. Med.* 70:899, 1981.
2. Bidwell, J. L., Lewis, D. A., and Reeves, D. S. A rapid single-colony lysate method for the selective visualization of plasmids in Enterobacteriaceae, including *Serratia marcescens. J. Antimicrob. Chemother.* 8:481, 1981.
3. Coetzee, J. N., Datta, N., and Hedges, R. W. R factors from *Proteus rettgeri. J. Gen. Microbiol.* 72:543, 1972.
4. Cohen, S. N. Transposable genetic elements and genetic evolution. *Nature* 263:731, 1976.
5. Datta, N. Plasmid Classification: Incompatibility Grouping. In Timmis, K. N., and Pichler, A. (Eds.), *Plasmids of Medical, Environmental, and Commercial Importance.* Amsterdam: Elsevier/North-Holland Biomedical Press, 1979, pp. 47–53.
6. Datta, N., Hughes, V. M., Nugents, M. E., and Richards, H. Plasmids and transposons and their stability and mutability in bacteria isolated during an outbreak of hospital infection. *Plasmid* 2:182, 1979.
7. Davies, J. E., and Courvalin P. Mechanisms of resistance to aminoglycosides. *Am. J. Med.* 62:868, 1977.
8. Eckhardt, T. Rapid method for identification of plasmid DNA in bacteria. *Plasmid* 1:584, 1978.
9. Elwell, L. P., Inamine, J. M., and Minshew, B. H. Common plasmid specifying tobramycin resistance found in two enteric bacteria isolated from burn patients. *Antimicrob. Agents Chemother.* 13:312, 1978.
10. Falkow, S. *Infectious Multiple Drug Resistance.* London: Pion-Limited, 1975.
11. Farrar, W. E. Gentamicin transposons. *J. Antimicrob. Chemother.* 6:4, 1980.
12. Forbes, B. A., and Schaberg, D. R. Transfer of resistance plasmids from *Staphylococcus epidermidis* to *Staphylococcus aureus:* Evidence for conjugative exchange of resistance. *J. Bacteriol.* 153:627, 1983.
13. Gerding, D. N., Buxton, A. E., Hughes, R. A., Cleary, P. P., Arbacyawski, J., and Stamm, W. E. Nosocomial multiply-resistant *Klebsiella pneumoniae:* Epidemiology of an outbreak apparent index case origin. *Antimicrob. Agents Chemother.* 15:608, 1979.
14. Kado, C. I., and Liu, S. T. Rapid procedure for detection and isolation of large and small plasmids. *J. Bacteriol.* 145:1365, 1981.
15. Knight, S., and Casewell, M. W. Dissemination of resistance plasmids from among gentamicin-resistant enterobacteria from hospital patients. *Br. Med. J.* 283:755, 1981.
16. McDonnell, R. W., Sweeney, H. M., and Cohen, S. Conjugational transfer of gentamicin resistance plasmids intra- and interspecifically in *Staphylococcus aureus* and *Staphylococcus epidermidis. Antimicrob. Agents Chemother.* 23:151, 1983.
17. Meyers, J. A., Sanchez, D., Elwell, L. P., and Falkow, S. Simple agarose gel electrophoretic method for the identification and characterization of plasmid deoxyribonucleic acid. *J. Bacteriol.* 127:1529, 1976.
18. O'Brien, T. F., Ross, D. G., Guzman, M. A., Madeiros, A. A., Hedges, R. W., and Botstein, D. Dissemination of an antibiotic resistance plasmid in hospital patient flora. *Antimicrob. Agents Chemother.* 17:537, 1980.
19. Radloff, R., Bauer, W., and Vinograd, J. A dye-buoyant-density method for the detection and isolation of closed circular DNA: The closed circular DNA in HeLa cells. *Proc. Acad. Sci. U.S.A.* 57:1514, 1967.
20. Rubens, C. E., Farrar, W. E., McGee, Z. A., and Schaffner, W. Evolution of a plasmid mediating resistance to multiple antimicrobial agents during a prolonged epidemic of nosocomial infections: A molecular biological investigation. *J. Infect. Dis.* 143:170, 1981.
21. Rubens, C. E., McNeill, W. F., and Farrar, W. E. Evolution of multiple antibiotic-resistance plasmids mediated by transposable deoxyribonucleic acid sequences. *J. Bacteriol.* 140:713, 1979.
22. Sadowski, P. L., Peterson, B. C., Gerding, D., and Cleary, P. P. Physical characterization of ten R plasmids obtained from an outbreak of nosocomial *Klebsiella pneumoniae* infections. *Antimicrob. Agents Chemother.* 15:616, 1979.
23. Schaberg, D. R., Tompkins, L. S., and Falkow, S. Use of agarose gel electrophoresis of plasmid deoxyribonucleic acid to fingerprint gram-negative bacilli. *J. Clin. Microbiol.* 13:1105, 1981.
24. Schaberg, D. R., Tompkins, L. S., Rubens, C. E., and Falkow, S. R plasmids and Nosocomial Infection. In Stuttard, C., and Royce, K. R. (Eds.), *Plasmids and Transposons: Environmental Effects and Maintenance Mechanisms.* New York: Academic, 1980, pp. 43–55.
25. Thomas, F. E., Jackson, R. T., Melly, M. A., and Alford, R. H. Sequential hospital-wide out-

breaks of resistant *Serratia* and *Klebsiella* infections. *Arch. Intern. Med.* 137:581, 1977.

26. Tompkins, L. S., Plorde, J. J., and Falkow, S. Molecular analysis of R factors from multiresistant nosocomial isolates. *J. Infect. Dis.* 141:625, 1980

27. Wise, E. M., and Abou-Donia, M. M. Sulfonamide resistance mechanism in *Escherichia coli*: R plasmids can determine sulfonamide-resistant dihydropteroate synthetases. *Proc. Natl. Acad. Sci. U.S.A.* 72:2621, 1975.

# 13 MEDICOLEGAL ASPECTS OF NOSOCOMIAL INFECTIONS

Karen Rose Koppel Kaunitz
Andrew Moss Kaunitz

Liability for nosocomial infections may be imposed on any health-care provider, including hospitals, physicians, and nurses [23,52,55]. The number of substantial awards from health-care providers as a result of nosocomial infections has grown in recent years as patients have become more sensitive to treatment complications, including infection [90]. A variety of legal theories may be used to impose liability, including negligence, warranty, and strict tort liability, as well as government statutes and regulations. Hospital liability for negligence arises under two different theories. The first theory is based on the doctrine of *respondeat superior* ("let the master answer"), arising from the negligence of one or more employees or agents. The second theory holds that a hospital corporation itself may be negligent if it fails to perform a legally recognized corporate duty—the corporate negligence theory. If a staff physician, resident, nurse, or other hospital employee is negligent with respect to a patient, negligence may be imputed to the hospital, and the patient may have a cause of action against both the employee and the hospital-employer [38].

## DOCTRINE OF RESPONDEAT SUPERIOR (AGENCY)

Under the classic principle of agency (*respondeat superior*), a master is liable for the actions of his servants. Accordingly, an employer may be held liable for the wrongful acts of an employee, even though the employer is itself without fault (vicarious liability) [93]. Hospitals in general are not liable for the wrongful conduct of private physicians working in the hospital as independent contractors. Recent case law using the corporate theory, however, has expanded the responsibilities of hospitals to monitor the activities of independent medical personnel within their facilities. Hospitals have been held liable for the torts of independent physicians under a theory of "apparent or ostensible agency." This theory holds that a hospital is responsible when a patient is led to believe he or she is being treated by an agent of the hospital,

Disclaimer: This chapter was written by Karen Rose Koppel Kaunitz and Andrew Moss Kaunitz in their private capacity. No official support or endorsement by the U.S. Department of Health and Human Services, the Office of General Counsel, or the Centers for Disease Control is intended or should be inferred. The material presented should not be viewed as legal advice; the reader should always consult an attorney for the latest information on laws, regulations, and case precedents of his or her own jurisdiction.

typically when specialists under contract with the hospital are furnished by the hospital rather than personally selected by the patient [79].

Even if an employer is found to be liable under the principle of agency, the employee who actually committed the tort can also be held personally liable for his or her wrongful act or omission [100]. The plaintiff may sue any such parties separately or all of them together. The plaintiff is not, however, permitted to collect judgment in full from two or more defendants. If the plaintiff collects the judgment from the employer, the employer may have a right of indemnification from the negligent employee. This right is most likely to be asserted when employer and employee are insured by different carriers.

## CORPORATE NEGLIGENCE THEORY

The second theory of liability, the corporate negligence theory, recognizes that hospitals owe certain duties and responsibilities imposed by courts or legislatures directly to patients, visitors, and employees. If by failing to meet these duties the hospital causes harm, the hospital itself may be held liable.

Under the traditional rule, enunciated in *Scoendorff v. Society of New York Hospital*, 105 N.E. 92 (N.Y. 1914), hospitals were not liable for torts committed by physicians because physicians, not hospitals, practice medicine. The landmark case of *Darling v. Charleston Community Memorial Hospital*, 211 N.E.2d 253 (Ill. 1965), cert. denied 383 U.S. 946, 86 S.Ct. 1204 (1966), departed from this rule and expanded the obligations of hospitals to monitor the quality of patient-care services in the following three ways:

1. The hospital must not allow an independent staff physician to violate a specific hospital requirement for patient safety.
2. The hospital must ensure that its employees will detect apparent dangers to the patient and bring such dangers to the attention of the hospital medical staff or surgical staff and the administration so that the administration can act to alleviate the danger.
3. The hospital must supervise the actions of independent staff physicians [81].

In *Darling*, an emergency-department patient with a fractured leg was assigned to a general practitioner on call who applied a cast. Despite easily recognizable signs that the leg had become ischemic, the physician failed to recognize or react to this complication. Although the nurses were aware that the patient was developing obvious complications, the hospital administration failed to take steps to obtain consultation as required by hospital bylaws. The plaintiff's leg became infected and was ultimately amputated. The court held the hospital liable for failing to ensure the provision of quality medical care. Mere reliance on self-regulation, according to the court, was inadequate.

Cases after *Darling*, particularly those in the area of medical staff selection and review, have expanded malpractice liability by recognizing the independent duty of hospitals to ensure the provision of quality medical care [29,54,70,72,87,95].

Case law, however, stops short of providing that hospitals are guarantors of the adequacy of medical care. The isolated acts of otherwise competent physicians, therefore, remain the sole responsibility of that physician [62]. Some cases have gone even farther than requiring careful selection and review, and suggest that a hospital has a duty to supervise the competency and quality of its physicians. In these cases, however, the defendant hospitals had actual or constructive knowledge of provision of substandard care but failed to intervene [32,79,104]. This theory, however, was rejected in *Schenck v. Gov't of Guam*, 609 F.2d 387 (9th Cir. 1979).

## CORPORATE OBLIGATIONS

Hospitals have been found to owe a variety of obligations directly to patients and the public. These obligations include:

(1) The duty to furnish and maintain proper equipment, supplies, and services and to exercise reasonable care in the selection and use of such equipment, supplies and services,
(2) The duty to exercise reasonable care in the selection and retention of appropriate personnel,
(3) The duty to exercise reasonable care with respect to the maintenance of buildings and grounds, including keeping the environment clean and sanitary with the aim of preventing infection, and
(4) The duty to comply with policies and procedures which, whether established by the hospital or by outside agencies, have as their objective the safety and well-being of patients and the public [47].

Because such duties include the obligation to promulgate and enforce rules to protect patients from infections, hospitals that fail to establish proper procedures, organizations, and techniques in infection control may be liable. In addition, hospitals may have a duty to monitor physician infection rates and to intervene if excessively high rates are noted [37,50].

## NEGLIGENCE

Negligence is legally defined as a violation of the duty to use care [26]. To establish liability, the four elements of the tort of negligence must be satisfied. The elements are (1) the existence of a standard or duty owed to the plaintiff, (2) the defendant's failure to perform that duty or satisfy the standard of care owed, (3) the plaintiff's demonstration that his or her injury resulted directly or proximately from the defendant's failure to perform the duty or to meet the standard of care, and (4) the occurrence of damages attributable to the injury [86].

To prevail in litigation when alleging damages due to a hospital infection, a plaintiff must therefore establish that an infection was contracted in the hospital, that the hospital breached its duty to the plaintiff through an act of negligence, and that this negligence directly caused both the infection and any damages sustained [59]. The test for negligence in an infection control case might be framed in the following way: "Was the hospital care or lack of care in some way responsible for the infection; and did the hospital act in a reasonable and prudent manner in recognizing, reporting, and trying to control the infection?" [6]. Negligence in the treatment of infection will also result in liability [25,27,48].

## STANDARD OF CARE AND BREACH OF THE STANDARD

A fundamental component of establishing liability involves delineating which particular duties hospitals and physicians have toward patients. In the health-care context, these "duties" translate to the "standard of care." To prevail in negligence actions, plaintiffs must establish that a provider has failed to meet such a standard of care. The standard of care required depends, in turn, on the circumstances of the particular case. Local, state, or national practices may determine a standard of care. The traditional rule, which was favorable to providers, provided that practices should conform to the standards of other providers in the same locality. Under this "customary practice" standard of the local community, or "locality rule," a provider's performance was measured against the level of care delivered by reasonably competent persons or institutions of equivalent skill in the same geographic community. The court's sole function, therefore, was to determine whether the provider did something that was not customary or failed to do something that was [57]. This standard was subsequently expanded to include those practices

common in similar communities; hence, the standard was "same or similar communities."

Recent trends have replaced the "same or similar locality custom standard" with a national standard. This standard of care is based on the assumption that there should be and is *one* prevailing level of care. The standard of care in the provider's locality, or in a similar locality, is simply one factor in determining whether the standard of care has been met [4,28,48]. National accreditation standards promulgated by the Joint Commission on Accreditation of Hospitals (JCAH) and state licensure requirements and guidelines such as those published by the Centers for Disease Control (CDC) and the American Hospital Association (AHA) have encouraged courts to hold providers to a national standard of care. The court in the *Darling* case explicitly recognized this concept, which has frequently been applied in situations in which a court considers the prevailing community standard of care to be too low.

*Standard of Care in Nosocomial Infection Cases*
Although hospitals have a duty to protect patients from injury due to infections, courts have never maintained that hospitals *guarantee* their patients will not acquire nosocomial infections. A hospital, however, may be liable for a patient's infection if it can be shown that the infection was caused by the negligence of the hospital or any of its agents. Hospitals' duties to monitor medical care include conducting infection control reviews. If a plaintiff establishes that an excessive number of infections has occurred at a defendant hospital, the hospital may have to prove that it could not have discovered the pattern any sooner and that on discovery measures were immediately undertaken to correct the problem. To minimize the risk of failing to meet the standard of care, hospitals should vigorously educate personnel in aseptic technique and infection control procedures and should institute surveillance mechanisms to establish that proper procedures are indeed being followed.

A spectrum of standards rather than a single standard of infection control applies to hospitals. In determining the standards of care within a hospital, courts have looked to various sources. One source is based on the hospital's own internal rules; these include protocols, procedures manuals, and bylaws. In *Robinson v. St. John's Medical Center, Joplin,* 508 S.W.2d 7 (Mo. 1974), for example, the hospital's operating procedure manual was used to establish nurses' duties in the operating room. This established the standard of care for which the hospital was subsequently liable. In *Helman v. Sacred Heart Hospital,* 381 P.2d 605 (Wash. 1963), there was evidence that hospital personnel moved from one patient to another without washing their hands, failing to follow hospital policy designed to prevent the spread of infection. The court, therefore, ruled that the hospital breached its duty to the patient. In *Kapuschinsky v. U.S., 248 F. Supp. 732, 259 F. Supp. 1* (D.S.C. 1966), the court cited the hospital's failure to follow the standard of care it voluntarily assumed in its own procedure manual. The procedure manual prohibited nurse's aides from working with preterm infants, and this was allowed in this case. (See Exposure to Contagious Personnel for details of this case.)

Failure to follow a hospital's own rules and procedures may lead to a liability claim against which it may be particularly difficult to defend:

... the hospital should be very careful to make sure that its own hospital regulations and procedures are followed assiduously. Because these items may be taken as the duties or standards of care incumbent upon a hospital, the failure to perform such duties or to meet such standards of care may allow a plaintiff to show the first two elements of negligence; then he would only have to show that such failure to perform the duty or failure to meet a standard of care was the direct cause of his injury and to show the amount of his damages [76].

In addition to promoting staff compliance with internal regulations, hospitals are well advised to be certain that procedures established in such internal manuals be as practicable as possible.

State laws and regulations governing hospitals may also establish standards of care. In most states, hospitals are subject to governmental rules regulating the practice of hospital infection control. These requirements vary considerably from state to state; hence, hospital administrators and counsel should consult their own state's regulations. Some states allow considerable latitude in procedures, providing little guidance. Other states, such as Illinois, set forth requirements specifically for infection control procedures [62]. In some cases, courts have ruled that these regulations establish guidelines for minimum standards of hospital care.

Plaintiffs alleging damages resulting from violations of state regulations may be able to establish negligence. For example, in *Suburban Hospital Association v. Hadary,* (22 Md. App. 186, 322 A.2d 258 (Md. 1974), the hospital's failure to comply with a licensing regulation requiring the segregation of sterile and nonsterile needles established the hospital's negligence. In the case of *Derrick v. Ontario Community Hospital,* 120 Cal. Rptr. 566, 47 Cal. App.3d 145 (1975), a state law requiring hospitals to report com-

municable diseases to the local health officer was cited by the plaintiff in establishing a cause of action against the hospital, which failed to report a particular communicable disease. Even though the court stated that it might be difficult to prove that the defendant hospital's failure to report a communicable disease to the local health officer resulted in the plaintiff's injury, it found that the statute imposed a duty on the hospital to report such a case. The appellate court reversed the trial court and concluded that at trial the plaintiffs would have to prove that the hospital violated its duty under the statute and that this violation was the proximate cause of the plaintiff's injuries.

Mere compliance with minimum statutory or regulatory standards and licensure provisions, however, may not preclude liability for negligence. Hospitals may be held to a higher degree of care due to local practices and requirements of good medical practice or because the court rejects an existing standard as inadequate to protect the public.

Government agencies such as the Health Care Financing Administration [69] and the CDC [16] issue regulations and guidelines for health care. Private organizations such as the JCAH, AHA, and professional associations also issue standards and recommendations. All these may play a role in establishing a particular standard of care.

In addition to expanding the parameters of corporate liability, the *Darling* decision also held that the standards of the JCAH along with the hospital's medical staff bylaws were admissible as evidence in determining negligence. The court found that the defendant hospital failed to abide by its own rules and failed to maintain JCAH standards. Hence, failure to comply with these standards may lead to liability [15].

Whereas accreditation standards have ordinarily applied only to accredited hospitals, these standards may receive such acceptance in a given community that the courts will accept the accreditation standards in determining negligence in nonaccredited hospitals as well. In its chapter on infection control, the JCAH lists the following standards:

Standard 1. There shall be an active hospitalwide infection control program.
Standard 2. Responsibility for monitoring the infection control program shall be vested in a multidisciplinary committee. The committee shall recommend corrective action based on records and reports of infections and infection potentials among patients and hospital personnel.

Standard 3. There shall be specific written infection control policies and procedures for all services throughout the hospital [52].

Each standard is followed by an interpretation section to assist hospitals in understanding the standards and their application.

The CDC *Guidelines for the Prevention and Control of Nosocomial Infections* [16] was developed to update and consolidate recommendations for infection surveillance and control. The guideline topics include prevention of catheter-associated urinary tract infections, environmental control of nosocomial infections, prevention of intravascular infections, prevention of surgical wound infections, prevention of respiratory tract infections, isolation techniques, role of the microbiology laboratory in infection surveillance and control programs, employee health services and objectives, and methods of surveillance. To assist infection control staff in critically assessing the value of the recommendations, a ranking scheme was developed consisting of three categories: category I—strongly recommended for adoption, category II—moderately recommended for adoption, and category III—weakly recommended for adoption. Category I recommendations "are judged to be applicable to the majority of hospitals—regardless of size, patient population, or endemic nosocomial infection rate, and are considered practical to implement" [16]. Category II recommendations "are not to be considered a standard of practice for every hospital" [16]. Although the CDC recommendations are likely to influence standards of care on a national basis, the standard of care is ultimately established on a case-by-case evaluation [64].

To summarize, courts look to a variety of sources, including national practices, local or national rules, and guidelines when determining the standard by which a defendant is judged.

*Proof of the Standard of Care*
When a plaintiff alleges a defendant has failed to meet a standard of care, the plaintiff must first establish the standard and then prove that it was breached. This proof is normally accomplished by the use of expert testimony. When negligence has been admitted, however, or in cases in which the negligence is obvious to laypersons, expert testimony may not be required. Other alternatives to expert testimony include the use of medical books, journals, state and federal laws, regulations, and guidelines as evidence to prove the standard; direct cross-examination of the provider; and use of the doctrine of *res ipsa loquitur*.

Application of a national standard of care has allowed the use of experts from outside the defendant's locality.

## THE DOCTRINE OF RES IPSA LOQUITUR

The doctrine of *res ipsa loquitur*, (*res ipsa*: "the thing speaks for itself") is related to the expert testimony requirement [31,45]. The case of *Ybarra v. Spangard,* 25 Cal.2d 486, 489, 154 P.2d 687 (1944), established that the use of *res ipsa* requires that three elements be established:

(1) The accident must be of a kind which ordinarily does not occur in the absence of someone's negligence,
(2) It must be caused by an agency or instrumentality within the exclusive control of the defendant, and
(3) It must not have been due to any voluntary action or contribution on the part of the plaintiff.

Because the main reason supporting the use of *res ipsa* is the plaintiff's inability to discover the cause of injury, some states have applied a fourth requirement that the defendant must have superior knowledge of the cause of the accident [62].

When circumstantial evidence indicates that the defendant's negligence is the most plausible explanation for the injury, despite the absence of direct evidence the doctrine of *res ipsa* may apply. The applicability of *res ipsa* is determined at the conclusion of trial. When applied, defendants lose the advantage of evidentiary barriers plaintiffs normally face in proving a breach of the professional standard of care. Use of *res ipsa* in health-care litigation increased during the mid-1960s as courts attempted to compensate for the legal system's barriers against plaintiffs' recoveries [98].

*Res Ipsa and Infection Cases*
Because infections may indeed occur in the absence of negligence, courts have infrequently applied *res ipsa* in cases in which plaintiffs attempt to establish liability for infections. Two recent cases reflect this principle: In *Roark v. St. Paul Fire & Marine Insurance Company, et al.,* 415 So.2d 295 (La. 1982), the court stated that a certain number of hospital patients will contract a staphylococcal infection regardless of the hospital's conduct. An essential element of *res ipsa* was absent, therefore, in that the plaintiff's infection could indeed have occurred without negligence. In *Wilson v. Stilwill,* 411 Mich. 587, 284 N.W.2d 773 (1981), the defendant hospital's postoperative infec-

tion rate was well below the national average. The plaintiff sought to apply *res ipsa* by establishing that the low incidence of infection at the hospital implied that infection did not ordinarily occur. The court, however, was not persuaded: "Although it is true that statistically infections did not ordinarily occur at the defendant hospital, this fact does not suggest that when an infection does occur, it is the result of negligence."

The doctrine of *res ipsa* has been held applicable, however, in other hospital infection cases. In *Southern Florida Sanitarium and Hospital v. Hodge,* 215 S.2d 753 (Fla. 1968), *res ipsa* was allowed because testimony established that thrombophlebitis would not have occurred if proper sterile technique had been maintained by the defendant hospital throughout an injection procedure. This testimony fulfilled the three required elements for *res ipsa*: (1) thrombophlebitis ordinarily should not occur in the absence of negligence, (2) the injection was performed by an agent or instrumentality under the control of the hospital, and (3) the thrombophlebitis was not caused by any voluntary action or contribution by the plaintiff.

As the case of *Sommers v. Sisters of Charity of Providence in Oregon,* 277 Or. 549, 561 P.2d 603 (1977) demonstrates, use of the *res ipsa* doctrine may involve certain pitfalls. In this case, a patient sued the hospital for negligence after a *Staphylococcus aureus* infection developed at the site of an intravenous cannula. The patient alleged that hospital nurses did not properly disinfect her skin before inserting the cannula. Medical experts testified that it was impossible to sterilize skin completely. They also stated that the patient had a poison oak rash that had large numbers of bacteria; hence, the patient was probably the source of her own infection. Had the plaintiff not relied on the doctrine of *res ipsa,* she might have been able to establish that a reasonably prudent nurse should not cannulate an area where a rash is present [22].

## CAUSATION AND DAMAGES AND INFECTION LIABILITY

To prevail in a negligence action, a plaintiff must prove that a provider's failure to exercise the required standard of care resulted in the plaintiff's injury [100]. If a patient can establish that he or she suffered injury due to an infection resulting from hospital and/or staff negligence, the hospital and/or its staff may be liable. A hospital's responsibility for the prevention and control of infections extends to patients, personnel, and visitors. As was discussed earlier, however, hospitals neither ensure nor guarantee patients' safety;

hence, liability is not established on mere proof that a plaintiff developed an infection, nor would *res ipsa* apply [100]. In *Rohdy v. James Decker Munson Hospital,* 170 N.W.2d 67 (Mich. 1969), for instance, a plaintiff alleged that the hospital was responsible for a staphylococcal infection occurring on the same arm as an injection received one month earlier. The court held, however, that *res ipsa* could not be applied because there was no certainty that the infection resulted from the injection.

Because nosocomial infections are common, unpredictable, and may be difficult to prevent, courts have recognized that such infections may occur despite reasonable care. In addition, it is often difficult or impossible to establish that a particular negligent act or omission *specifically* resulted in infection (the element of proximate causation) [33]. In *Wilson v. Stilwill,* 411 Mich. 587, 284 N.W.2d 773 (1981), the plaintiff alleged that the occurrence of an arm infection following hospital treatment indicated negligence. Because there was no testimony establishing that the treatment was negligent or contrary to any professional standard of conduct, however, the jury decided against the plaintiff. The court stated: "The mere occurrence of a postoperative infection is not a situation which gives rise to an inference of negligence when no more has been shown than the fact that an infection has occurred and that an infection is rare" [14,21,68,96].

A hospital was held liable in *St. Paul Fire & Marine Ins. Co. v. Prothro,* 590 S.W.2d 35 (Ark. 1979) when a patient developed an infection after a metal basket lowering him into a whirlpool bath broke, struck him, and reopened his surgical wound. The appeals court supported the plaintiff's assertion that the infection was caused by the fall into the bath.

It is unusual for patients to be awarded damages for hospital-acquired infections. As methods of typing microorganisms improve, however, the ability to trace the specific sources of infections proving proximate causation may improve. As discussed earlier, plaintiffs may also attempt to use the doctrine of *res ipsa* to establish negligence without proving proximate cause.

## MEDICAL STAFF OBLIGATIONS

The medical staff as well as the hospital have an obligation to prevent and control infections. Physician responsibilities include appropriate clinical care, in certain cases serving as a member of the Infection Control Committee or as a hospital epidemiologist or infection control officer, and in general setting a proper example in practicing medical asepsis. Physicians may incur liability for failure to adhere to appropriate standards of care. In addition, as the number of physicians specializing in infectious disease grows, liability may even be imposed for failure to consult with such a specialist [80].

## PATIENT NOTIFICATION OF THE PRESENCE OF INFECTION OR DISEASE

Some lawsuits have involved plaintiffs' allegations that they were not informed of the presence of hospital infections. In *Jones v. Sisters of Charity*, 173 S.W. 639 (Tex. 1915), the plaintiff alleged that his wife died from smallpox because the hospital failed to notify his wife that there was a case of this disease in the hospital. Because strict quarantine was maintained and there was no concealment, the court found for the defendant hospital. In *Robey v. Jewish Hospital of Brooklyn*, 20 N.E.2d 6 (N.Y. 1939), the court took a similar stand when damages for the infection of a newborn infant was alleged. In this case an expectant mother was not warned of infection currently affecting infants in the hospital; the court ruled, however, that the record failed to show any actionable negligence on the part of the hospital. In *Aetna Casualty and Surety Company v. Pilcher*, 244 Ark. 11, 424 S.W.2d 181 (1968), the hospital's failure to warn the plaintiff before surgery that pathogens existed in the hospital was not found to be the proximate cause of the infection.

Hospitals have an obligation to patients sharing a room with another patient with a contagious disease. It is recommended that physicians treating such patients be informed; the physicians can then determine appropriate care. The patient should be informed of exposure in such situations [85].

## NEGLIGENT HANDLING OF PATIENTS

Infections resulting from negligent handling of patients have resulted in liability. For example, in *Inderbitzen v. Lane Hospital*, 124 Cal. App. 462, 12 P.2d 744, 13 P.2d 905 (1932), the plaintiff, a woman in active labor, received vaginal examinations by two medical students with unsterilized hands; the plaintiff developed postpartum endometritis. Noting the risk of infection from receiving a vaginal examination with unsterilized hands while in labor, the court found the hospital liable.

In *Kirchoff v. St. Joseph's Hospital*, 260 N.W. 509 (Minn. 1935), a hospital was found liable after a nurse

gave a mother the wrong baby, which was infected with impetigo. The mother was infected by this infant and subsequently transmitted the disease to her own child.

A hospital was found negligent in *Helman v. Sacred Heart Hospital*, 62 Wn. 2d 136, 381 P.2d 605 (1963), for failing to prevent cross-infection of the plaintiff. The plaintiff contracted a staphylococcal infection after being placed in a room with a patient who had a staphylococcal infection; testimony indicated that the two patients were infected with the same strain of coagulase-positive *Staphylococcus aureus*. The court observed that the hospital attendants did not observe the sterile techniques prescribed by the hospital for infected cases nor did they wash their hands between administering to the patients. In addition, the court indicated that when the presence of an infected patient presented a serious risk to the well-being of another patient, the hospital may have a corporate duty to isolate the infected patient [78].

## EXPOSURE TO CONTAGIOUS PATIENTS

Liability may be imposed for failure to isolate patients with communicable diseases or for failure to guard against cross-infection. Hospital licensure regulations in most states require isolation facilities for patients with communicable disease. The JCAH provides that an infection control program must have "written policies defining the specific indications for isolation requirements in relation to the medical condition involved" [55].

Courts have held that defendants are liable should a patient contract an infection after being negligently exposed to a contagious patient. An early case involving patient-to-patient contact was *Gadsden General Hospital v. Bishop*, 96 So. 145 (Ala. 1923); in this suit, a patient's administrator alleged that the deceased patient died from smallpox acquired in the hospital. The court assumed that proper care and attention would include preventing a patient from being exposed to a contagious disease from another patient in the hospital. To recover damages the court ruled the following five elements would need to be established: (1) the patient died of smallpox, (2) he acquired the disease while a patient in the hospital, (3) the infection was transmitted to him from another patient in the hospital during the patient's stay, (4) hospital staff knew that the other patient had smallpox, and (5) hospital staff negligently exposed the deceased to the infected patient. The court ruled that the plaintiff did not meet all of these requirements. In *Bush v. Board of Managers of Binghamton City Hos-*

*pital,* 251 App. Div. 601, 297 N.Y.S. 991 (1937), the plaintiff alleged that his wife contracted fatal diphtheria because she was placed too close to patients with diphtheria at the defendant hospital. Although the lower court held for the plaintiff, the appellate division reversed the judgment; it found neither evidence of the defendants' failure to employ safe and suitable methods and equipment nor adequate proof that the decedent had in fact contracted diphtheria.

A hospital may avoid liability when it is not aware of a contagious patient. In *Gill v. Hartford Accident and Indemnity Co., et al.,* 337 So.2d 420 (Fla. App. 1976), for instance, a physician neglected to notify hospital personnel that a patient was contagious.

## EXPOSURE TO CONTAGIOUS PERSONNEL

Hospitals in most states are required to screen personnel for infectious disease by testing new employees and periodically screening existing personnel. For example, in Illinois periodic physical examinations are recommended, and personnel absent from work because of any communicable disease may not return to work until examined by a physician [51,62]. Medicare and Medicaid Conditions of Participation require that "a continuing process is enforced for inspection and reporting of any hospital employee with an infection who may be in contact with patients, their food, or laundry" [111]. The failure to recognize obvious symptoms of an employee's poor health and to remove such an employee from duty may also generate liability. Hospitals must minimize patient contact with staff who are carriers of infection. Detecting, reassigning, and even removing contagious staff from duty, therefore, are all parts of a hospital's duties. For example, routine screening of personnel working in dialysis units for hepatitis B markers is generally recommended at the present time. Liability related to hospital employee health is discussed in greater detail in a later section of this chapter.

Many suits have been brought alleging that patients contracted diseases resulting from negligent exposure to hospital staff. For example, in *Taaje v. St. Olaf Hospital,* 199 Minn. 113, 271 N.W. 109 (1937), the court held the hospital was negligent because a nurse with a severe cough, of which other nurses were aware, attended a newborn. The nurse was later found to have tuberculosis. The court found that the death of the infant from acute miliary tuberculosis was caused by contact with the nurse and that the hospital breached its duty by failing to take the infected nurse off duty [59]. In *Hurley v. Nashua Hospital Association,* 191 A. 649, 650 (N.H. 1937),

however, the plaintiff's evidence was insufficient to establish that the plaintiff's nosocomial pneumonia was caused by a nurse suffering from a severe cold.

Cases in which injury resulted because hospital policies or standards of care were blatantly violated appear most frequently to result in hospital liability. In *Kapuschinsky v. United States,* 248 F. Supp. 732, 259 F. Supp. 1 (D.S.C. 1966), hospital policy was violated when a nurses' aide was allowed to care for a sick premature infant. The infant developed a severe staphylococcal infection; subsequently, the aide's nose and throat were found to be colonized with *Staphylococcus aureus.* The court found the government, which operated the hospital, remiss in its duty in two respects, either one of which was sufficient to prevail:

(1) It permitted an inexperienced Corps Wave to come in "critical contact" with plaintiff whose susceptibility to infection was well known, in violation of proper medical standards; and (2) it permitted this "critical contact" without a complete physical examination of the Corps Wave, including appropriate laboratory tests, before she began to work in the premature nursery [73].

In the case of *Thompson v. Methodist Hospital,* 367 S.W.2d 134 (Tenn. 1962), an action was brought against a hospital based on injuries allegedly sustained by a newborn and his parents from a staphylococcal infection contracted by the baby. The baby allegedly transmitted the infection to his parents. Plaintiffs attempted to show that an intern who examined the plaintiff's mother when she was at the hospital was a carrier of the infection, that a practical nurse with a boil appeared in the hospital from time to time, and that there had been other failures to follow aseptic technique. The court dismissed the case, finding that there was no evidence that either the intern or the nurse in question had ever come in contact with the infant or that the alleged events had in fact occurred while the infant and his mother were patients in the hospital. The court stated that the infant's infection could be attributed to other causes and that the degree of care exercised by the hospital at the time met in every detail the local standard of care. The court concluded that if, under the evidence in this case, the hospital were held liable for the infection, then few hospitals could afford the financial risks of having a child born within their walls.

The case of *Peck v. Charles B. Towns Hospital,* 275 App. Div. 302, 89 N.Y.S.2d 190 (1949), is another example of the need to provide a higher standard of care in special situations. The plaintiff, a drug abuser, established that the skin of drug addicts is highly susceptible to infection. The court held that the hospital should have been aware of his unusual susceptibility to infection and therefore his skin should have been disinfected more carefully before placement of an intravenous catheter.

An outbreak of streptococcal infection demonstrates that maintaining the standard of care can minimize the potential for successful litigation. An operating room circulating nurse was found to be the source of an outbreak of ten postoperative wound infections due to group-A streptococci (GAS) during a four-month period. After penicillin eradicated the nurse's colonization with GAS, she was allowed to return to work. Five months later two additional cases of GAS postoperative wound infections occurred; the same nurse was subsequently found to be recolonized with this organism. The hospital had followed the CDC recommendations, and since there had been no previous case of a subsequent recolonization with GAS reported in the medical literature, the hospital may be able to defend itself from suits on the grounds of having satisfied the standard of care. This case, not yet adjudicated at this writing, raises questions regarding how hospitals should respond to similar situations in the future [8].

## CONTAGIOUS PATIENTS SEEKING PREMATURE HOSPITAL DISCHARGE

When a patient who is actively infected with a communicable disease seeks discharge from the hospital against medical advice, the general rule that a patient of sound mind may leave the hospital at any time he or she chooses does not apply. In such cases hospitals generally have the lawful authority to detain the patient. In fact many state public health laws provide the authority to restrain a contagious patient from leaving. Hospital legal counsel and public health authorities should be consulted immediately in such situations.

## INFORMED CONSENT

Patients should be fully informed of the risks of medical procedures, including the risk of contracting infection [3]. Decisions in some cases have suggested that because infection is an inevitable risk over which the physician and hospital have no control, there is no legal obligation to warn of its dangers, which are widely known to the public. For example, in *Butler v. Berkeley*, 25 N.C. App. 325, 213 S.E.2d 571, 582 (1975), the court ruled that risk of infection is known to any person of ordinary sophistication and that "the

probability of infection was not so great as to warrant advising plaintiff of the possibility." Failure to inform the plaintiff that an infection could have resulted from surgery did not result in liability in *Tripp v. Pate*, N.C. App. 271 S.E.2d 407 (1980), because the failure to inform the patient of the risk was not a proximate cause of the injury.

In another case involving a postoperative infection, *Contreras v. St. Luke's Hospital, et al.*, 78 Cal. App. 3d 919, 144 Cal. Rptr. 647, 653 (1978), the court found that the defendant physician, who informed the plaintiff before surgery that infections occurred in one out of one hundred operations, had complied with the disclosure rule. The court concluded, "It is a matter of common knowledge that infections may have serious consequences and at times are stubbornly resistant to treatment, and . . . the doctor was not required to calculate and give information as to how long the plaintiff might have to be hospitalized or as to what specific treatment might be required in the unlikely event that an infection occurred.

Decisions in the 1980s, however, have indicated that patients are entitled to all relevant information to assess risks associated with their medical care [50]. In *Harwell v. Pittman*, No. 82 CA. 0397, Court of Appeal of Louisiana, First Cir., Slip Opinion, Feb. 22, 1983, the court concluded that the patient was not adequately informed of the material risks of postoperative infection. The plaintiff underwent an elective cholecystectomy without being informed that the risks of infection were greater in his case due to his obesity. The plaintiff alleged that had he been so advised, he would not have consented to the proposed surgery.

To establish patients' awareness of hospital infections, some attorneys have suggested that hospital admission consent forms should state that infections are a risk associated with any hospitalization and that there is no assurance that the patient will not contract an infection. Operative consent forms in many hospitals state that infections are a possible complication of surgical procedures [75].

As discussed in the section Posttransfusion Infection and Litigation, the patient's risk of contracting hepatitis from blood products should be discussed, if appropriate, when obtaining informed consent. In the case of *Moore v. Underwood Memorial Hospital*, 371 A.2d 105 (N.J. App. 1977), a physician was sued for failing to warn the patient of the risks of posttransfusion hepatitis. The physician avoided liability because the patient had taken a course in hematology, was the son of a physician, and was presumed to be familiar with such risks. A federal appeals court, interpreting Tennessee law, found that the physician need not have warned the patient of the risk of contracting hepatitis because the likelihood at the defendant hospital of contracting this infection was remote (*Sawyer v. Methodist Hospital*, 522 F.2d 1102 [6th Cir. 1975]). Despite the finding in this case, warning patients of the risk of hepatitis associated with transfusions is appropriate for both the patient's information and the provider's protection.

## POSTOPERATIVE INFECTIONS

Malpractice claims filed against surgeons commonly involve infections [7,53]. As in all categories of potential liability, one key element in such suits is whether the provider met the standard of care. In *Fluhrer v. Ritter*, Sup. Ct., Nassau Co., 845-1956, N.Y.L.J. p. 12, col. 2, (Ap. 1962) [23], the plaintiff successfully sued the hospital because its employees negligently allowed him to contract a postoperative infection in the operating room. The testimony of a pathologist and an orthopedic surgeon established that they had performed a "clean" operation in the same operating room that had previously been used for a "dirty" (contaminated) operation, and that this was at variance with good hospital practice. In *Bartlett v. Argonaut Insurance Companies*, 258 Ark. 221, 523 S.W.2d 385 (1975), a malpractice action against a hospital was brought by a patient who had a postoperative staphylococcal infection. The court ruled that although hospital floors were not swept daily and some nurses wore their uniforms from home, there was no proof that these hospital activities, inappropriate as they were, caused the patient's infection. The court held that "one of the known hazards to hospitalization and to conducting surgical procedures is postoperative infection" and that the germ causing the infection "could have entered her body in many ways and from many sources." The court refused to apply *res ipsa*, stating, "It is impossible for a hospital to be in complete control of a staph germ which may be brought in by the patient."

In *Denneny v. Siegel*, 407 F.2d 433 (3rd Cir. 1969), the plaintiff alleged her infection occurred because she was wheeled into an operating room for emergency surgery by a person wearing street clothes rather than operating-room attire. This plaintiff lost the case because there was no evidence to prove a connection between the alleged negligence and the subsequent infection.

Organisms causing postoperative infections are those frequently present in many "normal" people. This observation has been used to counter plaintiffs' allegations of negligence in cases involving postoperative infections. For example, in *Roark v. St. Paul Fire & Marine Insurance Company, et al.*, 415 So.2d 295, 297 (La. 1982), a staphylococcal infection occurred at the plaintiff's surgical site. Evidence established that standard procedures were followed by the hospital to establish the sterility of the supplies and instruments and that the environment met or exceeded national standards. An expert testified that:

Most individuals who contract a staph infection after surgery had the bacteria on their skin prior to surgery. Since the bacteria is found within the subcutaneous sweat glands and hair follicles of some patients, the organism may survive the cleansing of the skin with antiseptics. The doctor also testified that susceptibility to staph infection varies from individual to individual. With the present state of medicine, there is no practical way to determine prior to surgery who may be more susceptible to staph infection or who may be a "carrier" of the staph bacteria.

The expert concluded that staphylococcal infections are an unavoidable risk of surgery.

Control of airborne contamination of operating rooms has been a particularly controversial area. Some experts recommend use of "laminar flow" ventilation or ultraviolet irradiation units to reduce the risk of infection during operations. It was feared that failure to install such systems would result in liability if postoperative infection developed. However, the important question is whether the standard of care has been satisfied, not the particular vehicle used to meet it. The CDC states that "the ventilation recommended for modern OR's . . . appears to be adequate to remove most airborne microorganisms. In addition, laminar flow units are very expensive, and although currently under study, they have not been subjected to an adequate trial of their efficacy (or cost-effectiveness) in preventing infections" [16]. Hence, whether or not laminar flow units or other air-quality devices should be installed in operating rooms is a matter of professional judgment.

## OBLIGATION TO INFORM PATIENTS OF NOSOCOMIAL INFECTION

Courts have been increasingly insistent that physicians have a duty to disclose fully all pertinent facts concerning their patient's condition, even if the physician is convinced that he or she is acting in the patient's best interest by remaining silent. This obligation exists regardless of whether the condition is the result of negligence of the physician, a colleague, or the hospital. Failure to inform patients in such situations may result in liability for fraud (constructive fraud or fraudulent concealment) and conspiracy, as well as negligence. Punitive as well as compensatory damages may be awarded in these situations. In addition, courts have held that allegation of fraud stops the running of the statute of limitations [65,107]. Hence, providers should inform patients when a nosocomial infection has occurred [19].

## INFECTIONS DUE TO MEDICAL EQUIPMENT AND DEVICES

As many as 45 percent of all nosocomial infections (or more than 850,000 per year) may be related to the patient's exposure to a medical device; the urinary catheter is the most common [101,105]. Infections caused by contaminated instruments, equipment, or appliances may result in liability when the hospital is responsible for their sterilization. Many such cases have involved the use of improperly sterilized needles or unclean catheters [56,71,84,94,99]. When presterilized supplies become contaminated, however, and the contamination is not the result of hospital negligence, hospital liability should not result unless it can be established that the hospital should have been aware of the contamination. In *Shephard v. McGinnis,* 131 N.W.2d 475 (Iowa 1964), for example, the court held the hospital and physician liable for an infection because they should have been aware that certain sutures were contaminated.

The reuse of disposable "single-use" medical devices can be problematic. Some providers have reused devices such as hemodialyzers. Although it is not illegal to reuse such devices, manufacturers often recommend against it. In addition, professional organizations, associations, and government agencies have policies against such reuse. The 1983 JCAH *Accreditation Manual,* for example, states that "disposable items should not be reused" [55]. A panel of health-care providers and manufacturers of medical instruments sponsored by Georgetown University's Institute for Health Policy Analysis met in early 1984 to study the economic, ethical, and medical considerations of reusing disposable devices, and warned hospitals to reuse with "great caution." They called for a national survey to collect information, and in the interim recommended that hospitals develop appropriate standards and quality-control measures and thoroughly educate health professionals involved in reuse. If disposable devices are being used, the patient should be told the reasons. Patients should, in addition, be informed of the risks associated with the reuse of disposable products [97]. Administering special consent forms may also be appropriate in this

situation [5]. One other precaution for providers reusing disposable devices is to obtain documentation that physicians are aware of and approve of such reuse. When reuse of certain disposable devices is acceptable to a substantial segment of the medical community, this practice may indeed become acceptable to courts.

## ANTIBIOTICS

When antibiotics are used inappropriately, litigation may result [30]. Suits alleging negligence have focused on the injudicious use of antibiotics for surgical prophylaxis, failure to perform indicated cultures before administering antibiotics, and prescription of antibiotics that are either not clinically indicated or actually contraindicated for a particular patient [80]. In addition, the emergence of organisms resistant to multiple antibiotics may increase litigation in this area.

In *Lewis v. Golden State Memorial Hospital, et al.,* Los Angeles County Superior Court No. NWC40143, a jury awarded a patient $1,225,000 in damages after gentamicin prescribed for a surgical infection resulted in renal failure. This jury found that the presence of preoperative albuminuria should have alerted the physicians to the increased risk of nephrotoxicity in the patient [41,44,86,108].

JCAH standards require that hospitals monitor antibiotic use in their quality-assurance audit programs. The 1983 JCAH *Accreditation Manual* in the chapter entitled "Medical Staff" states under "Antibiotic Usage Review":

The actual review of the clinical use of antibiotics is a function of the medical staff. Although the direction of the review shall be determined by the medical staff, it should include review of the prophylactic use of antibiotics for inpatients, ambulatory care patients, and emergency care patients. Criteria for the prophylactic and therapeutic use of antibiotics should be established in problem areas, and departures from these criteria should be reviewed in a timely manner [55].

In the chapter on infection control it is stated that the program must provide for coordination with the medical staff on action relative to the findings from the regular review of the clinical use of antibiotics [55].

*Medicare and Medicaid Conditions of Participation* state that "there are measures which control the indiscriminate use of preventive antibiotics in the absence of infection, and the use of antibiotics in the presence of infection is based on necessary cultures and sensitivity tests" [110].

Clinical review of hospital antibiotic use may be performed by the medical staff as a whole, by a medical staff committee, or by a hospital clinical department. Assessment should include a clinical review as well as a numerical summary of antibiotic use. Trends of pathogen resistance reported by the hospital microbiology laboratory and pharmacy data on antibiotic use are appropriate in making these assessments. Institutional observations, actions, and recommendations regarding hospital antibiotic use should be documented in writing. Should it be appropriate to restrict the use of a particular antibiotic, this decision should be implemented through the medical staff or departmental chairpersons.

## DUTIES TO NONPATIENTS

Providers' duties extend to persons other than their patients. A hospital visitor who visits during regular visiting hours and remains in those parts of the premises open to visitors is an invitee to whom the hospital owes the duty of exercising ordinary care for his or her safety [48]. Case law has established that if a third party develops an infection from a patient because of a provider's negligence, damages may be awarded to the third party. The provider, therefore, has a duty either to prevent such incidents or to warn third parties that they could contract an infection [50]. Visitors of isolation patients, for example, should be warned of the risk of contracting the disease, and documentation should be made indicating the visitor was so advised [34]. The AHA recommends that suitable regulations pertaining to visitors are imperative in the control of nosocomial infection, and states:

To visit a patient is basically a privilege. Visits often have therapeutic value—or the converse—and hence should be subject to the control of the attending physician. The rules and regulations regarding visiting should take into consideration such aspects as the areas of special risks of infection, the particular needs of individual patients, and the peak work periods of staff [2].

The case of *Livingston v. Gribetz,* 549 F. Supp. 238, (S.D.N.Y. 1982), is an example of litigation arising from alleged exposure to a contagious patient. In this case, a nurse alleged that she contracted herpes encephalitis because of contact with an infant suffering from herpes. The nurse sued the infant's pediatrician on the grounds that the pediatrician failed to institute or monitor proper isolation procedures for the child

and the nurse. The pediatrician prevailed, however, because the court held that there was no evidence of a duty owed to the nurse or breach of duty. Furthermore, proximate cause was not established since there was no proof that room placement, use of gloves, or donning of masks and gowns would have prevented the nurse from becoming infected with the virus.

## NEW LEGAL TRENDS: STRICT LIABILITY OR BREACH OF IMPLIED WARRANTY

Liability is usually based on finding fault, or negligence. Attorneys, however, have sought to assert that providers are liable on a theory of strict liability in tort or breach of implied warranty [13,42,82]. Under these theories, a plaintiff need not allege or prove a negligent act or omission to establish liability. The genesis of these theories is found in the Uniform Commercial Code concerning implied warranty of fitness for a particular purpose. The implied warranty of fitness provides that when a merchant knows that a product is purchased for a particular use and is relied on to provide the correct product, an implied-in-law warranty arises that the product provided should be suitable for the particular use.

Proponents of applying this theory to health-care litigation argue that the implied warranty applies to a hospital room and warrants that the room is infection-free. This argument has not prevailed to date. It has been suggested that an approach more successful for plaintiffs may be to establish that an implied contract, under which the hospital had infection control obligations, arose between a patient and the hospital at the time of admission. In *Hall v. City of Huntsville,* 278 S.2d 708, 710 (Ala. 1973), for example, the court found an implied contract, but only to ensure a reasonable degree of infection control. The plaintiff developed a hip infection after numerous injections. There was no proof, however, that the infection resulted from the defendant's failure to give proper care and attention to the plaintiff. The plaintiff was still obligated to establish negligence or nonperformance because "to charge an implied contract to keep the plaintiff safe from infection, and then to prove merely that an infection did occur, would amount to equating the hospital's duty to that of an insurer."

While efforts to establish liability without negligence have failed in many cases involving infections, courts have applied strict liability in tort and warranty liability in cases in which a patient contracted viral hepatitis following a blood transfusion [100].

## POSTTRANSFUSION INFECTION AND LITIGATION

Liability for negligence may be imposed when a patient contracts an infection from a blood transfusion [11,48,88,91,109]. Infections acquired through blood transfusions include viral hepatitis, syphilis, malaria, toxoplasmosis, brucellosis, cytomegalovirus [62], and acquired immunodeficiency syndrome (AIDS). As a general rule, to incur liability there must be a reliable test available to detect the particular infection in the donor blood. Since tests are available to detect the presence of syphilis, failure to do so has resulted in liability, such as in *Giambozi v. Peters,* 127 Conn. 380, 16 A.2d 833 (1940). Because posttransfusion viral hepatitis is not universally preventable by donor screening, however, acquisition of this disease per se does not imply negligence.

Early cases, such as *Perlmutter v. Beth David Hospital,* 308 N.Y. 100, 123 N.E.2d 792 (1954), rehearing denied, 308 N.Y. 812, 125 N.E.2d 869 (1955), held that a hospital was performing a "service" rather than a "sale" in furnishing blood to its patients; therefore no warranty of fitness was implied. Under this interpretation, hospitals could not incur liability related to administering blood without proof of negligence. The "sales-service" dichotomy has controlled most of the posttransfusion viral hepatitis case law subsequent to *Perlmutter* [60]. As a reaction to difficulty in establishing negligence in posttransfusion cases, some courts have categorized the administration of blood components as the sale of a product, using product liability or implied warranty of fitness theories to impose liability. As the following case attests, whether blood is classified as a "service" or "product" assumes importance.

*Cunningham v. MacNeal Memorial Hospital,* 266 N.E.2d 897 (Ill. 1970), held that because a transfused patient acquired hepatitis, the hospital was liable even though not negligent. This decision was made despite the lack of a reliable test for the presence of hepatitis virus in donor blood. The court apparently preferred to compensate the innocent patient rather than find for those who provided the blood for a fee [9]. In *Hoffman v. Misericordia Hosp. of Philadelphia,* 439 Pa. 501, 267 A.2d 867 (1970), a plaintiff successfully used a breach of implied warranty theory in a case regarding the transfusion of "impure" blood. Most decisions, however, have denied liability under the warranty theory.

Since the *Cunningham* decision, virtually every state has enacted remedial legislation that classifies blood transfusions as services (adopting the *Perlmutter* rule and precluding strict liability) in an attempt to limit liability for adverse effects to those unusual cases in which negligence can be demonstrated [10,67]. In many states, however, these statutes fail to state explicitly that blood banks and hospitals that administer blood components are immune from liability in the absence of negligence [100]. Some new lawsuits concerning transfusion-related AIDS are challenging state laws that protect blood transfusions from product liability claims. It has been suggested that the new AIDS litigation may force states to reexamine their laws on blood transfusions.

Efforts to apply *res ipsa* generally fail in posttransfusion hepatitis cases because the first criterion (the injury does not ordinarily happen without negligence) is not met. In *Morse v. Riverside Hospital,* 44 Ohio App.2d 422, 339 N.E.2d 846, 848 (1974), for instance, the court stated that "no presumption that the hospital is negligent can be drawn solely from the fact that the patient contracted hepatitis following a blood transfusion, and the patient cannot recover damages on the theory of *res ipsa loquitur.*" The case of *Mullins v. Bexar County Hospital District,* 535 S.W.2d 44, 45–46 (Tex. 1976), however, indicates that *res ipsa* in certain situations might be successful. In this case the plaintiff developed a posttransfusion infection caused by contamination of either the IV apparatus or the blood. Expert testimony was unable to establish which caused the infection, and the judge reversed a jury verdict for the plaintiff, stating, "Under these circumstances, the jury could do no more than guess or speculate as to which was, in fact, the cause of the infection, and it was improper to permit the jury to make the choice." If the burden had been shifted from the plaintiff to the defendant using *res ipsa,* another result might have occurred [47].

Established blood bank practices; accreditation standards; and state and federal statutes, regulations and guidelines may all play a role in establishing standards of care for transfusion services. Recent Public Health Service (PHS) recommendations for the prevention of AIDS [17], for example, might be scrutinized by a court seeking to establish the appropriate standard of care.

Although hospitals normally are not held responsible for contaminated blood obtained from community blood banks, hospitals have been required to scrutinize the sources from which they obtain blood. This includes ascertaining that the supplier is in fact screening donors in accordance with professional standards [46]. Federal requirements promulgated by the Food and Drug Administration provide that blood must be labeled "paid donor" or "volunteer donor" [20]. Many states also require such labeling.

A recent Oklahoma Supreme Court decision relates

to this practice. In *Gilmore v. St. Anthony Hospital, et al.*, 598 P.2d 1200 (Okl. 1979), the court ruled that a woman who contracted posttransfusion hepatitis could sue the blood bank for negligence because the bank may have failed to ensure safe sources. The observation that hepatitis occurs more frequently in a paid donor system determined the outcome of this case.

As discussed in the section Informed Consent, patients should be informed about the risks involved in the use of blood products.

## ROLE OF MEDICAL RECORDS IN HOSPITAL INFECTION LIABILITY

Statutes and regulations concerning medical records vary from state to state. Some states require that the record contain minimum categories of information. Other statutes stipulate that records should be "adequate," "accurate," or "complete." Other jurisdictions set out requirements for medical records in greater detail, addressing such concerns as timeliness, retention procedures, and requirements for maintenance, signature, and filing. Medicare and Medicaid regulations and the standards of the JCAH should be adhered to. In the context of infection control, the 1983 JCAH *Accreditation Manual* states:

Medical records must accurately reflect in the final diagnosis or list of complications all infections occurring during hospitalization. However, the medical staff should determine whether or not infection control report forms are to be subsequently filed in the patient's medical record [55].

Medical records are often critically important in defending against a charge of negligence. A complete and accurate record of the patient's care is among the best defenses in malpractice litigation. Failure to maintain accurate, complete, and current records has frequently enhanced plaintiffs' assertions of negligence. Speculative comments should not be included in the chart, nor should blame be assigned for an outbreak. The notation of "nosocomial infection," for instance, should be written in a chart only after such an infection is confirmed.

If a patient has been determined to pose a risk of spreading infection to other patients, recommendations of infection control practitioners should be recorded in the medical record and filed with the hospital administration [35].

Although it has been suggested that infection control reports in cases of nosocomial infection should not be included in the progress notes of the patient's chart, others feel that such reports should indeed appear in the physician's progress notes to establish that the managing physician knows of the report [49].

## INFECTION CONTROL COMMITTEE REPORTS

According to the JCAH, hospital infection control programs are to include a multidisciplinary committee that recommends "corrective action based on records and reports of infections and infection potentials among patients and hospital personnel" [55]. Plaintiffs' attorneys, not surprisingly, may be interested in the proceedings, records, and reports of these committees. Accordingly, protection of the patient's confidentiality, names of personnel involved in hospital infection surveillance, and the infection control reports themselves have become controversial issues. Whether or not these records may be disclosed is an unresolved issue. Courts have sought to balance the desire of infection control personnel to maintain confidentiality with plaintiffs' need for information to support their allegations. In response to court decisions that have found infection control program records discoverable, the majority of states have enacted statutes to protect such records.

Case law has shown that the protection these statutes offer varies considerably among states. In *Davidson v. Light*, 79 F.R.D. 137, 25 F.R. Serv.2d 137 (Colo. 1978), the defendant hospital was ordered to produce the infection control report of the hospital's Infection Control Committee. The court concluded that free discussion among hospital employees during committee meetings would be relatively unaffected by the discovery of factual data used in producing the committee's report.

In *Spears v. Mason*, 303 So.2d 260 (La. 1974), which concerned an alleged postoperative infection, the court ordered the defendant hospital to disclose hospital Infection Control Committee reports related only to the plaintiff's case and the period of his hospitalization. *Young v. King*, 136 N.J. Super. 127, 344 A.2d 792 (1975), involved a fatal staphylococcal infection. The plaintiff's subpoena for the records was allowed because the court held that the statutory privilege protecting the records of the Utilization Review Committee applied only to that committee. Records of other committees, even if they were also involved in quality review functions, were not held to be protected.

In a contrasting decision an Oklahoma court, in *City of Edmond v. Parr*, 587 P.2d 56, 57 (Okl. 1978), agreed that the records of the Hospital Infectious Disease Control Committee were protected by the statute that prevented disclosure of "all information, interviews, reports, statements, memoranda, or other data relating to the condition and treatment of any person . . . for the purpose of reducing morbidity or mortality . . . (by) . . . any in-hospital staff committee." In a broader opinion, *Texarkana Memorial Hospital, Inc. v. Jones,* 551 S.W.2d 33 (Tex. 1977), the Texas Supreme Court held that the Texas statute protected the records and proceedings of any hospital committee.

In *Lang v. Abbott Laboratories,* 59 A.D.2d 734, 398 N.Y.S.2d 577 (1977), the plaintiff alleged she contracted septicemia from contaminated intravenous fluids manufactured by the defendant. The plaintiff's attempt to obtain records documenting the incidence of septicemia during the years before and following her admission was denied by the lower court. Because the hospital and staff were not parties to the suit, however, the appellate court allowed release of the records.

By avoiding written speculation when recording observations, members of hospital Infection Control Committees can minimize potential medicolegal problems [74]. An infection control nurse's written observations on a *S. aureus* outbreak in a newborn nursery exemplify this type of written speculation: the nurse's report stated that the use of float personnel and inadequate facilities "contributed to" the outbreak. In the absence of data documenting the source of the outbreak, using the phrase "may have contributed" would be more accurate and less damaging to the hospital should litigation occur [49].

## EMPLOYEE HEALTH

Hospitals have a duty to protect the health of personnel as well as patients. In the absence of specific federal and state occupational safety and health laws and regulations, an employer is subject to the "general duty" to provide a safe workplace. Under federal law, 29 U.S.C. 654 (a)(1), the duty exists to furnish employment and place of employment "which are free from recognized hazards that are causing or are likely to cause death or serious physical harm." Some courts interpret this to mean that an employer must use all "feasible" means to abate hazards, while others look to industry practice. State laws also should be examined for employee safety requirements.

Transmission of infection both to and from employees has been described in hospital outbreaks of rubella, pertussis, hepatitis B, measles, and Legion-

naires' disease. The following publications address responsibilities of hospitals in the area of employee health and are likely sources of the applicable standard of care: the JCAH's *Accreditation Manual* [55], the CDC's *Guidelines for the Prevention and Control of Nosocomial Infections* [16], and the AHA's *Infection Control in the Hospital* (recommendations of the AHA's Committee on Infections within Hospitals) [2]. The JCAH's *Accreditation Manual* states that an infection control program must include "a practical system for reporting, evaluating, and maintaining records of infections among patients and personnel. This must include assignment of responsibility for the ongoing collection and analytic review of such data, as well as for required follow-up action . . . input into the content and scope of the employee health program . . . and orientation of all new employees as to the importance of infection control, personal hygiene, and their responsibility in the program, and documented in-service education for all departments and services relative to infection, prevention, and control" [55] (see Chapter 2).

### Medical Examination of Prospective Employees
Applicants for hospital employment should provide a medical history and undergo a physical examination. It may also be appropriate to evaluate the immune status of such persons. Hospital employee immunization is discussed in a later section.

### Surveillance of Personnel
Hospitals should maintain ongoing surveillance of infectious disease and carrier states in personnel. Special care should be taken to monitor staff in high-risk areas such as nurseries and hemodialysis units. Employees should be instructed to report to their supervisor or employee health service when ill [39].

The Study on the Efficacy of Nosocomial Infection Control (SENIC Project) included interviews with selected hospital personnel involved in infection surveillance and control in a sample of 433 hospitals. The authors' observations regarding hospital employees included the following:

The majority of U.S. hospitals are routinely performing the recommended tests to detect potentially contagious infections among their employees, and hospitals with employees at presumably higher risk of acquiring such infections (e.g., those with hemodialysis units) are more likely to be performing the appropriate screening tests. There appears to be, however, a sizable minority of hospitals in which the appropriate screening tests are not being offered and many in which unnecessary but expensive screening procedures (for example, routine culturing of employees) are continuing despite recommendations to the contrary [40].

*Immunization of Personnel*

Immunization of personnel is an important component of hospital infection control programs. Records of the immunization status of employees should be maintained. The PHS's Immunization Practices Advisory Committee (ACIP), the AHA's Committee on Infections within Hospitals, and some medical specialty organizations routinely issue immunization recommendations. A number of states also require particular immunizations. New York, New Jersey, and Rhode Island, for example, currently have regulations dealing with rubella immunization. The North Carolina Division of Health Services recently issued a letter to the North Carolina Hospital Association requesting that members make hepatitis B vaccine available to high-risk health care employees (as defined by the hospital) at the hospitals' expense [83]. This request was based on recommendations of the ACIP and the AHA's Advisory Committee on Infections within Hospitals. In preparing this request, North Carolina also relied on a section of the North Carolina General Statutes that provides that "each employer shall furnish to each of his employees conditions of employment and a place of employment free from recognized hazards that are causing or are likely to cause death or serious injury or serious physical harm to his employees." The Texas Department of Health has issued a policy statement on prevention of hepatitis B [106].

Some states have issued immunization recommendations. The Massachusetts Department of Public Health recommends an immunizations program for hospital employees younger than 30 years of age who provide patient care [58]. In the absence of state or local requirements, immunization recommendations issued by such groups as the ACIP, the AHA Advisory Committee on Infections, and medical specialty organizations are likely to establish a nationwide standard of care. Hospitals are thus well advised to monitor such recommendations. If a hospital decides not to follow such recommendations, the reasons for the decision should be fully documented. Unfortunately, however, recommendations in this controversial area may be conflicting. Whether hospitals indeed should have special obligations in the area of employee immunizations remains unresolved. For example, even though the CDC [18], the AHA Advisory Committee [89], and the American College of Obstetricians and Gynecologists [1] currently recommend rubella immunization of hospital employees, a recent study did not find an increased risk of rubella transmission to pregnant patients in the healthcare setting compared to the community. This study concluded that "rubella screening and immunization

of health-care personnel will escalate health-care costs without substantially decreasing the incidence of congenital rubella except in young female health-care workers who voluntarily consent to immunization" [43]. A debate among members of the Vanderbilt University Hospital Infection Control Committee on the issue of mandatory immunization of hospital staff articulates the spectrum of opinions in this area:

*Counterpoint.* In the absence of state or local laws or regulations, one can anticipate legal difficulties in requiring immunization of current and new employees, especially those who are not actual employees of the hospital (e.g., community physicians, volunteers, private duty nurses). Many believe immunization should remain a personal, not an institutional, decision.

*Point.* The question of whether hospitals may require serologic evidence of rubella immunity or immunization as a condition of employment or practice in the hospital should not be a major legal issue. Our society often has supported compliance with health requirements for certain groups. For example, food handlers must pass health examinations and children in most states must have certain immunizations before they may attend school. If the Infection Control Committee recommended evidence of rubella immunity for employment or practice in the hospital and the policy were adopted by the hospital's governing board, the decision very likely would be supported by the courts [92].

In the absence of relevant case law, administrators and attorneys advising hospitals formulating a staff immunization policy should consider the following areas:

1. Applicable state and local statutes and regulations,
2. Consent forms which specifically address potential side effects,
3. Potential liability arising from either hospital administration of the vaccine or the hospital requirement of immunization as a condition of employment,
4. Current hospital liability insurance coverage vis-à-vis the program,
5. Applicability of the state worker's compensation law to claims that may arise,
6. Potential religious objections that might be raised by requiring vaccination [89].

It is likely that a court would decide that the health and safety of the public outweighs any individual interests asserted by employees challenging hospital immunization policy. In the event that an employee in a critical patient contact area (e.g., an obstetric clinic) refuses rubella immunization, the employee should be offered transfer to a noncritical area. Publicizing requirements and maintaining open communications with employees, medical staff, and volunteers should be an important component of any hospital staff immunization program.

### When Employees Refuse to Care for Contagious Patients

Patients suffering from incurable infections such as Lassa fever, Jakob-Creutzfeldt disease, and AIDS have at times encountered difficulty in obtaining care. Private hospitals in general are under no obligation to accept nonemergency patients they do not desire. Once a hospital admits a patient, however, it is obligated to provide appropriate care. Hence if the hospital staff refuses to care for a patient with a contagious disease, the hospital has a responsibility to transfer the patient to another facility where appropriate care will be provided. By providing inservice education of personnel with regard to the disease, its transmission, and precautions to be taken; by giving staff an opportunity to ventilate their anxieties; and by taking all appropriate measures to minimize the risk of infection transmission to staff, hospitals can do much to encourage staff willingness to care for patients with these infections. These measures notwithstanding, if the staff persist in their refusal to care for patients with certain infections, the issue becomes a legal and administrative problem to be resolved on an individual basis [103]. The advice of legal counsel should be solicited in such situations. Some would consider terminating the employment of these persons [36].

### Hospital Employees Who Contract Nosocomial Infections

Infections acquired on the job by hospital employees are ordinarily covered under the states' workers' compensation laws [66]. California law, for instance, specifically extends disability benefits to individuals ordered not to work because they are infected with, or suspected of being infected with, a communicable disease. This law applies to hospital employees acquiring infections in the course of their work as well as to healthy convalescent carriers awaiting clearance to return to work. It is hoped that such legislation may deter employees with communicable diseases from returning to their jobs surreptitiously without clearance to avoid financial hardship [63].

When seeking coverage under workers' compensation laws, a hospital employee alleging he or she contracted an infection on the job must establish that the infection was not acquired outside the working environment. Such an employee may have to prove that the risk of acquiring the infection as a hospital employee was greater than the general public's risk [77].

In one such case, *Russell v. Camden Community Hospital,* 359 A.2d 607 (Me. 1976), a nurses' aide was awarded compensation after applying ointment to a tuberculous ulcer and subsequently developing tuberculosis. An electroencephalogram (EEG) technician in *Melamed v. Montefiore Hospital,* 182 Pa. Super. 482, 128 A.2d 129 (1956), alleging she developed tuberculosis from exposure to infected patients at work, was awarded compensation after it was established that several hundred people with tuberculosis had been inpatients during this woman's period of employment. That the technician had not performed EEGs on any of these patients did not influence the award. In *Evans v. Indiana University Medical Center,* 121 Ind. App. 679, 100 N.E.2d 828 (1951), a plumber who occasionally worked in an isolation ward and once in a room occupied by a patient with tuberculosis was denied compensation because his exposure to the disease was considered too uncertain.

Hospital employee infections other than tuberculosis have also resulted in litigation. In *Furchtsam v. Binghamton General Hospital,* 24 App. Div.2d 786, 263 N.Y.S.2d 746, 747 (1965), a general duty nurse who developed a staphylococcal middle ear infection was awarded compensation. The court held that ". . . the close contacts of a hospital nurse inherent in caring for infected patients enhances the risk of contracting the disease." Compensation was awarded to the wife of a laboratory technician who died after being exposed to viral hepatitis. The court in *Booker v. Duke Medical Center,* 256 S.E.2d 189 (N.C. 1979), ruled that even though viral hepatitis may be contracted by people outside the laboratory environment, the technician's job "exposed him to a greater risk of contracting the disease than members of the public or employees in general." In addition, there was no evidence that he was exposed to viral hepatitis outside of the laboratory or that he had received any previous injections or transfusions.

In *Sacred Heart Medical Center v. Department of Labor & Industries,* 600 P.2d 1015 (Wash. 1979), workers' compensation was awarded to a nurse who contracted hepatitis. There was no evidence to establish that she had contracted this disease at work. After examining her life-style, however, the court concluded it was most likely that she acquired hepatitis in the course of her employment. Entrance employee health evaluations may prove useful later should employees allege contraction of infection on the job. Detailed histories regarding previous infections and immunizations, preemployment tuberculin tests, chest radiographs, and serologic studies may be helpful in this context [77]. In addition, it may be useful to keep records of the room location of patients (for this purpose there is no need to use patient names) infected with contagious diseases to help determine possible exposure to a specific infection [77].

Workers receiving injuries resulting from mandatory hospital employee health examinations or immunizations are eligible for workers' compensation. Whether such examinations or immunizations are mandated by government authorities or specifically by the hospital has not influenced the awarding of workers' compensation [61].

In recent years the exclusive remedy doctrine, holding that negligence actions against employers are barred, has been eroded. The growing volume of such litigation reflects a trend away from strict interpretation of the exclusive remedy doctrine and appears to be at odds with the no-fault approach of the workers' compensation system [102]. In *McBroom v. Zevallos,* 145 Ga. 375, 244 S.E.2d 19 (1978), for example, a laboratory worker allegedly acquired coccidioidomycosis at work. Although workers' compensation benefits were granted, the worker's husband subsequently sued the laboratory director. The court held that it was a jury question as to whether the pathology department director was the "alter ego" of the hospital in relation to the circumstances that caused the death of the laboratory technician and thus was protected from suit as a third-party wrongdoer by the hospital's workers' compensation coverage.

## CONCLUSION

As long as hospital infections continue to occur, litigation is inevitable. Hospitals, their employees, and independent practitioners can minimize liability by monitoring and adhering to applicable standards of care in preventing and controlling infection.

## REFERENCES

1. American College of Obstetricians and Gynecologists. Rubella: A clinical update. *Technical Bulletin* No. 62, July 1981.
2. American Hospital Association. *Infection Control in the Hospital* (4th ed.). Chicago: American Hospital Association, 1979, pp. 39–40.
3. Annas, G. J. Informed Consent to Treatment. In *The Rights of Hospital Patients.* New York: Avon, 1975.
4. Annas, G. J., Glantz, L. H., and Katz, B. F. Malpractice Litigation. In *The Rights of Doctors, Nurses, and Allied Health Professionals: A Health Law Primer.* New York: Avon, 1981, p. 246.
5. Attorneys explain liability of hemodialyzer reuse. *Hosp. Infect. Control* 9:129, 1982.
6. Attorneys outline basics of IC malpractice cases. *Hosp. Infect. Control* 7:32, 1980.
7. Barnes, B. A. The challenge of cost containment, *Surg. Annu.* 14:392, 1982.
8. Berkelman, R. L., Martin, D., Graham, D. R., Mowry, J. L., and Allen, J. R. Streptococcal wound infections caused by a vaginal carrier. *J.A.M.A.* 247:2680, 1982.
9. Bernstein, A. H. *A Trustee's Guide to Hospital Law.* Chicago: Teach 'Em Inc., 1981, p. 59.
10. Bernstein, A. H. Legal implications of administering blood. *Hospitals* 55:43, 1981.
11. Bock, J. A. Liability for Injury or Death from Blood Transfusion. 59 ALR2d 768.
12. *Brannan v. Lankenau Hospital,* 417 A.2d 196 (Pa. 1980).
13. Carmichael, M. C. Liability of Hospital or Medical Practitioner under Doctrine of Strict Liability in Tort, or Breach of Warranty, for Harm Caused by Drug, Medical Instrument, or Similar Device Used in Treating Patient, 54 ALR3d 258.
14. *Carpenter v. Campbell,* 149 Ind. App. 189, 271 N.E.2d 163 (1971).
15. Castle, M. *Hospital Infection Control.* New York: Wiley, 1980, p. 233.
16. Centers for Disease Control. *Guidelines for the Prevention and Control of Nosocomial Infections. Introduction.* Springfield, VA: National Technical Information Service, U.S. Department of Commerce, 1981.
17. Centers for Disease Control. Prevention of acquired immune deficiency syndrome (AIDS): Report of the inter-agency recommendations. *Morbid. Mortal. Weekly Rep.* 32:101, 1983.
18. Centers for Disease Control. Rubella prevention. *Morbid. Mortal. Weekly Rep.* 30:37, 1981.
19. Chavigny, K. H., and Helm, A. Ethical dilemmas and the practice of infection control. *Law Med. Health Care* 10:169, 1982.
20. Classification Labeling Requirements, 21 C.F.R. 606.120 and 640.2, *et seq.*
21. *Contreras v. St. Luke's Hospital,* 78 Cal. App.3d 919; 144 Cal. Rptr. 647 (1978).
22. Cram, S. The hospital's obligation to protect patients from carriers of infectious diseases. *Medicolegal News* 7:11, 1979.
23. Creighton, H. Legal aspects of nosocomial infection. *Nurs. Clin. North Am.* 15:789, 1980.
24. Creighton, H. Nosocomial infections. *Supervisor Nurse* 12:60, 1981.
25. *Criss v. Angelus Hospital Ass'n of Los Angeles, et al.,* 13 Cal. App.2d 4 12, 56 P.2d 1274 (1936),

37 ALR2d 1290, Section 5.

26. Crook, G. B. Negligence. In 57 Am. Jur. 2d, Municipal, School, and State Tort Liability, Section 1.

27. Davis, R. P. Hospital's Liability for Injury or Death in Obstetrical Cases, 37 ALR2d 1284.

28. Drechsler, C. T. Physicians, Surgeons, and Other Healers. In 61 Am. Jur. 2d, Perpetuities and Restraints on Alienation, Section 219.

29. *Elam v. College Park Hospital,* 132 Cal. App.3d 332 (1982), opinion modified 122 Cal. App.3d 94a (1982).

30. Fifer, W. R. Infection control is quality control. *Am. J. Infect. Control* 9:121, 1981.

31. Frechette, A. L., and Swarthout, A. M. *Res Ipsa Loquitur* in Action Against Hospital for Injury to Patient, 9 ALR3d 1315.

32. *Fridena v. Evans,* 622 P.2d 463 (Ariz. 1980).

33. Frumer, L. R. (Ed.). *Personal Injury: Actions, Defenses, Damages, Hospitals and Asylums,* 1.06{5}. New York: Matthew Bender, 1982.

34. Griffith, J. L. Advise visitors of risks from isolated patients. *Hosp. Infect. Control* 7:53, 1980.

35. Griffith, J. L. Document recommendations in chart, with administration. *Hosp. Infect. Control* 8:111, 1981.

36. Griffith, J. L. Fire nurses who refuse to provide patient care. *Hosp. Infect. Control* 9:12, 1982.

37. Griffith, J. L. Hospitals have legal duty. *Hosp. Infect. Control* 9:52, 1982.

38. Griffith, J. L. Legal commentary. *Hosp. Infect. Control* 5:11, 1978.

39. Haley, R. W., and Emori, T. G. The employee health service and infection control in U.S. hospitals, 1976–1977. II. Managing employee illness. *J.A.M.A.* 256:962, 1981.

40. Haley, R. W., and Emori, T. G. The employee health service and infection control in U.S. hospitals, 1976–1977. I. Screening procedures. *J.A.M.A.* 246:847, 1981.

41. *Harris v. State through Huey P. Long Memorial Hospital,* 378 So.2d 383 (La. 1979).

42. Harrison, D. B. Application of Rule of Strict Liability in Tort to Person or Entity Rendering Medical Services, 100 ALR3d 1205.

43. Hartstein, A. I., Quan, M. A., Williams, M. L., Osterud, H. T., and Foster, L. R. Rubella screening and immunization of health care personnel: Critical appraisal of a voluntary program. *Am. J. Infect. Control* 11:8, 1983.

44. *Hawkes v. Mt. Sinai Hospital,* 426 N.Y.S.2d 745 (1980).

45. Henry, H. H. Physicians and Surgeons: *Res Ipsa Loquitur,* or Presumption or Inference of Negligence in Malpractice Cases, 82 ALR2d 1262.

46. *Hoder v. Sayet,* 196 So.2d 205 (Fla. App. 1967).

47. Horty, J. *Hospital Law.* Pittsburgh: Action-Kit for Hospital Law, 1978, 1981, pp. 2, 6.

48. Hospitals and Asylums, 40 Am. Jur. 2d, Highways, Streets, and Bridges, Sections 14.5, 26, 29, 33, 35.

49. Hospital records: Friends or foes in the courtroom? *Hosp. Infect. Control* 7:25, 1980.

50. Iffy, L., and Wecht, C. H. Medical-legal aspects of perinatal and surgical infections. *Legal Medicine 1980.* Philadelphia: Saunders, 1980, p. 177.

51. Illinois: Hospital Licensing Requirements, 1977 Sections 4-1.4 and 4-1.5.

52. Infection control in nursing care: Legalities. *Regan Report on Nursing Law* 22:1, 1982.

53. Infection therapy results in claims. *Hosp. Infect. Control* 8:14, 1981.

54. *Johnson v. Misericordia Community Hospital,* 301 N.W.2d 156 (Wisc. 1981).

55. Joint Commission on Accreditation of Hospitals. *Accreditation Manual for Hospitals.* Chicago: Joint Commission on Accreditation of Hospitals, 1983, pp. 70–74, 76, 104.

56. *Kalmus v. Cedars of Lebanon Hospital,* 132 Cal. App.2d 243, 281 P.2d 872, (1955).

57. Keeton, P. Medical negligence: The standard of care. *Tex. Tec L.R.* 10:351, 1979.

58. Klein, J. O. Management of infections in hospital employees. *Am. J. Med.* 70:920, 1981.

59. Kraut, J. Hospital's Liability for Exposing Patient to Extraneous Infection or Contagion, 96 ALR2d 1205.

60. Lance, P. Perlmutter and Its Progeny: Liability for Posttransfusion Serum Hepatitis. In Bertolet, M. M., and Goldsmith, L. S. (Eds.), *Hospital Liability Law and Tactics* (4th ed.). New York: Practicing Law Institute, 1980.

61. Larsen, A. *Workmen's Compensation for Occupational Injuries and Death.* New York: M. Bender, 1972, pp. 5–298.

62. Lasky, P. C. Principles of Liability. In Lasky, P. C. (Ed.), *Hospital Law Manual.* Rockville, Md.: Health Law Center, Aspen Systems Corporation 1983, pp. 4, 21, 37–38, 75.

63. Law gives disability to workers with communicable disease. *Hosp. Infect. Control* 5:17, 1978.

64. Lawyers predict new CDC guidelines will become standard of care. *Hosp. Infect. Control* 8:73, 1981.

65. LeBlang, T. R. Disclosure of injury and illness: Responsibilities in the physician-patient relationship. *Law Med. Health Care* 9:4, 1981.

66. Malone, W. S., and Plant M. L. *Cases and Materials on Workmen's Compensation.* St. Paul, Minn.:

West Publishing Co., 1963.

67. *McAllister v. American National Red Cross,* 240 S.E.2d 247 (Ga. 1977).

68. *McCall v. St. Joseph's Hospital,* 184 Neb. 1, 165 N.W.2d 85 (1969).

69. Medicare and Medicaid Conditions of Participation. 42 C.F.R. 405.1011 *et seq.*, Section 505.1022(c)(1)-(8).

70. *Mitchell County Hospital Authority v. Joiner,* 189 S.E.2d 412 (Ga. 1972).

71. *Moses v. St. Barnabas Hospital,* 130 Minn 1, 153 N.W. 128, (1915).

72. Nadel, A. G. Hospital's Liability for Negligence in Failing to Review or Supervise Treatment Given by Doctor, or to Require Consultation, 12 ALR4th 57.

73. Nottebart, H. C., Jr. Hospital-acquired staphylococcal infection transmitted by hospital personnel. *Infect. Control* 1:190, 1980.

74. Nottebart, H. C., Jr. Infection Control Committee reports. *Infect. Control* 1:47, 1980.

75. Nottebart, H. C., Jr. The law and infection control: The myth of negligence. *Infect. Control* 2:158, 1981.

76. Nottebart, H. C., Jr. Legal Aspects of Infection Control. In Cundy, K. R., and Ball, W. (Eds.), *Infection Control in Health Care Facilities: Microbiological Surveillance.* Baltimore: University Park Press, 1977, p. 199.

77. Nottebart, H. C., Jr. Nosocomial infections acquired by hospital employees. *Infect. Control* 1:257, 259, 1980.

78. Nottebart, H. C., Jr. Staphylococcal infection in hospital roommates. *Infect. Control* 1:105, 1981.

79. O'Brien, J. P. Emerging malpractice trends. *Hospitals* 57:60, and Note 17, 1983.

80. Olson, M. Nosocomial infections next target for malpractice suits. *Hosp. Med. Staff* 10:19, 22, 1981.

81. Orlikoff, J. E., Fifer, W. R., and Greeley, H. *Malpractice Prevention and Liability Control for Hospitals.* Chicago: American Hospital Association, 1981, p. 9.

82. Peters, B. M. The application of reasonable prudence to medical malpractice litigation: The precursor to strict liability? *Law Med. and Health Care* 9:21, 1981.

83. Peterson, R. N. Order requires North Carolina to pay Hepatitis B vaccination costs. *Health Law Vigil* 6:3, 1983.

84. *Posthuma v. Northwestern Hospital,* 197 Minn 304, 267 N.W. 221, (1936).

85. Practitioner outlines isolation problems. *Hosp. Infect. Control* 7:70, 1980.

86. Prosser, W. L. *Handbook of The Law of Torts* (3d ed.). St. Paul, Minn.: West Publishing Co., 1964, p. 146.

87. *Purcell v. Zimbelman,* 500 P.2d 335 (Ariz. App. 1972).

88. Purver, J. M. Liability for Injury or Death from Blood Transfusion, 45 ALR3d 1364.

89. Recommendations from AHA Office of the General Counsel. Hospital rubella control alert: Immunization recommendations, May 1981. *Infect. Control* 2:410 and Appendix A, 1981.

90. Salman, S. L., and Click, N. Risk manager must interact with infection control expert. *Hospitals* 54:52, 1980.

91. Shafer, N., Wilkenfeld, M., and Shafer, R. Blood Transfusion Reactions. In Wecht, C. (Ed.), *Legal Medicine 1980.* Philadelphia: Saunders, 1980, p. 207.

92. Schaffner, W., and Evans, M. E. Rubella immunization of hospital personnel: A debate. *Infect. Control* 2:389, 1981.

93. Shaw, J. W., Jr. Hospital's Liability for Negligence in Selection or Appointment of Staff Physicians or Surgeons, 51 ALR3d 981.

94. *Sheehan v. Strong,* 257 Mass 525, 154 N.E. 253, (1926).

95. Shipley, W. E. Hospital's Liability for Negligence in Failing to Review or Supervise Treatment Given By Individual Doctor, or to Require Consultation, 14 ALR3d 873.

96. *Shurpit v. Brah,* 30 Wis.2d 388; 141 N.W.2d 266 (1966).

97. Single-use devices should not be reused. *Hospitals* 54:157, 1980.

98. Slaven, T. How courts measure the standard of care. *Hosp. Med. Staff* 7:27, 1978.

99. *Sommers v. Sisters of Charity of Providence in Oregon.* 561 P.2d 603 (Ore. 1977).

100. Southwick, A. *The Law of Hospital and Health Care Administration.* Ann Arbor, Mich.: Health Administration Press, 1978, pp. 128, 351–352, 355, 358.

101. Stamm, W. E. Nosocomial infections due to medical devices. *Qual. Rev. Bull.* 5:23, 1979.

102. Stander, I. Current trends in workers' compensation. *Law Med. and Health Care* 10:71, 1982.

103. Stickler, B. K. Labor Law and Liability Considerations of Acquired Immune Deficiency Syndrome. Handout prepared by Wood, Lucksinger, & Epstein, 444 North Michigan Avenue, Suite 1150, Chicago, IL 60611.

104. *Tucson Medical Center v. Misevch,* 545 P.2d 958 (Ariz. 1976).

105. Valenti, W. M. Infection control in perspective:

Infections due to medical equipment and devices. *Infect. Control* 2:305, 1981.

106. Venable, Baetjer, and Howard. Legal Aspects of Preventive Health Care for Hospital and Health Care Workers: The Hepatitis B Vaccine. Handout prepared by Constance H. Baker, 2 Hopkins Plaza, 1800 Mercantile Bank and Trust Building, Baltimore, MD 21201.

107. Vogel, J., and Delgado, R. To Tell the Truth: Physicians' Duty To Disclose Medical Mistakes, 28 U.C.L.A. L. Rev. 52-94 (1980).

108. *Zito v. Friedman,* 430 N.Y.S.2d 78, 77 A.D.2d 514 (1980).

109. Zitter, J. M. Liability of Hospital, Physician, or Other Individual Medical Practitioner for Injury or Death Resulting from Blood Transfusion, 20 ALR4th 136.

110. 42 C.F.R. 405.1022(c)(6).

111. 42 C.F.R. 405.1022(c)(8).

# 14 THE INANIMATE ENVIRONMENT

Frank S. Rhame

The hypothesis that environmental microorganisms cause human disease readily arises from two incontestable observations: (1) our interaction with the inanimate environment is constant and close, and (2) environmental objects are usually contaminated, often with important human pathogens. Microbes are remarkably efficient at becoming dispersed to virtually all unprotected niches. Where there is moisture and at least small amounts of organic material, proliferation to large numbers occurs. Even on dry, infertile surfaces, microbes survive in various relatively inactive states. Unfortunately, while it is relatively easy to assess the prevalence of microorganisms in the environment, it is relatively hard to establish the role of the organisms in these environments as causes of human disease. Evaluating the evidence bearing on this matter is the fundamental task of this chapter.

Although the division of the world into the animate and the inanimate is sharper than most dichotomies, there are borderline situations. For instance, platelets awaiting transfusion, which are maintained under physiologic conditions so that active metabolism maintains their essential properties, might be considered either living or nonliving. Some would argue that viable viruses, when not infecting cells, are not alive. A "brain-dead" human maintained on a respirator to sustain organs for donation would not generally be considered part of the inanimate environment. Pus, while in a patient's wound or on the unwashed hands of a hospital worker, would not be considered part of the inanimate environment, but as soon as it is deposited on a fomite* it would.

Tradition is a factor in this issue. In the context of hospital infection control, there is a variety of living items that usually have been considered in discussions of the inanimate environment: potted plants, cut flowers, and fresh fruits. (In fact, if the inanimate environment were completely inanimate, it would not require consideration in this book!) Other problems often included in discussions of the inanimate environment are insect infestation and problems associated with animal visitation to patients. There is also a large number of inanimate objects and ma-

*The word *fomite*, although sometimes in disfavor, remains quite useful. A fomite is an inanimate object that may be contaminated with microorganisms and serve in their transmission. The word arose as a backformation from "fomites," which is the latin plural of *Fomes*. *Fomes* is a genus of fungus that was used as tinder. The dried fungus is porous and thus was considered "capable of absorbing and retaining contagious effluvia" [10].

The author thanks Jo Kill for typing and Su Reaney for proofreading.

terials that usually have not been considered. These are items that have a clear-cut potential for causing infection when contaminated; the need to achieve and maintain sterility is widely accepted (e.g., surgical instruments). Here too there are some borderline situations: the internal surfaces of respirator and anesthesia breathing circuits, water in humidifier reservoirs, endoscopes passed through nonsterile cavities, and pressure transducer heads. These items are considered in other chapters of this book.

The fomites to be discussed in this chapter include a large number of items of which the infection-causing potential, in routine circumstances, is not established. Determination of the proper management of these items produces a series of vexatious questions that frequently confront infection control personnel. It is not appropriate simply to dismiss these concerns with the assertion that no infection hazard has been fully demonstrated. Environmental objects may be heavily contaminated with recognized human pathogens. These objects may bring these organisms into close approximation to potential portals of entry. Even those skeptical of the infection-causing potential of ordinary patient-care objects and environmental surfaces advocate processing and cleaning methods [125] requiring decisions that may have considerable financial impact.

The simplistic black-or-white view that we generally apply to sterilization is not applicable to the items to be discussed. Rather, we have to contend with the difficulty of determining the appropriate degree of contamination. Rigorous research is hampered in this context because speciation of contaminating organisms becomes relevant. In some cases standards exist (e.g., dialysis water), but for the most part, no standards have been set and there is little rational basis for setting them.

We must also recognize that procedures for processing environmental items rest in part on aesthetic and achievability considerations. Carpets may not usually constitute an infection hazard, but fecal stains are unacceptable. We may be quite convinced that microorganisms on the walls and floors play no role in causing human disease, but the lay public's perception is exactly the contrary; in an era of increasing attention to marketing, visible dirt is undesirable. When standards have been set, formally or informally, they are often based on recognition of what reductions in microbial content can be consistently achieved with moderate effort rather than what levels are required to prevent infection. Some objects may be sterile as a by-product of manufacture. For instance, the protected outside surfaces of IV-bottle

stoppers are usually sterile, although manufacturers do not make the claim of sterility because it is burdensome to prove it to regulatory agencies. There are items that are not marketed as sterile but usually are and arguably should be. When contaminated, these items have been responsible for outbreaks: elastic bandages have caused *Rhizopus* [94] and *Clostridium perfringens* [106] skin infections; contaminated blood collection tubes have caused pseudobacteremias [69] and true bacteremias [121]; contaminated hand-care products have been implicated as a cause of infection [105]. Clinicians often perceive products that come in closed containers as sterile and use them as such even when they are not so marketed [33]. Most would find surprising the frequency of contamination of oral medications (especially those of animal origin), ointments, nasal sprays, and lotions [72].

The occurrence of outbreaks of nosocomial infection due to contaminated inanimate objects is often invoked as a basis for concern about the inanimate environment as a cause of endemic nosocomial infection. In fact, most outbreaks of nosocomial infection are associated with person-to-person spread or due to contamination of an item that should be sterile [87, 128]. Such an item often can be traced ultimately to a contaminated reservoir. Such outbreaks contribute to our understanding of the pathophysiology of nosocomial infection, but they do not constitute a significant numerical contribution to the problem of nosocomial infection. These outbreaks stimulate us to seek improved methods of achieving or maintaining sterility of objects that should be sterile (a matter not considered additionally in this chapter), but are not a substantial basis for concern about environmental contamination.

## ENVIRONMENTALLY ALTERED MICROORGANISMS

It seems paradoxical that environmental objects can frequently be contaminated by human pathogens while only rarely contributing to human infection. A potential explanation lies in the concept of "environmentally damaged organisms." This concept has been rigorously demonstrated for *Streptococcus pyogenes* by Rammelkamp, Perry, and their colleagues. In a classic series of experiments, they studied streptococcal transmission in army barracks. Air, dust, and personal effects such as blankets were more often contaminated by streptococci when recruits had streptococcal illness or pharyngeal colonization. However, recruits who had been issued freshly laundered, *Strep-tococcus*-free blankets acquired streptococcal infection or pharyngeal colonization just as often as barracks-mates issued highly contaminated blankets [108]. These workers directly assessed the infectious potential of naturally contaminated barracks dust. Dust samples were repeatedly dispersed in small enclosures (air samples showed between 1 and 1,600 streptococci per cubic foot) without producing pharyngeal colo-nizations or infection in volunteers within the enclo-sures. Six volunteers had seventeen direct inoculations of dust containing 1,800 to 42,000 streptococci onto the posterior pharynx. There resulted only transient colonization lasting no more than 30 minutes [107]. Hypothesizing that dryness was responsible for the inability of the streptococci to produce colonization, they assessed the infectious potential of oropharyngeal secretions that were mixed with sterile dust. Infection followed inoculation of wet dust or direct transfer of secretions to volunteers. When the inoculated dust was permitted to dry for 4 to 8 hours, however, during which time there was no decrease in the num-ber of recoverable organisms on artificial media, it did not cause infection [112]. The designation of this phenomenon as "environmental damage" reflects a rather anthropocentric perspective. The streptococci presumably have shifted their metabolism to meet their current needs. The physiologic basis of bacterial adaptation to desiccation has been explored [84] and involves substantial shifts in internal constituents.

The Perry-Rammelkamp streptococcal studies set a pattern recently confirmed by Maki, et al [88]. Much of the time the direction of transfer of organ-isms is from humans to the environment rather than vice versa. Thus even when an association is dem-onstrated between human disease and an increased prevalence of an organism in the environment, the causative role of environmental organisms cannot be considered established.

The loss of human pathogenicity associated with adaptation to the environment has been established for desiccated *Streptococcus pyogenes*. It seems plausible that other species have different adaptations to various environmental situations that would also reduce their pathogenicity for humans. For some organisms, how-ever, it is reasonable to speculate that the required adaptations are less debilitating. "Water bacteria" in moist environments might be in metabolic states less different from their most pathogenic state. Vi-ruses are probably either viable or not. *Clostridium difficile* as an environmental spore is more durable and might be more infectious than as a vegetative organ-ism. These matters are, at present, largely unexplored.

## METHODS OF STUDY

With the above generalities in mind, we confront the methodologic inadequacies that characterize most published studies asserting a causative role of inan-imate objects in human disease. There are six classes of evidence suggesting that a fomite has a role in causing disease due to a particular pathogen. They are ordered here by the rigor with which they estab-lish the point. Each argument is strengthened when subspecies or strain analysis of the implicated patho-gen shows similarity between human and environ-mental isolates.

1. *The organism can survive after inoculation onto the fomite.* This is the weakest form of evidence, yet good journals allocate space to these studies, which sometimes achieve widespread attention from the press. A case in point is the recent demonstration that herpes simplex virus can survive when inoc-ulated on hot-tub seats [102]. The finding was published despite the cogent words of the accom-panying editorial [47] pointing out the inconclu-siveness of the observation. At present, it is not possible to provide firm generalizations on the du-ration of survival required for significance.

2. *The pathogen can be cultured from in-use fomites.* This element is a sine qua non of the association but only a first step. When there is a demonstration that the pathogen is present more frequently or in higher concentration in association with infected humans this element is marginally strengthened. But, as mentioned previously, this association is as likely to arise from the patient infecting the environment as vice versa. When the pathogen cannot be cultured, other markers may be used (e.g., HBsAg in the case of hepatitis B [83]). When it is suspected that environmental adapta-tion may reduce pathogenicity, it is desirable that the detection method simulate the natural infec-tion (e.g., animal inoculation).

3. *The pathogen can proliferate in the fomite.* Whether proliferation must be demonstrated is largely a function of the size of the inoculum required to cause infection. For instance, this element is im-portant in the case of contaminated IV solution: most IV-fluid contamination is at low concentra-tions, and humans ordinarily tolerate a few or-ganisms given intravenously. For IV-fluid contam-ination to be a hazard, the organisms must have the ability and time to proliferate. In general, contaminated objects do not cause infection unless the contaminating organism can proliferate in the

contaminated environment or the contamination is heavy and occurs shortly before exposure.

4. *Some fraction of acquisition cannot be accounted for by other recognized methods of transmission.* An example of this type of evidence is found in the last in a series of studies that began with the classic demonstration of the importance of hands and contact in nursery acquisition by newborns of *Staphylococcus aureus*. In the final study of the series, Mortimer and colleagues [98] went to great lengths to eliminate contact transmission in a nursery in which index babies were colonized by *S. aureus*. At least 9 of 158 contact-protected babies became colonized. This (along with other observations) was taken as evidence that air was the vector of transmission.

This element may appear to be present simply because of the vicissitudes of biologic systems. It is inevitable that it will be difficult to account for all transmissions by any given mechanism. Implication of a fomite by exclusion of alternatives should be considered weak evidence unless a large fraction of transmissions cannot otherwise be accounted for. This line of logic can also lead to false exoneration of important mechanisms of transmission when several valid mechanisms, all operating at the steep portion of the dose-infection curve, are present [25].

5. *Case-control studies show an association between exposure to the contaminated fomite and infection.* Most well-studied epidemics implicating fomites include this element. One must always be cautious about projecting conclusions derived from the epidemic situation to conclusions about endemic infections. Case-control methodology is discussed in Chapter 5.

6. *Prospective studies isolating exposure to the contaminated fomite as the only perturbation show an association between the exposure and infection.* Ideally, the exposed group is selected randomly.

Only evidence from categories 5 and 6 should be considered strong enough to implicate a fomite. Unfortunately, the bulk of published studies of fomite transmission presents evidence of types 1 or 2. Accordingly, chapters such as this one often appear to be a litany of inconclusiveness.

Whenever possible in this chapter we eschew data of type 1 or 2 in favor of higher levels of evidence. We continue with an analysis of a variety of potential fomites that are usually nonsterile but are plausible enough causes of nosocomial infection to warrant discussion. We discuss the ultimate extension of concern about the inanimate environment: ultraclean protective environments for immunosuppressed patients. We conclude with sections on disinfection and sterilization and a rational routine program of microbiologic monitoring of inanimate objects in the hospital.

## AIR

There has probably been concern about air as a vehicle for transmission of infection for as long as there has been recognition of the transmissibility of disease. Surely more data have been generated for this fomite than for any other. Entire books [48,80] have been devoted to the subject, suggesting that concise summarization is difficult. As an indication of trends in this area, there were six articles dealing with airborne spread presented at the initial International Conference of Nosocomial Infections in 1970 and an estimate by Brachman [24] that between 10 and 20 percent of endemic nosocomial infections resulted from the airborne route. At the Second International Conference on Nosocomial Infections in 1982, however, only one presentation dealt with airborne organisms [86], and it dealt with the operating room. Air-quality standards and the treatment of air for operating rooms is discussed in Chapter 20.

Despite concern about air as a vector of disease, there are surprisingly few general surveys of the microbial content of hospital air with complete identification of the organisms recovered. This lack no doubt results from the formidable obstacles to such an undertaking. There is not yet a consensus on the optimal sampling method. (For a concise discussion of the available methods, see Groschell [59].) It is not even clear whether volumetric sampling is better than settling techniques. Volumetric sampling produces quantitative data that are more readily conceptualized; this technique is probably more relevant to situations in which a pathogen is inhaled. Settling techniques may be more relevant to infections that result from settling organisms (e.g., wound infections). Because the concentration of certain organisms in the air is small compared to the volumes that can be conveniently assessed, culturing air is often subject to considerable sampling error. Furthermore, there is tremendous variation in the microbial content of air, depending on location in the hospital, ventilation systems, concurrent human activity, and proximity to sources of organisms. Finally, the broadest based survey available [55,56] was performed over 20 years ago, which raises questions about its current applicability.

In the previously mentioned general survey, Greene and colleagues [55,56] found a mean organism count of roughly 10 to 20 organisms per cubic foot.* The highest counts were in waste storage and disposal areas, and slightly higher counts were in laundry handling areas. The lowest counts were in operating and delivery rooms. Roughly one-third of the organisms recovered were gram-positive cocci, roughly one-third gram-positive bacilli, and the remainder gram-negative bacilli or fungi. Gram-positive cocci constituted a higher proportion of the organisms in operating rooms; gram-positive bacilli (presumably mostly *Bacillus* species) constituted a higher proportion of the organisms in the laundry and waste storage areas; and gram-negative bacilli were relatively high in corridors.

More detailed consideration of air as a fomite is best made by specific organism. Airborne[†] person-to-person transmission of *Mycobacterium tuberculosis*, varicella-zoster virus, smallpox, influenza, and measles has been convincingly established and probably constitutes the major mechanism of spread. The epidemiology of rubella and mumps suggests they have similar transmission mechanisms. However, control of these infections in hospitals consists mainly of identifying patients with active infection and promptly placing them in isolation rooms with proper air control. Influenza control is a bit more complicated because infectious patients and personnel may have subtle or no respiratory symptoms during community outbreaks [15]. Preventing nosocomial influenza during community influenza outbreaks is one of the few solid rationales for human traffic control within hospitals.

*Staphylococcus Aureus*

There is a solid theoretical basis for concern about the importance of airborne transmission of *S. aureus*. Noble, probably the most avid student of this matter, summarizes information bearing on the origin of airborne *S. aureus* as follows [104]: Humans liberate approximately $3 \times 10^8$ squames per day. Because the size distribution of airborne particles containing *S. aureus* (about 4 to 25 $\mu$ in diameter) is approximately that of squames and well above the diameter of naked, single *S. aureus* cells (approximately 1 $\mu$

in diameter), it is presum[...] *S. aureus* organisms are c[...] (There is great variation [...] production by humans, b[...] the province of this chap[...] airborne.) Since particles [...] on the nasal turbinates, [...] satisfying closed loop may occur: proliferation of *S. aureus* on nasal mucosa, hand transfer of *S. aureus* to the skin, liberation on squames, airborne transport of squames, and impaction on the nasal mucosa. Hospital air contains approximately 0.02 *S. aureus* cfu per cubic foot of air [123].

Outbreaks of *S. aureus* (and *S. pyogenes*) surgical wound infection have been solidly linked to airborne spread from dispersers in the operating room (see Chapter 27). In this context surgical gowns make direct contact improbable, and masks make droplet spread improbable. However, the importance of air for endemic *S. aureus* transmission in other settings is less clear. The strongest positive evidence is that of Mortimer and coworkers [98], who studied acquisition of staphylococcal colonization in newly born infants housed in a special nursery that was also used for the care of known colonized infants. Extraordinary measures were undertaken to eliminate contact transfer of *S. aureus* from the index babies to the study babies. Nevertheless, at least 9 of 158 newborns became colonized. The authors offered as evidence that these acquisitions were airborne the following points: contact transmission did not occur, index strains of *S. aureus* were recovered on settling plates throughout the nursery, the infants were at least 2.1 m apart, making large-droplet transmission unlikely, and the study infants tended to be colonized in the nose first, whereas in previous studies infants acquiring *S. aureus* by physical transfer tended to be colonized at the umbilicus first. Wenzel and colleagues [133] have critically analyzed nine additional articles published between 1966 and 1976 purporting to show airborne transmission of *S. aureus*. None of these additional studies provides even strongly suggestive evidence of airborne spread. A bit of negative evidence with respect to endemic operating room acquisition of *S. aureus* came from the National Academy of Sciences–National Research Council study of the influence of ultraviolet radiation on postoperative wound infection [38] (see Chapter 20). In the study high-intensity ultraviolet light in the operating room reduced airborne bacterial counts, as measured on settling plates, by 52 or 63 percent, depending on the ultraviolet intensity used. At neither intensity was there a similar reduction in postoperative wound infection rates.

---

*Organisms per cubic foot is the unit used in this section because most published articles have used this unit (1 ft$^3$ = 28.3 l = .0283 m$^3$ · 1 m$^3$ = 1000 l = 34.9 ft$^3$).

[†]In the context of infection transmission, *airborne* means "borne on the air" rather than "transported through the air." Large droplets travel up to 1 to 2 m through the air but are not borne on it. Large-droplet transmission is considered a type of contact spread.

### ...ative Bacilli

...etric sampling of ordinary hospital air with ...tification of Enterobacteriaceae and nonfermen...rs has been rare. Available studies tend to focus on specialized areas of the hospital (especially operating rooms), to use settling-plate methods, to assess outbreak situations, or to provide incomplete microbiologic identification. In a 1973 study Turner and Craddock [130] found 20 percent of air samples positive for *Klebsiella*. Settling plate studies for *Pseudomonas* generally have not yielded the organism [37], although there are exceptions [44].

Clinicians have been particularly concerned about spread of *Pseudomonas aeruginosa* from or to hospitalized patients with cystic fibrosis. In one study [19], the organism was recovered on settle plates near the patients with cystic fibrosis. In another study, however, [89] 1740 children were hospitalized during 1981 on a university hospital pediatrics ward. During this interval, 28 cystic fibrosis patients with gentamicin-resistant *P. aeruginosa* colonization were hospitalized. During the entire interval, only one nosocomial acquisition of a gentamicin-resistant *P. aeruginosa* infection occurred among the noncystic patients. The proximate source of the *P. aeruginosa* organisms colonizing cystic fibrosis patients appears to be environmental—even the ultimate source does not appear to be other cystic fibrosis patients [73].

Two studies have described an association between airborne gram-negative bacilli and endemic nosocomial infection. The first and more convincing situation resulted from a very unusual circumstance. The newly constructed Hines VA Hospital had a novel chute hydropulping waste disposal system that introduced malodorous bacteria-laden air throughout the hospital. Air sampling near the system showed greater than 160 *Pseudomonas* and Enterobacteriaceae cfu per cubic foot (unfortunately the relative amounts were unspecified) [57]. Concurrent continuous surveillance indicated that the nosocomial bacteremia rate approximately doubled coincident with moving to the new hospital and fell to the baseline level after the chute hydropulping system was closed down. In a second study, carried out over a five-year interval by Kelsen and McGuckin [74], there was a significant positive correlation between the monthly rate of nosocomial respiratory tract infection in patients hospitalized in an ICU and the average bacterial content of the ICU air in a particular month (see Chapter 18). During periods of heavy air contamination, the authors found an unusually high concentration of airborne gram-negative bacilli ranging up to a *P. aeruginosa* content of 30 per cubic foot and *Klebsiella* con-

tent of 9 per cubic foot. As the authors point out, the association may not imply that airborne gram-negative rods directly cause nosocomial respiratory tract disease. It is possible that airborne bacteria seeded nebulizers [75] or another intermediate reservoir. The association may have resulted from a third factor affecting both bacterial content of the air and the nosocomial infection rate. Finally, it is possible that the air may reflect patient illness rather than vice versa.

Ultimately the best evidence that endemic nosocomial infection does not often result from airborne gram-negative bacilli probably arises from the repeated failure to recover such organisms in air cultures obtained during epidemic investigations. Although these situations may be atypical, as negative evidence they are convincing. This context may be expected to be the situation most likely to produce positive air cultures. The widespread belief that gram-negative bacilli do not survive for prolonged periods when airborne may provide additional evidence if it is true. Here the experimental support is more tenuous than one might wish. Under certain conditions of humidity, temperature, and physiologic state, *Escherichia coli* can sustain up to 100 percent survival for one-half hour in microaerosols [40]. In general, *E. coli* survives better when aerosols are generated using broth cultures of organisms in relatively inactive states. In summary, although there is insufficient evidence that airborne gram-negative bacilli constitute a source of endemic nosocomial infection to warrant changes in our current practices, situations that lead to high airborne concentrations of gram-negative bacilli should be avoided. This includes the use of aerosol-generating room humidifiers, which have been shown to cause considerable dissemination of *Pseudomonas* [58] and *Acinetobacter* [126].

### Legionella

In at least some outbreaks, *Legionella pneumophila* transmission by the airborne route has occurred (see Chapter 26). For nosocomial legionellosis, however, the strongest associations have been with contamination of the potable water supply, as discussed in the next section.

### Aspergillus

Several lines of evidence strongly suggest that airborne *Aspergillus fumigatus* spores cause aspergillosis in immunosuppressed patients [114]: (1) *Aspergillus* spores are always present in unfiltered air and the organism is highly adapted to airborne spread; (2) most nosocomial aspergillosis appears first as pneumonia. Even if there is an intermediate step of nasopharyngeal colonization, airborne spores would be the ultimate source; (3) two hospitals have reported a decrease in endemic nosocomial aspergillosis coincident with moving to new facilities with improved air filtration systems; (4) in all six reported outbreaks of nosocomial aspergillosis, there has been an implicated airborne source; (5) nosocomial aspergillosis arising in a patient cared for in a high efficiency particulate air (HEPA) air-filtered room has not been described; and (6) in one hospital, reductions in airborne *Aspergillus* spores coincided with a lowered rate of nosocomial aspergillosis in bone marrow transplant recipients. It is likely that other fungal organisms, such as *Mucor*, *Fusarium*, and *Petriellidium*, also are transmitted to patients through the air. Hospitals caring for highly immunosuppressed patients should probably strive to maintain air free from fungal spores. Wet organic materials used in hospital construction, such as fire proofing should be treated with a fungicide [114].

## WATER

### Potable Water

Achievement of potability of water is a major public health activity and beyond the scope of this book. Standard works may be consulted for details of water treatment and examination [7]. Verification of ordinary potability is of importance to infection control personnel only in hospitals with private water supplies in which certification of the water supply is a hospital responsibility. It should be noted that federal drinking water regulations [132] call for only one microbiologic assessment: a coliform count (acceptable levels depend on sampling frequency but must average less than 1 per 100 ml). Even for community water this sole criterion is probably inadequate considering the variety of water sources, potential contaminants, and uses of water [54]. Additional considerations are appropriate in the hospital because of its specialized water uses.

Potable water supply systems must be protected by vacuum breakers or other devices, which add expense. Accordingly, some building designers plan separate potable and nonpotable water systems. These systems should not be interconnected. Common sense and the Joint Commission on Accreditation of Hospitals (JCAH) [71] require that in hospitals the potable water system be used for all hand-washing, patient bathing, cooking, washing of foods and utensils for cooking and eating, food preparation or processing, and laundry. Given the few valid uses for

nonpotable water in the hospital and the difficulty in forever preventing cross-connection, it is doubtful that hospitals should be designed with separate nonpotable water systems.

### Dialysis Water

Detailed standards for hemodialysis water have been prepared by the Association for the Advancement of Medical Instrumentation (AAMI) and accepted by the American National Standards Institution [13]. The standard specifies that water used to prepare dialysate shall have a total microbial count of less than 200 per milliliter and the dialysate itself have less than 2000 per milliliter (see Chapter 17). The rationale for the AAMI standard lies in studies carried out in the 1970s indicating that pyrogenic reactions did not occur when dialysate had fewer than 2000 organisms per milliliter [42,50]. Bacteria do not cross an intact dialysis membrane, but endotoxin may. The viable bacterial concentration is a rough measure of the endotoxin concentration. The rationale for the stricter (<200 organisms per milliliter) standard for water used to prepare dialysate is that organism multiplication may occur within the dialyzer. This is a more important problem for recirculating systems than for single pass systems [82], a distinction not recognized in the AAMI standard. In recirculating systems, dialyzed materials can provide nutrition to contaminating bacteria.

There are many types of water treatment devices for use in preparing dialysate. A brief discussion is available in Appendix B to the AAMI standard [13]. A more detailed discussion is available in an FDA Technical Report [77].

### Hydrotherapy Pools and Tanks

A number of features of hydrotherapy tanks produce concern that they may be causes of infection: patients using them may have active infection, which may introduce hazardous bacteria and organic debris, or patients may be incontinent of feces; warm temperature, water agitation, and a high number of patients per unit volume of water reduce available chlorine; the internal channels of agitators are difficult to disinfect; and highly contaminated water may be brought into close contact with potential portals of entry such as pressure sores, Foley catheters, or percutaneous devices (see Chapter 31). An outbreak of *P. aeruginosa* wound infections has been reliably linked to these tanks [93]. Since a wide variety of other human pathogens such as coliforms, staphylococci, and fungi have been isolated from immersion tanks [131], there is a broader potential of transmission. Indeed, in a burn center, where the infection potential of hydrotherapy tanks may be most severe, Mayhall and colleagues [91] have reported a bacteremia outbreak due to *Enterobacter cloacae*, which may have been associated with hydrotherapy transmission. To the extent that hydrotherapy tanks are similar to hot tubs and whirlpool spas, there is a more ominous possibility. Contamination of these water sources has resulted in *P. aeruginosa* folliculitis [61], urinary tract infections [117], and even pneumonia [116]. The danger of in-hospital hydrotherapy tanks is probably mitigated by higher standards of disinfection: in the outbreaks of community-acquired *P. aeruginosa* skin infections, rudimentary standards of water maintenance were not in effect [61].

The Centers for Disease Control (CDC) published recommendations for disinfection of hydrotherapy pools and tanks in 1974 [31]. For immersion tanks the CDC recommended maintaining a free chlorine residual of 15 mg/l with a pH of 7.2 to 7.6, draining tanks between each patient use, scrubbing out the tank with a germicidal detergent, and circulating chlorine solution through the agitator of the tank at least 15 minutes at the end of each treatment day. For hydrotherapy pools the CDC favored continuous filtration and the maintenance of free chlorine residuals of 0.4 to 0.6 mg/l. In the absence of continuous filtration, the CDC recommended potassium iodide and chloramine.

### High-Purity Water

Distillation apparatus, reverse osmosis devices, and ion-exchange resin beds are all subject to contamination. Some hospital personnel erroneously presume this type of water is sterile. Distilled water, even if subsequently sterilized, may contain endotoxin. Febrile reactions caused by exposure to items rinsed in endotoxin containing distilled water have occurred [32].

### Water Bacteria

"Water bacteria," or more loosely, "water bugs," are organisms that proliferate in relatively pure water. The most adept species is *Pseudomonas cepacia* [29]. Carson and colleagues found *P. cepacia* strains that could multiply to levels of $10^7$ per milliliter and remain at these high levels for weeks in distilled water of very high resistivity. *P. aeruginosa* follows closely behind in this ability [49]. Furthermore, *P. aeruginosa* strains adapted to distilled water are relatively resistant to disinfectants [28]. *Acinetobacter calcoaceticus* seems particularly well adapted to highly aerated water sources. An enrichment technique for isolation of *Acinetobacter* from environmental samples using

vigorous aeration has been described [14]. This feature of *Acinetobacter* presumably accounts for its increased relative frequency as a cause of humidifier or other respiratory-device contamination. Other water bacteria include *Flavobacterium meningosepticum* [113], other *Pseudomonas* species, *Achromobacter* species, *Aeromonas hydrophila*, and certain nontuberculous mycobacteria. The last are also relatively resistant to various disinfectants [30] including formaldehyde [67]. Virtually every unprotected wet area in a hospital should be considered contaminated at high levels with one or more water bacteria. These sources include tap water, drains and sinks, water baths, shower heads, flower water, ice machines, and water carafes.

### Legionella

*L. pneumophila* has been isolated repeatedly from natural and man-made water sources. The latter include cooling towers, hot water tanks, and potable water distribution systems. Since person-to-person transmission of *L. pneumophila* is either very rare or nonexistent [136], *L. pneumophila* is an organism for which control of environmental contamination is the main preventive measure (see Chapter 26). Less is known about other *Legionella* species. *L. micdadei* has been isolated from potable water systems and presumably has similar transmission mechanisms to *L. pneumophila*.

Most of the early *L. pneumophila* outbreaks, particularly those occurring in nonhospital settings, were associated with adjacent excavation or contaminated air-handling systems. However, hospital outbreaks have most often been linked with contamination of potable water systems [114]. At the Wadsworth VA Hospital in Los Angeles, where a large outbreak of nosocomial legionellosis occurred over a period of several years, improvements in the air-handling system preceded efforts to eliminate *Legionella* from the potable water system. Only the latter was followed by reductions in cases [12,96]. *L. pneumophila* most often contaminates the hot water side of potable water systems. Since the most common presentation of legionellosis is pneumonia, it is logical to conclude that inhalation is the most significant portal of entry. The organism has been found repeatedly in shower heads, leading to the hypothesis that aerosolization and subsequent inhalation occurs. However, case-control analyses in outbreaks have not established the mechanism by which the organism reaches patients.

A consensus that all hospital potable water systems should be free from *Legionella* contamination has not yet emerged. It may be that nosocomial *Legionella* pneumonia often goes unrecognized unless avidly sought [99], making it difficult to assess the overall magnitude of this problem or for any one hospital to be comfortable with its *Legionella* situation. There is, however, at least one hospital (RH in reference [110]) in which contamination of the potable water system was present and, in spite of rigorous detection efforts, practically no nosocomial legionellosis could be documented.

The problem of persistent colonization of hospital potable water systems by *L. pneumophila* arises, at least in part, because the organism can tolerate low levels of chlorine for relatively long periods of time [79]. One study has suggested that hospitals maintaining hot water storage temperatures at 40°C to 45°C (104°F to 113°F) have *L. pneumophila* contamination, while hospitals maintaining hot water storage at 58°C to 60°C (136°F to 140°F) do not [111]. In hospitals in which nosocomial legionellosis is occurring, the water system should be assessed for *Legionella* contamination. If nosocomial *Legionella* cases and water system contamination are both present, efforts to disinfect the water system should be undertaken. Two methods have been used successfully, although both have disadvantages. Hyperchlorination may corrode pipework, and periodic overheating of the water (to as high as 77°C [170°F]) may cause scalding of patients or personnel.

## WALLS, FLOORS, AND OTHER SMOOTH SURFACES

Maki and his infection control group performed a landmark study assessing the relation between organisms on environmental surfaces and nosocomial infection [88]. During 1979 the University of Wisconsin Hospital moved to a new facility. There was no change in the rate of nosocomial infection at any patient site or due to any pathogen associated with this change. Cultures of floors, walls, and other surfaces (as well as air, water, faucets, and sink drains) showed very similar organism profiles in the old facility and, after 6 to 12 months of occupancy, in the new facility. In contrast, corresponding cultures taken in the new facility before occupancy were relatively devoid of common nosocomial pathogens. The constancy of infection rates provides strong evidence that the association between hospital environmental organism content and nosocomial infection arises because patients infect the environment, not vice versa. It is important to realize some limitations of the Maki study: the two pathogens for which environmental content is of primary importance (*Aspergillus* and *Legionella*) were not assessed; neither were the environmental cultures processed for anaerobes or viruses.

This study virtually rules out the environment as a significant vector for the assessed organism-object combinations and severely undercuts the rationale for concern about other combinations in the absence of specific data to the contrary. In fact, one is forced to question seriously even such relatively modest recommendations as the use of antimicrobial detergents in hospital cleaning, terminal disinfection of isolation rooms, special cleaning of objects removed from isolation rooms, and the wearing of gowns and gloves when entering the room of patients in classic strict isolation when no direct patient contact is anticipated.

### Respiratory Syncytial Virus

One pathogen clearly transmissible in the hospital by fomites is respiratory syncytial virus (RSV) (see Chapter 35). Indirect evidence suggests that RSV transmission occurs by contact: inoculation of the RSV onto nasal or eye membranes causes infection quite efficiently [65]. RSV survives for several hours on smooth surfaces [64]. Direct evidence of fomite transmission is now available [63]: volunteers entering a hospital room recently vacated by an RSV-infected patient, after handling objects in the room and touching their eyes and nose, became infected with RSV more than half as often as volunteers who cuddled RSV-infected babies. Volunteers sitting in the room with an RSV-infected baby did not contract the illness. The relative importance of hand and fomite transmission in "natural" infection is unknown, but it is of interest that RSV survives about ten times better on smooth surfaces than on skin [64].

### Clostridium Difficile

Sophisticated strain analysis techniques have unequivocally established that in-hospital transmission of *C. difficile* can occur [134]. Endemic in-hospital *C. difficile* transmission would provide a satisfactory explanation for the apparent wide variation in rates of *C. difficile* colitis in different hospitals. As is the case for many nosocomial pathogens, increased environmental presence of *C. difficile* is associated with infected patients [51]. What is different about *C. difficile* is its ability to form spores, with the consequent prolonged survival of the organism in the environment and the plausibility that the spores retain full infectiousness. At present, these concerns are largely hypothetical. No special environmental cleaning techniques for *C. difficile* contamination have been formally advocated.

### Hepatitis B Virus

Hemodialysis units and clinical laboratories, areas with frequent contamination of the environment by blood, are foci of hepatitis B virus transmission (see Chapters 7 and 17). Many ward-acquired and an even larger fraction of laboratory-acquired hepatitis B cases occur without recognized percutaneous inoculation of blood. HBsAg may be antigenically detected on surfaces in hospital areas likely to have been blood-contaminated [83]. Even surfaces not visibly contaminated with blood may yield HBsAg. Hepatitis B virus in blood survives desiccation at room temperature up to one week [23]. Very high dilutions of hepatitis B virus–containing blood can transmit hepatitis B. The CDC has advocated special techniques for environmental decontamination after HBsAg-positive blood spills [22].

While a needle contaminated with blood or a collection tube containing blood is arguably a fomite, the more difficult issue is the hazard of hepatitis B–containing blood on an environmental surface. The historical evolution of nosocomial hepatitis B provides suggestive evidence. Sharp increases in nosocomial hepatitis B among hospital workers and patients occurred in the early and mid-1970s as hemodialysis became more prevalent. Widespread recognition of the hazard of needle stick occurred early. Yet declines in the incidence of nosocomial hepatitis did not occur until the late 1970s and early 1980s (notably, before the introduction of hepatitis B vaccine). Coincident with this decline were efforts to segregate HBsAg-positive patients, use gowns and gloves while dialyzing these patients, and eliminate or decontaminate environmental blood. Most observers feel that a general "respect" for the hazard of blood has been an important part of hepatitis B prevention, implying a concern about environmental surfaces.

## OTHER ENVIRONMENTAL OBJECTS

### Carpets
Ordinary carpets increase the microbiologic content per unit of floor surface by about four orders of magnitude [9]. Contaminating organisms include *S. aureus*, *E. coli*, and more rarely, *Pseudomonas*. After removal from hospital environments, carpet content of *S. aureus* remains stable for over a month, and of other organisms for up to six months. In the best controlled study, however, the total bacterial content of air is apparently unaffected by whether the sampled area was carpeted [122]. For areas with carpets, air content was also not significantly influenced by vacuuming frequency (daily, every other day, or every third day) [122]. The infection hazard of carpets may

be more important when there is direct contact of patients with carpeting (e.g., in pediatric areas) or when patients use wheelchairs. However, there has yet to be a demonstration that any nosocomial infection has arisen from a carpet. In recent years, manufacturers have marketed carpets with antimicrobial substances. As yet, these have not been rigorously assessed in independent studies.

### Air-Fluidized Beds
Designed to prevent pressure sores by "flotation," air-fluidized beds have a number of unprecedented design features posing novel questions with respect to infection transmission (see Chapter 18). Flotation is accomplished by driving air up through a 25-cm-deep layer of silicon-coated, soda lime glass microspheres 50 to 150 $\mu$ in diameter. The microspheres are held in the bed by a monofilament polyester filter sheet with openings of approximately 37 $\mu$, through which the microspheres cannot pass. Disinfection of the beds is accomplished by sieving organic debris—bead clumps and desiccation.

The two best studies on the microbiology of air-fluidized beds present seemingly contradictory data. However, neither of these studies affords much help in the assessment of the infection hazard posed by air-fluidized beds. In one [124], the microbial challenge is quite dissimilar to the in-use situation. The other [118] contains too few data.

Details of the kinetics of microbial content after natural contamination during the course of sieving and fluidization are unknown. The relation between organisms on the microspheres within the air-fluidized bed and delivery to the patient in the rising air are unknown. Persistence of organisms that tolerate desiccation, such as *C. difficile*, other *Clostridium* species, or *Mycobacterium tuberculosis*, has not been assessed. In fact, no data on anaerobic organisms are available. Whether or not the air fluidization process can render airborne organisms that usually remain harmlessly attached to surfaces (e.g., *M. tuberculosis*) is unknown.

### Soap
Given the emphasis on hand-washing, it is surprising that the problem of soap contamination is not better studied. That the problem is largely theoretical is suggested by the paucity of reported outbreaks attributed to contaminated soap. The outbreak most often cited [97] is relatively unconvincing. Recently, however, clinical illness has been securely attributed to an antiseptic soap [105]. It is reasonable to postulate that it is advantageous to hand-wash with ster-

ile soap (liquid or leaf) dispensed from forearm- or leg-operated dispensers that are resistant to contamination.

Data confirming the expected contamination of in-use bar soap have been widely disseminated in the promotion of dispensed liquid soap [68]. However, data comparing the microbial burden on hands washed using a contaminated soap bar with that using uncontaminated nonmedicated soap are unavailable. At the least, it seems prudent to reduce the microbial content of soaps by using disposable liquid soap containers, thoroughly cleaning reusable liquid soap containers, or if bar soap is used, purchasing small bars and providing soap racks that permit water drainage. The relative merits of these alternatives await additional study.

*Flowers*

Flowers pose two theoretical infection hazards: vase water inevitably contains large concentrations of potential nosocomial pathogens, and any decaying organic matter may provide a substrate for fungal growth. Although there are no data establishing vase water as a common cause of nosocomial infections, many hospitals bar flowers from the rooms of immunosuppressed patients and intensive care units. If vase water were disposed of gently, and patients, personnel, and visitors washed their hands after touching the water, little danger should arise. Unfortunately, achieving uniform compliance with these precautions is improbable.

## ANIMAL VISITATION

Sanctioned animal contact with hospital patients is of several types: blind patients or personnel may be accompanied by seeing eye dogs, family members may bring pets to visit sick children, volunteer groups may bring animal acts to entertain patients, and animals used in research may be housed in areas near patient care units. Although Q fever is the only zoonosis shown to have caused epidemics in health-care facilities, over 100 organisms infect both humans and other animals [2]. Knowledge of transmission mechanisms of these organisms suggests several prudent measures.

Seeing eye dogs may be used by personnel, visitors, or patients. Patient use should occur infrequently since patients are usually escorted to places within the hospital. However, some blind patients may desire the companionship of their animal or may be physically capable of walks outside the hospital even though there is a requirement for continued hospitalization. Minimum reasonable requests in these situations include assurance that the dog is vaccinated against rabies, free of ectoparasites, and healthy (in particular, ringworm should not be present). The patient should make arrangements for someone to walk the dog and assume responsibility for disposal of animal excreta. There are effective vaccines for dog leptospirosis, although it seems unlikely that patient contact with dog urine would occur. The remaining dog vaccines are for pathogens that are not transmitted to humans. There are numerous enteric pathogens that may spread from dogs to humans, but attention to proper disposal of dog feces should eliminate this hazard.

Several outbreaks of Q fever have been reported resulting from exposure to pregnant ewes used in research centers [66]. Hospitalized patients have not been affected in these outbreaks. However, airborne transmission has occurred to personnel with no direct contact with the pregnant ewes. The hazard appears to be most severe at or near parturition [1]. The magnitude of this phenomenon is unclear because Q fever is not clinically distinctive, and *Coxiella burnetii* serologic studies are infrequently performed. It seems prudent to bar all direct contact between patients and pregnant ewes and to be sure that pregnant ewes used for research are never, even during transportation, in areas from which airborne spread to patients can occur. More stringent recommendations for protection of personnel working with pregnant ewes have been published [16].

Certain animal contacts with children seem inadvisable in any circumstance: turtles cannot be reliably certified free of salmonellosis; wild carnivores (e.g., skunks, raccoons) and bats pose an unacceptably high risk of rabies; and sick birds of virtually any species may transmit psittacosis. Any contact with animal urine should be followed by hand-washing, and if appropriate, more extensive disinfection procedures because of the possibility of leptospirosis. Contact with mouse or hamster urine is also hazardous to the immunocompromised patient because of the possibility of transmission of lymphocytic choriomeningitis virus.

## LINEN

*Soiled Linen*

Soiled linen is heavily contaminated with human pathogens (see Chapter 15). Total aerobic bacteria colony forming unit counts are about $10^3$ cfu per square centimeter for sheets and about $10^6$ cfu per square centimeter for terry cloth items. Of these organisms, about 70 percent are gram-negative bacilli and 20 percent are gram-positive cocci. Among common nosocomial pathogens, *E. coli*, other Enterobacteriaceae, and *P. aeruginosa* occur frequently, and *S. aureus* is occasionally found [18].

Despite this frequent contamination, reports of transmission of infection to laundry workers are restricted to Q fever, smallpox [11] and hepatitis A [35]. The infection hazard to laundry workers can be divided into that due to pathogens for which patients are normally placed in isolation and that due to fecal contamination from patients who are unrecognized excreters of enteric pathogens. Mitigation of the infection hazard from isolation laundry is largely accomplished by the use of hot water–soluble bags, which may be placed in washing machines without being opened. Although single bagging with such bags should suffice, most hospitals prefer to add an impervious, more tear-resistant outer bag. The CDC isolation guideline appears to suggest that all linen from every patient in any form of isolation precaution should be specially handled [53]. This is probably unnecessary, but the educational effort required to acquaint all appropriate personnel with the necessary distinctions is probably not worth it.

The infection hazard due to unrecognized enteric pathogens in stool is often overlooked. In fact, most pathogens resulting in isolation are of relatively little threat to healthy laundry workers. In contrast, enteric pathogens are quite adept at piercing normal host defenses. The two most straightforward solutions to this problem are disposal of all fecally contaminated laundry as "isolation laundry" and the elimination of "presorting"—sorting before washing. The latter is impractical, however, since different wash cycles are appropriate for different laundry items and sorting damp laundry (postsorting) is less efficient.

The infection hazard posed to patients by soiled laundry appears to be practically nonexistent. Handling soiled linen gently to reduce the dispersal of microorganisms in patient-care areas seems prudent and requires little extra effort. Beyond that, there is little basis for special procedures. Given the improbability that soiled laundry reposing in a partially filled hamper causes infection (or even adds organisms to the environment), it is difficult to understand the emphasis that hospital inspection agencies have placed on soiled-linen hampers. Through 1979, individual JCAH surveyors often cited hospitals for open, partially filled laundry hampers, although the written standards were ambiguous: "Soiled linen . . . should be placed in impervious bags or containers that are properly closed at the site of collection" [70, pp. 69,70]. In 1980 the standard was made more rational. The 1984 version states: "As soon as they are filled and prior to further transport, the bags or containers should be properly closed" [71, p. 76]. Unfortunately, state hospital licensing agencies and agencies establishing that hospitals meet the conditions of participation in Federal Medicare programs still sometimes cite hospitals for uncovered soiled laundry hampers.

### Clean Laundry

Existing recommendations for cleaning laundry were formulated almost half a century ago at a time when cleaning agents required hot water for effectiveness, and energy conservation was of less concern [18]. The American Hospital Association recommends the use of water above 71°C (160°F) for 25 minutes for all laundered items except delicate fabrics [5, p. 66]. Lower temperatures probably suffice, however [18]. Studies of naturally contaminated hospital laundry washed at 22°C (72°F) in bulk hospital washer-extractors reveal that a 3 log reduction in total organisms occurs as a result of agitation, dilution, and drainage alone. Adding laundry chemicals, including bleach, produces an additional 3 log reduction. Flatwork ironers, which expose sheets to a temperature above 175°C (347°F), are highly lethal to bacteria. Tumble dryers, used for terry cloth items, also effect a reduction in bacterial content. After complete cold-water processing, sheets have a total aerobic colony forming unit count of about .2 cfu per cubic centimeter, and terry cloth items about 2 cfu per cubic centimeter. The profile of contaminating organisms (*Bacillus* species 58 percent, coagulase-negative staphylococci 25 percent, *Corynebacterium* species 18 percent) is markedly changed from the prewash profile. Pathogenic species are quite rare. These counts and identities are not different from those on laundry washed at 71°C (160°F).

Proper handling of clean linen during transportation and storage is probably the most important determinant of the microbial content at the time of patient use. Meyer and colleagues [95] studied newborn intensive care laundry that had been washed at 75°C (167°F), dried at 96°C (205°F), and carefully handled. Rodac contact plates showed no organisms one third of the time and greater than ten colonies per contact plate only 9 percent of the time. Linen near the top of the stack had a higher incidence of positivity and a greater number of colonies per plate than linen in the middle of the stack, suggesting that handling was the source of organisms.

The AHA recommends autoclaving linen for patients "particularly susceptible to infections," such as burned patients, and for the nursery [5, p. 67]. The American Academy of Pediatrics [3, pp. 118–119] supported this recommendation until 1983, when they softened their stand [4, p. 116]. Data to support autoclaving any linen are lacking. One set of arguments against autoclaving linen arises after consideration of the panoply of techniques ordinarily employed to maintain sterility until point of use. Applying these procedures to autoclaved nursery linen would be quite burdensome and costly.

Only one outbreak has been attributed to cleaned linen [17]. The outbreak consisted of *Bacillus cereus* umbilical colonization without clinical signs of infection in normal neonates and neonates in a special baby care unit. The cause was considered to be contaminated, cleaned diapers because the implicated *B. cereus* type was found in washed diapers and the laundry machine. Since the implicated *B. cereus* type was also recovered from the hands of nursing staff, this attribution is unconvincing.

## ULTRACLEAN PROTECTIVE ENVIRONMENTS

The ultimate expression of concern that environmental organisms pose an infection hazard is the ultraclean protective environment. When fully developed, these efforts at reducing patient exposure to microorganisms include HEPA air filtration with horizontal or vertical laminar air flow; sterile or low-organism-content food; frequent disinfection of walls, floors, and other environmental surfaces; sterile linen and drinking water; toilet water disinfection; use of sterile booties, gowns, caps, and gloves for personnel and visitors entering the room; and elaborate protective garb when patients leave the room. Patients placed in such an environment are generally given oral nonabsorbable, topical, and/or systemic antimicrobials. This package of protective measures has been termed the *total protective environment, life island, protected environment*, or *barrier isolation*.

It has long been recognized that these special efforts can produce environmental surfaces and ambient air with markedly reduced organism content [127]. More important, it appears that this package of patient-care techniques produces a statistically significant reduction in the incidence of infection. Of ten random allocation trials of various forms of ultraclean protective environments (Table 14-1), five showed a statistically significant reduction in overall, severe, and/or fatal infections. Of the remaining studies three showed a trend to fewer infections in the protected

patients, and one did not report infection rates. This infection prevention effect generally occurs after the second week, consistent with the view that there is a lag between becoming colonized with a nosocomial pathogen and subsequent infection.

However, the use of ultraprotective environments remains controversial for a number of reasons:

1. *Expense.* In new hospital construction the capital cost of laminar air flow rooms is not great, especially when amortized over the life of a building. Modular units are commercially available. However, depending on what additional features are incorporated into the protective package, substantial ongoing expenses may be incurred.

2. *Deleterious effects.* During periods of severe illness, seeing only masked, gowned people, being served relatively unpalatable food, remaining confined to a small room, and consuming foul-tasting, diarrheogenic antibiotics must aggravate the psychologic stress of having a potentially fatal condition. Premature withdrawal from protected environments may predispose to gut colonization and subsequent disease caused by environmental pathogens.

3. *Difficulty in apportioning benefit* among the various features of protected environments. With few exceptions [120], the studies summarized in Table 14-1 deal with the impact of the total package versus conventional patient management. If infections are prevented, it is difficult to factor out which component is responsible. It is even possible that the beneficial effect results from enhanced adherence to standard infection control procedures (e.g., cannula or Foley catheter management) in protected environments.

4. *Doubts about study design.* Diagnosis of infection in highly complicated, very immunosuppressed patients is problematic. The physicians providing direct care of the patients, who are in the best position to make the assessment, are also the least blinded with respect to study group. All of these studies are described as using random allocation. However, the vicissitudes of room availability at the time of patient admission and the many factors involved in assignment of patients to rooms make true randomization awkward. Only six of the studies provide detailed information about comparability of the patient groups. The studies from the M. D. Anderson Hospital [21,115] have a troublesome design feature: the protected patients received more intensive chemotherapy. The investigators proceeded on the unproven but logical presumption that subsequent courses of induction

TABLE 14-1. Controlled trials of ultraclean protective environments for immunosuppressed patients

| First author and reference | Diagnosis | Groups[a] | Room[b] | Food[c] | Antibiotics[d] Oral | Topical | Infections/PT[e] All | Severe | Fatal | Remission[e] | Survival[e] |
|---|---|---|---|---|---|---|---|---|---|---|---|
| Levine [85] | Leukemia | GR 1 | PE | L | GVN | Y | | .36 | 0* | .45 | .91 — At 100 days |
| | | GR 2 | N | N | GVN | N | | .79 } | .24* | .42 | .66* |
| | | GR 3 | N | N | N | N | | .78 | .21 | .43 | .61 |
| Yates [135] | Acute myelogenous leukemia | Convent | N | N | N | N | | .86[f] | | No diff | No diff |
| | | Rev Iso,GS | PI | L,S | GVN | Y | | .72[f] | | | |
| | | Isolator | PE | L,S | N | N | | .32[f] | | | |
| | | Isolator,GS | PE | L,S | GVN | Y | | .27[f] | | | |
| Klastersky [78] | Acute leukemia | Iso + Dec | PE | S | MULT | Y | 1.2 | .62 | .34 | No diff | No diff |
| | | Decontam | PI | S | MULT | Y | 1.3 | .50 | .33 | | |
| | | Control | PI | S | N | N | 1.2 | .69 | .31 | | |
| Schimpff [120] | Acute myelogenous leukemia | LAF+A | PE | L | GVN | Y | 1.1* | .17* | .17 | .54 | .52 — At 100 days |
| | | W+A | N | N | GVN | N | 1.7 | .37* | .32* | .63* | .67 |
| | | W | N | N | N | N | 3.0 | 1.0 | .52 | .24 | .24 |
| Dietrich [45] | Acute leukemia | A | PE | S | MULT | Y/N | | .83 | .09 | .69 | No diff |
| | | B | PE | S | N | N | | 1.02 | .11 | .61 | |
| | | C | W | N | N | N | | 1.06 | .16 | .49 | |
| Schimpff [119] | Acute nonlymphocytic leukemia | GR I | H,PI,A | L | GVN | N | .9 | .45 | .18 | .73 | 322+ — Median days |
| | | GR II | H,PI | L | GVN | N | 1.4 | .70 | .20 | .70 | 357+ |
| | | GR III | H,N | L | GVN | N | 1.2 | .62 | .19 | .81 | 179+ |

| Study | Disease | Room type | Room | Food | Oral | Topical | | | | | | Time |
|---|---|---|---|---|---|---|---|---|---|---|---|---|
| Rodriguez [115] | Acute leukemia | PEPA+PESA | PE | S | MULT | Y | | .52 >** | .13 >* | .71 >** | .97 >** | At 6 wks |
| | | PA+SA+SA | N | N | N | N | | .84 | .28 | .43 | .82 | |
| Buckner [26] | Bone marrow transplant | IN | PE | S | MULT | Y | .44 >** | .29 | .02 | .96 | .14 | At an unspecified date |
| | | OUT | S | N | N | N | 1.39 | 1.02 | .04 | .82 | .41 | |
| Bodey [21] | Lymphoma | PEPA | PE | S | GVN | Y | | .07 >* | 0 | .77 | .74 | At 1 yr |
| | | Control | S | N | N | N | | .36 | .04 | .71 | .67 | |
| Storb [129] | Aplastic anemia | LAF | PE | S | Mult | Y | | | | | .86g | * |
| | | No LAF | S | N | N | N | | | | | .69g | |

[a] The abbreviations from the original articles are used to name the groups.

[b] Room

PE = protected environment; PI = conventional protective isolation; S = single room; N = no special room; H = supply air HEPA filter and at positive pressure relative to hall; A = air filtration unit (Med-Aire).

[c] Food

S = "sterile"; L = low in bacteria; N = no special food.

[d] Antibiotics

Oral: GVN = gentamicin, vancomycin, nystatin; MULT = multiple; N = no prophylactic antibiotics.

Topical: Y = topical antibiotics; N = no topical antibiotics.

[e] Probability

*p < .05

**p < .01

[f] Approximate values (taken from a figure) for only those patients not infected at randomization, p value not presented.

[g] Graft take.

could be more intensive in patients with no previous infection. The improved survival may have resulted from the more intensive therapy, which may have been administrable to the more often previously infected control patients.

5. *Doubts about the larger significance of a real difference in infection rates.* In many of the studies, the lower infection rate provided only a brief postponement of death; longevity was more strongly influenced by severity of underlying illness. The reduction in infection, if real, may be most meaningful for patients undergoing potentially curative therapies, such as children with acute lymphocytic leukemia or patients undergoing bone marrow transplantation.

Which components of the ultraprotective package are most likely to be responsible for the presumed real reduction in infection rate? Attention is often focused on specialized air purification systems. It is important to consider separately several features of these systems: fineness of filtration, location of filters, air change rate, and laminar air flow. Top-of-the-line bag filters probably remove nearly all fungal spores, but many hospitals prefer HEPA filters because they add relatively little capital expense and meet standards more directly related to microbial filtration [114]. Placing filters at the point of entrance of air into the patient's room permits safe maintenance while the room is otherwise unoccupied by patients. Malfunction or maintenance of central systems may cause patient exposure to unfiltered usual air unless the entire supplied area can be freed of patients. Increasing the air change rate three- to fivefold will reduce potential patient exposure to airborne organisms bypassing the filter (e.g., through incompletely sealed windows) or be brought into the rooms by personnel or on objects. Laminar air flow can be produced in empty chambers by a series of baffles and diffusers and approximated in patient rooms. Horizontal and vertical units have been employed, but the former seem to have prevailed in the most recently constructed units. These units provide additional increases in air change rate ($>100$ air changes per hour) and have the following marginal advantage: organisms with rapid settling velocities shed by personnel leaning over the patient would be washed away horizontally before reaching the patient.

There are problems associated with other efforts to eliminate patient exposure to environmental organisms. Even low-organism food is unpalatable. Organisms on surfaces that do not come in contact with the patient probably are harmless. Elimination of environmental organisms can be very difficult. In one ultraprotective unit there was a prolonged struggle to eliminate an unusual *Pseudomonas* species from toilet bowl water. Notably, although the organism was present for 20 months, no instance of infection or colonization due to the organism was recognized [103].

In summary, ultraprotective environments are promising but not yet established infection control measures. Even their advocates do not feel they are securely indicated except for patients undergoing bone marrow transplantation or intensive chemotherapy likely to produce more than 25 days of granulocytopenia [109]. What is critically needed is analysis of the relative benefit of the components of the protective package.

## DISINFECTION AND STERILIZATION

### Definitions

*Sterilization* means the complete elimination of all viable microorganisms. *Nonviable* is best taken to mean the irreversible loss of the ability to propagate indefinitely [41]. Ultraviolet light, although lethal, does not interrupt germination and temporary growth. Conversely, seemingly killed, mercury-treated microorganisms can be resurrected by compounds that displace mercury from sulfhydryl groups. *Disinfection* implies the removal of all life forms capable of causing disease. As a practical matter, this is accomplished by elimination of all viable microorganisms except bacterial spores. *Sanitization* refers to a substantial reduction in microbial content without elimination of all vegetative forms. *Antisepsis* is the application of compounds to skin or mucous membranes to substantially reduce microorganism content.

### Kinetics of Microbial Killing

It is generally presumed, although not always supported by experimental evidence, that most microbial inactivation processes follow a "one hit" killing curve and that all of the organisms in the population are equally susceptible to the process. These presumptions can be restated mathematically as follows: the number of microorganisms killed is proportional to the number present and the proportion does not change as the population of remaining organisms decreases. When the log of the concentration of organisms is displayed on the vertical scale and time on the horizontal scale, this relation results in the familiar straight-line killing curve. The steepness of the killing curve is the measure of the rapidity of organism destruction. It is most often expressed as the "decimal reduction time," the time interval required to bring the concentration of organisms to one-tenth its previous concentration (i.e., 90 percent destruction).

The difficulty in validating one-hit kinetics arises because of technical obstacles to experimentally ruling out that a very small fraction of the starting population of organisms is relatively more resistant to killing. The potential difficulty in killing the last few (possibly more resistant) contaminating organisms is one basis for the overkill prescribed in most sterility standards.

The above kinetics analysis establishes the importance of exposure time in accomplishing microbial destruction. A perfectly acceptable disinfection process will fail if not applied for sufficient time. If extremely high numbers of organisms must be inactivated with a very high probability that no survivors remain (e.g., vaccine manufacture), prolonged disinfection times may be required. Furthermore, a given process may be sanitizing, disinfecting, or sterilizing, depending on the length of time it is applied.

*Microbial Safety Index*
The kinetics analysis additionally establishes the inescapable reality that "sterility" is a probabilistic assertion, not an all-or-nothing phenomenon [76]. This fact has led to the recommendation that the label "sterile" should be supplemented by a microbial safety index (MSI) [27], defined as the absolute value of the logarithm of the probability that the item is contaminated. For example, an item with an MSI of 3 would have a probability of 1 in 1000 of containing a viable microorganism. As a practical matter, establishment that an item in a lot has an MSI in excess of 3 is extremely difficult by direct microbiologic assessment. With even the most rigorous culture technique, it is difficult to avoid introducing contamination at a level less than 1 per 1000 cultured items. Furthermore, the mathematics of sterility testing are quite unfavorable. For instance, to establish with 95 percent confidence that a lot containing 10,000 items is contaminated at a rate of less than 1 per 1000, almost 3000 of the items must be cultured and found sterile.

*Reuse of Disposable Items*
The relevant standard-setting organizations have lined up fairly solidly against reuse of disposable items. The JCAH flatly states: "disposable items should not be reused" [71, p. 74]. The CDC recommends that "no disposable object designed for sterile, single-use should be resterilized" [125]. The FDA policy guide [52] assigns full responsibility to the hospital when disposable medical devices are reused. Product liability law concurs in this assignment: if an item malfunctions due to a design defect and the hospital did not use the item in the way specified by the manufacturer, the hospital may be at increased risk because the manufacturer may contend that the malfunction arose from the improper use (see Chapter 13). However, the FDA guide explicitly sanctions the reuse of disposable items when the facility can establish that the item can be cleaned and sterilized adequately, its "physical characteristics or quality are not adversely affected by their reprocessing," and, somewhat redundantly, the product remains safe and effective for its intended use.

None of the above standards wrestle with the issue of resterilization of an unused item. Occasionally an item is removed from its package or the package is damaged, but the item has not been used. To be consistent with the above reuse dicta, proscription of resterilization of unused items would seem to be required. Yet the above standards seem to permit such resterilization.

The key question, begged by all the above bodies, is: "How do you determine if an item is disposable?" Currently the manufacturer makes the determination: most hospital personnel consider an item disposable if it comes in a package labeled with the words "disposable," "single use only," or the like. Some manufacturers have added such language to packages of products previously marketed with resterilization instructions. Indeed, manufacturers have little incentive, at least in the short run, to do otherwise. Labeling an item "single use" minimizes their liability and maximizes sales volume. Disposability of needles, syringes, and so on, is not the problem; much more expensive items, many of which appear quite sturdy, are now marked "disposable." At a multidisciplinary conference held in May 1983, the reuse issue was thoroughly explored, and some relaxation of the absolute proscription can be expected.

The most compelling case for reuse of disposable items has been made for dialyzers. First use of hollow fiber dialyzers may be more often associated with mechanical failure and systemic reactions (fever, chest pain, transient fall in white blood cell count) due to chemicals leaching out of the membrane [43] or increased complement activation by new dialysis membranes [62]. Newer sterilants, such as peracetic acid, and highly automated dialyzer reprocessors may reduce the potential for toxic reactions due to residual formaldehyde in reprocessed dialyzers. Since resterilization of an item costs a hospital between $10 and $20, depending on the time required to clean and package it and the sterilization method required, the impetus to reuse only occurs for such expensive items. At the University of Minnesota Hospitals we reuse some items marked "single use" (e.g., lumenless cardiac electrophysiology probes, which can cost up

TABLE 14-2. Methods of sterilization and disinfection (CDC)

| Object | Sterilization | | High-level Disinfection | Low-level Disinfection |
|---|---|---|---|---|
| | Will enter tissue or vascular system or blood will flow through | | Will come in contact with mucous membranes but not enter tissue or vascular system | Will not come in contact with mucous membranes or skin that is not intact |
| | Procedure | Exposure time (hr) | Procedure (exposure time 10 to 30 min)[a] | Procedure (exposure time < 10 min) |
| Smooth, hard surface | A | mfr. rec. | D | J |
| | B | mfr. rec. | E | L |
| | C | 10 | F | M |
| | D | 18 | G | N |
| | E | 6 | H | P |
| | | | I | |
| | | | J | |
| | | | Q | |
| Rubber tubing and catheters[b] | A | mfr. rec. | E | |
| | B | mfr. rec. | F | |
| | E | 6 | H | |
| | | | I | |
| | | | Q | |
| Polyethylene tubing and catheters[b,c] | A | mfr. rec. | D | |
| | B | mfr. rec. | E | |
| | C | 10 | F | |
| | D | 18 | H | |
| | E | 6 | I | |
| | | | J | |
| | | | Q | |
| Lensed instruments | B | mfr. rec. | E | |
| | C | 10 | Q | |
| | E | 6 | | |
| Thermometers (oral & rectal)[d] | B | mfr. rec. | K | |
| | C | 10 | | |
| | D | 18 | | |
| | E | 6 | | |
| Hinged instruments | A | mfr. rec. | | |
| | B | mfr. rec. | | |
| | C | 10 | | |
| | E | 6 | | |

*Key*

A = Heat sterilization including steam or hot air (see manufacturer's recommendations).

B = Ethylene oxide gas (for time, see manufacturer's recommendations).

C = Glutaraldehyde (2%).

D = Formaldehyde (8%)-alcohol (70%) solution (corrosion inhibitor needed if formulated in hospital).

E = 6% stabilized hydrogen peroxide (will corrode copper, zinc, and brass).

F = Wet pasteurization at 75°C for 30 minutes after detergent cleaning.

G = Sodium hypochlorite (1000 ppm available chlorine) (will corrode metal instruments).

H = Phenolic solutions (3% aqueous solution of concentrate).

I = Iodophor. Use only a product approved for disinfection by the Environmental Protection Agency (EPA), and follow the product label for use dilution.

J = Ethyl or isopropyl alcohol (70%–90%).

K = Ethyl alcohol (70%–90%).

to $500, and of which several may be used in a single patient study). Our policy requires that each model type be individually considered by the Infection Control Committee after the development of a detailed protocol for reprocessing. These protocols must include a procedure for testing the safety and functional integrity of the item, a method of numbering each individual item, and the use of a log book to record the test outcomes and number of times the item is reprocessed. Note that it is not necessary to reprocess any item very many times. After 20 reuses, the capital cost per use of even very expensive items approaches the reprocessing cost.

*Disinfection-Sterilization Methods*
There are many physical modalities and chemical agents that are useful in various contexts for disinfection or sterilization [20]. A concise summary of methods appropriate for various uses was first published by the CDC in 1970 as an appendix to the first version of the CDC isolation manual. This summary has been updated periodically. The final version was published in July 1982 (Table 14-2). Unfortunately this table, which has been used by a generation of infection control practitioners, will not be reissued. The CDC has been forced to refrain from tying recommendations so closely to particular products. The new CDC environmental guideline discusses disinfectants-sterilants in a more general way.

Regarding selection of a specific brand of disinfecting agent, there has been, until recently, a good basis for reliance on a product's EPA registration label. Although most promotional material is relatively unregulated, a product label containing an EPA registration number established that the product met a highly specified EPA-performed test. Recently the EPA suspended intramural testing, and the basis for labeling disinfectants is less clear [8,60]. Before this change, there was little basis for choosing among marketed formulations of a disinfectant type as long as they had achieved EPA registration.

## ROUTINE MICROBIOLOGIC SURVEILLANCE OF INANIMATE OBJECTS

"Environmental sampling" has accounted for a large fraction of nosocomial infection control efforts in the United States for at least two decades. As late as 1976, 74 percent of hospitals with 50 beds or more conducted routine environmental culturing [90]. This activity was underway in the face of explicit statements by the CDC in 1970 [34] and the American Hospital Association [6] in 1973 recommending sharp circumscription of routine environmental culturing. These statements advocated abandonment of routine cultures of floors, walls, linens, and air but left open the possibility of epidemiologically indicated cultures, spot-checking of critical hospital equipment items (e.g., respiratory care equipment), routine microbial evaluation of hospital-prepared infant formula, and verification of sterilization procedures. Only the last, however, was deemed necessary.

Possible grounds for routine culture of inanimate objects include prevention of infection, education of personnel, and response to statements from a welter of organizations and governmental agencies. To contribute to the prevention of infection, the culture must, at the least, have an interpretable result. When sterility is the goal, this criterion is met. Culturing may also be of value, however, when the need for sterility is not established (e.g., the internal surfaces of breathing circuits) or not required (e.g., infant formula, dialysis water). Perhaps the best operational definition of interpretability is that particular results lead to specific actions. An additional, less commonly articulated criterion is that the cultured object have

---

L = Sodium hypochlorite (100 ppm available chlorine).
M = Phenolic germicidal detergent solution.
N = Iodophor germicidal detergent.
P = Quaternary ammonium germicidal detergent solution.
Q = Glutaraldehyde (a 2% solution has been customary for high-level disinfection and has been shown to be effective for high-level disinfection of respiratory therapy tubing by in-use testing. A glutaraldehyde-phenate formulation also has been shown to be effective for high-level disinfection of respiratory therapy tubing at a glutaraldehyde concentration of 0.13%. Caution should be exercised with all glutaraldehyde formulations when further in-use dilution is anticipated).

*Notes*
[a]The longer the exposure to a disinfectant, the more likely it is that all bacteria will be eliminated. Ten minutes' exposure may not be adequate to disinfect many objects, especially those that are difficult to clean because they have narrow channels or other areas that can harbor organic material and bacteria.
[b]Tubing must be completely filled for disinfection.
[c]Thermostability should be investigated when indicated.
[d]Do not mix rectal and oral thermometers at any stage of handling or processing.
Source: Modified from Simmons, B. P. *Infect. Control* 2:131, 1981 (rev. July 1982, available from CDC, Atlanta, GA 30333).

a high enough probability of contamination, with a severe enough consequence if contaminated, to justify the culture. Routine culturing of purchased sterile supplies isn't justified because of the very low chance of a positive culture.

The educational value of culture of inanimate objects is limited but may be a valid adjunct to other teaching efforts. Care must be taken to prevent such efforts from growing beyond the bounds of a specific educational objective.

Responding to the statements of various organizations quickly becomes an arcane and talmudistic exercise. First, these bodies have considerably varied standings. One *must* comply with the rules of regulatory agencies such as the FDA or the Federal End-Stage Renal Dialysis (ESRD) program. Any hospital with a training program must meet the standards of the JCAH. However, the degree of compulsion diminishes for the recommendations of the many respected governmental (e.g., CDC) and nongovernmental (e.g., Association for the Advancement of Medical Instrumentation [AAMI]) agencies.

A second problem in formulating a hospital's response to these various statements is that statements themselves are sometimes frankly inconsistent. For instance, the CDC's Guideline for Prevention of Intravenous Therapy—related Infection [36] makes no mention of culturing hospital-compounded infusion solutions. In contrast, the JCAH seems to require such culturing.

A third problem—ambiguity—is illustrated by the JCAH statement indicating that solutions "manufactured" in the hospital "should be examined on a sampling basis." We can only presume that this examination should be microbiologic.

A fourth problem is lack of regular updating. Although some agencies, such as the JCAH and AAMI, have formal updating mechanisms that include specific rescissions of previous statements, others such as the CDC do not, and some bodies have actually disbanded (e.g., the USP-FDA-sponsored National Coordinating Committee on Large-Volume Parenterals (NCCLVP)).

A fifth complexity involves interlocking uses of these dicta. The AAMI dialysis water culturing protocol is explicitly intended to be flexible. However, the Federal ESRD program appears to require exact compliance (although no ESRD official will state that in writing). The American Society of Hospital Pharmacists [100] has formally accepted the NCCLVP recommendations, giving them a longevity beyond their creator. In spite of these complexities, infection control personnel must consider the statements of these bodies in decisions about culturing inanimate objects. If nothing else, these statements can assume substantial medicolegal importance.

A general problem arising in considering culture protocols for any product is when in the preparation-use sequence to perform the culture. Generally it is logistically simpler to obtain the culture at the point of preparation. But more relevant to any patient-care implication is the status of the product at the time of patient use. If cultures are positive at the end of the preparation-use sequence, efforts may be undertaken to determine the sources of contamination. However, the impetus to culture patient-care items often comes from the quality-control effort of the department preparing them.

Some unusual biologic items probably should be routinely cultured. Organs, including corneas, bone, kidneys, livers, hearts, pancreases, and bone marrow for transplantation may become contaminated in procurement, transportation, or storage. Positive cultures can have therapeutic implications in addition to suggesting the need for improved sterile technique. A biologic product that probably does not need routine culture is banked, expressed human milk: it is administered orally and inevitably frequently contaminated [81]. Consensus on two possible recommendations may soon emerge: routine culture of hospital water for *Legionella* and of air for fungi. The latter would only be relevant in hospitals with highly immunosuppressed patients. Additional specific items are discussed in the following sections.

### Dialysis Water

The AAMI standard and its adequately convincing rationale have been presented. Sampling frequency is not specified but probably should be at least monthly. It is preferable to sample system water just before a disinfection cycle. Machine water should be taken from different machines to be sure all defects are identified.

### Hospital-Compounded Infusion Solutions

A 1980 NCCLVP statement "endorses the concept of hospital pharmacies using sterility testing of IV admixtures as a method for monitoring the performances of pharmacy equipment and personnel" [102]. The rationale is explicitly stated to avoid the requirement that sterility testing be completed before administering the solutions. The JCAH also appears to require culturing of infusion solutions [71, p. 136].

These recommendations may be challenged on several grounds. Currently, the bulk of infusion-caused infection arises from organisms ascending along the tissue-cannula interface rather than by fluid contamination (see Chapter 36). Much of the contamination of in-use infusion fluid probably arises during administration rather than compounding. Even the need for sterility of infusion fluid is arguable. Most in-use fluid contamination is at very low concentrations, due to relatively nonpathogenic strains and is not associated with patient illness.

The least irrational program of infusion fluid culturing would focus on the in-use product, would use culture methods that don't yield positive cultures with very low levels of contamination, but would involve organism speciation to identify properly the few hazardous species capable of proliferating in the product.

### Respiratory Therapy–Anesthesia Equipment

Although the CDC and American Hospital Association view culturing respiratory therapy equipment as potentially rational, there appears to be no organizational statement actually favoring it. Advocates of routine culture of breathing circuits must surmount two counterarguments: first, that there is no secure demonstration that small numbers of organisms on internal surfaces of breathing circuits cause patient disease, and second, that in-use breathing circuits frequently become contaminated with the patient's organisms even if they start out sterile [39]. Liquids to be administered by nebulizers clearly should be sterile. Any program of routine culture of these fluids should cope with the logistic problem of examining the most relevant specimens: those actually being administered to patients.

### Laminar Air Flow Hoods

The JCAH states [71, page 135]: "When laminar air flow hoods are used, quality control requirements shall include . . . microbiological monitoring as determined by the Infection Control Committee . . . at least every 12 months." Presumably the periodic use of settle plates meets this interpretation. Since HEPA filters do develop leaks, routine periodic evaluation is indicated. However, dioctyl phthalate testing is more reliable than settle plates or other microbiologic assessment [101].

### Infant Formula

Through 1977 successive editions of *Standards and Recommendations for Hospital Care of Newborn Infants*, published by the American Academy of Pediatrics [3], recommended routine culture of hospital-manufactured formula obtained from nursing units. Plate counts exceeding 25 organisms per milliliter were deemed to indicate that technique was faulty and immediate corrective action required. A 1983 American Academy of Pediatrics and American College of Obstetricians and Gynecologists publication, *Guidelines for Perinatal Care*, [4], has superseded the former series. The *Guidelines for Perinatal Care* is silent with respect to culturing hospital-manufactured formula. Similarly, recent relevant statements by the CDC, AHA [5], and JCAH contain no reference to this issue. Abandonment of this recommendation, which had previously been widely accepted—even by those skeptical of environmental culturing [92]—probably reflects a perception that most hospitals have switched to commercially prepared formulas. While this is true of routine infant care, there is an increase in the development of hospital-prepared specialized enteral feeding for which specific guidelines may need to be developed.

Clearly it is necessary for infant formula to be free of enteric pathogens and organisms capable of generating enterotoxins (e.g., *S. aureus*). It seems desirable that infant formula be free of high concentrations of potent nosocomial pathogens. Neonatal *Klebsiella* bacteremia has followed oral ingestion of *Klebsiella*-contaminated breast milk [46]. Freedom from *Aspergillus flavus* is probably desirable for all foodstuffs because of the potential of aflatoxin production. But previous recommendations call for no organism identification, and it is unclear that even large numbers of organisms, excluding those mentioned above, constitute any hazard.

Establishing protocols for culturing infant formula leads to many questions: (1) which of the many formulas hospitals now make must meet the standard? The usual age break point for infants is one year. But it is likely that a contaminated enteral formula poses a greater hazard to an immunocompromised adult than a relatively healthy 11-month-old baby; (2) what culture methods should be used? Since dry formula powder may contain high concentrations of spores, culture techniques that promote thermophilic organism growth frequently produce excessive counts from nonhazardous formulas; (3) if counts exceed 25 organism per milliliter, what actions should be taken? Hospitals producing many small batches of highly individualized enteral formulas find it very burdensome to use sterile blenders and, when possible, sterile formula components. Blenders are difficult to sanitize because of the crevices in the blade housing. Many specialized supplements rapidly lose nutritional value at 100°C (212°F), precluding postpreparation treatment.

The least irrational routine culture program would focus on formula to be given to the most debilitated neonates or other patients, would use culture methods yielding only human pathogens—perhaps only enteric pathogens—and would be considered only a marginal supplement to general sanitary measures.

## REFERENCES

1. Abinanti, F. R., Welsh, H. H., Lennette, E. H., and Brunetti, O. Q fever studies. XVI. Some aspects of the experimental infection induced in sheep by the intratracheal route of inoculation. *Am. J. Hygiene* 57:170, 1953.
2. Acha, P. N., and Szyfres, B. *Zoonoses and Communicable Diseases Common to Man and Animals.* Scientific Publication No. 354. Washington, D.C.: Pan American Health Organization, 1980.
3. American Academy of Pediatrics. *Standards and Recommendations for Hospital Care of Newborn Infants* (6th ed.). Evanston, Ill.: American Academy of Pediatrics, 1977.
4. American Academy of Pediatrics and American College of Obstetricians and Gynecologists. *Guidelines for Perinatal Care.* Evanston, Ill.: American Academy of Pediatrics, 1983.
5. American Hospital Association. *Infection Control in the Hospital* (4th ed.). Chicago: American Hospital Association, 1979.
6. American Hospital Association. Statement on microbiological sampling in the hospital. *Hospitals* 48:125, 1974.
7. American Public Health Association. *Standard Methods for the Examination of Water and Wastewater* (15th ed.). Washington, D.C.: American Public Health Association, 1980.
8. American Society for Microbiology, Public and Scientific Affairs Board. PSAB questions EPA testing of disinfectants. *ASM News* 49:441, 1983.
9. Anderson, R. L. Biological evaluation of carpeting. *Appl. Microbiol.* 18:180, 1969.
10. Anonymous. *Oxford English Dictionary.* Glasgow: Oxford University Press, 1971.
11. Anonymous. Smallpox (editorial). *Br. Med. J.* 1:288, 1951.
12. Anonymous. Waterborne *Legionella. Lancet* 2:381, 1983.
13. Association for the Advancement of Medical Instrumentation. *American National Standard for Hemodialysis Systems.* Association for the Advancement of Medical Instrumentation, Arlington, Va., 1981.
14. Baumann, P. Isolation of *Acinetobacter* from soil and water. *J. Bacteriol.* 96:39, 1968.
15. Bean, B., Rhame, F. S., Hughes, R. S., Weiler, M. D., Peterson, L. R., and Gerding, D. N. Influenza B: Hospital activity during a community epidemic. *Diagn. Microbiol. Infect. Dis.* 1:177, 1983.
16. Bernard, K. W., Parham, G. L., Winkler, W. G., and Melmick, C. G. Q fever control measures: Recommendations for research facilities using sheep. *Infect. Control* 3:461, 1982.
17. Birch, B. R., Perera, B. S., Hyde, W. A., et al. *Bacillus cereus* cross-infection in a maternity unit. *J. Hosp. Infect.* 2:349, 1981.
18. Blaser, M. J., Smith, P. F., Cody, H. J., Wang, W. L., and LaForce, F. M. Killing of fabric-associated bacteria in hospital laundry by low-temperature washing. *J. Infect. Dis.* 149:48, 1984.
19. Blessing-Moore, J., Maybury, B., Lewiston, N., and Yeager, A. Mucosal droplet spread of *Pseudomonas aeruginosa* from cough of patients with cystic fibrosis. *Thorax* 34:429, 1979.
20. Block, S. S. ed *Disinfection, Sterilization and Preservation* (3d ed.). Philadelphia: Lea & Febiger, 1983.
21. Bodey, G. P., Rodriguez, V., Cabanillas, F., and Freireich, E. J. Protected environment—prophylactic antibiotic program for malignant lymphoma: Randomized trial during chemotherapy to induce remission. *Am. J. Med.* 66:74, 1979.
22. Bond, W. W., Favero, M. S., Petersen, N. J., and Ebert, J. W. Inactivation of hepatitis B virus by intermediate-to-high-level disinfectant chemicals. *J. Clin. Microbiol.* 18:535, 1983.
23. Bond, W. W., Favero, M. S., Petersen, N. J., Gravelle, C. R., Ebert, J. W., and Maynard, J. E. Survival of hepatitis B virus after drying and storage for one week. *Lancet* 1:550, 1981.
24. Brachman, P. S. Nosocomial Infection—Airborne or Not? In *Proceedings of the International Conference on Nosocomial Infections,* Center for Disease Control, Atlanta, Ga., August 3–6, 1970. American Hospital Association, pp. 189–92.
25. Briscoe, J. Intervention studies and the definition of dominant transmission routes. *Am. J. Epidemiol.* 120:449, 1984.
26. Buckner, C. D., Clift, R. A., Sanders, J. E., Meyers, J. D., Counts, G. W., Farewell, V. T., Thomas, E. D., and the Seattle Marrow Transplant Team. Protective environment for marrow transplant recipients: A prospective study. *Ann. Intern. Med.* 89:893, 1978.
27. Campbell, R. W. Sterile is a sterile word. *Radiat. Phys. Chem.* 15:121, 1980.
28. Carson, L. A., Favero, M. S., Bond, W. W., and Petersen, N. J. Factors affecting comparative resistance of naturally occurring and subcultured *Pseudomonas aeruginosa* to disinfectants. *Appl. Microbiol.* 23:863, 1972.
29. Carson, L. A., Favero, M. S., Bond, W. W., and Petersen, N. J. Morphological, biochemical, and growth characteristics of *Pseudomonas cepacia*

from distilled water. *Appl. Microbiol.* 25:476, 1973.

30. Carson, L. A., Petersen, N. J., Favero, M. S., and Aguero, S. M. Growth characteristics of atypical mycobacteria in water and their comparative resistance to disinfectants. *Appl. Environ. Microbiol.* 36:839, 1978.

31. Centers for Disease Control. *Disinfection of Hydrotherapy Pools and Tanks.* Hospital Infections Program, Center for Infectious Diseases, Centers for Disease Control, Atlanta, Ga., 1974, reprinted 1982.

32. Centers for Disease Control. Endotoxic reactions associated with the reuse of cardiac catheters—Massachusetts. *Morbid. Mortal. Weekly Rep.* 28:25, 1979.

33. Centers for Disease Control. Guidelines for prevention of intravascular infections. *Infect. Control* 3:61, 1982.

34. Center for Disease Control. *Microbial Environmental Surveillance in the Hospital.* National Nosocomial Infections Study Report, June 1970.

35. Centers for Disease Control. Outbreak of viral hepatitis in the staff of a pediatric ward—California. *Morbid. Mortal. Weekly Rep.* 26:77, 1977.

36. Centers for Disease Control. *Pseudomonas cepacia* colonization—Minnesota. *Morbid. Mortal. Weekly Rep.* 30:610, 1981.

37. Chadwick, P. Relative Importance of Airborne and Other Routes in the Infection of Tracheostomized Patients with *Pseudomonas aeruginosa.* In Hers, J. F. Ph., and Winkler, K. C. (Eds.), *Airborne Transmission and Airborne Infection.* New York: Wiley, 1973, pp. 481–486.

38. Committee on Trauma, Division of Medical Sciences, National Academy of Sciences—National Research Council. Postoperative wound infections: The influence of ultraviolet irradiation of the operating room and of various other factors. *Ann. Surg.* 160(Suppl.):1, 1964.

39. Craven, D. E., Goularte, T. A., and Make, B. J. Contaminated condensate in mechanical ventilation circuits: A risk factor for nosocomial pneumonia? *Am. Rev. Respir. Dis.* 129:625, 1984.

40. Dark, F. A., and Callow, D. S. The Effect of Growth Conditions on the Survival of Airborne *E. Coli.* In Hers, J. F. Ph., and Winkler, K. C. (Eds.), *Airborne Transmission and Airborne Infection.* New York: Wiley, 1973, pp. 97–99.

41. Davis, B. D., and Dulbecco, R. Sterilization and Disinfection. In Davis, B. D., Dulbecco, R., Eilsen, H. N., and Ginsberg, H. S. (Eds.), *Microbiology* (3d ed.). Hagerstown, Md.: Harper & Row, 1980, pp. 1263–1274.

42. Dawids, S. G., and Vejlsgaard, R. Bacteriological and clinical evaluation of different dialysate delivery systems. *Acta Med. Scand.* 199:151, 1976.

43. Deane, N. Dialyzer reuse and therapeutic effect. In *AAMI Technology Assessment Report. Reuse of Disposables: Implications for Quality Health Care and Cost Containment*, pp. 24–28. Association for the Advancement of Medical Instrumentation, Arlington, Va., 1983. Reprinted in *Contemp. Dialysis,* July 1984, pp. 40–46.

44. Dexter, F. *Pseudomonas aeruginosa* in a regional burn center. *J. Hyg.* 69:179, 1971.

45. Dietrich, M., Gaus, W., Vossen, J., vanvder Waaij, D., and Wendt, F. Protective isolation and antimicrobial decontamination in patients with high susceptibility to infection: A prospective cooperative study of gnotobiotic care in acute leukemia patients. I. Clinical results. *Infection* 5:107, 1977.

46. Donowitz, L. G., Marsik, F. J., Fisher, K. A., and Wenzel, R. P. Contaminated breast milk: A source of *Klebsiella* bacteremia in a newborn intensive care unit. *Rev. Infect. Dis.* 3:716, 1981.

47. Douglas, J. M., and Corey, L. Fomites and herpes simplex viruses: A case for nonvenereal transmission? *J.A.M.A.* 250:3093, 1983.

48. Edmonds, R. L. (Ed.). *Aerobiology: The Ecological Systems Approach.* Stroudsburg, Pa.: Dowden, Hutchinson & Ross, 1979.

49. Favero, M. S., Carson, L. A., Bond, W. W., and Petersen, N. J. *Pseudomonas aeruginosa:* Growth in distilled water from hospitals. *Science* 173:836, 1971.

50. Favero, M. S., Petersen, N. J., Carson, L. A., Bond, W. W., and Hindman, S. H. Gram-negative bacteria in hemodialysis systems. *Health Lab. Sci.* 12:321, 1975.

51. Fekety, R., Kim, Y. -H., Brown, D., Batts, D. M., Cudmore, M., and Silva, J., Jr. Epidemiology of antibiotic-associated colitis: Isolation of *Clostridium difficile* from the hospital environment. *Am. J. Med.* 70:906, 1981.

52. Food and Drug Administration Compliance Policy Guide #7124.23. Chapter 24. *Devices: Reuse of Medical Disposal Devices.* Washington, D.C.: EDRO, Division of Field Operations, 1977.

53. Garner, J. S., and Simmons, B. P. *CDC Guideline for Isolation Precautions in Hospitals.* National Technical Information Service, U.S. Department of Commerce, Springfield, Va. Reprinted in *Infect. Control* 49(Suppl.):245, 1983.

54. Geldreich, E. E. Current status of microbiological water quality criteria. *ASM News* 47:23, 1981.

55. Greene, V. W., Vesley, D., Bond, R. G., and Michaelsen, G. S. Microbiological contamination of hospital air. I. Quantitative studies. *Appl. Microbiol.* 10:561, 1962.

56. Greene, V. W., Vesley, D., Bond, R. G., and Michaelsen, G. S. Microbiological studies of hospital air. II. Qualitative studies. *Appl. Microbiol.* 10:567, 1962.

57. Grieble, H. G., Bird, T. J., Nidea, H. M., and Miller, C. A. Chute-hydropulping waste disposal system: A reservoir of enteric bacilli and *Pseudomonas* in a modern hospital. *J. Infect. Dis.* 130:602, 1974.

58. Grieble, H. G., Colton, F. R., Bird, T. J., Toigo, A., and Griffith, L. G. Fine-particle humidifiers: Source of *Pseudomonas aeruginosa* infections in a respiratory-disease unit. *N. Engl. J. Med.* 282:531, 1970.

59. Groschell, D. H. M. Air sampling in hospitals. *Ann. N.Y. Acad. Sci.* 353:230, 1980.

60. Groschell, D. H. M. Caveat emptor—Do your disinfectants work? *Infect. Control* 4:144, 1983.

61. Gustafson, T. L., Bank, J. D., Hutcheson, R. H., Jr., and Schaffner, W. *Pseudomonas* folliculitis: An outbreak and review. *Rev. Infect. Dis.* 5:1, 1983.

62. Hakim, R. M., Breillatt, J., Lazarus, J. M., and Port, F. K. Complement activation and hypersensitivity reactions to dialysis membranes. *N. Engl. J. Med.* 311:878, 1984.

63. Hall, C. B., and Douglas, R. G., Jr. Modes of transmission of respiratory syncytial virus. *J. Pediatr.* 99:100, 1981.

64. Hall, C. B., Douglas, R. G., Jr., and Geiman, J. M. Possible transmission by fomites of respiratory syncytial virus. *J. Infect. Dis.* 141:98, 1980.

65. Hall, C. B., Douglas, R. G., Jr., Schnabel, K. C., and Geiman, J. M. Infectivity of respiratory syncytial virus by various routes of inoculation. *Infect. Immun.* 33:779, 1981.

66. Hall, C. J., Richmond, S. J., Caul, E. O., Pearce, N. H., and Silver, I. A. Laboratory outbreak of Q fever acquired from sheep. *Lancet* 1:1004, 1982.

67. Hays, P. S., McGiboney, D. L., and Band, J. D., and Feeley, J. C. Resistance of *Mycobacterium chelonei*–like organisms to formaldehyde. *Appl. Environ. Microbiol.* 43:722, 1982.

68. Heinze, J. E. Bar soap and liquid soap (letter). *J.A.M.A.* 251:3222, 1984.

69. Hoffman, P. C., Arnow, P. M., Goldmann, D. A., Parrott, P. L., Stamm, W. E., and McGowan, J. E., Jr. False-positive blood cultures: Association with nonsterile blood collection tubes. *J.A.M.A.* 236:2073, 1976.

70. Joint Commission on Accreditation of Hospitals. *Accreditation Manual for Hospitals* (1979 ed.). Chicago: Joint Commission on Accreditation of Hospitals, 1978.

71. Joint Commission on Accreditation of Hospitals. *AMH/84 Accreditation Manual for Hospitals.* Chicago: Joint Commission on Accreditation of Hospitals, 1983.

72. Kallings, L. O. Contamination of Therapeutic Agents. In *Proceedings of the International Conference of Nosocomial Infections,* Atlanta, Ga., August 3–6, 1970, pp. 241–245.

73. Kelly, N. M., Fitzgerald, M. X., Tempany, E., O'Boyle, C. O., Falkiner, F. R., and Keane, C. T. Does *Pseudomonas* cross-infection occur between cystic fibrosis patients? *Lancet* 2:688, 1982.

74. Kelsen, S. G., and McGuckin, M. The role of airborne bacteria in the contamination of fine-particle nebulizers and the development of nosocomial pneumonia. In Kundsin, R. B. (Ed.), Airborne contagion. *Ann. N.Y. Acad. Sci.* 353:218, 1980.

75. Kelsen, S. G., McGuckin, M., Kelsen, D. P., and Cherniack, N. S. Airborne contamination of fine-particle nebulizers. *J.A.M.A.* 237:2311, 1977.

76. Kelsey, J. C. The myth of surgical sterility. *Lancet* 2:1301, 1972.

77. Kesmaviam, P., Luehmann, D., Shapiro, F., and Comty, C. Investigation of the risks and hazards associated with hemodialysis systems. (Technical report, Contract #223-78-5046). FDA Bureau of Medical Devices, June 1980.

78. Klastersky, J., Debusscher, L., Weerts, D., and Daneau, D. Use of oral antibiotics in protected environment units: Clinical effectiveness and role in the emergence of antibiotic-resistant strains. *Pathol. Biol.* (Paris) 22:5, 1974.

79. Kuchta, J. M., States, S. N., McNamara, A. M., Wadowsky, R. M., and Yee, R. B. Susceptibility of *Legionella pneumophila* to chlorine in tap water. *Appl. Environ. Microbiol.* 46:1134, 1983.

80. Kundsin, R. B. (Ed.). Airborne contagion. *Ann. N.Y. Acad. Sci.* 353:1, 1980.

81. Larson, E., Zuill, R., Zier, V., and Berg, B. Storage of human breast milk. *Infect. Control* 5:127, 1984.

82. Lauer, J., Steifel, A., Kjellstrand, C., and DeRoos, R. The bacteriological quality of hemodialysis solution as related to several environmental factors. *Nephron* 15:87, 1975.

83. Lauer, J. L., Van Drunen, N. A., Washburn, J. W., and Balfour, H. H., Jr. Transmission of hepatitis B virus in clinical laboratory areas. *J. Infect. Dis.* 140:512, 1979.

84. LeRudulier, D., Strom, A. R., Dandekar, A. M., Smith, L. T., and Valentine, R. C. Molecular biology of osmoregulation. *Science* 224:1064, 1984.

85. Levine, A. S., Siegel, S. E., Schreiber, A. D., Hauser, J., Preisler, H., Goldstein, I. M., Seidler, F., Simon, R., Perry, S., Bennett, J. E., and Henderson, E. S. Protected environments and prophylactic antibiotics: A prospective controlled study of their utility in the therapy of acute leukemia. *N. Engl. J. Med.* 288:477, 1973.

86. Lidwell, O. M. Airborne bacteria and surgical infection. *Am. J. Med.* 70:693, 1981.

87. Maki, D. G. Epidemic nosocomial bacteremias. In Wenzel, R. P. (Ed.), *CRC Handbook of Hospital Acquired Infections.* Boca Raton, Fla.: CRC Press, 1981, pp. 371–512.

88. Maki, D. G., Alvarado, C. J., Hassemer, C. A., and Zilz, M. A. Relation of the inanimate hospital environment to endemic nosocomial infection. *N. Engl. J. Med.* 307:1562, 1982.

89. Maki, D. G., and Zilz, M. Minimal transmissibility of gentamicin-resistant *Pseudomonas aeruginosa* from cystic fibrosis patients. Presented at the 9th Annual Conference of the Association of Practitioners in Infection Control, May, 1982, New Orleans, La., poster 40.

90. Mallison, G. F., and Haley, R. W. Microbiological sampling of the inanimate environment in U.S. hospitals, 1976–1977. *Am. J. Med.* 70:941, 1981.

91. Mayhall, C. G., Lamb, V. A., Gayle, W. E., Jr., and Haynes, B. W., Jr. *Enterobacter cloacae* septicemia in a burn center: Epidemiology and control of an outbreak. *J. Infect. Dis.* 139:166, 1979.

92. McGowan, J. E., Jr. Environmental factors in nosocomial infection: A selective focus. *Rev. Infect. Dis.* 3:760, 1981.

93. McGuckin, M. B., Thorpe, R. J., and Abrutyn, E. An outbreak of *Pseudomonas aeruginosa* wound infections related to Hubbard tank treatments. *Arch. Phys. Med. Rehabil.* 62:283, 1981.

94. Mead, J. H., Lupton, G. P., Dillavon, C. L., and Odom, R. B. Cutaneous *Rhizopus* infection. Occurrence as a postoperative complication associated with an elasticized adhesive dressing. *J.A.M.A.* 242:272, 1979.

95. Meyer, C. L., Eitzen, H. E., Schreiner, R. L.,

Gfell, M. A., Moye, L., and Kleiman, M. B. Should linen in newborn intensive care units be autoclaved? *Pediatrics* 67:362, 1981.

96. Meyer, R. D. *Legionella* infections: A review of five years research. *Rev. Infect. Dis.* 5:258, 1983.

97. Morse, L. J., Williams, H. L., Grenn, F. P., Jr., Eldridge, E. E., and Rotta, J. R. Septicemia due to *Klebsiella pneumoniae* originating from a hand-cream dispenser. *N. Engl. J. Med.* 277:472, 1967.

98. Mortimer, E. A., Jr., Wolinsky, E., Gonzaga, A. J., and Rammelkamp, C. H., Jr. Role of airborne transmission in staphylococcal infections. *Br. Med. J.* 1:319, 1966.

99. Muder, R. R., Yu, V. L., McClure, J. K., Kroboth, F. J., Kominos, S. D., and Lumish, R. M. Nosocomial legionnaires' disease uncovered in a prospective study: Implications for underdiagnosis. *J.A.M.A.* 249:3184, 1983.

100. National Coordinating Committee on Large Volume Parenterals: Recommended guidelines for quality assurance in hospital centralized intravenous admixture services. *Am. J. Hosp. Pharm.* 37:645, 1980.

101. National Sanitation Foundation. *Standard No. 49 for Class II (Laminar Flow) Biohazard Cabinetry.* Ann Arbor, Mich.: National Sanitation Foundation, 1976, p. B4.

102. Nerurkar, L. S., West, F., Madden, D. L., and Sever, J. L. Survival of herpes simplex virus in water specimens collected from hot tubs in spa facilities and on plastic surfaces. *J.A.M.A.* 250:3081, 1983.

103. Newman, K. A., Tenney, J. H., Oken, H. A., Moody, M. R., Wharton, R., and Schimpff, S. C. Persistent isolation of an unusual *Pseudomonas* species from a phenolic disinfectant system. *Infect. Control* 5:219, 1984.

104. Noble, W. C. Dispersal of Microorganisms from Skin. In *Microbiology of Human Skin* (2d ed.). London: Lloyd-Luke Ltd., 1981, pp. 79–85.

105. Parrott, P. L., Terry, P. M., Whitworth, E. N., Frawley, L. W., Coble, R. S., Wachsmuth, I. K., and McGowan, J. E., Jr. *Pseudomonas aeruginosa* peritonitis associated with contaminated poloxamer-iodine solution. *Lancet* 2:683, 1982.

106. Pearson, R. D., Valenti, W. M., and Steigbigel, R. T. *Clostridium perfringens* wound infection associated with elastic bandages. *J.A.M.A.* 244:1128, 1980.

107. Perry, W. D., Siegel, A. C., and Rammelkamp, C. H., Jr. Transmission of group-A

streptococci. II. The role of contaminated dust. *Am. J. Hyg.* 66:96, 1957.

108. Perry, W. D., Siegel, A. C., Rammelkamp, C. H., Jr. Wannamaker, L. W., and Marple, E. C. Transmission of group-A streptococci. I. The role of contaminated bedding. *Am. J. Hyg.* 66:85, 1957.

109. Pizzo, P. A. The value of protective isolation in preventing nosocomial infections in high risk patients. *Am. J. Med.* 70:631, 1981.

110. Plouffe, J. F., Para, M. F., Maher, W. E., Hackman, B., and Webster, L. Subtypes of *Legionella pneumophila* serogroup 1 associated with different attack rates. *Lancet* 2:649, 1983.

111. Plouffe, J. F., Webster, L. R., and Hackman, B. Relationship between colonization of hospital buildings with *Legionella pneumophila* and hot water temperatures. *Appl. Environ. Microbiol.* 46:769, 1983.

112. Rammelkamp, C. H., Jr., Morris, A. J., Catanzaro, F. J., Wannamaker, L. W., Chamovitz, R., and Marple, E. C. Transmission of group-A streptococci. III. The effect of drying on the infectivity of the organism for man. *J. Hyg.* (Lond.) 56:280, 1958.

113. Ratner, H. *Flavobacterium meningosepticum.* *Infect. Control* 5:237, 1984.

114. Rhame, F. S., Streifel, A. J., Kersey, J. H., Jr., and McGlave, P. B. Extrinsic risk factors for pneumonia in the patient at risk. *Am. J. Med.* 76(5A):42, 1984.

115. Rodriguez, V., Bodey, G. P., Freireich, E. J., McCredie, K. B., Gutterman, J. U., Keating, M. J., Smith, T. L., and Gehan, E. A. Randomized trial of protected environment—prophylactic antibiotics in 145 adults with acute leukemia. *Medicine* 57:253, 1978.

116. Rose, H. D., Franson, T. R., Sheth, N. K., Chusid, M. J., Macher, A. M., and Zeirdt, C. H. *Pseudomonas* pneumonia associated with use of a home whirlpool spa. *J.A.M.A.* 250:2027, 1983.

117. Salmen, P., Dwyer, D. M., Vorse, H., and Kruse, W. Whirlpool-associated *Pseudomonas aeruginosa* urinary tract infections. *J.A.M.A.* 260:2025, 1983.

118. Scheidt, A., and Drusin, L. M. Bacteriologic contamination in an air-fluidized bed. *J. Trauma* 23:241, 1983.

119. Schimpff, S. C., Green, W. H., Young, V. M., Fortner, C. L., Jepsen, L., Cusack, N., Block, J. B., and Wiernik, P. H. Infection prevention in nonlymphocytic leukemia: Laminar air flow room reverse isolation with oral,

nonabsorbable antibiotic prophylaxis. *Ann. Intern. Med.* 82:351, 1975.

120. Schimpff, S. C., Hahn, D. M., Brouillet, M. D., Young, V. M., Fortner, C. L., and Wiernik, P. H. Comparison of basic infection prevention techniques with standard room reverse isolation or with reverse isolation plus added air filtration. *Leukemia Res.* 2:231, 1978.

121. Semel, J. D., Trenholm, G. M., Harris, A. A., Jupa, J. E., and Levin, S. *Pseudomonas maltophilia* pseudosepticemia. *Am. J. Med.* 64:403, 1978.

122. Shaffer, J. G. Microbiology of hospital carpeting. *Health Lab. Sci.* 3:73, 1966.

123. Shaffer, J. G., and Key, I. D. A three-year study of carpeting in a general hospital. *Health Lab. Sci.* 6:215, 1969.

124. Sharbaugh, R. J., Hargest, T. S., and Wright, F. A. Further studies on the bactericidal effect of the air-fluidized bed. *Am. Surg.* 39:253, 1973.

125. Simmons, B. P. Guideline for hospital environmental control. *Infect. Control* 2:131, 1981 (revision of July 1982, available from CDC, Atlanta, GA 30333).

126. Smith, P. W., and Massanari, R. M. Room humidifiers as the source of *Acinetobacter* infections. *J.A.M.A.* 237:795, 1977.

127. Solberg, C. O., Matsen, J. M., Vesley, D., Wheeler, D. J., Good, R. A., and Meuwissen, H. J. Laminar airflow protection in bone marrow transplantation. *Appl. Microbiol.* 21:209, 1971.

128. Stamm, W. E., Weinstein, R. A., and Dixon, R. E. Comparison of endemic and epidemic nosocomial infections. *Am. J. Med.* 70:393, 1981.

129. Storb, R., Prentice, R. L., Buckner, C. D., Clift, R. A., Appelbaum, F., Deeg, J., Doney, K., Hansen, J. A., Mason, M., Sanders, J. E., Singer, J., Sullivan, K. M., Witherspoon, R. P., and Thomas, E. D. Graft-versus-host disease and survival in patients with aplastic anemia treated by marrow grafts from HLA-identical siblings: Beneficial effect of a protective environment. *N. Engl. J. Med.* 308:302, 1983.

130. Turner, A. G., and Craddock, J. G. *Klebsiella* in a thoracic ICU. *Hospitals* 47:79, 1973.

131. Turner, A. G., Higgins, M. M., and Craddock, J. G. Disinfection of immersion tanks (Hubbard) in a hospital burn unit. *Arch. Environ. Health* 28:101, 1974.

132. U.S. Environmental Protection Agency. National interim primary drinking water regulations. *Fed. Reg.* 40:59566, 1975.

133. Wenzel, R. P., Veazey, J. M., Jr., and Towns-end, T. R. Role of the Inanimate Environment in Hospital-Acquired Infections. In Cundy, K. R., and Ball, W. (Eds.), *Infection Control in Health Care Facilities: Microbiological Surveillance.* Baltimore: University Park Press, 1977, pp. 71–98.

134. Wüst, J., Sullivan, N. M., Hardegger, U., and Wilkins, T. D. Investigation of an outbreak of antibiotic-associated colitis by various typing methods. *J. Clin. Microbiol.* 16:1096, 1982.

135. Yates, J. W., and Holland, J. F. A controlled study of isolation and endogenous microbial suppression in acute myelocytic leukemia patients. *Cancer* 32:1490, 1973.

136. Yu, V. L., Zuravleff, J. J., Gavlik, L., and Magnussen, M. H. Lack of evidence for person-to-person transmission of legionnaires' disease. *J. Infect. Dis.* 147:362, 1983.

# 15 CENTRAL SERVICES AND LINENS AND LAUNDRY

George F. Mallison

## CENTRAL SERVICES

The central services department (CSD) in a hospital processes, stores, and dispenses the supplies and equipment required for all aspects of patient care, including diagnosis and treatment [2]. In carrying out these functions, a CSD removes or destroys infectious contamination on reusable items and redistributes them; it also distributes safe single-use items. The role of the CSD in the prevention of nosocomial disease is clear: nonsterilized or improperly disinfected reusable items, including endoscopic equipment, thermometers, bedpans and urinals, respiratory therapy and anesthesia supplies, equipment for aspiration and suction, pressure transducers, and surgical instruments, have been directly responsible for the transmission of infection.

For economic reasons, efficiency of operations, and maintenance of high standards, hospitals have found it preferable for all reusable supplies and equipment requiring special cleaning, disinfection, or sterilization to be handled centrally whenever possible; it is also preferable, for the same reasons, for prepackaged supplies purchased for patient care to be handled centrally [7,21].

Precleaning reusable supplies and equipment in patient-care areas is almost never indicated. Such cleaning is inefficient, expensive, unsafe, and clearly unnecessary with central processing. Rather, items for reprocessing should simply be packaged, clearly marked for contents (if not obvious), and returned to the CSD. If they are potentially contaminated with infectious material, items should be placed in impervious plastic bags labeled "contaminated." Items for reprocessing should be placed in designated areas for pickup and subsequent transfer to the CSD. To prevent the risk of viral hepatitis or other infections to personnel, used surgical instruments should never be cleaned by hand. Rather, they should be processed through a washer-sterilizer in the operating room before being sent to the CSD. Reusable linens should be returned to the laundry, not to the CSD.

Details of the requirements and recommendations for the disinfection and sterilization processes to be carried out in a CSD are described in Chapter 14 and by Simmons and colleagues [21].

### Design of a CSD

A CSD should have separate receiving areas for new single-use items and for soiled reusable items that have been returned for reprocessing. Separate decontamination and disinfection, sterilization (steam and ethylene oxide), and packaging areas and facilities also are required. A storage area should be provided for clean or disinfected nonsterile items that are ready for reuse, such as carts, stands, lamps, heaters, wheelchairs, ice mattresses, and so on. Additionally, a storage area is necessary for sterile items, both new and hospital-processed. Finally, an area for dispensing items and an administrative area are necessary in a well-organized CSD [21,25].

In the design of a new hospital or major renovation of an old one, the CSD should be planned to provide efficiency and safety of operation. In planning, consideration should be given to the location of the CSD in relation to major areas in which goods are received or distributed, such as the loading dock, laundry, operating and obstetric suites, emergency rooms, respiratory therapy and intensive care units, and major patient-care areas. The best location for the CSD is one that minimizes the costs of construction and operation of the entire hospital.

Highly sophisticated, "automated" handling systems for supplies that have been installed in some hospitals in the last decade have not been economical in terms of total costs (i.e., space required, costs of installation and maintenance, and cost of replacement services during downtime). The use of wheeled carts moved by hospital ancillary personnel remains the most efficient and economical means for the transfer of supplies from the CSD to patient areas.

## Initial Processing of Supplies

SORTING AND DECONTAMINATION Sorting and decontamination (the preliminary processing required to make items safe for subsequent handling with reasonable care) should be carried out in a room that is under negative air pressure (i.e., air movement into the room from surrounding areas). Furthermore, the room should be ventilated by at least six air changes per hour; and all air should be exhausted directly to the outdoors [25].

Decontamination by vigorous physical scrubbing, using either a detergent or disinfectant-detergent solution in hot water, and preferably by machine, greatly reduces microbial contamination on the surfaces of items. Sometimes, decontamination processing is sufficient, and no additional processing is necessary. Some items need only be scrubbed with detergent before being stored for reuse (e.g., heating lamps, carts, wheelchairs, crutches, and headboards). However, patient-care items that are contaminated with excretions or secretions, become wet in use (e.g., ice mattresses and flotation pads), have been used by or for patients who are under one or several isolation procedures, or may have had significant direct skin con-

tact with patients while in use (e.g., perineal lamps, toys, and portable commodes) should be scrubbed with a fresh disinfectant-detergent solution, and rinsed and dried before being stored for reuse.

### Washer-Sterilizers and Ultrasonic Cleaners
Washer-sterilizers, which are recommended for the initial decontamination of surgical instruments, provide an agitated, high-temperature, detergent bath followed by steam sterilization. The washing and sterilization of a load of unwrapped, used instruments are possible in about 20 minutes. After processing in a washer-sterilizer, surgical instruments should be additionally processed through an ultrasonic cleaner in the CSD; dried, inspected, and cleaned additionally by hand if necessary; assembled into appropriate packs; wrapped; and terminally steam-sterilized in trays with a mesh bottom or the equivalent. Unless there is an urgent need for the instruments, the trays should be sterilized and dried thoroughly before being removed from the sterilizer.

### Linen Packs
Linen packs should be assembled in the hospital laundry and transferred to the CSD for sterilization. These packs should weigh no more than 5.5 kg (12 pounds) and be no larger than 30 by 30 by 50 cm (12 by 12 by 20 inches). Cotton cloth, paper, and cellophane wrappers have been used for linen and other packs that have been sterilized by steam; only tape should be used to seal packs. Textile wrappers for packs should not have more than 20 percent of their surface area occluded by heat-sealed patches [12]. Sterilization and quality control of sterilization is discussed in the CDC Guidelines for Hospital Environmental Control [21].

### Storage of Sterile Goods
STORAGE AREAS Storage areas for hospital-processed or other sterile items should be ventilated with at least two air changes per hour, and the temperature should be maintained at between 18°C and 25°C (64°F and 77°F). Prevention of excessive humidity in storage areas is also necessary to preclude any possibility of condensation of water on cold surfaces (e.g., inside surfaces of outside walls) that could wet packages of sterile goods, as well as to prevent mold or mildew growth. A relative humidity of 80% or less must be maintained in areas in which sterile goods are stored. Low humidity is also undesirable, because excessive drying may result in fabric damage due to superheating of outdated linen packs during resterilization; if a relative humidity above 30% is maintained, it is not necessary to disassemble, relaunder, and repack outdated linen packs for resterilization. Relative hu-

midity should be measured continuously, and the measuring device should be checked at least monthly using a sling psychrometer. All storage of sterile goods should be at least 30 cm (12 inches) above floor level; no sterile items should ever be placed on the floor. A thorough, continuous program for insect and rodent exclusion and control is essential in an area for sterile storage. No hanging steam, potable-water, or waste-water pipes should be permitted in a room used for sterile storage. Light levels of at least 110 lumens per square meter (10 foot-candles) should be present in all locations in a sterile storage area.

SAFE STORAGE TIMES   Some types of wrappers used for packs sterilized in hospitals have not been tested under carefully controlled, comparable conditions. It is recommended that most types of packs sterilized in hospitals, whether by gas or steam, be double-wrapped with cotton muslin, with each wrapper consisting of two fabric layers (a total of four layers). Such a wrapper will maintain sterility of the pack contents for three weeks when stored on open shelves (Table 15-1). The use of single-wrapped muslin packs (one or two layers) is not recommended [12]. All sterile packs wrapped in pervious wrappers should be handled as little as possible to reduce the opportunity for microbial contamination of the contents.

Closed-cabinet storage clearly is preferable to storage on open shelves, but the extra labor required to move supplies in and out of closed cabinets and the extra cost for the cabinets should be considered when weighing the advantages against those of open-shelf storage for short periods of time. Long-term (at least nine months) sterile storage is possible (open or closed cabinet storage) if packs are sealed in sterile, 3-mil

polyethylene bags [18]. Long storage times may be uneconomical, however, even if the storage is safe, because they reflect an unused inventory of sterile items. Nonetheless, a hospital may wish to maintain in storage a supply of sterile, single-use, nonwoven fabric packs for emergency use in the event of laundry or sterilizer problems or disasters. Routine use of such packs is not recommended, however, because of excessive costs [5].

A pack should not be considered sterile if it becomes wet, if it has been dropped on the floor, or if the tape seal has been broken. An expiration date should be marked clearly on each pack immediately after sterilization. There should be an ongoing procedure for review of all hospital-sterilized and commercially sterilized packs and items in storage to ensure reprocessing (or disposal) of outdated sterile supplies [13].

### Single-Use Items

There are several types of small, single-use (disposable) items that are reliable and cost less than reusable supplies. Examples include surgical caps and shoe covers, gauze sponges, surgical masks and gloves, and syringes and needles [15]. Such disposables must be discarded after use, however, because manufacturers have not guaranteed that they are safe for reuse even if decontaminated or sterilized [26]. Manufacturers generally do not indicate to hospitals the safe time of storage for unused items (i.e., with respect to microbial contamination and/or deterioration of quality). If such items are stored at a relative humidity less than 80%, kept in the original shipping carton, and prevented from becoming wet, the items should remain in satisfactory condition for at least

TABLE 15-1. Storage times during which *hospital-sterilized* packs remained sterile

| Wrapping | Duration of sterility* | |
| --- | --- | --- |
| | In closed cabinet | On open shelves |
| Single-wrapped muslin (two layers) | 1 week | 2 days |
| Double-wrapped muslin (each two layers) | 7 weeks | 3 weeks |
| Single-wrapped two-way crepe paper (single layer) | At least 8 weeks | 3 weeks |
| Tightly woven pima cotton (single layer) over single wrapped muslin (two layers) | — | 8 weeks |
| Two-way crepe paper (single layer) over single-wrapped muslin (two layers) | — | 10 weeks |
| Single-wrapped muslin (two layers) sealed in 3-mil polyethylene | — | At least 9 months |
| Heat-sealed paper or plastic pouches | — | At least 1 year |

*Sterility was checked daily for the first week of storage and weekly thereafter.
Source: From Mallison, G. F., and Standard, P. G. *Hospitals* 48:77, 1974, and Simmons, G. P., et al. *Guidelines for Hospital Environmental Control.* NTIS, U.S. Department of Commerce, Springfield, VA 22161, 1982.

three years. Clear dates indicating when such materials were received and when the products should be discarded if unused should be placed on each carton.

## Inhospital Sterilization of Fluids

A small number of U.S. hospitals (estimated at 400 to 500 in 1980) still sterilize water for patient-care purposes. But these hospitals may not test their sterilized products as recommended by the United States Pharmacopeia (USP). The USP requires that ten bottles from each autoclave load be sterility-tested and ten more bottles be tested for freedom from pyrogens. There are additional personnel costs and potential for injury in loading and unloading. Additionally, the cost of testing 20 bottles from each sterilizer load makes it uneconomical for a hospital to sterilize its own fluids. Hospitals should be encouraged to use commercially manufactured fluids [17].

## LINENS AND LAUNDRY

The purpose of a hospital laundry is to process soiled and/or contaminated linens into clean linen that contributes to patient comfort and care and is not a vehicle of infection or irritation. An estimated 5 billion pounds of soiled linens are produced in U.S. hospitals annually. Most of these linens are potentially contaminated with microbial pathogens that could be the source of infections for patients or the hospital staff, particularly persons who handle them. Linens are handled throughout the hospital by many people, and when they reach the laundry, complex handling and processing operations are necessary to prepare them for reuse.

A review of scientific literature reveals at least four documented instances in which hospital employees handling soiled linens have acquired infectious disease from these linens; one instance involved Q fever [20] and the others, salmonellosis [8,20,23]. Fungal infections can be spread from contaminated fabrics in the hospital; for example, wool socks washed at low temperatures without a disinfectant added to the wash water have spread "ringworm" of the feet in an extended-care hospital [9]. Urinary catheters contaminated by direct contact with patient linens have caused patient infections [14]. Heavily contaminated linens (as well as hands) have caused transfer of staphylococcal colonization to exposed infants [11]. Other episodes of infections due to contamination of linens with pathogens may have occurred in hospitals, but because of lack of recognition of an association or failure of reporting, may not have been investigated and/or published in the scientific literature.

Linens may cause noninfectious problems in hospitals as well. Dermal irritation may occur in employees who handle glass-fiber fabrics or patients who use linens that have been washed with glass-fiber fabrics. Linens inadequately rinsed after washing also may irritate skin. Residues of aniline dyes and phenols on diapers have caused illness and death in newborns [3].

There is a potential for transmission of pathogens by soiled linens. The actual occurrence of disease related to contaminated fabrics in hospitals apparently is very rare, even among hospital staff who have direct and frequent contact with soiled linens as a part of their work. This low rate of transmission may be related to the care given to following procedures designed to reduce the risk of such transmission. Adequate procedures for the collection, transportation, processing, and storage of hospital linens are essential, not only to limit the possibility of disease in patients who may be unusually susceptible or in hospital employees who may handle soiled linens, but also for aesthetic reasons.

## Transportation

Soiled linens should be transported in rolling carts or hampers that are used exclusively for this purpose. The carts or hampers need not be covered. The linings of hard-surfaced carts should be cleaned frequently; if a hospital uses cloth liners in carts or cloth bags on rolling hamper frames, the linens or bags should be laundered daily. If laundry chutes are used, all soiled linens so transported should be bagged to reduce contamination of hands and chutes and to help eliminate clogging of chutes. Chutes should be cleaned on a regular basis. Charging doors and receiving areas for chutes should be located in well-ventilated, fireproof rooms, preferably, not on corridors [25]. Laundry chutes should be continuously ventilated (preferably to roof level) to reduce airborne microbial contamination when the chute doors are opened [25].

Linens known to be contaminated with infectious microorganisms—particularly linens from strict and respiratory isolation areas and from enteric and drainage-secretion precaution areas [10]—should be clearly labeled and handled with special care. Impervious bags are recommended, and hot-water-soluble bags are particularly useful because they can be placed into the washing machine without sorting the contents [10]; however, they are expensive.

## Sorting

Soiled linens should be handled and sorted as little as practical, and linens from infected patients should not be sorted. If any sorting is done, it should be in a room separate from the main laundering area. Consideration should be given to the wearing of protective clothing and gloves by laundry personnel who sort soiled linens before washing. There is no evidence that masks are necessary, and few persons who sort linens are willing to wear even comfortable surgical masks. Frequent hand-washing by persons who sort soiled linens is essential; thus hand-washing facilities must be convenient to laundry personnel. Cloth bags for soiled linens require the same laundering as their contents each time the bags are used.

## The Laundry Process

WASHING AND RINSING  A hospital laundry should be designed to wash seven days' worth of soiled linens within the work week of the laundry. There is no evidence that "continuous-flow" washers or "pass-through" washer-extractors [24] reduce contamination of linens or reduce the risk of disease to laundry workers. The floor and all equipment in a hospital laundry should be cleaned at the end of each work day, and a regular schedule should be established to clean the overhead and hard-to-reach areas of the laundry. The flow of ventilating air in the laundry should be from the cleanest to the dirtiest areas [22].

Thorough washing action using hot water and effective detergents is essential to highly efficient removal of soil and microbial contamination in the laundering process. An accurate thermometer should be used to measure water temperatures. Water temperatures above 71°C (160°F) for 25 minutes kill nearly all microorganisms other than spores; such temperatures have been recommended for decades for all but delicate fabrics. Laundering at lower temperatures has been considered to result in lower effectiveness in the removal of microbial contamination. However, data from a controlled study conducted by the U.S. Veterans Administration appears to show comparable microbial reductions with water temperatures of 50°C (122°F) [6].

The use of hypochlorite bleach in the laundering process provides additional reduction of microbial contamination beyond the effects of washing alone. Although some recontamination of washed linens may occur during extraction, drying and ironing ultimately reduce microbial contamination of well-processed hospital linens to insignificant levels for routine patient use.

It is recommended that all heavily soiled launderable items (e.g., web-footed wet mops or the "step-off mats" placed just inside the outdoor entrances to hospitals) be washed in separate machines used only for these items. Mops must be thoroughly dried after laundering or they are likely to become heavily contaminated with microorganisms before reuse [16].

USE OF ADDITIVES  There are a number of advantages to treating linens with safe and effective combination textile softeners and bacteriostatic agents that are incorporated in the laundry process. Softeners make the linen easier to wash and handle and softer for the patient, and reduce linting. Effective bacteriostatic agents help prevent putrefaction in soiled and wet linen, thus increasing its useful life. Such agents also help to prevent the growth of potentially pathogenic microorganisms in soiled, wet linen and may reduce the incidence of ammonia dermatitis.

STERILIZATION OF LINENS  It is recommended that surgical gowns and linens used in or on patients in operating and delivery rooms be sterilized by steam autoclaving after laundering. However, neither the American Academy of Pediatrics (AAP) nor the Centers for Disease Control requires the use of sterile nursery linens; also, the AAP has stated that the use of clean disposable diapers should be satisfactory for normal, well infants. Diapers and other soiled linens from hospital nurseries should be washed separately from all other hospital linen. Thorough rinsing after washing is essential to prevent any risk of carry-over of laundry chemicals.

STORAGE OF LINENS  To minimize microbial contamination after washing and ironing, clean linen should be handled as little as possible and stored wrapped or covered. The clean linen storage rooms should be separate from the main laundering area, and personnel who work with clean linens should have this as their exclusive activity. Storage in enclosed or covered linen carts that are wheeled to patient areas should minimize handling (and lower costs), and the covering helps to protect linens from contamination by dust. Shelves of carts or closets where clean linens are stored should be cleaned on a regular basis; cleaning at least weekly is suggested.

## Disposable Linens

Disposable sheets, mattress covers, drapes, gowns, curtains, and the like are available in good quality for use in hospitals. However, evaluations have shown that most disposable items (except for small items such as sponges, masks, diapers, and caps) usually are considerably more expensive than reusable linens. Sanitary techniques are necessary for the handling (and disposal) of soiled disposable linens.

## REFERENCES

1. American Academy of Pediatrics. *Hospital Care of Newborn Infants* (6th ed.). Evanston, Ill: American Academy of Pediatrics, 1977.
2. American Hospital Association. *Hospital Laundry Manual of Operation.* Chicago: American Hospital Association, 1949.
3. Armstrong, R. W., Eichner, E. R., Klein, D. E., Barthel, W. F., Bennett, J. V., Jonsson, V., Bruce, H., and Loveless, L. E. Pentachlorophenol poisoning in a nursery for newborn infants. II. Epidemiologic and toxicologic studies. *J. Pediatr.* 75:317, 1969.
4. Arnold, L. A sanitary study of commercial laundry practices. *Am. J. Public Health* 28:839, 1938.
5. Badner, B., Zelner, L., Merchant, R., and Laufman, H. Costs of linen vs. disposable OR packs, *Hospitals* 47:76, 1973.
6. Blaser, M. J., Smith, P. F., Cody, H. J., Wang, W. L., and LaForce, F. M. Killing of fabric-associated bacteria in hospital laundry by low-temperature washing. *J. Infect. Dis.* 149:48, 1984.
7. Committee on Infection Control. *Infection Control in the Hospital* (4th ed.). Chicago: American Hospital Association, 1979.
8. Datta, N., Pridie, R. B., and Anderson, E. S. An outbreak of infection with *Salmonella typhimurium* in a general hospital. *J. Hyg. (Camb.)* 58:229, 1960.
9. English, M. P., Wethered, R. R., and Duncan, E. H. L. Studies in the epidemiology of tinea pedis. VIII. Fungal infection in a long-stay hospital. *Br. Med. J.* 3:136, 1967.
10. Garner, J. S., and Simmons, B. P. CDC Guidelines for isolation precautions in hospitals. *Infect. Control* (Suppl.) 4:245, 1983.
11. Gonzaga, A. J., Mortimer, E. A., Jr., Wolinsky, E., and Rammelkamp, C. H., Jr. Transmission of staphylococci by fomites. *J.A.M.A.* 189:711, 1964.
12. Greene, V. W., Borland, G. M., and Nelson, E. Effects of patching on sterilization of surgical textiles. *A.O.R.N. J.* 33:1249, 1981.
13. Joint Commission on Accreditation of Hospitals. *Accreditation Manual for Hospitals.* Chicago: Joint Commission on Accreditation of Hospitals, 1983.
14. Kirby, W. M. M., Corpron, D. O., and Tanner, D. C. Urinary tract infections caused by antibiotic-resistant coliform bacilli. *J.A.M.A.* 162:1, 1956.
15. Laufman, H., Riley, L., Badner, B., and Zelner, L. Use of disposable products in surgical practice. *Arch. Surg.* 111:20, 1976.
16. Mallison, G. F. Housekeeping in operating suites, *A.O.R.N. J.* 21:213, 1975.
17. Mallison, G. F., and Danielson, N. E. Inhospital production of sterile water. *Hospitals* 54:66, 1980.
18. Mallison, G. F., and Standard, P. G. Safe storage times for sterile packs. *Hospitals* 48:77, 1974.
19. Oliphant, J. W., Gordon, D. A., Meis, A., and Parker, R. R. Q fever in laundry workers, presumably transmitted from contaminated clothing. *Am. J. Hyg.* 49:76, 1949.
20. *Salmonella typhi. Can. Epidemiol. Bull.* 16:128, 1972.
21. Simmons, B. P., Hooten, T. M., and Mallison, G. F. *Guidelines for Hospital Environmental Control,* February 1981, rev. July, 1982. NTIS, U.S. Department of Commerce, Springfield, VA 22161.
22. Simmons, B. P., Hooten, T. M., and Mallison, G. F. *Guidelines for Hospital Environmental Control.* Laundry Services, 2 pp. October 1981. NTIS, U.S. Department of Commerce, Springfield, VA 22161.
23. Steere, A. C., Craven, P. J., Hall, W. J., III, Leotsakis, N., Wells, J. G., Farmer, J. J., III, and Gangarosa, E. J. Person-to-person spread of *Salmonella typhimurium* after a hospital common-source outbreak. *Lancet* 1:319, 1975.
24. U.S. Department of Health, Education, and Welfare. *The Hospital Laundry.* Washington, D.C.: U.S. Government Printing Office, DHEW Publ. No. 930-D-24, 1966.
25. U.S. Department of Health, Education, and Welfare. *Minimum Requirements of Construction and Equipment for Hospital and Medical Facilities,* 1982 ed. Hyattsville, Md.: DHEW, 1982.
26. U.S. Department of Health and Human Services. *F.D.A. Compliance Policy Guide* 7124.23, Transmittal No. 77-55. Reuse of Medical Disposable Devices, p. 1.
27. U.S. Department of Health and Human Services. *A Manual for Hospital Central Services.* Washington, D.C.: U.S. Government Printing Office, DHEW Publ. No. (ARA) 74-4012, 1975.

# 16 HOSPITAL FOOD SERVICES: ROLE IN PREVENTION OF NOSOCOMIAL FOODBORNE DISEASE

James M. Hughes
Eugene J. Gangarosa

For a foodborne disease outbreak to occur, food must first become contaminated with pathogenic organisms or toxins. In the case of bacterial foodborne pathogens, food must then be mishandled in a way that permits the organisms to proliferate. Finally, the food must be ingested by susceptible persons. Hospital food-service departments face all the problems of other large food-service establishments—problems associated with handling large amounts of raw food, serving large quantities of food throughout the day, preparing food for many different diets, preparing and handling food before serving, delays in serving, and tight budgets; in addition, hospital food-service departments serve many patients who are at high risk for foodborne disease. Because of these problems, prevention of foodborne disease should be a serious concern in hospitals.

Foodborne disease outbreaks related to hospital food services may affect patients [38,43], hospital personnel [13], and visitors [10,26] and may involve food prepared in the hospital [38] and food prepared elsewhere but served in the hospital [11,36]. Hospitalized patients are generally at increased risk for diseases transmitted by food because of host factors (e.g., malignancy, achlorhydria, and advanced age) or iatrogenic factors (e.g., antibiotics, immunosuppressive agents, antacids, and gastric surgery). Persons ill enough to be hospitalized are more likely not only to acquire disease when exposed to foodborne agents but also to develop various sequelae associated with such diseases. Small inocula of enteric pathogens that might be innocuous to most healthy people can cause disease and even death in highly susceptible hospitalized patients.

Secondary transmission of foodborne pathogens may also occur when patients or hospital personnel become infected, and they, in turn, unknowingly expose other patients or personnel as a consequence of poor personal hygiene or faulty patient-care technique (see Chapter 32). Two outbreaks vividly illustrate the potential for such secondary transmission in the hospital setting. In 1963 a serious nosocomial *Salmonella derby* outbreak occurred, in which organisms were initially transmitted by ingestion of raw and undercooked eggs and then secondarily transmitted to other patients by hospital personnel [30]. In 1973 a *Salmonella typhimurium* outbreak caused by contaminated egg nog affected patients initially, and secondary transmission to hospital personnel subsequently occurred [37]. Secondary transmission may extend even farther to visitors or others, such as family members, outside the hospital setting. Foodborne disease outbreaks affecting large numbers of hospital personnel have led to staffing problems [10,13] and could hinder delivery of optimal patient care.

The problems of hospital food or dietetic services generally parallel those of a large restaurant or catering firm but are even more complex [17]. Hospital food services typically operate 12 to 18 hours a day, 7 days a week. There is a need to purchase and rapidly process quantities of food that require large working surfaces, numerous utensils, and many working hands. There is also pressure to adhere to tight schedules and ensure rapid preparation and safe storage of a variety of foods. Besides these common issues, hospital food services have additional unique problems created by the need for a wide variety of special diets. Meals and supplemental feedings must be provided from a central kitchen and sometimes from decentralized kitchens on wards. Finally, food must often be transported from a central preparation area throughout the hospital. Delays between preparation and service present the opportunity for proliferation of foodborne pathogens if food is not held at correct temperatures.

## EPIDEMIOLOGIC ASPECTS OF FOODBORNE DISEASES

The epidemiology of foodborne disease outbreaks has been reviewed extensively elsewhere [19,20]. During 1973–77 50 foodborne disease outbreaks were reported from hospitals in Scotland; 31 (62 percent) were caused by *Clostridium perfringens*, 11 (22 percent) were caused by *Salmonella* species, 3 (6 percent) were caused by staphylococcal enterotoxins, and 5 (10 percent) were of unknown cause [33]. In England and

Wales during 1973–75, 202 (32 percent) of 632 reported outbreaks of salmonellosis and food poisoning occurred in hospitals; 157 (78 percent) were caused by *Salmonella* species, 44 (22 percent) by *C. perfringens*, and 1 by staphylococcal enterotoxins [41]. Of the 44 salmonellosis outbreaks in which the mode of transmission was identified, 20 (45 percent) were foodborne.

According to reports of foodborne illness throughout the United States received at the Centers for Disease Control (CDC) during the period 1979–81, the bacterial agents most often responsible for foodborne outbreaks were *Salmonella* species, staphylococcal enterotoxins, and *C. perfringens* (Table 16-1). Transmission of each of the common foodborne bacterial pathogens is typically associated with certain food vehicles; the sources of contamination vary for the different pathogens (Table 16-1). During 1979–81, outbreaks in hospitals and nursing homes accounted for 3.3 percent of all reported foodborne outbreaks, 6.3 percent of all reported cases, and 39.4 percent of all reported deaths (Table 16-2). The fact that only 19 foodborne disease outbreaks in hospitals were reported during this three-year period may be misleading, however, since the foodborne disease outbreak surveillance system is a passive one that requires that the outbreak be recognized, investigated, and reported to a state health department before it can be reported to the CDC; therefore, the problem is almost certainly greater than reported figures suggest. During 1979–81 outbreaks in hospitals and nursing homes were more likely to be caused by bacterial agents and less likely to be caused by viruses, parasites, or chemicals than were outbreaks in other settings (Table 16-3). Although no viral or parasitic foodborne disease outbreaks were reported during this time, foodborne outbreaks of hepatitis A have oc-

TABLE 16-1. Foods commonly involved and usual source of contamination in foodborne outbreaks of bacterial etiology, United States, 1979–81

| Cause | Number of outbreaks | Typical foods | Usual source of contamination | | |
|---|---|---|---|---|---|
| | | | Raw food | Food-handler | Food preparation environment |
| *Salmonella* species | 149 | Beef, poultry, eggs, dairy products | + | − | + |
| *Staphylococcus aureus* | 105 | Ham, poultry, egg salads, pastries | − | + | − |
| *Clostridium perfringens* | 73 | Beef, poultry | + | − | − |
| *Clostridium botulinum* | 32 | Vegetables, fruit, fish | + | − | − |
| *Shigella* species | 27 | Egg salads | − | + | − |
| *Bacillus cereus* | 17 | Fried rice, beef, poultry | + | − | − |
| *Campylobacter jejuni* | 15 | Raw milk, poultry | + | − | + |
| *Vibrio parahaemolyticus* | 8 | Crab | + | − | + |

TABLE 16-2. Reported foodborne outbreaks, cases, and
deaths in hospitals and nursing homes, United States, 1979–81

|  | Hospitals[a] | | Nursing homes[b] | | All other locations | | All outbreaks | |
|---|---|---|---|---|---|---|---|---|
|  | Total | Confirmed etiology | Total | Confirmed etiology | Total | Confirmed etiology | Total | Confirmed etiology |
| Number of outbreaks | 19 | 13 | 35 | 18 | 1,586 | 612 | 1,640 | 643 |
| Number of cases | 1,024 | 638 | 1,566 | 935 | 38,840 | 22,320 | 41,430 | 23,893 |
| Number of deaths | 1 | 1 | 27 | 23 | 43 | 27 | 71 | 51 |
| Deaths/1,000 cases | 1.0 | 1.6 | 17.2 | 24.6 | 1.1 | 1.2 | 1.7 | 2.1 |

[a]Excludes three outbreaks in which food prepared outside the hospital was contaminated but not served by hospital food services.
[b]Includes two outbreaks in state psychiatric hospitals and one outbreak in a state hospital affecting patients on medical, surgical, and geriatric units.

TABLE 16-3. Causes of reported foodborne outbreaks of confirmed
etiology related to hospitals and nursing homes, United States, 1979–81

| Cause | Hospitals or nursing homes | | Other locations | |
|---|---|---|---|---|
|  | No. of outbreaks | % of total | No. of outbreaks | % of total |
| Bacterial | | | | |
| *Salmonella* | 12 | 39 | 137 | 22 |
| *Staphylococcus aureus* | 8 | 26 | 97 | 16 |
| *Clostridium perfringens* | 6 | 19 | 67 | 11 |
| *Vibrio parahaemolyticus* | 1 | 3 | 7 | 1 |
| *Shigella* | 1 | 3 | 26 | 4 |
| Other bacteria | 0 | 0 | 78 | 13 |
| Subtotal | 28 | 90 | 412 | 67 |
| Viral | 0 | 0 | 24 | 4 |
| Parasitic | 0 | 0 | 26 | 4 |
| Chemical | | | | |
| Scombroid | 2 | 7 | 46 | 8 |
| Other | 1 | 3 | 104 | 17 |
| Subtotal | 3 | 10 | 150 | 25 |
| Total | 31 | 100 | 612 | 100 |

curred in hospitals [26], and parasitic disease (e.g., trichinosis) transmission is theoretically possible.

Salmonellosis is the most well-documented disease transmitted by food in hospital settings. In a review of the problem of institutional salmonellosis covering the period 1963–72, Baine and coworkers [2] found that 112 (28 percent) of 395 outbreaks of salmonellosis in the United States reported to the CDC occurred in institutions (hospitals, mental institutions, and nursing homes); 3496 cases in patients and staff were associated with these 112 outbreaks. Institutions ranked second to private homes in frequency of reported outbreaks of salmonellosis. Outbreaks on adult wards were more likely to be due to contaminated common vehicles, while those in the nursery and pediatric setting were more likely to result from contact (person-to-person) transmission. In England

and Wales 6 (11 percent) of 55 reported outbreaks of salmonellosis occurring in hospitals during a two-year period resulted from foodborne transmission; foodborne outbreaks affected more persons, on the average, than cross-infection outbreaks [27].

During 1979–81, 71 patients who became ill in reported foodborne disease outbreaks died (Table 16-4). Only 1 death occurred in hospital outbreaks, but 27 (38 percent) of the 71 deaths occurred in nursing home outbreaks. *Salmonella* species accounted for over half the deaths. The potential severity of foodborne salmonellosis is also underscored by an outbreak due to *Salmonella enteritidis* in a nursing home, in which 25 of 104 affected patients died—constituting an unusually high case-fatality ratio of 24 percent [12].

Reported data can help elucidate the relative importance of various factors that contribute to the oc-

TABLE 16-4. Causes of deaths associated with foodborne disease outbreaks in hospitals and nursing homes, United States, 1979–81

| Cause | Total deaths | Deaths in hospital outbreaks | | Deaths in nursing home outbreaks | |
|---|---|---|---|---|---|
| | | No. | % of total | No. | % of total |
| *Salmonella* | 26 | 1 | 4 | 14 | 54 |
| *Clostridium perfringens* | 7 | 0 | 0 | 7 | 100 |
| *Staphylococcus aureus* | 2 | 0 | 0 | 2 | 100 |
| Other known cause | 16 | 0 | 0 | 0 | 0 |
| Unknown cause | 20 | 0 | 0 | 4 | 20 |
| Total | 71 | 1 | 1.4 | 27 | 38 |

TABLE 16-5. Food-handling errors in reported foodborne outbreaks, United States, 1979–81

| Error[a] | Hospital or nursing home outbreaks (n = 28)[b] | | Outbreaks in other locations (n = 679)[b] | |
|---|---|---|---|---|
| | No. | % | No. | % |
| Improper holding temperatures | 19 | 68 | 461 | 68 |
| Inadequate cooking | 6 | 21 | 150 | 22 |
| Poor personal hygiene | 5 | 18 | 255 | 38 |
| Contaminated equipment | 3 | 11 | 165 | 24 |
| Food from unsafe source | 3 | 11 | 67 | 10 |
| Other | 5 | 18 | 73 | 11 |

[a]Multiple errors noted in some outbreaks.
[b]Outbreaks for which errors were reported.

currence of foodborne disease outbreaks. In the period 1979–81, there were 28 foodborne outbreaks in hospitals or nursing homes in which the factors responsible for the outbreaks were identified (Table 16-5). Food-handling errors contributing to outbreaks in hospitals and nursing homes were generally similar to errors that contributed to outbreaks elsewhere. Holding food at improper temperatures (reported in 68 percent of all outbreaks) was the leading contributing factor in outbreaks in hospitals, nursing homes, and other locations. Other errors occurring with similar frequency in hospitals, nursing homes, and other settings included inadequate cooking and using food from unsafe sources. Poor personal hygiene of foodhandlers and use of contaminated equipment were reported less frequently in hospital and nursing home outbreaks than in outbreaks in other locations. Clearly, training personnel in proper food-handling practices and careful planning of food preparation and service can eliminate these contributing factors and thereby prevent outbreaks.

Food served from a hospital kitchen can be contaminated before, during, or after preparation. Raw poultry and red meat are often already contaminated with organisms such as *Salmonella* species, *C. perfringens*, or *Campylobacter jejuni* when purchased. In several surveys of dressed poultry collected from poultry-processing plants or from retail markets, the frequency of *Salmonella* contamination was as high as 50 percent [6]. Even higher frequencies of *C. jejuni* contamination of poultry have been reported [4,35]. Raw fish may be contaminated with such pathogens as *Vibrio parahaemolyticus* and *C. perfringens*. Fecal matter on the surface of unprocessed eggs is often contaminated with *Salmonella* species. Food may also become contaminated while being processed; organisms may come from hands, coughing, and sneezing as well as from contaminated equipment such as meat slicers or working surfaces [23]. Finally, bacteria may grow while food is in storage (e.g., when cooked foods are stored in direct contact with raw foods or when foods are held at inadequate temperatures).

The hazard of cross-contamination of food is illustrated by an outbreak of salmonellosis in a Missouri hospital. Fifteen cases of diarrhea occurred intermittently among patients and staff in a seven-week period, suggesting contact (person-to-person) transmission, but epidemiologic and microbiologic evidence incriminated tuna fish salad and macaroni salad as the vehicles of infection. Additional studies demonstrated that raw meat was the source of contamination. The salad was prepared in an area of the kitchen where frozen raw meat was thawed [18]. This outbreak underscores the potential hazard of cross-contamination of food in the hospital kitchen and the fact that the distribution of cases in outbreaks due to a common vehicle may occasionally resemble that seen in cross-infection outbreaks [32].

## FOODS AND THE COMPROMISED HOST

Certain foods, especially fruits, vegetables, and dairy products, can be contaminated with gram-negative bacteria [15,34]. Data suggest that in a hospital setting, some foods may serve as a vehicle of transmission for organisms that rarely cause disease in healthy persons but can cause disease in a compromised host. Although the gastrointestinal tract is normally quite resistant to colonization, this resistance is substantially diminished by antimicrobial therapy [40]. Organisms that have colonized the gastrointestinal tract may cause systemic infection in such patients [14,31]. However, the importance of dietary items as a source of organisms that subsequently cause systemic infection is uncertain.

Kominos and colleagues [24] found *Pseudomonas aeruginosa* of the same pyocin type in clinical specimens and on raw vegetables from a kitchen in a general hospital and concluded that the vegetables were the source of the pathogens for the patients. Organisms such as *Escherichia coli* or *Klebsiella* species that are common contaminants of a variety of foods may subsequently colonize patients, particularly those receiving antimicrobial agents to which the ingested strain is resistant, and infections of the urinary, respiratory, and other systems result [3,9]. Some authorities recommend that immunosuppressed patients not be served salads [29]. Others feel that patients who may be extremely susceptible to infection (e.g., leukemia patients receiving immunosuppressive therapy) should receive a sterile or semisterile diet as a component of the "total protected environment" [28]. Whether or not sterile or semisterile diets in combination with other prophylactic measures actually help reduce infection rates in compromised hosts remains to be determined.

Enteral feeding solutions are being used with increasing frequency to provide nutritional support to seriously ill patients. Such solutions are often prepared in food-service departments. Adherence to appropriate food-handling practices to minimize bacterial contamination during preparation and proliferation during storage of these solutions is essential since these solutions have been reported to be the source of organisms causing systemic infections [7–9,16].

## PREVENTION OF FOODBORNE TRANSMISSION

The Joint Commission on Accreditation of Hospitals (JCAH) has requirements and the American Hospital Association (AHA) has recommendations for food-service (dietetic) departments in hospitals (Table 16-6). The Infection Control Committee of each hospital has an important responsibility in the prevention of foodborne disease in hospitals (see Chapter 3). The Infection Control Committee is responsible for cooperating with the food-services department in developing written policies and procedures and for reviewing these policies at least annually [22]. Prevention efforts should be focused mainly in two directions: food hygiene (i.e., food preparation, storage, and distribution) and personal health and hygiene of food-service personnel. Prevention—limiting contamination and destroying or inhibiting the growth of potential pathogens—is simple in principle but may be difficult in practice; approaches to preventing foodborne disease have been reviewed elsewhere [5]. A dietician with special training in food-service sanitation, a sanitarian, or both should be consulted about formulating and monitoring food-handling operations and procedures. Compliance with state and local regulations and standards concerning food-service personnel, food sanitation, and waste disposal is necessary. Consultants should be available from local or state health departments.

### Food Hygiene

A critical factor in preventing bacterial foodborne disease is holding food at appropriate temperatures, that is, keeping hot food above 60°C (140°F) and cold food below 7°C (45°F), and avoiding cross-contamination of cooked food by raw food. In addition, items such as raw milk and cracked or ungraded eggs should not be used. Food must be purchased from reliable sources. Microbial contaminants on some raw foods must be kept from multiplying during processing; proper storage practices and adequate heat treatment must be used. Since work surfaces, knives, slicers, pots, pans, and other kitchen equipment can serve as a means of conveying bacteria from contam-

TABLE 16-6. Summary of requirements and recommendations of the Joint Commission on Accreditation of Hospitals (JCAH) and American Hospital Association (AHA) for food (dietetic) services

| JCAH | AHA |
|---|---|
| Principle:<br>Dietetic services shall meet the nutritional needs of patients<br>Standards:<br>  I. Organized to provide optimal nutritional care and quality food service<br>  II. Appropriate training of personnel<br>  III. Written policies and procedures<br>  IV. Safe, sanitary, and timely provision of food to meet nutritional needs<br>  V. Diet in accord with physician's order<br>  VI. Quality and appropriateness regularly evaluated | General responsibilities of food service department:<br>1. Develop and maintain clean and sanitary work areas, storage areas, and equipment<br>2. Develop written standards and procedures for daily operation<br>3. Prepare purchasing specifications for food equipment, serviceware, and cleaning supplies<br>4. Develop written procedures for cleaning and sanitizing trays and tableware<br>5. Develop procedures that comply with local health department regulations in collection and disposal of waste<br>6. Develop training programs in food hygiene for personnel |

Source: From Joint Commission on Accreditation of Hospitals. *Accreditation Manual for Hospitals,* 1983 ed. Chicago: JCAH, 1982, and American Hospital Association. *Infection Control in the Hospital* (4th ed.). Chicago: AHA, 1979, pp. 61–65.

inated food to other foods, all food-contact surfaces of equipment and utensils must be cleaned and decontaminated after use. All workers must thoroughly wash their hands when they enter the food-processing area after using bathrooms and after handling raw poultry, meat, and fish. Spilled food should be cleaned up immediately. Equipment and kitchen layout should be designed to promote rapid processing to minimize chances for cross-contamination; to avoid producing aerosols, sprays, or splashing during processing; and to facilitate cleaning and sanitizing operations [39]. Contamination by insects, birds, rodents, sewage backflow, or drips must be prevented by screening, proper storage (including separating raw meats from processed foods), and adequate plumbing. Garbage from hospital kitchens and wards should be enclosed, protected from insects and rodents, and transported or disposed of in a sanitary manner according to state and local regulations.

The chances of cross-contamination can be minimized by adopting standard techniques for cleaning work surfaces and kitchen utensils and by ensuring that raw foods are processed in areas of the kitchen and on work surfaces that are not subsequently used for cooked foods. These procedures should be reviewed periodically and when physical changes are made in the kitchen or new equipment is put into use. New personnel should receive prompt training in good food-handling practices. All food-service personnel should receive regular inservice training stressing the epidemiology of foodborne diseases and appropriate food-handling practices (see Chapter 3).

Some common mistakes that have caused foodborne diseases result from poor planning or simply a lack of understanding of appropriate food-handling practices. A typical example is not allowing enough time for poultry to thaw, or assuming that thawing is complete, before cooking. This problem can result in undercooking and can be compounded by keeping undercooked food in the oven after the heat has been shut off, providing ideal incubation conditions for bacteria that survived the initial cooking. Potentially harmful bacteria in foods must be destroyed by thorough cooking or reheating to internal temperatures that reach 74°C (165°F); internal meat temperatures should be measured by bayonet-type thermometers. Cooked foods should be served hot—at or above 60°C (140°F)—or cold—at or below 7°C (45°F). Periodically, the internal temperature of foods in serving lines should be checked.

In some outbreaks, even when refrigerator temperatures were adequate, the center temperature of perishable foods was warm enough to permit bacteria to grow or toxin to be produced. When cooked foods are kept at room temperature (or are refrigerated in large quantities) for a period of four hours or more, certain pathogens remaining in the food may be able to multiply to a high enough level or produce enough toxin to cause disease. The usual reasons for keeping cooked foods at room temperature long enough for potential pathogens to replicate are inadequate refrigerator space, poor use of kitchen facilities, or failure to perceive the importance of refrigeration. In general, food that requires refrigeration should be stored at 7°C (45°F) or below in shallow containers so the food is no more than four inches deep.

In the past, problems have arisen because of preferences for raw or undercooked foods, such as eggnog. Eggnog prepared from undercooked or raw eggs was an important cause of foodborne salmonellosis before the regulation requiring pasteurization of eggs that are to be dried or frozen. An outbreak of diarrhea was caused by *S. typhimurium* in 1973 in a hospital that prepared eggnog from fresh eggs purchased directly from a farm [37]. Such direct farm purchases of eggs may be economically expedient but can be dangerous, as demonstrated by this outbreak.

Storage is a particular problem when food must be delivered from a central kitchen to peripheral areas of the hospital or other buildings by either truck or food carts. A *C. perfringens* foodborne outbreak affecting 49 patients related to a "meals-on-wheels" operation in England illustrates the kind of problem that can result when food is not held at appropriate temperatures before serving [21]. Procedures for transporting food must include facilities for keeping hot food hot and cold food cold. Thermometers used to measure holding temperatures should be standard equipment in such conveyances. Standby equipment should be on hand or alternative plans formulated to handle emergency conditions arising from equipment failure. Food delivered to a kitchen or ward should be stored to prevent growth of bacteria, and it should be distributed with minimum handling by ward personnel. In the event that ward personnel must handle food, they should be carefully supervised to ensure that the same high standards required of kitchen personnel are maintained.

### Personal Health and Hygiene

Supervision of food-service personnel requires attention to work habits, personal hygiene, and health. Hands of food-service personnel may become contaminated by organisms not only from raw foods (*Salmonella* species, *C. perfringens*, and *C. jejuni*) but also from human excreta (*Salmonella* species, *Shigella* species, *C. perfringens*, and hepatitis A virus). Handwashing facilities should be easily accessible in all food preparation and service areas, and soap dispensers and single-use paper towels should be available.

Various strategies have been used in an attempt to monitor the health of food-service personnel. Such approaches have often included stool examinations for ova and parasites, for certain enteric bacterial pathogens, or for both. These measures are not cost-effective with respect to preventing foodborne diseases. It is particularly important to recognize that one stool culture is often not sufficient to detect the small number of organisms in the stool of a person who does not have diarrhea but is infected with enteric pathogens. McCall and coworkers [25] found, for example, that one rectal swab detected only 47 percent of chronic *S. derby* carriers and that seven consecutive daily swabs were needed to detect 95 percent of known carriers. Clearly such extensive culturing is impractical and costly. Furthermore, a person may not be infected on the day the culture specimen is taken, but the same person may later acquire infection. Also, a carrier may excrete organisms intermittently, so sporadic sampling for culture tests may never reveal the true carriage status. Finally, cultures of nose and throat secretions and the feces of many persons may reveal potential foodborne pathogens such as *S. aureus*, but this carriage may be of no danger to others; that is, the carrier is usually not disseminating the organisms. *Thus such routine laboratory testing should not be performed since there is no scientific justification, and it is not cost-effective.*

Laboratory monitoring of food-handlers may actually be counterproductive by giving the food-handler a false sense of security. Negative culture reports are likely to be interpreted by the employee to mean that he or she is not capable of contaminating food with potential foodborne pathogens. From the management standpoint, laboratory monitoring of food-handlers may convey the false impression that food safety is being enhanced.

The proper approach is to establish and pursue a policy of training food-service managers and workers. The hospital Infection Control Committee should ensure that a program exists that includes an initial comprehensive training course in the appropriate languages for all new employees as well as inservice training at regular intervals for all food-service personnel (see Chapter 3). Such courses should include the basic principles of personal and food hygiene and emphasize the need for good hand-washing practices.

Courses should emphasize why food-handlers should wash their hands after using the toilet and after handling such foods as raw poultry, fish, and meats. They should emphasize the importance of informing supervisors of acute intestinal diseases, boils, and any skin infection, particularly on the fingers and hands. In addition to these personal aspects of hygiene, the principles of food sanitation should be stressed. Emphasis must be on rapid and effective cooling, holding of hot foods at appropriate temperatures, and sufficient reheating of foods.

### Surveillance

Responsibility for preventing, detecting, and investigating foodborne disease outbreaks rests with the hospital Infection Control Committee and the infection control nurse (see Chapter 3). The personnel health service should inform infection control personnel of acute illnesses among food service workers that could potentially be transmitted by food. It is important that an atmosphere be created that does not penalize food-handlers for reporting illness. Any policy for work restriction should be designed to encourage personnel to report their illnesses or exposures and not penalize them with loss of wages, benefits, or job status [42].

Appropriate culture specimens should be taken and processed during such illnesses (see Chapter 2). Rectal swab or fecal specimens promptly inoculated onto appropriate laboratory media are recommended in cases of acute diarrhea. Workers should not be permitted to return to their assigned jobs until their diarrhea has resolved. If stool cultures reveal an enteric pathogen, the individual should not return to work until two stool cultures obtained at least 24 hours apart are negative (see Chapter 32). If antimicrobial agents are used, the follow-up cultures should be obtained after treatment has been completed. Personnel with boils, open sores, or cellulitis of the fingers, hands, and face should be excluded until they are adequately treated. The personnel health service's judgment should prevail in deciding when the worker can return to work.

Routine surveillance of patients and employees should detect any cases of gastrointestinal disease related to the hospital's food service. Temporal clustering of such cases should alert the infection control nurse to the possibility of an outbreak. Any cluster should be investigated promptly and reported to the appropriate public health authorities.

# REFERENCES

1. American Hospital Association. *Infection Control in the Hospital* (4th ed.). Chicago: American Hospital Association, 1979, pp. 61–65.
2. Baine, W. B., Gangarosa, E. J., Bennett, J. V., and Barker, W. H., Jr. Institutional salmonellosis. *J. Infect. Dis.* 128:357, 1973.
3. Bettelheim, K. A., Cooke, E. M., O'Farrell, S., and Shooter, R. A. The effect of diet on intestinal *Escherichia coli. J. Hyg. (Camb.)* 79:43, 1977.
4. Blaser, M. J. *Campylobacter jejuni* and food. *Food Technology.* 36:89–92, 1982.
5. Bryan, F. L. Prevention of foodborne diseases in food-service establishments. *J. Environ. Health* 41:198, 1979.
6. Bryan, F. L. What the sanitarian should know about staphylococci and salmonellae in nondairy products. II. Salmonellae. *J. Milk Food Technol.* 31:131, 1968.
7. Casewell, M. W. Bacteriological hazards of contaminated enteral feeds. *J. Hosp. Infect.* 3:329, 1982.
8. Casewell, M. W., Cooper, J. E., and Webster, M. Enteral feeds contaminated with *Enterobacter cloacae* as a cause of septicaemia. *Br. Med. J.* 282:973, 1981.
9. Casewell, M. W., and Phillips, I. Food as a source of *Klebsiella* species for colonisation and infection of intensive care patients. *J. Clin. Pathol.* 31:845, 1978.
10. Centers for Disease Control. Hospital-associated outbreak of *Shigella dysenteriae* type 2: Maryland. *Morbid. Mortal. Weekly Rep.* 32:250, 1983.
11. Centers for Disease Control. Multistate outbreak of salmonellosis caused by precooked roast beef. *Morbid. Mortal. Weekly Rep.* 30:391, 1981.
12. Centers for Disease Control. Salmonellosis: Baltimore, Maryland. *Morbid. Mortal. Weekly Rep.* 19:314, 1970.
13. Centers for Disease Control. Shigellosis in a children's hospital: Pennsylvania. *Morbid. Mortal. Weekly Rep.* 28:498, 1979.
14. Chow, A. W., Taylor, P. R., Yoshikawa, T. T., and Guze, L. B. A nosocomial outbreak of infections due to multiply resistant *Proteus mirabilis:* Role of intestinal colonization as a major reservoir. *J. Infect. Dis.* 139:621, 1979.
15. Cooke, E. M., Sazegar, T., Edmondson, A. S., Brayson, J. C., and Hall, D. *Klebsiella* species in hospital food and kitchens: A source of organisms in the bowel of patients. *J. Hyg. (Camb.)* 84:97, 1980.
16. de Vries, E. G. E., Mulder, N. H., Houwen, B., and de Vries-Hospers, H. G. Enteral nutrition by nasogastric tube in adult patients treated with intensive chemotherapy for acute leukemia. *Am. J. Clin. Nutr.* 35:1490, 1982.
17. Food poisoning in hospitals (editorial). *Lancet* 1:576, 1980.
18. Gunn, R. A. Personal communication, 1976.
19. Horwitz, M. A. Specific diagnosis of foodborne disease. *Gastroenterology* 73:375, 1977.
20. Hughes, J. M. Food Poisoning. In Mandell, G. L., Douglas, R. G., Jr., and Bennett, J. E. (Eds.), *Principles and Practice of Infectious Diseases* (2nd ed). New York: Wiley, 1985, pp. 680–691.
21. Jephcott, A. E., Barton, B. W., Gilbert, R. J., and Shearer, C. W. An unusual outbreak of food-poisoning associated with meals-on-wheels. *Lancet* 2:129, 1977.

22. Joint Commission on Accreditation of Hospitals. *Accreditation Manual for Hospitals, 1983 ed.* Chicago: Joint Commission on Accreditation of Hospitals, 1982.

23. Jordan, M. C., Powell, K. E., Corothers, T. E., and Murray, R. J. Salmonellosis among restaurant patrons: The incisive role of a meat slicer. *Am. J. Public Health* 63:982, 1973.

24. Kominos, S. D., Copeland, C. E., Grosiak, B., and Postic, B. Introduction of *Pseudomonas aeruginosa* into a hospital via vegetables. *Appl. Microbiol.* 24:567, 1972.

25. McCall, C. E., Sanders, W. E., Boring, J. R., Brachman, P. S., and Wikingsson, M. Delineation of Chronic Carriers of *Salmonella Derby* within an Institution for Incurables. Antimicrobial Agents and Chemotherapy, 1964. *Proceedings of the Fourth Interscience Conference on Antimicrobial Agents and Chemotherapy.* Ann Arbor, MI: American Society for Microbiology, 1965, pp. 717–721.

26. Meyers, J. D., Frederic, J. R., Tihen, W. S., and Bryan, J. A. Foodborne hepatitis A in a general hospital: Epidemiologic study of an outbreak attributed to sandwiches. *J.A.M.A.* 231:1049, 1975.

27. Palmer, S. R., and Rowe, B. Investigation of outbreaks of *Salmonella* in hospitals. *Br. Med. J.* 287:891, 1983.

28. Pizzo, P. A. The value of protective isolation in preventing nosocomial infections in high risk patients. *Am. J. Med.* 70:631, 1981.

29. Remington, J. S., and Schimpff, S. C. Please don't eat the salads. *N. Engl. J. Med.* 304:433, 1981.

30. Sanders, E., Sweeney, F. J., Jr., Friedman, E. A., Boring, J. R., Randall, E. L., and Polk, L. D. An outbreak of hospital-associated infections due to *Salmonella derby*. *J.A.M.A.* 186:984, 1963.

31. Schimpff, S. C., Young, V. M., Greene, W. H., Vermeulen, G. D., Moody, M. R., and Wiernik, P. H. Origin of infection in acute nonlymphocytic leukemia. *Ann. Intern. Med.* 77:707, 1972.

32. Schroeder, S. A., Aserkoff, B., and Brachman, P. S. Epidemic salmonellosis in hospitals and institutions: A five-year review. *N. Engl. J. Med.* 279:674, 1968.

33. Sharp, J. C. M., Collier, P. W., and Gilbert, R. J. Food poisoning in hospitals in Scotland. *J. Hyg. (Camb.)* 83:231, 1979.

34. Shooter, R. A., Faiers, M. C., Cooke, E. M., Breaden, A. L., and O'Farrell, S. M. Isolation of *Escherichia coli, Pseudomonas aeruginosa,* and *Klebsiella* from food in hospitals, canteens, and schools. *Lancet* 2:390, 1971.

35. Simmons, N. A., and Gibbs, F. J. *Campylobacter* spp. in oven-ready poultry. *J. Infect.* 1:159, 1979.

36. Spitalny, K. C., Okowitz, E. N., and Vogt, R. L. Salmonellosis outbreak at a Vermont hospital. *South Med. J.* 77:168, 1984.

37. Steere, A. C., Craven, P. J., Hall, W. J., III, Leotsakis, N., Wells, J. G., Farmer, J. J., III, and Gangarosa, E. J. Person-to-person spread of *Salmonella typhimurium* after a hospital common-source outbreak. *Lancet* 1:319, 1975.

38. Thomas, M., Noah, N. D., Male, G. E., Stringer, M. F., Kendall, M., Gilbert, R. J., Jones, P. H., and Phillips, K. D. Hospital outbreak of *Clostridium perfringens* food poisoning. *Lancet* 1:1046, 1977.

39. U.S. Department of Health, Education, and Welfare. *Food Service Sanitation Manual.* Washington, D.C.: Public Health Service, Food and Drug Administration, 1976.

40. van der Waaij, D., Berghuis, J. M., and Lekkerkerk, J. E. C. Colonization resistance of the digestive tract of mice during systemic antibiotic treatment. *J. Hyg. (Camb.)* 70:605, 1972.

41. Vernon, E. Food poisoning and *Salmonella* infections in England and Wales, 1973–75: An analysis of reports to the public health laboratory service. *Public Health (Lond.)* 91:225, 1977.

42. Williams, W. W. Guideline for infection control in hospital personnel. *Infect. Control* 4:326, 1983.

43. Yamagishi, T., Sakamoto, K., Sakurai, S., Konishi, K., Daimon, Y., Matsuda, M., Gyobu, Y., Kubo, Y., and Kodama, H. A nosocomial outbreak of food poisoning caused by enterotoxigenic *Clostridium perfringens. Microbiol. Immunol.* 27:291, 1983.

# 17 DIALYSIS-ASSOCIATED DISEASES AND THEIR CONTROL

Martin S. Favero

In the last 15 years our knowledge and application of chronic dialysis has increased dramatically. In 1967 there were about 1,000 patients on maintenance dialysis. In 1973, when Medicare included coverage of end-stage renal disease, there were approximately 11,000 patients undergoing dialysis in private or hospital-based centers and in homes in the United States; this number has increased almost sixfold in ten years, and the trend is likely to continue. In 1983 there were approximately 72,000 patients undergoing chronic maintenance dialysis, and there were 25,000 staff members in over 1,200 dialysis centers throughout the United States.

In the early 1960s hemodialysis was used almost exclusively for the treatment of acute renal failure. Subsequently, the development of the arterial-venous shunt and other ancillary technologic advances in dialysis equipment allowed maintenance or chronic hemodialysis to become a common procedure. In the 1970s the primary mode for dialysis treatment was hemodialysis accomplished with various types of artificial kidney machines. In recent years peritoneal dialysis, accomplished by automated machines or by intermittent cycling, has increased in use. Over the last several years continuous ambulatory peritoneal dialysis (CAPD) has become popular, because patients can perform this procedure at home and are not tied to either a center or a home machine. Approximately 13 percent of all dialysis patients currently are undergoing some form of peritoneal dialysis.

The purpose of this chapter is to delineate the major infectious diseases that are associated with hemodialysis centers, and describe the important epidemiologic and environmental considerations and control procedures. There is also included a brief review of dialysis dementia and other noninfectious complications of hemodialysis.

## BACTERIAL INFECTIONS

Patients undergoing chronic dialysis have a compromised immune system and other disorders that make them susceptible to a number of infectious diseases. In this chapter, only infectious diseases acquired in the dialysis unit are discussed.

### High Levels of Gram-Negative Bacteria in Hemodialysis Systems

Technical development and clinical use of hemodialysis systems improved dramatically in the late 1960s and early 1970s. However, a number of microbiologic parameters were not taken into consideration in the design of many hemodialysis machines or their respective water supply systems. As a result, there are many situations in which types of gram-negative water bacteria can persist and actively multiply in aqueous environments associated with hemodialysis equipment. This can result in the production of massive levels of gram-negative bacteria, which can directly or indirectly affect patients by causing septicemia or endotoxemia [20,21,26].

In general a hemodialysis system consists of a water supply, a system for mixing water and concentrated dialysis fluid, and a machine to pump the dialysis fluid through the artificial kidney. This kidney (dialyzer) is connected to the patient's circulatory system to remove waste products from the patient's blood. There are several factors that can influence microbial contamination in hemodialysis systems (Table 17-1).

The gram-negative water bacteria can be significant contaminants in hemodialysis systems (Table 17-2), and virtually all disinfection and sterilization strategies are targeted to this group of bacteria. Gram-negative water bacteria have the capability not only of surviving, but also of multiplying rapidly in all

TABLE 17-1. Factors influencing microbial contamination in hemodialysis systems

| Factors | Comments |
| --- | --- |
| Water supply | |
| Source of community water | |
| 1. Ground water | Contains endotoxin and bacteria |
| 2. Surface water | Contains high levels of endotoxin and bacteria |
| Water treatment at dialysis center | |
| None | Not recommended |
| Filtration | |
| 1. Prefilter | Particulate filter—to protect dialysis machine; does not remove microorganisms |
| 2. Absolute filter (depth or membrane) | Removes bacteria but unless changed frequently and/or disinfected, bacteria will accumulate and grow through filter; acts as significant reservoir of bacteria |
| 3. Activated carbon filter | Removes organic material and available chlorine; significant reservoir of water bacteria |
| Water treatment devices | |
| 1. Ion-exchange softener | Both softeners and deionizers are significant reservoirs of bacteria and do |
| 2. Deionization | not remove endotoxin |
| 3. Reverse osmosis | Removes bacteria and endotoxin, but must be disinfected; operates at high water pressure |
| 4. Ultraviolet light (UV) | Kills some bacteria, but there is no residual, and UV-resistant bacteria can develop |
| 5. Ultrafilter | Removes bacteria and endotoxin; operates on normal line pressure; can be positioned distal to deionizer |
| Water and dialysate distribution system | |
| Distribution pipes | |
| 1. Size | Oversized diameter and length increase bacterial reservoir for both treated water and centrally prepared dialysate |
| 2. Construction | Rough joints, dead ends, and unused branches can act as bacterial reservoirs |
| 3. Elevation | Outlet taps should be located at highest elevation to prevent loss of disinfectant |
| Storage tanks | Undesirable because they act as reservoir of water bacteria; if present must be routinely disinfected |
| Dialysis machines | |
| Single pass | Disinfectant should have contact with *all* parts of the machine |
| Recirculating–single pass or recirculating (batch) | Recirculating pumps and machine design allow for massive contamination levels if not properly disinfected. Overnight chemical germicide treatment is recommended |

TABLE 17-2. Water microorganisms
found in dialysis systems

Gram-negative water bacteria
   Pseudomonas
   Flavobacterium
   Acinetobacter
   Alcaligenes
   Achromobacter
   Aeromonas
   Serratia

Nontuberculous mycobacteria
   Mycobacterium chelonei
   M. fortuitum
   M. gordonae
   M. scrofulaceum
   M. kansasii
   M. avium
   M. intracellulare

types of waters, even those containing relatively small amounts of organic matter, such as water treated by distillation, softening, deionization, or reverse osmosis. These organisms can attain levels ranging from $10^3$ to $10^6$ per milliliter of water, and under certain circumstances can be a health hazard for patients undergoing dialysis; they constitute a direct threat of septicemia, and they contain bacterial endotoxin (lipopolysaccharide), which can cause pyrogenic reactions [21,26,30]. It should be emphasized that virtually any gram-negative water bacterium that can grow in water systems represents a potential problem in a hemodialysis unit.

These organisms are able to grow rapidly in water and even more rapidly in treated water mixed with a salt solution. This mixture results in dialysis fluid that is both a balanced salt solution and a growth medium almost as fertile as conventional nutrient broth [26]. Gram-negative water bacteria growing in distilled, deionized, or reverse-osmosis water can reach levels of $10^5$ to $10^7$ per milliliter, but these cell populations are not turbid. On the other hand, these same bacteria growing in dialysis fluids can achieve levels of $10^8$ to $10^9$ per milliliter and are quite often associated with turbidity.

The strategy for controlling the potentially massive accumulation of gram-negative water bacteria in dialysis systems primarily involves preventing their growth. This can be accomplished by proper disinfection of the water treatment system and the artificial kidney machines. Gram-negative water bacteria and their associated lipopolysaccharides (bacterial endotoxins) ultimately come from the community water supply, and levels of these bacteria can be amplified

by the water treatment systems, dialysate distribution systems, type of dialysis machine, and method of disinfection (Table 17-1).

*Water Supply*

Dialysis centers use water from a public supply, which may be derived from either surface or ground waters. The source of the supply may be significant in terms of bacterial endotoxin content, since surface sources frequently contain endotoxin from gram-negative water bacteria as well as certain types of blue-green algae. Endotoxin levels are not significantly reduced by conventional water treatment processes and can occur at levels high enough to cause pyrogenic reactions in patients undergoing dialysis [29].

Essentially all water supplies are contaminated with gram-negative water bacteria, and consequently the water treatment and distribution systems and the dialysis machine are challenged repeatedly with continuous inoculation of these ubiquitous bacteria. Even adequately chlorinated water supplies commonly contain low levels of these microorganisms. While chlorine and other disinfectants added to water may prevent high levels of contamination, the presence of these chemicals in dialysis fluids is considered undesirable because of possible adverse effects on patients being dialyzed. Also, some of the water treatment systems described below effectively remove chlorine, allowing for growth of water microorganisms.

*Water Treatment Systems*

Water used for the production of dialysis fluid must be treated to remove chemical contaminants. The Association for the Advancement of Medical Instrumentation (AAMI) has recently published a list of chemical guidelines for the quality of water used to prepare dialysis fluid [4]. Depending on the area of the United States, a variety of different water treatment systems are used, but most of them are associated with amplification of gram-negative water bacteria (Table 17-1). The most common type of treatment is ion exchange with water softeners and deionizers. Neither of these processes removes endotoxins or bacteria, and both provide sites of significant gram-negative water bacterial multiplication [42]. The most effective means of treating water for dialysis currently is reverse osmosis (RO), which is usually used in conjunction with deionization. RO possesses the singular advantage of being able to remove both bacterial endotoxins and bacteria from supply water. However, low numbers of gram-negative water bacteria can either penetrate this barrier or by other means colonize the downstream portion of the RO unit. Consequently, RO systems must be disinfected routinely (usually weekly).

There are a variety of filters used ostensibly to control bacterial contamination in water and dialysis fluids. Most of these are inadequate, especially if they are not changed frequently and disinfected. Particulate filters, commonly called prefilters, operate by depth filtration and do not remove bacteria or bacterial endotoxins. These filters can become colonized with gram-negative water bacteria, resulting in amplification of the levels of both bacteria and endotoxin in the filter effluent. Absolute filters, including the membrane types, temporarily remove bacteria from passing water. However, some of these filters tend to clog, and gram-negative water bacteria can "grow through" the filter matrix and colonize the downstream surface of the filters within a couple of days. Also, absolute filters do not reduce levels of endotoxin present in the effluent water. These types of filters should be changed regularly and disinfected in the same manner and at the same time as the dialysis system.

Activated carbon filters are used to remove certain organic chemicals and available chlorine from water, but they too significantly increase the level of gram-negative water bacteria and do not remove bacterial endotoxins.

Ultraviolet irradiation (UV) is sometimes used to reduce bacterial contamination in water. This approach is not recommended, however [26], because certain populations of gram-negative water bacteria appear to be far more resistant to UV than others, resulting in instances in which significant numbers of bacteria survive theoretically adequate treatment. This problem is accentuated in recirculating dialysis systems in which repeated exposures to UV are used to ensure adequate disinfection. Resistance to UV is enhanced because of the multiplication of those microorganisms surviving initial exposure. In addition, bacterial endotoxin is not affected.

As mentioned previously, the most effective means of treating water for dialysis is by the correct use of RO systems. The Centers for Disease Control (CDC) has recommended a water treatment system that produces chemically adequate water without massive levels of microbial contamination [17]. This system is well suited for hard water and involves the following procedure: community-supplied water is subjected to softening and passed through an RO unit and then a deionization unit. Through these phases the water progressively becomes chemically pure, but the level of bacterial contamination may increase. To compensate, an ultrafilter is included in the final step

of the system to remove bacteria and bacterial endotoxins. The ultrafilter consists of the same type of membranes as an RO unit but can be operated at ordinary water line pressure. This entire system can be augmented with other water treatment devices, such as activated carbon, depending on the chemical quality of the water in question. If this system is adequately disinfected with formaldehyde or by other means, the microbial content of the water should be well within the recommended guidelines discussed in Disinfection Procedures.

### Distribution Systems

Dialysis centers use one of two general systems for delivering dialysis fluids to patients. In some, incoming supply water is treated and distributed to individual free-standing dialysis stations. At each station, the water is mixed with a concentrated dialysate by automatic proportioning. A second type of system, usually found in large dialysis centers, involves the automatic mixing of treated water and concentrated dialysate at a central location, followed by distribution of the warmed dialysis fluid through insulated pipes to individual dialysis stations. In both designs, the distribution system consists of plastic pipes (usually, polyvinyl chloride) and appurtenances.

These distribution systems can contribute to microbial contamination in two ways. Dialysis systems are frequently made of larger diameter pipes than are necessary to handle the required fluid flow, and they often use longer links of pipe than are necessary. This increases both the total fluid volume and the wetted surface area of the system. Gram-negative bacteria in fluids left standing in pipes overnight multiply rapidly and colonize the wetted surfaces of the pipes, producing bacterial populations and endotoxin quantities in proportion to the volume and surface area.

Because pipes can constitute a source of gram-negative water bacteria in a distribution system, routine disinfection must be performed at least weekly. To ensure that the disinfectant cannot drain from pipes by gravity before adequate contact time is achieved, distribution systems should be designed with the outlet taps at equal elevation and at the highest point of the system. Furthermore, the system should be free of rough joints, dead-end pipes, and unused branches and taps. Fluid trapped in such stagnant areas can serve as reservoirs of gram-negative bacteria capable of continuously inoculating the entire volume of the system [37].

Incorporation of a storage tank in a distribution system greatly increases the volume of fluid available to act as a reservoir for the multiplication of gram-negative water bacteria. Storage tanks should not be used in dialysis systems unless they are frequently drained and adequately disinfected.

## Type of Dialysis System

There are two basic types of hemodialysis machines: single pass and recirculating single pass. It has been shown that by the nature of their design, the recirculating dialysis machines contribute to a relatively high level of gram-negative bacterial contamination in dialysis fluid. Single pass dialysis machines tend to respond to adequate cleaning and disinfection procedures and in general have lower levels of bacterial contamination in their dialysis fluid than recirculating machines. Levels of contamination in single pass machines depend primarily on the bacteriologic quality of the incoming water and on the method of machine disinfection [21,26].

A frequent error in disinfecting single pass systems involves introducing the disinfectant in the same manner and through the same port as the concentrated dialysate. The incoming water (about two-thirds of the liquid volume of the system) is not exposed to a disinfectant; it therefore provides an environment in which bacteria can proliferate and acts as a constant reservoir of contamination. Consequently, for adequate disinfection of a single pass system, the disinfectant must reach all pertinent parts of the fluid pathways of the dialysis system.

## Types of Dialyzer

In most instances the dialyzer (artificial kidney) is not an important factor contributing to bacterial contamination. A noteworthy exception is the large Kiil dialyzer, in which dead spaces can occur between plates, allowing gram-negative water bacteria to proliferate in the dialysate. Currently virtually all dialysis centers use dialyzers that are disposable: hollow fiber dialyzers, plate (parallel flow) dialyzers, or coil dialyzers. These types of dialyzers do not tend to amplify bacterial contamination in the dialysis systems.

## Disinfection Procedures

The objective of a disinfection procedure for a dialysis system is to inactivate bacteria in the fluid pathways associated with the dialysis system and to prevent these organisms from growing to significant levels once the system is in operation. Routine disinfection of isolated components of a dialysis system frequently produces inadequate results, in which the hazard to the patient persists. Consequently the total dialysis system (water treatment system, distribution system, and dialysis machine) needs to be considered when selecting and applying disinfection procedures.

Chlorine-based disinfectants such as sodium hypochlorite solutions are convenient and are effective in most parts of the dialysis system when used at the manufacturer's recommended concentration. Also, the test for residual available chlorine to confirm adequate rinsing is simple and sensitive. Because of the corrosive nature of chlorine, however, the disinfectant is usually rinsed from the system after a short exposure time—usually 30 to 45 minutes. This practice commonly negates the disinfection procedure because the rinse water invariably contains gram-negative water bacteria, which immediately resume multiplication, and if permitted to stand overnight will result in a significant microbial contamination level. Therefore, chlorine disinfectants are most effective when used just before use of the dialysis system rather than at the end of the daily operation. In some large centers with multiple shifts, it may be reasonable to use sodium hypochlorite disinfection between shifts and, as described in subsequent sections, formaldehyde disinfection at the end of the day.

Aqueous formaldehyde solutions tend to produce the best disinfection results. They are not as corrosive as hypochlorite solutions and can be allowed to remain in the dialysis system for long periods when the system is not operational; this prevents the growth of bacteria in the system. Formaldehyde contains good penetrating characteristics but is associated with irritating qualities that are objectionable to staff members. There are several commercial tests on the market for testing formaldehyde in water.

There are two commercially available glutaraldehyde-based disinfectants for dialysis systems. When used according to the manufacturer's recommendations, these disinfectants are not corrosive to machines and are good germicides [38,45]. Furthermore, they are not associated with the irritating qualities of formaldehyde.

Some dialysis systems use hot water disinfection for the control of microbial contamination. In this type of system, water in excess of 90°C (194°F) is passed through all proportioning, distribution, and patient-monitoring devices before use. This is an excellent system for eliminating bacterial contamination.

## DISEASE SURVEILLANCE

Pyrogenic reactions and gram-negative sepsis are the most common complications associated with high levels of gram-negative bacterial contamination of dialysis fluid. The former results from the passage of pyrogenic substances of bacterial origin, presumably endotoxins, across the dialysis membrane, and the latter from the direct inoculation of bacteria into the bloodstream.

The higher the level of bacteria and endotoxin in dialysis fluid, the higher is the probability that bacteria or endotoxin will pass through the dialysis membrane. It has been shown in an outbreak of febrile reactions among patients undergoing dialysis that the attack rates were directly proportional to the level of bacterial contamination in the dialysis fluid [26]. Gram-negative sepsis appears to occur much less frequently than pyrogenic reactions.

In 1982 11 percent of the hemodialysis centers in the United States reported pyrogenic reactions in patients undergoing dialysis. An active surveillance system is essential for the early detection and control of these complications (see Chapter 4). Clinical reactions should be defined as they occur, since this may be the first clue that a problem exists. In addition, the dialysis system should be bacteriologically monitored periodically by methods described below.

Pyrogenic reactions in patients undergoing dialysis are associated with a characteristic set of signs and symptoms. Shaking chills, fever, and hypotension are the most common clinical manifestations. Depending on the type of dialysis system and level of initial contamination, the onset of chills can occur 1 to 5 hours after the initiation of the dialysis and usually is associated with a decrease in systolic blood pressure of 30 mm Hg or greater. Temperature elevation usually follows in 1 to 2 hours. Other less frequent but characteristic symptoms include headache, myalgia, and nausea and vomiting. Specific criteria have been used to define cases of pyrogenic reactions during outbreak investigations (Table 17-3) [26].

Differentiating gram-negative sepsis from a pyrogenic reaction can be difficult, since initially the signs and symptoms of the two are identical. The most reliable means of detecting sepsis is by culturing blood samples taken at the time of the reaction. Because the results of these cultures take at least 18 to 24 hours, however, and since therapy for sepsis should not be withheld for this length of time, other less reliable criteria must be used. Most pyrogenic reactions are not associated with bacteremia, and the above signs and symptoms generally abate within a few hours after dialysis has been stopped. With gram-negative sepsis, fever and chills may persist, and hypotension is more refractory to therapy [29,30].

The early detection of pyrogenic reactions or gram-negative sepsis depends on the thorough understanding of signs and symptoms of these entities by the dialysis staff and on the careful charting of symptoms of the patient, as well as changes in blood pressure

TABLE 17-3. Criteria used in case definition of pyrogenic reactions during hemodialysis

Major criteria
  Objective chill reaction (i.e., visible rigors)
  Elevated temperature while on dialysis (< 1.1°C [2°F]) with absolute > 38°C [100°F]

Minor criteria
  Subjective chill (i.e., patient complains of chills)
  Isolated temperature > 38°C (100°F)
  Myalgia
  Nausea and vomiting
  Decrease in systolic blood pressure > 30 mm Hg

Definite case
  Two major criteria
  One major criterion and two minor criteria

Probable case
  One major alone or one major criterion and one minor criterion
  Two or more minor criteria

Possible case
  Subjective chill alone
  Isolated temperature > 38°C (100°F) alone

and temperature. The following diagnostic procedures are recommended for patients who meet the criteria of a definite or probable pyrogenic reaction:

1. A thorough physical examination to rule out other causes of chills and fever (e.g., pneumonia, shunt or fistula infection, urinary tract infection)
2. Cultures of blood samples taken at the time of reactions and cultures of any additional body fluids or secretions indicated by the physical examination to be likely sources of infection
3. Collection of dialysis fluid downstream from the dialyzer for quantitative and qualitative bacteriologic assays
4. If available, collection of dialysis fluid and plasma samples for endotoxin analysis by the *Limulus* lysate assay procedure [10]

In addition to disease surveillance, periodic bacteriologic assays of water and dialysis fluids should be performed. It has been recommended that the levels of microbial contamination in water used to prepare dialysis fluid not exceed 200 organisms per milliliter and that contamination levels not exceed 2000 organisms per milliliter in dialysis fluids [4,25]. These particular quantitative guidelines are based on epidemiologic investigations [25].

The bacteriologic assay is quantitative rather than qualitative, and a standard technique for enumeration should be used. Water samples should be collected at the point at which water enters a proportioner or where it enters mixing tanks, depending on the type of system used to prepare dialysis fluids. Samples should be assayed at least monthly. Repeat samples should be collected when bacteriologic counts exceed 200 organisms per milliliter and after disinfection changes have been instituted. Dialysis fluid samples should be taken at the end of a treatment from a site where the dialysis fluid leaves the dialyzer or, in the case of recirculating systems, from the periphery of the recirculating cannister containing the coil dialyzer. These types of samples should also be taken once a month.

Samples should be assayed within 30 minutes or refrigerated and assayed within 24 hours of collection. Total viable counts (standard plate counts) are the objective of the assays, and conventional laboratory procedures such as the pour plate, spread plate, or membrane filter technique can be used. Suitable culture media are trypticase-soy agar or standard methods agar. Colonies should be counted after 48 hours of incubation at 37°C (98.6°F).

In the event of an outbreak investigation, the assay may need to be qualitative as well as quantitative, and there might be concern for nontuberculous mycobacteria in water (Table 17-2). In this instance, plates should be incubated 5 to 14 days. Nontuberculous mycobacteria are discussed in the following section.

*Dialysis and Infections*

As mentioned previously, the number of patients in the United States treated by peritoneal dialysis has increased significantly in the past five years, and continuous ambulatory peritoneal dialysis (CAPD), especially, is gaining in popularity. In peritoneal dialysis, the patient's peritoneal membrane is used to accomplish blood exchange. In the mid-1970s, the development of automated peritoneal dialysis systems helped make intermittent peritoneal dialysis an alternative to hemodialysis for long-term management of patients with end-stage renal disease. Currently this type of approach has been replaced by continuous cyclic peritoneal dialysis (CCPD), in which presterilized dialysis fluid is introduced by gravity into a patient's peritoneal cavity continuously and by CAPD. In CAPD a plastic bag is filled with sterile dialysis fluid, which is self-administered by the patient, who has a surgically placed catheter. The exchanges are done every four hours, and the patient can be mobile between exchanges. The most persistent problem in

the management of patients treated by peritoneal dialysis is peritonitis.

With automated peritoneal dialysis systems, the machines must be cleaned and maintained properly, or they may provide a reservoir of pathogenic microorganisms. The machines are designed to sterilize and desalinate large quantities of tap water for subsequent mixture with a dialysate concentrate. Ostensibly the incidence of peritonitis should be reduced, because the machine functions as a closed system. However, automated peritoneal dialysis machines may themselves provide a reservoir for pathogens, which may cause peritonitis. Several outbreaks of bacterial peritonitis among patients receiving chronic intermittent peritoneal dialysis have been reported, and the causative agents have included *Mycobacterium chelonei*–like organisms and *Pseudomonas cepacia* [5,7]. Both of these organisms are capable of growing in water, and in the investigation of these outbreaks it was found that machines were inadequately cleaned and disinfected and that the product water and dialysis fluid contained the microorganisms responsible for peritonitis [39]. In addition, one group of organisms, the nontuberculous mycobacteria such as *M. chelonei*, is significantly and extraordinarily resistant to the commonly used disinfectants [11]. Berkelman and colleagues [6] have recommended a set of guidelines that can ensure the production of sterile dialysis fluid and reduce the likelihood of outbreaks of peritonitis for dialysis centers using automated peritoneal dialysis machines. It was pointed out that if not cleaned and maintained properly, the machines may provide a reservoir for pathogenic microorganisms. The precise details and protocols differ for each machine type, and the reader is referred to Berkelman's paper [6].

Clinical symptoms suggestive of peritoneal infection usually appear 12 to 36 hours after bacterial contamination of the peritoneal cavity. Symptoms include nausea, vomiting, and abdominal pain. Later, vague abdominal tenderness may progress to severe, diffuse, or localized pain associated with fever, abdominal distention, and gastrointestinal dysfunction. The clinical diagnosis needs to be confirmed by bacteriologic analysis of the peritoneal fluid. Cloudy peritoneal fluid is often the first sign suggestive of infection.

The causative agents of peritonitis are usually *Staphylococcus epidermidis* and other gram-positive bacteria, which collectively account for 40 to 60 percent of instances, while gram-negative organisms such as Enterobacteriaceae, *Pseudomonas aeruginosa*, *P. cepacia*, and *Acinetobacter*, and in a few cases, fungi, account for 20 to 40 percent [32,35]. The primary control procedure for peritonitis in this setting is to prevent contamination of the dialysis fluid that enters the peritoneal cavity. This involves (1) proper manipulation of the sterile, disposable plastic lines leading into the abdominal catheter, which deliver the dialysis fluid into the peritoneal cavity, and (2) a system for aseptic connection of the sterile dialysis fluid and the patient's catheter.

## DIALYSIS DEMENTIA

Dialysis encephalopathy, or dialysis dementia, is a disorder that affects dialyzing patients who for a variety of reasons are subjected to water that has a relatively high amount of aluminum, such as community water supplies treated with alum. This complication was first described in 1972 by Alfrey and colleagues [1], and the role of aluminum as a significant contributing factor in this disorder was shown by Schreeder and colleagues [40] in an epidemiologic study. Case definitions of dialysis encephalopathy include three different groups of objective findings:

1. Speech impairment (stuttering, stammering, dysnomia, hypofluency, mutism)
2. Seizure disorder (generalized tonic-clonic, focal, or multifocal seizures)
3. Motor disturbance (myoclonic jerks, motor apraxia, immobility)

Schreeder showed that patients were at increased risk of dialysis dementia when aluminum content of water was high. The number of cases of dialysis dementia reported to the CDC in 1980 was 229, an incidence of 0.4 percent. The case fatality ratio was 34.9 percent [3]. The control of this disorder revolves around adequate water treatment systems and invariably requires the use of reverse osmosis, either alone or with deionization [40].

## TOXIC REACTIONS

There are instances in which chemicals in water or as residual in dialysis systems adversely affect dialyzing patients. Certain chemicals in water may not be toxic when ingested by humans, but the hemodialysis patient may be exposed directly to 150 L of water per treatment. A few examples will illustrate this problem.

Occasionally suppliers of community water change water disinfection patterns by increasing chlorine dosages or using chloramines. These changes usually occur without the knowledge of the dialysis staff. Chloramines in water must be removed, or the patient will experience acute hemolysis. If the correct water treatment system (activated carbon) is not used in the dialysis center, patients will be exposed to this chemical. In November 1979 the water treatment plant in Annapolis, Maryland, accidentally fed excessive levels of fluoride into the community water supply, resulting in the death of one patient and acute illness in several other patients in a hemodialysis center receiving this community water supply. The center's water treatment system was not adequate to remove excessive fluoride from water [13].

In both of the above examples, a water treatment system consisting of activated carbon filtration, reverse osmosis, deionization, and ultrafiltration would have prevented toxic reactions.

There also have been instances in which a disinfectant such as formaldehyde was not sufficiently removed from dialysis systems, and patients were exposed to this chemical. This can be prevented by monitoring the system for complete rinsing, using a chemical assay sensitive to the chemical.

## REUSE OF HEMODIALYZERS

In the early 1960s the most common dialyzer used in dialysis centers was the Kiil plate dialyzer, which was cleaned and disinfected after each patient use and supplied with a new set of cuprophane membranes. The dialyzer housing, however, was reused each time. With the development of disposable coil and hollow fiber dialyzers, use of the Kiil dialyzer was discontinued. Disposable dialyzers are medical devices that are supplied in a sterile state and meant for one-time use. In recent years, as a cost-saving effort, many centers have been reusing dialyzers on the same patient after an appropriate disinfection procedure. This practice has caused some controversy but is currently performed in almost 52 percent of all dialysis centers and with more than 60,000 patients in the United States. The CDC has made no specific recommendations for or against reusing dialyzers. In a response to an outbreak investigation, however, the CDC has recently recommended a specific disinfection procedure, which is discussed in this section.

The reuse of all types of disposable medical devices will not be discussed; instead, a brief description will be given of the important factors involved in reusing dialyzers. The procedures used in a dialysis center are not sterilization procedures; they are high-level disinfection procedures [19]. If the technique is correctly performed according to established protocols, however, there appear to be no harmful effects on dialysis patients. Indeed, in performing surveillance of dialysis-associated diseases in centers in the United States, the CDC has determined that the risk of acquiring viral hepatitis type B among dialysis patients and staff members is not affected by the practice of reusing hemodialyzers [3,22]. In terms of both the incidence and the prevalence of this disease, there is no significant difference between patients and staff in dialysis centers that do not reuse dialyzers and those that do. Similarly, there has been no difference in the occurrence of reported pyrogenic reactions between patients in hemodialysis centers that reuse dialyzers and those that do not [3].

Although a variety of disinfectants and procedures has been described for disinfecting dialyzers, by far the most commonly used agent is formaldehyde. Most centers in the United States have used 2% formaldehyde with a contact time of approximately 36 hours for the high-level disinfection of dialyzers. Although this regimen appears to be satisfactory against the presumed microbiologic challenge of gram-negative water bacteria, it may be inadequate for the highly germicide-resistant nontuberculous mycobacteria. The CDC investigated an outbreak of infections caused by nontuberculous mycobacteria during which 27 cases of infection occurred among 140 patients with end-stage renal disease [14]. The source of the nontuberculous mycobacteria appeared to be the water used in processing the dialyzers. Furthermore, it was evident that 2% formaldehyde did not effectively inactivate these organisms in 36 hours. Tests have shown that 4 percent formaldehyde with a minimum contact of 24 hours can inactivate high numbers of nontuberculous mycobacteria, and as a consequence 4% formaldehyde is recommended as a minimum for disinfection if dialyzers are reused [19].

## VIRAL HEPATITIS

A concomitant of the significant increase in the number of dialysis centers, patients, and staff members in the United States was the realization that viral hepatitis can be a major complication of maintenance hemodialysis (see Chapter 35). The CDC, which has been conducting surveillance of viral hepatitis in dialysis centers since 1969, reported that in the period between 1972 and 1974, the incidence of hepatitis B surface antigen (HBsAg) positivity among patients and staff increased by more than 100 percent to 6.2 percent and 5.2 percent, respectively [41]. In a separate survey of 15 hemodialysis centers during the same two-year period, Szmuness and colleagues [44] showed that the point prevalence of HBsAg was 16.8

percent among patients and 2.4 percent among staff. This time period correlated with a significant increase in the number of dialysis centers, patients, and staff members due to the Federal Government's decision to pay for treatment of patients with end-stage renal disease.

The primary strategy for controlling viral hepatitis in dialysis units has centered around disease and serologic surveillance of patients and staff members and separation of HBsAg-positive patients from susceptible patients [12,33,34]. In 1976 the CDC's surveillance system was expanded through collaboration with the Health Care Financing Administration (HCFA), and during the HCFA's annual facility survey for the calendar years of 1976, 1980, and 1982, a questionnaire from the CDC was included. The response rate was over 95 percent. In general the data showed that incidence and prevalence of HBsAg positivity among patients and staff in this time period decreased significantly and that this reduction appeared to be due to better infection control practices (Table 17-4). These practices included complete segregation of HBsAg-positive patients and their dialysis equipment in conjunction with rapid identification of patients seroconverting to HBsAg by the use of better serologic surveillance [3]. By 1983 the average hemodialysis center in the United States, although still considered a relatively high-risk environment for acquiring hepatitis B infection, was no longer considered to be an "extraordinarily" high-risk environment.

There have also been outbreaks of dialysis-associated non-A, non-B hepatitis [27]. The primary or reactivated infections with such viruses as herpesvirus, Epstein-Barr virus, and cytomegaloviruses have been observed in renal transplant recipients and other immunologically suppressed persons (see Chapter 37) [15,31], but they are not considered as important in dialysis centers as hepatitis B. Viral hepatitis type A, which is spread by the fecal-oral route rather than blood, has not been reported to occur in hemodialysis units.

### Modes of Transmission

A person who is in the acute phase of hepatitis B infection or is a chronic carrier of HBsAg and is also HBeAg-positive has an extraordinary amount of hepatitis B virus (HBV) circulating in the blood—approximately $10^8$ per milliliter. With titers this high, excretions and secretions that contain serum may also contain HBV [23]. Blood can be diluted until it is no longer visible or chemically detectable and still contain $10^2$ to $10^3$ infectious HBV per milliliter. Furthermore, HBV is relatively stable in the envi-

TABLE 17-4. Incidence and prevalence of HBsAg in hemodialysis patients and staff, 1972–82, United States

| | Year | Number tested | Incidence[a] (%) | Number tested | Prevalence[b] (%) |
|---|---|---|---|---|---|
| Patients | 1972 | 8,709 | 2.8 | ND | |
| | 1974 | 15,382 | 6.2 | ND | |
| | 1976 | 33,875 | 3.0 | 22,876 | 7.8 |
| | 1980 | 62,723 | 1.0 | 43,796 | 3.8 |
| | 1982 | 66,326 | 0.5 | 49,275 | 2.7 |
| Staff | 1972 | 2,523 | 1.9 | ND | |
| | 1974 | 5,408 | 5.8 | ND | |
| | 1976 | 15,946 | 2.6 | ND | |
| | 1980 | 24,853 | 0.7 | 20,399 | 0.7 |
| | 1982 | 25,260 | 0.4 | 21,139 | 0.4 |

ND = Not done.
[a]Percentage who converted to HBsAg-positive during the calendar year.
[b]Percentage who were HBsAg-positive during the last week of December.

ronment and has been shown to remain viable for at least seven days on environmental surfaces at room temperature [9]. These factors cause environments in which there is a good deal of blood exposure to have a high risk for potential HBV transmission if proper control measures are not practiced. This is especially true of hemodialysis units.

HBV infection may be acquired by patients in a dialysis unit by transfusion of infective blood or blood products. This is less likely now since all blood is screened for HBsAg, and patients who are already HBsAg-positive are so identified at admission. Dialysis patients, once infected, frequently become chronic asymptomatic HBsAg carriers who in turn become sources of HBV contamination for many environmental surfaces. Indeed, during the early 1970s hepatitis B infection in dialysis units tended to become endemic because of the presence of chronic carriers who were asymptomatic and because of the absence of sufficient disease and serologic surveillance systems.

Given the extraordinarily high level of HBV in blood, one can categorize the various modes of hepatitis B transmission as follows:

1. Direct percutaneous inoculation by needle of contaminated serum or plasma or transfusion of infective blood or blood products
2. Percutaneous transfer of infected serum or plasma, such as may occur through cuts, scratches, abrasions, or other breaks in the skin
3. Introduction of infected serum or plasma onto mucosal surfaces such as may occur through inadvertent introduction of these materials into the mouth or eyes

4. Introduction of other known infectious secretions, such as saliva and peritoneal fluid, onto mucosal surfaces
5. Indirect transfer of serum or plasma via inanimate environmental surfaces [23]

There is no epidemiologic evidence to suggest airborne transmission of HBV [36] and no disease transmission occurs by the intestinal circuit. Splashes of infective blood that enter the oral cavity may result in HBV infection, because the virus enters the vascular system through the buccal cavity but not the intestinal tract.

There are various routes of hepatitis B transmission that may occur in hemodialysis units (Table 17-5). Staff members in hemodialysis units may become infected with HBV through accidental needle punctures or breaks in their skin or mucous membranes. These staff members have frequent and continuous contact with blood and blood-contaminated surfaces. Dialysis patients may acquire HBV infection in several ways, including:

1. Internally contaminated dialysis equipment such as venous pressure gauges or venous pressure isolators or filters (used to prevent reflux of blood into gauges) that are not routinely changed after each use
2. Injections if the site of injection is contaminated with HBV
3. Breaks in skin or mucous membranes when in contact with contaminated objects

There is no epidemiologic documentation that HBV has been transmitted from infected hemodialysis staff

TABLE 17-5. Routes of hepatitis B transmission in hemodialysis centers

| Route | Comment |
|---|---|
| Transfused blood and blood products → patient | Uncommon for hepatitis B due to HBsAg screening; possible for transmission of NANB hepatitis |
| Patient → staff member | Transmitted by needle sticks—inapparent percutaneous exposure |
| Patient → dialysis system → staff member | Transmitted by HBV-contaminated blood on devices, tubes, and environmental surfaces |
| Patient → dialysis system external surfaces → → staff member hands → patient | Frequently touched dialysis machines or associated environmental surfaces may be reservoirs of HBV; transmitted by staff with contaminated gloves or hands |
| Staff member → patient | Rare; has never been reported in a dialysis center |

NANB = non-A, non-B; HBV = hepatitis B virus.

members to dialysis patients. Hypothetically, this route of transmission is possible but not likely, because infectious blood and body fluids of dialysis personnel are not readily accessible to patients. However, dialysis staff members may physically carry HBV from infected patients to susceptible patients by means of contaminated hands, gloves, and other objects.

Environmental surfaces in the hemodialysis center may play a major role in HBV transmission. It has been shown that although HBsAg, which can be considered a footprint of HBV, has never been detected in the air of hemodialysis centers [36], environmental surfaces, especially those often touched, can be contaminated frequently even in the absence of visible blood staining [24]. For example, HBsAg has been detected on clamps, scissors, dialysis machine control knobs, door knobs, and other surfaces in the dialysis center. If these surfaces or objects are not cleaned or disinfected frequently and are shared among patients on the same or neighboring machines, an almost unnoticeable infection transmission route is created. Although dialysis staff members may routinely change gloves after caring for each patient, a new pair of gloves can become contaminated when the staff member touches surfaces previously contaminated with blood from an HBsAg-positive patient. HBV can be transmitted to a patient when a staff member, wearing the contaminated gloves, searches for the patient's best site of injection by applying finger pressure or by contaminating that site before injection. The proper procedure here is for a staff member, when donning a pair of new gloves, to refrain from touching any environmental surfaces before injecting the patient.

It is this mode of disease transmission, rather than any phenomenon dealing with internal contamination of dialysis machines, that is the rationale for separating HBsAg-positive patients from others.

## INFECTION CONTROL STRATEGIES IN DIALYSIS CENTERS

### Surveillance*

Routine surveillance of HBsAg and antibody (anti-HBs) must be performed in a dialysis center as part of a comprehensive surveillance and control program to determine if transmission of hepatitis B is occurring (see Chapter 4). This surveillance can identify patients and staff as either potential sources of infection (i.e., HBsAg-positive), immune (anti-HB-positive), or susceptible (negative for HBsAg and anti-HBs). Patients and staff members should be screened for HBsAg and anti-HBs when they enter the unit to determine their serologic status. The HBsAg status of visiting and home patients should be known at the time of admission. HBsAg positivity in staff members does not preclude employment in a dialysis center, because disease transmission from dialysis staff members to patients has not been reported, and these persons may be assigned preferentially to care for HBsAg-positive patients.

There are many commercially available tests that can be used to assay for various markers of HBV infection. Besides HBsAg and anti-HBs, there are tests for the assay of anti-core (anti-HBc) and for e antigen and its antibody (HBeAg and anti-HBe). It should be kept in mind that major infection control decisions in dialysis centers are associated almost exclusively with the HBsAg status of patients. Consequently, other tests are not necessary for infection control purposes. There are times when non-A, non-B hepatitis may be suspected in a dialysis staff member or patient, and in this circumstance, in addition

*Strategies for serologic surveillance, use of the hepatitis B vaccine, and immune prophylaxis are discussed in a recent CDC report: Centers for Disease Control, Hepatitis Surveillance Report No. 49. Issued January 1985.

to testing for HBV markers, one should also test for acute hepatitis A infection, specifically, anti-HAV, IgM-specific.

The infection control staff or the director of the dialysis center should make sure that the most sensitive test methods available for HBsAg and anti-HBs are used. These tests are commercially available and are primarily methods of radioimmunoassay (RIA) or enzyme immunoassay (EIA).

Patients and staff who are susceptible to HBV infection (HBsAg- and anti-HBs-negative) should receive hepatitis B vaccine (see discussion below and Chapters 2 and 35). Susceptible patients and staff who have not yet received vaccine, are in the process of being vaccinated, or have not adequately responded to vaccination should be tested regularly for HBsAg and anti-HBs. Patients should be tested once a month for HBsAg, and at least once every three months for anti-HBs. Staff members should be tested every three months for HBsAg and anti-HBs.

Patients and staff who are confirmed as HBsAg-positive (on two consecutive tests) should be tested once every three months or perhaps more frequently if clinically indicated or deemed necessary for other reasons. Only when they become HBsAg-negative, should they be tested for anti-HBs. Patients and staff who remain HBsAg-positive for six months should be tested annually for HBsAg since a small percentage of HBsAg carriers (1 percent to 2 percent per year) may become HBsAg-negative.

Unvaccinated patients and staff who are found to have anti-HBs on two consecutive tests at a level of at least 10 sample ratio units (SRU) by RIA or who are positive by EIA need only be tested for anti-HBs

annually to verify their immune status. If anti-HBs decreases to less than 10 SRUs by RIA or becomes undetectable, such persons should be considered susceptible and vaccinated.

Patients and staff who are in the process of receiving hepatitis B vaccine, but have not received the complete series, should continue to be routinely screened as susceptible. Between one and three months after the third dose, all vaccinees should be tested for anti-HBs to confirm their response to the vaccine. Those persons who have a level of anti-HBs of at least 10 SRUs by RIA or who are positive by EIA are considered adequate responders to vaccine. Patients in this category should be tested for anti-HBs semiannually to verify their immune status. Staff who have adequate response to vaccine need only be tested for anti-HBs annually. Patients and staff who have low-level or no response to the vaccine are susceptible to HBV infection and should continue to be routinely screened as susceptible.

There is no specific serologic test for the diagnosis of non-A, non-B hepatitis. Patients should be screened monthly for alanine aminotransferase (ALT or SGPT) and/or aspartate aminotransferase (AST or SGOT) to identify persons who may potentially be infected. Criteria used to diagnose non-A, non-B hepatitis includes values of ALT and AST greater than two and one-half times the upper limit of normal on two determinations at least one week apart and the exclusion of other possible causes of liver injury or infections.

Table 17-6 contains a summary of recommendations for serologic surveillance in chronic hemodialysis centers.

TABLE 17-6. Recommendations for serologic surveillance in chronic hemodialysis centers

| Screening for | Test and screening interval | | | |
| | HBsAg | | Anti-HBs | |
| | Patients | Staff | Patients | Staff |
|---|---|---|---|---|
| Hepatitis B | | | | |
| Unvaccinated | | | | |
|   Susceptible | Monthly | Quarterly | Quarterly | Quarterly |
|   HBsAg carrier | Annually | Annually | None | None |
|   Anti-HBs-positive | None | None | Annually | Annually |
| Vaccinees | | | | |
|   Anti-HBs-positive | None | None | Semiannually | Annually |
|   Low level or no anti-HBs | Monthly | Quarterly | Quarterly | Quarterly |
| | ALT/AST | | | |
| Hepatitis non-A, non-B | Monthly | None | | |

## Record-keeping

As part of the surveillance system, the infection control staff should ensure that the patient's dialysis records be properly kept. These should include the lot number of all blood and blood products used; all mishaps such as blood leaks, blood spills, and dialysis machine malfunctions; the location, name, or number of the dialysis machine used for each dialysis; and the names of staff members who connect and disconnect the patient to and from a machine. In addition, a log should be maintained to record all hepatitis serologic results. Another log should contain records of all accidental needle punctures and similar accidents sustained by staff members and patients, including time, place, patient, and staff involved, and prophylactic measures if any were taken.

## Specific Infection Control Recommendation

Patients who are HBsAg-positive should be dialyzed in a separate room designated only for HBsAg-positive patients. If this is impossible, they should be separated from hepatitis B seronegative patients in an area removed from the mainstream of activity. Anti-HBs-positive patients may undergo dialysis in the same area as HBsAg-positive patients, or they may serve as a geographic buffer between HBsAg-positive and seronegative patients. The same hemodialysis equipment should not be used for both HBsAg-positive and seronegative patients.

Outpatients should have specific dialysis stations assigned to them, and chairs and beds should be cleaned after each use. Sharing of ancillary supply equipment such as trays, blood pressure cuffs, clamps, scissors, and other nondisposable items should be avoided. Nondisposable items should be autoclaved or appropriately disinfected between use.

Dialysis staff members should not care for both HBsAg-positive and seronegative patients during the same shift but can care for HBsAg-positive and anti-HBs-positive patients during the same shift. Staff members who are HBsAg-positive or anti-HBs-positive may be assigned preferentially to care for HBsAg-positive patients. If for some reason a staff member must care for both HBsAg-positive and seronegative patients during the same shift, he or she should, ideally, change gowns between patients, and more important, change gloves and wash hands to prevent cross-contamination. Disposable gloves can be worn by staff personnel for their own protection when handling patients or dialysis equipment and accessories. Gloves should be worn when taking blood pressure, injecting saline or heparin, or touching dialysis machine knobs to adjust flow rates. For the patient's

protection, the staff member should use a fresh pair of gloves with each patient to prevent cross-contamination. Gloves also should be used when handling blood specimens.

Staff members may wish to wear protective eyeglasses or surgical-type masks for procedures in which spurting or spattering of blood may occur, such as cleaning of dialyzers or centrifugation of blood. Staff members should wear gowns, scrub suits, or equivalent garb at all times while working in the unit and should discard this clothing at the end of each day.

At the end of each dialysis treatment or dialysis shift, nondisposable equipment should be cleaned and disinfected or sterilized. Special attention should be given to control knobs on the dialysis machines and other surfaces that are frequently touched and potentially contaminated with patients' blood.

In single pass artificial kidney machines, the internal fluid pathways that supply dialysis fluid to the dialyzer are not subject to contamination with blood. Although the fluid pathways that exhaust dialysis fluid from the dialyzer may become contaminated with blood in the event of a dialyzer leak, it is unlikely that this blood contamination will reach a subsequent patient. In the absence of microbiologic or epidemiologic evidence incriminating these fluid pathways, the disinfection and rinsing procedure should be designed to control effectively microbial contamination problems other than those associated with hepatitis. In kidney machines that use a recirculating system, a blood leak in a dialyzer, especially a massive leak, can result in contamination of a number of surfaces that will contact the dialysis fluid of subsequent patients. However, the procedures involving draining, rinsing, and disinfection that are normally practiced after each use will reduce the level of contamination to below infectious levels. Consequently if a blood leak does occur with either type of dialysis machine, the standard disinfection procedure used in the dialysis center is appropriate, whether it be the use of sodium hypochlorite, formaldehyde, or glutaraldehyde-based chemical germicides. External surfaces of the dialysis machine also should be cleaned and disinfected. Venous pressure isolators or in-line filters should be used to prevent blood contamination of venous pressure monitors. These isolators or filters should not be reused.

The staff members in a hemodialysis unit should not smoke, eat, or drink in the dialysis treatment area or in the laboratory. There should be a separate lounge for this purpose. On the other hand, patients may be served meals even if they are HBsAg-positive and are being treated in a separate area. The glasses, dishes, and other utensils may be cleaned in the usual manner by the hospital staff. No special care of these items is needed.

Crowding of patients and overtaxing of staff may increase the likelihood of hepatitis B transmission in dialysis units. To minimize transmission, each patient's station with its attendant equipment should have sufficient space to permit easy movement of a staff member completely around the patient without interfering with the neighboring station. This will allow for adequate cleaning and proper patient care.

Blood and other specimens such as peritoneal fluid from HBsAg-positive persons should be labeled as such, and the charts of these persons should be flagged (e.g., hepatitis B or blood precautions).

Peritoneal fluid has been shown to contain high levels of HBsAg and HBV and should be handled in the same manner as an infected patient's blood. Consequently if the center performs peritoneal dialysis only, the same criteria for separation of HBsAg-positive patients who are undergoing hemodialysis will apply to those undergoing peritoneal dialysis.

*Housekeeping*

In general housekeeping in the dialysis center serves two purposes: (1) to remove soil and waste on a regular basis, thereby preventing the accumulation and concentration of potentially infectious material in the patient-staff environment, and (2) to maintain an environment that is conducive to better patient care (see Chapter 14). These two purposes are of particular importance in a hemodialysis center because of the critical nature of the procedures performed. The requirement for aseptic access to a patient's blood supply at least twice in each dialysis procedure makes the hemodialysis unit more similar to a surgical suite than to a conventional patient room. Yet because of crowding and the presence of complex hemodialysis machines with multiple wires, tubes, and hoses, the dialysis unit frequently receives an inferior level of cleaning. If good housekeeping is to be achieved, it is necessary to have adequate space in which to work, as well as special instructions and training for the staff regarding the cleaning of hemodialysis equipment and stations. Although allotted space is often limited, much can be done to use it more efficiently. Elimination of unneeded items, orderly arrangement of required items, and removal of excess lengths of tubes, hoses, and wires from the floor are steps that can provide more accessibility for cleaning.

All disposable items should be placed in bags strong enough to contain the weight of discarded dialyzers and other items. The bags should be thick enough so they do not leak, or double bagging should be practiced. Bags should not be overfilled, requiring the staff to compact the contents by hand to make room for additional waste. Since bags may become contaminated on the outside before they leave the unit, they should be placed in another bag in a "clean" area in the unit before they are picked up. All used needles and syringes should be discarded without being separated in puncture-proof containers. Wastes from a hemodialysis center that are actually or potentially contaminated with blood should be considered infectious and handled accordingly. Eventually these items of solid wastes should be disposed of properly by incineration or sanitary landfill, depending on local ordinances.

Nondisposable items such as linen, especially if contaminated with blood, also should be considered potentially infectious and handled accordingly (see Chapter 15). These items should be bagged properly, laundry personnel should wear gloves while handling them, and personnel should not work with them in the same area as clean linen.

## CLEANING, DISINFECTION, AND STERILIZATION

Good cleaning and adequate disinfection procedures are an important part of a hemodialysis center's efforts to control and prevent cross-contamination of viral hepatitis type B. Although many of the procedures do not differ from those recommended for medical devices in hospitals and for inanimate surfaces [16,18], the hemodialysis environment is somewhat unique. In the dialysis procedure there is an extraordinary amount of blood contamination and concern for an infectious disease—viral hepatitis B—in which the infectious agent occurs in very high amounts in blood and is relatively stable in dried blood and serum. However, the basic approach is the same one used in other health-care environments: there should be a thorough mechanical cleaning step before any sterilization or disinfection treatment, and, depending on the compatibility of materials—especially medical devices—a sterilization treatment should be chosen over a disinfection treatment.

Hepatitis B virus has not been grown on tissue cultures, and without a simple viral assay system, studies on the precise resistivity of this virus to various chemical germicides and heat have not been done. In the absence of firm data, some investigators have considered the HBV to be extremely resistant and have recommended unreasonably long decontamination and sterilization protocols and use of corrosive chemicals. These recommendations are counterproductive because health professionals do not use them. It should be kept in mind that the HBV is a virus, and its resistance to heat and chemical germicides may at best reach the resistance of some other viruses and bacteria but certainly not that of the bacterial endospore. Furthermore, recent studies have shown that the HBV is not especially resistant to chemical germicides [8].

A physical or chemical treatment known to exhibit sporicidal activity also should be virucidal for HBV. Standard autoclave cycles of 121°C (250°F) for 15 minutes or ethylene oxide cycles can be used to inactivate HBV. In many instances, however, it is decontamination that is needed and not sterilization. For example, in the hemodialysis unit blood spills can be adequately decontaminated without using special procedures and corrosive chemical germicides. Immediately after a blood spill, the area should be thoroughly cleaned with a towel soaked in an appropriate disinfectant. The staff member doing the cleaning should wear gloves, and the towel can be placed in a bucket. After all visible blood is cleaned, a second application of disinfectant using a cloth or towel containing approximately 500 to 1000 ppm of sodium hypochlorite can be used. Other high-level disinfectants can be used, but they may be too expensive or corrosive for this type of application. Some of the generic disinfectants that can be considered for use, either on environmental surfaces or on medical devices that are contaminated with blood spills, include glutaraldehyde preparations, sodium hypochlorite, iodophor disinfectants, and formaldehyde [16, 18]. Actual concentrations and contact times can be determined by the manufacturer's recommendations.

When routinely cleaning frequently touched environmental surfaces in a dialysis unit to prevent cross-contamination with HBV, these surfaces can be physically cleaned initially by using a good detergent or detergent germicide. After this step, a cloth soaked with an appropriate chemical germicide, such as sodium hypochlorite (500 to 1000 ppm), can be used. Low-level chemical germicides such as quaternary ammonium compounds should not be used, and antiseptics such as formulations with povidone-iodine, hexachlorophene, or chlorhexidine should not be used, because these are antiseptics formulated for use on skin and not disinfectants designed for use on hard surfaces.

## ACTIVE AND PASSIVE IMMUNITY TO HEPATITIS B

Temporary passive immunity to hepatitis B infection may be acquired by the proper use of hyperimmune B globulin (HBIG) and active immunity by the administration of the recently licensed subunit hepatitis B vaccine (see Chapters 2 and 35).

As mentioned previously, the risk of acquiring hepatitis B infection for patients and staff members in hemodialysis centers has decreased significantly in the United States in the past 10 years. These infection control activities make the dialysis center a rather unique health-care environment when designing strategies for the application of a hepatitis B vaccination program. In a hospital only staff members in occupations considered high risk for hepatitis B infection are advised to receive the hepatitis B vaccine. In many dialysis centers in the United States, hepatitis B infection currently is not a problem, and the expense of administering the hepatitis B vaccine may be questioned. However, the hemodialysis center is the only health-care environment in which routine serologic screening for hepatitis B infection is recommended; this screening is frequent and costly but necessary to a dialysis center's infection control strategy for viral hepatitis. Vaccination of staff members and patients should pay for itself within 1 to 2 years because most serologic screening can then be eliminated [2].

In the case of vaccinated dialysis patients, the development of anti-HBs should be confirmed no sooner than one month after the third dose of vaccine and thereafter annually. If a patient has not developed anti-HBs after the administration of three doses of hepatitis B vaccine, he or she may be immunologically incompetent to do so and should, therefore, be considered and treated as susceptible.

HBIG should be considered for use in a hemodialysis unit when a susceptible staff member or patient is exposed to HBsAg-positive blood or potentially infectious blood (see Chapter 35).

When percutaneous, ocular, or mucous membrane exposure to a known HBsAg-positive source occurs in patient or staff member who has received one or more doses of the vaccine, the need for additional prophylaxis will depend on the exposed person's antibody response to the vaccine. The exposed person should be tested promptly for anti-HBs. If testing for anti-HBs has already been done within one year, these results may be used for decision-making and testing need not be repeated. Adequate antibody response to the vaccine is defined as anti-HBs at a level of at least 10 SRUs by RIA or positive by EIA. Low-level antibody response (less than 10 SRUs by RIA) is not considered adequate for protection.

1. Partially vaccinated persons (less than three doses): Sera should be tested for anti-HBs; if adequate

antibody levels are present, no HBIG is necessary and the vaccine series should be completed as scheduled. If anti-HBs is low or absent, the exposed person should be given a single dose of HBIG and the vaccine series completed as scheduled.

2. Fully vaccinated persons never tested for anti-HBs after vaccination: Sera should be tested for anti-HBs; if adequate antibody levels are present, no treatment is necessary. If anti-HBs is low or absent, one dose of HBIG should be given immediately and a second dose one month later.

3. Fully vaccinated persons known to have developed adequate antibody: Sera should be retested for anti-HBs only if previous testing more than one year ago; if adequate antibody levels are present, no treatment is necessary. If anti-HBs is found to be low or absent, one dose (20 $\mu$g) of vaccine should be given.

4. Fully vaccinated persons known to be nonresponders: If the exposed person has been fully vaccinated but is known to have had low or no anti-HBs on postvaccination testing, that person should be treated as a vaccine nonresponder and given two doses of HBIG one month apart.

## NON-A, NON-B HEPATITIS

There are at least two types of non-A, non-B hepatitis that are bloodborne and potentially transmissible in the hemodialysis environment. The diagnosis of non-A, non-B hepatitis is one of exclusion and involves testing for hepatitis B markers of infection, acute hepatitis A infection, as well as cytomegalovirus and Epstein-Barr viral infection. If clinical signs and symptoms are consistent with hepatitis and not associated with the other types of viral infections, a presumptive diagnosis of non-A, non-B hepatitis can be made. Since the epidemiology of non-A, non-B hepatitis is quite similar to that of hepatitis B, virtually all the infection control strategies that have been discussed in this chapter for viral hepatitis type B can be applied directly to non-A, non-B hepatitis.

Currently there is no direct serologic test for non-A, non-B hepatitis, and the presumptive diagnosis based on the exclusion of hepatitis A and B and the presence of elevated liver enzymes lacks specificity and sensitivity. Consequently, a diagnosis of non-A, non-B hepatitis can never be definite. Patients who are suspected of having non-A, non-B hepatitis can be dialyzed under normal conditions in the regular area of the dialysis center and do not require isolation. Furthermore, the practice of good environmental control, disinfection and cleaning strategies, and the use

of blood precautions should significantly help prevent transmission of non-A, non-B hepatitis in this setting.

## ACQUIRED IMMUNODEFICIENCY SYNDROME

When a patient has or is suspected of having the acquired immunodeficiency syndrome (AIDS), the same infection control strategies used for the control and prevention of hepatitis B infection should be used (see Chapter 35). One way this disease is transmitted is by blood, although probably not as efficiently as is hepatitis B. This suggests that the titer of the infectious agent is not as high as that of HBV in infected patients or that more of the causative agent is needed to produce an infection. In any case, proper blood precautions are recommended. It would also be good practice to dialyze AIDS patients in a separate room using a separate dialysis machine. If this is not possible a separate machine should be used, and frequently touched environmental surfaces should be cleaned and disinfected as described previously. Extreme use of isolation precautions or disinfectants is not indicated. Problems such as blood spills and contaminated surfaces can be managed as described for HBV contamination.

Disposable hemodialyzers should not be reused with AIDS patients.

## REFERENCES

1. Alfrey, A. C., Mishell, J. M., Burks, J., et al. Syndrome of dyspraxia and multifocal seizures associated with chronic hemodialysis. *Trans. Am. Soc. Artif. Intern. Organs* 18:257, 1972.
2. Alter, M. J., Favero, M. S., and Francis, D. P. Cost benefit of vaccination for hepatitis B in hemodialysis centers. *J. Infect. Dis.* 148:770, 1983.
3. Alter, M. J., Favero, M. S., Petersen, N. J., Doto, I. L., Leger, R. T., and Maynard, J. E. National surveillance of dialysis-associated hepatitis and other diseases. *Dialysis Transplant.* 12:860, 1983.
4. Association for the Advancement of Medical Instrumentation. *American National Standard for Hemodialysis Systems.* Arlington, VA: Association for the Advancement of Medical Instrumentation, 1981.
5. Band, J. D., Ward, J. I., Fraser, D. W., Petersen, N. J., Hayes, P. W., Silcox, V. A., et al. Peritonitis due to a *Mycobacterium chelonei*-like

organism associated with intermittent chronic peritoneal dialysis. *J. Infect. Dis.* 145:9, 1982.

6. Berkelman, R. L., Band, J. D., and Petersen, N. J. Recommendations for the care of automated peritoneal dialysis machines: Can the risk of peritonitis be reduced? *Infect. Control* 5:85, 1984.

7. Berkelman, R. L., Godley, J., Weber, J. A., Anderson, R. L., Lerner, A. M., Petersen, N. J., et al. *Pseudomonas cepacia* peritonitis associated with contamination of automatic peritoneal dialysis machines. *Ann. Intern. Med.* 96:456, 1982.

8. Bond, W. W., Favero, M. S., Petersen, N. J., and Ebert, J. W. Inactivation of hepatitis B virus by intermediate-to-high-level disinfection chemicals. *J. Clin. Microbiol.* 18:535, 1983.

9. Bond, W. W., Favero, M. S., Petersen, N. J., Gravelle, C. R., Ebert, J. W., and Maynard, J. E. Survival of hepatitis B virus after drying and storage for one week. *Lancet* 1:550, 1981.

10. Carson, L. A., Petersen, N. J., and Favero, M. S. Use of the *Limulus* Amoebocyte Lysate Assay System for Detection of Bacterial Endotoxin in Fluids Associated with Hemodialysis Procedures. In *Biomedical Applications of the Horseshoe Crab (Limulidae).* New York: Alan R. Liss, 1979, pp. 453–464.

11. Carson, L. A., Petersen, N. J., Favero, M. S., and Aguero, S. M. Growth characteristics of atypical mycobacteria in water and their comparative resistance to disinfection. *Appl. Environ. Microbiol.* 36:839, 1978.

12. Centers for Disease Control. *Control Measures for Hepatitis B in Dialysis Centers.* Viral Hepatitis Investigations Control Series, November 1977.

13. Centers for Disease Control. Fluoride intoxication in a dialysis unit: Maryland. *Morbid. Mortal. Weekly Rep.* 29:134, 1980.

14. Centers for Disease Control. Nontubercular mycobacterial infections in hemodialysis patients: Louisiana. *Morbid. Mortal. Weekly Rep.* 32:244, 1983.

15. Corey, L., Stamm, W. E., Feorino, P. M., Bryan, J. A., Wesley, S., Gregg, M. B., et al. HB$_s$Ag hepatitis in a hemodialysis unit: Relation to Epstein-Barr virus. *N. Engl. J. Med.* 293:1273, 1975.

16. Favero, M. S. Sterilization, Disinfection, and Antisepsis in the Hospital. In *Manual of Clinical Microbiology* (3d ed.). Washington, D.C.: American Society for Microbiology, 1980, pp. 952–959.

17. Favero, M. S. *Microbiological Contaminants.* Proceedings of the Association for the Advancement of Medical Instrumentation Technological Assessment Conference: Issues in Hemodialysis 1981, pp. 30–33.

18. Favero, M. S. Chemical Disinfection of Medical and Surgical Materials. In Block, S. S. (Ed.), *Disinfection, Sterilization, and Preservation.* Philadelphia: Lea & Febiger, 1983, pp. 469–492.

19. Favero, M. S. Distinguishing Between High-Level Disinfection, Reprocessing, and Sterilization. In Association for the Advancement of Medical Instrumentation. *Reuse of Disposables: Implications for Quality Health Care and Cost Containment.* Arlington, VA: AAMI Technological Assessment Report 6, 1983, pp. 19–20.

20. Favero, M. S., Carson, L. A., Bond, W. W., and Petersen, N. J. *Pseudomonas aeruginosa:* Growth in distilled water from hospitals. *Science* 173:836, 1971.

21. Favero, M. S., Carson, L. A., Bond, W. W., and Petersen, N. J. Factors that influence microbial contamination of fluids associated with hemodialysis machines. *Appl. Microbiol.* 28:822, 1974.

22. Favero, M. S., Deane, N., Leger, R. T., and Sosin, A. E. Effect of multiple use of dialyzers on hepatitis B incidence in patients and staff. *J.A.M.A.* 245:166, 1981.

23. Favero, M. S., Maynard, J. E., Leger, R. T., Graham, D. R., and Dixon, R. E. Guidelines for the care of patients hospitalized with viral hepatitis. *Ann. Intern. Med.* 91:872, 1979.

24. Favero, M. S., Maynard, J. E., Petersen, N. J., Boyer, K. M., Bond, W. W., Berquist, K. R., et al. Hepatitis B antigen on environmental surfaces. *Lancet* 2:1455, 1973.

25. Favero, M. S., and Petersen, N. J. Microbiologic guidelines for hemodialysis systems. *Dialysis Transplant.* 6:34, 1977.

26. Favero, M. S., Petersen, N. J., Carson, L. A., Bond, W. W., and Hindman, S. H. Gram-negative water bacteria in hemodialysis systems. *Health Lab. Sci.* 12:321, 1975.

27. Galbraith, R. M., Dienstag, J. L., Purcell, R. H., Gower, P. H., Zuckerman, A. J., and Williams, R. Non-A, non-B hepatitis associated with chronic liver disease in a haemodialysis unit. *Lancet* 1:951, 1979.

28. Gazenfeldt-Gazit, E., and Elaihou, H. E. Endotoxin antibodies in patients on maintenance hemodialysis. *Isr. J. Med. Sci.* 5:1032, 1969.

29. Hindman, S. H., Favero, M. S., Carson, L. S., Petersen, N. J., Schonberger, L. B., and Solano, J. T. Pyrogenic reactions during haemodialysis caused by extramural endotoxin. *Lancet* 2:732, 1975.

30. Kantor, R. J., Carson, L. A., Graham, D. R., Petersen, N. J., and Favero, M. S. Outbreak of pyrogenic reactions at a dialysis center. *Am. J. Med.* 74:449, 1983.

31. Lang, D. J., and Daniels, C. A. Herpesvirus Hepatitis in Transplant Recipients and Hemodialysis Patients. In Touraine, J. L., Traeger, J., Betuel, H., Brocher, J., Dubernard, J. M., Revillard, J. P., et al. (Eds.), *Transplantation and Clinical Immunology* vol. 10. Amsterdam: Excerpta Medica, 1979, pp. 18–26.

32. Legrain, M. (Ed.). *Continuous Ambulatory Peritoneal Dialysis.* Amsterdam: Excerpta Medica, 1980.

33. Marmion, B. P., Burrell, C. J., Tonkin, R. W., and Dickson, J. Dialysis-associated hepatitis in Edinburgh, 1969–1978. *Rev. Infect. Dis.* 4:619, 1982.

34. Najem, G. R., Louria, D. B., Thind, I. S., Lavenhar, M. A., Gocke, D. J., et al. Control of hepatitis B infection: The role of surveillance in an isolation hemodialysis center. *J.A.M.A.* 245:153, 1981.

35. Nolph, K. D., and Prowant, B. Complications During Continuous Ambulatory Peritoneal Dialysis. In Legrain, M. (Ed.), *Continuous Ambulatory Peritoneal Dialysis.* Amsterdam: Excerpta Medica, 1980, pp. 258–262.

36. Petersen, N. J. An assessment of the airborne route in hepatitis B transmission. *Ann. N.Y. Acad. Sci.* 353:157, 1980.

37. Petersen, N. J., Boyer, K. M., Carson, L. A., and Favero, M. S. Pyrogenic reactions from inadequate disinfection of a dialysis fluid distribution system. *Dialysis Transplant.* 52:57, 1978.

38. Petersen, N. J., Carson, L. A., Doto, I. L., Aguero, S. M., and Favero, M. S. Microbiologic evaluation of a new glutaraldehyde-based disinfectant for hemodialysis systems. *Trans. Am. Soc. Artif. Intern. Organs* XXVIII:287, 1982.

39. Petersen, N. J., Carson, L. A., and Favero, M. S. Microbiological quality of water in an automatic peritoneal dialysis system. *Dialysis Transplant.* 6:38, 1977.

40. Schreeder, M. T., Favero, M. S., Hughes, J. R., Petersen, N. J., Bennett, P. H., and Maynard, J. E. Dialysis encephalopathy and aluminum exposure: An epidemiologic analysis. *J. Chron. Dis.* 36:581, 1983.

41. Snydman, D., Bryan, J., and Hanson, B. Hemodialysis-associated hepatitis in the United States: 1972. *J. Infect. Dis.* 132:109, 1975.

42. Stamm, J. M., Engelhard, W. E., and Parsons, J. E. Microbiological study of water softener resins. *Appl. Microbiol.* 18:376, 1969.

43. Szmuness, W., Dienstag, J. L., Purcell, R. H., Prince, A. M., Stevens, C. E., and Levine, R. W. Hepatitis type A and hemodialysis: A seroepidemiologic study in 15 U.S. centers. *Ann. Intern. Med.* 87:8, 1977.

44. Szmuness, W., Prince, A. M., Grady, G. F., et al. Hepatitis B infection: A point prevalence study in 15 U.S. hemodialysis centers. *J.A.M.A.* 227:901, 1974.

45. Townsend, T. R., Siok-Bi, W., and Bartlett, J. Disinfection of hemodialysis machines: An evaluation of three disinfectants. *Dialysis Transplant.* 14:274, 1985.

# 18 THE INTENSIVE CARE UNIT

R. Michael Massanari
Walter J. Hierholzer, Jr.

Specialized patient-care units providing a focus for the technologic "rescue" of critically ill patients have become the hallmark of modern medicine during the past 25 years. These units are characterized by small groups of severely ill patients with compromised host defenses, the routine use of multiple medical devices and therapies with significant inherent side effects, and high ratios of specially trained medical personnel. Intensive care units are frequently subspecialized into pediatric, neonatal, medical, cardiac, respiratory, surgical, or mixed facilities, depending on the needs and expertise of the hospital.

More than 95 percent of acute-care hospitals in the United States currently support one or more such units, including 16 percent of 222 hospitals with less than 25 beds who responded to a survey [2]. Approximately 8 percent of nonpsychiatric, acute-care beds in the United States in 1983 were devoted to these units. While the efficacy and efficiency of intensive care units are still under discussion, it is clear that for selected patients, mortality and morbidity have been significantly reduced by application of these techniques and methods [7,10].

The typical patient admitted to intensive care is at an extreme of age and suffers one or more serious illnesses. Pulmonary, cardiovascular, and neurologic diseases, and drug overdose are frequent underlying conditions [10]. Although the average length of stay is short (two to five days), the cost of intensive care is estimated to contribute 15 to 20 percent of the total dollars expended on hospital care [13,49].

Mortality in intensive care units (ICUs) may exceed 25 percent. Over one-third of the patients admitted to these units experience unexpected complications of medical care. Mortality in the group with complications exceeds 40 percent [1]. Nosocomial infection is one of the most frequent medical complications affecting patients in intensive care.

Nosocomial infections in intensive care patients comprised approximately 20 percent of nosocomial infections reported in one study of 33 hospitals. These infections included more than one-third of all bacteremias reported and accounted for one-third of all aminoglycoside-resistant gram-negative rods isolated. In the university hospital included in this report, all nosocomial epidemics recognized over a two-year period occurred in ICUs [87].

Control of nosocomial infections is complicated by the fact that 15 percent of the patients are readmissions, over one-half have had surgery, 25 percent are from the emergency service, and 2 to 11 percent are direct transfers from other hospitals. More than 50 percent of patients admitted to intensive care are already colonized with the pathogen that subsequently causes their nosocomial infection [67].

The interactions of extremes of age, multiple comorbid conditions, severity of disease, transfers from multiple patient sources, geographic clustering, multiple medical devices, multiple interventions with high potentials for side effects, and high rates of contact with medical personnel in emergent situations conribute to the high rates of mortality, morbidity, and cost reported in association with nosocomial infections in these units [15,27,87].

## HOST FACTORS

In contrast to conditions in the healthy host, the patient admitted to intensive care is highly susceptible to infection, due in part to compromised host defenses (see Chapter 1). These alterations in the integrity of the defense network often accompany the underlying disease. The problem is compounded following admission to the unit because of inadequate nutrition, introduction and insertion of an assortment of devices for monitoring and treating the patient, and administration of a variety of medications for purposes of diagnosis and treatment.

### Disease Effects
The risk of nosocomial infection is positively associated with the severity of the underlying illness. Although methods for determining severity of illness are poorly standarized, Britt and associates [6] stratified patients according to whether the underlying disease was fatal, ultimately fatal, or nonfatal, and observed increasing rates of infections among patients with more severe illnesses. These observations were confirmed in the Study on the Efficacy of Nosocomial Infection Control (SENIC) project [35]. Intensive care units, by design, serve patients with severe illnesses—illnesses that compromise host defense. Each patient must be assessed individually to determine how the underlying illness may interfere with host defense mechanisms.

### Nutrition
The integrity of the body's defenses depends on proper nutrition. Although the association between malnutrition and nosocomial infections has never been properly confirmed, inferences regarding the importance of nutrition have been drawn from observations in malnourished children in underdeveloped countries. Children with severe protein-calorie malnutrition are more susceptible to severe, life-threatening

infections and exhibit a variety of defects in host defense mechanisms [46]. The prevalence of malnutrition has been estimated to be as high as 50 percent in some U.S. hospitals [5]. That malnutrition enhances susceptibility to nosocomial infections has been suggested by observations that poor nutrition was one of several predisposing factors for postoperative pneumonia [24] and by observations that it was associated with impaired delayed hypersensitivity, which was in turn associated with risk of postoperative complications [59]. Because intensive care patients often take nothing by mouth and are catabolic from the underlying disease, obstacles to maintaining adequate nutrition are apparent. Although the relative importance of malnutrition to risk of nosocomial infection is uncertain, it seems reasonable to assume that nutritional disturbances compound existing problems with the host defense.

### Medical Devices
Objectives of intensive care include concurrent monitoring of vital functions and physiologic support of failing organ systems. The technology required to achieve these objectives frequently requires introduction of foreign materials into body orifices or insertion of cannulas percutaneously, often directly into the circulatory system (see Chapter 36). Vascular cannulas traverse mechanical skin barriers and provide a direct portal of entry to the bloodstream (see Chapters 36 and 38). Insertion of tubes and catheters into airways (see Chapter 26) and into the urinary tract (see Chapter 25) circumvents local defense mechanisms. Nasotracheal tubes may obstruct the normal flow of secretions from paranasal sinuses and predispose to sinusitis. Insertion of cannulas into sterile cavities such as the intracranial cavity for monitoring CSF pressure (see Chapter 38) or the peritoneal cavity for dialysis (see Chapter 17) exposes otherwise sterile, internal environments to exogenous and endogenous microorganisms.

### Medical Therapy
Medical therapy, while administered for its beneficial effects, is often accompanied by adverse effects on host defense. These detrimental effects may be local or systemic. Cimetidine administered to reduce gastric secretion alters both the qualitative and quantitative flora of the stomach [70]. Alterations in this important chemical barrier have implications for both respiratory and gastrointestinal infections.

The adverse effects of cancer chemotherapeutic agents and immunosuppressive therapy are multifarious (see Chapter 37). Some agents are locally toxic to mucosal cells lining the gastrointestinal tract and disrupt mechanical barriers to bacterial invasion. Many agents interfere with synthesis of new phagocytic and immunocompetent cells, significantly impairing the phagocytic and immune systems.

Less appreciated are the potential adverse effects of other commonly used agents. Several investigators have reported in vitro evidence for the adverse effects of antimicrobial agents on phagocytic cells [88] and on immune responses [37]. Whether these observations in vitro reflect significant impairment of host defense in vivo is still uncertain.

In summary, assessment of the risk of nosocomial infections in the ICU must consider the host and the integrity of the body's defenses against infection. The patient admitted to an intensive care until will be compromised by the existing disease that precipitated the admission. These marginal defenses will be additionally impaired by poor nutrition and by procedures and medications administered during the patient's stay in the unit.

## INFECTIOUS AGENTS

More than 50 percent of infections documented in adult intensive care are associated with aerobic gram-negative bacilli [21,61]. Organisms isolated in neonatal intensive care also show high frequencies of gram-negative bacilli (Table 18-1), but *Staphylococcus aureus,* isolated from superficial sites is equally prevalent [18,39]. Approximately one-third of all aminoglycoside-resistant gram-negative bacilli isolated in nosocomial infections are found in patients in intensive care units [87]. The species of nosocomial pathogens in ICUs are often identical to those found elsewhere in the institution except for the antibiotic resistance patterns. The unusual frequency of infections mainly reflects the perilous condition of the host

rather than enhanced inherent virulence of the pathogens causing infections in intensive care units.

### Virulence Factors
Although patients in the ICU are susceptible to common virulent community pathogens, nosocomial infections are usually associated with microbes found in host or hospital environmental flora. Nosocomial pathogens are usually less virulent factors and are therefore infrequent causes of infection in otherwise healthy individuals. The risk of infection, therefore, depends on impaired host defenses and on introduction of a sufficient number of organisms to establish a nidus for infection. Although nosocomial pathogens are not exceptionally virulent, they often exhibit properties that enable survival and multiplication in the hospital environment.

### Persistence and Multiplication of Pathogens
IMBALANCE IN ENDOGENOUS FLORA   The proper balance of endogenous microflora is essential for symbiotic relationships between host and microbes. Alterations in this relationship by therapeutic intervention eliminates selected organisms from the niche and upsets the balance of nutrients. Untoward growth of *Candida* species on mucosal surfaces is usually inhibited by bacterial flora, which compete for nutrients and binding sites [47,55]. Elimination of selected flora by administration of antibiotics predisposes to local infection (see Chapter 11). *Clostridium difficile* pseudomembranous colitis is also associated with an apparent imbalance in endogenous flora (see Chapter 32) [84]. Thus normal florae capable of surviving selective pressures on the ecologic niche become potential pathogens as their numbers increase.

LATENCY   The ability of some organisms to produce latent or chronic subclinical infections provides op-

TABLE 18-1. Microbiology of nosocomial infections in pediatric intensive care

| Organism | Hemming, et al. (%) | Daschner, et al. (%) |
|---|---|---|
| *Staphylococcus aureus* | 47.3 | 41.8 |
| Enterococcus | 5.4 | 3.5 |
| *Staphylococcus epidermidis* | — | 7.0 |
| *Escherichia coli* | 27.0 | 13.4 |
| *Klebsiella pneumoniae* | 7.7 | 7.6 |
| *Pseudomonas aeruginosa* | 5.4 | 14.5 |
| *Candida* species | 3.6 | 4.1 |
| Other GNRs | 4.5 | 4.6 |

GNR = gram-negative rod.
Source: Adapted from Hemming, V. G., et al. *N. Engl. J. Med.* 294:1310, 1976, and Daschner, F. D., et al. *Intensivelechandllung* 6:81, 1981.

portunity for reactivation and transmission to other susceptible patients in the unit. Viral infections are particularly problematic in this respect (see Chapter 35). Herpesvirus infections, hepatitis B, and hepatitis non-A, non-B, as well as tuberculosis, toxoplasmosis, and pneumocystis, are infections that may remain chronic and inapparent until the host is severely compromised. Some of these latent or inapparent infections such as tuberculosis or hepatitis B present a significant risk to nonimmune health-care personnel working in ICUs (see Chapter 2).

TRANSMISSIBILITY   Some potential pathogens produce alternative biologic forms such as spores that enhance transmission from patient to patient or environment to patient. Production of stable spores by the obligate anaerobe *C. difficile* may account for clusters of pseudomembranous colitis that have occurred mainly in ICUs [84]. The ubiquitous fungus *Aspergillus* produces conidia that can be aerosolized and inhaled. Other pathogens are shed in droplets in such large numbers that they spread with facility to susceptible persons. Several respiratory viruses including rhinoviruses, respiratory syncytial virus, and influenza viruses have been introduced into ICUs in this manner [83].

ANTIMICROBIAL RESISTANCE   Extensive use of antibiotics and antiseptics in ICUs exerts selective pressures on endogenous and exogenous microflora (see Chapter 11). An organism that carries and expresses resistance to these toxic agents is ensured survival in this otherwise hostile milieu. Multiply resistant organisms often emerge as the predominant endemic pathogen in this setting [32,34,72,81] (see Chapters 10, 11, 12). The capacity of microbes to transmit this vital information via transfer of plasmids ensures continued survival as long as the selective pressures persist. In addition to antimicrobial resistance, organisms have been identified in ICUs that are resistant to antiseptics [44] and heavy metals [66]. Plasmid-mediated antimicrobial resistance is a trait shared by many nosocomial pathogens recovered in the ICU.

## EPIDEMIOLOGY

Since nosocomial infections are not reported in routine community surveillance systems, and national studies including the National Nosocomial Infection Study (NNIS) have not separated intensive care data from other patient-care infection data, there are no recognized norms for nosocomial infections in these units. However, a growing body of data from individual institutions has been published. The comparability of these data has been hampered by the different characteristics of the units studied (surgical, surgical trauma, medical, coronary care, pediatric, neonatal, and mixed) and by the methods used.

Most investigators have used infection criteria based on standard Centers for Disease Control (CDC) guidelines and reported either the number of patients infected per 100 at risk or the number of nosocomial infections per 100 patients admitted or discharged. Since the relative length of stay reported for these units is short relative to other patient-care areas (2 to 5 days vs. 7 to 9 days), this rate-determining method tends to underestimate relative nosocomial risk [23,40]. Methods using a time-weighted denominator (patient days of risk) and adequate controls for severity of illness, comorbidity, and other potentially biasing factors have rarely been used [6,23,30].

Most reports can be stratified by patient age (adult, pediatric, or neonatal) and by service (medical, surgical, or mixed). A few studies based on subspecialty services are available (e.g., coronary care, trauma). Examples of data and rates from investigators using CDC methodology to determine the incidence of nosocomial infections in adult and pediatric intensive care units are summarized in Tables 18-2 and 18-3, respectively. In adult units, nosocomial infection rates from 10.3 to 50.9 percent have been reported. All nosocomial rates reported for intensive care units exceed those for routine inpatient care by five- to tenfold.

Pediatric units have been additionally subspecialized into newborn and general pediatric intensive care, the latter devoted to care of children beyond the neonatal period. Rates in neonatal intensive care units are reported to be from 7.7 to 35.5 nosocomial infections per 100 children admitted. In these studies, an inverse relation between low birth weight and high nosocomial infection rate has been a consistent finding [30]. Nosocomial infections in intensive care units for older pediatric patients have been studied less frequently; however, an investigation in 1984 reported a nosocomial infection rate in such a unit of 11.0 per 100 admissions [85].

The most frequently reported sites and types of nosocomial infections in adult intensive care units are the lower respiratory tract, urinary tract, bacteremias, and wounds (Table 18-4). In pediatric units, superficial sites (skin, umbilicus, conjunctiva) and bacteremias predominate (Table 18-5). Conjunctivitis is a complication reported in both adult and pediatric units [41]. This potentially serious infection follows inoculation with excretions from tracheal suction catheters carelessly passed over the orbit. Meningitis plays a much more prominent role in pediatric than

TABLE 18-2. Nosocomial infection rates in adult intensive care units

| Author [reference] | Year | Service | Rate* | Country |
|---|---|---|---|---|
| Caplan [11] | 1977–78 | Surgical Trauma | 50.9 | U.S.A. |
| Daschner [17] | 1976–79 | Surgical Combined | 26.8 12.4 | West Germany |
| Egoz [21] | 1975–76 | Coronary | 25.3 | Israel |
| Kollisch [48] | 1981 | Medical Surgical | 23.0 36.0 | U.S.A. |
| McGuckin [56] | 1973–78 | Surgical | 10.3 | U.S.A. |
| Munzinger [61] | 1981 | Surgical | 42.5 | Switzerland |
| Northey [63] | 1973 | Surgical | 23.4 | U.S.A. |
| Preston [67] | 1973–79 | Mixed | 15.0 | U.S.A. |

*Rate expressed as number of infections per 100 admissions.

TABLE 18-3. Nosocomial infections in pediatric intensive care units

| Author [reference] | Year | Service | Rate* | Country |
|---|---|---|---|---|
| Daschner [18] | 1976–80 | Neonatal | 24.6 | West Germany |
| Egoz [21] | 1975–76 | Premature | 35.5 | Israel |
| Goldmann [29] | 1974–78 | Neonatal | 7.7 | U.S.A. |
| Hemming [39] | 1970–74 | Neonatal | 24.6 | U.S.A. |
| Welliver [85] | 1980–81 | Pediatric | 11.0 | U.S.A. |
|  | 1980–81 | Neonatal | 22.2 | U.S.A. |
| Wenzel [86] | 1972–75 | Neonatal | 24.0 | U.S.A. |

*Rate expressed as number of infections per 100 admissions.

TABLE 18-4. Comparative frequency of sites of nosocomial infections in adult intensive care units

| Author [reference] | Type of Infection (%) | | | | |
|---|---|---|---|---|---|
|  | Resp | UTI | Wnd | Bact | Other |
| Craig [15] | 33.0 | 29.0 | 11.0 | 10.6 | 16.4 |
| Daschner [17] | 16.0 | 27.0 | 7.0 | 22.0 | 28.0 |
| Munzinger [61] | 28.8 | 15.4 | 40.4 | 8.7 | 6.7 |
| Northey [63] | 44.0 | 39.0 | — | — | 17.0 |

Resp = respiratory; UTI = urinary tract infection; wnd = wound; bact = bacteremia.

TABLE 18-5. Comparative frequency of sites of nosocomial infections in pediatric intensive care units

| Author [reference] | Type of Infection (%) | | | | | | |
|---|---|---|---|---|---|---|---|
|  | Resp | UTI | Wnd | Surf | Bact | Mening | Other |
| Daschner [17] | 3.7 | 0.6 | 6.8 | 44.7 | 14.3 | — | 29.9 |
| Hemming [39] | 29.3 | 4.5 | 8.2 | 40.0 | 14.0 | 4.0 | — |
| Wenzel [86] | 7.3 | 22.0 | 1.0 | — | 15.8 | — | 53.9 |

Resp = respiratory; UTI = urinary tract infection; wnd = wound; surf = surface; bact = bacteremia; mening = meningitis.

in adult units. One report suggests that virus-induced respiratory and gastrointestinal infections may present risks heretofore unrecognized in pediatric units [85].

Primary and secondary bloodstream infections have been repeatedly studied and reported as increased in frequency in intensive care units. Forty-five percent of all bacteremias reported in one major study were found in the ICU. Rates from the different subspecialty intensive care units showed 8 bacteremias per 100 patients at risk in the newborn ICU (NICU), 7 per 100 in the surgical ICU (SICU), and 1.0 per 100 in the coronary care unit (CCU) at a time when the general hospital rate was 0.76 per 100 admissions [87]. In a study involving 33 hospitals [87], one-third of all bacteremias occurred in ICUs. Eleven percent of these bacteremias were related to hyperalimentation therapy. Other authors have noted equally high or higher bacteremia rates in intensive care units [15,17,21,61]. In a study of intensive care patients in West Germany, Daschner and colleagues [17] noted secondary bacteremias in 31 percent of nosocomial UTIs, 36 percent of pneumonias, 47 percent of wounds, and 78 percent of IV sites with phlebitis. Several studies in neonatal intensive care units report bacteremias as one of the two most frequent sites of infection [18,39,87].

The respiratory tract is another frequently reported site of nosocomial infection. The rates are highest in subspecialty units devoted to respiratory intensive care [56], but usually exceed 25 percent for all nosocomial infections in adult units. SENIC investigators estimated that respiratory care increased the risk of pneumonia by 21-fold and of bacteremia by 16-fold [35]. In the 33-hospital study from Virginia, 9 percent of nosocomial penumonias were related to respiratory care [86]. In the university hospital included in that study, 3.4 percent of patients requiring the use of ventilators had an associated nosocomial pneumonia.

## SOURCES OF EXOGENOUS ORGANISMS

### Reservoirs of Special Importance

Control of nosocomial infections in intensive care units requires an understanding of the ecology of the unit. Potential reservoirs for nosocomial pathogens, in particular bacteria and fungi, are numerous. As medical devices become more complex and difficult to clean and sterilize, the number of reservoirs increases.

EXOGENOUS—ANIMATE  Any person entering the ICU, whether patient, employee or visitor, consti-

tutes a potential exogenous reservoir for nosocomial pathogens. The most significant of these sources relative to cross-over between patients are health-care workers (see Chapter 2). Physicians and nursing personnel may, unknowingly, harbor and shed S. aureus or group A streptococci from the nares or perineum. Active dermatitis predisposes to carriage and shedding of large numbers of organisms, including unusual environmental organisms such as Acinetobacter [8].

HOSPITAL ENVIRONMENT  Air in modern hospitals contains few organisms. Dispersion of dust during construction or aerosolization of water particles may significantly increase spores and aquaphilic bacteria in inspired air (see Chapter 14). Relative to other reservoirs, air is only infrequently a source of nosocomial pathogens in an ICU, possibly because modern ICUs are equipped with high-efficiency air filtration systems [45,63] (see Chapter 26). Potable water, on the other hand, is an important reservoir (see Chapter 14). Outbreaks due to Pseudomonas aeruginosa [80], Flavobacterium [20], and Legionella pneumophila [38] have been traced to tap-water reservoirs. Food also serves as a reservoir, not only for enteric pathogens, but for antibiotic-resistant hospital flora too (see Chapter 16). Utilities in the ICU such as telephones have been reported to harbor hospital flora [14]; however, the significance of this observation for risk of nosocomial infections is uncertain.

MEDICAL EQUIPMENT  Medical devices are among the more important reservoirs in an ICU because they are used so frequently. Once a device is identified as a reservoir, however, solving the problem is relatively simple. Respiratory therapy equipment and devices for assessing respiratory functions, particularly those that contains water reservoirs, can be contaminated with nosocomial pathogens [12] (see Chapter 26). Nebulizers [69], humidifiers [75], and ventilatory circuits [16] provide niches in which bacteria reside. Liquid reservoirs are also involved in equipment used to monitor and manage arterial lines. Pressure transducers [79,54] and stopcocks [79] may be contaminated and support growth of microorganisms (see Chapter 38). Additional reservoirs include equipment for collecting and handling human secretions and excretions, such as breast pumps [19] and urinometers [71]. Common to many of these devices is a complex instrument that is difficult to clean and disinfect. To compound the problem, some instruments contain delicate components that will not tolerate standard sterilization procedures (see Chapter 14).

DRUGS AND SUPPLIES  Medications and antiseptics used for skin preparation and hand-washing are usually assumed to be free of microorganisms. Occasionally products are contaminated and serve as reservoirs for nosocomial pathogens. Use of multidose medication vials increases the risk of contamination and potential for multiple infections [9] (see Chapter 38). Contamination of antiseptics [44] and hand lotions [60] also provides a reservoir from which organisms may be disseminated to patients. In short any reusable product is susceptible to contamination and may serve as a reservoir for nosocomial pathogens. Microorganisms that contaminate these products are often unusual aerobic gram-negative bacilli, and infection problems related to such sources are most likely to occur in ICU patients.

The air-fluidized bed, a recent addition to the medical paraphernalia of ICUs, is an example of new technology for which adequate standards for cleaning are still wanting (see Chapter 14). Air under pressure is forced through a tank of latex beads or into Gortex bags, which provide uniform support for body surfaces when patients are confined to beds. Many patients placed on these units have extensive burns or decubitus ulcers. Because it is difficult to clean and disinfect the unit, beds become reservoirs from which organisms may be spread directly to other patients [73]. Furthermore, airflow across the patient's skin may be sufficient to create microbial aerosols.

FOOD AND WATER  Transmission of nosocomial pathogens by food is of minor significance in the ICU since many patients are unable to eat (see Chapter 16). Similarly, water may serve as a reservoir of nosocomial pathogens but is usually not directly involved in the transmission of organisms except when aerosolized [38,69].

## PATHOGENESIS

Colonization of patients with the offending organism and replication to sufficient numbers is a necessary prerequisite to infection [25,42]. When infection results from endogenous flora present on admission to the unit, colonization may simply reflect changes in the balance and constituents of flora following therapeutic interventions (e.g., administration of antibiotics) [78]. Exogenous flora is often introduced into the patient. The frequency and rapidity of colonization with hospital flora is a function of several factors, including site of colonization and presence of a foreign body. In the presence of a tracheostomy, colonization of the upper respiratory tract occurs within 48 hours of insertion [63]. On the other hand, infants receiving antibiotics and admitted to the NICU may not be colonized for several days following admission to the unit [26,31]. Ultimately, the longer the patient remains in the unit, the greater the risk of colonization with exogenous hospital flora.

Since normal host flora interferes with the growth of many exogenous pathogens [77], colonization is augmented by disturbances or eradication of host flora. Furthermore, some underlying diseases may be accompanied by changes in binding sites on epithelial cells, which enhance binding by aerobic gram-negative rods [43]. Once colonization is established, we and others [26] have noted that this multiresistant flora often persists as resident flora for years following hospitalization. Thus the patient becomes a reservoir of nosocomial pathogens when introduced to different wards in the same hospital or when admitted to other institutions.

Infection follows an event that introduces a critical number of organisms into host tissues. The event may be the introduction of medical devices, medical therapy, or a sequela of the underlying disease (see preceding discussion). The pathogenesis of nosocomial infections is a function of the parasite, host, and site of infection. Discussions of the pathogenesis of specific infections and the host responses to that infection may be found elsewhere in this text.

## CONTROL AND PREVENTION

### Surveillance

The recognition of important risk areas and resultant nosocomial infections in intensive care units depends on the availability of adequate, accurate data (see Chapter 4). Feedback of such data to medical personnel is central to the concept of surveillance and critical to the formation, implementation, and evaluation of control efforts necessary to continue safe care. The multiplicity of risks and the high costs of intensive care demand continued attention to the documentation of events as they occur. Recommended CDC surveillance methods or modifications thereof, have been repeatedly reported as successful in determining the causal events leading to increased nosocomial infection rates. Presumed successful interventions should be followed by continued monitoring to ensure their efficacy. Failure to follow nosocomial events closely may lead to subtle endemic problems or to large, disastrous epidemics.

*Structural Design*

Structural designs for the control of nosocomial infections should take advantage of information from studies showing the superiority of single-patient cubicles over common multipatient rooms in controlling the spread of infection from patient to patient [30,45,63]. In some studies, provision of a higher level of environmental control through filtered air conditioning, use of doors, and the addition of ventilated anterooms has reduced both the airborne counts of microorganisms and the recorded risk of nosocomial infection [45,63]. However, this observation is difficult to separate from the effect provided by an additional barrier to hand-contact transmission [57,76].

Structures should be built to allow control of traffic. Intensive care units should be placed in cul-de-sacs to prevent passage of non-unit personnel or visitors through the unit except for emergencies.

Clean function and storage should be physically separate from dirty function and waste disposal (see Chapter 14). Housekeeping facilities and equipment should be designated specifically for the unit and stored separately from clean and dirty utilities.

Hand-washing sinks should be placed near entrances and exits and at convenient locations throughout larger units. The placement of sinks at the head of the bed or on outer walls will discourage or prevent use since access to these areas is frequently obstructed by medical equipment. Separate, designated sinks should be provided for cleaning equipment.

Adequate floor space should surround each bed to allow access to the patient, provide room for large, bulky equipment, and discourage immediate contact with the next patient without hand-washing. Standard guidelines for multibed units suggest at least 7 feet between beds and at least 120 square feet of floor space per bed [82].

Isolation rooms should be available in sufficient numbers to serve the expected patient population requiring strict or respiratory isolation. These rooms should be equipped with nonrecirculated, controlled air conditioning and maintained at negative pressure to the surrounding facility (see Chapter 9). The addition of an anteroom with separate airflow may increase effectiveness in controlling airborne pathogens. The anteroom should be provided with a sink for hand-washing and clean storage, including gowns, gloves, and other pertinent equipment. The patient room should be equipped with a sink and toilet to allow on-site disposal of liquid wastes and excretions.

The efficacy of routine protective isolation techniques in immunocompromised patients in preventing acquisition of nosocomial infection has not been documented [62,67] (see Chapter 9). Life island, complete laminar flow, and similar highly technical isolation techniques may have a role in selected patients when combined with prophylactic antibiotics, sterile water, and cooked food [65]. However, the cost and interference with routine patient care make these programs impractical in the usual intensive care environment.

Recent outbreaks related to water [38] and food in special care patients may force reconsideration of routine policies for use of potable water and of routine diet in certain patient groups.

*Staffing Requirements*

The extent and severity of illnesses in intensive care patients necessitate a high level of nursing care. The high rate of nosocomial infections mandates strict application of rigid barrier nursing techniques to control potential transmission. Breakdown in these techniques during periods of understaffing or overcrowding has been associated with recurrent outbreaks of nosocomial infection [33]. A nurse-to-patient staffing ratio of 1:1 has been recommended to reduce breaks leading to hand transmission in intensive care [86].

*Patient Placement—Isolation*

It is estimated that more than 50 percent of patients admitted to intensive care units are already colonized with the organism responsible for subsequent infection [67]. Patients who are readmitted may carry and transmit resistant organisms acquired during past hospitalization. Not infrequently, unrecognized infection contributes to the decision for entry into the unit and the early diagnosis of potentially transmissible disease requires a high index of suspicion. Patients with suspected communicable disease should be appropriately segregated at the time of admission. The degree of isolation should be geared to the site of infection, mode of transmission, amount of secretion or excretion, and virulence and resistance of the infecting organism. The isolation guidelines published by the CDC are extremely useful in this respect [74] (see Chapter 9). Strict and respiratory isolation are rarely required. The basic barrier to hand-contact transmission is simple hand-washing. Patients sharing common pathogens may be cohorted into designated areas with designated staffing.

Patients with pneumonia or significant respiratory colonization and who require mechanical respiratory assistance are potential reservoirs from which organisms may be widely disseminated. Suction catheters for these patients should be sterile, rinsed with sterile fluids, stored dry, and discarded frequently, During the endotracheal suctioning process, care should be taken not to contaminate the surrounding environment with infected secretions or to allow contamination of other sites (e.g., the eye) [41]. For patients housed in multibed rooms, care should be taken to provide adequate exit filtration on their respirators. Aerosolization from these devices may travel significant distances providing airborne and contact transmission to other patients.

It should be recognized that as the duration of stay increases, patients frequently are heavily colonized with resistant microflora and become animate reservoirs for transmission to susceptible patients entering the area (see Chapter 10). It may be wise to separate these patients from the high-flow, short-stay patients making up the major portion of the population in the unit. This may be accomplished by moving chronically ill patients to single rooms or relocating groups of patients to a physically separate portion of the unit, preferably with a dedicated nursing staff. Frequent movement of patients through various levels of intensive care and out of the unit to general patient wards provides one of the most difficult reservoirs of resistant microorganisms to control in a tertiary care hospital. These patients are important animate reservoirs of resistant microorganisms during interinstitutional transfers and probably account epidemiologically for the spread of methicillin-resistant *S. aureus* [34,81]. Recognition of these patients as reservoirs and reporting of this information to receiving units and facilities through adequate medical-record notations and other alert devices is extremely important for the successful control of these agents [81].

## Control of Medical Devices

The engineering design of medical devices contributes significantly to the staff's ability to clean and disinfect them for serial patient care. During periods of economic constriction, there is increased incentive to acquire less expensive devices of which the design may prevent easy cleaning and disinfection. During the past 20 years, an increasing number of medical devices have been introduced for single-patient use. The cost of "disposable" devices and the potential danger and liability in reuse has engendered extensive discussions among representatives of governmental regulating agencies, medical providers, and industry [3] (see Chapter 14).

The routine application of guidelines for the use of medical devices could contribute significantly to the control of nosocomial infections [52,53]. Guidelines for the use and control of urinary tract catheters and collection systems (see Chapter 25), intravascular devices (see Chapter 36), respiratory devices (see Chapter 26), and other products have been published and distributed by the CDC [74].

## Human Factors

OCCUPATIONAL HEALTH   The medical care worker is both an animate reservoir and a frequent final common pathway in the transmission of nosocomial infections (see Chapter 2). Principles of occupational health may be more important for intensive care workers than for employees in any other area of the hospital. The opportunities for stress, trauma, and exposure to communicable disease exceed those of coworkers in other areas of the hospital. The use of multiple new and sophisticated devices, drugs, and techniques in emergent situations offers potential for human error.

The extensive education required to work in these units, high activity levels, incessant demands for services, and high professional standards contribute to a high level of responsibility and *esprit de corps* in these workers. Unfortunately, this *esprit* may be perversely translated into an ill-founded perception that one's function in the unit is irreplaceable, even when prudence dictates medical absence. Attempts to "stick it out" often coincide with the most infectious periods of acute communicable disease [36]. It is important that workers in these units understand their responsibility in preventing transmission of communicable diseases. It is equally important that the hospital provide adequate staffing to cover medical absences and personal benefits that do not punish persons who are responsible enough to avoid working when ill.

POLICY, PROCEDURES, AND COMPLIANCE   Intensive care workers are among the most highly trained individuals in acute medical care. Technical education programs compete regularly with recommended orientation and inservice educational programs on infection control topics. This problem is compounded by stress-related "burn-out" syndromes responsible for high rates of employee turnover in special care units. Loss of highly skilled medical care workers requires an extensive training effort for the replacement workers, including careful attention to appropriate priorities for infection control. It is not difficult to document nosocomial epidemics initiated by a change in staff and resulting from unrecognized modifications in infection control procedure. Provision of a routine surveillance system, with an attentive, experienced infection control practitioner, is an important method of ensuring appropriate infection control education (see Chapter 4). Unfortunately, knowledge is not always uniformly applied. In this highly sophisticated, crisis-oriented environment, it may be difficult to maintain appropriate priorities in the routine application of infection control methods, even those of indisputable worth.

HAND-WASHING  Routine hand-washing before and between patient contact is, without question, the most important feature of infection control. Virtually all medical care workers are aware of and agree with this concept [50,51,58]. It is dismaying, therefore, to see repeated reports of low levels of compliance with this simple and inexpensive technique. Several reasons have been suggested for this low level of compliance [28], including (1) lack of priority over other required procedures, (2) lack of sufficient time to accomplish hand-washing, (3) inconvenient placement of hand-washing sinks or other hand-washing tools, (4) allergy to unpleasant character of the hand-washing solutions, (5) lack of leadership of the senior medical staff in personally demonstrating the routine importance of hand-washing and demanding its priority, (6) lack of personal commitment to the routine application of the hand-washing procedure.

OTHER METHODS  The use of protective equipment in intensive care units is a frequent source of discussion but has little documentation or support. The carriage of potential pathogens on the gowns and uniforms of nurses and medical care workers in special care units has been repeatedly studied [63,68]. Isolation of microorganisms from clothing has been confirmed, and indeed increases with time. However, the risk of clothing as a causative factor in nosocomial transmission has been convincingly documented for some pathogens only; for most, including the gram-negative bacilli, it has not been documented. It appears prudent nonetheless to avoid contamination of uniforms with organisms. Wearing protective gowns and aprons to prevent contamination appears wise [22,74]. There is no evidence, however, that the addition of special surgical scrubs and/or caps improves infection control.

Gloves should probably be reserved for prevention of gross soiling of the hands when cleaning infected sites or orifices (e.g., patients with hepatitis B). There is no evidence that the addition of gloves in the routine intensive care situation has any benefit over routine hand-washing in control of infections.

The use of shoe covers, special "antimicrobial" floor mats, or other protective environmental materials increases costs without demonstrated effects on nosocomial risk [4].

SPECIAL UNITS—SPECIAL PROBLEMS  Each subspecialty unit uses unique administrative and medical methods that are in turn associated with speical risks. Consequently, each unit develops unique endemic and epidemic nosocomial problems. These unique and varied risks will only be recognized with active surveillance systems in each unit. Effective surveillance allows for early interception of problems and for efficacious, focused interventions.

## UNRESOLVED PROBLEMS

The complex ecology of intensive care units, with the numerous potential reservoirs for nosocomial pathogens and multiple modes of transmission, makes it difficult to pinpoint the specific epidemiology of nosocomial infections in ICUs. Many theoretically sound general control procedures are often impractical to apply routinely in ICUs, and infections stemming from the lack of their application may become the basis for doubt concerning their appropriateness and efficacy in control of nosocomial infections. Continued attention to specific controls and procedures that tend to be cost-effective is imperative. Personal commitment on the part of medical care leadership to the practice of recognized successful interventions is essential to the success of control efforts.

## REFERENCES

1. Abramson, N. S., Silvasy, K., Grenvik, A. N. A., Robinson, D., and Snyder, J. V. Adverse occurrences in intensive care units. *J.A.M.A.* 244:1582, 1980.
2. American Hospital Association. *Hospital Statistics* (1984 ed.). Chicago: American Hospital Association. 1984.
3. Association for the Advancement of Medical Instrumentation. *Reuse of Disposables: Implications for quality health care and cost containment.* Arlington, Va: Association for the Advancement of Medical Instrumentation, 1983.
4. Ayliffe, G. A. F., Collins, B. J., Lowburg, E. J. L., et al. Ward floors and other surfaces as reservoirs of hospital infection. *J. Hyg. (Lond.)* 65:515, 1967.
5. Bistrain, R. B., Blackburn, G. L., Vitale, J., Cochran, D., and Naylor, J. Prevalence of malnutrition in general medical patients. *J.A.M.A.* 235:1567, 1976.
6. Britt, M. R., Schleupner, C. J., and Matsumiya, S. Severity of underlying disease as a predictor of nosocomial infection. *J.A.M.A.* 239:1047, 1978.
7. Budetti, P. P., and McManus, P. Assessing the

effectiveness of neonatal intensive care. *Med. Care* 20:1027, 1982.

8. Buxton, A. E., Anderson, R. L., Werdegar, D., and Atlas, E. Nosocomial respiratory tract infection and colonization with *Acinetobacter calcoaceticus:* Epidemiologic characteristics, *Am. J. Med.* 65:507, 1978.

9. Cabrera, H. A., and Drake, M. A. An epidemic in a coronary care unit caused by *Pseudomonas* species. *Am. J. Clin. Pathol.* 64:700, 1975.

10. Campion, E. W., Malley, A. G., Goldstein, R. L., Barnett, G. O., and Theibault G. E. Medical intensive care for the elderly. *J.A.M.A.* 246:2052, 1981.

11. Caplan, E. S., Hoyt, N., and Cowley, R. A. Changing patterns of nosocomial infections in severely traumatized patients. *Am. Surg.* 45:204, 1979.

12. Castle, M., Tenney, J. H., Weinstein, M. P., and Eickhoff, T. C. Outbreak of a multiply resistant *Acinetobacter* in a surgical intensive care unit: Epidemiology and control. *Heart Lung* 7:641, 1978.

13. Chassen, M. R. Costs and outcome of medical intensive care. *Med. Care* 20:165, 1982.

14. Cozanitis, D. A., Grant, J., and Makela, P. Bacterial contamination of telephones in an intensive care unit. *Anaesthesist* 27:439, 1978.

15. Craig, C. P., and Connelly, S. Effect of intensive care unit nosocomial pneumonia on duration of stay and mortality. *Am. J. Infect. Control* 12:233, 1984.

16. Craven, D. E., Connolly, M. G., Lichtenberg D. A., et al. Contamination of mechanical ventilators with tubing changes every 24 or 48 hours. *N. Engl. J. Med.* 306:1505, 1982.

17. Daschner, F. D., Frey, P., Wolff, G., et al. Nosocomial infections in intensive care wards: A multicenter prospective study. *Intensive Care Med.* 8:5, 1982.

18. Daschner, F. D., Saal, E., and Pringsheim, W. Krankenhausenfektionen in einer neugeborenen intensivpfligestation. *Intensivelehandlung* 6:81, 1981.

19. Donowitz, L. G., Marsik, F. J., Fisher, K. A., and Wenzel, R. P. Contaminated breast milk: A source of *Klebsiella* bacteremia in a newborn intensive care unit. *Rev. Infect. Dis.* 3:716, 1981.

20. Du Moulin, G. C. Airway colonization by *Flavobacterium* in an intensive care unit. *J. Clin. Microbiol.* 10:155, 1979.

21. Egoz, N., and Michaeli, D. A program for surveillance of hospital-acquired infection in a university hospital: A two-year experience. *Rev. Infect. Dis.* 3:649, 1981.

22. Evans, H., Alepatu, S. O., and Buki, A. Bacteriologic and clinical evaluation of gowning in a premature nursery. *J. Pediatr.* 78:883, 1976.

23. Freeman, J., and McGowan, J. E., Jr. Risk factors for nosocomial infection. *J. Infect. Dis.* 138:811, 1978.

24. Garibaldi, R. A., Britt, M. R., Coleman, M. L., Reading, J. C., and Pace, N. L. Risk factors for postoperative pneumonia. *J.A.M.A.* 70:677, 1981.

25. Garibaldi, R. A., Burke, J. P., Dickman, M. L., and Smith, C. B. Factors predisposing to bacteriuria during indwelling urethral catheterization. *N. Engl. J. Med.* 291:215, 1974.

26. Goldmann, D. A. Bacterial colonization and infection in the neonate. *Am. J. Med.* 70:279, 1981.

27. Goldmann, D. A. Nosocomial infection: A hazard of newborn intensive care (editorial). *N. Engl. J. Med.* 294:1342, 1976.

28. Goldmann, D. A. Nosocomial transmission of gram-negative bacilli and the effect of hand-washing. *Br. J. Clin. Pract.* 25:(Suppl.)39, 1982.

29. Goldmann, D. A., Durbin, W. A., and Freeman, J. Nosocomial infections in a neonatal intensive care unit. *J. Infect. Dis.* 144:449, 1981.

30. Goldmann, D. A., Freeman, J., and Durbin, W. A. Nosocomial infection and death in a neonatal intensive care unit. *J. Infect. Dis.* 147:635, 1983.

31. Goldmann, D. A., Leclair, J., and Macone, A. Bacterial colonization of neonates admitted to an intensive care environment. *J. Pediatr.* 93:288, 1978.

32. Graham, D. R., Clegg, H. W., Anderson, R. L., et al. Gentamicin treatment associated with later nosocomial gentamicin-resistant *Serratia marcescens* infections. *Infect. Control* 2:31, 1981.

33. Haley, R. W., and Bregman, D. A. The role of understaffing and overcrowding in recurrent outbreaks of staphylococcal infection in a neonatal special-care unit. *J. Infect. Dis.* 145:875, 1982.

34. Haley, R. W., Hightower, A. W., Khabbaz, R. F., et al. The emergence of methicillin-resistant *Staphylococcus aureus* infections in United States hospitals. *Ann. Intern. Med.* 97:297, 1982.

35. Haley, R. W., Hoston, T. M., Culver, D. H., Stanley, R. C., and Emori, T. G. Nosocomial infection in U.S. Hospitals, 1975–76: Estimated frequency by selected characteristics of patients. *Am. J. Med.* 70:947, 1981.

36. Hall, C. B. The shedding and spreading of res-

piratory syncytial virus. *Pediatr. Res.* 11:236, 1977.

37. Hauser, W. E., and Remington, J. S. Effect of antibiotics on the immune response. *Am. J. Med.* 72:711, 1982.

38. Helms, C. M., Massanari, R. M., Zeitler, R., et al. Legionnaires' disease in Iowa: A cluster of 24 nosocomial cases. *Ann. Intern. Med.* 99:172, 1982.

39. Hemming, V. G., Overall, J. C., and Britt, M. R. Nosocomial infections in a newborn intensive care unit: Results of forty-one months of surveillance. *N. Engl. J. Med.* 294:1310, 1976.

40. Hierholzer, W. J., Jr., Streed, S. A., and Rasley, D. A. *Comparison of Nosocomial Infection Risk with Varying Denominators at a University Medical Center.* Abstracts of Poster Presentation, Second International Conference in Nosocomial Infections, Atlanta, Ga., 1980.

41. Hilton, E., Adams, A. A., Uliss, A., et al. Nosocomial bacterial eye infections in intensive care units. *Lancet* 1:1318, 1983.

42. Johanson, W. G., Jr., Pierce, A. K., Sanford, J. P., and Thomas, G. D. Nosocomial respiratory infections with gram-negative bacilli: The significance of colonization of the respiratory tract. *Ann. Intern. Med.* 77:701, 1979.

43. Johanson, W. G., Jr., Woods, D. E., and Chaudhuri, T. Association of respiratory tract colonization with adherence of gram-negative bacilli to epithelial cells. *J. Infect. Dis.* 139:667, 1979.

44. Kahan, A., Philippon, A., Paul, G., et al. Nosocomial infections by chlorhexidine solution contaminated with *Pseudomonas picketti* (Biovar. VA-1). *J. Infect.* 7:256, 1983.

45. Kallings, L. P. Program for surveillance and intervention in specific problem areas of nosocomial infections. *Rev. Infect. Dis.* 3:721, 1981.

46. Keusch, G. T. Nutrition as determinant of host response to infection and the metabolic sequelae of infectious diseases. In Weinstein, L., and Fields, B. N. (Eds.), *Seminars in Infectious Disease.* New York: Stratton Intercontinental Medical Book Corp., 1979.

47. Knight, L., and Fletcher, J. *Candida*: Colonization in the face of antibiotics. *J. Infect. Dis.* 123:371, 1971.

48. Kollisch, N. R., Kunches, L. M., and Craven, D. E. *A Prospective Analysis of Nosocomial Infections Occurring in the Intensive Care Units at Boston City Hospital.* An abstract presented at the Ninth Annual Conference of the Association for Practitioners in Infection Control, New Orleans, La. May 9–13, 1982.

49. Kraus, W. A., Wagner, D. P., Draper, E. A., Lawrence, D. E., and Zimmerman, J. E. The range of intensive care service today. *J.A.M.A.* 246:2711, 1981.

50. Larson, E. Current handwashing issues. *Infect. Control* 5:15, 1984.

51. Larson, E., and Killien, M. Factors influencing handwashing behavior of patient care personnel. *Am. J. Infect. Control* 10:93, 1982.

52. Maki, D. G. Preventing infusion-related infection. *Drug Therapy (Hosp.)* 2:37, 1977.

53. Maki, D. G., Goldmann, D. A., and Rhame, F. S. Infection control in intravenous therapy. *Ann. Intern. Med.* 79:867, 1973.

54. Maki, D. G., and Hassemer, C. A. Endemic rate of fluid contamination and related septicemia in arterial pressure monitoring. *Am. J. Med.* 70:733, 1981.

55. Marrie, T. J., and Costerton, J. W. The ultrastructure of *Candida albicans* infections. *Can. J. Microbiol.* 72:1156, 1981.

56. McGuckin, M. B., and Kelsen, S. G. Surveillance in a surgical intensive care unit: Patient and environment. *Infect. Control* 2:21, 1981.

57. McKendrick, G. D., and Emand, R. T. D. Investigation of cross-infection in isolation wards of different designs. *J. Hyg.* (Camb.) 76:23, 1976.

58. McLane, C., Chenelly, S., Sylwestrak, M. L., and Kirchhoff, K. T. A nursing practice problem: Failure to observe aseptic technique. *Am. J. Infect. Control* 11:178, 1983.

59. Meakins, J. L., Pietsch, J. B., Bubenick, O., Kelly, R., Rode, H., Gordon, J., and Maclean, L. D. Delayed hypersensitivity: Indicator of acquired failure of host defenses in sepsis and trauma. *Ann. Surg.* 186:241, 1977.

60. Morse, L. J., and Schonbeck, L. E. Hand lotions: A potential nosocomial hazard. *N. Engl. J. Med.* 278:376, 1968.

61. Munzinger, J., Buhler, M., Geroulanos, S., Luthy, R., and von Graevenitz, A. Nosokomiale infektionen in einem universitatsspital. *Schwerz Med. Wschr.* 113:1787, 1983.

62. Nauseff, W. M., and Maki, D. G. A study of the value of simple protective isolation in patients with granulocytopenia. *N. Engl. J. Med.* 304:448, 1981.

63. Northey, D., Adess, M. L., Hartsuck, J. M., et al. Microbial surveillance in a surgical intensive care unit. *Surg. Gynecol. Obstet.* 139:321, 1974.

64. Nystrom, B. The contamination of gowns in an intensive care unit. *J. Hosp. Infect.* 2:167, 1981.

65. Pizzo, P. A. The value of protective isolation in

preventing nosocomial infections in high risk patients. *Am. J. Med.* 70:631, 1981.

66. Poster, F. D., Silver, S., Ong, C., and Nakahara, H. Selection for mercuried resistance in hospital settings. *Antimicrob. Agents Chemother.* 22:852, 1982.

67. Preston, G. A., Larson, E. L., and Stamm, W. E. The effect of private isolation rooms on patient care practices: Colonization and infection in an intensive care unit. *Am. J. Med.* 70:641, 1981.

68. Ransjo, U. Attempts to control clothes-borne infections in a burn unit. *J. Hyg.* (Camb.) 82:369, 1979.

69. Reinarz, J. A., Pierce, A. K., Mays, B.B., and Sanford, J. P. The potential role of inhalation therapy equpiment in nosocomial pulmonary infection. *J. Clin. Invest.* 44:831, 1965.

70. Ruddell, W. S., Axon, A. T., Bartholomew, B. A., Hill, M. J., and Findley, J. M. Effect of cimetidine on the gastric bacterial flora. *Lancet* 1:672, 1980.

71. Rutala, W. A., Kennedy, V. A., Loflin, H. B., and Sarubbi, F. A. *Serratia marcescens* nosocomial infections of the urinary tract associated with urine measuring containers and urinometers. *Am. J. Med.* 70:649, 1981.

72. Saravolatz, L. D., Arking, L., Pohlod, D., et al. An outbreak of gentamicin-resistant *Klebsiella pneumoniae:* Analysis of control measures. *Infect. Control* 5:79, 1984.

73. Scheidt, A., and Drusin, L. M. Bacteriologic contamination in an air-fluidized bed. *J. Trauma* 23:241, 1983.

74. Simmons, B. P., and Wong, E. S. Guideline for Prevention of Nosocomial Pneumonia. In Centers for Disease Control, *Guidelines for Prevention and Control of Nosocomial Infections.* Atlanta, Ga.: U.S. Department of Health and Human Services, 1981.

75. Smith, P. W., and Massanari, R. M. Room humidifiers as the source of *Acinetobacter* infections. *J.A.M.A.* 237:795, 1977.

76. Snyder, H. G., Davidson, A. I. G., MacDonald, A., and Smith, G. Ward design in relation to postoperative wound infection. Part I. *Br. Med. J.* 1:67, 1971.

77. Sprunt, K., Leidy, G., and Redman, W. Abnormal colonization of neonates in an intensive care unit: Means of identifying neonates at risk of infection. *Pediatr. Res.* 12:998, 1978.

78. Sprunt, K., and Redman, W. Evidence suggesting importance of role of interbacterial inhibition in maintaining balance of normal flora. *Ann. Intern. Med.* 68:579, 1968.

79. Tamotsu, S., Deane, R. S., Mazuzan, J. E., et al: Bacterial contamination of arterial lines. *J.A.M.A.* 249:223, 1983.

80. Teres, D., Schweers, P., Bushnell, L. S., Hedley-Whyte, J., and Feingold, D. S. Sources of *Pseudomonas aeruginosa* infection in a respiratory/surgical intensive-therapy unit. *Lancet* 2:415, 1973.

81. Thompson, R. L., Cabezudo, I., and Wenzel, R. P. Epidemiology of nosocomial infections caused by methicillin-resistant *Staphylococcus aureus. Ann. Intern. Med.* 97:309, 1982.

82. U.S. Department of Health and Human Services. PHS, Health Resource Administration. *Minimum Requirements of Construction and Equipment for Hospital and Medical Facilities.* Washington, D.C.: U.S. Government Printing Office, DHEW (HRA) Publ. No. 79-14500, 1978.

83. Valenti, W. M., Clarke, T. A., Hall, C. B., et al. Concurrent outbreaks of rhinovirus and respiratory syncytial virus in an intensive care nursery: Epidemiology and associated risk factors. *J. Pediatr.* 100:722, 1982.

84. Walters, B. A., Stafford, R., Robert, R. K., and Seneviratne, E. Contamination and cross-infection with *Clostridium difficile* in an intensive care unit. *Aust. N.Z. J. Med.* 12:255, 1982.

85. Welliver, R., and McLaughlin, S. Unique epidemiology of nosocomial infection in a children's hospital. *Am. J. Dis. Child.* 138:131, 1984.

86. Wenzel, R. P., Osterman, C. A., Donowitz, L. G., Hoyt, J. W., Sande, M. A., et al. Identification of procedure-related nosocomial infections in high-risk patients. *Rev. Infect. Dis.* 3:701, 1981.

87. Wenzel, R. P., Thompson, R. L., Landry, S. M., et al. Hospital-acquired infections in intensive care unit patients: An overview with emphasis on epidemics. *Infect. Control* 4:371, 1983.

88. Yourtee, E. L., and Root, R. K. Effect of Antibiotics on Phagocytic-Microbe Interactions. In Root, R. K., and Sande, M. A. (Eds.), *New Dimensions in Antimicrobial Therapy.* New York: Churchill Livingstone, 1984.

# 19 THE NEWBORN NURSERY
James R. Allen

## NOSOCOMIAL NURSERY INFECTIONS

Striking changes have occurred in the medical and surgical care provided for neonates during the last two decades. While standards have continued to improve for infants in term newborn nurseries, the quality and sophistication of care provided in neonatal intensive care units (NICU) for premature and sick infants have improved manyfold. These advances, however, have been accompanied by significant risks of nosocomial infection. The impact of these infections may be more significant given the regional organization of tertiary medical care facilities for sick and premature infants. Organisms resistant to multiple antibiotics may be disseminated inadvertently to other hospitals, and a regional NICU forced to close because of an epidemic may have a major impact in the area on the delivery of health-care services for sick infants [42].

In contrast to these developments in the care of the smallest and sickest newborns, family-centered birth facilities have been emerging in a variety of settings for birth of infants carried to term. These birth centers are acceptable alternatives if they are able to provide quality care with rapid access to emergency facilities if required. Although sufficient information is not available regarding all aspects of these birth methods, they do not seem to be associated with any increase in infections for either mother or infant if practitioners follow carefully established operating procedures.

### Predisposing Factors
Neonates are particularly susceptible to infection for several reasons. Before birth, most fetuses live in sterile environments. During the hours and days following birth, infants are exposed to numerous organisms that readily colonize the open umbilical wound, circumcision site, skin, nares, throat, and gastrointestinal tract. Colonization of most healthy infants occurs without difficulty, but without the inhibition provided by a balanced normal flora, a small number of microbial species, including highly virulent strains, may selectively colonize infants and increase the risk of infection [26]. The immune system of infants, particularly pre-term (premature) or sick infants, is not fully developed. All neonates have physiologic dysgammaglobulinemia. Maternal immunoglobulin G (IgG) crosses the placenta readily, but IgM and IgE pass in miniscule amounts and IgA not at all. In addition, the polymorphonuclear leukocytes of an infant, particularly those of a stressed

neonate, are less functional at phagocytizing and killing organisms than are those of an older person. Other factors, including opsonins and chemotactic factors, may also be depressed in the neonate. Infants in an NICU frequently are extremely ill with complicated medical and surgical problems, including prematurity, respiratory disease, cardiovascular disease, or poor nutritional status. These high-risk infants require invasive diagnostic, monitoring, and therapeutic procedures, all of which are associated with increased risk of infection.

*Classification*
Infections in neonates are acquired from one of four sources:

1. A small percentage of infections are acquired transplacentally, such as congenital syphilis or rubella.
2. Some infections, such as gonococcal ophthalmia and early-onset group-B streptococcal disease, are acquired from the mother during labor and delivery.
3. Most infections are produced by organisms acquired in the hospital, although it is often difficult to determine whether the organism was originally acquired from maternal or hospital sources.
4. A small proportion of infections are acquired before admission to the nursery in infants born outside the hospital or in those who are readmitted to the nursery from home.

Because the majority of infants are born in a hospital, and because it frequently is highly impractical (if not impossible) to determine whether an organism causing infection in an infant is acquired from maternal or hospital sources, the Centers for Disease Control National Nosocomial Infections Study (NNIS) has chosen to define all neonatal infections—acquired either intrapartum or during hospitalization—as nosocomial.

*Incidence*
Using this broad definition, NNIS hospitals have reported a combined nosocomial infection rate of 1.2 percent for all infants discharged from the newborn nursery service (term plus NICU) for the years 1980–82. The majority of the infants were discharged from community or community teaching hospitals, with a reported neonatal nosocomial infection rate of approximately 1 percent. In contrast, the NICUs of some university medical centers have reported nosocomial infection rates as high as 24 percent [32,65], with over 15 percent of the infants in

one NICU developing one or more infections [32]; other NICUs have reported lower rates [25].

*Pathogens*
About 39 percent of the infections reported by the NNIS hospitals (Table 19-1) were caused by *Staphylococcus aureus*, most of which were superficial cutaneous or eye infections (conjunctivitis) (see Chapter 31). *Escherichia coli* caused almost 9 percent of the reported infections, including many of the urinary tract infections; surprisingly, few enteric infections have been reported with this pathogen during the early 1980s. Group-B *Streptococcus* was the most frequent cause of primary bacteremia; it was isolated from 23 percent of cases. Other prominent causes of bacteremia were *S. aureus, Staphylococcus epidermidis*,

TABLE 19-1. Frequency of selected pathogens causing nursery-associated nosocomial infections, 1980–82

| Pathogen[a] | Rate of isolation[b] | Relative frequency of isolation (%) |
|---|---|---|
| *Staphylococcus aureus* | 451.6 | 38.9 |
| *Staphylococcus epidermidis* | 106.4 | 9.2 |
| *Escherichia coli* | 101.4 | 8.7 |
| *Streptococcus* (group B) | 82.4 | 7.1 |
| *Streptococcus* (group D) | 69.9 | 6.0 |
| *Klebsiella* species | 68.5 | 5.9 |
| *Streptococcus* (not group B or D) | 48.1 | 4.1 |
| *Candida* species | 47.0 | 4.0 |
| *Enterobacter* species | 34.0 | 2.9 |
| *Pseudomonas* species | 28.2 | 2.4 |
| Other gram-negative bacteria | 21.0 | 1.8 |
| *Serratia* species | 14.1 | 1.2 |
| *Proteus* species | 13.5 | 1.2 |
| *Hemophilus* species | 13.5 | 1.2 |
| *Streptococcus pneumoniae* | 11.3 | 1.0 |
| Anaerobic bacteria | 14.9 | 1.3 |
| *Citrobacter* species | 6.6 | 0.6 |
| Other gram-positive bacteria | 7.7 | 0.7 |
| Other fungi | 7.5 | 0.6 |
| Viruses | 6.4 | 0.5 |
| Miscellaneous pathogens | 8.0 | 0.7 |
| No culture | 147.9 | — |
| No pathogen isolated | 66.9 | — |

[a]Reported by hospitals in the National Nosocomial Infections Study; 4,207 pathogens isolated, 535 infections not cultured, 242 infections with no pathogen isolated, 361,788 infants discharged. Hospitals were requested to report only isolates responsible for disease; in some instances, colonizing or contaminating organisms may have been reported.
[b]Per 100,000 infants discharged.

group-D *Streptococcus, E. coli,* and species of both *Klebsiella* and *Enterobacter.* Although *S. epidermidis* has often been cited as a contaminant of blood cultures from infants, reports in the literature have confirmed the significance of this organism as an opportunistic pathogen [17,45]. *E. coli* or group-B *Streptococcus* was isolated from almost 44 percent of neonatal meningitis cases. *Pseudomonas* species, *Klebsiella* species, *S. aureus,* and group-B *Streptococcus* caused most of the pneumonia and other lower respiratory tract infections in this series.

Nosocomial viral and fungal infections as well as those with onset of clinical expression after the infant is discharged from the hospital are incompletely reported through NNIS hospital surveillance.

Several marked changes in the pattern of pathogens causing nursery-associated nosocomial infections in NNIS hospitals have occurred over the last decade. Compared with the mid-1970s, the pattern for 1980–82 shows a 40 percent decline in the proportion of all infections caused by *E. coli,* a 23 percent decline in the proportion caused by *Klebsiella,* and over a 50 percent decline in those caused by *Pseudomonas* and *Proteus.* In contrast, the proportion of group-B streptococcal infections has increased 140 percent and the proportion caused by *Enterobacter* has increased 25 percent. The proportion of infections caused by *Candida* has declined by 31 percent.

### Patterns of Infection

Cutaneous and conjunctival infections are the most common nursery-associated infections in both term and premature infants (Table 19-2). Premature newborns in an NICU, particularly those that are acutely ill or have multiple medical or surgical problems, are much more likely than term infants to develop bacteremia, pneumonia, and other clinically significant infection. Compared with the frequency of nursery-associated infections reported by NNIS hospitals during the mid-1970s, the actual frequency of infections reported from 1980–82 shows a decrease at many sites. In contrast, however, the actual frequency of lower respiratory tract infections increased 26 percent over the last 10 years; the proportion of all infections at this site increased sharply to 9.3 percent of the total. The actual frequency of both primary bacteremias and central nervous system infections did not change markedly over this time, but the relative proportion of infections at these sites increased 22 percent and 38 percent, respectively. Enteric (gastrointestinal tract) infections during this same period decreased 58 percent in actual frequency.

Most clinical infections in nurseries develop as spo-

TABLE 19-2. Frequency of nursery-associated nosocomial infections by site of infection, 1980–82

| Site of infection[a] | Rate of isolation[b] | Relative frequency of isolation (%) |
|---|---|---|
| Cutaneous[c] | 553.6 | 40.2 |
| Blood (primary infection) | 143.7 | 10.4 |
| Lower respiratory tract | 127.4 | 9.3 |
| Genitourinary tract | 60.5 | 4.4 |
| Surgical wound | 55.6 | 4.0 |
| Central nervous system | 45.6 | 3.3 |
| Cardiovascular system | 36.8 | 2.7 |
| Gastrointestinal tract | 26.3 | 1.9 |
| Intraabdominal | 25.7 | 1.9 |
| Upper respiratory | 17.7 | 1.3 |
| Other[d] | 283.6 | 20.6 |

[a]Reported by hospitals in the National Nosocomial Infections Study. Hospitals were requested to report only those infections causing disease.
[b]Per 100,000 infants discharged.
[c]"Cutaneous" includes umbilicus, external genitalia, and breast.
[d]Includes conjunctivitis and superficial ocular infections.

radic or endemic disease rather than as an epidemic problem. In part, this occurs because the majority of infants who become colonized with a particular organism do not develop disease with that organism. This is the case not only with colonization of the umbilicus or nares with *S. aureus,* but also with colonization of the gastrointestinal tract with *Klebsiella* species of *Pseudomonas* species. Because of the potential presence of a large reservoir of asymptomatic infants who are colonized with pathogenic organisms, it is important to evaluate carefully even the small clusters of infectious disease within a nursery that appear to be nosocomial.

In addition, infections acquired within the hospital may not become clinically manifest until after discharge of the infant. The median age of infants developing staphylococcal skin disease, for example, is usually seven to ten days. A small cluster of infants with disease in the hospital may therefore portend that a large number of infants recently discharged from the nursery will have nosocomial infection.

Many infections in infants can be diagnosed more rapidly, and precautionary steps can be taken to prevent additional transmission of the organism within the nursery if there is close cooperation between the obstetric and the neonatal or pediatric medical personnel. It is important for the nursery to be informed of a suspected or diagnosed infection in a mother, such as gonorrhea, salmonellosis, or shigellosis. Similarly, if an obstetric procedure is causing morbidity in infants, such as infections following the use of scalp electrodes for fetal monitoring, it is important that the obstetric personnel be informed of the problem and steps be taken jointly to solve it.

## MANAGEMENT OF SPECIFIC PROBLEMS IN THE NURSERY

### Staphylococcal Infection

Although staphylococcal infections are still common in infants (see also Chapter 31), most infections with this pathogen during the last decade have been less serious than those occurring during the pandemic years of the mid-1950s through the early 1960s, when phage-group-I S. aureus, particularly phage-type 80/81, was prevalent. Many staphylococcal infections currently seen in neonates are caused by phage-group-II staphylococci; these occasionally result in exfoliative infections.

Infants during the first few days of life frequently become colonized at one or more skin sites with one of the strains of S. aureus prevalent in the nursery; the umbilicus, groin, or circumcision site is usually the first site to become colonized [34]. The most common means of transmission of staphylococcus in the nursery is from infant to infant on the inadequately washed hands of personnel; only rarely is an outbreak of disease in the nursery traced to an asymptomatic carrier (see Chapter 31). If the strains of S. aureus prevalent in the nursery are of low virulence, disease rates will usually be low compared with the frequency of colonization, and they will display a sporadic pattern. The prevalence of S. aureus colonization of infants in the nursery fluctuates, and may at times be higher than 50 percent; nurseries with good infection control programs often are able to achieve colonization rates of 20 percent or less.

### Group-B Streptococcal Infection

Group-B streptococcal disease continues to be a major problem for infants [33]. Estimates of the neonatal colonization rate with group-B Streptococcus range from 5 to 35 percent; the disease rate is approximately 0.3 percent. Most disease with onset during the first several days of life probably results directly from in-utero or intrapartum acquisition of the organism. The source of organisms that cause disease with later onset is less certain; colonization and subsequent clinical infection in at least some infants occur as the result of infant-to-infant transmission of the organism on the hands of nursery personnel. The role that the colonization of personnel plays in the transmission of infection to infants has not been determined.

Screening programs to identify infants who are colonized with group-B streptococci are costly and not sufficiently useful for disease prevention to be justified except during an epidemic. Routine care of infants in the nursery with all personnel washing their hands carefully between handling infants is usually sufficient to prevent transmission of this organism. The relative efficacy of various agents (e.g., triple dye) that are applied to the umbilical stump to prevent or eliminate colonization of infants with group-B streptococci is unknown. Attempts to use systemic or topical antibiotics to eradicate colonization and prevent neonatal infection with this organism have not been uniformly successful, and no routine use of antibiotics for this purpose is justified at this time [56].

### Gram-Negative Bacterial Infection

Much information remains to be learned about the biology and epidemiology of gram-negative bacillus infections in infants. E. coli is the most common organism causing serious neonatal infections; most strains of this organism are acquired from the infants' mothers. The majority of other gram-negative bacilli that cause neonatal infection are probably acquired within the nursery [47]. Contaminated fomites play an important role in some common-source epidemics, but the most important source of gram-negative organisms are the inadequately washed hands of nursery personnel [15]. Although nursery personnel occasionally are colonized with the same strains of enteric bacteria as those causing infections within a nursery, personnel carrying these organisms at intestinal or other sites other than the hands rarely are the source of a problem within a nursery [10]. The usual pattern of infection is for an infant to become heavily colonized in the intestinal tract, upper respiratory tract, umbilical stump, or skin with a gram-negative organism that is prevalent in the nursery [11,31,41]; subsequent procedures or manipulation of the infant allow invasion of the organism to occur and disease to develop [60].

### Neonatal Conjunctivitis and Gonococcal Infection

Gonorrhea, caused by Neisseria gonorrhoeae, remains a common infection, particularly among young adults. Gonococcal infection during pregnancy is associated with an increased risk of perinatal morbidity and mortality, and intrapartum gonococcal infection can result in neonatal conjunctivitis or infection at other sites, including fetal sepsis or scalp abscess from intrauterine monitoring. Cogent reasons for providing prophylaxis against gonococcal conjunctivitis for all newborns include the prevalence of asymptomatic genital gonococcal infection in pregnant women, the incidence of gonococcal ophthalmia in over 25 percent of infants born to infected women, and the severe and permanent sequelae of ocular infection (corneal ulceration or perforation with visual impairment or blindness) if treatment is delayed or inappropriate.

Prevention of perinatal gonococcal infection starts with obtaining endocervical cultures during early pregnancy (at the first prenatal visit) from women at risk of infection, and treating those with infection. Women at high risk of infection should be cultured a second time late in the third trimester. With the exception of tetracycline, drug regimens of choice are those for uncomplicated gonorrhea.

Transmission of gonococcal infection to newborns is generally by direct inoculation of the conjunctivae and oropharynx during passage through the birth canal. Onset of disease with periorbital edema, erythema, and purulent discharge occurs one to three days later, although the inflammatory response may be mild [50]. Less often, intrauterine infection occurs, especially after prolonged rupture of the amniotic membranes, or postnatal infection occurs by direct inoculation of the infant from the hands or secretions of its infected mother. Ocular prophylaxis at the time of birth may not prevent infection by these means of transmission. Gonococci do not survive well in the inanimate environment, and nonhuman reservoirs are not important.

Ocular prophylaxis for infants consists of a single application into the conjunctival sac of sterile ophthalmic ointment with 1% tetracycline or 0.5% erythromycin in single-dose tubes, or 1% silver nitrate solution in single-dose ampules. None of these medications should be flushed from the eye because flushing may reduce efficacy and probably does not reduce the chemical conjunctivitis that occurs with silver nitrate prophylaxis. Erythromycin [30] and tetracycline ointments may also provide prophylaxis against *Chlamydia trachomatis* ophthalmia. The efficacy of all these prophylactic agents may be reduced against penicillinase-producing strains of gonococcus [14]. Ocular prophylaxis should be administered as soon after birth of the infant as possible, but a delay of an hour may not diminish efficacy and allows infant-parent contact (bonding) to be initiated. Because of the potential for ascending infection in the mother (even though small), infants born by cesarean delivery also should receive ocular prophylaxis against gonococcal infection.

Infants born to mothers with proven or suspected gonococcal infection, particularly with prolonged rupture of membranes, should have eye, pharyngeal, and rectal cultures obtained and be managed appropriately. Because of the potential for disseminated infection, topical ocular prophylaxis alone is not adequate treatment for infants born to mothers with recognized gonococcal infection. These infants should also receive a single injection of 50,000 units of aqueous crystalline penicillin G (low-birth-weight infants should receive 20,000 units).

Infants with clinical ophthalmia or complicated or disseminated infection should be treated in the hospital with an appropriate antibiotic and supportive regimen. Since some strains of *N. gonorrhoeae* produce penicillinase, specimens for culture must be obtained (preferably from both mother and infant) and isolates tested for penicillin resistance [14]. The clinical response to therapy should be monitored closely. Ophthalmologic consultation is recommended.

Although nosocomial transmission of gonococcal infection is rare, gonococcal ophthalmia is contagious, and infected infants should be managed with contact isolation for 24 hours after initiation of therapy—including use of gloves for contact with infectious material.

*Herpes Simplex Virus Infection*
The appropriate management in the nursery of infants exposed to herpes simplex virus infection continues to be strongly debated (see also Chapter 35). Although onset of disease may occur as long as a month after birth, most infants develop infection during the first two weeks. The majority of diseased infants have vesicular skin lesions as an overt manifestation of illness, but suspecting and documenting the correct diagnosis in infants without skin lesions is difficult and often occurs only at autopsy. Most infants are exposed to herpes simplex virus at the time of birth during passage through an infected birth canal; cesarean birth appears to decrease the risk of exposure markedly if the amniotic membranes are intact or have been ruptured for only a few hours at the time of birth. Occasionally transmission of herpes simplex virus to an infant will occur from nursery personnel [64], another adult [38], or another infected infant [22,29]. The precise means of transmission during these episodes is not usually known, although the most likely means is on the hands of personnel; airborne transmission has not been suspected.

Most experts agree that an infant born by vaginal delivery to a woman with active genital herpes simplex infection is at highest risk of becoming infected and should be managed with contact isolation (an isolation room is not essential to accomplish this). Personnel working with the infant must be meticulous in technique, particularly hand-washing.

In contrast, an infant born by cesarean delivery before rupture of the amniotic membranes is at low risk of infection and can be managed in the nursery with few special precautions.

Since early signs of herpes simplex infection in the newborn may be subtle and nonspecific, a high index of suspicion should be maintained for known exposed infants. They should be managed as though they had infection until proved otherwise, including physical segregation from the rest of the nursery and contact isolation, with gowns and gloves used for direct contact with the infant. Infected infants should be managed in a tertiary care facility, and expert advice should be sought regarding antiviral drug therapy.

A mother with herpes simplex virus infections should be counseled about her infection and taught means of preventing postnatal transmission to her infant. She should put on a clean gown and wash her hands carefully each time before touching her baby. The baby of a mother with genital infection can room-in with its mother after she has learned the preventive measures; this is one acceptable means of segregating the infant from others in the nursery. A mother may breast-feed her infant if she has no vesicular lesions in the area and all active cutaneous lesions are covered. Labial herpes lesions (cold sores) should be covered with a disposable surgical mask when the mother is with her baby until the lesions have crusted and dried; she should be counseled about not kissing or nuzzling her baby until the lesions have cleared.

## Hepatitis B: Perinatal Transmission and Postexposure Prophylaxis

Hepatitis B virus (HBV) is transmitted efficiently from mothers to their infants during birth, particularly if the mother is seropositive for both surface antigen (HBsAg) and e antigen (HBeAg). A high proportion of these infants will become chronic HBV carriers and will be at risk of early death from cirrhosis or primary hepatocellular carcinoma. The appropriate, concurrent use of hepatitis B vaccine and hepatitis B immune globulin (HBIG) for infants born to mothers with HBV infection reduces the risk of this infection to the infant by almost 90 percent, reducing the risk of both acute clinical infection and chronic HBV carriage [7,69].

The Public Health Service Immunization Practices Advisory Committee recommends that all infants born to mothers with HBV infection receive 0.5 ml HBIG by intramuscular injection within 12 hours of birth and 0.5 ml hepatitis B vaccine by injection within seven days of birth* (see Chapter 35) [35]. The second and third doses of vaccine should be given one and six months after the first dose. Since the effectiveness of this prophylaxis depends on administering HBIG within hours of birth, it is imperative that HBsAg-positive mothers be identified before birth of their infants. Mothers belonging to groups known to be at high risk of HBV infection should be screened for HBsAg during a prenatal visit. If this has not been done prenatally, they should be screened at or as soon as possible after delivery.

To protect hospital and medical personnel against HBV infection and to ensure that infants born to seropositive mothers receive HBIG as rapidly as possible, obstetric and pediatric-nursery staff should be notified about pregnant HBsAg-positive women and the pending birth of their infants.

### Necrotizing Enterocolitis

Necrotizing enterocolitis is a disease defined pathologically or by a symptom complex that includes abdominal distention, gastrointestinal bleeding, ileal and gastric retention, and pneumatosis intestinalis on abdominal radiograph. The illness predominantly affects premature newborns during the first few weeks of life. The etiology and pathophysiology of the disease remain poorly defined despite numerous studies and investigations. Although the disease may well be multifactorial, an infectious component to the problem is highly likely [52]. Cases often occur in clusters, and infants colonized with specific bacterial strains often appear more likely to develop disease than do those not colonized. Microbial species most often associated with necrotizing enterocolitis include *Klebsiella pneumoniae, E. coli,* and *Clostridium difficile.*

Although an infectious cause for this disease is not certain, taking precautions to prevent potential spread of the disease may be justified. Infants with suspected or definite necrotizing enterocolitis should be managed with enteric precautions, including the use of gowns and gloves when working directly with the infant or with items contaminated with feces. A cohort of affected infants and of personnel to work with them may be required if a cluster of cases occurs, particularly one associated with colonization with a single species of bacterium.

Prophylactic oral or systemic antibiotics have been tried but have not been clearly or consistently useful; they are not recommended on a routine basis.

---

*The first dose of hepatitis B vaccine can be given at the same time as the HBIG dose but at a separate site.

# GENERAL PREVENTION AND CONTROL MEASURES

## Nursery Design

Until relatively recently, most nurseries were designed with special rooms, separate from the regular nursery, called "suspect nurseries." These were used to house infants with suspected infection or an increased potential for developing infection, such as the infant of a mother with prolonged rupture of the membranes. Because of the inconvenience of caring for them, the infants at increased risk of illness often received poorer care and less frequent observation than the nonsuspect babies. Infants with proved infection were immediately removed from the nursery and frequently placed in isolation on the pediatric ward, where they did not receive the special medical and nursing care they needed. The current design of NICUs has changed this in many hospitals by providing graded care facilities, including an observation unit, an intensive care unit, and an intermediate-care or long-term growth unit. In general, infants with many types of infections can be managed successfully in these relatively open units if techniques to prevent transmission of organisms from one infant to the next are meticulously followed. Adequate space must be provided for each infant, including those requiring special procedures such as ventilatory assistance; recommendations for minimum floor space and facilities per infant have been published [2]. The intensive care unit especially should be designed to be flexible in use to allow optimal care to be provided for varying numbers of infants and to meet the special needs of each [54,63].

## Isolation Procedures

The general principles of isolation technique (see Chapter 9) apply to the nursery, although unique problems and circumstances in this area require amplification of the established procedures [2]. Infants with most types of infection can be managed within the nursery area or NICU, as can infants who are born under nonsterile conditions or who are considered to be at increased risk of developing an infection. Factors that must be considered in each individual case include the type of infectious agent, the site of infection, the source of the infection, and the mode of transmission of the infection. In practice, infants with deep bacterial infections usually can be managed safely within the nursery area. Infants with gastroenteritis or draining skin lesions also can be managed safely in these areas, if necessary, provided that enteric or drainage-secretion precautions (see Chapter 9), including meticulous hand-washing, are strictly followed. Successful patient management requires adequate staffing and space, uncrowded facilities, and support for isolation procedures [25,28]. Infants with infections that can be spread by the airborne route, however, must be separated from the other infants, preferably by moving them out of the nursery area.

In the past, it has been felt that enclosed incubators with access to the infant through portholes provided adequate isolation, both for the protection of the infant from disease as well as for the prevention of spread of infection. No clinical studies have confirmed either hypothesis. Although many enclosed incubators manufactured today use high-efficiency intake air filters, opening and closing of the units to provide care for the infant effectively nullify the value of this filtration. Air leaving the incubators is not filtered. Manipulation of the units can allow cross-contamination, and at least one epidemic has been traced to contamination of the porthole covers of the incubators [5]. Open incubators using radiant heat as the warming source have become increasingly popular, because they allow easy access to infants requiring intensive care. These units do not provide any isolation from the airborne spread of organisms. Although an experimental open incubator has been constructed that provides forced air isolation (air curtain) through high-efficiency particulate air (HEPA) filters [46], this system has not been extensively evaluated for isolation purposes and is not in commercial production.

## Prophylactic Antibiotics

Signs of serious infection in newborns are nonspecific and extremely subtle, and the mortality rate from infections is high [32]. Because infants in an NICU are frequently seriously ill, have had invasive procedures performed, and are at high risk of developing an infection, a large proportion of them (frequently 50 percent or greater) are given broad-spectrum "prophylactic" antibiotics. Very few controlled, double-blind studies have been conducted to demonstrate the efficacy of this approach to prevention. Antibiotics, for example, are not useful in preventing infections from venous catheters for total parenteral nutrition or from umbilical vessel catheters for monitoring and fluid therapy [4,9], although they may be useful in preventing colonization and clinical infection in a selected group of high-risk infants with endotracheal intubation and respiratory support [31].

The frequent use of antibiotics in an NICU enhances the emergence of organisms resistant to the antibiotics and increases the likelihood that the infants will be colonized with the resistant strains [12]. Infants heavily colonized with resistant bacteria are probably at greater risk of developing clinical infections caused by their endogenous flora, particularly if they have had a complicated course and have been subjected to invasive procedures [26]. Similarly, with the exception of group-A streptococcal outbreaks and some enteric bacterial gastroenteritis outbreaks, the use of prophylactic systemic antibiotic therapy for all neonates in a unit has not been an effective way of dealing with nursery epidemics. Prophylactic systemic antibiotics should not, therefore, be given as a routine procedure following prolonged rupture of the maternal membranes, insertion of an umbilical vessel catheter, or following exchange transfusion.

### Employee Health

Employee health services should function to protect the infant from being exposed to infectious diseases carried by nursery personnel as well as to protect personnel from infections carried by infants (see Chapter 2). In addition to the well-described problems of staphylococcal and streptococcal disseminators among personnel, reports have described the transmission of pertussis [39], tuberculosis [62], and influenza [6] from nursery personnel to infants.

A person with acute respiratory tract infection (including pharyngitis), nonspecific febrile illness, gastroenteritis, or open or draining skin lesions should not work in the nursery for the duration of the illness. Persons with chronic dermatitis should be evaluated carefully to determine whether they can safely work in the nursery.

Appropriate policy for managing nursery personnel with active herpes simplex virus infections continues to be debated [2]. Although personnel with active lesions such as cold sores are able, under some circumstances, to transmit infection to newborns, the risk is generally low if correct procedures are followed at all times [64]. Personnel with genital herpes infections probably pose little risk to infants; those with labial herpes (cold sores) may pose a somewhat greater risk, although it is probably acceptably small if precautions are taken to avoid practices or procedures that might allow transmission of virus to the infant [64]. Personnel with herpetic hand infections (herpetic whitlow) should not provide direct patient care until the lesions have healed. The probability that errors will occur or that patient care will be compromised if personnel are excluded from the nursery during the active stage of herpes infection must be weighed against the small risk of transmitting infection to infants if essential personnel are allowed to continue working.

All personnel susceptible to rubella should be vaccinated [2,51]. In particular, female personnel of childbearing age should have a rubella antibody titer obtained and, if susceptible, be vaccinated before they become pregnant or are exposed to infected infants. Rubella vaccination is contraindicated for any woman who is pregnant or might become pregnant within three months of vaccine administration.

Female personnel should also be warned about the potential transmission of cytomegalovirus from infected infants [70,73] and the potential danger of contact during the first trimester of pregnancy with any virus-infected infant. A routine program of serologic testing of nursery personnel for susceptibility to cytomegalovirus is not recommended.

Personnel working with infants with the acquired immunodeficiency syndrome (AIDS) are not at increased risk of acquiring this disease from the infants if they follow appropriate procedures, including using blood-body fluid precautions for the infants and laboratory specimens (see Chapter 35).

### Surveillance for Infections

A surveillance program using multiple techniques to detect infections and problems within a nursery is essential to detect as rapidly as possible any pattern of infections that could indicate a break in patient-care practices or herald an epidemic (see Chapter 4). The potential usefulness of obtaining routine or periodic nasal cultures for staphylococci from infants in the nursery to detect lapses in patient-care techniques [67] must be balanced against the time and expense required for such surveillance. Routine culture testing of nursery personnel is not useful and is to be discouraged.

An active and continuing inservice educational program is essential to remind personnel of the problems that can arise in the nursery and to review the correct techniques for using all equipment and performing all procedures. The hospital epidemiologist as well as the physicians responsible for the nursery must be constantly sensitive to changes in frequency and patterns of infections and to changes in antimicrobial sensitivity of bacteria causing infections. Since infections may first become apparent after the patients are discharged from the nursery, it is imperative to establish good contact with pediatricians in the community to learn rapidly about infections that may be nosocomial in origin. Postdischarge surveillance by hospital personnel to obtain this information from mothers is effective but time-consuming.

### Evaluation of New Procedures

As new procedures and techniques are introduced into the nursery, each needs to be critically evaluated for its efficacy and safety, including its risk of introducing nosocomial infection. Examples of infectious hazards associated with minor procedures include staphylococcal enterocolitis developing in infants who had an indwelling nasoduodenal feeding catheter passed through nares colonized with *S. aureus* [27], cutaneous abscesses developing at the site where needle leads were inserted for electrocardiographic monitoring [32], and scalp abscesses or skull osteomyelitis developing at the site where the intrauterine fetal-monitoring lead was attached to the scalp [48,68].

## SPECIFIC NURSERY ROUTINES TO PREVENT INFECTIONS

Many nursery routines have been developed over the years and frequently have been incorporated into state codes for nursery operation. A number of these nursery routines are little more than ceremonial, as has been clearly shown by Williams and Oliver [67]. These investigators demonstrated that nasal colonization with *S. aureus* in neonates was unaffected by discontinuing the use of caps and masks, delaying the initial bath after birth until thermal homeostasis was achieved, discontinuing the use of hairnets, allowing medical students into the nursery, permitting parents to enter the nurseries and handle their infants provided they used good hand-washing techniques, discontinuing the use of brushes in initial hand-washing, and discontinuing the use of gowns except when handling an infant outside a closed incubator. Others have confirmed these results [16,21]. Procedures or routines found through controlled studies to be unnecessary or ineffective should be eliminated, not only because they may be expensive and time-consuming, but also because they may discourage personnel from giving optimal care to ill infants and may dilute the emphasis given to effective procedures [57].

### Gowns, Caps, Masks, and Linen
Caps, beard-bags, and masks are not necessary for routine nursery activities, but they are recommended for special procedures such as catheterization of an umbilical vessel. Gowns should be used for handling infected or possibly infected infants outside of incubators and bassinets. The clothing and unscrubbed skin areas of nursery personnel should not come into contact with the infants.

Linen used in the admission-observation nursery, the NICU, and other special care areas of the nursery traditionally has been sterile (autoclaved). The effectiveness of such sterilization in preventing infection in neonates has not been studied, however, and is under debate [43]. Sterile linen is probably not necessary for normal newborn care if hospital laundry facilities are satisfactory.

### Hand-Washing
The major mode of transmission of organisms to an infant is on the hands of personnel [44]. Hand-washing is therefore the most crucial element in infection control in the nursery [61]. Although transient surface bacteria can be largely eliminated simply by washing one's hands in tap water for 15 seconds with vigorous rubbing [58], even careful hand-washing with antiseptic compounds is not always adequate to eliminate all organisms on the hands that can be transmitted to infants [15].

Antiseptic agents should be used by nursery personnel for all hand-washing. Preferably, these should contain either 3% hexachlorophene, an iodophor, or 4% chlorhexidine. Persons sensitive to these agents should use plain soap or detergent compounds. Personnel coming on duty should use an initial two-minute scrub to the elbows. Immediately *before* and *after* handling each infant or after handling contaminated objects, the hands should be washed for 15 seconds.

### Gloves
Any infant with diarrhea or with a draining skin infection should be considered potentially infective regardless of whether a pathogenic organism has been identified. Such an infant should receive the appropriate enteric or drainage-secretion precautions, both of which require gloves for direct handling of the patient (see Chapter 9).

### Cohort Programs
For the purposes of hospital epidemiology, a *cohort* is a group of patients kept together to minimize contact between members of the cohort and other patients (cohorts) or personnel to decrease opportunities for the transmission of infectious agents. The success of a cohort porgram at limiting the spread of infectious disease depends significantly on the willingness of hospital personnel to cooperate fully with its objectives (see Chapter 35).

Some hospitals, particularly those with large nurseries, routinely establish cohorts of neonates to minimize the risk of transmission of *S. aureus* or other infectious agents to noninfected infants. The common characteristic of the infants in any given cohort is that they have been born within the same 24- or 48-hour period. The group of infants is admitted to one room of the nursery, and following the end of the admitting period for that cohort, no additional infants are admitted to that nursery room until all the infants have been discharged and the room has undergone thorough cleaning. The most successful cohort programs are those in which personnel during any one shift work only with one group of infants and do not work even temporarily with any infants other than those in their assigned cohort. Separate facilities should be provided for handling any infant who needs special observation or care or who will be remaining in the hospital longer than other members of his cohort.

During a nursery epidemic, establishing cohorts of infants and personnel frequently can provide effective isolation of infected infants from noninfected infants. The success of the separation depends heavily on the rapidity and thoroughness with which different aspects of the program are conducted. All infants who have overt clinical disease or who are colonized with the epidemic organism must be identified and placed in the cohort of infected infants. If rapid identification of infected infants is not possible, then all exposed and potentially infected infants should be placed in a cohort separate from new admissions to the nursery. Regular nursery personnel should be assigned to work with only one cohort and should not be permitted to work even temporarily with other groups. Physicians, laboratory technicians, and other transient personnel in the nursery must either work only with one cohort or take meticulous precautions to prevent transmission of infection between groups; if they are to handle more than one infant on a single visit, they should move from the noninfected cohort to the infected cohort. If the infection can be transmitted from asymptomatic colonized personnel to infants, personnel may need to be screened, and those who are found to be infected assigned to care only for the group of infants already infected.

Term nurseries that have sufficient admissions to justify the program should be arranged so that infants can be placed into a cohort routinely; nurseries that are being constructed or remodeled may be designed to facilitate this. Routine cohorts for infants in an NICU are not usually practical. The technique may be used during epidemics, however, by forming groups in different rooms of the NICU or simply by establishing groups of infected and noninfected infants and providing physical separation within a common room with strict assignment of personnel and equipment to each group. NICUs that have sufficient floor space for each infant and that are flexible in arrangement facilitate the implementation of this system. Diseases that are spread by the airborne route cannot be controlled effectively in this manner.

### Care of Equipment

Bassinets, incubators, nebulization and humidification equipment, resuscitation equipment, oxygen hoods, and any other equipment used directly with infants must be dismantled, thoroughly cleaned to remove all organic material, and then sterilized or disinfected (see Chapter 14). Diagnostic instruments such as stethoscopes and otoscopes should be disinfected with alcohol or an iodophor compound before use on each infant. Preferably, each infant in the NICU will be assigned specific equipment, such as a stethoscope, so that these instruments will not be carried from infant to infant.

One of the most serious problems affecting nurseries is what Wheeler has described as "water bugs in the bassinet" [66]. Any container or device filled with water or a solution may potentially be contaminated with organisms that thrive in water. Such devices include nebulization and humidification equipment, plastic squeeze bottles used for eyewashes or eye rinsing, and bowls used for bath or rinse water. All such devices should be cleaned and sterilized or disinfected at frequent intervals. Unit-dose medications and drugs should be used if possible. Water or other solutions used should be sterile (distilled water is not synonymous with sterile water). Once opened, bottles of sterile water should no longer be considered sterile. No container such as that used for an infant bath or for moistening sponges for wiping an infant's buttocks should be allowed to remain standing; the water must be discarded and the container cleaned, disinfected, and dried before its next use.

### Infant Bathing and Cord Care

Numerous studies have demonstrated the effectiveness of routine bathing of infants with a 3% hexachlorophene preparation in reducing the rate of colonization of infants with *S. aureus* [23]. Bathing infants with this agent has also been useful as an adjunctive control measure in stopping epidemics of staphylococcal disease. Because of the neuropathologic toxicity of hexachlorophene [40,55], which can be absorbed percutaneously, the current recommendation is that this agent not be used for routine bathing of infants [2]. Its usefulness as an adjunctive measure in controlling an epidemic of staphylococcal disease must be weighed against its potential toxic effects (see Chapter 31).

No other topical preparations for bathing infants have been proved unequivocally to be both safe and effective in reducing colonization and disease with *S. aureus* or other organisms. In view of this, the American Academy of Pediatrics has recommended that it is best to handle the infant's skin as little as possible by using a technique known as "dry skin care" [2].

Numerous methods of caring for the umbilical stump have been recommended, but no one method has proved to be clearly superior at preventing colonization or disease with *S. aureus*. Trials with bacitracin ointment [23,37] and triple dye [49] applied to the umbilical cord stump suggest that these agents are effective in preventing colonization. The potential toxicity of triple dye has not been adequately studied, however. Alcohol also has frequently been applied to the umbilical stump, both for its antiseptic effect as well as to hasten drying of the cord; it is not highly effective, however, in preventing colonization and disease [37]. Iodophor solutions for skin and umbilical stump care have not been widely studied, but they do not appear to be useful for this purpose. Chlorhexidine gluconate is poorly absorbed through intact skin; its efficacy and safety for skin and umbilical stump care of infants are under study.

## SPECIAL CONSIDERATIONS INVOLVING NEONATAL INTENSIVE CARE UNITS

### Equipment and Procedures

The equipment used to care for infants in the NICU is extremely sophisticated and expensive. The diagnostic, monitoring, or therapeutic procedures associated with the use of such equipment are frequently invasive and associated with a high risk of infection. It is imperative that these procedures be conducted using aseptic technique and that the devices, when in use, be regularly inspected and cared for. Examples of such equipment include ventilators, humidifiers, and other equipment used in respiratory therapy or ventilatory support; pressure transducers and lines for monitoring intraarterial pressures; umbilical vessel catheters for fluid therapy, blood-gas monitoring, or other reasons; or central venous catheters for total parenteral nutrition. Procedures employing any of these devices can be safely conducted if the correct techniques are carefully followed. The rapid introduction of new types of equipment, modification to procedures, and new therapeutic agents ensures a dynamic pattern of nosocomial infections. The availability of some medications or therapeutic agents only in large-volume packages not suitable for infants demands close cooperation with pharmacy personnel to ensure that dosages and methods of delivery are safe and not liable to contamination [36].

Transfusion of red blood cells and other blood components to premature infants is common. Blood components from a seropositive donor may transmit cytomegalovirus [1], and infants born to mothers seronegative for this virus are at high risk for serious morbidity or death if they are infected. Evidence is accumulating to suggest that screening blood components for antibody against cytomegalovirus reduces risk of infection and subsequent complications, including death, in premature infants [71,72].

Blood components may also be contaminated with human T-lymphotropic virus, type III (HTLV-III), the virus that causes AIDS. This disease has been transmitted to infants through transfusion [3]. Although the risk of HTLV-III transmission and the subsequent development of AIDS is unknown, the potential severity of the disease has resulted in donor screening programs to prevent donation of blood by those at risk for AIDS; the availability of serologic screening tests against HTLV-III should additionally increase the safety of blood component therapy.

The demand within a nursery for available equipment, particularly for expensive items, will occasionally exceed the supply, but it is extremely important that the equipment be carefully cleaned and sterilized between use on each patient. Many of the sophisticated devices available for use have not been adequately tested for their ease of cleaning and sterilization or for their safety from a microbiologic viewpoint. These factors must be considered when equipment is being evaluated before purchase. New equipment being developed may decrease the risk of nosocomial infection by reducing the frequency of invasive procedures. Transcutaneous oxygen electrodes, for example, should reduce the need for indwelling arterial cannulas and blood sampling for monitoring blood gases.

### Human Milk

The increased interest in breast feeding of infants in recent years has been accompanied by interest in providing human milk for premature infants in hospital nurseries. Although the psychologic benefits of encouraging families to interact with and support their premature infant are important, the nutritional benefits of human milk (particularly donor human milk) for feeding premature infants is uncertain. The immunologic benefits also have not been clearly defined [24]. Several investigators have suggested that fresh human milk may help prevent necrotizing enterocolitis from developing in infants, but this has not been demonstrated in controlled clinical trials [52].

Fresh human milk contains multiple components or factors, including immunoglobulins and active leukocytes, that enhance the resistance of infants to infection and that promote heavy intestinal colonization with *Lactobacillus* rather than with a mixed bacterial flora, predominantly *E. coli* [8,24].

Potential risks of feeding human milk to premature infants also exist. Milk frequently is contaminated with skin bacteria at the time of collection; although this is not a significant problem for an infant who is nursing or if the milk is used promptly, prolonged or inadequate storage of the milk can result in proliferation of the bacteria to levels that might cause adverse effects. Outbreaks of *Salmonella kottbus* and *Klebsiella* infections have been traced to contamination of human milk collected to feed premature infants [13,53]. Human milk also may transmit cytomegalovirus infection to infants [59].

The potential risks for premature infants from human milk can be reduced or prevented by freezing or pasteurizing the milk before storing it or feeding it to an infant. Such treatment methods will destroy living cells, and additionally, heat treatment may denature protective proteins in the milk [20]. By processing the milk to make it safer for the infants, therefore, the protective antimicrobial and immunologic factors in the milk may be destroyed. Frozen or heat-processed human milk has not been demonstrated to be protective against septicemia or gastroenteritis in neonates or premature infants.

Methods for collecting, transporting, storing, processing, and feeding of human milk from donors to premature infants in a nursery have not been standardized [18,19]. Collection of fresh human milk from a mother for feeding to her own premature infant appears to be safe and may be beneficial. The mother must be instructed in the careful collection and storage of the milk; even with refrigeration, it should be fed to the infant within 24 hours of collection. Until standards have been established for operating a non-related donor milk bank, however, and until it is known whether or not processed human milk enhances the resistance of premature infants to infection, hospitals are discouraged from establishing this complex service without giving extremely careful consideration to all aspects of operating a human milk bank and to the benefits that are expected to accrue to the infants.

## REFERENCES

1. Adler, S. P., Tattamangalam, C., Lawrence, L., and Baggett, J. Cytomegalovirus infections in neonates acquired by blood transfusions. *Pediatr. Infect. Dis.* 2:114, 1983.

2. American Academy of Pediatrics and American College of Obstetricians and Gynecologists. *Guidelines for Perinatal Care.* Evanston, Ill.: American Academy of Pediatrics, 1983.

3. Ammann, A. J., Cowan, M. J., Wara, D. W., et al. Acquired immunodeficiency in an infant: Possible transmission by means of blood products. *Lancet* 1:956, 1983.

4. Anagnostakis, D., Kamba, A., Petrochilou, V., Arseni, A., and Matsaniotis, N. Risk of infection associated with umbilical vein catheterization. *J. Pediatr.* 86:759, 1975.

5. Barrie, D. Incubator-borne *Pseudomonas pyocyanea* infection in a newborn nursery. *Arch. Dis. Child.* 40:555, 1965.

6. Bauer, C. R., Elic, K., Spence L., and Stern, L. Hong Kong influenza in a neonatal unit. *J.A.M.A.* 223:1233, 1973.

7. Beasley, R. P., Hwang, L.-Y., Lee, G. C., et al. Prevention of perinatally transmitted hepatitis B virus infections with hepatitis B immune globulin and hepatitis B vaccine. *Lancet* 2:1099, 1983.

8. Beer, A. F., and Billingham, R. E. Immunologic benefits and hazards of milk in maternal-perinatal relationship. *Ann. Intern. Med.* 83:865, 1975.

9. Bhatt, D. R., Hodgman, J. E., and Tatter, D. Evaluation of prophylactic antibiotics during umbilical catheterization in newborns (abstract). *Clin. Res.* 18:217, 1970.

10. Burke, J. P., Ingall, D., Klein, J. O., Gezon, H. M., and Finland, M. *Proteus mirabilis* infections in a hospital nursery traced to a human carrier. *N. Engl. J. Med.* 284:115, 1971.

11. Christensen, G. D., Korones, S. B., Reed, L., Bulley, R., McLaughlin, B., and Bisno, A. L. Epidemic *Serratia marcescens* in a neonatal intensive care unit: Importance of the gastrointestinal tract as a reservoir. *Infect. Control* 3:127, 1982.

12. Crosson, F. J., and Moxon, E. R. Factors influencing kanamycin resistance in gram-negative enteric neonatal sepsis. *Pediatrics* 61:488, 1978.

13. Donowitz, L. G., Marsik, F. J., Fisher, K. A., and Wenzel, R. P. Contaminated breast milk: A source of *Klebsiella* bacteremia in a newborn intensive care unit. *Rev. Infect. Dis.* 3:716, 1981.

14. Doraiswamy, B., Hammerschlag, M. R., Pringle, G. F., and du Bouchet, L. Ophthalmia neonatorum caused by beta-lactamase-producing *Neisseria gonorrhoeae*. *J.A.M.A.* 250:790, 1983.

15. Eisenoch, K. D., Reber, R. M., Eitzman, D. V., and Baer, H. Nosocomial infections due to

kanamycin-resistant, (R)-factor-carrying enteric organisms in an intensive care nursery. *Pediatrics* 50:395, 1972.

16. Evans, H. E., Akpata, S. O., and Baki, A. Bacteriologic and clinical evaluation of gowning in a premature nursery. *J. Pediatr.* 78:883, 1971.

17. Fleer, A., Senders, R. C., Visser, M. R., Bijlmer, R. P., Gerards, L. J., Kraaijeveld, C. A., and Verhoef, J. Septicemia due to coagulase-negative staphylococci in a neonatal intensive care unit: Clinical and bacteriological features and contaminated parenteral fluids as a source of sepsis. *Pediatr. Infect. Dis.* 2:426, 1983.

18. Fomon, S. J. Human milk in premature infant feeding: Report of a second workshop. *Am. J. Public Health* 67:361, 1977.

19. Fomon, S. J., et al. Human milk in premature infant feeding: Summary of a workshop. *Pediatrics* 57:741, 1976.

20. Ford, J. E., Law, B. A., Marshall, V. M. E., and Reiter, B. Influence of the heat treatment of human milk on some of its protective constituents. *J. Pediatr.* 90:29, 1977.

21. Forfar, J. O., and MacCabe, A. F. Masking and gowning in nurseries for the newborn infant: Effect on staphylococcal carriage and infection. *Br. Med. J.* 1:76, 1958.

22. Francis, D. P., Herrmann, K. L., MacMahan, J. R., et al. Nosocomial and maternally acquired *Herpesvirus hominis* infections: A report of four fatal cases in neonates. *Am. J. Dis. Child.* 129:889, 1975.

23. Gezon, H. M., Thompson, D. J., Rogers, K. D., Hatch, T. F., Rycheck, R. R., and Yee, R. B. Control of staphylococcal infections and disease in the newborn through the use of hexachlorophene bathing. *Pediatrics* 51(Suppl.):331, 1973.

24. Goldman, A. S., and Smith, C. W. Host resistance factors in human milk. *J. Pediatr.* 82:1082, 1973.

25. Goldmann, D. A., Durbin, W. A., and Freeman, J. Nosocomial infections in a neonatal intensive care unit. *J. Infect. Dis.* 144:449, 1981.

26. Goldmann, D. A., LeClair, and Macone, A. Bacterial colonization of neonates admitted to an intensive care environment. *J. Pediatr.* 93:288, 1978.

27. Gutman, L. T., Idriss, Z. H., Gehlbach, S., and Blackmon, L. Neonatal staphylococcal enterocolitis: Association with indwelling feeding catheters and *S. aureus* colonization. *J. Pediatr.* 88:836, 1976.

28. Haley, R. W., and Bregman, D. A. The role of understaffing and overcrowding in recurrent outbreaks of staphylococcal infection in a neonatal special-care unit. *J. Infect. Dis.* 145:875, 1982.

29. Hammerberg, O., Watts, J., Chernesky, M., Luchsinger, I., and Rawls, W. An outbreak of herpes simplex virus type 1 in an intensive care nursery. *Pediatr. Infect. Dis.* 2:290, 1983.

30. Hammerschlag, M. R., Chandler, J. W., Alexander, E. R., et al. Erythromycin ointment for ocular prohylaxis of neonatal chlamydial infection. *J.A.M.A.* 244:2291, 1980.

31. Harris, H., Wirtschafter, D., and Cassady, G. Endotracheal intubation and its relationship to bacterial colonization and systemic infection of newborn infants. *Pediatrics* 58:816, 1976.

32. Hemming, V. G., Overall, J. C., and Britt, M. R. Nosocomial infections in a newborn intensive-care unit: Results of forty-one months of surveillance. *N. Engl. J. Med.* 294:1310, 1976.

33. Howard, J. B., and McCracken, G.H. The spectrum of group B streptococcal infections in infancy. *Am. J. Dis. Child.* 128:815, 1974.

34. Hurst, V. Colonization in the Newborn. In Maibach, H. I., and Hildick-Smith, G. (Eds.), *Skin Bacteria and their Role in Infection*. New York: McGraw-Hill, 1965, pp. 127–141.

35. Immunization Practices Advisory Committee, Centers for Disease Control. Postexposure prophylaxis of hepatitis B. *Morbid. Mortal. Weekly Rep.* 33:285, 1984.

36. Jarvis, W. R., Highsmith, A. K., Allen, J. R., and Halcy, R. W. Polymicrobial bacteremia associated with lipid emulsion in a neonatal intensive care unit. *Pediatr. Infect. Dis.* 2:203, 1983.

37. Johnson, J. D., Malachowski, N. C., Vosti, K. L., and Sunshine, P. A sequential study of various modes of skin and umbilical care and the incidence of staphylococcal colonization and infection in the neonate. *Pediatrics* 58:354, 1976.

38. Linnemann, C. C., Light, I. J., Buchman, T. G., et al. Transmission of herpes simplex virus type 1 in a nursery for the newborn: Identification of viral isolates by DNA "fingerprinting." *Lancet* 1:964, 1978.

39. Linnemann, C. C., Ramundo, N., Perlstein, P. H., Minton, S. D., Englender, G. S., McCormick, J. B., and Hayes, P.S. Use of pertussis vaccine in an epidemic involving hospital staff. *Lancet* 2:540, 1975.

40. Lockhart, J. D. How toxic is hexachlorophene? *Pediatrics* 50:229, 1972.

41. Mayhall, C. G., Lamb, V. A., Bitar, C. M., et

al. Nosocomial *Klebsiella* infection in a neonatal unit: Identification of risk factors for gastrointestinal colonization. *Infect. Control* 4:239, 1980.

42. McKee, K. T., Cotton, R. B., Stratton, C. W., et al. Nursery epidemic due to multiply resistant *Klebsiella pneumoniae:* Epidemiologic setting and impact on perinatal health care delivery. *Infect. Control* 3:150, 1982.

43. Meyer, C. L., Eitzen, H. E., Schreiner, R. L., et al. Should linen in newborn intensive care units be autoclaved? *Pediatrics* 67:362, 1981.

44. Mortimer, E. A., Lipsitz, P. J., Wolinski, E., Gonzaga, A. J., and Rammelkamp, C. H. Transmission of staphylococci between newborns: Importance of hands of personnel. *Am. J. Dis. Child.* 104:289, 1962.

45. Munson, D. P., Thompson, T. R., Johnson, D. E., Rhame, F. S., Van Drunen, N., and Ferrieri, P. Coagulase-negative staphylococcal septicemia: Experience in a newborn intensive care unit. *J. Pediatr.* 101:602, 1982.

46. Musch, B., Adams, J. L., and Sunshine, P. An air curtain incubator for use in an intensive-care nursery. *J. Pediatr.* 79:1024, 1971.

47. Noy, J. H., Ayliffe, G. A. J., and Linton, K. B. Antibiotic-resistant gram-negative bacilli in the faeces of neonates. *J. Med. Microbiol.* 7:509, 1974.

48. Overturf, G. D., and Balfour, G. Osteomyelitis and sepsis: Severe complications of fetal monitoring. *Pediatrics* 55:244, 1975.

49. Pildes, R. S., Ramamurthy, R. S., and Vidyasagar, D. Effect of triple dye on staphylococcal colonization in the newborn infant. *J. Pediatr.* 82:987, 1973.

50. Podgore, J. K., and Holmes, K. K. Ocular gonococcal infection with minimal or no inflammatory response. *J.A.M.A.* 246:242, 1981.

51. Polk, B. F., White, J. A., DeGirolami, P. C., and Modlin, J. F. An outbreak of rubella among hospital employees. *N. Engl. J. Med.* 303:541, 1980.

52. Rotbart, H. A., and Levin, M. J. How contagious is necrotizing enterocolitis? *Pediatr. Infect. Dis.* 2:406, 1983.

53. Ryder, R. W., Crosby-Ritchie, A., McDonough, B., and Hall, W. J. Human milk contaminated with *Salmonella kottbus:* A cause of nosocomial illness in infants. *J.A.M.A.* 283:1533, 1977.

54. Segal, S. Neonatal intensive care: A prediction of continuing development. *Pediatr. Clin. North Am.* 13:1149, 1966.

55. Shuman, R. M., Leech, R. W., and Alvord, E.

D. Neurotoxicity of hexachlorophene in humans. II. A clinicopathological study of 46 premature infants. *Arch. Neurol.* 32:320, 1975.

56. Siegel, J. D., McCracken, G. H., Threlkeld, N., et al. Single-dose penicillin prophylaxis against neonatal group B streptococcal infections. *N. Engl. J. Med.* 303:769, 1980.

57. Silverman, W. A., and Sinclair, J. C. Evaluation of precautions before entering a neonatal unit. *Pediatrics* 40:900, 1967.

58. Sprunt, K., Redman, W., and Leidy, G. Antibacterial effectiveness of routine handwashing. *Pediatrics* 52:264, 1973.

59. Stagno, S., Reynolds, D. W., Pass, R. F., et al. Breast milk and the risk of cytomegalovirus infection. *N. Engl. J. Med.* 302:1073, 1980.

60. Stamm, W. E., Kolff, C. A., Dones, E. M., Javariz, R., Anderson, R. L., Farmer, J. J., and de Quinones, H. R. A nursery outbreak caused by *Serratia marcescens:* Scalp-vein needles as a portal of entry. *J. Pediatr.* 89:96, 1976.

61. Steere, A. C., and Mallison, G. F. Handwashing practices for the prevention of nosocomial infections. *Ann. Intern. Med.* 83:683, 1975.

62. Steiner, P., Rao, M., Victoria, M. S., Rudolph, N., and Buynoski, G. Miliary tuberculosis in two infants after nursery exposure: Epidemiologic, clinical, and laboratory findings. *Am. Rev. Respir. Dis.* 113:267, 1976.

63. Tyne, M. D. Concepts for improved nursery design. *Hospitals* 48:66, 1974.

64. Van Dyke, R. B., and Spector, S. A. Transmission of herpes simplex virus type 1 to a newborn infant during endotracheal suctioning for meconium aspiration. *Pediatr. Infect. Dis.* 3:153, 1984.

65. Wenzel, R. P., Osterman, C. A., and Hunting, K. J. Hospital-acquired infections. II. Infection rates by site, service, and common procedures in a university hospital. *Am. J. Epidemiol.* 104:645, 1976.

66. Wheeler, W. E. Water bugs in the bassinet (editorial). *Am. J. Dis. Child.* 101:273, 1961.

67. Williams, C. P. S., and Oliver, T. K., Jr. Nursery routines and staphylococcal colonization of the newborn. *Pediatrics* 44:640, 1969.

68. Winkel, C. A., Snyder, D. L., and Schaerth, J. B. Scalp abscess: A complication of the spiral fetal electrode. *Am. J. Obstet. Gynecol.* 126:720, 1976.

69. Wong, V. C. W., Ip, H. M. H., Reesink, H. W., et al. Prevention of the HBsAg carrier status in newborn infants of mothers who are chronic carriers of HBsAg and HBeAg by administration

of hepatitis B vaccine and hepatitis B immuno-globulin: Double-blind randomized placebo-controlled study. *Lancet* 1:921, 1984.

70. Yeager, A. S. Longitudinal serological study of cytomegalovirus infections in nurses and in personnel without patient contact. *J. Clin. Microbiol.* 2:448, 1975.

71. Yeager, A. S. Transmission of cytomegalovirus to mothers by infected infants: Another reason to prevent transfusion-acquired infections. *Pediatr. Infect. Dis.* 2:295, 1983.

72. Yeager, A. S., Grumet, F. C., Hafleigh, E. B., Arvin, A. M., Bradley, J. S., and Prober, C. G. Prevention of transfusion-acquired cytomegalovirus infection in newborn infants. *J. Pediatr.* 98:281, 1981.

73. Yow, M. D., Lakeman, A. D., Stagno, S., Reynolds, R. B., and Plavidal, F. J. Use of restriction enzymes to investigate the source of a primary cytomegalovirus infection in a pediatric nurse. *Pediatrics* 70:713, 1982.

# 20 THE OPERATING ROOM

Harold Laufman

Critical analysis of the operating-room environment in recent years has given rise to basic principles of architecture and engineering on the one hand, but has exposed misdirected and expensive developments on the other. Despite a host of existing codes and guidelines directed at minimizing hazards, these hazards until recently have been ill-defined and, in some cases, exaggerated. Identifiable operating-room hazards include infection, power failure, electrical and mechanical malfunctions, flame, and explosion. Inherent in all these hazards in the physical environment is the pervading effect of human failure. The danger associated with unskilled, poorly trained, or untrustworthy personnel who may abuse an otherwise satisfactory environment constitutes an insidious, but perhaps the most important, aspect of hazard control in the operating room. Human failure is strongly related to the problem of infection control.

It is impossible to discuss a single factor such as architectural design without acknowledging its relation to the other interdependent factors in the complex mosaic of surgical infection control. For the sake of convenience, the five main categories of factors involved in surgical infection control have been classified into "five D's": discipline, defense mechanisms, drugs, design, and devices [14]. Table 20-1 demonstrates, without attempting to quantify, the relationship between architectural design and the other factors.

## ENVIRONMENTAL DESIGN OF THE SURGICAL SUITE

Design and equipment of a surgical suite can affect utilization patterns, material handling, and traffic and commerce in and around the suite. To a certain extent, design and equipment have an influence on the effectiveness of people, of machines, and of the various systems in which there is interaction between people and things. Insofar as there is an interrelationship between design, efficiency, methods, economy, and the human element, the architectural configuration and the equipment of a surgical suite indirectly affect the incidence of surgical infection [12].

From an architectural point of view, a number of design concepts have arisen that are directed at the control of surgical infection. Most planners of surgical suites acknowledge that people rather than things are the chief problem in the control of wound infection. Although both surgeons and planners agree that the

315

TABLE 20-1. The five D's of surgical infection control

| Discipline | Defense mechanisms | Drugs | Design | Devices |
|---|---|---|---|---|
| Surgeon's technique | Type of patient | Antibiotics | Configuration of surgical suite | Aseptic barriers |
| Type of operation | Age | Prophylactic | Central core | Gloves |
| Length of operation | Immune mechanisms | Preventive | Peripheral corridor | Clothing |
| Contact errors | Anatomic operative site | Therapeutic | Cluster plan | Drapes |
| OR team breaks | Obesity | Skin preparation | Central corridor | Masks |
| Scrub-procedure breaks | Malnourishment | Irrigation solutions | Location of CSR | Mechanical devices |
| Touch-contamination | Anemia | | On-site recycling | Air handling |
| Overall technique breaks | Type of operation | | Ceiling design | HVAC |
| Anesthesiologist | Foreign body implant | | Presence of tracks | Gases and vacuum |
| Breaks | Organ transplant | | Location of services | Anesthesia equipment |
| Attire and preparation | Effects of immunosuppressive drugs | | Air grilles | Sterilization devices |
| Technique | Effects of irradiation | | Lighting | High vacuum |
| Errors contributing to airborne transmission | Bacterial type, virulence, and number | | Ambient | Steam |
| Faulty containment | | | Surgical | Gas—EO |
| Hair and skin | | | Cabinetry | Transport mechanisms |
| Carrier potential | | | Ventilation | Case carts vs. supply carts |
| Shedding potential | | | Pass-through | On-site inventory |
| Support services | | | Open vs. closed | |
| Sterilization techniques | | | Materials and surfaces | |
| Maintenance and repair | | | Storage space | |
| Standards and policies | | | Amount | |
| Infection control nurse | | | Location | |
| Infection Control Committee | | | Internal design | |
| Infection reporting and recording | | | Traffic patterns | |
| Statistics keeping | | | | |

CSR = central supply room; HVAC = heating, ventilating, air-conditioning; EO = ethylene oxide; prophylactic = antibiotics given before surgery without evidence of the presence of infection; preventive = antibiotics given during or after surgery without evidence of the presence of infection.

environmental approach cannot be ignored, proof of the effects of architecture on infection is almost impossible to obtain. It is widely agreed that the surgical suite should be located to provide isolation from the mainstreams of common corridor traffic.

An effort at developing traffic patterns that would separate "clean" from "dirty" traffic in a surgical suite has resulted in the architectural concepts known as the "clean central core" and the "peripheral corridor." Although these concepts were experimented with by American architects since the late 1920s, British architects developed them in the post–World War II years. In principle, these concepts were developed on the proposition that the site of the operation in the center of each operating room is the cleanest spot, the periphery of the room less clean, the corridors of the surgical suite less clean, and so on, toward the periphery of the suite. The central core of the suite serves as the supply center and therefore is supposedly cleanest of all. The clean core and inner corridors are designated for use by clean traffic (patients before elective, clean operations, as well as surgeons and nurses before operating), whereas the peripheral corridors are designated for so-called dirty traffic (patients after operation, as well as surgeons and nurses after operating). If the patient is considered infected before operation, he or she is brought in and taken out of the operating room through the dirty corridors.

A number of suites now in use have been the subject of criticism. Observations made in them reveal that, unfortunately, almost none is being used as planned [10]. The existing traffic pattern does not conform with the one conceived by the architect. People tend to take the shortest distance between two points, rather than a roundabout way. Moreover, in those suites being used almost as planned, no notable reduction in infection rates has been observed over previous rates or over those found with other architectural designs. The peripheral corridors, occupying thousands of square feet of otherwise valuable space, have become long storage halls for expensive floor-standing equipment that should have been accorded legitimate storage space inside the suite.

The clean core in its pure form is intended to be an area of the surgical suite that is virtually as clean as any operating room, where only such clean activities as clean storage, instrument packing, and autoclaving are done, or that serves as a supply port for adjacent operating rooms. All traffic from this area is intended to be in the direction of the operating rooms, and all traffic out of the operating rooms is intended to be in the direction of the peripheral corridor. In practice, however, we have observed that personnel working in the clean-core area do not usually wear masks and are not confined to the clean core. Clean storage in this area may contain cartons that often come directly off the truck that delivered them to the hospital. In this area, short sleeve clothing is commonly worn by the personnel. The shedding of bacteria-carrying squamae from exposed skin is well documented. Of necessity, people go into and come out of the operating rooms into the clean core in the course of their work. This unavoidable activity, plus the other abuses mentioned, give one pause to ponder the validity of the clean-core concept, as well as to wonder about the absence of studies concerned with it.

The architectural configurations of surgical suites fall into four categories, each with variations: (1) the central corridor or hotel plan with "L" or "T" variations; (2) the double central corridor, multiple corridors, or clean-core plan; (3) the grouping or cluster plan, and (4) the peripheral corridor, ring, or racetrack plan. A partial or complete peripheral corridor may be designed for any of these plans.

The fact that equally good surgery can be done in any of these suites at equally low risk and with equally good results, provided the surgery is done well and is supported by efficient support personnel who do not abuse their environment, may mean one of three things: (1) traffic patterns within the surgical suite are not important as long as clean internal traffic is effectively segregated from the so-called dirty traffic outside the suite; (2) traffic patterns are important, but architects are not planning them realistically; or (3) current ideas on designing surgical suites and traffic patterns are in need of revision in concept. One is inclined to see a bit of truth in all three possibilities.

*Recovery Areas*

Recovery areas have emerged from their original designation as a place for a patient to recover from anesthesia to a place where intensive nursing care can be given to a critically ill patient postoperatively. Especially since the advent of open-heart surgery, organ transplantation, and other types of major surgery, the recovery "room" has become an intensive care suite of windowed cubicles. Patients with severe infections can be given care as good as that given to patients whose defense mechanisms may be suppressed, and all patients are under close surveillance. Thus the open, Florence Nightingale–type of recovery room, although still in wide use, is giving way to a recovery area of isolation cubicles, located immediately adjacent to, or as part of, the surgical suite.

### Transfer Areas

A transfer area is ordinarily considered desirable. In this area, the patient is transferred from the "outside" cart to an "inside" cart, ostensibly to prevent the tracking of hospital dirt into the surgical suite. Although this practice is acknowledged to have theoretical validity, no hard evidence is available that traces surgical infections to the wheels of carts. Some costly devices are available for patient transfer, including mechanical transfer-board arrangements. The same procedure, however, can be simply, effectively, and economically carried out at any counter-height barrier. Many hospitals continue to bring the hospital cart into the operating room and to transfer the patient directly to the operating table. No reported infections thus far have been traced to this practice.

### Other Areas

A conference room, nurses' offices, a scheduling area, holding and preparation areas, an adequate vestibular area, and appropriately sized and located locker rooms and lounges are all considered essential to an up-to-date surgical suite. All require significant space in terms of square footage, but a good case can be made for them on the basis of hazard control alone. At the entrance to a surgical suite, for example, the frequent opening and closing of the doors to the common corridor or to a bank of elevators causes an inevitable influx of unfiltered air, regardless of the pressurizing of the air in the operating rooms. For this reason, a well-ventilated, generously proportioned vestibular space, preferably demarcated by a second set of doors, will permit appropriate dilution of airborne contamination and thus serve as a sort of airlock. Opening on this vestibular space are the offices mentioned previously, the transfer area, surgeons' lockers, the scheduling desk, and other spaces requiring an outside and inside interface. Through such an arrangement, these spaces need not open directly to a common corridor.

### Number of Operating Rooms

The number of operating rooms is relevant to hazard control only as it relates to the economy of scheduling, housekeeping practices, and staffing. For most hospitals, the "five-percent formula" works quite well: the number of operating rooms should be 5 percent of the total number of surgical beds. Thus for a hospital with 100 surgical beds utilized by all surgical specialties combined, there should be five or six operating rooms. Of course, this number must be adjusted according to the volume of lengthy versus short operations: upward if a large proportion of operations are lengthy, downward if most operations are of short

duration. Accurate programming is based on careful analysis of data and sound predictions. Cystoscopy and endoscopy rooms are additional. Overuse of operating rooms gives rise to the risk of personnel fatigue and incomplete cleansing practices.

### Size of Operating Rooms

The size of operating rooms that is considered optimal for most operations is 20 by 20 feet and 10 feet high. Although some procedures—such as those in ophthalmology, otolaryngology, and cystoscopy—can be done comfortably in smaller rooms, the primary requisite regarding size is that all maneuvers, including gowning and draping, the circulation of personnel, and the use of equipment, should be executable without the risk of contact contamination. Because of the space requirements of the extracorporeal pump, the pump team, and other additional people, a somewhat larger room—for example, 24 by 26 feet—is recommended for open-heart surgery. When one dimension of a room exceeds 30 feet, however, something is lost in personnel efficiency.

## METHODS OF INFECTION CONTROL

### Operating-Room Surfaces

In general, the harder and less porous the floor, walls, ceilings, and other surfaces, the more dirt-resistant the surface will be and the easier it will be to clean. Ceramic tile has been criticized because the rough surfaces of grouting may attract bacteria. A new grouting material is now available, however, that has a surface as smooth as ceramic tile itself. Other wall materials suitable for operating-room use include laminated polyester with an epoxy finish, hard vinyl coverings that can be heat-sealed at the seams, and other hard building materials such as formica.

Tacky mats with replaceable sheets have been widely promoted and used in front of the doors leading to the surgical suite on the pretext that they prevent the tracking in of dirt from common corridors. Our test results have shown that these mats do not remove bacteria but in fact transfer tagged bacteria to new contacts [12]. Yet in a recent survey, Garner and coworkers [9] found that almost half of 433 hospitals were routinely using the useless tacky mats, and of the users only 29 percent changed the mat more often than once a day. Wet-mopping of hard-surfaced floors with a phenolic solution between each patient in the operating room, as well as every several hours during the working day in the corridors of the suite, with wet-vacuuming at night, is an unsurpassed method of keeping the floors clean.

*Air-Handling Systems*

Most conventional operating rooms are, or should be, ventilated by efficient, well-maintained, bag-filtered or high-efficiency particulate air-filtered (HEPA) systems. The environment of such operating rooms suffers only by abuse, but otherwise it has been shown to be virtually as effectively clean as that of costly special chambers. Defective air-handling systems, on the other hand, may be considered hazardous under special circumstances.

The significance of airborne contamination as a cause of wound infection has gone through several cycles of argument. Today's consensus holds that airborne organisms assume a significant role in causing wound infections only when (1) an air-handling system is grossly contaminated [8], (2) an otherwise effective air-handling system is abused, or (3) in occasional instances of highly specialized procedures in which a large foreign body is implanted (the last point is still controversial). Additionally, an occasional infection in clean surgical wounds occurs in which the route of infection appears to have been the air, but that is unassociated with any of these three factors. The infrequency of this occurrence probably is the result of the low numbers of airborne bacteria and the attention paid to the air in operating rooms.

It must be emphasized that no matter how clean the air may be in an operating room and no matter what direction it is blown toward, the air system will not have any effect on contact contamination from the patient himself or from the surgical team.

Abuse of the operating-room environment by personnel includes such practices as leaving a door open to the corridor during operative procedures; permitting unrestricted opening and closing of the operating-room doors as people come and go; not covering long hair, sideburns, or beards; and allowing technical, nursing, and anesthesia-administering personnel to circulate in and out of operating rooms while wearing short-sleeved shirts. No matter how particulate-free the air may be that is blown into a room, the particulate biologic matter that inevitably is circulated around the room is quantitatively in direct proportion to the number and movement of people in the room and the amount of exposed hair and skin. Shed particles tend to mount exponentially when excessive numbers of improperly covered visitors are present and when unnecessary activity of people occurs, including the flapping of drapes, towels, and gowns as well as any other maneuver that may unsettle previously shed particles from horizontal surfaces.

Current U.S. Public Health Service and National Fire Protection Association (NFPA) minimum requirements for operating-room air call for a minimum of 25 changes per hour, positive pressure compared with corridors, temperatures between 18°C and 24°C (65°F and 75°F), humidity of 50 to 55 percent, and depending on the locality, up to 80 percent recirculation with the use of effective filtering. In some states, 100 percent outside air with no recirculation is still required. Recently engineers have been suggesting an upgrading of these requirements for new hospitals in which high-risk surgery is to be performed. They are specifying that air be supplied into the operating room through ceiling panels (approximately 10 by 10 feet) directly over the operating table at 60 feet per minute face velocity. This high-flow system delivers 6000 cubic feet of air per minute and would result in one and a half air changes per minute (or 90 per hour) in a room 20 by 20 by 10 feet. When the air flow is this great, an important feature is adequate exhaust; this should be located on the walls above the baseboard to maintain some directionality and prevent great turbulence. If the inflow is reduced to 30 feet per minute face velocity, it will result in 45 air changes per hour, a figure considered highly satisfactory by many authorities.

We believe that the air in the entire surgical suite—including closets, storage areas, personnel areas, and recovery-room areas—should be as well filtered and ventilated as the air in the operating room. This design of the air system would minimize the number of areas of contaminated air in the suite.

Several questions remain unanswered with respect to laminar flow in the operating room. These questions relate largely to whether this method of diffusing air has any effect on infection control, and whether it is relevant at all to hospital use. The term *laminar* is being applied or misapplied to many types of unidirectional air-blowing systems, ranging from virtually any type of ceiling or wall diffuser to a variety of "curtain effect" air systems. The use of the term, erroneous though it may be, appears to be here to stay. So-called laminar flow can be delivered in a horizontal or vertical direction. Although there are proponents of each, neither method has been shown to be superior to the other; indeed, it has not been shown whether either is superior to nonlaminar flow. The British surgeon, Charnley, gave impetus to the promotion of laminar-flow chambers by claiming that his reduction of wound infections following hip replacement operations from 9 percent to 1 percent was due to the use of the chamber [4]. Charnley's critics point out that this improvement in results over the six-year study period could well have been the result of several other changes in technique that he employed, including the use of a coverall surgical gown as well as changes in a number of technical maneuvers [13].

Most bacteria are in the 0.5 to 5.0 $\mu$ diameter range. Thus, if HEPA filtering is used, the first air downstream from the filter is virtually bacteria-free. HEPA-filtered air, however, is often confused with laminar air flow. One is a filtering capability; the other, a method of diffusion or distribution of air into a space in a more or less unidirectional manner. Thus laminar flow may be imparted to air that is either filtered or unfiltered, and HEPA-filtered air can be delivered by any type or size of diffusing method, laminar or nonlaminar, high speed or low speed. It must be remembered that HEPA filtering does nothing to filter particles produced in the room; it merely produces almost particle-free first air as it leaves the diffuser.

Although ambient bacterial counts can be reduced by large-volume unidirectional air flow, no evidence has been presented to show that this *alone* has a significant effect on the incidence of surgical wound infections or whether unidirectional flow is or is not superior to a well-functioning, properly installed, conventional nonlaminar system in this respect.

In a multicenter study of sepsis after total hip or knee replacement in England, Scotland, and Sweden, 8000 records were studied [19]. In the patients whose prostheses were inserted in an operating room ventilated by an ultraclean-air system, the incidence of joint sepsis confirmed at reoperation within the next one to four years was about half that of patients who had the operation in a conventionally ventilated room at the same hospital. When whole-body exhaust suits were worn by the operating team in an operating room ventilated by an ultraclean-air system, the incidence of sepsis was about one-quarter that found after operations performed with so-called conventional ventilation. When all groups in the trial were considered together, the analysis showed an incidence of 1.5 percent deep infections after operations in the control group, and 0.6 percent in the ultraclean-air groups. The design of the study did not include a strictly controlled test of the effect of prophylactic antibiotics, but their use was associated with a lower incidence of sepsis than found in patients who received no antibiotic prophylaxis (0.6 vs. 2.3 percent).

This study, the largest and best controlled of the studies thus far published on the subject, demonstrates that ultraclean air is preferable to so-called conventional air. The problem in transferring these results to American experiences is the difference in what is called "conventional" air supply in the United States compared with that in England, Scotland, and Sweden. A code-accepted, properly installed and maintained conventional air system in American operating rooms is basically a vertical-flow, unidirectional air system, delivering a minimum of 25 changes per hour of HEPA-filtered air into an operating room. The air is exhausted low on the walls with an active exhaust system, which helps to maintain unidirectionality. Joint replacement operations done in such conventional operating rooms and with good barrier containment of the surgical team carry equally low infection rates to those found in the British study. Although the British study was otherwise well designed, it provides no information matching the types of airborne bacteria with those found in the infected wounds. Also, only imprecise information is presented on the possibilities of contact contamination in the infected cases (see Chapter 29).

The fact that the coverall exhaust-ventilation suit worn by the surgical team additionally lowered the incidence of infection a full 50 percent from that resulting from operations performed in ultraclean-air rooms with so-called conventional clothing makes one wonder what the incidence of infection would be if the surgeons wore coverall exhaust-ventilated suits in a conventional-air operating room. The study did not isolate the effect of barrier containment alone.

A number of American orthopedic surgeons who have performed thousands of hip replacement operations in conventional operating rooms without laminar-flow chambers report a combined two-year infection rate of 0.45 percent, a figure as low as or lower than that reported by surgeons with comparable numbers of operations performed in laminar-flow chambers [13]. The bacteria cultured from wound infections following hip replacement surgery have been shown to correlate poorly with those found in the air of the room or chamber [15].

Air is only one of several possible sources of microorganisms; others include endogenous sources, person-to-person transmission, and the inanimate environment (equipment and the like) [21].

## Use of Ultraviolet Light

The bactericidal effect of ultraviolet (UV) light is undeniable. Many European hospitals use UV in the empty operating room, either overnight or during protracted periods of nonuse of the room. The use of UV is limited by the possibility of burns as well as by the fact that, because it is a ray, it can only strike exposed surfaces. In a large, rather well-controlled study, the use of UV was not shown to influence the overall incidence of wound infection [1], although it did appear to have an effect on the incidence of infection in clean procedures.

## Cleaning Methods

Every major surgical operation is now considered to be "dirty," because evidence is available to show that saprophytic organisms previously considered harmless may occasionally be responsible for severe sepsis. Also, viral hepatitis type B may be unsuspectedly carried in the blood of any surgical patient. Therefore, the current recommendation is for terminal sterilization of all instruments on completion of an operation. If the instruments must leave the operating room to be terminally sterilized, they must be placed in containers, as should all other used materials. Only after terminal sterilization are instruments to be handled and examined by personnel. These points speak in favor of an on-site instrument-processing operation in the surgical suite, rather than in a distant central supply area.

There remains some difference of opinion regarding the virtues of ultrasonic cleaning over other methods, but many hospitals use commercially available ultrasonic devices, either as a separate operation or in combination with automatic washing of instruments.

The contaminated or "dirty" case is commonly considered as one in which frank pus was encountered during the operation. In a few hospitals, it is still the practice to clean the room thoroughly where such an operation was performed and keep it sealed for up to 48 hours before another operation is permitted in it. This practice is no longer considered necessary, provided the appropriate clean-up techniques are used and the air-handling system is adequate [20]. Even with a minimum of 12 air changes per hour, the air in an operating room is exchanged every five minutes. Therefore, the usual clean-up period of 20 or 30 minutes should allow four to six complete air changes, provided the doors are kept closed. This should be adequate to dispose of any airborne bacteria that may have resulted from the contaminated case. The air systems of many modern operating rooms provide 25, 30, or more changes of air per hour, thus ensuring faster clean-out of any residual airborne contamination.

The technique of cleaning a "contaminated" room consists of wet mopping or flooding with a good phenolic detergent, wiping down all metal furniture and plastic surfaces with a germicidal detergent or with 70% alcohol, and changing all rubber or plastic tubing in the room [20]. It is not considered necessary any longer to clean the walls any more than what is provided by the usual routine at the end of each day, unless, of course, direct contamination such as splashing has occurred. One of the common defects in cleaning methods is to scrub walls unnecessarily while neglecting to clean the anesthesia equipment. The instruments, linen, and waste should be placed separately and carefully in containers before they are taken from the room. All gowns, masks, and shoe covers used during the procedure and in the cleanup must be left in the room to be put in containers [11].

## Scheduling of Operations

Scheduling practices also may have a bearing on infection hazard, especially in terms of the type of case scheduled to follow another. In some hospitals, it is the policy to schedule all "dirty" operations at the end of the day. In others, a septic room is set aside for such cases. Some surgeons believe the risk of wound infection in an otherwise "clean" case is greater if the operation is performed late in the day.

It is no longer deemed advisable to set aside a room for septic surgery. Current thinking considers every case to be potentially, if not actually, infected. Clean-up techniques have made such separate, low-usage facilities unnecessary. Nonetheless, on doctrinaire grounds, an open-heart operation would not be scheduled to follow the drainage of an abscess in the same room if it could be avoided. Many times, however, a "clean" emergency operation must of necessity be performed late in the day or following a septic case. With appropriate clean-up techniques, there is no evidence of increased risk of infection in such instances.

## OPERATING-ROOM PERSONNEL

Routine culture testing of specimens from the nasopharynx or other sites of personnel who work in operating rooms is not considered mandatory or necessary [20]. In tracking down possible sources of infection, however, it is necessary to review not only the microbiologic contribution of such sources as the nasopharynx, hair [7], skin, and occasionally respiratory and gastrointestinal tracts of all concerned personnel, but also all applicable cleaning methods and routines as well. An additional factor involves the personal integrity and work ethics of the personnel. All duties may be well performed while under surveillance but some may be poorly done or even omitted when employees are on their own. Clean-up methods should be checked for efficacy at regular intervals [11] (see Chapter 2).

Personnel may be the source of organisms that cause disease when transmitted to patients. These personnel may be classified as carriers or disseminators (shedders). A *carrier* is an infected person who harbors a specific infectious agent but shows no evidence of clinical disease. If this individual sheds these organisms, he or she is referred to as a *shedder* or *disseminator,* and if disease results in another individual, then the shedder may be referred to as a *dangerous disseminator* (see Chapter 1). Organisms can be disseminated on skin squamae, from the oral or nasal pharynx, in the blood, and in secretions or excretions.

Nasopharyngeal droplets expelled by talking, coughing, or yawning are usually entrapped in the mask, but a certain portion will manage to escape around the mask or through a damp or defective mask. Face masks should therefore cover the nose and mouth snugly. Permeation of moisture and bacteria through the mask will depend on the barrier qualities of the material of the mask. Moreover, face masks should not be allowed to hang under the chin when not in place, since they may be a disseminating source. A mask should not be reused after being used once and then carried under the chin.

There are many different types of surgical masks that have been developed for use in the operating room. The literature on their evaluations is voluminous and difficult to summarize. The best universal recommendation is to use a high-efficiency filter mask that is properly worn at all times while in the operating room.

*Operating-Room Garb*
The purpose of operating-room clothing is primarily to provide a barrier to contamination that may pass from personnel to patient as well as from patient to personnel. Traditional garb consists of gowns, caps, masks, and shoe covers, made of either woven launderable materials or nonwoven disposable materials. Impermeability to moisture is an important property of any barrier material, because the wicking effect tends to transmit bacteria. Surgical gowns reinforced on the front and sleeves with a tightly woven material (Barbac) and treated with waterproofing have been shown to be impermeable at the areas of reinforcement through up to 100 launderings, averaging 75 [2]. Drapes reinforced with this material are equally impermeable. Among the nonwoven materials, however, very few stand up to the stresses of stretch, pressure, and friction common to operating-room usage without becoming permeable to a moist contaminant unless reinforced with a plastic laminate or a plastic impregnation [16–18]. Equally disturbing is the fact that manufacturing standards for surgical gloves permit at least two holes per hundred gloves. Gloves are only spot-checked for holes, and therefore many more defective gloves are used than are realized by surgeons.

In an effort to prevent shedding at its source—that is, the skin of personnel—a variety of coverall hoods and gowns are available that are used in conjunction with a plastic mask or helmet and are designed to cover the entire head and body of the surgeon and his team members. These outfits are highly effective in eliminating shedding. Because of the discomfort due to retained heat under such outfits, however, it is necessary to use vacuum to exhaust the space between wearer and uniform to keep the wearer comfortable [5]. Such precautions may be more than what is required for everyday surgery, except for types of surgery in which the risk of contamination may be exceptionally great, as in the implantation of large devices (e.g., joint replacements).

Hoods rather than caps are now being recommended for all operating-room personnel. Since it is known that hair may acquire and might shed bacterial particles, it is recommended that all hair on the face and head be covered in the operating room.

The usual practice of wearing white shoes with dried secretions on the leather is condemned as unsanitary for a number of reasons, one of which is the tendency for flakes to come off with motion and enter the general environment. Thus shoe covers are recommended for use in the surgical suite. Disposable, easy to put on, and equipped with a conductive strip, nonwoven shoe covers should be put on fresh every time a person enters the surgical suite from the outside.

The search goes on for the ideal material for operating-room garb, both disposable and reusable. Materials sought are those that are impervious to bacteria and moisture; resistant to the stresses of stretch, pressure, and friction; relatively nonretentive of heat; flame retardant; low in static; and economical. None of the disposable materials now in use fulfills all these requirements.

*The Scrub and Skin Preparation*
The surgeon's hands and forearms, as well as those of his or her assistants and scrub nurse, must be washed before an operation. Experience has shown that this "scrub" should take at least 10 minutes and should consist of constant friction, soaping, and repeated rinsings. Scrubbing much longer will often result in raising bacteria from deep dermal layers to the surface and lead to higher bacterial counts on the surface. Although scrubbings for shorter periods than 10 minutes have been shown to be virtually as effective, the full period is still advocated for scrubbing. The lubricating material may be soap or a detergent that contains either iodophor or hexachlorophene. In recent years, hexachlorophene has been shown to be absorbed under certain circumstances into the blood, fat cells, and brain cells. The Food and Drug Admin-

istration has therefore banned its routine use for new-born infants (see Chapter 19); however, it can still be used by surgeons and other hospital personnel for washing their hands. Soap and detergent dispensers have been shown at times to support the growth of gram-negative bacteria. Hence the most expedient and safest scrub technique today consists of using a disposable brush or sponge impregnated with detergent that contains iodophor solution. For iodine-sensitive surgical personnel, 3% hexachlorophene or chlorhexidine may be used [21].

Scrub sinks are traditionally fitted with foot, knee, or elbow pedals to allow operation of the sink without using one's hands. New sinks are activated either with an electric eye or electrical field of flux for no-touch operation. They have additional features such as no-splash streams, controlled water temperature, and filtered water. If sprinklers or aerators are used, they should be periodically washed in a high-temperature washer or autoclaved.

The skin of the patient is prepared by shaving the operative site, if necessary, as short a time as possible before surgery. Alexander and colleagues [2] have recently shown that clipping hair rather than shaving is the preferred method of hair removal when it must be done preoperatively. Just before surgery, the operative site should be scrubbed with soap and water or a detergent solution, dried with a sterile towel, and then painted with an iodophor or tincture of chlorhexidine.

The skin preparation ritual is followed by appropriate draping to protect the clean field from the unprepared parts of the patient.

## RECORD KEEPING

Guidelines of the Joint Commission on Accreditation of Hospitals contain standards requiring the existence of an Infection Control Committee in all hospitals (see Chapter 3). In large hospitals, there may be a separate committee or subcommittee on surgical infections. The purpose of such committees is not only to define, monitor, and investigate all infections within its purview, but also to keep a careful record or log of such infections. Unfortunately, the methods used by hospitals in complying with these standards vary greatly. Surgeons do not always agree on the definition of a wound infection, for example. Some anesthetists are unwilling to ascribe postoperative fever accompanying pulmonary "congestion" to a respiratory tract infection acquired during anesthesia administration and therefore do not gather follow-up statistics. In many cases, the infection of a wound

does not become evident until after the patient leaves the hospital and so is lost to the record. If the patient is readmitted with an established infection, the infection is rarely recorded as a complication, especially if the original operation was performed at another hospital. For these reasons and others, a standard method should be formulated and adopted by all hospitals. Amazingly, no such standard exists.

## REFERENCES

1. Ad Hoc Committee on Trauma, NAS-NRC. Postoperative wound infections. *Ann. Surg.* 160(Suppl.):August, 1964.
2. Alexander, J. W., Fischer, J. E., Boyajian, M., et al. The influence of hair-removal methods on wound infections. *Arch. Surg.* 118:347, 1983.
3. Badner, B., Zelner, L., Merchant, R., and Laufman, H. Costs of linen *vs.* disposable OR packs. *Hospitals* 47:78, 1973.
4. Charnley, J., and Eftekhar, N. Postoperative infection in total prosthetic replacement arthroplasty of the hip joint. *Br. J. Surg.* 56:641, 1969.
5. Charnley, J., and Eftekhar, N. Penetration of gown material by organisms from the surgeon's body. *Lancet* 1:175, 1969.
6. Cruse, P. J. E., and Foord, R. The epidemiology of wound infection: A ten-year prospective study of 62,939 wounds. *Surg. Clin. North Am.* 60:27, 1980.
7. Dineen, P., and Drusin, L. Epidemics of postoperative wound infections associated with hair carriers. *Lancet* 2:1157, 1973.
8. Gage, A. A., Dean, D. C., Schimert, G., and Minsky, N. *Aspergillus* infection after cardiac surgery. *Arch. Surg.* 101:384, 1970.
9. Garner, J. S., Emori, T. G., and Haley, R. W. Operating room practices for the control of infection in U.S. hospitals. *Surg. Gynecol. Obstet.* 155:873, 1982.
10. Laufman, H. What's wrong with our operating rooms? *Am. J. Surg.* 122:332, 1971.
11. Laufman, H. Cleanup techniques in the operating room. *Med. Surg. Rev.* October–November, 1971, pp. 1–4.
12. Laufman, H. Surgical hazard control: Effect of architecture and engineering. *Arch. Surg.* 107:552, 1973.
13. Laufman, H. Current status of special air handling systems in operating rooms. *Med. Instrum.* 7:7, 1973.
14. Laufman, H. The control of operating room infection: Discipline, defense mechanisms, drugs,

design, and devices. *Bull. N.Y. Acad. Med.* 54:465, 1978.

15. Laufman, H. Airflow effects in surgery: Perspective of an era. *Arch. Surg.* 114:826, 1979.
16. Laufman, H., Eddy, W. W., Vandernoot, A. M., et al. Strike-through of moist contamination by woven and nonwoven surgical materials. *Ann. Surg.* 181:857, 1975.
17. Laufman, H., Montefusco, C., Siegal, J. D., and Edberg, S. C. Scanning electron microscopy of moist bacterial strike-through of surgical materials. *Surg. Gynecol. Obstet.* 150:165, 1980.
18. Laufman, H., Siegal, J. D., and Edberg, S. C. Moist bacterial strike-through of surgical materials: Confirmatory tests. *Ann. Surg.* 189:68, 1979.
19. Lidwell, O. M., Lowburg, E. J. L., Whyte, W., Blowers, R., Stanley, S. J., and Lowe, D. Effect of ultraclean air in operating rooms on deep sepsis in the joint after total hip or knee replacement: A randomised study. *Br. Med. J.* 285:10, 1982.
20. Mallison, G. F. Housekeeping in operating suites. *A.O.R.N. J.* 21:213, 1975.
21. Simmons, B. P. CDC *Guideline for Prevention of Surgical Wound Infections.* March 1982. Republished in *A.O.R.N. J.* 37:556, 1983.

# 21 AMBULATORY CARE SETTINGS

Marguerite M. Jackson
Patricia Lynch

The vast majority of physician-patient contacts are in ambulatory care facilities. About 75 percent of the population see a physician in a given year, whereas only 10 percent of the population are hospitalized. Annually, there are about four times as many visits to physicians on an ambulatory basis as there are hospital days of care [14].

Because of the millions of patient visits in these settings annually, questions frequently arise about the risk for nosocomial infection and about interventions to reduce these risks. Infection risk associated with care in an ambulatory setting is probably quite low, although it has not been studied extensively. The majority of patients seen in these settings present with nonurgent problems and are not admitted to hospitals. A substantial proportion of the infections seen in ambulatory care settings are viral respiratory infections and probably carry with them risks of transmission similar to the risks of transmission in the community.

Nosocomial infection risk increases with the number of devices or procedures to which the patient is exposed. Except for emergent and some urgent visits to hospital emergency departments, few ambulatory care patients are exposed to invasive devices or procedures that are known to pose significant infection risk. In addition the duration of the patient's visit to the facility is usually limited, which is also a factor in reduced risk for nosocomial infection.

This chapter discusses the various types of ambulatory care settings (ACS), general infection risks associated with these settings, and interventions known or suspected to reduce infection risks for patients seen there.

## AMBULATORY CARE SETTINGS

Ambulatory care may be delivered in various settings, ranging from a single physician's private office to a comprehensive emergency medical services system. The most common types of ACS are described below.

### Emergency Medical Services System

The emergency medical services system (EMSS) was developed partly in response to results from a National Academy of Sciences study of accidental death and disability, conducted in the early 1960s [17]. The Federal EMSS Act, enacted in 1973, outlined 15 separate components, defined seven patient categories (trauma, burns, spinal cord injuries, poisoning, cardiac, neonatal, behavioral), and provided for

325

a national EMSS framework. At the same time communities increased emphasis on the timely delivery of care to patients with serious injuries, beginning before arrival at the hospital [24].

PREHOSPITAL CARE  Prehospital care incorporates all emergency rescue, medical, and transportation services provided to ill or injured patients before they reach the hospital.

The functional unit of prehospital care includes the hospital-based emergency department, personnel there who advise the field team, the field team for emergency transport, and the transport vehicle. In addition some systems incorporate fire department personnel, community-based services, and volunteers.

EMERGENCY DEPARTMENT OF A HOSPITAL  The emergency department of a hospital may provide three major services: (1) care of critically ill or injured patients, most of whom are subsequently admitted to the facility; (2) offices where physicians can examine their own patients (e.g., after office hours or when more sophisticated care is necessary than a physician's office can provide); (3) care for persons who are not critically injured or ill but who do not use any other organized ambulatory service or physician's office. Patients in the latter two categories usually are not admitted to the hospital.

Weinerman and colleagues [29] define three categories used by *providers* to describe requirements for emergency care:

1. *Nonurgent.* Care does not require resources of an emergency service; referral for routine medical care may or may not be needed; disorder is nonacute or minor in severity. Few of these patients require hospital admission.
2. *Urgent.* Condition requires medical attention within the period of a few hours; there is possible danger to the patient if medically unattended; disorder is acute but not necessarily severe. Some of these patients will require hospital admission.
3. *Emergent.* Condition requires immediate medical attention; time delay is harmful to the patient; disorder is acute and possibly threatening to life or function. Many of these patients will require hospital admission and may require intensive care management.

Jonas and colleagues [13] studied 678 patient visits in the summer of 1970 to the emergency department of a 331-bed hospital in New York City. The average distribution by category among patients seen in the

emergency department was approximately 53 percent nonurgent; 37 percent urgent; and 5 percent emergent. The distribution will vary among hospitals according to the specific nature of the facility; however, this and other studies have consistently reported the majority of visits to be nonurgent in nature.

In two recent studies of hospital emergency department visits [11,21], the two most common responses from patients regarding factors associated with their decision to visit the emergency department were expediency (e.g., available hours or comprehensive care) and immediacy. The patient's perception of these factors may be different from that of the provider. The patient is scheduling care at his or her convenience, often because the emergency department is always open; also, third-party reimbursements may cover emergency department visits but not the same care in a physician's office.

TRAUMA UNITS  Trauma units are inpatient facilities that provide immediate and continuing care for patients with severe injuries. Some hospitals admit patients directly into the trauma unit. Infection risks associated with trauma units and the patient care provided there are discussed in Chapter 18.

*Emergicenters*
Emergicenters are usually freestanding facilities that care for patients with urgent or nonurgent problems. These centers are able to operate at considerably less cost than are emergency departments attached to hospitals because of the limited and exclusive nature of their function. The emergicenter functions like a physician's office with extended hours and may make referrals for more extensive care.

*Surgicenters*
Surgicenters or ambulatory surgery centers are defined as centers that handle on a "same-day basis" those surgical procedures that cannot properly be performed in a physician's office or hospital outpatient department but that can be scheduled and performed so that the patient does not need to remain in a hospital overnight. These centers may be freestanding or part of the hospital facility. Administratively they may be under the jurisdiction of the hospital's operating room or function independently.

*Outpatient Diagnostic and Treatment Facilities*
Outpatient diagnostic and treatment facilities provide care outside the usual inpatient institutional setting. This may include individual physicians' offices, clinics attached to teaching hospitals, specialty clin-

ics, and clinics or office practices administered by groups of physicians or health maintenance organizations (HMOs). Visits are usually scheduled at the request of the patient and convenience of the care provider and are usually elective in nature.

### Hospital Admitting Departments

A visit to the hospital admitting department is the usual first stop for patients with scheduled elective admissions and a prehospitalization step for many patients admitted directly from clinics or emergency departments. Although emergency admissions interact with admitting departments for billing and organizational purposes, many emergency admissions go directly from the emergency department to a nursing unit or intensive care unit and do not visit the admitting department personally.

## NOSOCOMIAL INFECTIONS

A nosocomial infection associated with an ACS can be defined as one that is associated temporally with the visit, with the care provided during the visit, or with an event that took place during the visit (e.g., an inadvertent exposure to a communicable disease while in the waiting room). In other words, it is an infection associated with medical intervention.

Patients seen in an ACS usually leave the facility after the visit and often are not followed up. If an infection develops associated with the visit, it may not be identified to the hospital or facility. The true incidence of these infections is not known, although several reports from ambulatory surgery settings have been published [5,18].

### Risk of Nosocomial Infection in the ACS

Risk of nosocomial infection in the ambulatory care setting has been demonstrated to be associated with the interaction between host defenses and exposure to potentially infectious agents in a dose sufficient to cause infection (see Chapter 1).

Factors of an ACS that are different from the hospital setting include the following:

1. Large numbers of patients are seen in rapid succession.
2. Few procedures are performed in which access to the vascular system (e.g., intravenous therapy) or mucous membranes (e.g., intubation, laryngoscopy) is necessary.
3. A wide variety of ailments may be seen by the same care provider during a single day.

4. Most patients seen in an ACS, including emergency departments, outpatient clinics, or physicians' offices, do not require admission to the hospital.

In summary, most patients in the ACS are seeking care for relatively minor illnesses or injuries that have not compromised their host defenses. The duration of contact with the facility is brief, and contact with potentially infectious agents usually depends on instrumentation. The likelihood of all three factors being sufficient to result in infection is quite low.

It is widely accepted that approximately 5 percent of hospitalized patients develop nosocomial infections, primarily of four major types: urinary tract, surgical wound, lower respiratory, and bacteremia. Several investigators have estimated that the proportion of these infections that are potentially preventable is about 25 to 40 percent [2] and that most of those are related to devices and procedures. The remaining 60 to 75 percent are often judged unavoidable because of the patient's underlying disease combined with other factors such as the duration of hospitalization (see Chapter 24).

The incidence and preventability of nosocomial infections in the ACS has not been investigated adequately. It is reasonable to assume that most nosocomial infections in these settings are largely preventable because the duration of contact with the facility is brief, and those that do occur are usually related to medical devices and procedures.

To answer some of the questions raised about incidence of infection following ACS visits, several investigators have concentrated on patients in ambulatory surgery settings. Complications associated with ambulatory surgery were studied prospectively in 13,433 patients during a four-year period by Natof [18]. Surgical procedures included tonsillectomy and/or adenoidectomy, augmentation mammoplasty, submucous resection, and a variety of genitourinary procedures, primarily performed on young, healthy hosts. Only 10 of 13,433 patients developed infections that could be associated with the ambulatory surgery procedure (three wound infections, three gynecologic infections, two pneumonias, and two upper respiratory infections). The frequency of infectious complications following ambulatory surgery in this series was less than one infection per 1000 patients (<0.1 percent).

Craig [5] summarized results of several studies of postoperative infections among ambulatory surgery patients. Despite several differences in study design, when patients and physicians responded to written questionnaires or telephone calls, the infection rate in all studies was no more than 2 percent and usually substantially lower.

When the incidence of nosocomial infection is so low, the benefit of an intensive surveillance system is likely to be exceeded by the cost. That is, the time required to follow all patients makes the cost to identify each infection quite high; however, the consequences of some nosocomial infections associated with the ACS have been serious [3].

## PERSONNEL WORKING IN THE ACS

The key to prevention of nosocomial infections in an ACS may lie in the combination of skill in performing procedures and use of aseptic practices. As in any patient care area, personnel in the ACS should not work when they have infectious diseases and should follow the facility's program for personnel health, immunizations, and exposures to communicable diseases (see Chapter 2). Facilities that are not attached to hospitals can also use these guidelines to develop programs.

The training of personnel in aseptic practices and ensuring that skills and knowledge of invasive procedures are current is also essential in the ACS. Training patients and home-care givers is increasingly important with the trend toward managing patients with indwelling devices at home. Several reports have described programs for administration of outpatient intravenous antibiotic therapy [1,8,15,22,26,27,28], home parenteral nutrition [9,12], and ambulatory dialysis [4,10,19,25]. An integral component of all these programs is training for the patient or home-care giver in aseptic practices and recognition of complications. The reported incidence of infectious complications varies with the type of device, reason for and duration of therapy, host susceptibility, and many other factors.

## THE INANIMATE ENVIRONMENT

### Cleaning, Disinfection, and Sterilization
The principles of cleaning, disinfection, and sterilization of equipment and devices used in the ACS are the same as in the hospital setting (see Chapter 14). However, the proportion of patients experiencing device-related procedures is much smaller than in the inpatient setting. When a procedure involves contact with the vascular system or with mucous membranes, it is reasonable to expect similar risk in ambulatory patients as in hospitalized patients. There may be differences, however, in the duration of exposure to the device (e.g., intravenous therapy, urinary catheterization) and conditions under which the device is inserted (e.g., starting intravenous therapy without adequate preparation of the insertion site).

Devices that are in contact with the vascular system should be sterile (e.g., instruments used to close lacerations, intravascular devices). Instruments that are in contact with mucous membranes should be sterile or receive high-level disinfection before use (e.g., vaginal specula, sigmoidoscopes, tonometers).

In general articles and instruments that touch intact skin should be as clean as articles that are readily available in commercial establishments such as restaurants. Proper cleaning includes removal of all soil and body substances and the use of disinfectant agents appropriate to the situation. The more distant and peripheral an article is to any patient, the less infection risk there is associated with it. For example, chairs in the waiting room, cabinets in examining rooms, and curtains present virtually no infection risk.

Because of the possibility of examining tables being soiled by patient secretions, excretions, or blood, there is a common practice in the ACS to provide some barrier between the patient and the table. This is often accomplished by rolls of paper sheets or by linen sheets that are changed between patients. Unless there is soilage of the table surface, disinfection between patients is not necessary. Examination tables, counter tops, floors, and other articles in the treatment areas should be cleaned on a regular schedule consistent with need in the facility.

Cleanliness of the physical facility, in general, is most easily accomplished when the number of examination rooms is sufficient and the flow of patients, personnel, and supplies can be accomplished easily.

### Ventilation Systems
Airborne transmission of potentially infectious agents via ventilation systems has been studied extensively, and data show that very few agents persist in the air for extended periods of time. The most common organism that persists in the air for extended periods is *Mycobacterium tuberculosis*. To transmit tuberculosis requires that the host be susceptible and in contact with a large enough dose of droplet nuclei for a sufficient time to become infected. Riley and colleagues [23] studied the infectiousness of a series of treated and untreated patients with tuberculosis by experiments in which air from rooms of tuberculosis patients was conducted to an exposurer chamber in which guinea pigs in cages were located. Of 61 untreated patients with drug-susceptible organisms, eight patients were responsible for all of the transmissions to

guinea pigs; a patient with tuberculous laryngitis was the most infectious. Riley and colleagues concluded that untreated patients were much more infectious than treated patients and that infectivity was also related to the number of air changes per hour in the room.

Although an ACS may provide the opportunity for the susceptible host to come in contact with a potentially infectious tuberculosis patient, the time interval of contact is usually insufficient to transmit the agent effectively. Whether or not an examining room in which multiple tuberculosis patients are seen in succession can sustain sufficient droplet nuclei to transmit tuberculosis depends on several factors: the number of infectious patients seen in a short time interval; aerosolization of droplet nuclei by the infectious patients (i.e., the efficiency of dissemination); number of air changes in the examining room per unit of time, whether or not the air is vented directly to the outside, whether filters or ultraviolet lights are in the ventilation system, and what type of filters they are; and finally, the presence of susceptible patients and/or personnel in the examination room during or after the same time interval. These factors tend to have an additive effect, and risk is increased accordingly; however, the actual risk is unknown (see Chapter 26).

Although diseases that are spread by droplet contact are seen in the ACS (e.g., varicella, rubella, and other childhood diseases), the droplets that are potentially infectious to the susceptible host do not remain suspended in the air for extended periods of time, as droplet nuclei do. Accordingly, it is probably not necessary to restrict subsequent use of an examining room after patients with these infections are seen. More important, when a patient presents to an ACS with a fever, skin rash, or other signs characteristic of infection that may be spread by droplet contact, expeditious placement in a treatment room alone will reduce the risk to susceptible persons of contact with droplets that may be sneezed or coughed into the patient's immediate environment. In addition, most of these viral agents are transmitted most effectively by direct contact, and hand-washing will best reduce the risk of transmission to others (see Chapter 35).

### Potentially Infectious Body Substances

Potentially infectious agents may be present in all body substances (e.g., blood, secretions, excretions), and all body substances should be handled as if they are infectious. The implementation of these practices, in reality, is often made difficult because personnel may believe that only patients with diagnosed communicable diseases present a risk of infection. Accordingly, they may not take precautions until a diagnosis is established. Table 21-1 presents general precautionary measures, described according to body substance, that are applicable to the ACS. Additional information about specific diseases may be found in Chapter 9.

## THE INFECTION CONTROL NURSE

### Hospital-Based Settings

Infection control nurses (ICNs) who work in hospitals usually have responsibility for infection control in the emergency department, admitting department, and ambulatory care clinics [6,20] (see Chapter 3). These responsibilities include education of personnel about measures that reduce infection risks associated with emergency care; cleaning, disinfection, and sterilization; isolation precautions; management of needlestick injuries and other exposures; and orientation for new personnel. The ICN may also act as a consultant for the development of policies and procedures. Policies and education programs should be specifically tailored for each department.

### Freestanding Settings

Most freestanding settings (e.g., surgicenters, emergicenters, physicians' offices) do not have a designated ICN. Consultation about infection control in these settings can frequently be obtained from the local health department and ICNs in hospitals in the community.

### Reportable Diseases

State and local health departments require that certain communicable (notifiable) diseases be reported to them. Designation of a person responsible for this task is essential in both the hospital-based and the freestanding ACS. In many hospitals, this is a responsibility of the ICN. In addition, local health departments may provide follow-up for contacts of patients with many infectious diseases (e.g., syphilis, gonorrhea, salmonellosis, viral hepatitis, meningococcal disease).

## PATIENT AND PERSONNEL RISKS FOR NOSOCOMIAL INFECTIONS

### Emergency Medical Services System

The risks to patients and personnel in the EMSS are increased by the urgency of the patient situation and the need for prompt and efficient patient manage-

TABLE 21-1. General precautionary measures for handling potentially infectious body substances

| Body substance | Examples of infectious agents | Precautions for personnel in direct contact with substance | Precautions for patients or personnel in same room |
|---|---|---|---|
| Blood (e.g., uncontrolled bleeding; lacerations, GI bleed) | Hepatitis B, NANB; acquired immunodeficiency syndrome (AIDS) | Gloves; cover gowns for large amounts | No direct contact, no risk |
| Saliva, sputum (e.g., purulent sputum, oral secretions) | Viral agents; mixed gram-positive and gram-negative bacteria | Gloves* | No direct contact, no risk* |
| Feces (e.g., diarrhea, fecal incontinence) | Enteric pathogens; viral agents; other gram-negative bacteria | Gloves; cover gowns for large amounts | No direct contact, no risk |
| Urine (e.g., incontinence) | Gram-negative bacteria | Gloves | No direct contact, no risk |
| Wound drainage (e.g., wound infections, abscesses, impetigo) | Gram-positive and gram-negative bacteria | Gloves; cover gowns for large amounts | No direct contact, no risk |

Note: Hand washing is usually sufficient to remove soil and potentially infectious agents from hands; however, regardless of diagnosis, when contact with these substances is anticipated, personnel should glove their hands to reduce the quantity of hand contamination and wash their hands after glove removal. Unless there is direct soilage of articles in the environment, there is no need to restrict the room or perform special cleaning procedures.

*For pediatric or other patients who may have a disease spread by droplet contact (e.g., chickenpox, measles, rubella, mumps), personnel with negative or unknown history of the disease or immunization should not examine the patient. Droplets generally travel a distance of about a meter from the patient and rapidly settle on a horizontal surface; accordingly, observers at a greater distance are not generally at risk.

ment. As the urgency for intervention increases (e.g., to provide an airway, control bleeding, stabilize a fracture, provide intravenous fluids), the situation becomes less easily controlled and adherence to aseptic practices by personnel generally decreases.

PREHOSPITAL CARE    Risks to patients in the prehospital care phase are generally related to aseptic practices. It is important to recognize that the need for careful aseptic practices must be balanced against the patient's need for prompt management. The duration of contact with the field situation is often brief; however, the devices inserted there and the procedures done to stabilize the patient carry with them certain infection risks.. Training programs for personnel working in these situations should include information about and practice in using aseptic practices. When the urgency of the field situation is such that aseptic practices may be difficult to employ, the decision to compromise them is made *for* the patient and should reflect his or her best interests rather than personnel convenience. When the patient is stabilized, devices inserted under less than optimal conditions should be replaced aseptically and in a timely

fashion. Communication among the field team, personnel in the emergency department, and ultimately, the health-care providers in the nursing unit where the patient is admitted, will help maintain this continuity of care.

Risks to personnel depend on contact with body substances (e.g., blood, feces, saliva) that may be contaminated with an infectious agent. Infection precautions may include the use of barrier techniques (e.g., gloves) to prevent substances from soiling personnel hands, clothing, and supplies. Personnel reduce the risk of transmitting infectious agents to patients or of acquiring infections themselves by using these barrier techniques along with hand-washing (or antiseptic foams when sinks are not available).

The risks to personnel are rarely known at the onset of a transport situation, and the patient's diagnosis may never be known to the transport personnel. Accordingly, the development of standard procedures including aseptic practices when possible is appropriate in any transport situation.

When communicable diseases are diagnosed, transport personnel should be included in any exposure workups and should receive prophylaxis when indicated. These personnel should follow the same immunization and tuberculin skin testing routines as hospital personnel (see Chapter 2).

The transport vehicle, whether an ambulance, van, or helicopter, should be cleaned on a regular schedule; articles soiled with body substances should be cleaned and disinfected before being used for another patient. Although the patient area of the transport vehicle is a small, closed space, ventilation is easily accomplished, and it is unnecessary to provide extended ventilation times or special decontamination procedures (e.g., fumigation) before the transport of another patient.

EMERGENCY DEPARTMENT OF A HOSPITAL Risks to patients who present to an emergency department of a hospital are related to the patient's underlying condition and the procedures performed for the patient in the emergency department. Few procedures are generally performed for patients in the nonurgent category, and they are at little risk for nosocomial infection; patients in the urgent category undergo more procedures and are at somewhat greater risk; patients in the emergent category may undergo numerous procedures and are at the greatest risk. Additionally, it is for these patients that asepsis is most often compromised.

A survey of patient visits to emergency departments has been reported by Moffet [16], who studied 1145 randomly selected visits to an urban hospital emergency department in 1977. Of these visits, 47 percent were for trauma and 28 percent for infections. The majority of the visits for infections were by patients under the age of 18 years; 70 percent of the infections were respiratory infections. Only 1.9 percent of the patients with infections were hospitalized.

Respiratory infections reflect seasonal and community incidence, and are usually viral. Risk to emergency-department personnel of exposure to many of these infections is probably similar to that in nonhospital settings in which numbers of people are together who may be in the prodromal or acute phase of a viral illness (e.g., schools, offices, stores); however, the concentration of such persons may be greater in an emergency department.

Emergency-department personnel are at greater risk for exposure to hepatitis B than are many other hospital workers due to their frequent exposure to blood. In a recent study, Dienstag and Ryan [7] surveyed 624 health workers in an urban hospital in Boston. These personnel represented a spectrum of exposure to blood and to patients. Of the 30 emergency-department nurses studied, 30 percent were positive for one or more serologic markers for hepatitis B. Among

the groups surveyed, this was the group with the highest prevalence for hepatitis B seropositivity. Dienstag and Ryan conclude that emergency-department personnel are exposed to the most severely ill patients (including those with uncontrolled bleeding), that emergency department *nurses* are often the first personnel to encounter such patients, and that these nurses generally do not wear gloves or protective gowns when providing such care (see Chapter 35).

### Emergicenters

Seriously injured and ill patients are not generally seen in emergicenters; most of the visits are by patients with nonurgent problems. Procedures performed in these facilities are similar to those performed in hospital emergency departments (e.g., laceration repairs, incision and drainage of abscesses, and other minor surgical procedures). The same principles of asepsis apply in this setting as in the hospital emergency department.

### Surgicenters

The care of instruments and the quality of aseptic practices should be the same in surgicenters as it is in hospital operating rooms. Written policies and procedures for care of instruments, cleaning of operating rooms, and personnel health practices should be developed following guidelines for hospital operating rooms (see Chapters 2 and 20).

Preoperative assessment of the patient should include screening for infection and for presence of communicable disease. Preparation and aftercare management of patients should emphasize prevention of nosocomial infection (e.g., wound care, pre- and postoperative pulmonary management). Patients should be instructed regarding signs of infection (e.g., fever, redness, pain, swelling, drainage) and whom to contact if questions arise.

It is generally accepted that cleaning after all cases should remove all soil and body substances, and that special cleaning after "dirty cases" is not necessary. Cleaning routines and preparation for subsequent cases should follow the same guidelines that are used for hospital operating rooms (see Chapter 20).

### Outpatient Diagnostic and Treatment Facilities

Risk for nosocomial infection in these settings is generally quite low. In some special situations such as oncology or pediatric clinics or physician's offices, it may be important to identify patients whose compromised immune status may place them at increased risk of infection, especially to the droplet-spread viral respiratory infections. These patients may benefit from reduced contact with other patients in the waiting room. Some pediatric clinics or physicians' offices also have separate waiting rooms for children seeking well care and for those who are ill. Some treatment rooms also have doors that open directly to the outside, permitting selected patients to bypass the office waiting room entirely.

### Hospital Admitting Department

Generally infection risk in the admitting department is quite low. Inadvertent exposures to communicable diseases may occur there because persons with unknown exposure or disease status may be together in the same waiting area for varying lengths of time. This is particularly true in pediatric facilities or hospitals with large pediatric units.

The admitting department can serve a useful purpose in reducing the risk of transmission of infectious agents between hospitalized patients by being attentive to the room and bed assignments for newly admitted patients and for patients who develop infections while in the hospital. In many hospitals the ICN conveys information about potentially infectious patients (i.e., patients requiring isolation precautions) to the admitting department and serves as a consultant for patient placement.

## REFERENCES

1. Antoniskis, A., Anderson, B. C., Van Volkinburg, E. J., Jackson, J. M., and Gilbert, D. N. Feasibility of outpatient self-administration of parenteral antibiotics. *West. J. Med.* 128:203, 1978.
2. Bennett, J. V. Human infections: Economic implications and prevention. *Ann. Intern. Med.* 89(Part 2):761, 1978.
3. Centers for Disease Control. Amebiasis associated with colonic irrigation: Colorado. *Morbid. Mortal. Weekly Rep.* 30:101, 1981.
4. Chan, M. K., Chuau, P., Raftery, M. J., Baillod, R. A., Sweny, P., Varghese, Z., and Moorhead, J. F. Three years' experience of continuous ambulatory peritoneal dialysis. *Lancet* 1:1409, 1981.
5. Craig, C. P. Infection surveillance for ambulatory surgery patients: An overview. *Qual. Rev. Bull.* (QRB) 9:107, 1983.
6. Crow, S. Infection control in the emergency room. *Nurs. Clin. North Am.* 15:869, 1980.
7. Dienstag, J. L., and Ryan, D. M. Occupational exposure to hepatitis B virus in hospital personnel: Infection or immunization? *Am. J. Epidemiol.* 115:26, 1982.
8. Frame, P. T. Outpatient intravenous antibiotic therapy (letter). *J.A.M.A.* 248:356, 1982.
9. Gaffron, R. E., Fleming, C. R., Berkner, S., McCallum, D., Schwartau, N., and McGill, D. B. Organization and operation of a home parenteral nutrition program with emphasis on the pharmacist's role. *Mayo Clin. Proc.* 55:94, 1980.
10. Harrison, J. T. Chronic ambulatory peritoneal dialysis (letter). *N. Engl. J. Med.* 306:670, 1982.
11. Jacoby, L. E., and Jones, L. S. Factors associated with ED use by "repeater" and "nonrepeater" patients. *J. Emerg. Nurs.* 8:243, 1982.
12. Jeejeebhoy, K. N., Langer, B., Tsallas, G., Chu, R. C., Kuksis, A., and Anderson, G. H. Total parenteral nutrition at home: Studies in patients surviving 4 months to 5 years. *Gastroenterology* 71:943, 1976.
13. Jonas, S., Flesh, R., Brook, R., and Wassertheil-Smoller, S. Monitoring utilization of a municipal hospital emergency department. *Hosp. Top.* 54(1):43, 1976.
14. Jonas, S., and Greifinger, R. Ambulatory Care. In Jonas, S. (Ed.), *Health Care Delivery in the United States* (2d ed.). New York: Springer, 1981.
15. Kind, A. C., Williams, D. N., Persons, G., and Gibson, J. A. Intravenous antibiotic therapy at home. *Arch. Intern. Med.* 139:413, 1979.
16. Moffet, H. L. Common infections in ambulatory patients. *Ann. Intern. Med.* 89(Part 2):743, 1978.
17. National Academy of Sciences, National Research Council. *Accidental Death and Disability: The Neglected Disease of Modern Society.* Washington, D. C.: National Academy of Sciences, 1966.
18. Natof, H. E. Complications associated with ambulatory surgery. *J.A.M.A.* 244:1116, 1980.
19. Nolph, K. D., Sorkin, M., Rubin, J., Arfania, D., Prowant, B., Fruto, L., and Kennedy, D. Continuous ambulatory peritoneal dialysis: Three-year experience at one center. *Ann. Intern. Med.* 92:609, 1980.
20. Owens, K. S. W. Section I: The Admitting and Outpatient Departments. In Bennett, J. V., and Brachman, P. H. (Eds.), *Hospital Infections* (1st ed.). Boston: Little, Brown, 1979.
21. Pisarcik, G. Why patients use the emergency department. *J. Emerg. Nurs.* 6(2):16, 1980.
22. Poretz, D. M., Eron, L. J., Goldenberg, R. I., Gilbert, A. F., Rising, J., Sparks, S., and Horn, C. E. Intravenous antibiotic therapy in an outpatient setting. *J.A.M.A.* 248:336, 1982.
23. Riley, R. L., Mills, C. C., O'Grady, F., Sultan, L. V., Wittstad, F., and Shivpuri, D. N. Infectiousness of air from a tuberculosis ward. Ul-

traviolet irradiation of infected air: Comparative infectiousness of different patients. *Am. Rev. Respir. Dis.* 85:511, 1962.

24. Secord-Pletz, B. Prehospital Emergency Care and Transportation. In Kravis, T. C., and Warner, C. G. *Emergency Medicine: A Comprehensive Review.* Rockville, MD: Aspen Systems Corp., 1983.

25. Sewell, C. M., Clarridge, J., Lacke, C., Weinman, E. J., and Young, E. J. Staphylococcal nasal carriage and subsequent infection in peritoneal dialysis patients. *J.A.M.A.* 248:1493, 1982.

26. Stiver, H. G., Telford, G. O., Mossey, J. M., Cote, D. D., Van Middlesworth, E. J., Trosky, S. K., McKay, N. L., and Mossey, W. L. Intravenous antibiotic therapy at home. *Ann. Intern. Med.* 89(Part 1):690, 1978.

27. Swenson, J. P. Training patients to administer intravenous antibiotics at home. *Am. J. Hosp. Pharm.* 38:1480, 1981.

28. Swenson, J. P. Outpatient intravenous antibiotic therapy (letter). *J.A.M.A.* 249:592, 1983.

29. Weinerman, E. R., Ratner, R. S., Robbins, A., et al. Yale studies in ambulatory medical care. V. Determinants of use of hospital emergency services. *Am. J. Public Health* 56:1037, 1966.

# 22 THE CLINICAL LABORATORY

Marie B. Coyle
Fritz D. Schoenknecht

The clinical laboratory is an area of special concern for nosocomial infection, both because it is a focus for the handling and processing of potentially hazardous materials from infectious patients and because it generates a considerable volume of pathogenic organisms in its microbiologic work. The risks are greatest for the laboratory personnel, but visitors and messengers carrying specimens to the laboratory area may also be exposed to infectious organisms. Poor design and operation can allow accidentally generated aerosols to extend beyond the confines of the laboratory and, at least potentially, present a hazard to other areas of the institution.

This chapter considers the nature and extent of these problems and practical means of controlling them. In particular, we discuss infection control in the clinical microbiology laboratory and the more general problem of the control of hepatitis B infections in all areas of clinical laboratory work. We do not deal with the special problems associated with diagnostic virology laboratories or the large-scale handling of pathogenic microorganisms in research or manufacturing facilities. The role of the clinical laboratory in surveillance, investigation, and control of nosocomial infections is described in Chapters 4 and 5.

## EXTENT OF THE PROBLEM

The incidence of clinical laboratory–acquired infections is unknown, because many are unrecognized and most are probably never recorded. The literature contains numerous reports of individual infections and occasionally small outbreaks of infections, and certain organisms are recognized as especially likely to produce severe or fatal disease in laboratory workers or as having unusual infectivity. Valuable information on laboratory–acquired infections has been tabulated by Pike [26] and Sulkin [32] from questionnaires, reports in the literature, and personal communications. They have compiled data from over 4000 cases of laboratory-associated infections, with an overall case fatality rate of 4.3 percent [27]. Many of these infections, however, occurred in research departments rather than clinical laboratories.

The overall pattern that emerges from these reports and other published literature is that infections sufficiently severe to be recognized or reported usually involve a small group of infectious organisms. These include *Mycobacterium tuberculosis*, *Brucella* species, *Francisella tularensis*, *Coxiella burnetii*, various other

335

*Rickettsia, Coccidioides immitis, Salmonella typhi, Shigella,* and hepatitis B virus. These have the common characteristic of being able to initiate infections in the susceptible subject with a relatively small challenge dose. The potential for infection exists with all pathogenic species, however, and it may be realized following a laboratory accident involving the introduction of an unusually large number of organisms.

## SOURCES AND ROUTES OF SPREAD

Pike's review [26] showed that only about 20 percent of laboratory–acquired infections were preceded by a known accident (Table 22-1). Self-inoculation with a needle and syringe and aspiration while pipetting by mouth accounted for over one-third of the known accidents but only about 9 percent of all laboratory-associated infections.

The identities of the agents most commonly involved in these laboratory infections suggest that the inhalation of aerosols produced during routine laboratory manipulations and the ingestion of pathogenic microorganisms were the most common means by which they were acquired. Only 17 percent of all the respondents, however, associated their infections with a specific aerosol-generating procedure (see Table 22-1). The manipulation of liquids always results in some aerosol production, but the amount is highly dependent on the particular procedure used as well as on the adequacy of the technique of the individual worker. Table 22-2 contains some data of Reitman and Wedum [28, 34] comparing aerosol production during some commonly used bacteriologic procedures. Considerable dissemination may occur and most of the droplets produced are between 2 and 5 $\mu$ in diameter [22]. Particles of this size are capable of bypassing the defenses of the upper respiratory tract, and they can be drawn into the alveoli [6] where fewer organisms may be required to establish an infection [16].

These data emphasize the need for special safety procedures when dealing with agents known to be highly infective. Whenever it becomes apparent from a suspected clinical diagnosis or from the laboratory workup of a specimen that such an agent may be present, additional safety precautions appropriate for the suspected agent should be employed.

Recommended "biosafety levels" for specific microbiologic agents, depending on the aerosol potential of the procedure, have been prepared by a panel of eminent microbiologists and published as an excellent monograph entitled *Biosafety in Microbiological and Biomedical Laboratories* [29]. This document recommends that clinical laboratories dealing with moderate-risk agents use biosafety level 2, which corresponds to a conventional laboratory that conducts routine work on an open bench top but uses a biologic safety cabinet for procedures with high aerosol potential. Greater containment, biosafety level 3, is

TABLE 22-1. Sources of laboratory infections

| Known accident | Number of infections | Percentage of total* |
|---|---|---|
| Cut, bite, or scratch | 207 | 6.6 |
| Spill or spatter | 188 | 6.0 |
| Syringe and needle | 177 | 5.6 |
| Pipetting | 92 | 2.9 |
| All other | 39 | 1.2 |
| Subtotal | 703 | 22.3 |
| No known accident, most likely source | | |
| Working with agent | 827 | 26.2 |
| Animal, egg, or arthropod | 659 | 20.9 |
| Aerosol | 522 | 16.6 |
| Clinical specimen | 287 | 9.1 |
| Human autopsy | 75 | 2.4 |
| Discarded glassware | 46 | 1.5 |
| Other | 35 | 1.1 |
| Subtotal | 2451 | 77.8 |
| Total* | 3154 | 100.1 |

*Excluding infections with unknown accident status and source.
Source: Modified from Pike, R. M. *Health Lab. Sci.* 13:105, 1976.

TABLE 22-2. Bacteria recovered by air-sampling within two feet of the site of common bacteriologic procedures

| Procedure | Colonies obtained per operation |
|---|---|
| Removing tight cover of standard blender immediately after mixing cultures | Too numerous to count |
| Opening lyophilized culture tube | 86 |
| Decanting centrifuged fluid into flask | 17 |
| Inserting hot loop in culture flask | 9 |
| Removing dry cotton plug from shaken culture flask | 5 |
| Pipetting 1 ml of inoculum to poured agar in Petri plate | 3 |
| Pipetting 1 ml of culture into 50 ml of broth | 1 |

Source: Adapted from Wedum, A. G. *Public Health Rep.* 76:619, 1964, and Reitman, M., and Wedum, A. G. *Public Health Rep.* 71:659, 1956.

recommended for any manipulation of cultures of such high-risk organisms as *C. immitis, M. tuberculosis, M. bovis, F. tularensis,* and *Brucella* species. With the exception of liquefaction and concentration of sputa and other specimens for *M. tuberculosis,* however, the new biosafety monograph would permit the initial processing and inoculation of specimens containing this group of organisms to be conducted in a biosafety level 2 facility without the protection of a biologic safety cabinet. In general, our recommendations are more stringent than those proposed in this valuable resource.

## GENERAL CONTROL MEASURES

### Education and Training
There is little doubt that the most important factors in preventing laboratory–acquired infections are the knowledge, training, and techniques of the individual laboratory worker. The other methods and procedures discussed in this section are adjunctive and may be rendered ineffective by carelessness and lack of understanding of the hazards and routes of infection.

It is critical, as in hospital infection control generally, that examples of good technique and safe practices be provided by those in supervisory positions and that the operating regulations be rigidly enforced. A laboratory director who smokes, eats, or drinks in the laboratory or who fails to wash his or her hands and change coats before leaving the laboratory area encourages an environment in which accidents are more likely to occur. Training must be supplemented with a written manual that details the routine and emergency procedures to be employed as well as with continuing programs of safety education and monitoring of the effectiveness of equipment designed to contain infection. Excellent training materials are available from the Centers for Disease Control [5, 11].

### Laboratory Design
From the point of view of microbiologic safety, the microbiology laboratory ideally would be a self-contained unit isolated from the rest of the hospital environment. This is impractical if important consultative interactions between the laboratory and clinical staffs are to be maintained. Within the laboratory, however, work areas can be set up to minimize the risk of spread of infectious particles. Some form of partitioning of such work spaces has two advantages: it prevents traffic patterns passing behind the technologist and creating unnecessary air currents, and it

helps to contain any aerosols that may be produced by accidents. Certain spaces should be set aside for particularly hazardous operations, such as handling *M. tuberculosis* and *C. immitis.* These should be self-contained, provided with sterilizing equipment and hand-washing facilities, and equipped with the appropriate safety hood to prevent dispersion of organisms into the general laboratory environment.

The general plan for the laboratory should include provisions for an adequate number and placement of autoclaves, adequate disposal containers, and an adequate number and placement of sinks. Surfaces should be nonporous, without cracks, and easy to clean.

The overall ventilation system of the laboratory should be capable of diluting aerosols and ensuring a flow of air from "clean" to "dirty" zones. Ideally, the ventilation system for laboratories should be completely separate from that of the rest of the hospital, and air should be vented at least 25 feet from any windows, doors, or air intakes.

Laboratories should be designed to prevent overcrowding and avoid needless personnel movement, which may in itself contribute to accidents.

Specific regulations and recommendations governing procedures for particular classes of pathogenic agents [8, 29] have been and are being developed at both national and state levels. It is essential that laboratory directors become acquainted through their state health departments with the current requirements.

## SPECIALIZED EQUIPMENT

For reasons presented later in this chapter, biologic safety cabinets (BSC) should be available for the initial processing and inoculation of routine specimens as well as for handling especially hazardous cultures such as those involved in the diagnosis of tuberculosis or containing conidia of the systemic fungi. The best safety cabinets for clinical laboratories are class II cabinets that depend on high-efficiency particulate air (HEPA) filters. The entrances for hands into the working space should be kept at a minimum and yet be sufficiently large to permit easy manipulation, and there should be an air flow rate of 50 to 75 linear feet per minute through this area [7]. Ideally the exhaust from the hood should be vented through the HEPA filter to the outside.

The efficacy of safety cabinets depends on proper construction to eliminate all leakage around seams, gaskets, fans, filters, and other component parts. Cabinets and HEPA filters must be tested for leakage and certified annually as well as immediately after they have been moved to ensure that they are operating effectively and that there is no discharge of potentially contaminated material into the laboratory environment. Only persons with formal training in BSC certification procedures should attempt this hazardous, highly technical task that requires expensive, specialized equipment. Routine quality-control procedures are also needed for ultraviolet lamps in safety cabinets. These cannot be considered germicidal just because they are emitting blue light; they must be routinely cleansed to avoid any dirt or grease that may be deposited and checked for germicidal efficiency. The CDC has published a brochure on maintaining both biologic safety cabinets and ultraviolet lamps [7].

Other laboratory equipment also needs regular inspection and monitoring to avoid accidents. Autoclave temperatures, pressures, and times of sterilization should be routinely recorded. They may be tested on a weekly basis for the capacity to kill spores during a routine cycle by using commercially available products (see Chapter 7). Autoclave tape serves to ensure that items have gone through an autoclave cycle, but it is not designed to indicate sterility (see Chapter 7). Deep freezes should be organized into well-labeled compartments that permit easy identification of the vials of infected materials or cultures sought. This permits shorter search periods and less chance of breakage. Gloves and a surgical mask should be worn while cleaning freezers that may contain vials of infectious material.

An effective way to detect aerosols produced during centrifugation is to process a methylene blue solution as if it were a specimen, including decanting and recentrifuging. A strip of white paper taped to the inner surface of the centrifuge wall serves as a sensitive detector of aerosol production. Centrifuges used to process hazardous specimens or cultures should have safety cups that can be transferred to a biologic safety cabinet before the covers are opened. Centrifuging within a safety cabinet will not prevent dissemination of high-velocity aerosols unless the manufacturer specifically designed the cabinet to accommodate a centrifuge.

### Routine Prophylaxis

Specific immunization of laboratory personnel will reduce the risk of infection with some of the pathogenic organisms that may be encountered (see Chapter 2). Personnel working in clinical microbiology laboratories should have up-to-date tetanus and diphtheria immunizations. The current recommendation of the Immunization Practices Advisory Committee is for a Td booster every 10 years [12]. Laboratory

workers should also be immunized for any other infectious disease for which adult immunization in the community is recommended. Laboratory personnel who are processing blood or blood products should be immunized with the hepatitis B virus (HBV) vaccine [13]. All persons who handle specimens that may contain *M. tuberculosis* should receive a skin test with purified protein derivative (PPD) of tuberculin, to be repeated annually if their initial test is negative. If a skin test is positive, a yearly chest roentgenogram is recommended. If reactivity is primarily to PPD-S, skin test converters should be medically evaluated for currently recommended prophylaxis (see Chapter 26).

Immunization against typhoid fever should be required if the disease is endemic in the area. The frequency of laboratory-associated infections due to proficiency testing with *S. typhi* in this country suggests that many technologists do not give sufficient attention to the simple laboratory techniques that minimize risk of contracting this infection [1, 2].

## SPECIFIC TECHNICAL ROUTINES

### Biologic Safety Cabinet for
### Inoculating Routine Specimens

The major hazards from infectious aerosols in a clinical microbiology laboratory usually occur during the initial specimen processing that may include homogenizing, decanting, pipetting, and transferring with a needle and syringe. With good technique, routine inoculation on the open bench top should generate insignificant amounts of aerosol. Personnel who do this processing, however, particularly part-time employees on evening and weekend shifts, are the least likely to have the scientific background or training that would enable them to develop the best techniques. In addition many laboratories have students and residents working in the setup area as part of their laboratory training. A biologic safety cabinet for routine inoculation of all specimens provides protection for all these persons and eliminates the need for numerous decisions regarding the relative hazard of unusual specimens submitted to the laboratory.

Additional reasons in support of having a biologic safety cabinet available for routine setup procedures are as follows:

1. Newer products for blood cultures increase the probability of aerosols since needles and syringes are used with vials or tubes that may contain vacuums.

2. The transmissible stage of many diseases (including AIDS) may precede the symptomatic stage by an unknown time period (see Chapter 35).

3. Since the diagnosis of tuberculosis may not be suspected or simply not indicated on the request slip, it is possible for routine sputa, CSF, urine, and tissues to contain large numbers of acid-fast bacilli, particularly in a laboratory that receives a number of smear-positive specimens each month.

*Standard Precautions*

Certain routines and procedures are mandatory to reduce the risk of laboratory–acquired infections. These are stated below as specific guidelines. Other lists have been prepared by other authors [14,16,17,32]. Laboratories engaged in mycobacteriology should follow the guidelines specified by the CDC [33].

1. Personnel hygiene in the laboratory
   a. No eating, drinking, or smoking should be allowed.
   b. Personnel should wash hands before leaving the laboratory.
   c. Personnel should remove laboratory coats before leaving the laboratory area.
   d. No food should be stored in refrigerators that contain specimens or serum products.
2. Routine culture procedures
   a. Pipetting by mouth—including *all* solutions—should be prohibited.
   b. While pipetting, bubble production should be avoided.
   c. A cool inoculating loop should be used.
   d. Cylindric electric burners should be used when culturing tuberculosis specimens.
   e. Petri dishes should be inoculated without striking their walls.
   f. Before flaming loops with excess material, they should be precleaned in a container of alcohol and sand.
   g. When removing rubber stoppers from Vacutainers, the tops should be covered with an alcohol pad.
   h. Stool isolates should be suspended in a saline solution containing mercuric iodide for agglutination tests with *Salmonella* or *Shigella* antisera [25].
3. Hazardous procedures that should be carried out in biologic safety cabinet
   a. Opening lyophilized cultures (a safe and simple procedure has been reported that greatly reduces the risk of dispersal [20]).
   b. Decanting supernatants.
   c. Homogenizing with a mortar and pestle or high-speed blender. Wait at least five minutes after the blender has come to a complete stop before opening the cover. If blender is opened too soon, aerosols of high velocity can penetrate the cabinet air barrier and contaminate the laboratory. The Stomacher method is a safe alternative for homogenizing specimens [15].
4. Centrifugation
   a. Centrifuge should be operated in a well-ventilated room that can be closed off in case of accident (see Major Spills Outside a Biological Safety Cabinet).
   b. Careful balancing is critical.
   c. Sturdy plastic screw-top tubes are recommended.
5. Syringes and needles
   a. Only needle-locking syringes may be used.
   b. An alcohol pad should be placed around the stopper and needle when withdrawing the needle from a rubber-stoppered vial.
   c. Excess air and bubbles should be expelled into an alcohol pad.
   d. Animals should be swabbed with antiseptic both before and after inoculation.
   e. Used needles should not be cut or resheathed before placing them in a narrow-mouthed puncture-proof container for disposal.
6. Discarding contaminated materials
   a. All contaminated materials should be autoclaved.
   b. All contaminated slides and pipettes should be placed in a jar of disinfectant until they are autoclaved.
   c. Open metal containers should be used for disinfectants and autoclaving; plastic prevents effective heat transfer [30].
   d. All specimens—including urine and those for immunoserologic study—should be autoclaved before they are discarded.
   e. Heat-resistant plastic bags prevent autoclave steam from penetrating. Double bagging, overfilling, or complete closure prevents sterilization of materials in the bag [18,30].
   f. Autoclaving should be done for at least 30 minutes. Each laboratory should do periodic sterility tests on their autoclaved waste to ensure sterilization [30].
   g. Stools should be collected in a separate, lined container and incinerated.
7. Shipping specimens to reference laboratories. Postal regulations described by Richardson and Barkley should be observed [29].

## AIDS Precautions

Transmission of the HTLV-III virus which is etiologically associated with acquired immunodeficiency syndrome (AIDS) appears to have a pattern similar to that of hepatitis B; therefore, the precautions presented in the following section for hepatitis B should be used in clinical laboratories processing specimens from known or suspected AIDS patients (see Chapter 35). It is assumed that recommendations listed previously in the section Specific Technical Routines will also be followed. Precautions for persons performing laboratory tests on clinical specimens from known or suspected AIDS patients have been published by the CDC [9]. The specific recommendations that go beyond the routine procedures employed by most clinical microbiology laboratories include (1) gloves for processing the specimens and (2) using a biologic safety cabinet and other primary containment devices such as centrifuge safety cups for procedures that have a high potential for creating aerosols or infectious droplets. These include centrifuging, blending, sonicating, vigorous mixing, and harvesting infected tissues from animals or embryonated eggs. For reasons already presented in this chapter, we recommend that the initial processing of specimens from all patients be done in a biologic safety cabinet and that additional workup of specimens and cultures from AIDS patients that involves decanting, transferring with needle and syringe, or pipetting also be performed in a safety cabinet.

## Hepatitis B Precautions

Hepatitis has long been recognized as a special hazard for laboratory workers, particularly those working with blood or serum samples (see Chapters 2 and 35). Thus the risk has been greatest for those working in hematology, biochemistry, and serology laboratories. Several episodes of hepatitis B infection involving a number of laboratory workers have been recorded. One outbreak in a university hospital involved 74 cases of viral hepatitis, including one fatality, within a four-year period [35]. Almost half the cases were associated with the clinical laboratories, but no cases occurred among laboratory personnel who did not routinely handle blood specimens.

Hepatitis B virus (HBV) can be acquired by the alimentary or conjunctival route as well as by the respiratory route and transdermal inoculation through cuts and needle punctures. The infectivity of specimens can be very high. There should be special identification and flagging of all blood and urine samples from patients with hepatitis, patients known to be hepatitis B antigen-positive, and patients from high-risk groups such as drug addicts, recipients of multiple transfusions, and renal transplant patients. Over 50 percent of blood-specimen containers from patients who are positive for hepatitis B surface antigen (HBsAg) can be contaminated on their outer surface [23]. Specimens from such patients should be double-bagged on collection and handled with special care within the laboratory. The risk, however, is not restricted to these specimens, because any serum sample may be infective and pose a hazard. Thus laboratory personnel should not develop a false sense of security in handling unflagged specimens. Some measures that may reduce the risk of infection are listed below:

1. Laboratory workers who have frequent contact with blood or serum should receive three doses of hepatitis B virus vaccine [13] (see Chapter 2).
2. Personnel working with blood or serum should wear specially colored gowns that may not be worn outside the laboratory area.
3. The contamination of hands with blood should be avoided, as should all mouth pipetting. Rubber gloves should be worn when specimens of known hazard are being processed or when contamination is unavoidable.
4. Gloves should be removed or dipped in disinfectant before touching telephones, pens, and other items that may be handled by others.
5. Rubber stoppers should be covered with alcohol-soaked pads and removed by gentle twisting to avoid aerosol production.
6. All sera should be transferred by bulb suctioning. Aerosols can be reduced by avoiding bubbles and not forcing the last drop from the pipette.
7. All spills should be cleaned up immediately with a 1% solution of hypochlorite (1:5 solution of Clorox). A recent study that assayed for viable hepatitis viruses rather than the surface antigen found that *10-minute exposures* to 70% isopropyl alcohol or a commercial iodophor preparation also inactivates the HBV [4].
8. All discarded blood samples, clots, and sera and the glassware or other equipment used in processing should be autoclaved. Disposable glass or plastic pipettes and tubes should be used whenever possible. These may be incinerated rather than autoclaved if preferred.
9. Stringent regulations should be enforced to ensure that hands are washed and outer protective clothing such as gowns and coats changed before workers leave the laboratory area. Eating, drinking, or smoking in the laboratory should be totally prohibited.
10. Accident documentation
    a. An employee who sustains any cut or needle-

puncture wound or who swallows any blood or blood product should report it to the supervisor immediately.

b. A baseline blood sample for hepatitis B antigen testing should be drawn.

c. Information should be sought concerning the person from whom the blood products were obtained.

d. Postexposure prophylaxis for an individual sustaining an accidental needle-stick, ocular, or mucosal exposure to blood known to contain HBsAg is dependent on previous HBV vaccine history. If not previously vaccinated, the individual should receive hepatitis B immune globulin (HBIG) and be vaccinated. If the person has been previously vaccinated and demonstrates an adequate anti-HBs titer, neither HBIG nor additional doses of vaccine are necessary; if anti-HBs is low or absent, HBIG is recommended as is one booster dose of vaccine. If the previous vaccine series was incomplete, the series should be completed and, if anti-HBs is low or absent, one dose of HBIG should be given [10].

## PROCEDURES FOR SPILLS AND ACCIDENTS

### Minor Spills
Spills involving small volumes of moderate-risk agents are regular occurrences in many overcrowded clinical laboratories. A wash bottle of disinfectant should be kept at hand to carry out decontamination of such spills. Phenolics are most useful in clinical laboratories that do not culture for viruses, while hypochlorites are recommended when contamination by viruses is expected. Some references on disinfectants are listed [3,21,31].

### Major Spills Outside a Biologic Safety Cabinet
Any spill or accident involving *M. tuberculosis, C. immitis, F. tularensis,* or *Brucella* species should be considered a major hazard. Accidents with cultures of moderate-risk agents that have the potential for generating large quantities of aerosol, such as breakage in a centrifuge, should also be handled with precautions designed to minimize inhalation of airborne infectious agents—the following recommendations were adapted with minor modifications [19,24]:

1. Hold your breath, leave the room immediately, and close the door.
2. Warn others not to enter the contaminated area.

3. Remove contaminated garments and place them in a container for autoclaving; thoroughly wash hands and face.
4. Wait at least 30 minutes to allow reduction of aerosols created by the spill.
5. Prepare in advance a "spill kit" containing leakproof autoclavable containers, forceps, paper towels, sponges, disinfectant, long-sleeved gowns, industrial safety masks, rubber gloves, and plastic shoe covers.
6. Before reentering the room, don the protective clothing stored in the "spill kit" as described in item 5.
7. Use disinfectants that are two to three times more concentrated than those routinely employed in the laboratory, because the volume of the spill may reduce their concentration.
8. Pour the disinfectant around the spill and allow it to flow into the spill. Paper towels soaked with disinfectant may be used to cover the area. To minimize aerosolization, avoid pouring disinfectant directly on the spill.
9. Allow 20 minutes contact time.
10. Use paper towels to wipe up disinfectant and spill, working toward the center of the spill. Discard towels into an autoclavable container as they are used.
11. Using an autoclavable dust pan and squeegee, transfer broken glass and other debris to an autoclave pan.
12. Wipe the outside of the discard container, especially the bottom, with disinfectant.
13. Place protective clothing, dust pan, and squeegee in container and autoclave them.

### Major Spills in a Biologic Safety Cabinet
If a spill is confined to the interior of the cabinet it should not be hazardous; however, the following disinfection procedures should be initiated at once while the cabinet continues to operate to prevent escape of contaminants:

1. Wear gloves and gown for the cleanup.
2. Spray or wipe walls, work surfaces, and equipment with a disinfectant. A disinfectant containing a detergent offers an advantage since extraneous organic substances interfere with the activity of some compounds.
3. Use sufficient disinfectant to flood the top work surface tray and, if a class II cabinet, the drain pans and catch basins below the surface. Allow to stand 15 minutes.
4. See your biologic safety cabinet manual for procedure to disinfect drain pans and catch basins.

5. It should not be necessary to disinfect the filters, blowers, and air ducts of a cabinet that is certified for nonleakage. Only a specially trained person should attempt this procedure.

6. Autoclave disinfectant, gloves, towels, and sponges before discarding.

*Accident and Illness Reporting*
Medical records of infectious diseases, including hepatitis, should be maintained for all personnel. It is a wise precaution to file a sample of serum from each laboratory worker annually. In the event of subsequent illness, a rising titer may be rapidly detected, which will facilitate diagnosis and recognition of the source of the infection.

It is the responsibility of the hospital to provide sufficient funds and appoint competent supervisory staff to ensure the safe operation of clinical microbiology laboratories. Laboratory supervisors should maintain a high index of suspicion of possible job-related infections when employees become ill and, when indicated, ensure that appropriate steps are taken to evaluate this possibility. Infections that are job-related should not result in financial penalty to the employee.

There should be a policy of reporting all accidents to the employee health clinic regardless of how minor they might seem to be (see Chapter 2). This is beneficial because (1) it permits appropriate prophylaxis, (2) a review of reports can lead to the recognition of special hazards and the introduction of safer techniques and equipment, and (3) reports provide the data for an accurate assessment of the hazards of various pathogens and attack rates.

## CONCLUSIONS

Laboratory infections pose a particular risk to the staff of the clinical microbiology laboratories and to those handling discarded materials, whereas hepatitis B antigen poses a serious hazard to all laboratories handling blood specimens. The frequency of laboratory infections in clinical laboratories is unknown, and prospective studies to compare sickness rates with matched groups in less potentially hazardous occupations would be desirable.

Good training, ongoing educational programs, and scrupulous technique are the main factors protecting against laboratory infection. Special attention to laboratory design can reduce the risk, as can the use of adequate safety cabinets. Routine immunization and tuberculin testing is mandatory, and health and accident records must be maintained. Significant ac-cidental exposure to pathogens should be considered a medical emergency and a basis for consideration of prophylactic chemotherapy or immunotherapy.

Stringent procedures, infrequently used until this time, are needed in biochemistry and hematology laboratories to lessen the risk of hepatitis B infections, which have increased substantially with the increase in immunosuppressive therapy and drug abuse.

## REFERENCES

1. Blaser, M. J., Hickman, F. W., Farmer, J. J., III, Brenner, D. J., Balows, A., and Feldman, R. A. *Salmonella typhi*: The laboratory as a reservoir of infection. *J. Infect. Dis.* 142:934, 1980.

2. Blaser, M. J., and Lofgren, J. P. Fatal salmonellosis originating in a clinical microbiology laboratory. *J. Clin. Microbiol.* 13:855, 1981.

3. Block, S. S. *Disinfection, Sterilization, and Preservation* (3d ed.). Philadelphia: Lea & Febiger, 1983.

4. Bond, W. W., Favero, M. S., Petersen, N. J., and Ebert, J. W. Inactivation of hepatitis B virus by intermediate- to high-level disinfectant chemicals. *J. Clin. Microbiol.* 18:535, 1983.

5. Brooks, P. *Guide to Educational Resources for Laboratorians*. U.S. Department of Health and Human Services, Centers for Disease Control Laboratory Improvement Program Office, Atlanta, GA 30333, 1981.

6. Brown, J. H., Cook, K. M., Ney, F. G., and Hatch, T. Influence of particle size upon retention of particulate matter in the human lung. *Am. J. Public Health* 40:450, 1950.

7. Center for Disease Control. *Biological Safety Cabinet*. Atlanta, GA 30333, 1971.

8. Center for Disease Control, Office of Biosafety. *Classification of Etiologic Agents on the Basis of Hazard* (4th ed.). U.S. Dept. of Health, Education and Welfare, Public Health Service, Atlanta, GA 30333, 1974.

9. Centers for Disease Control. Acquired immune deficiency syndrome (AIDS): Precautions for clinical and laboratory staff. *Morbid. Mortal. Weekly Rep.* 31:577, 1982.

10. Centers for Disease Control. *Hepatitis Surveillance Report, No. 49*. January, 1985, p. 2.

11. Centers for Disease Control. *Laboratory Training and Consultation Division Training Aids*. U.S. Department of Health and Human Services, Centers for Disease Control, Atlanta, GA 30333.

12. Centers for Disease Control. Recommendation of

the immunization practices advisory committee. Diphtheria, tetanus, and pertussis: Guidelines for vaccine prophylaxis and other preventive measures. *Morbid. Mortal. Weekly Rep.* 30:392, 1981.

13. Centers for Disease Control. Recommendation of the immunization practices advisory committee: Inactivated hepatitis B virus vaccine. *Morbid. Mortal. Weekly Rep.* 31:317, 1982.

14. Collins, C. H. Laboratory-acquired infections. *Med. Lab. Sci.* 37:291, 1980.

15. Collins, C. H., and Lyne, P. M. *Microbiological Methods* (4th ed.). London: Butterworths, 1976, pp. 23, 58.

16. Darlow, H. M., Safety in the Microbiological Laboratory. In Norris, J. R., and Ribbons, D. W. (Eds.), *Methods in Microbiology,* vol. 1. New York: Academic, 1969.

17. Darlow, H. M. Safety in the Microbiological Laboratory: An Introduction. In Shapton, D. A., and Board, R. G. (Eds.), *Safety in Microbiology.* (The Society for Applied Bacteriology, Technical Series No. 6.) New York: Academic, 1972.

18. Dole, M. Warning on autoclave bags. *ASM News* 44:293, 1978.

19. Environmental Health and Safety Department and the Biohazard Safety Committee of the University of Washington. *Biohazard Safety Manual.* University of Washington, Seattle, WA 98195, 1978.

20. Grief, D. Safe procedure for opening evacuated glass ampoules containing dried pathogens. *Appl. Microbiol.* 18:130, 1969.

21. Hugo, W. B. *Inhibition and Destruction of the Microbial Cell.* New York: Academic, 1971.

22. Kenny, M. T., and Sabel, F. L. Particle size distribution of *Serratia marcescens* aerosols created during common laboratory procedures and simulated laboratory accidents. *Appl. Microbiol.* 16:1146, 1968.

23. Lauer, J. L., Van Drunen, N. A., Washburn, J. W., and Balfour, H. H., Jr. Transmission of hepatitis B virus in clinical laboratory areas. *J. Infect. Dis.* 140:513, 1979.

24. Office of Research Safety, National Cancer Institute and the Special Committee of Safety and Health Experts. *Laboratory Safety Monograph: A Supplement to the NIH Guidelines for Recombinant DNA Research.* Bethesda, Md.: National Institutes of Health, 1979.

25. Paik, G. Reagents, stains, and miscellaneous test procedures, p. 1004. In Lennette, E. H., Balows, A., Hausler, W. J., and Truant, J. P. (Eds.), *Manual of Clinical Microbiology* (3d ed.). Washington, DC: American Society for Microbiology, 1980.

26. Pike, R. M. Laboratory-associated infections: Summary and analysis of 3921 cases. *Health Lab. Sci.* 13:105, 1976.

27. Pike, R. M. Past and present hazards of working with infectious agents. *Arch. Pathol. Lab. Med.* 102:33, 1978.

28. Reitman, M., and Wedum, A. G. Microbiological safety. *Public Health Rep.* 71:659, 1956.

29. Richardson, J. H., and Barkley, W. E. *Biosafety in Microbiological and Biomedical Laboratories.* U.S. Dept. of Health and Human Services, Public Health Services, Centers for Disease Control, Atlanta, Georgia. National Institutes of Health, Bethesda, Maryland, 1984. Available from Centers for Disease Control, Biosafety Office, 1600 Clifton Road, Atlanta, GA 30333.

30. Rutala, W. A., Stiegel, M. M., and Sarubbi, F. A. Decontamination of laboratory microbiological waste by steam sterilization. *Appl. Environ. Microbiol.* 43:1311, 1982.

31. Spaulding, E. H. Chemical disinfection and antisepsis in the hospital. *J. Hosp. Res.* 9:7, 1972.

32. Sulkin, S. E., Long, E. R., Pike, R. M., Sigel, M. M., Smith, C. E., and Wedum, A. G. Laboratory Infections and Accidents. In Harris, A. H., and Coleman, M. B. (Eds.), *Diagnostic Procedures and Reagents* (4th ed.). New York: American Public Health Association, 1963.

33. Vestal, A. L. Procedures for the Isolation and Identification of Mycobacteria. Centers for Disease Control, Atlanta, GA 30333, 1981.

34. Wedum, A. G. Laboratory safety in research with infectious aerosols. *Public Health Rep.* 76:619, 1964.

35. Williams, S. V., Huff, J. C., Feinglass, E. J., Gregg, M. B., Hatch, M. H., and Matsen, J. M. Epidemic viral hepatitis type B in hospital personnel. *Am. J. Med.* 57:904, 1974.

# 23  INFECTIONS IN NURSING HOMES

Richard A. Garibaldi

It has been estimated that approximately 5 percent of persons 65 years of age and older in the United States (1,122,000 persons) presently reside in nursing homes [10]. The Bureau of the Census projects that by the year 2050, the total U.S. population will be one-third larger. However, the subgroup of the population that is 65 years of age or older will increase by two and one-half times, and the subgroup 85 years of age or older will be six and one-half times greater than in 1982. In numerical terms, the number of persons 85 years of age or older will increase from 2.5 million people to 16 million people over the next 70 years.

As the population of elderly persons continues to grow, it is anticipated that more and more will require temporary or permanent placement in extended-care facilities. In 1977 4.8 percent of persons aged 65 years or greater and 22 percent aged 85 years or greater required nursing-home care [13]. In the years ahead, it is reasonable to expect that a similar percentage of the aged population will be as frail and alone as their 1977 counterparts and require institutionalized care. Our challenge as health-care providers is to ensure that these patients receive high-quality medical care and maintain productive lifestyles without exposing them to the additional risks of diseases associated with institutionalization.

This challenge is directed especially toward the infection control practitioner. Many nursing-home patients are at increased risk for infection because of underlying, debilitating conditions, which make them more susceptible to infection. These include diseases that alter immunologic reactivity, cause dysfunctions in specific organ systems, and prompt the use of medications that may additionally decrease resistance. In addition, the nursing-home setting itself affords a unique opportunity for the acquisition and transmission of infectious diseases. In the nursing home, aged patients are clustered together in a relatively confined environment, encouraged to partake in group activities, and cared for by a relatively small group of professional and nonprofessional persons who may have limited training in the techniques of infection control. The combination of a susceptible population and a setting in which infections may be readily spread makes nursing-home patients vulnerable to serious infectious disease.

Despite the potential seriousness of the problem, physicians, administrators, and infection control practitioners in nursing homes have little information regarding the rates or types of infections in their institutions. Few comprehensive studies are available that attempt to delineate the magnitude of the problem or to identify specific risk factors that predispose these patients to infections. Published studies offer limited generalizable information because of the small numbers of patients who have been surveyed and methodologic problems that make their results difficult to interpret. The few guidelines available to nursing homes for infection control have been adapted from policies or procedures for the care of patients in acute-care hospitals.

This chapter reviews the epidemiology of infections in nursing homes and identifies risk factors that are known to enhance the likelihood of acquisition or transmission of these infections. Attention is given to both the common types of endemic infections and occurrences of epidemic infections. An approach to disease prevention is presented, based on an understanding of the epidemiology of disease transmission, host risk factors that predispose patients to infection, and the unique features of the nursing-home setting that contribute to the transmission of disease.

## EPIDEMIOLOGY

### Nursing-Home Patients

The majority of patients who reside in nursing homes are elderly and moderately debilitated. The median age of nursing-home patients ranges between 80 and 85 years. In some surveys as many as 20 percent of patients are 90 years of age or older. There are generally two to three times as many women as men at each nursing home. Most nursing homes provide a broad range of services for an unselected spectrum of patients who require some degree of medical and/or social supervision. The median duration of residence for patients ranges from 12 to 18 months. In our survey of patients in seven nursing homes in Salt Lake City, approximately one-third of the patients had been institutionalized for less than six months, one-third for six months to two years, and one-third for more than two years [5].

Exceptions to these generalizations occur in nursing homes that specialize in providing long-term care for selected subpopulations, such as veterans, patients with psychiatric diseases, patients requiring rehabilitative services, and the mentally retarded. The demographic characteristics of these nursing homes vary according to the population for whom care is provided. Many nursing homes select patients according to the level of care. Thus an entire nursing home or specified section of a nursing home may provide skilled care for residents who require close supervision, or lesser levels of care for patients who are relatively independent and require less assistance. In addition selected patients may be admitted to nursing homes for special reasons. Some homes specialize in rehabilitative or recuperative services, while others provide long-term, domiciliary care or comfort for the terminally ill. The type and frequency of infections vary greatly according to the characteristics of the nursing home.

Nursing-home patients often have extensive problems including chronic diseases involving multiple sites. The average patient has more than three diagnoses recorded in the medical record. Organic brain syndrome and organic heart disease are the two most common diagnostic categories recorded, each affecting between 35 and 40 percent of institutionalized patients. Approximately 20 to 25 percent of patients have a history of cerebral vascular accident or other central nervous system disease, hypertension, arthritis, or old fractures. In our study, 15 percent of patients had diabetes mellitus; of these, 25 percent (4 percent of the total population) were receiving insulin [5]. The ambulatory status of the patient often reflects the extent of his or her debility. In skilled nursing facilities 50 to 60 percent of the total population are ambulatory, 35 to 45 percent are confined to bed and chair, and 0 to 5 percent are bedridden. In our study two-thirds of the patients had stable, long-standing medical conditions, while the other one-third had either a deteriorating or a terminal status. As many as 50 percent of nursing-home residents are incontinent of urine, and 30 to 40 percent are also incontinent of feces. The majority of incontinent patients have substantial cognitive impairments and limitations in mobility. Between 5 and 10 percent of patients require chronic urinary drainage despite the hazards of long-term catheterization and attempts by many nursing homes to avoid catheterization if possible. Relatively few patients in nursing homes have intravenous lines, tracheostomies, gastrostomies, or nasogastric tubes because most chronic-care facilities do not admit patients who require this level of care.

Nursing-home patients often receive a large number of medications for a variety of purposes. Drugs are prescribed to treat underlying disease states, regulate body functions, control behavior, modulate sleep, and prevent the acquisition of infections. A prevalence survey conducted in 1974 by the Office of Long-Term Care, U.S. Public Health Service, involving more than 3000 nursing-home residents, reported an average of 6.1 medication orders per patient. Cathartics, analgesics, and tranquilizers were the most common drugs prescribed. Antimicrobials accounted for only 3 percent of all prescriptions; however, these drugs were prescribed for 16 percent of the study population. As might be expected in a prevalence survey, long-term, antiinfective therapies used for the suppression of chronic urinary tract infection accounted for a large proportion of these orders. In our prevalence survey of 532 nursing-home residents in 1980–81, approximately 50 percent of patients were receiving sedative or tranquilizer medications; systemic antimicrobials were prescribed for 10 percent of patients [5]. Trimethoprim-sulfamethoxazole and cephalosporin derivatives were the most commonly prescribed antimicrobials. In most nursing homes, the decision to immunize patients is left to the discretion of the attending physician. Even though immunization with influenza and pneumococcal vaccines is generally recommended for geriatric patients with multisystem diseases, we were able to find documentation of influenza immunization for only 40 percent of patients and of pneumococcal vaccination for only 17 percent of patients in our prevalence survey. We found no records of tuberculin skin test results in our review of patients' charts, although annual skin testing was required by state regulations and presumably had been done.

The characteristics that describe the typical features of nursing-home patients also describe host factors that predispose to infection. Thus the physiologic process of aging, multiplicity and severity of underlying diseases, loss of control of body functions, exposure to invasive devices, and receipt of medications that alter mental status or inhibit the growth of normal bacterial flora all increase the susceptibility of the nursing-home patient to infection. With age, the immune system is altered and the ability to respond to stress is diminished. The deterioration of immunologic function involves immune lymphocytes and is reflected by a decrease in skin-test responsiveness. In addition, certain natural barriers to infection break down in the elderly. In the lung, for instance, some of the specialized defenses against bacterial invasion are impaired, including coughing, localized immunoglobulin production, and ciliary action. The loss of gastric acid with aging greatly increases the susceptibility of patients to potentially pathogenic bacteria that are swallowed. Patients with gastric achlorhydria acquire gastrointestinal infection with *Salmonella* or *Shigella* at much lower inocula than patients with normal gastric acidity (see Chapter 32). Thus infectious diarrhea, including epidemic outbreaks, occurs relatively frequently among nursing-home residents. In the urinary tract, incomplete emptying of the bladder, impaired generation of acid urine, and poor perineal hygiene secondary to fecal or urinary incontinence can predispose to infection. Diminished levels of activity or immobility in chronically ill elderly patients encourages the development of skin infections. Nonambulatory patients are more likely than ambulatory patients to be incontinent, require urinary catheterization, and develop pressure sores. Thus physiologic changes that occur with aging and are unrelated to specific disease processes may enhance the susceptibility of these patients to infection.

Specific disease processes also predispose patients to infectious complications. Patients with neurologic disorders such as organic brain syndrome, dementia, mental retardation, previous cerebral vascular accidents, and multiple sclerosis may be unable to care for themselves properly. These patients may be unable to feed themselves, communicate, move in bed, or sense danger, and are at increased risk for infection. Patients with impaired central nervous system function are also likely to be incontinent of urine or feces and to be treated with long-term indwelling urinary catheterization. Oftentimes these patients become agitated and require sedative or tranquilizing medications that additionally diminish their physiologic responsiveness and increase their risk for aspiration pneumonia or bed sores.

In addition to primary central nervous system diseases, institutionalized nursing-home patients may have other chronic conditions that interfere with their ability to resist infections. Patients with chronic pulmonary disease are susceptible to respiratory infections because they are unable to clear bacteria or viruses from their airways and because they have depressed immunocytologic responsiveness. Similarly, patients with pulmonary congestion secondary to heart failure are also prone to lower respiratory tract infections. Certain cancers, chronic renal failure, chronic liver disease, and other long-term illnesses predispose to infection by interfering with immunologic reactivity and white blood cell function. Sometimes, patients require therapy with antimetabolic drugs that additionally depress immunocytologic defenses. In addition, these chronically ill patients have some degree of protein-calorie malnutrition. In fact prevalence surveys have shown that between 30 and 40 percent of nursing-home patients are malnourished, using such markers as serum albumin determinations, serum transferrin levels, triceps skin fold measurements, and height-weight ratios. Malnourished patients frequently are unable to respond to skin test antigens, suggesting that they have significant impairments in cell-mediated immunity. Moreover, elderly patients with depressed cell-mediated immunity have an extremely high mortality rate (48 percent) during the six-month period following testing, compared with patients who react (13 percent) [12].

Finally, the use of medications and other iatrogenic

devices also increases the patient's risk for acquiring infections. Sedative-tranquilizer medications predispose to the aspiration of oropharyngeal contents and the subsequent development of pulmonary infection. Antibiotic agents alter the indigenous microflora of the gastrointestinal tract, oropharynx, and perineal area. Patients who are treated with antibiotics are frequently colonized with antibiotic-resistant bacteria and are at increased risk for infection with these organisms. Medications that interfere with gastric acidity or gastrointestinal motility predispose to enteric infections. Antidepressant drugs and other atropine-containing medications can cause mucous surfaces to become dry and lose their local barrier effects. Fortunately, invasive procedures are prescribed infrequently for nursing-home patients with the exception of indwelling urinary catheters. As yet there are no data to show that alternatives to chronic indwelling urinary catheterization such as condom drainage, intermittent catheterization, or suprapubic drainage are less likely to cause infection. Intravenous catheters, tracheal tubes, and nasogastric tubes are uncommon among nursing-home residents. If present, however, each of these invasive therapies is associated with an increased risk of infection.

## THE NURSING-HOME ENVIRONMENT

In 1977 there were approximately 19,000 nursing homes that provided care for 1,300,000 nursing-home patients. Without doubt, both the number of available nursing homes and the number of patients who require institutionalization has increased since that time and will continue to increase over the next several decades. Some nursing homes are closely affiliated with, or under contract to, organizations such as the Veterans Administration or state programs for the mentally retarded. Some nursing homes have a close working agreement with acute-care hospitals that facilitate the exchange of patients between institutions; hospitalized patients are transferred to the nursing-home unit for less intensive, lower cost care or rehabilitative services; nursing-home patients are transferred to the hospital unit for emergent medical problems or diagnostic evaluations.

More than three-quarters of nursing homes are proprietary. In some regions private corporations have emerged that have consolidated the administrative and fiscal operations of several nursing homes and function on a "for-profit" basis. Reimbursement for nursing-home care is borne either by the patient and his or her family or by the federal government. In fiscal year 1979, the federal-state Medicaid program spent $8.8 billion for nursing-home care [6]. This represented 49 percent of the total spending for nursing homes. Sources of third-party reimbursement other than Medicaid are extremely limited. Nearly 50 percent of the costs of nursing-home care are financed through out-of-pocket expenditures by patients and families. Many patients are admitted to facilities as private patients but qualify for Medicaid after they have exhausted their assets. Nursing-home care is expensive. For example, in New York State in 1981, daily reimbursement rates ranged roughly from $50 to $100, depending on the home's location and range of services it provided [11]. Financial issues have an impact on the types of patients who can afford nursing-home services as well as on the availability and quality of facilities in the community. Costs of care and quality of service do not always go hand in hand. Many nursing homes provide first-class care at relatively low costs, whereas some more expensive homes provide poor-quality care. Nursing homes are small, autonomous institutions in which the skills and personalities of individual operators and nursing directors have an overriding influence on the quality of care.

The nursing-home setting more closely resembles that of an acute-care hospital than an individual family unit. Nursing homes are self-contained environments that provide total daily care for large groups of patients. The bed capacities range from less than 50 to more than 300; the majority have between 100 and 150 beds. Occupancy rates are generally high. In most homes, more than 85 percent of beds are filled; in some homes, there is a waiting list for prospective residents. The daily activities of residents are usually conducted within the walls of the institution. Generally, patients occupy semiprivate rooms with one or two roommates. Private rooms are available to some. Infrequently, a ward with multiple occupants comprises a basic living unit. Patients who are ambulatory usually share a common clean-up area that contains a sink and toilet. Bathing facilities are often communal. In some facilities, the clean-up area may be shared by patients from several rooms. Nonambulatory patients require the assistance of nursing-home employees or family members to provide them with personal services such as washing, bathing, toileting, and eating. These services are carried out in the patient's room or bed. Nursing aides or orderlies often move directly from patient to patient to complete specified service assignments. These contacts may provide opportunities for the transmission of infectious diseases.

In addition, nursing-home residents are encouraged to participate in group activities. Ambulatory patients usually eat in a common cafeteria, participate in physical and occupational therapy sessions, and are grouped together in recreational programs. These activities are designed to encourage social interactions. Patients with mild upper respiratory illnesses, diarrhea, or conjunctivitis may not be excluded from these group activities. Thus within the nursing home, there is a markedly increased likelihood for patient-to-patient contact and a potential for disease transmission. These risks are much greater for institutionalized patients than for elderly home-care patients in the community.

Nursing-home patients are similar to hospitalized patients in their propensity to serve as reservoirs for certain unique infectious agents. These patients are more likely than noninstitutionalized persons to be harboring or infected with antibiotic-resistant bacteria. For instance, the urinary tracts of patients with chronic, indwelling urethral catheters are virtually always colonized with one or more species of bacteria. Catheterized patients with asymptomatic bacteriuria serve as reservoirs for antibiotic-resistant, gram-negative bacilli within the nursing-home environment. Patient-to-patient spread of infection may occur by direct contact or by indirect contact through unwashed hands of personnel who may serve as vectors for the passive transfer of organisms. This is especially true when patients with indwelling catheters reside in the same room or are clustered together in close proximity with each other in group activities (see Chapter 25). Objects such as urine collection vessels, bedpans, and nondisposable equipment may also become contaminated with bacteria and serve as inanimate reservoirs for epidemic, common-source transmission.

Person-to-person transmission of infectious agents in the nursing-home setting is additionally enhanced by the difficulties in diagnosing actual infections when they occur. The clinical presentations of infections in elderly, chronically diseased patients are often atypical and difficult to diagnose. Signs and symptoms usually associated with infections may be absent or diminished, which may result in delays in diagnosis. The detrimental effects of delayed diagnosis are twofold: the initiation of effective treatment may be late in the course of infection, and the spread of infection may occur before the clinical manifestations of the disease are recognized. A relative nonavailability of clinical microbiology laboratories may additionally delay the diagnosis of an infectious problem. Cultures are ordered infrequently, transportation of specimens to the laboratory may be slow, reliability of test results may be inconsistent, and results may be reported irregularly. These limitations lead the physician to diagnose and treat possible infections on an empirical basis. Thus antibiotics may be prescribed more frequently than clinically indicated and broader spectrum drugs may be chosen to initiate therapy. These actions encourage the selection of antibiotic-resistant bacteria for colonization in the treated patient and alter the general patterns of bacterial flora in the nursing-home setting.

Other factors in the nursing-home setting that contribute to the acquisition and spread of infections include employee staffing patterns, levels of staff education, and administrative decisions that have an impact on infection control practices. In general, there is a relatively low awareness of the hazards of infection or the risks of epidemic spread in nursing homes. Most extended-care facilities have infection control programs and a designated infection control practitioner. Infection control programs are usually mandated by state law. In most nursing homes, however, the designated infection control practitioner has other responsibilities in addition to infection control. Usually, these responsibilities are administrative or supervisory rather than direct nursing activities. Most practitioners have had no specific training in infection control practices or epidemiologic techniques. Most nursing homes do not have trained physicians or epidemiologists to oversee their infection control activities. Many nursing homes have regularly scheduled meetings to discuss institutional infections, but few perform systematic surveillance to identify rates of infection, monitor patient-care practices, or conduct training programs in infection control techniques on a regular basis. As a result, most of the personnel with direct nursing-care responsibilities have little awareness of the epidemiology of disease transmission or knowledge of methods of control.

In most skilled-care facilities, patients are cared for by orderlies or aides who have little formal training in nursing techniques. Registered nurses and licensed practical nurses are often relegated to supervisory positions. The number of nurses available per patient for each shift and the level of training vary greatly from facility to facility. In our survey of nursing homes in Salt Lake City, an average of 17 aides, five licensed practical nurses, and three registered nurses were on duty during a 24-hour period in facilities with an average census of 80 patients [5]. The ratio of patients to staff during each shift varied from 6 : 1 during the daytime hours to 15 : 1 during the night. In these nursing homes, there was an extremely high turnover of staff at all levels of training. In the three months previous to our survey, the average nursing home had hired 15 new aides, two new licensed practical nurses, and one new registered nurse.

This high rate of staff turnover may reflect local factors related to an urban setting, economic conditions at the time, and the high job mobility that is seen among nonprofessional staff. Within the period of a year, we saw complete turnovers of supervisory staff positions as well as multiple turnovers of nonprofessional employees. High rates of employee turnover, understaffing, high ratios of nonprofessional to professional staff, and limited training in health-care practices have been cited by other investigators as important problems in nursing homes. These factors contribute to the spread of infections and make it extremely difficult to establish and maintain efficient programs for infection control.

The difficulty in establishing effective programs for infection control is compounded by the fact that there are no standardized guidelines for infection control practices that focus on the unique problems of the nursing-home setting. Some states have adapted regulations from guidelines devised for patients in acute-care hospitals. Most states mandate that patients and employees be tested for tuberculosis at the time of admission or employment and yearly thereafter. However, there are no national recommendations for tuberculin skin testing or for immunizations against influenza, pneumococcal infection, or other infectious agents for either residents or nursing-home staff. No regulations exist to establish minimum staffing requirements or minimum levels of education in health-related subjects for nursing-home employees. Most nursing homes have no formal guidelines for monitoring health status of employees at the time of hiring or during the performance of their job activities. Most homes have no formal policies to deal with sick employees. Usually there is no compensation for sick time; thus employees with acute infections might be forced to work rather than remain at home, and thereby may introduce a community infection into the closed nursing-home environment.

## ENDEMIC INFECTIONS

As yet there are no well-defined, comprehensive studies that use standard methodology to document the rate of endemic infections among nursing-home residents. The published data available give inconsistent results from survey to survey. Overall prevalence rates vary from 2.7 to 17 percent. The differences in rates reflect differences in patient populations, prevalence periods, definitions of infection, case identification methodology, and surveillance techniques. Lower rates are reported in surveys that include nursing homes that agree to participate, use chart reviews as the sole method for case-finding, define infections strictly, and limit surveillance to specific sites. Higher rates are observed when chart reviews are augmented by patient examinations, definitions are less strict, infections at all sites are included, and asymptomatic as well as symptomatic patients are counted. In our survey of seven Salt Lake City nursing homes, we documented a prevalence rate of infection of 16.2 percent [5]. In this study, patient examinations were performed, infections were defined by the documentation of purulence or the acknowledgment of the attending physician that an infection was present, and all types of infections including conjunctivitis and diarrhea were added to the case count. An earlier study of 18 Connecticut nursing homes revealed a prevalence of infection of only 2.4 percent [3]. In this study, however, only nursing homes whose administrators agreed to participate were included in the survey; infections were defined by chart reviews, and the diagnosis of infection was restricted to only three sites. There are no studies that compare the prevalence of infections in different types of nursing-home facilities. Two studies that have attempted to define incidence rates of infections among nursing-home residents report that 7 to 10 percent of patients acquire new infections each month [2,9].

### Urinary Tract Infections
Most studies report that urinary tract infections are the most common types of institutionally acquired infection (see Chapter 25). In prevalence surveys the rates of urinary tract infection range between 1.2 and 3.1 percent of nursing-home residents. Rates are higher in nursing homes in which a relatively large segment of the population is being treated with long-term, indwelling urinary catheters and in studies in which asymptomatically colonized patients are included. In most nursing homes, between 5 and 10 percent of the population is catheterized. In some nursing homes that treat more debilitated patients, however, as many as 50 percent of the population may be catheterized. In a study of infections in a long-term care facility that was affiliated with a Veterans Administration Medical Center, 58 of 398 patients developed asymptomatic bacteriuria or urinary tract infections over a two-month period [9]. Of these, 83 percent had been treated with urethral catheterization or condom drainage during the period of surveillance. In this institution, urinary tract infections accounted for 71 percent of all infections that were identified during the two-month period.

In our survey in Salt Lake City, we identified 14 symptomatic urinary tract infections among 532 institutionalized patients for a rate of 2.6 percent [5].

In these nursing homes, 63 of the 532 patients were chronically catheterized. Catheterized patients were more likely than noncatheterized patients to be non-ambulatory, have deteriorating clinical conditions, be incontinent of feces, and have decubitus ulcers. We found that 85 percent of urine specimens taken from this group of chronically catheterized patients revealed bacteriuria with at least $10^5$ cfu per milliliter of urine. The rate of bacteriuria was similar in patients receiving chronic suppressive therapy to those who were not. An average of two bacterial isolates were recovered from each positive urine specimen. The most common isolates were enterococci, *Proteus vulgaris, Escherichia coli, Proteus mirabilis,* and *Providencia stuartii.* Two-thirds of the bacterial isolates were resistant to ampicillin, two-thirds to cephalothin, one-third to trimethaprim-sulfamethoxazole, and one-fifth to gentamicin.

Other studies of chronically catheterized nursing-home residents have revealed results similar to those just described. In one study in which weekly cultures were collected, the prevalence of bacteriuria approached 100 percent, and a mean of 2.6 organisms was identified in each specimen [14]. In these patients changes in bacterial strain were detected every two weeks. Episodes of bacteriuria with *P. stuartii, P. mirabilis, E. coli,* and *Pseudomonas aeruginosa* were commonly identified. However, the persistence of colonization varied with different organisms. For instance, when *P. stuartii* gained access to the urinary tract, it persisted for an average of ten weeks; some durations of bacteriuria with this organism lasted as long as 36 weeks. On the other hand, most gram-positive organisms, with the exception of enterococci, were recovered in only a single weekly culture. Other gram-negative organisms persisted for two to five weeks. Thus it appears that bacterial colonization of the chronically catheterized urinary tract is in a constant state of flux. Sequential cultures reveal a constantly changing array of bacterial isolates. The constantly changing patterns of urinary colonization undermine any rationale for collecting routine urine surveillance cultures. It is imperative for physicians to obtain a fresh urinary culture before treating symptomatic urinary tract infections in these patients.

### Skin Infections

Rates of skin and subcutaneous infections vary from 1.1 to 6 percent in prevalence surveys (see Chapter 31). Two studies in which the prevalence of superficial skin infections was 5 percent and 6 percent used clinical criteria to define an infection [5,8]. Studies that have reported lower rates have used stricter definitions. No study has used the technique of quantitative wound cultures to define these infections. Skin infections usually occur in sites of decubitus ulcers. Oftentimes it is difficult to distinguish uninfected pressure sores from superficial skin infections. Decubitus ulcers are frequently present in debilitated elderly patients who may be unable to respond to infection with typical signs or symptoms. These patients are often immobile, fecally incontinent, diabetic, and malnourished, factors that also predispose these patients to infection.

### Respiratory Tract Infections

Respiratory tract infections are reported to be present in between 0.3 and 3.6 percent of nursing-home residents (see Chapter 26). Approximately half of these infections involve the lower respiratory tract and half involve the upper respiratory tract. In some areas of the country, the prevalence of respiratory tract infections may vary according to the time of year and prevalence of infections in the community. In the nursing home, the diagnosis of respiratory tract infections is often ambiguous. Objective verification of infections is rare. X-rays are not usually ordered, and physical examination findings are often not included in the medical record. Cultures are obtained infrequently; when they are available, they are often difficult to interpret. In our prevalence survey, 11 of the 532 patients (2.1 percent) had lower respiratory tract infections and 8 (1.5 percent) had upper respiratory tract infections [5]. It is noteworthy that 6 of the 8 patients with upper respiratory tract infection resided in the same nursing home and were thought to be part of an epidemic cluster that was occurring at the time of the prevalence survey. In our survey, we noted an association between lower respiratory tract infections and the receipt of sedative or tranquilizing medications. However, this association was not statistically significant. The prevalence of lower respiratory tract infection was 3.1 percent in patients who received these medications, and 1.1 percent in those who did not. We noted no decrease in the prevalence of lower or upper respiratory infections in patients who had received pneumococcal or influenza vaccine. However, documentation of the immunization status of patients was frequently absent from the patient record. Thus the apparent lack of impact of immunizations may have reflected poor charting practices.

Patients in nursing homes who develop pneumonia are infected with pathogens similar to those recovered from hospitalized patients with nosocomial pneumonias; these organisms are quite unlike those isolated from patients with community-acquired pneumonias. Institutionalized patients are more likely than community patients to have received antibiotics before the onset of pneumonia and to be infected with such pathogens as *Klebsiella pneumoniae* and *Staphylococcus aureus* [4]. Thus with respiratory tract infections as well as with urinary tract infections, there appears to be an increased incidence of infections with relatively antibiotic-resistant pathogens. For this reason, appropriate cultures should be obtained before initiating therapy. If empirical therapy is warranted after cultures are collected, broad-spectrum antimicrobials should be used.

### Other Infections

In most surveys, infections at other sites occur less frequently than in sites mentioned so far. Sporadic cases or case clusters of conjunctivitis, diarrhea, wound infections, and other gastrointestinal infections have been noted occasionally. Clusters of cases of diarrhea or conjunctivitis may occur relatively commonly among nursing-home patients but go unreported.

## EPIDEMIC INFECTIONS

A small number of reports of epidemic infections in nursing-home residents have appeared in the literature. It is likely that the majority of case clusters or epidemic occurrences in nursing homes go unreported because they are not thoroughly investigated or reports are not submitted for publication.

### Respiratory Infections

The most common site of epidemic infection is the respiratory tract (see Chapter 26). These infections are easily disseminated in the nursing-home setting where elderly, susceptible patients are in close contact with each other. Outbreaks of influenza A, influenza B, parainfluenza, respiratory syncytial virus, and tuberculosis have been reported. These infections can be quite severe in debilitated nursing-home residents. In one outbreak of influenza A, the case fatality ratio was 30 percent [7]. Many of the epidemics involve nursing-home staff as well as patients. Epidemic influenza infections frequently occur concurrently with community outbreaks. In nursing homes, clinical attack rates of influenza range between 25 and 40 percent; in one outbreak an attack rate of 85 percent was observed among unvaccinated patients. Unfortunately, vaccine has not been as effective as hoped among institutionalized patients: in this epidemic, the attack rate of influenza for vaccinated patients was 48 percent, resulting in a calculated rate of vaccine efficacy for preventing clinical illness of only 43 per-

cent [1]. However, vaccination does appear to reduce substantially the risk of dying from influenza.

### Gastroenteritis

Occurrences of other types of epidemic infections among nursing-home patients are reported less commonly. Epidemics of diarrhea have been attributed to infections with *Salmonella* and rotaviruses (see Chapter 32). Both foodborne and person-to-person transmission have been implicated as possible modes of spread. It is likely that most case clusters of gastroenteritis or diarrheal disease go unreported.

### Urinary Tract Infections

Scattered outbreaks of epidemic catheter-associated urinary tract infections have been described (see Chapter 25). These reports have been generated from specialty-oriented chronic-care facilities in which there are groups of patients who require chronic, indwelling urinary catheters. Infection is thought to be transmitted from patient to patient by passive carriage of bacteria on the hands of personnel. These outbreaks are characterized by high rates of infection or colonization with unusual bacterial isolates such as *P. stuartii* or *Proteus rettgeri*, which are also resistant to multiple antibiotics.

In our prevalence survey, we noted apparent clusterings of infections at several of the nursing homes [5]. For instance six of the eight patients that we identified with upper respiratory tract infections were residents of a single nursing home. This nursing home was surveyed in the fall when there was a community outbreak of upper respiratory tract infections. The prevalence of respiratory infections in this home was 8.8 percent, compared with a rate of 0.4 percent in the six other homes that we surveyed. In addition, five of seven patients whom we identified with diarrhea were residents of another home; the prevalence of diarrhea among patients in this home was 9.8 percent, compared with a rate of 0.4 percent at all other homes. We also observed clusters of lower respiratory tract infections and conjunctivitis in individual nursing homes. We found that case clusters accounted for 20 percent of all infections that we identified in our prevalence survey.

Clustering of bacterial isolates also occurred in urine specimens from patients who were being treated with chronic indwelling urethral catheterization. Certain isolates were recovered frequently in one nursing home but were only infrequently isolated from patients in other homes. For instance, *P. stuartii* was recovered from the majority of catheterized patients in one home but isolated very infrequently from patients outside this home. Similarly, isolates of *P. mirabilis, P. aeruginosa,* and *Enterobacter cloacae* were observed at individual nursing-home facilities but were rarely recovered at other nursing homes.

## THE INFECTION CONTROL PROGRAM

The basic elements for an effective infection control program have been clearly defined for acute care hospitals (see Chapter 3). The major components of such a program include the identification and active participation of personnel interested in infection control issues, a system of surveillance to identify problems, and the implementation of strategies to prevent the acquisition of infections or control their transmission. The primary goal of any program is disease prevention. This implies that an effective infection control program must be action-oriented. The major goals and objectives of the infection control program in nursing homes are similar to those of the acute-care hospital. However, some of the specific problems and their solutions may be different.

### The Infection Control Committee
The cornerstone of an effective infection control program is the Infection Control Committee. An effective infection control committee must have a strong and supportive chairperson. In most nursing homes, this position is delegated to the medical director or an attending physician with an interest in infectious diseases. The installation of an attending physician as committee chairperson adds to the credibility and authority of the committee and enables the committee to deal more effectively with other physicians or administrators.

The core group of the Infection Control Committee should include the infection control physician, infection control nurse, nursing-home administrator, and director of nurses. To carry out an effective program, the infection control nurse needs the active support of the nursing-home administration. Financial resources must be made available for salary support, infection control supplies, educational materials, and other items needed for the daily operation of the program. The administrator provides the committee with realistic expectations of the ability of the home to comply with the committee's recommendations. He or she is a key person in the communication, implementation, and enforcement of facility-wide decisions. The remaining members of the Infection Control Committee should reflect the multidisciplinary nature of infection control activities.

Representatives from the pharmacy, dietetic, housekeeping, and maintenance departments, and the local health department are often included.

The infection control nurse must be able to perform several roles effectively, including those of surveillance officer, teacher, educational consultant, clinical evaluator, and epidemiologic investigator (see Chapter 3). To do this a basic understanding of infectious diseases, microbiology, epidemiology, and public health is required, as well as in-depth knowledge of nursing techniques and aseptic practices. Most important, excellent communicative skills, respect of the staff, and a desire to become educated in the discipline of infection control are needed.

### Surveillance
To identify problems, the infection control nurse must make regularly scheduled ward rounds and talk with nursing personnel regarding infectious disease problems and preventive practices (see Chapter 4). Surveillance activities need not be limited to the identification of infections in institutionalized patients. They should also include surveillance of infections among employees and monitoring to ensure the proper use or implementation of infection control practices. Rates of infections should be determined by periodic surveys of disease incidence or prevalence. The exact methods of the surveillance activity may vary from institution to institution; however, it is important that the same methodologic techniques for data collection be repeated in each survey, including standard definitions of infections, procedures for case identification, and calculation of rates. Thus results from multiple surveys can be compared, and disease trends or patterns can be identified. The nurse must work closely with attending physicians and nurses to document each infection with bacteriologic cultures. The surveillance system should characterize the epidemiology of institutionally acquired infections by site, room location, date of onset, and relation to iatrogenic manipulations. Surveillance activities in the nursing home may require techniques different from those required in the hospital setting. Chart reviews and reviews of microbiology laboratory results cannot be relied on to document the occurrence of infections. Even the monitoring of daily temperature elevations may not identify infected patients because temperatures may not be recorded on a regular basis and because elderly patients may not respond to infection with a febrile reaction. On the other hand regular rounds with nursing personnel who provide direct patient care and chart reviews of nursing notes may provide more accurate clues to identify the in-

fected patients. Floor personnel should be encouraged to report patients with newly diagnosed infections. Surveillance of new prescriptions for antibiotic treatments might also identify newly infected patients. The routine collection of surveillance cultures from environmental sources or patients, even urine from chronically catheterized patients, is not recommended. It is the responsibility of the infection control nurse to report the results of surveillance and control activities on a regular basis to the Infection Control Committee.

When an unusual clustering of cases is noted, the infection control nurse should initiate an epidemiologic investigation (see Chapter 5). This investigation should include the identification of the problem; a case count that documents the number of patients involved; and an analysis of cases by time, place, and person. In most instances, this type of investigation will reveal the extent of the epidemic and the epidemiology of disease transmission. With this information, the infection control nurse can recommend appropriate control measures to the Infection Control Committee. On rare occasions, however, the extent of the problem may be great or seemingly appropriate control measures may be ineffective. In these situations, the nursing-home administrator or medical director should be alerted and outside help obtained. Sources of outside help include the local health department, infectious disease practitioners from the area, and consultation with epidemiologists at the state department of health.

*Infection Control Techniques*
Once an infectious disease problem is identified, it becomes the infection control nurse's responsibility to implement effective intervention. The problem may be an increased frequency of a specific type of infection, a breakdown in aseptic technique, a failure to institute proper isolation precautions, or a possible epidemic occurrence of infections. In each of these instances, it is likely that the infection control nurse will intervene by initiating some type of educational program. In addition to organizing educational programs, the infection control nurse should routinely orient new employees to the risks of infections in nursing homes and the techniques of infection control and observe new personnel in patient-care activities to monitor their appreciation, knowledge, and performance of infection control practices. For old employees, a series of seminars to review new techniques in infection control and reemphasize the proper application of old techniques should be scheduled. These sessions should emphasize the importance of infection

control practices in daily patient care. They may also serve as problem-solving exercises in which issues raised by employees can be discussed.

One of the major focuses of the infection control nurse's educational efforts must be to emphasize the importance of hand-washing. Hand-washing remains the single most important factor in effective infection control. Appropriate facilities for hand-washing should be available in every patient's room. All personnel should be trained in proper hand-washing technique. By frequently reinforcing techniques and practices that are known to reduce the likelihood of disease transmission, the infection control practitioner can lower the rates of institutionally acquired infections.

Both patients and employees with communicable diseases should be identified early and isolated in some manner to avoid the spread of infection within the institution (see Chapters 2 and 9). Ill employees should remain at home. Guests with symptoms of acute infections should not be allowed to visit patients in the facility. Patients with infectious diseases should have their activities restricted. However, the type and severity of isolation precautions must be individualized according to the type of infection and the patient's total needs. Logic and knowledge of the epidemiology of disease transmission will dictate the specific precautions that may be recommended (see Chapter 9). Each decision must take into account the psychologic and health-care needs of the patient as well as the total health-care responsibilities of the institution.

*Employee Health*
The surveillance and control of infections in employees is as important as the prevention of infection in patients (see Chapter 2). Nursing homes should have some mechanism for evaluating the health of their personnel. At the time of employment, all new employees should be evaluated to rule out the presence of any acute or chronic infectious disease. Their immunization status should be checked and updated. These screens can be conducted by the employee's private physician or by the infection control nurse, who may serve as the employee health nurse. Even though their size may limit their ability to provide a formal employee health program, nursing homes should maintain a file of health-related problems for each of their employees and provide a means to evaluate acutely ill employees who might be infected. Employees who develop acute infections should be encouraged to seek early medical evaluation to determine their infectivity. Infected personnel should be given time off from work without being penalized.

*Administrative Considerations*

An effective infection control program requires more than surveillance and control activities by an infection control nurse. Each nursing home must address deficits in its administration of patient-care resources. For instance, nursing homes must provide a professional staff of adequate size during each shift to care for patients and maintain sound infection control practices. These staff members should have an educational background that provides them with a basic understanding of techniques to prevent disease transmission. Staff who are genuinely interested in patient care and empathetic to patient needs should be recruited whenever possible. Appropriate financial or fringe-benefit incentives must be offered to attract professionally trained personnel and reverse the trend of high employee job turnover. A stable, conscientious, well-educated team of patient-care providers is likely to have good infection-control practices and respond to educational efforts. This type of employee, together with a competent infection control nurse, will have a great impact on diminishing the spread of infections within the nursing home.

# REFERENCES

1. Centers for Disease Control. Impact of influenza on a nursing home population: New York. *Morbid. Mortal. Weekly Rep.* 32:32, 1983.
2. Checko, P. J. *A Study of Infection Control Programs in Skilled Nursing Facilities in Connecticut: Suggested Alternatives for Surveillance and Criteria of Infection* (thesis). New Haven, Conn.: Yale University, 1981.
3. Cohen, E. D., Hierholzer, W., Jr., Schilling, C. R., and Snydman, D. R. Nosocomial infections in skilled nursing facilities: A preliminary survey. *Public Health Rep.* 94:162, 1979.
4. Garb, J. L., Brown, R. B., Garb, J. R., et. al. Difference in the etiology of pneumonias in nursing home and community patients. *J.A.M.A.* 240:2169, 1978.
5. Garibaldi, R. A., Brodine, S., and Matsumiya, S. Infections among patients in nursing homes: Policies, prevalence, and problems. *N. Engl. J. Med.* 305:731, 1981.
6. Gibson, R. National health expenditures, 1979. *Health Care Finance Rev.* 2(1):1, 1980.
7. Goodman, R. A., Orenstein, W. A., Munro, T. F., et. al. Impact of influenza A in a nursing home. *J.A.M.A.* 247:1451, 1982.
8. Lester, M. R. Looking inside 101 nursing homes. *Am. J. Nurs.* 64:111, 1964.
9. Magnussen, M. H., and Robb, S. S. Nosocomial infections in a long-term care facility. *A.P.I.C. J.* 8:12, 1980.
10. Rabin, D. L. Physician care in nursing homes. *Ann. Intern. Med.* 94:126, 1981.
11. Rango, N. Nursing home care in the United States. Prevailing conditions and policy implications. *N. Engl. J. Med.* 307:883, 1982.
12. Shaver, H. J., Loper, J. A., and Lutes, R. A. Nutritional status of nursing home patients. *J.P.E.N.* 4:367, 1980.
13. United States National Center for Health Statistics. *The National Nursing Home Survey: 1977 Summary for the United States.* Hyattsville, Md: National Center for Health Statistics, 1979. (Vital and health statistics. Series 13, No. 43. DHEW publication no. [PHS] 79-1794.)
14. Warren, J. W., Tenney, J. H., Hoopes, J. M., Muncie, H. L., and Anthony, W. C. A prospective microbiologic study of bacteriuria in patients with chronic indwelling urethral catheters. *J. Infect. Dis.* 146:719, 1982.

# II ENDEMIC AND EPIDEMIC HOSPITAL INFECTIONS

# 24 INCIDENCE AND NATURE OF ENDEMIC AND EPIDEMIC NOSOCOMIAL INFECTIONS

Robert W. Haley

One of the central concepts of modern infection control is that one must have a thorough knowledge of the occurrence of infection problems to control them most effectively. Although there is no substitute for timely information on the current infection situation in one's own hospital from ongoing surveillance, a valuable perspective can be gained from studying the incidence and nature of nosocomial infections in the nation as a whole and in hospitals similar to one's own. Such information not only points out national infection problems and trends that are likely to be mirrored in local situations, but also alerts infection control personnel to potentially useful concepts and techniques that can be adopted and to potential pitfalls that can be avoided.

The problem of nosocomial infections is usually discussed in two different contexts: epidemics of infections and endemic occurrences. Epidemics have been very important in the development of the modern approach to hospital infection control by presenting emergency situations that have focused concern and effort on the problem; consequently epidemics of infections have received much attention from infection control personnel and have been the focus of much of the scientific literature on the subject. Since, however, only about 2 to 4 percent of nosocomial infections occur as part of epidemics [25,54], descriptions of nosocomial infections reflect almost entirely the nature of endemic infections and give little insight into epidemic problems. This does not mean that epidemics are not important, for when they are recognized they often provoke crises that call for intensive investigation and decisive control measures. It does mean, however, that an adequate description of nosocomial infections must deal with endemic and epidemic infections separately.

The purpose of this chapter is, first, to describe the nationwide incidence and distribution of endemic nosocomial infections in U.S. hospitals from several studies recently completed; second, to characterize the nature of epidemics and trends in their occurrence, including the troublesome problem of pseudoepidemics; and third, to discuss methods of estimating the adverse consequences of these problems in terms of prolongation of hospital stay, extra costs, and death.

## ENDEMIC NOSOCOMIAL INFECTIONS

### Overall Infection Rates

The effort to estimate rates of nosocomial infections began with surveillance studies of the prevalence [31] and incidence [11, 49] of infections in individual hospitals. The first effort to estimate the magnitude of the problem on a wider scale was made by the Centers for Disease Control (CDC) in a collaborative study of eight community hospitals known as the Comprehensive Hospital Infections Project (CHIP) [11]. Performed in the late 1960s and early 1970s, this contract-supported study involved very intensive surveillance efforts to detect both nosocomial and community-acquired infections. Validation studies were performed by CDC epidemiologists who visited the hospitals on a regular basis to estimate the percentage of infections detected by the hospitals' surveillance personnel. Based on an overall rate of 3.2 infected patients per 100 discharges and an adjustment for the percentage of true infections detected, it was estimated that in 1970 approximately 5 percent of patients in community hospitals developed one or more nosocomial infections (the "infection percentage"—see Chapter 4) [4], an estimate that was subsequently widely held to be the national rate of nosocomial infection.

In 1970 the CDC studies were extended to a group of approximately 80 volunteer hospitals of diverse sizes and types and called the National Nosocomial Infections Study (NNIS). Although the same general surveillance methods were used, the quality-control techniques used in CHIP were not feasible in the NNIS; however, the advantages of the NNIS were that the group contained a substantial number of hospitals representing the major types of hospitals in the United States, and the system could continue reporting data over a number of years. The overall infection rates reported from the NNIS hospitals, unadjusted for completeness of ascertainment, have remained relatively stable at about 3.2 infections per 100 discharges (the "infection ratio"—see Chapter 4) from 1970 through 1982, although some interesting secular trends have been observed and are described in this section and in Secular Trends below. Assuming that the completeness of ascertainment of infections in the NNIS was similar to that in CHIP, we could derive an estimate of the nationwide infection rate in the same range as the 5 percent figure estimated from CHIP. Although the design of these two surveillance studies limited the precision of the estimates, they gave the first consistent estimates of the order of magnitude of the problem.

One of the objectives of the Study on the Efficacy of Nosocomial Infection Control (SENIC) Project (see Chapter 3) was to derive a more precise estimate of the nationwide nosocomial infection rate from a statistical sample of U.S. hospitals [22]. On the basis of direct estimates made in 338 randomly selected general medical and surgical hospitals with 50 beds or more and statistically derived extrapolations to groups of small and specialty hospitals, the report from the SENIC Project estimated that at least 2.1 million nosocomial infections occurred among the 37.7 million admissions to the 6449 acute-care U.S. hospitals in a 12-month period in 1975–76 [17]. Thus nationwide there were approximately 5.7 nosocomial infections per 100 admissions (the infection ratio), and approximately 4.5 percent of hospitalized patients experienced at least one nosocomial infection (the infection percentage). Given that patients stayed a total of almost 299 million days in U.S. hospitals in 1976, the incidence-density of infections was approximately seven infections per 1000 patient-days (see Chapter 4).

These figures should be considered lower-bounds estimates of the current infection rates for at least three reasons. First, the methods used in most studies of nosocomial infections appear to underestimate infection rates to some degree. Although the standardized procedures used in the SENIC Project were intended to minimize this bias, some underestimation is possible. Second, the fact that the nationwide infection rate appears to have increased by approximately 10 percent from 1970 to 1975–76 [18] suggests that infection rates in the 1980s can be expected to be higher than those estimated by the SENIC Project in the mid-1970s unless substantial improvement in hospitals' surveillance and control activities counterbalances this trend.

Third, since the estimates from the SENIC Project applied specifically to the 6449 acute-care U.S. hospitals, they do not account for a substantial number of additional institutional infections that occur each year in chronic-care hospitals and nursing homes (see Chapter 23). On the basis of the one study from which incidence rates in nursing homes can be estimated, as many as 3.3 infections per 1000 resident-days may be occurring, an incidence-density about half that in acute-care hospitals [17,33]. Since there are somewhat more total institutional days spent by residents in nursing homes than by patients in hospitals (approximately 451 million versus 299 million), nursing homes may be accounting for as many as 1.5 million institutional infections per year. If these figures and the secular trends are reasonably accurate, the total number of nosocomial and other institutional infections in the 1980s may exceed 4 million per year, a number substantially larger than the total number of yearly hospital admissions for all cancers, accidents, and acute myocardial infarctions combined [50].

### Rates by Site of Infection

Nosocomial infections involve diverse anatomic sites, but the risks of these various types of infections, and consequently their relative frequency, appear to be very similar in most hospitals. Table 24-1 lists the estimated nationwide infection rates and the relative frequency of the most common sites found in the SENIC Project [17]. These estimates, as well as those from past studies, support the following conclusions: nosocomial urinary tract infections make up about one-half of all nosocomial infections; surgical wound infections, about one-quarter; respiratory tract infections, about one-eighth; bacteremia, about one-sixteenth; and all other types of nosocomial infections collectively account for the remainder. Although these data are expected to vary from hospital to hospital, they have been remarkably consistent in most reported studies.

### Rates by Pathogen

Currently the best source of information for gaining insight into the nationwide patterns of microorganisms involved in nosocomial infections is the NNIS. In the report of data from 1980–82, the epidemiology of the various nosocomial pathogens was particularly well analyzed [29]. Cultures were obtained in 90 percent of reported nosocomial infections, and in 85 percent at least one causative pathogen was isolated (a single pathogen in 65 percent and more than one in 20 percent). Among these infections of known cause, 91 percent involved aerobic bacteria; 2 percent, anaerobic bacteria; 6 percent, fungi; and the remaining 1 percent, a miscellaneous group of viruses, protozoa, and parasites. On the basis of other studies [26,51], it appears that viral nosocomial infections are substantially underreported in the NNIS, a fact that mirrors the underrecognition of viral infections in hospitals generally.

The relative frequency of the 12 most commonly isolated pathogens is shown for each of the four major sites of infection in Figure 24-1. In nosocomial urinary tract infections, *Escherichia coli* was by far the most commonly isolated pathogen, and this held true on all services. The second most common urinary pathogen was the enterococcus (*Streptococcus faecalis*), although it was slightly exceeded by *Pseudomonas* in surgical patients and by *Klebsiella* in pediatric patients, and was uncommonly seen in urinary tract infections of newborns.

In surgical wound infections *Staphylococcus aureus*

TABLE 24-1. Rates and relative frequencies of the major types of nosocomial infections, SENIC Project 1975–76

|  | Nationwide infection rates[a] | Percentage distribution |
|---|---|---|
| Urinary tract infection | 2.39 | 42 |
| Surgical wound infection | 1.39[b] | 24 |
| Lower respiratory infection | 0.60 | 11 |
| Bacteremia[c] | 0.27 | 5 |
| Other sites | 1.07 | 18 |
| All sites | 5.72 | 100 |

[a]Ratio of number of infections to number of admissions multiplied by 100 (i.e., number of nosocomial infections per 100 admissions). From Haley, R. W., et al. *Am. J. Epidemiol.* 121:159, 1985.
[b]The ratio of surgical wound infections to total operations was 2.79 per 100 operations.
[c]Includes primary and secondary bacteremias.

was the most common because of its predominance on adult and pediatric surgical services. On the obstetric and gynecology services, however, *S. aureus* was far exceeded by wound infections with *E. coli*, the enterococcus, and *Bacteroides;* group-B streptococci also played a substantial role in wound infections on obstetrics services.

In lower respiratory infections *S. aureus, Pseudomonas aeruginosa,* and *Klebsiella* were encountered with about equal frequency overall, and the variation by service was not great. In cutaneous infections *S. aureus* strongly predominated, with little variation by service.

The microbiology was somewhat more complex for primary bacteremia (i.e., culture-documented bloodstream infections in which no other site of infection was found to be seeding the bloodstream with organisms). *S. aureus* and *E. coli* predominated overall and constituted between approximately 9 and 15 percent of primary bacteremias on all services. Coagulase-negative staphylococci made up about 10 percent of infections on all services, except pediatrics, on which they predominated (17 percent) and obstetrics, on which they were uncommonly isolated. *Bacteroides* predominated on gynecology services (24 percent), and along with other anaerobes were relatively common on obstetrics services but uncommonly isolated on the other services. Group-B streptococci were the most commonly isolated pathogens from primary bacteremia on obstetrics (16 percent) and newborn (25 percent) services but were virtually unseen on the other services. It should be noted that some primary bacteremias are in fact cases of secondary bacteremias in which the primary site of infection was never ascertained.

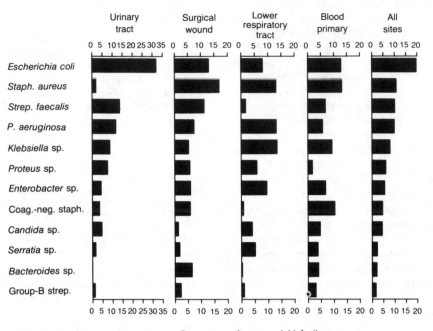

FIG. 24-1. Percentage distribution of nosocomial infections by primary pathogen at the major sites of infection, National Nosocomial Infection Study, 1980–82.

It is interesting that on the basis of its microbiology secondary bacteremia (not included in Fig. 24-1) appears to be a different disease from primary bacteremia. The risk of secondary bacteremia is highest following cardiovascular infections (e.g., endocarditis of a prosthetic valve), postoperative infections of the central nervous system, intraabdominal wound infections, and burns. Complication of infection by secondary bacteremia is most common on the newborn and pediatric services, of intermediate likelihood on the medical and surgical services, and least likely on the obstetrics and gynecologic services. Secondary bacteremia is also more likely in large teaching hospitals. The organisms most commonly involved are *Bacteroides* (12 percent); *Serratia* and *S. aureus* (each about 10 percent); group-B streptococci and coagulase-negative staphylococci (7 percent); and *Klebsiella, Enterobacter, Pseudomonas, Candida,* and *Acinetobacter* (each about 5 to 6 percent).

*E. coli* is the most commonly isolated pathogen from all nosocomial infections regardless of site because of its predominance in urinary tract infections and its substantial role in infections at all other sites. *S. aureus* is the second most commonly isolated pathogen overall, because of its frequent involvement in all types of infections except those of the urinary tract where it is uncommonly found. The high frequency of enterococci, the third leading pathogen, has per-

haps not been well enough appreciated in the past. The important role of *Pseudomonas* as the fourth most common pathogen is not surprising because of its well-known involvement in all types of nosocomial infections. Improvements in surveillance and laboratory techniques are needed to clarify the roles of coagulase-negative staphylococci, anaerobic bacteria, and viruses, whose true frequencies have probably been misjudged, and perhaps more attention should be given to the endogenous mechanisms and nosocomial transmission of group-B streptococci in the obstetric and newborn areas.

### Patient Risk Factors

The strongest determinants of the risk of nosocomial infection are the characteristics and exposures of patients that predispose them to infection. Like the so-called chronic diseases, such as coronary heart disease and cancer, nosocomial infections arise from the complex interactions of multiple causal factors, and these factors interact differently in predisposing to the different types of infection (see Chapter 1). Much epidemiologic and clinical research has been devoted to studying the characteristics associated with the occurrence of nosocomial infection [7,9,10,13,14,16, 20,27,28,32,35,47]. It has not always been clear whether the associations are truly causal, however, and these characteristics are often referred to as "risk factors," that is, factors associated with, but not necessarily causing, infection. Undoubtedly, some of these risk factors are true causes of infection; others are only coincidentally associated with infection because they frequently follow infection or occur along with the truly causal factors. Complicating matters additionally is the fact that two or more risk factors often occur simultaneously in the same patient, sometimes exerting additive, or even synergistic, effects. In this respect it is said that these risk factors are strongly intercorrelated.

To design strategies for preventing infections, it is important to try to differentiate among coincidental indicators of risk, independent causal factors, and synergistic interactions of causal factors. There have been several attempts to study multiple risk factors using modern techniques of multivariate statistical analysis. Much of this work can be illustrated by the results of analyses of risk factors performed on a group of 169,526 patients who made up a representative sample of patients admitted to acute-care U.S. hospitals in 1975–76 as part of the SENIC Project [16, 20,27]. In an initial descriptive analysis, population estimates of infection rates for each of the four major types of infection were calculated within each category of exposure to between 10 and 20 separate risk factors [20]. A striking finding was that all of the risk factors were associated with infection at all four sites. At first this seems surprising since one would not expect a direct causal association between being treated on a respirator, for example, and acquiring a urinary tract infection. The explanation, of course, is that some of the associations are indicative of direct causal relationships; others are indicative of partial causal relationships, potentiated or diminished by other concurrent influences; and others (such as that between respirators and urinary tract infection) represent largely coincidental associations (most patients on respirators also have indwelling urinary catheters that predispose them to urinary tract infection).

The two factors that appeared to exert the strongest causal influences in all four sites of infection were indicators of the degree of the patient's underlying illness: (1) in surgical patients, the duration of the patient's operation and (2) an index of the number and type of distinct diagnoses and surgical procedures recorded (intrinsic risk index). After these, several factors were strongly associated with infections at one or two sites but not with all four. Having a combined thoracic-abdominal operation was strongly associated

with pneumonia and surgical wound infection; undergoing a "dirty" or "contaminated" operation was associated with surgical wound infection; having an indwelling urinary catheter was linked to urinary tract infection; being on a respirator, with pneumonia and bacteremia; previous nosocomial infection, with bacteremia; and receiving immunosuppressive therapy, with bacteremia. Examples of risk factors that had weaker associations with all four sites were age, sex, previous community-acquired infection, and length of preoperative hospitalization.

Another way of viewing these complex multivariate associations is to hypothesize that there are two general categories of causes: those that allow microorganisms access to vulnerable areas of the patient (e.g., operations, catheters, and endotracheal tubes) and those that reduce the patient's capacity for resisting the multiplication and injurious effects of the microorganisms (e.g., immunosuppressive therapy and metabolic sequelae of lengthy operations). In a later multivariate analysis of the SENIC data, this concept was tested using surgical wound infection as an example [16]. The resulting multivariate model indicated that 2 factors—the familiar surgical wound classification [2] and undergoing an abdominal operation—both represent the likely degree of contamination of the operative wound. These measured a portion of the risk of surgical wound infection largely separate from that measured by the other two factors—the duration of the operation and the number of diagnoses recorded. These later 2 factors represent the patient's degree of susceptibility to infection. Moreover, one might infer that the degree of contamination of the wound and the patient's susceptibility were of about equal importance in the genesis of surgical wound infections because each of these four factors was about equally important in the multivariate model.

Although multivariate modeling of risk factors for nosocomial infection is still in an early stage, several conclusions appear reasonable, pending additional research. The risk of infection is primarily determined by definable causal factors reflecting the patient's underlying susceptibility to infection or the degree to which microorganisms have access to vulnerable body sites. Modification of one or more of these factors can alter a patient's risk. Multivariate statistical models can be developed to predict accurately a patient's risk of nosocomial infection from measurable risk factors. The aggregate infection risk of a hospital, or of a subgroup of patients in a hospital—measured by its overall nosocomial infection rate—is primarily determined by the mix of patients, that is, by the causal factors present when patients are admitted and to which they are exposed in diagnosis and treatment. These conclusions form the basis for understanding much of the variation in nosocomial infection rates described in the following sections.

### Rates by Service

Differences in the average risk of infection among groups have been most readily noticed in relation to the well-known differences in infection rates of different services, or specialty areas. Analyses of the SENIC data showed that surgical patients were not only at highest risk of surgical wound infections but also had rates of infection for the other main sites almost three times higher than medical patients (approximately four times higher for pneumonia and approximately one and one-half times higher for urinary tract infection and bacteremia). Moreover, even though surgical patients constituted only 42 percent of general medical and surgical patients, they accounted for 71 percent of nosocomial infections of the four major types (virtually all surgical wound infections, 74 percent of pneumonias, 56 percent of urinary tract infections, and 54 percent of bacteremias) [20]. Analyses of data collected in the NNIS from 1980–82 showed a stepwise decrease of nosocomial infection rates by service from surgical to medical, to gynecology and obstetrics, with the lowest rates on pediatric and newborn services [30]. Other investigators have quantitated the inordinately high risks of patients in special care units (see Chapter 18).

### Rates by Type of Hospital

It has long been apparent that overall nosocomial infection rates differ substantially from one hospital to another. In the midnineteenth century Sir James Y. Simpson found that the rate of death from infection of amputated extremities varied directly with the size of the hospital in which the operation was performed (with larger hospitals having higher rates), a phenomenon he called "hospitalism" [46]. The rates of surgical wound infection in the five hospitals participating in the National Research Council's prospective evaluation of ultraviolet light were found to vary from 3.2 to 11.0 percent [28]. The average infection rates of hospitals participating in the NNIS were reported to vary from 1.7 percent in small community hospitals to over 11 percent in chronic disease hospitals [4].

A multivariate analysis of the SENIC data was performed to determine what institutional characteristics of the hospitals best predicted their nosocomial infection rates. Of the many characteristics studied, those found to differentiate best were affiliation with a medical school (teaching vs. nonteaching), size of the hospital (indicated by the number of beds), type of control or ownership of the hospital (municipal, nonprofit, investor-owned), and region of the country [21]. The overall nosocomial infection rates averaged 3.7 percent in small (< 200 beds) nonteaching hospitals, 5.1 percent in large (≥ 200 beds) nonteaching ones, 7.6 percent in nonprofit teaching hospitals, and 8.5 percent in the municipal teaching hospitals. These relationships tended to be consistent for each of the four major sites of infection. Since nonprofit teaching hospitals tend to have fewer than 500 beds, and municipal teaching hospitals tend to have more than 500, teaching hospitals could be subclassified almost as well by size as by ownership-control. In addition, within these four hospital groups rates of urinary tract infection, surgical wound infection, and bacteremia were generally higher in the northeast and north central regions, whereas rates of pneumonia were higher in the West. A similar analysis of NNIS data from 1980–82 found the lowest rates in nonteaching hospitals, intermediate levels in teaching hospitals with less than 500 beds, and highest rates in teaching hospitals with 500 beds or more [29]. This relationship held consistently for infection rates at each site, on every service, and for all pathogens.

To test the hypothesis that these differences were largely due to differences in the mix of patients typically treated in the different types of hospitals, the SENIC data were additionally analyzed to try to explain the differences. Indeed, indexes of the patients' risk factors explained the greatest part of the interhospital differences, and after controlling for indexes of patients' risk factors, average length of stay, and measures of the completeness of diagnostic workups for infection (e.g., culturing rates), the differences in the average infection rates of the various hospital groups virtually disappeared. These findings indicate that much of the difference in observable infection rates of different types of hospitals is due to differences in the intrinsic degree of illness of their patients and related factors, and because of this the overall infection rate per se usually gives little insight into whether the hospital's infection control efforts are effective.

### Trends Over Time

The occurrence of nosocomial infections is a dynamic process. Changes are constantly occurring in the types of patients admitted to hospitals, risk factors to which they are exposed, character of the pathogens predominating in the hospital milieu, quality of patient care, thrust of infection control efforts, and other important factors. Two indicators of the dynamic nature of the problem are the seasonality of certain types of nosocomial infections and the long-term secular trends that may occur.

SEASONALITY  Analysis of the data from NNIS has repeatedly shown seasonal variations in the occurrence of nosocomial infections involving certain gram-negative rods [1,29,39]. The report of the 1980–82 results shows clear seasonal peaks of infections in the summer and early fall with certain gram-negative bacteria, specifically—*Klebsiella, Enterobacter, Serratia,* and *Acinetobacter* species as well as *P. aeruginosa.* In contrast to the seasonal occurrence of pyogenic infections in the community [3], staphylococcal and streptococcal infections show no significant seasonal variation in the hospital. There also seems to be no seasonality of infections with other common bacteria, such as *E. coli,* enterococcus, *Enterobacter,* and anaerobes. Nosocomial viral respiratory infections occur mostly during the seasons in which they occur in the community (e.g., influenza and respiratory syncytial virus infections in the winter and early spring) [26].

SECULAR TRENDS  Changes in nosocomial infection rates over time are difficult to study. In prevalence studies performed over several decades, the relatively small sample sizes have hampered the detection of secular changes. An analysis of secular trends in the NNIS from 1970–79 suggested that surgical wound infections may have decreased slightly over the decade, bacteremias may have increased, and other types of infections remained unchanged [1]. The inability to control these analyses for other factors that could have accounted for the changes, however, rendered these findings difficult to interpret.

To address this issue, the rates from the two time periods of the SENIC Project, 1970 and 1975–76, were compared after controlling for the most likely biasing factors [18]. After controlling for changes in levels of patient risk, length of stay, and completeness of ascertainment of infections, overall nosocomial infection rates in acute-care hospitals were found to have increased by a statistically significant 10 percent over the five-year period. Additional analysis, however, revealed three contrasting trends in different groups of hospitals. In the group that established no substantial infection surveillance and control programs, the overall infection rate increased by 18 percent; in the group in which moderately intensive programs were established, the rates tended to show no significant change; and in the group that established very intensive programs for preventing infections at all four of the major sites, the overall rate

decreased by 36 percent. These findings suggest strongly that the overall nationwide trend of a 10 percent increase was really the result of two forces that were affecting the nationwide rate in opposite directions: (1) the continuing introduction of more invasive and immunocompromising techniques into the care of hospitalized patients, which tended to increase the infection rates and (2) the efficacy of newly established infection surveillance and control programs, which tended to decrease them. This indicates that future secular trends in the rates of endemic nosocomial infections could be in either direction, depending strongly on the balance that hospitals achieve between technologic innovations in patient care, and investments in infection surveillance and control programs.

## EPIDEMIC NOSOCOMIAL INFECTIONS

### Incidence, Recognition, and Control
While many scientific articles have been written to describe individual outbreaks of nosocomial infections, very little work has been done to estimate the frequency of these epidemics. The earliest study on this subject was performed in the CDC's CHIP study in the early 1970s [25]. Among seven community hospitals participating in CHIP during 12 months in 1972–73, a computerized threshold program screened the regularly reported cases of nosocomial infection for clusters of infection that might indicate an outbreak, and a CDC epidemiologist additionally analyzed the data to eliminate purely coincidental clusters. Then CDC staff members visited the hospitals that had potential outbreaks to confirm the nature of the problem and suggest control measures if needed. From these data it was estimated that one true outbreak occurred for every 10,000 hospital admissions and that outbreaks accounted for somewhere in the range of 2 percent of patients with nosocomial infections. More recently, Wenzel and colleagues [54] estimated that 3.7 percent of nosocomial infections in a large university-affiliated referral hospital occurred in outbreaks. Although confined to a relatively small number of hospitals, these estimates appear to confirm the prevailing view that outbreaks account for a relatively small proportion of nosocomial infections.

Besides the attention often provoked by outbreaks, one of the main reasons for infection control personnel to be concerned about them is that, if recognized and investigated, control measures can often stop them, thus bringing about demonstrable reductions in morbidity and mortality. In the CHIP investigations, despite the fact that the seven hospitals had very active surveillance systems, one-third of the clusters had not been recognized before the CDC visit. This fact points out the difficulty of recognizing outbreaks even in the best of circumstances and suggests the usefulness of inventive computerized systems to screen surveillance data for potential epidemics (see the Role of Computers in Surveillance, Chapter 4). It also suggests that hospitals that appear never to have outbreaks may simply be failing to recognize them.

The CHIP investigations also demonstrated that 40 percent of the outbreaks appeared to have resolved spontaneously, while the remaining 60 percent continued until control measures were instituted [25]. Half of the outbreaks that continued were controlled by measures taken by the hospitals' infection control staff and the other half were completely resolved only after measures suggested by the outside investigators. While the rate of spontaneous resolution explains the origin of opinions against surveillance expressed by some persons, if these figures are representative of community hospitals in general—and it must be recalled that these were hospitals with very active infection surveillance systems—then a large number of outbreaks may currently be going unrecognized and uncontrolled, despite the advanced state of infection surveillance and control programs.

*Characteristics of Epidemics*

To recognize, investigate, and control epidemics most effectively, it is helpful to understand their nature, likely problems, and mechanisms. Although there are many reports of individual outbreak investigations, the only body of information large enough to study the characteristics of epidemics is the series of investigations performed by the CDC in response to hospitals that request assistance. Recently reviewed by Stamm and colleagues [48], this series included 252 hospital investigations performed between 1956 and 1979. Since various factors influence the types of investigations undertaken by the CDC, this series should be considered only an approximate reflection of the mix of outbreaks that occur routinely in U.S. hospitals. The studies probably reflect the types of problems that infection control personnel find particularly urgent, perplexing, or difficult to control.

In the early phase of these investigations—1958 through 1962—the outbreak investigations were divided between epidemics of gastrointestinal disease—mainly due to *Salmonella* and enteropathogenic *E. coli*—and outbreaks of staphylococcal infections. Almost all these problems were centered in newborn nurseries. From the mid-1960s on, investigations of

staphylococcal infections diminished abruptly down to an occasional yearly episode, and by the early 1970s, outbreaks of gastroenteritis similarly diminished to a continuing low level. From the late 1960s until the present, there has been an increasing trend toward involvement of gram-negative pathogens, bacteremia, and surgical wound infections in outbreaks, and toward problems related to intensive care and newly introduced medical devices and related technologies. For example, during the 1970s the type of infection most commonly investigated was bacteremia. Also noteworthy was an increase in investigations of hepatitis outbreaks that peaked in 1975 and 1976. Other interesting groupings included outbreaks of necrotizing enterocolitis in nurseries and sternal wound infections following open-heart surgery—both beginning in the mid-1970s—and outbreaks of legionnaires' disease, about half of which occurred in hospitals. From the late 1960s on, an increasingly important issue in many of these investigations was the resistance of epidemic pathogens to multiple antimicrobial agents, particularly resistance of gram-negative bacilli to aminoglycosides and of *S. aureus* to methicillin and/or gentamicin.

One of the most striking characteristics of the epidemics was that the percentage distribution of types of infections and pathogens involved bore little resemblance to the percentage distributions in endemic infections. Eight types of nosocomial infections occurred with roughly the same frequency in the CDC-investigated epidemics, whereas three or four major types predominate in endemic infections (Table 24-2). Moreover, except for *S. aureus,* which constituted about 10 to 12 percent of both endemic and epidemic infections, the pathogens found most commonly in the CDC-investigated epidemics—*Salmonella,* hepatitis B, *Serratia,* and *Enterobacter*—were among the least common pathogens in endemic infections (Table 24-2). This interesting relationship probably reflects in part the fact that outbreaks occur by epidemiologic mechanisms different from those that cause endemic infections. It may also be due to the greater likelihood that clusters of unusual pathogens or site-pathogen combinations will be recognized by infection control personnel, and conversely that outbreaks of infections similar to the most common endemic infections are not as easily recognized. The selection factors that get the CDC involved in investigations also undoubtedly contribute to this profile of epidemic problems.

Of most practical value is the information that this investigatory experience provides for identifying the modes of transmission of future outbreaks. The outbreaks can be classified into five groups according to the most likely mode of transmission: (1) common-source, (2) human transmitter (carrier), (3) person to person (cross-infection), (4) airborne (microorganisms traveling more than a few feet), and (5) uncertain mode of transmission. After outbreaks were classified in this manner, it became apparent that certain site-pathogen combinations, sometimes specific to a patient group, could be rather specifically identified with particular modes of transmission. These combinations are listed in Table 24-3.

Knowledge of these unique combinations can be useful in focusing on the most likely mode of transmission early in an outbreak investigation. For example, outbreaks of *Salmonella* gastroenteritis among adult patients are most likely to be spread by a common source (e.g., food), whereas a similar outbreak in a newborn nursery is most likely to be spread by person-to-person contact, although the roles of hospital-prepared formula or breast-milk banks must be

TABLE 24-2. Comparison of types of infections and pathogens involved in endemic and epidemic infections

|  | Endemic infections[a] (%) | Epidemic infections[b] (%) |
|---|---|---|
| Type of infection |  |  |
| Urinary tract infection | 38 | 10 |
| Surgical wound infection | 27 | 9 |
| Pneumonia | 16 | 12 |
| Cutaneous infection | 6 | 11 |
| Bacteremia | 4 | 16 |
| Meningitis | <1 | 6 |
| Gastroenteritis | <1 | 17 |
| Hepatitis | <1 | 12 |
| Other | 8 | 7 |
| Total | 100 | 100 |
|  |  |  |
| Pathogen |  |  |
| *Escherichia coli* | 19 | 3 |
| Enterococcus | 10 | <1 |
| *Staphylococcus aureus* | 10 | 12 |
| *Pseudomonas* | 9 | 4 |
| *Proteus* | 8 | <1 |
| *Klebsiella* | 8 | 3 |
| *Enterobacter* | 4 | 7 |
| Group-A streptococci | 2 | 3 |
| *Serratia* | 2 | 8 |
| *Salmonella* | <1 | 11 |
| Hepatitis B virus | <1 | 10 |
| Total | 100 | 100 |

[a]National Nosocomial Infection Study, 1975 through 1978.
[b]1971 through 1979.
Source: Adapted from Stamm, W. E., et al. *Am. J. Med.* 70:393, 1981.

ruled out (see Chapter 32). Similarly, outbreaks of hepatitis A are most likely to be due to a common source, whereas outbreaks of hepatitis B are most likely to be caused by either a human disseminator (e.g., a surgeon who is a carrier) or person-to-person spread (e.g., poor blood-handling techniques) (see Chapter 35). Surgical wound infections caused by the group-A streptococci are very likely to be related to a human disseminator (e.g., an anal carrier), whereas wound infections due to *S. aureus* may be due to a human disseminator or other factors (see Chapter 27). It is noteworthy that no human disseminator was implicated in 68 outbreaks involving gram-negative bacilli. Perhaps half the outbreaks of staphylococcal infections in nurseries can be attributed to cross-infection and about one-quarter to human disseminators (see Chapter 19). Outbreaks of bacteremia due to gram-negative bacilli, particularly if they occur in intensive care units, are very likely to be due to a common source (e.g., contaminated devices), whereas outbreaks involving other types of infections with gram-negative bacilli (particularly urinary tract infections) are most likely to be due to cross-infection (e.g., inadequate care of urinary catheters) (see Chapter 18). The types of outbreaks likely to involve airborne spread are varicella infections, *Aspergillus* infections, and legionnaires' pneumonia, particularly in immunosuppressed patients (see Chapter 37), and pulmonary tuberculosis, particularly in hospital personnel working in emergency rooms (see Chapter 2).

*Multihospital Epidemics*

An issue of increasing concern is the involvement of multiple hospitals in an epidemic. This occurs most commonly by interhospital spread and less commonly through the nationwide distribution of products that cause or predispose to infection. First, a pathogen involved in an epidemic in one hospital may be introduced into the patient population of another hospital, generally by one of three modes of transmission: (1) transfer of infected or colonized patients, particularly those with burns or decubitus ulcers [38,40, 41,44,53], (2) transfer of colonized or infected medical house staff [45,51], and (3) transient colonization of hands of nurses and technicians who alternate working at different hospitals [42]. Since the transfer of house staff and seriously ill patients occurs primarily among large, university-affiliated, tertiary referral hospitals, interhospital spread appears to occur most frequently in these and less commonly among smaller community hospitals [19]; however, the increasing trend of nurses and technicians toward working in cooperatives serving several hospitals may encourage more interhospital spread.

TABLE 24-3. Likely modes of transmission of the most common types of nosocomial infection epidemics

| Mode of transmission | Site or type of infection | Pathogen | Service or patient group | CDC investigations[a] Number[b] | (%) |
|---|---|---|---|---|---|
| Common source | Gastroenteritis | *Salmonella* | Adults | 11/13 | 85 |
| | Hepatitis | Hepatitis A virus | Any | 3/3 | 100 |
| | Urinary tract or bacteremia | *Pseudomonas cepacia* | Any | 4/4 | 100 |
| | Pulmonary | *Pseudomonas aeruginosa* | Any | 4/5 | 80 |
| | Bacteremia | Gram-negative bacilli | Any | 10/13 | 77 |
| Human disseminator | Bacteremia | Any | ICU | 6/7[c] | 86 |
| | Surgical wound | Group-A streptococci | Any | 5/6 | 83 |
| | Surgical wound | *Staphylococcus aureus* | Surgery | 3/8 | 38 |
| | Cutaneous | *S. aureus* | Nursery | 5/24 | 20 |
| | Hepatitis | Hepatitis B virus | Any | 3/12 | 25 |
| Cross-infection | Gastroenteritis | *Salmonella* or enteropathic *Escherichia coli* | Nursery | 16/17 | 94 |
| | Cutaneous | *S. aureus* | Nursery | 12/24 | 50 |
| | Urinary tract | Gram-negative bacilli | Any | 10/14 | 71 |
| | Hepatitis | Hepatitis B virus | Any | 8/12 | 67 |
| Airborne | Varicella | V-Z virus | Any | — | ? |
| | Pulmonary | *Aspergillus* | Any | — | ? |
| | Pulmonary | *Mycobacterium tuberculosis* | Any | — | 100 |
| | Pulmonary | *Legionella* | Any | — | ? |

V-Z = varicella-zoster; ICU = intensive care unit.
[a]From Stamm, W. E., et al. *J. Infect. Dis.* 136(Suppl.)S151, 1977.
[b]Of the 13 outbreaks of gastroenteritis due to *Salmonella* among adults, 11 were transmitted by the common-source mode.
[c]From Wenzel, R. P., et al. *IC Infect. Control* 4:371, 1983.

Interhospital transmission of outbreaks has been observed primarily in epidemics involving pathogens with important antimicrobial resistance patterns, such as multiply resistant *Serratia* [42], aminoglycoside-resistant gram-negative bacilli [53], and methicillin-resistant *S. aureus* [19] (see Chapter 12). This association could be due to the genetic colinkage of antimicrobial resistance with factors that facilitate spread. For example, strains of diverse genera that are prevalent in nosocomial infections have been shown to share the genetic information that confers resistance to important antimicrobial agents [43]. Similarly, the diversity of phage types involved in epidemiologically clear outbreaks of methicillin-resistant *S. aureus* infections suggests the spread of genetic information among different strains that have strong predispositions to infect hospital patients. Alternatively, the association could be due merely to the fact that resistance provides a dramatic marker that increases the likelihood that an epidemic will be recognized. If so, as infection control personnel in hospitals develop more sensitive means for recognizing outbreaks and more effectively share surveillance data with their counterparts in other local hospitals (e.g., through area-wide surveillance systems supported by local health departments), interhospital transmission of infection will probably be recognized more commonly.

In the second type of multiple-hospital involvement, a widely distributed product used in patient care may cause infections in many hospitals simultaneously, due to either intrinsic contamination of the product in the factory [34] or design flaws or common usage errors that encourage in-use contamination in the hospitals [5,8] (see Chapters 36 and 38). After a series of nationwide epidemics due to intrinsically contaminated products in the early 1970s, it appeared that intrinsic product contamination would become a common problem [34]. Subsequent experience has shown, however, that in-use contamination is a far more common explanation for infections related to newly introduced products and devices.

*Pseudoepidemics*

Not all clusters of reported nosocomial infections constitute true epidemics of disease. In the prospective study of outbreaks in the CDC's CHIP project, about 80 percent of the clusters of infection identified statistically by a computerized threshold program were judged to be coincidental, illustrating the need for epidemiologic evaluation of surveillance data to detect outbreaks [25]. More important, of those clusters that appeared to represent real outbreaks epidemiologically, approximately one-third (37 percent) were found not to be true outbreaks after thorough investigations. Most of these pseudoepidemics were traced to systematic errors or changes in clinical diagnosis of infections or in reporting of infections by the infection surveillance staff; systematic errors in the microbiology laboratory explained fewer than one-quarter of them. In the series of epidemic investigations performed by the CDC, pseudoepidemics accounted for only 11 percent of the presumed outbreaks for which hospitals requested epidemiologic assistance, and about one-half of these were attributed to processing errors in the microbiology laboratories [48,52].

The difference in results between these two studies is probably due to the more extensive investigation usually done by hospital personnel to rule out artifactual problems before the CDC epidemiologists undertake a formal investigation. Consequently in the routine practice of infection control in most hospitals, the majority of pseudoepidemics may be due to diagnostic and reporting errors as reflected by the CHIP investigation, although truly perplexing pseudoepidemics may more often be traced to contaminated equipment or errors in the microbiology laboratory, as reflected in the CDC investigations (see Chapter 5).

## ADVERSE CONSEQUENCES OF NOSOCOMIAL INFECTIONS

In reading the scientific literature on the subject of nosocomial infections, one is struck by the disproportionately large number of articles on the adverse consequences—prolongation of hospital stay, extra hospital costs or charges, and deaths—of these infections. The importance of these studies stems from two factors: first, in contrast to most other hospital services, hospitals have not traditionally been able to charge patients or their insurance carriers directly for the costs of their infection surveillance and control programs; and second, it has been difficult to demonstrate how many nosocomial infections these programs prevent. Consequently it has been necessary, or at least very helpful, in many hospitals to demonstrate how costly the infections are for the patients to justify the expenditures of mounting and sustaining a preventive program.

Estimates of extra costs attributable to nosocomial infections must be interpreted with some caution. Because the actual costs of hospitals are difficult to study, their charges to patients are usually used as a substitute for their actual costs. However, hospitals commonly redistribute charges among different cost centers to recover costs not fully reimbursed by public and private reimbursement agencies, so charges to the patient may not accurately represent the hospital's costs of treatment [12]. In addition, estimates expressed in dollars must be constantly adjusted for inflation to be meaningful in the current context.

The studies on this subject have used one of three methods to estimate the prolongation of hospital stay, extra charges, and number of deaths attributable to nosocomial infections: concurrent assessments of infected patients, unmatched comparisons of infected and uninfected patients, and matched comparisons [24]. Each approach has its own strengths and weaknesses, which may lead to a biased estimate.

The concurrent assessment method relies on a physician to visit each infected patient frequently enough to enumerate all extra days and extra services that were performed to treat the infection but would not have occurred if the infection had not supervened. By applying the routine per diem room charge to each extra day and the actual charge for each ancillary service from the patient's hospital bill, the physician can estimate directly the total extra charges attributable to the nosocomial infection. The advantage of this method is that the identifiable charges are directly itemized; the disadvantage is that, by relying on the physician's clinical judgment to determine what days and services are attributable, the results may be biased in either direction depending on how conservative the judgments are. For example, for some days or services the circumstances are too ambiguous to make a clear determination; if the ambiguous circumstances are always considered nonattributable to infection, the final results will be underestimates.

In the unmatched comparison approach, the average extra stay (or charge) is estimated after the completion of a study by subtracting the average total length of stay (or total hospital charges) of uninfected patients from that of infected patients. This method always substantially overestimates the attributable extra stay (and charges) because of a strong selection bias: patients who contract nosocomial infections tend strongly to have been more seriously ill at the beginning of hospitalization (and thus more strongly predisposed to long hospital stays, higher charges, and death) than those who are likely to be discharged without an infectious complication.

The matched comparison approach is similar to the comparison approach except that for each infected patient the investigator selects one or more uninfected patients who are similar to their match on several selected characteristics. The advantage of this approach, like the unmatched comparison, is that it avoids use of clinical judgment to decide what is attributable to infection. The disadvantage is that it is extremely difficult to match uninfected patients with infected patients closely enough to overcome the powerful selection bias. To the degree that the matching fails to control for this underlying noncomparability of infected and uninfected patients, the study will overestimate the magnitude of extra stay, extra charges, or deaths attributable to infection.

One fundamental reason that the matched comparison studies performed to date have failed to control for the large disparity in degree of underlying illness is that they have generally matched infected and uninfected patients on the wrong characteristics. These studies have used as matching criteria such predictors of infection risk as age, sex, service, first diagnosis, and first surgical procedure. To control for the underlying predisposition to an extended hospital stay, the matching characteristics should include the major factors that determine prolonged hospital stay (or death), which are not necessarily the same as those that predispose to nosocomial infection. For example, it was pointed out in one of the earliest concurrent assessment studies that some of the main factors that increase length of stay apart from nosocomial infection include severe underlying illness, development of unexpected complications such as venous thrombosis or pulmonary embolism, and social factors that delay discharge [6]; these appear frequently to be colinked with the severity-of-illness factors that also predispose to nosocomial infections. For matching comparisons to be useful, it must be shown that the matching characteristics are sufficiently complete predictors of prolonged hospital stay, high total hospital costs, or the probability of death to control completely for the bias caused by the greater complexity of the infected patients' underlying conditions.

In a study comparing all three methods in the same cohort of patients, the estimates were lowest by the concurrent assessment, intermediate for the matched approach, and highest for the unmatched approach [24]. Published estimates of the prolongation of stay for surgical wound infections by the concurrent assessment method have ranged from 1.5 to 11 days;

by the matched comparison approach, from 7 to 18 days; and by the unmatched comparison approach, from 5 to 26 days.

Nationwide estimates of the number of deaths attributable to nosocomial infections have varied even more widely. By combining data from the SENIC project [17] and from a concurrent assessment of mortality performed in NNIS [30], 19,000 deaths nationwide per year were estimated to be directly attributable to nosocomial infections, and in 58,000 more deaths nosocomial infections contributed but were not the only cause (Table 24-4). At the other extreme, a recent study using multivariate logistic regression techniques, with the same drawbacks as the matched comparison approach, estimated 300,000 deaths per year nationwide attributable to nosocomial urinary tract infections alone [37]. Regardless of which estimates are used, however, the large number of deaths from nosocomial infections is a cause for concern. Counting only the 19,000 deaths directly caused by nosocomial infections—the lowest estimate derived from NNIS and SENIC—would place it just below the tenth leading cause of death in the U.S. population; whereas, if one also counts the 58,000 deaths to which nosocomial infections contribute but are not the only cause, it would rank as the fourth leading cause of death, just behind heart disease, cancer, and stroke. These figures indicate the need for an accurate counting of nosocomial infections in our national systems for vital and health statistics [17].

Until the serious methodologic problems are solved, it seems prudent to use the more conservative estimates derived from concurrent assessments even though they may underestimate the magnitude of the problem. Table 24-4 lists the estimates of extra days and costs derived from concurrent assessments in the SENIC pilot studies [23] and estimates of deaths derived from the NNIS [30] and SENIC [17]. In view of the new strategies of prospective reimbursement for hospital care and the evidence for the efficacy of infection surveillance and control programs, it is likely that the direct cost reductions produced by infection control will be sufficiently obvious even if derived from the most conservative estimates.

*Preventability*

That large numbers of endemic as well as epidemic nosocomial infections are preventable has periodically been reaffirmed by milestone reports such as that of Semmelweis, studies on the effects of proper care of urinary catheters and respirators, and the virtual elimination of epidemic bacteremia caused by intrinsic contamination of commercial intravenous solu-

TABLE 24-4. Estimated extra days, extra charges, and deaths attributable to nosocomial infections annually in U.S. hospitals

| | Extra days | | Extra charges | | | Deaths | | | |
| | | | | | | Infections directly causing death | | Infections contributing to death | |
| | Avg. per infection[a] | Est. U.S. total[b] | Avg. extra charges per infection in 1975 dollars[a] | Avg. extra charges per infection in 1985 dollars[c] | Est. U.S. total in 1985 dollars[b] | Percent[d] | Est. U.S. total[b] | Percent[d] | Est. U.S. total[b] |
|---|---|---|---|---|---|---|---|---|---|
| Surgical wound infection | 7.3 | 3,726,000 | $838 | $2,734 | $1,395,000,000 | 0.64 | 3,251 | 1.91 | 9,726 |
| Pneumonia | 5.9 | 1,339,000 | $1,511 | $4,947 | $1,123,000,000 | 3.12 | 7,087 | 10.13 | 22,983 |
| Bacteremia | 7.4 | 762,000 | $935 | $3,061 | $315,000,000 | 4.37 | 4,496 | 8.59 | 8,844 |
| Urinary tract infection | 1.0 | 903,000 | $181 | $593 | $535,000,000 | 0.10 | 947 | 0.72 | 6,503 |
| Other site | 4.8 | 1,946,000 | $430 | $1,408 | $571,000,000 | 0.80 | 3,246 | 2.48 | 10,036 |
| All sites | 4.0[e] | 8,676,000 | $560[e] | $1,833[e] | $3,939,000,000 | 0.90[e] | 19,026 | 2.70[e] | 58,092 |

[a]Adapted from Haley, R. W., et al. Am. J. Med. 70:51, 1981, by pooling data from the three SENIC pilot study hospitals.

[b]Estimated by multiplying the total number of nosocomial infections estimated in the SENIC Project (Haley, R. W., et al. Am. J. Epidemiol. 121:159, 1985) by the average extra days, average extra charges, or percentage of infections causing or contributing to death, respectively.

[c]1985 dollars estimated from Haley, R. W., et al. Am. J. Med. 70:51, 1981, by pooling data from the three hospitals and adjusting for the annual rate of inflation of hospital expenses from 1976 to 1985 (range 4.9 to 19.1 percent) obtained from the American Hospital Association's National Panel Survey.

[d]Unpublished analyses of data reported to the National Nosocomial Infections Study (NNIS) in 1980–1982 (Hughes, J. M., et al. Abstracts of the Twenty-Second Interscience Conference on Antimicrobial Agents and Chemotherapy, 1982).

[e]Nationwide estimate obtained by summing the products of the site-specific estimate of the average extra days, average extra charges, or the percentage of infections causing or contributing to death, respectively, from the SENIC pilot studies (Haley, R. W., et al. Am. J. Med. 70:51, 1981), and the nationwide estimate of the proportion of nosocomial infections affecting the site from the main SENIC analysis (Haley, R. W., et al. Am. J. Epidemiol. 121:159, 1985).

tions. Yet when a representative sample of infection control program heads were asked to estimate the percentage of nosocomial infections presently occurring in U.S. hospitals that are preventable, the responses varied from 1 percent to 100 percent, with a mean of approximately 50 percent; the program heads who had served in their positions longer and who were more knowledgeable about infection control tended to give lower estimates [15]. There are at least two reasons for this lack of agreement among those working most closely with the problem. First, it is difficult to demonstrate that infections have been prevented or to infer whether active infections were preventable [36]. Second, because new risk factors for infection are constantly appearing, necessary control measures are continually evolving, and ability to manage the patient-care behavior of hospital personnel is changing, the true percentage of infections that are preventable probably changes from time to time.

Consequently the only meaningful way of framing the preventability question is to ask what percentage of nosocomial infections can be prevented by maintaining an intensive infection surveillance and control program that continually adjusts to the new risks and attempts to manage patient-care behavior. Since this was precisely the question framed in the SENIC Project, there is an approximate answer. Among U.S. hospitals in the 1970s, approximately one-third of all nosocomial infections were preventable by maintaining infection surveillance and control programs with particular characteristics [18] (see Chapter 3). The fact that the approaches found to be effective were general preventive strategies aimed at managing infection control (i.e., surveillance and control programs), rather than individual preventive practices (e.g., catheter care), suggests that the SENIC estimate of preventability will remain reasonably accurate for the foreseeable future.

## REFERENCES

1. Allen, J. R., Hightower, A. W., Martin, S. M., and Dixon, R. E. Secular trends in nosocomial infections: 1970–79. *Am. J. Med.* 70:389, 1981.
2. Altemeir, W. A., Burke, J. F., Pruitt, B. A., et al. (Eds.). *Manual on the Control of Infection in Surgical Patients.* Philadelphia: Lippincott, 1976, pp. 29–30.
3. Benenson, A. S. Staphylococcal Disease. In Benenson, A. S. (Ed.), *Control of Communicable Diseases in Man* (14th ed.). Washington, DC: American Public Health Association, 1985, pp. 358–366.
4. Bennett, J. V., Scheckler, W. E., Maki, D. G., and Brachman, P. S. Current National Patterns: United States. In *Proceedings of the International Conference on Nosocomial Infections,* August 3–6, 1970. Chicago: American Hospital Association, 1971, pp. 42–49.
5. Centers for Disease Control. Nosocomial Bacteremia from Intravascular Pressure Monitoring Systems. *National Nosocomial Infections Study Report,* 1977, issued 1979, pp. 31–36.
6. Clarke, S. Sepsis in surgical wounds with particular reference to *Staphylococcus aureus. Br. J. Surg.* 44:592, 1957.
7. Cruse, P. J. E., and Foord, R. The epidemiology of wound infection: A 10-year prospective study of 62,939 wounds. *Surg. Clin. North Am.* 60:27, 1980.
8. Donowitz, L. G., Marsik, F. J., Hoyt, J. W., and Wenzel, R. P. *Serratia marcescens* bacteremia from contaminated pressure transducers. *J.A.M.A.* 242:1749, 1979.
9. Dukes, C. Urinary infections after excision of the rectum: Their cause and prevention. *Proc. R. Soc. Med.* 22:259, 1928.
10. Ehrenkrantz, N. J. Surgical wound infection occurrence in clean operations: Risk stratification for interhospital comparisons. *Am. J. Med.* 70:909, 1981.
11. Eickhoff, T. C., Brachman, P. S., Bennett, J. V., and Brown, J. F. Surveillance of nosocomial infections in community hospitals. I. Surveillance methods, effectiveness, and initial results. *J. Infect. Dis.* 120:305, 1969.
12. Finkler, S. A. The distinction between costs and charges. *Ann. Intern. Med.* 96:102, 1982.
13. Freeman, J., and McGowan, J. E., Jr. Risk factors for nosocomial infection. *J. Infect. Dis.* 138:811, 1978.
14. Garibaldi, R. A., Britt, R. A., Coleman, M. L., Reading, J. C., and Pace, N. L. Risk factors for predicting postoperative pneumonia. *Am. J. Med.* 70:677, 1981.
15. Haley, R. W. The "hospital epidemiologist" in U.S. hospitals, 1976–1977: A description of the head of the infection surveillance and control program. *Infect. Control* 1:21, 1980.
16. Haley, R. W., Culver, D. H., Morgan, W. M., White, J. W., Emori, T. G., and Hooton, T. M. Identifying patients at high risk of surgical wound infection: A simple multivariate index of patient susceptibility and wound contamination. *Am. J. Epidemiol.* 121:206, 1985.
17. Haley, R. W., Culver, D. H., White, J. W., Morgan, W. M., and Emori, T. G. The nation-

wide nosocomial infection rate: A new need for vital statistics. *Am. J. Epidemiol.* 121:159, 1985.

18. Haley, R. W., Culver, D. H., White, J. W., Morgan, W. M., Emori, T. G., Munn, V. P., and Hooton, T. M. The efficacy of infection surveillance and control programs in preventing nosocomial infections in U.S. hospitals. *Am. J. Epidemiol.* 121:182, 1985.

19. Haley, R. W., Hightower, A., Khabbaz, R. F., Thornsberry, C., Martone, W. J., Allen, J. R., and Hughes, J. M. The emergence of methicillin-resistant *Staphylococcus aureus* infections in United States hospitals: Possible role of the house staff–patient transfer circuit. *Ann. Intern. Med.* 97:297, 1982.

20. Haley, R. W., Hooton, T. M., Culver, D. H., et al. Nosocomial infections in U.S. hospitals, 1975–1976: Estimated frequency by selected characteristics of patients. *Am. J. Med.* 70:947, 1981.

21. Haley, R. W., Morgan, W. M., Culver, D. H., and Schaberg, D. R. Differences in nosocomial infection rates by type of hospital: The influence of patient mix and diagnostic medical practices. (Unpublished data presented at Interscience Conference on Antimicrobial Agents and Chemotherapy. Miami, Fla., October 4, 1982.)

22. Haley, R. W., Quade, D. H., Freeman, H. E., and the CDC SENIC Planning Committee. Study on the efficacy of nosocomial infection control (SENIC Project): Summary of study design. *Am. J. Epidemiol.* 111:472, 1980.

23. Haley, R. W., Schaberg, D. R., Crossley, K. B., Von Allmen, S. D., and McGowan, J. E., Jr. Extra days and prolongation of stay attributable to nosocomial infections: A prospective interhospital comparison. *Am. J. Med.* 70:51, 1981.

24. Haley, R. W., Schaberg, D. R., Von Allmen, S. D., and McGowan, J. E., Jr. Estimating the extra charges and prolongation of hospitalization due to nosocomial infections: A comparison of methods. *J. Infect. Dis.* 141:248, 1980.

25. Haley, R. W., Tenney, J. H., Lindsey, J. O. II, Garner, J. S., and Bennett, J. V. How frequent are outbreaks of nosocomial infection in community hospitals? *Infect. Control* 6:233, 1985.

26. Hall, C. B. Nosocomial viral respiratory infections: Perennial weeds on pediatric wards. *Am. J. Med.* 70:670, 1981.

27. Hooton, T. M., Haley, R. W., Culver, D. H., White, J. W., and Morgan, W. M. The joint associations of multiple risk factors with the occurrence of nosocomial infection. *Am. J. Med.* 70:960, 1981.

28. Howard, J. M., Barker, W. F., Culbertson, W. R., et al. Postoperative wound infections: The influence of ultraviolet irradiation of the operating room and of various other factors. *Ann. Surg.* 160(Suppl.):1, 1964.

29. Hughes, J. M., Culver, D. H., White, J. W., et al. Nosocomial infections surveillance, 1980–1982. *Morbid. Mortal. Weekly Rep.* 32:1SS, 1983.

30. Hughes, J. M., Munn, V., Jarvis, W., Culver, D. H., and Haley, R. W. Mortality Associated with Nosocomial Infections in the United States, 1975–1981. *Abstracts of the Twenty-Second Interscience Conference on Antimicrobial Agents and Chemotherapy,* October 4–6, 1982, Miami Beach, Florida, p. 189.

31. Kislak, J. W., Eickhoff, T. C., and Finland, M. Hospital-acquired infections and antibiotic usage in the Boston City Hospital. *N. Engl. J. Med.* 271:834, 1964.

32. Lidwell, O. M. Sepsis in surgical wounds: Multiple regression analysis applied to records of postoperative hospital sepsis. *J. Hyg. (Camb.)* 59:259, 1961.

33. Magnussen, M. H., and Robb, S. S. Nosocomial infections in a long-term care facility. *Am. J. Infect. Control* 2:12, 1980.

34. Maki, D. G., Rhame, F. S., Mackel, D. C., and Bennett, J. V. Nationwide epidemic of septicemia caused by contaminated intravenous products. I. Epidemiologic and clinical features. *Am. J. Med.* 60:471, 1976.

35. McCabe, W. R., and Jackson, G. C. Gram-negative bacteremia. I. Etiology and ecology. *Arch. Intern. Med.* 110:847, 1962.

36. McGowan, J. E., Jr., Parrott, P. L., and Duty, V. P. Nosocomial bacteremia: Potential for prevention of procedure-related cases. *J.A.M.A.* 237:2737, 1977.

37. Platt, R., Polk, B. F., Murdock, B. S., et al. Mortality associated with nosocomial urinary tract infection. *N. Engl. J. Med.* 307:637, 1982.

38. Price, E. H., Brain, A., and Dickson, J. A. S. An outbreak of infection with a gentamicin- and methicillin-resistant *Staphylococcus aureus* in a neonatal unit. *J. Hosp. Infect.* 1:221, 1980.

39. Retailliau, H. F., Hightower, A. W., Khabbaz, R. F., et al. *Acinetobacter calcoaceticus:* A nosocomial pathogen with an unusual seasonal pattern. *J. Infect. Dis.* 139:371, 1979.

40. Sapico, F. L., Montgomerie, J. Z., Canawati, H. N., and Aeilts, G. Methicillin-resistant *Staphylococcus aureus* bacteriuria. *Am. J. Med. Sci.* 281:101, 1980.

41. Saraglou, G., Cromer, M., and Bisno, A. L. Methicillin-resistant *Staphylococcus aureus:* Interstate spread of nosocomial infections with emergence of gentamicin-methicillin-resistant strains. *Infect. Control* 1:81, 1980.

42. Schaberg, D. R., Alford, R. H., Anderson, R., Farmer, J. J., Melly, M. A., and Schaffner, W. An outbreak of nosocomial infection due to multiply resistant *Serratia marcescens:* Evidence of interhospital spread. *J. Infect. Dis.* 134:181, 1976.

43. Schaberg, D. R., Rubens, C. R., Alford, R. H., Farrar, E. D., Schaffner, W., and McGee, Z. A. Evolution of antimicrobial resistance and nosocomial infection: Lessons from the Vanderbilt experience. *Am. J. Med.* 70:445, 1981.

44. Shanson, D. C. Antibiotic-resistant *Staphylococcus aureus. J. Hosp. Infect.* 2:11, 1981.

45. Shanson, D. C., and McSwiggan, D. A. Operating theatre–acquired infection with a gentamicin-resistant strain of *Staphylococcus aureus:* Outbreaks in two hospitals attributable to one surgeon. *J. Hosp. Infect.* 1:171, 1980.

46. Simpson, J. Y. Our existing system of hospitalism and its effects. Part I. *Edinburgh Med. J.* 14:816, 1869.

47. Stamm, W. E., Martin, S. M., and Bennett, J. V. Epidemiology of nosocomial infections due to gram-negative bacilli: Aspects relevant to development and use of vaccines. *J. Infect. Dis.* 136(Suppl.):S151, 1977.

48. Stamm, W. E., Weinstein, R. A., and Dixon, R. E. Comparison of endemic and epidemic nosocomial infections. *Am. J. Med.* 70:393, 1981.

49. Thoburn, R., Fekety, F. R., Cluff, L. E., and Melvin, V. B. Infections acquired by hospitalized patients. *Arch. Intern. Med.* 121:1, 1968.

50. United States National Center for Health Statistics. *Utilization Patterns and Financial Characteristics of Nursing Homes in the United States: 1977 National Nursing Home Survey.* Hyattsville, MD: National Center for Health Statistics, 1981. (Data from the National Health Survey, Series 13, No. 53. DHHS publication no. [PHS]81-1714.)

51. Valenti, W. M., Meneges, M. A., Hall, C. B., et al. Nosocomial viral infections: Epidemiology and significance. *Infect. Control* 1:33, 1980.

52. Weinstein, R. A. Pseudoepidemics in hospital. *Lancet* 2:862, 1977.

53. Weinstein, R. A., and Kabins, S. A. Strategies for prevention and control of multiple drug-resistant nosocomial infection. *Am. J. Med.* 70:449, 1981.

54. Wenzel, R. P., Thompson, R. L., Landry, S. M., Russell, B. S., Miller, P. J., Ponce de Leon, S. P., and Miller, G. B. Hospital acquired infections in intensive care unit patients: An overview with emphasis on epidemics. *Infect. Control* 4:371, 1983.

55. Winn, R. E., Ward, T. T., Hartstein, A. I., et al. Epidemiological, bacteriological, and clinical observations on an interhospital outbreak of nafcillin-resistant *Staphylococcus aureus. Curr. Chemother.* 2:1096, 1979.

# 25 NOSOCOMIAL URINARY TRACT INFECTIONS

Walter E. Stamm

## INCIDENCE

According to data from numerous hospitals [1,35, 47,51] and from multihospital collaborative studies [9,10], nosocomial urinary tract infections have consistently been responsible for 35 to 45 percent of all hospital-acquired infections. Thus approximately 2 per 100 patients admitted to acute-care hospitals in the United States, or more than 0.8 million patients per annum, acquire nosocomial bacteriuria. In the National Nosocomial Infection Study (NNIS), urinary tract infections have consistently accounted for 40 percent of all hospital-acquired infections, with little change evident over the period 1970–83. In this survey, the proportion of nosocomial bacteriuria cases associated with or contributing to mortality was less than 3 percent.

## ENDEMIC VERSUS EPIDEMIC INFECTIONS

Endemic acquisition accounts for the majority of nosocomial urinary tract infections, but numerous examples of epidemic transmission have been reported [58,65]. Epidemics of nosocomial bacteriuria have resulted from inadequately disinfected cystoscopes, nonsterile irrigating solutions used on multiple patients, contaminated disinfectants in catheter-insertion trays, and most commonly, person-to-person transmission on crowded hospital wards where aseptic catheter-care practices were not being used [58,65]. Frequent catheter irrigation appeared to be an important causal factor in several epidemics. Multiply drug-resistant strains of *Serratia, Proteus, Klebsiella,* and *Pseudomonas* possessing unique antimicrobial susceptibility patterns have afforded opportunities to trace the epidemiology of nosocomial urinary tract infections in the epidemic setting. Most often, epidemic investigations have demonstrated transmission of organisms from one catheterized patient to another via the hands of hospital personnel. In several epidemics, patients with unrecognized asymptomatic bacteriuria lasting for weeks or even months served as an important reservoir, with temporal and spatial clustering of subsequent cases in proximity to these "source" patients.

Most likely, a proportion of infections classified as endemic actually result from clusters or microepidemics of cross-infection on hospital wards. Using tertiary marker systems (e.g., pyocin typing, serotyping, and phage typing) to trace cross-infection attributable to common organisms such as *Escherichia coli*, Schaberg and coworkers [57] demonstrated that approximately 15 percent of endemic nosocomial infections occur in clusters suggestive of cross-infection. *Pseudomonas* and *Serratia* infections were most often clustered, and *E. coli* infections least often. Thus attention to the same factors that prevent or terminate epidemics of nosocomial bacteriuria (see the section Prevention) presumably would prevent some endemic infections as well.

## RISK FACTORS

Nearly all nosocomial urinary tract infections occur in patients with indwelling urinary catheters (about 80 percent) or after other types of transient urologic instrumentation (about 20 percent). Specific host factors associated with an increased risk of infection during or after instrumentation include female sex, older age, and an increasing degree of underlying illness (Table 25-1). The risk of developing nosocomial bacteriuria in women exceeds the risk in men by approximately twofold in each decade of life [29, 64], but men more often manifest secondary bacteremia. For both men and women, the risk of catheter-associated bacteriuria increases with age [29,64]. In addition, 95 percent of deaths and 83 percent of bacteremic episodes occur in patients over 50 years of age [64].

In addition to host factors (which for the most part cannot be altered), the risk of urinary infection relates directly to the type and duration of urologic instrumentation. After a single in-and-out catheterization, between 1 and 20 percent of patients acquire bacteriuria [61,71]; lower rates occur in healthy outpatients and higher rates in older hospitalized patients. Indwelling urethral catheters draining into an open collecting vessel result in bacteriuria in 100 percent of patients within 4 days [32]. With the sterile closed collecting systems used in most hospitals today, bacteriuria occurs on the average in 10 to 25 percent of catheterized patients [15,39,70]. In hospitals with active prevention programs, rates less

TABLE 25-1. Risk factors associated with infection during catheterization

| Alterable factors | Unalterable factors |
| --- | --- |
| Indications for catheterization | Female sex |
| Length of catheterization | Older age |
| Catheter-care techniques | Severe underlying illness |
| Type of drainage system | Meatal colonization |

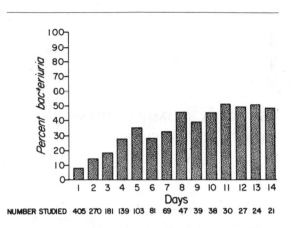

FIG. 25-1. Percent of catheterized patients with bacteriuria by day of catheterization. (From Garibaldi, R.A., Burke, J.P., Dickman, M.L., and Smith, C.B. Factors predisposing to bacteriuria during indwelling urethral catheterization. *N. Engl. J. Med.* 291:216, 1974. Reprinted by permission of The New England Journal of Medicine.)

than 10 percent have been reported [18]. The per day risk of developing bacteriuria appears comparable throughout catheterization (3 to 6 percent), but the cumulative risk increases with duration of catheterization [16,18]. Thus about 50 percent of hospitalized patients catheterized longer than 7 to 10 days develop bacteriuria [18,39] (Fig. 25-1).

## ETIOLOGY

Aerobic gram-negative rods account for the vast majority of catheter-associated urinary tract infections. In recent data collected by the National Nosocomial Infection Study (Table 25-2), Enterobacteriaceae and pseudomonads accounted for over 80 percent of all culture-positive infections. Of the gram-positive organisms, group-D streptococci accounted for approximately 14 percent, while staphylococci collectively caused about 5 percent. Increasingly, the aerobic gram-negative rods causing nosocomial bacteriuria have been characterized by multiple antimicrobial resistance, often mediated by transmissible plasmids [42].

The relative proportion of infections accounted for by an individual species, as well as their antimicrobial susceptibility patterns, vary widely from hospital to hospital, and fluctuate with time in each hospital. In two studies [37,64], *E. coli* and *Proteus* accounted for a progressively smaller percentage of nosocomial urinary tract infections as the period of hospitalization and catheterization lengthened. Conversely, *Serratia*

TABLE 25-2. Pathogens causing
nosocomial urinary tract infections*

| Pathogen | Percent |
|---|---|
| *Escherichia coli* | 31.9 |
| Group-D streptococci | 14.4 |
| *Pseudomonas aeruginosa* | 11.5 |
| *Klebsiella* | 8.8 |
| *Proteus mirabilis* | 6.7 |
| *Candida* species | 4.4 |
| *Enterobacter* | 4.1 |
| *Staphylococcus epidermidis* | 3.4 |
| *Staphylococcus aureus* | 1.9 |
| *Serratia* | 1.6 |
| Group-B streptococci | 1.2 |
| *Pseudomonas* species | 1.1 |
| *Morganella* | 0.9 |
| Others | 8.1 |
| Total | 100.0 |

n = 54,940 infections.
*Source: National Nosocomial Infections Study 1981–1982 (Haley,
R. W., et al. *Am. J. Epidemiol.* 121:159, 1985).

and *Pseudomonas aeruginosa* accounted for a progressively greater proportion of infection as hospitalization increased. These observations suggest that a proportion of catheter-associated infections are, in fact, not newly acquired, but may represent recognition of previous covert bacteriuria after insertion of a urinary catheter.

## PATHOGENESIS

Occasionally nosocomial urinary tract infections result from direct introduction of urethral microorganisms at the time of catheterization, other instrumentation (usually cystoscopy), or surgery. Based on time of onset, however, most catheter-associated infections arise later in the period of catheterization. Microorganisms causing these infections enter the catheterized urinary tract either through the lumen of the catheter (intraluminal route) or along its external surface in the mucous sheath between the catheter and urethral mucosa (transurethral route) (Fig. 25-2). Women appear to be at greater risk than men of transurethral infection. In a recent study about two-thirds of women who developed catheter-associated bacteriuria were shown to have previous urethral and rectal colonization with their infecting strain, compared with only one-third of men [11]. Thus the pathogenesis of catheter-associated infections in many women resembles the pathogenesis of noncatheter-associated infections. Studies of community-acquired

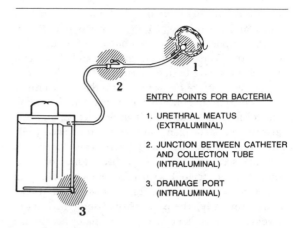

FIG. 25-2. Entry points for bacteria causing catheter-associated urinary tract infection.

bacteriuria in women suggest that fecal organisms establish introital, vaginal, and urethral colonization before urinary tract infection with these strains occurs [44,60]. Since only one-third of men who develop catheter-associated bacteriuria can be demonstrated to have antecedent urethral and rectal colonization, the urethral route of entry may be less important in men. In either sex, however, establishment of urethral colonization with a gram-negative rod apparently confers an increased risk of subsequent infection. Garibaldi and coworkers [16] showed that the increased risk of subsequent nosocomial bacteriuria associated with a positive meatal culture was approximately fourfold in women and twofold in men.

Bacteriuria may also result from microorganisms that enter the collecting system and ascend through the lumen of the urinary catheter into the bladder (intraluminal route). In studies assessing this mode of entry, approximately 15 to 20 percent of infected patients can be demonstrated to have their infecting organism in the collecting bag before entry into the bladder [17]. Retrograde spread of the organism from the collecting bag to the bladder occurs within 24 to 48 hours in nearly all such patients [17]. Thus contamination of the collecting bag or introduction of organisms by disconnection of the distal catheter and proximal collection tube can allow entry of organisms that produce nosocomial bacteriuria. Rarely, nosocomial bacteriuria arises secondary to hematogenous seeding of the genitourinary tract or as a complication of surgical procedures involving the urinary tract or adjacent structures.

Neither specific virulence factors common to strains producing nosocomial bacteriuria nor specific host factors important in conferring protection against such infections have been extensively studied. Petersdorf, Turck and coworkers [33,79] reported that *E. coli* strains responsible for nosocomial bacteriuria belonged to specific serotypic groups, and these serotypic groups have been associated with virulence factors characteristic of *E. coli* organisms that cause urinary tract infections in noncatheterized patients, including dulcitol fermentation, hemolysin production, a greater quantity of k antigen, and serum resistance [63]. However, specific virulence properties associated with organisms causing nosocomial bacteriuria, or more important, associated with bacteremia secondary to catheter-associated bacteriuria, deserve additional study. Similarly, the propensity of some patients to develop catheter-associated bacteriuria or bacteremia may be related to host factors. In noncatheterized patients, the ability of the uroepithelial cells to support bacterial adherence, the urinary pH, intrinsic urinary antibacterial activity, and intrinsic bladder wall antibacterial activity have been related to risk of infection [59]. Studies aimed at delineating similar factors associated with catheter-associated bacteriuria should be undertaken.

While catheter-associated bacteriuria has been clearly linked to subsequent bacteremia, the mechanism through which such bacteremia occurs has not been elucidated. Bacteremia could occur secondary to mucosal ulcerations resulting from bladder wall damage during catheterization. Cystoscopic examination of catheterized patients and animals suggests such ulcerations are common after seven days of catheterization [30,51]. Alternatively, the well-known association of bacteremia with either insertion or withdrawal of urinary catheters or other urologic instruments suggests that bacteremia may result from the mucosal trauma associated with these events [67]. Finally, as in non-catheter-associated urinary tract infections, bacteremia may result when infection ascends beyond the bladder to involve the kidney, prostate, or other portions of the upper urinary tract.

At present, the various mechanisms through which bacteremia may develop have not been distinguished in studies of catheter-associated bacteriuria. To address this issue, localization of the site of infection in patients with catheter-associated bacteriuria requires additional study. Certainly, few patients with unobstructed urinary tracts develop characteristic clinical evidence of renal infection. The antibody-coated bacteria (ACB) test has been used in patients with catheter-associated bacteriuria to assess the frequency of asymptomatic renal involvement and in some studies has suggested the presence of clinically inapparent upper tract infection in 15 to 20 percent of those with bacteriuria [20,69]. However, comparison of the ACB test with other localization tests in catheterized patients has not been carried out, and thus the actual significance of a positive result has not been established.

## SEQUELAE

From the short-term clinical perspective, most catheter-associated urinary tract infections appear benign. Because only 20 to 30 percent cause symptoms, most episodes can be classified as asymptomatic bacteriuria [25,52]. Pyuria accompanies most episodes of catheter-associated bacteriuria, however, suggesting host invasion rather than simple bladder colonization [53, 62]. Not many patients with catheter-associated bacteriuria have undergone localization studies, and thus the proportion of patients with bladder, prostate, or kidney infections has not been determined. In studies using the ACB test, as many as one-quarter of episodes of catheter-associated bacteriuria were positive, suggesting upper tract infection [20,69]. Clinically recognized ascending infection, including prostatitis, epididymitis, seminal vesiculitis, and renal infection may arise from bacteriuria originating during catheterization, but their frequency remains ill-defined. In general, these complications arise primarily in patients with long-term indwelling catheters, and are rare in patients whose catheterization lasts less than ten days.

The major systemic complication of catheter-associated bacteriuria has been secondary bacteremia. Although the risk of secondary bacteremia is small in any given patient, taken collectively bacteremia arising from catheter-associated bacteriuria accounts for a large proportion of all nosocomial bacteremias. Most series of hospitalized patients with gram-negative bacteremia demonstrate that 30 to 40 percent of all gram-negative bacteremias acquired in the hospital originate in the urinary tract [13,36,66,78], making this the most commonly recognized source of gram-negative sepsis. Estimates of the frequency of secondary bacteremia associated with catheterization range from 1 per 50 to 1 per 150 catheterized bacteriuric patients. In one prospective study, however, 8 percent of patients had bacteremia after urinary catheterization [67]. Bacteremia thus may occur more often than is recognized clinically, especially on insertion, withdrawal, manipulation, or obstruction of the catheter.

Recent studies have associated nosocomial bacteriuria with an increased mortality [55]. After adjustment for other factors, such as type of underlying disease, severity of illness, age, and sex, an approximately threefold relative increase in risk of death was observed by Platt and colleagues [55]. The mechanism through which bacteriuria may produce increased mortality has not been elucidated. To date, catheter-associated bacteriuria has not been associated with long-term renal damage, but the natural history of this condition has not been studied prospectively.

Several authors have attempted to estimate whether increased hospital stay results from nosocomial urinary tract infection [19,21,54]. In a case-controlled study, Givens and Wenzel [19] found that urinary infections occurring in surgical patients resulted in 2.4 days of increased hospitalization and a cost of $558 per patient. Other estimates of increased hospitalization attributable to catheter-associated infection have ranged from 1 to 4 days and estimates of increased costs have ranged from none to $1100 [21, 54].

## CLINICAL MANIFESTATIONS

Only 25 to 35 percent of patients with catheter-associated bacteriuria experience symptoms attributable to infection, and thus most cases can be classified as asymptomatic bacteriuria [52]. When present, symptoms include dysuria, urgency, frequency, and hematuria. Fever, flank pain, or other clinical manifestations of pyelonephritis develop in less than 1 percent of patients with catheter-associated bacteriuria [53,62]. Thus despite the absence of symptoms in most patients with catheter-associated bacteriuria, the presence of pyuria suggests host invasion and actual infection rather than simple bladder colonization. Clinical findings characteristic of gram-negative bacteremia accompany bacteremia secondary to bacteriuria. Interestingly, the onset of bacteremia usually occurs within 24 hours of the onset of bacteriuria except for *Serratia marcescens* infections, in which bacteremia most commonly originates days after the onset of bacteriuria [37].

## DIAGNOSIS

Most physicians diagnose catheter-associated bacteriuria by obtaining a urine specimen for culture via needle aspiration of the distal catheter or via aspiration through a sampling port on the catheter itself. Since specimens so collected presumably represent actual bladder urine, contamination is infrequent. In recent studies, catheter aspiration corresponded with cultures obtained by suprapubic aspiration in at least 90 percent of cases [3]. Because the bladder is normally sterile, the presence of any bacteriuria in such a specimen probably signifies the presence of bacteriuria in the bladder itself. Quantitative culture results may demonstrate organisms ranging in quantity from 10 to more than $10^5$ cfu per milliliter. Various authors have used quantitative bacterial counts ranging from at least $10^2$ to at least $10^5$ cfu per milliliter to define infection in catheterized patients. However, prospective studies to establish a specific quantitative level as more or less indicative of infection have not been carried out. For clinical purposes, bacteriuria of $10^3$ cfu per milliliter or more, especially when associated with pyuria, can probably be taken as evidence of bladder infection. Catheter-tip cultures should not be used to diagnose urinary infection [22].

## TREATMENT

Since most patients with catheter-associated bacteriuria lack associated symptoms, treatment need not be undertaken unless the patient is at high risk for complications such as bacteremia or renal infection. Thus treatment may be useful in patients with neutropenia, obstructed urinary tracts, renal transplants, or other specific situations in which bacteriuria in and of itself may be of significant risk. In most patients without such complicating clinical features, however, treatment of bacteriuria should not be undertaken. In such patients, bacteriuria often resolves spontaneously with removal of the catheter; if one anticipates removal of the catheter, treatment should be postponed until that time. After catheter removal, the patient can either be observed for a period of time and subsequently treated if the bacteriuria does not resolve spontaneously, or treated empirically after the catheter has been removed. Treatment with the catheter in place often results in emergence of resistant strains, and eradication of bacteriuria in the presence of an indwelling catheter has been largely unsuccessful [8]. Since the antimicrobial susceptibility patterns of strains causing catheter-associated bacteriuria vary widely, choice of a specific antimicrobial agent should be guided by the in vitro antimicrobial sensitivities of the infecting organisms.

## PREVENTION

Guidelines for prevention of catheter-associated bacteriuria have been published by the Centers for Disease Control [80]. Until more has been learned about the pathogenesis of nosocomial bacteriuria, preventive efforts must be focused largely on aseptic care of the urinary catheter (Table 25-3). These measures are directed primarily at preventing entry of bacteria into the sterile closed drainage system and have been most effective when the period of catheterization is less than seven days. Probably the single most effective preventive measure is to avoid use of the indwelling catheter whenever possible. Indications for continued catheterization should be reviewed on a daily basis, since the risk of bacteriuria associated with catheterization can be markedly reduced by removing catheters as soon as possible. Catheters should be inserted aseptically under sterile conditions. In addition, the closed drainage system should be considered a sterile site, and aseptic precautions should be observed when manipulating any portion of the system. Inadvertent or purposeful disconnection of the catheter and collecting system predisposes to bacteriuria, as does use of nonsterile technique when emptying urine from the collecting vessel. Continuous downhill gravity flow drainage should be maintained at all times. Both hospital personnel and catheterized patients should be taught the importance of these principles.

Many technologic improvements in catheters and drainage systems have been proposed as means of preventing bacteriuria. These include polymeric silicone (Silastic) rather than rubber catheters; baffles, vents, or other devices for preventing reflux or retrograde infection; instillation of antimicrobial or antiseptic agents into the catheter bag; culture vents on the side of the urinary catheter; permanent junctions between the distal catheter and collecting system; and antimicrobial substances impregnated into the catheter itself. Most of these technologic improvements make sense from the standpoint of the pathogenesis of these infections, but it has been difficult in controlled trials to prove the effectiveness of most such innovations. Since opening the closed collecting system has been clearly shown to predispose to infection, sampling ports that permit cultures to be obtained without opening the system are pre-

TABLE 25-3. Methods for
prevention of catheter-associated infections

Avoid catheterization.
Decrease duration of catheterization.
Use intermittent catheterization.
Insert catheters aseptically.
Use a closed sterile drainage system.
Use a condom catheter in cooperative patients.
Maintain gravity drain.
Apply topical meatal antimicrobials in women.
Separate infected and uninfected patients.

ferred. Although sometimes inconvenient, drainage systems marketed as a single unit extending from the bladder catheter to the collecting bag prevent inadvertent disconnection of the catheter and collecting system and may reduce infection rates.

More controversial has been the value of using antimicrobial substances such as hydrogen peroxide or chlorhexidine in the collecting bag. In one study Maizels and Schaeffer [43] demonstrated that hydrogen peroxide in the collecting bag successfully eradicated microorganisms introduced into the collecting system and prevented retrograde infection. In another study, use of hydrogen peroxide in the drainage spigot prevented retrograde infection [12]. On the other hand, some studies have failed to find benefit attributable to either system [56,68]. In part the potential benefit of such a system relates to the proportion of infections acquired via the intraluminal route. In previous studies an estimated 15 to 20 percent of infections occurred in this manner [50], and thus the majority of infections may not be preventable through control measures aimed at interrupting this route of bacterial ingress. Such measures may, however, reduce reservoirs of organisms available for transfer from one catheterized patient to another on the hands of personnel. In hospitals in which technique is not optimal and intraluminal infection occurs more often, these preventive approaches may have greater benefit.

Since many infections acquired during catheterization arise following urethral and meatal colonization with the infecting strain, topical application of antiseptic agents to these areas has been advocated as a preventive measure. In a large and careful study addressing this topic, Garibaldi and coworkers [5] were unable to ascribe benefits to twice-daily application of povidone-iodine solution followed by povidine-iodine ointment. In a subsequent study Burke and colleagues [6] demonstrated reduced infection rates using a twice-daily polyantimicrobial ointment applied at the meatal-catheter junction; however, the benefit was seen only in a specific high-risk group: women with previous meatal colonization. Thus although the overall efficacy of this approach remains in doubt, it is apparently effective in some patients. Alternative means of blocking urethral colonization and ascension of organisms from the urethral meatus surface should be investigated. Many years ago, antimicrobial impregnation of catheters was assessed [7]. Although the technique was not successful in those studies, newer approaches using other antibiotics or methods of application might be warranted. Irrigation of the bladder with antimicrobial solutions is another technique used to prevent catheter-associated bacteriuria. Martin and Bookrajian [2,45] first reported prevention of infections using acetic acid or a neomycin-polymyxin B irrigant in an open collecting system. Instillation of chlorhexidine into the bladder has also been reported as efficacious [34]. However, Warren and colleagues [76], in a carefully controlled trial, were unable to ascribe any benefits to continuous irrigation with polymyxin-neosporin and found that patients on irrigation developed infections with more resistant organisms.

Systemic antibiotic agents have been demonstrated to decrease the likelihood of bacteriuria during the first five to seven days of catheterization [5,6,39, 52,76]. In addition, in one controlled trial systemic antimicrobials were associated with a decreased rate of catheter-associated bacteriuria [4]. Thus systemic antimicrobial agents probably reduce the likelihood of bacteriuria developing during short-term catheterization. However, whether the risks, side effects, and costs of such antimicrobials warrant their use for this purpose requires additional study. In patients with long-term urinary catheterization, continued antimicrobial use results in the emergence of resistant strains and probably should be avoided [74]. Antimicrobial prophylaxis has been of clear benefit in preventing postoperative urinary infection among men with sterile urine undergoing urologic surgery [14, 27].

Daily culture monitoring of catheterized patients to detect bacteriuria before onset of symptoms or bacteremia has been advocated [39]. However, Garibaldi and colleagues [18] found monitoring to be of little benefit since most symptomatic infections and bacteremias occurred within 24 hours of the onset of bacteriuria. Alternative methods of urinary drainage such as condom drainage, suprapubic catheterization, or intermittent catheterization (see following section) may be preferable in selected patients. Condom catheters have been most successfully used in alert, cooperative patients receiving meticulous skin care to prevent meatal ulceration [26]. In this setting condom catheters used for 2 to 4 weeks appear to have an infection risk less than that of indwelling catheters. In uncooperative patients who manipulate the condom catheter, however, infections occur at least as frequently as in comparable patients with indwelling catheters [69]. Suprapubic catheterization has been largely used by gynecologists and urologists for short-term catheterization after surgical procedures. Reported experience suggests that this technique may be less often associated with bacteriuria than is indwelling urethral catheterization, but a direct prospective comparison of the two techniques has not been published [28,46]. Suprapubic catheterization eliminates the urethral route of infection and thus might be expected to cause less bacteriuria than urethral catheterization.

## CHRONIC CATHETERIZATION

Bacteriuria occurs in essentially all patients who require chronic catheter drainage because of spinal cord injury or other causes of neurogenic bladder [72]. Prospective evaluation of such patients has shown that they experience multiple sequential episodes of bacteriuria, usually with a different species each episode (reinfection), but occasionally with a single persisting species [49,77]. Polymicrobial infections commonly occur. The vast majority of bacteriuric episodes are asymptomatic, but bacteremia, pyelonephritis, epididimitis, and renal calculi occur with sufficient frequency to be of major concern [49,75,77]. These conditions probably contribute in part to deterioration in renal function, a major cause of death in this population [76].

Prevention of infection has been difficult in patients with chronic indwelling catheters. Aseptic techniques applied to patients with short-term catheterization have not been successful in those with longer term catheterization. Antimicrobial treatment of asymptomatic bacteriuric episodes had no apparent impact on the frequency or natural history of infection according to one study, and instead selected for antibiotic-resistant strains [77]. Similarly, antimicrobial prophylaxis or the use of urinary antiseptics has not been successful in these patients [73]. Most bacteriuria in these patients is accompanied by pyuria, suggesting that more than simple bladder colonization has occurred, but studies to localize such infections to the lower or upper urinary tract have been largely unsuccessful [38,49]. Patients with chronic catheterization should probably receive antibiotic treatment only for clinically apparent pyelonephritis, epididymitis, or bacteremia—not for asymptomatic bacteriuria. Treatment should be guided by in vitro sensitivities, since these patients develop infections with multiply resistant hospital-acquired strains.

Recent experience suggests that intermittent catheterization, even if done in a nonsterile fashion, may be a significant advance over chronic indwelling catheterization. Infection reportedly can be avoided altogether in some patients and occurs periodically in others on intermittent catheterization [23,41]. In addition, low-dose continuous antimicrobial prophylaxis may be effective in patients with intermittent catheterization [76], but it is generally not effective in patients with indwelling catheters.

# REFERENCES

1. Barrett, F. F., Casey, J. I., and Finland, M. Infections and antibiotic use among patients at Boston City Hospital. *N. Engl. J. Med.* 278:5, 1968.

2. Bastable, J. R. G., Peel, R. N., Birch, D. M., and Richards, B. Continuous irrigation of the bladder after prostatectomy: Its effect on post-prostatectomy infections. *Br. J. Urol.* 49:689, 1977.

3. Bergquist, D., Bronnestam, R., Hedelin, H., and Stahl, A. The relevance of urinary sampling methods in patients with indwelling Foley catheters. *Br. J. Urol.* 52:92, 1980.

4. Britt, M. R., Garibaldi, R. A., Miller, W. A., et al. Antimicrobial prophylaxis for catheter-associated bacteriuria. *Antimicrob. Agents Chemother.* 11:240, 1977.

5. Burke, J. P., Garibaldi, R. A., Britt, M. R., Jacobson, J. A., Conti, M., and Alling, D. W. Prevention of catheter-associated urinary tract infections: Efficacy of daily meatal care regimens. *Am. J. Med.* 70:655, 1981.

6. Burke, J. P., Jacobson, J. J., Garibaldi, R. A., Conti, M. T., and Alling, D. W. Evaluation of daily meatal care with poly-antibiotic ointment in prevention of catheter-associated bacteriuria. *J. Urol.* 129:331, 1983.

7. Butler, H. K., and Kunin, C. M. Evaluation of polymyxin catheter lubricant and impregnated catheters. *J. Urol.* 100:560, 1968.

8. Butler, H. K., et al. Evaluation of specific systemic antimicrobial therapy in patients on closed catheter drainage. *J. Urol.* 100:567, 1968.

9. Center for Disease Control. *Nosocomial Infections in Community Hospitals.* Report No. 3, July 1967–June 1968. March 1969, pp. 16–17.

10. Center for Disease Control. *National Nosocomial Infections Study Report.* Atlanta: Center for Disease Control, Nov. 1979, pp. 2–14.

11. Daifuku, R., and Stamm, W. E. Association of rectal and urethral colonization with urinary tract infection in patients with indwelling catheters. *J.A.M.A.* 252:2028, 1984.

12. Desautels, R. E., Chibaro, E. A., and Lang, R. J. Maintenance of sterility in urinary drainage bags. *Surg. Gynecol. Obstet.* 154:838, 1982.

13. Dupont, H. L., and Spink, W. W. Infections due to gram-negative organisms: An analysis of 860 patients with bacteriuria at the University of Minnesota Medical Center 1958–1966. *Medicine* 48:307, 1969.

14. Falkiner, F. R., Ma, P. T., Murphy, D. M., Cafferkey, M. T., and Gillespie, W. A. Antimicrobial agents for the prevention of urinary tract infections in transurethral surgery. *J. Urol.* 129:766, 1983.

15. Finkelberg, Z., and Kunin, C. M. Clinical evaluation of closed urinary drainage systems. *J.A.M.A.* 207:1657, 1969.

16. Garibaldi, R. A., Burke, J. P., Britt, M. R., Miller, W. A., and Smith, C. B. Meatal colonization and catheter-associated bacteriuria. *N. Engl. J. Med.* 303:316, 1980.

17. Garibaldi, R. A., Burke, J. P., Dickman, M. L., et al. Factors predisposing to bacteriuria during indwelling urethral catheterization. *N. Engl. J. Med.* 291:215, 1974.

18. Garibaldi, R. A., Mooney, B. R., Epstein, B. J., and Britt, M. R. An evaluation of daily bacteriologic monitoring to identify preventable episodes of catheter-associated urinary tract infections. *Infect. Control* 3:466, 1982.

19. Givens, C. D., and Wenzel, R. P. Catheter-associated urinary tract infections in surgical patients: A controlled study on the excess morbidity and costs. *J. Urol.* 124:646, 1980.

20. Gonick, P., Falkner, B., Schwartz, A., and Pariser, R. Bacteriuria in the catheterized patient: Cystitis or pyelonephritis? *J.A.M.A.* 233:253, 1975.

21. Green, M. S., Rubinstein, E., and Amit, P. Estimating the effects of nosocomial infections on the length of hospitalization. *J. Infect. Dis.* 145:667, 1982.

22. Gross, P. A., Harlzavy, L. M., Barden, G. E., and Kerstein, M. Positive Foley catheter tip cultures: Fact or fancy. *J.A.M.A.* 228:72, 1979.

23. Guttman, L., and Frankel, H. The value of intermittent catheterization in the early management of traumatic paraplegia and tetraplegia. *Paraplegia* 4:63, 1966.

24. Haley, R. W., Culver, D. H., White, J. W., Morgan, W. M., and Emori, T. G. The nationwide nosocomial infection rate: A new need for vital statistics. *Am. J. Epidemiol.* 121:159, 1985.

25. Hartstein, A. I., Garber, S. B., Ward, T. T., Jones, S. R., and Morhland, V. H. Nosocomial urinary tract infection: A prospective evaluation of 108 catheterized patients. *Infect. Control* 2:380, 1981.

26. Hirch, D. D., Fainstein, V., and Musher, D. M. Do condom catheter collecting systems

cause urinary tract infections? *J.A.M.A.* 242:340, 1979.

27. Hirschmann, J. V., and Inui, T. S. Antimicrobial prophylaxis: A critique of recent trials. *Rev. Infect. Dis.* 2:1, 1980.

28. Hodgkinson, C. P., and Hodrari, A. A. Trocar suprapubic cystostomy for postoperative bladder drainage in the female. *J. Obstet. Gynecol.* 96:773, 1966.

29. Hooton, T. M., Haley, R. M., Culver, D. H., et al. The joint association of multiple risk factors with the occurrence of nosocomial infections. *Am. J. Med.* 70:960, 1981.

30. Isaacs, J. H., and McWhorter, D. M. Foley catheter drainage systems and bladder damage. *Surg. Gynecol. Obstet.* 132:889, 1971.

31. Johnson, E. T. The condom catheter: Urinary tract infection and other complications. *South. Med. J.* 76:579, 1983.

32. Kass, E. H. Asymptomatic infections of the urinary tract. *Trans. Assoc. Am. Physicians* 69:56, 1956.

33. Kennedy, R. P., Plorde, J. J., and Petersdorf, R. G. Studies on the epidemiology of *E. coli* infections. IV. Evidence for a nosocomial flora. *J. Clin. Invest.* 44:193, 1965.

34. Kirk, D., Bullock, D. W., Mitchell, J. P., and Hobbs, S. J. F. Hibitane bladder irrigation in the prevention of catheter-associated urinary infections. *Br. J. Urol.* 51:528, 1979.

35. Kislak, J. W., Eickhoff, T. C., and Finland, M. Hospital-acquired infection and antibiotic usage in the Boston City Hospital. *N. Engl. J. Med.* 271:834, 1964.

36. Kreger, B. E., Craven, D. E., Carling, P. C., and McCabe, W. R. Gram-negative bacteremia. III. Reassessment of etiology, epidemiology, and ecology in 612 patients. *Am. J. Med.* 68:332, 1980.

37. Krieger, J. N., Kaiser, D. L., and Wenzel, R. P. Urinary tract etiology of bloodstream infections in hospitalized patients. *J. Infect. Dis.* 148:57, 1983.

38. Kuhlemeier, K. V., Lloyd, L. K., and Stover, S. L. Localization of upper and lower urinary tract infections in patients with neurogenic bladders. *Sci. Digest* 4:29, 1982.

39. Kunin, C. M. *Detection, Prevention, and Management of Urinary Tract Infections* (3d ed.). Philadelphia: Lea & Febiger, 1979.

40. Kunin, C. M., and McCormack, R. C. Prevention of catheter-induced urinary tract infections by sterile closed drainage. *N. Engl. J. Med.* 274:1155, 1966.

41. Lapides, J., Diokno, A. C., Lowe, B. S., and Kalish, M. D. Followup on unsterile, intermittent self-catheterization. *J. Urol.* III:184, 1974.

42. Levy, S. B. Antibiotic resistance. *Infect. Control* 4:195, 1983.

43. Maizels, M., and Schaeffer, A. J. Decreased incidence of bacteriuria associated with periodic instillations of hydrogen peroxide into the urethral catheter drainage bag. *J. Urol.* 123:841, 1980.

44. Marsh, F. P., Murray, M., and Panchamia, P. The relationship between bacterial cultures of the vaginal introitus and urinary infection. *Br. J. Urol.* 44:368, 1972.

45. Martin, C. M., and Bookrajian, E. N. Bacteriuria prevention after indwelling urinary catheterization. *Arch. Intern. Med.* 110:703, 1962.

46. Mattingly, R. F., Moore, D. E., and Clark, D. O. Bacteriologic study of suprapubic bladder drainage. *Am. J. Obstet. Gynecol.* 114:732, 1972.

47. McNamara, M. J., Hill, M. C., Balows, A., et al. A study of bacteriologic patterns of hospital infections. *Ann. Intern. Med.* 66:486, 1967.

48. Merritt, J. L., Erickson, R. P., and Opitz, J. L. Bacteriuria during followup in patients with spinal cord injury. II. Efficacy of antimicrobial suppressants. *Arch. Phys. Med. Rehabil.* 63:413, 1982.

49. Merritt, J. L., and Keys, T. F. Limitations of the antibody-coated bacteria test in patients with neurogenic bladders. *J.A.M.A.* 247:1723, 1982.

50. Milles, G. Catheter-induced hemorrhagic pseudopolyps of the urinary bladder. *J.A.M.A.* 193:196, 1965.

51. Moody, M. L., and Burke, J. P. Infections and antibiotic use in a large private hospital. *Arch. Intern. Med.* 130:261, 1972.

52. Mooney, B. R., Garibaldi, R. A., and Britt, M. R. Natural History of Catheter-Associated Bacteriuria (Colonization, Infection, Bacteremia): Implication for Prevention. In Nelson, J. D., and Grassi, C. (Eds.), *Current Chemotherapy and Infectious Diseases*, vol. II. Washington, DC: American Society of Microbiology, 1980, pp. 1083–1084.

53. Musher, D. M., Thorsteinsson, S. B., and Airola, V. M. Quantitative urinalysis. Diagnosing urinary tract infection in men. *J.A.M.A.* 236:2069, 1976.

54. Pinner, R. W., Haley, R. W., Blumenstein, B. A., Schaberg, D. R., VonAllmen, S. D., and McGowan, J. E. High cost nosocomial infections. *Infect. Control* 3:143, 1982.

55. Platt, R., Polk, B. F., Murdock, B., and Rosner,

B. Mortality associated with nosocomial urinary tract infection. *N. Engl. J. Med.* 307:637, 1982.

56. Sarubbi, F. A., Rutala, W. A., and Samsa, G. Hydrogen peroxide instillations into the urinary drainage bag: Should we or shouldn't we? *Am. J. Infect. Control* 10:72, 1982.

57. Schaberg, D. R., Haley, R. W., Highsmith, A. K., Anderson, R. L., and McGowan, J. E. Nosocomial bacteriuria: A prospective study of case clustering and antimicrobial resistance. *Ann. Intern. Med.* 93:420, 1980.

58. Schaberg, D. R., Weinstein, R. A., and Stamm, W. E. Epidemics of nosocomial urinary tract infection caused by multiply resistant gram-negative bacilli: Epidemiology and control. *J. Infect. Dis.* 133:363, 1976.

59. Sobel, J. D., Kaye, D. Host factors in the pathogenesis of urinary tract infection. *Am. J. Med.* (Suppl.)76:122, 1984.

60. Stamey, T. A., Timothy, M., Millar, M., et al. Recurrent urinary infection in adult women: The role of introital enterobacteria. *Calif. Med.* 155:1, 1971.

61. Stamm, W. E. Guidelines for prevention of catheter-associated urinary tract infections. *Ann. Intern. Med.* 82:386, 1975.

62. Stamm, W. E. Measurement of pyuria and its relationship to bacteriuria. *Am. J. Med.* (Suppl.)75:53, 1983.

63. Stamm, W. E. Recent developments in the diagnosis and treatment of urinary tract infections. *West. J. Med.* 137:213, 1982.

64. Stamm, W. E., Martin, S. M., and Bennett, J. V. Epidemiology of nosocomial infections due to gram-negative bacilli: Aspects relevant to development and use of vaccines. *J. Infect. Dis.* 136S(Suppl.):S151, 1977.

65. Stamm, W. E., Weinstein, R. A., and Dixon, R. E. Comparison of endemic and epidemic nosocomial infections. *Am. J. Med.* 70:393, 1981.

66. Steere, A. C., Stamm, W. E., Martin, S. M., and Bennett, J. V. Gram-negative Rod Bacteremia. In Bennett, J. V., and Brachman, P. S. (Eds.), *Hospital Infections.* Boston: Little, Brown, 1979, pp. 507–518.

67. Sullivan, N. M., Sutter, V. L., Mims, M. M., Marsh, V. H., and Finegold, S. M. Clinical aspects of bacteremia after manipulation of the genitourinary tract. *J. Infect. Dis.* 127:49, 1973.

68. Thompson, R. L., Haley, C. E., Groschel, D. M., Gillenwater, J. Y., Kaiser, D. L., and Wenzel, R. P. *Effect of Periodic Instillation of Hydrogen Peroxide (H₂O₂) into Urinary Drainage Systems in the Prevention of Catheter-Associated Bacteriuria.* Program and Abstracts of the Twenty-Second Interscience Conference on Antimicrobial Agents and Chemotherapy. October 4–6, 1982, No. 769.

69. Thorley, J. D., Barbin, G. K., and Reinarz, J. A. The prevalence of antibody-coated bacteria in urine. *Am. J. Med. Sci.* 275:75, 1978.

70. Thornton, G. F., and Andriole, V. T. Bacteriuria during indwelling catheter drainage. II. Effect of a closed sterile drainage system. *J.A.M.A.* 214:339, 1970.

71. Turck, M., Goffee, B., and Petersdorf, R. G. The urethral catheter and urinary tract infection. *J. Urol.* 88:834, 1962.

72. Turck, M., and Stamm, W. E. Nosocomial infection of the urinary tract. *Am. J. Med.* 70:651, 1981.

73. Vainrub, B., and Musher, D. M. Lack of effect of methanimine in suppression of or prophylaxis against chronic urinary infections. *Antimicrob. Agents Chemother.* 12:625, 1977.

74. Warren, J. W., Anthony, W. C., Hoopes, J. M., and Muncie, H. L. Cephalexin or susceptible bacteriuria in afebrile, long-term catheterized patients. *J.A.M.A.* 248:454, 1982.

75. Warren, J. W., Muncie, H. L., Bergquist, E. J., and Hoopes, J. M. Sequelae and management of urinary tract infection in the patient requiring chronic catheterization. *J. Urol.* 125:1, 1981.

76. Warren, J. W., Platt, R., Thomas, K. J., et al. Antibiotic irrigation and catheter-associated urinary tract infections. *N. Engl. J. Med.* 299:570, 1978.

77. Warren, J. W., Tenney, J. H., Hoopes, J. M., Muncie, H. L., and Anthony, W. C. A prospective microbiologic study of bacteriuria in patients with chronic indwelling urethral catheters. *J. Infect. Dis.* 146:719, 1982.

78. Wenzel, R. P., Osterman, C. A., and Hunting, K. J. Hospital-acquired infections. I. Infection rates by site, service, and common procedures in a university hospital. *Am. J. Epidemiol.* 104:645, 1976.

79. Winterbauer, R. H. Turck, M., Petersdorf, R. G. Studies on the epidemiology of *E. coli* infections. V. Factors influencing acquisition of specific serologic groups. *J. Clin. Invest.* 46:21, 1967.

80. Wong, E. S., and Hooton, T. M. Guidelines for prevention of catheter-associated urinary tract infections. *Infect. Control* 2:125, 1982.

# 26 LOWER RESPIRATORY TRACT INFECTIONS

Jay P. Sanford

## NATURE OF LOWER RESPIRATORY TRACT INFECTIONS

### Classification

Nosocomial respiratory infections are those that develop in hospitalized patients in whom the infection was either not present or not incubating at the time of admission (see Chapter 1). Nosocomial infections are usually not manifest in the first 72 hours of hospitalization. For some lower respiratory infections, the recognition that incubating infections should not be classified as nosocomial is of importance; for example, the patient who develops influenzal pneumonia 24 hours after admission to a hospital or the patient who may have aspirated oropharyngeal materials several days before admission and who then goes on to develop a necrotizing pneumonia with community-acquired organisms after hospitalization should not be classified as having nosocomial pneumonia. Similarly, it is important to recognize that nosocomial infections may be incubating at the time of discharge from the hospital; hence they may be initially recognized at the time of outpatient follow-up. Although the delayed appearance of disease is more frequent with infections involving other sites than the lung, such delay may occur with nosocomial respiratory infections, such as nosocomial varicella pneumonia or tuberculosis. When the incubation period is unknown, infections are classified as nosocomial if they develop at any time after admission. An infection present on admission can be classified as nosocomial *only* if it is directly related to or is the residual of a previous admission. All infections that fail to satisfy these requirements should be classified as community-acquired.

### Incidence

Standardized criteria for diagnosis (reviewed in a subsequent section) have not been employed in most of the reported studies. The figures presented represent a mixture of prevalence data and "incidence" per hospitalized patients or number of admissions; the duration of hospitalization, and hence the time "at risk," is usually not estimated. The data relate almost exclusively to rapidly growing aerobic bacterial agents that occur endemically. Data seldom are presented that include viral, fungal, or parasitic agents or that correct for the occurrence of sporadic outbreaks. Nosocomial pneumonia represents 8 to 33 percent of the total nosocomial infections, and the rate of nosocomial pneumonia varies from 0.5 to 5.0 percent of all

TABLE 26-1. Incidences of nosocomial pneumonia and lower respiratory tract infections by hospital service

| Hospital service | Incidence per 1000 Discharges | |
|---|---|---|
| | 1970–1973 | 1980–1982 |
| Surgical | 6.5 | 7.5 |
| Medical | 6.1 | 7.0 |
| Obstetric | 0.2 | 0.4 |
| Gynecologic | 1.0 | 1.0 |
| Pediatric | 1.7 | 1.6 |
| Newborn | 0.4 | 1.0 |
| *Totals* | 4.3 | 5.1 |

Source: Data from National Nosocomial Infections Study (NNIS). (See Chapter 24.) 1970–73 data based on 14,772 lower respiratory infections among 3,456,000 discharges from January 1970 through August 1973. 1980–82 data based on 18,382 lower respiratory infections among 3,572,686 discharges from January 1980 through December 1982.

admissions (discharges). The incidence (expressed as the number of occurrences per 1000 admissions or discharges) in community hospitals [20] generally has been two to ten times lower than in university-affiliated teaching hospitals. The highest rates for university hospitals are based on prevalence studies, however, and these measurements tend to produce higher rates than incidence studies (see Chapter 4); thus the true difference in incidence of pneumonia

between community and university hospitals is likely to be less than tenfold but still higher for university hospitals. These differences may reflect social factors. University hospitals tend to be tertiary care centers to which the more sick, complicated patient is referred, and in which support procedures may be more advanced. Also, university-affiliated teaching hospitals often have individuals involved in patient care who are students and who may be less knowledgeable and skilled in those aspects of care important in the prevention of nosocomial infections.

Figures derived from the National Nosocomial Infections Study (NNIS) encompass data collected from 1980 through 1982: among 3,572,686 discharges, there were 116,444 patients who developed infections (3.1 percent). Of these infections, (15.8 percent) were reported as involving the lower respiratory tract. From these data, the incidence of pneumonia and lower respiratory infection was 5.1 per 1000 discharges.

As in most bacterial nosocomial infections, overall figures reflect composites of different patient groups who are at differing risks, depending on host factors such as age and type of illnesses for which they are admitted to hospitals. These differences are illustrated in Table 26-1, which provides incidence figures according to hospital service.

Over the ten-year interval between 1970–73 and 1980–82, despite advances in the institution of in-

TABLE 26-2. Etiology of nosocomial pneumonias by clinical epidemiologic group

| Microbial cause | Clinical-epidemiologic group (percentage) | | | | |
|---|---|---|---|---|---|
| | Community hospital[a] | VA hospital[b] | Immunosuppressed leukemia/lymphoma patients[c] | Renal transplant patients[d] | NNIS Study[e] |
| Viral | NR | NR | 4 | 46 | <1 |
| Bacterial | 83 | 82 | 16 | 13 | 94 |
| *Staphylococcus aureus* | 6 | 0 | 4 | 2 | 13 |
| *Streptococcus pneumoniae* | 6 | 3 | 0 | 0 | 4 |
| Gram-negative aerobes | 27 | 22 | 12 | 2 | 64 |
| *Hemophilus influenzae* | 17 | 0 | 0 | 2 | 6 |
| Legionellaceae | 13 | 47 | NR | NR | <1 |
| Aspiration | 6 | 9 | 0 | 6 | NR |
| Other | 6 | 0 | 0 | 4 | 8 |
| Fungal | 17 | NR | 12 | 10 | 6 |
| *Pneumocystis carinii* | NR | NR | 12 | NR | <1 |
| Polymicrobial | NR | NR | NR | 31 | 1 |
| Unknown—no specific diagnosis | 17 | 18 | 56 | NR | 0 |

NR = not reported.
[a]30 episodes in 28 patients. Muder, R. R. et al. *J.A.M.A.* 249:3184, 1983.
[b]32 patients. Muder, R. R. et al. *J.A.M.A.* 249:3184, 1983.
[c]24 patients. Singer, C. et al. *Am. J. Med.* 66:110, 1979.
[d]52 episodes. Peterson, P. K. et al. *Medicine* 61:360, 1982.
[e]82 hospitals, 18,676 isolates (many multiple isolations from same patient) (see Chapter 24).

fection control practices and inhalation and antimicrobial therapy, the incidence of nosocomial pneumonia has certainly not decreased (Table 26-1).

Pneumonia accounts for 10 to 20 percent of all hospital-associated infections. While nosocomial pneumonias are less prevalent than nosocomial urinary tract and surgical wound infections, nosocomial pneumonia is the leading cause of death due to nosocomial infections [29]. Because of its frequency and case fatality ratio—up to 50 percent in some reports [85]—nosocomial pneumonia remains a major infection control problem.

*Causative Agents*
A large number of microorganisms have been incriminated as the causative agents in nosocomial respiratory tract infections; broadly, these include aerobic gram-positive cocci, aerobic gram-negative bacilli, anaerobes, mycobacteria, nocardial species, and viral, chlamydial, fungal, and parasitic agents.

The patient's underlying disease and treatment are major factors in determining the cause of nosocomial pneumonias. Unique environmental conditions may impose additional important etiologic considerations; for example, legionnaires' disease is far more prevalent in some hospitals than in others, and aspergillosis is a more common cause of nosocomial pulmonary infections on oncology units than on other services. These differences are illustrated in Table 26-2; from

TABLE 26-3. Frequency of bacterial species isolated, reported by NNIS

| Bacterial species | Percentage of isolates |
|---|---|
| Gram-positive cocci | 25 |
| *Staphylococcus aureus* | 14 |
| *Streptococcus pneumoniae* | 4 |
| *Streptococcus faecalis* | 2 |
| Others | 5 |
| Gram-negative aerobic bacilli | 72 |
| *Hemophilus influenzae* | 8 |
| *Escherichia coli* | 8 |
| *Klebsiella* species | 14 |
| *Enterobacter* species | 10 |
| *Proteus, Morganella, Providencia* | 7 |
| *Pseudomonas* species | 15 |
| *Serratia* species | 6 |
| Anaerobes | <1 |
| Miscellaneous | 3 |

Source: Data from National Nosocomial Infections Study (NNIS), 1980–82, based on 17,609 bacterial isolates reported from 82 hospitals. Multiple isolates from the same specimen tabulated individually (see Chapter 24).

these data it is apparent that generalizations are difficult.

Data submitted under the National Nosocomial Infections Study are summarized in Table 26-3.

Aerobic gram-negative bacilli account for almost three-quarters of the isolates, while gram-positive cocci, predominantly *Staphylococcus aureus* and *Streptococcus pneumoniae*, account for the remaining one-quarter. Very few anaerobic bacteria and viruses were reported, probably because obtaining appropriate specimens for culture and isolating and identifying these organisms are difficult and not usually attempted.

## DIAGNOSTIC CRITERIA

*Clinical Criteria*
Establishing a diagnosis of nosocomial pneumonia may be difficult. The disease is most common in critically ill patients who may not be able to report symptoms accurately and in whom the primary disease may mask or simulate the occurrence of bacterial pneumonia. In the intensive-care-unit setting, many patients have fever and leukocytosis from their primary disease process. Antecedent densities in the chest radiograph and purulent sputum also are common. Gram-negative bacillary pathogens are found in the sputum in a high fraction of patients with or without pneumonia. For this reason the diagnosis of pneumonia or lower respiratory tract infection depends on clinical observations, including radiographic findings, rather than based solely or predominantly on microbiologic findings; as reviewed subsequently, however, microbiologic procedures are being evolved that will provide better correlation between clinical and microbiologic features.

Different clinicians and investigators have employed differing criteria for the diagnosis of lower respiratory tract infections. Wenzel and associates at the University of Virginia [97] have used the finding of infiltrate on chest radiography not present on admission and associated with new sputum production as a criterion for nosocomial pulmonary infections. Johanson and colleagues [41] used more stringent criteria and classified infections as "definite" or "probable" according to four determinants: (1) the radiographic appearance of a new or progressive pulmonary infiltrate, (2) fever, (3) leukocytosis, and (4) purulent tracheobronchial secretions. A diagnosis of "definite" infection required the occurrence of all four determinants. A diagnosis of "probable" infection was based on three criteria: (1) fever, (2) leukocytosis, and (3) either a new or progressive pulmonary infiltrate shown radiographically or the presence of purulent secretions. Results of culture tests were not used in making these determinations.

The Hospital Infections Program of the Centers for Disease Control (CDC), which monitors the National Nosocomial Infections Study, uses the following criteria for nosocomial pneumonia. In adults there must be either onset of purulent sputum production more than 48 hours after admission in a patient with no preceding pulmonary infection, or increased production of purulent sputum with recrudescence of fever in a patient admitted with pulmonary disease. In addition at least one of the following must also be present: (1) infiltration seen on chest roentgenography or characteristic physical findings of pneumonia in the absence of a chest roentgenogram or (2) cough, fever, and pleuritic chest pain. Diagnosis of pneumonia in a child can be made in the absence of purulent sputum if both of the latter criteria are satisfied. A diagnosis of pneumonia by the attending physician is accepted even when the above criteria are incompletely fulfilled. Other conditions that may result in similar signs or symptoms (e.g., congestive heart failure, postoperative atelectasis, pulmonary embolism, adult respiratory distress syndrome) may be differentiated from pneumonia by the clinical course of the patient, although this may be difficult.

Andrews and colleagues [2] undertook a clinical-pathologic correlative study to determine the reliability of clinical findings in diagnosing bacterial pneumonia in the patient with the adult respiratory distress syndrome (ARDS). The following clinical variables were examined: underlying disorder, age, duration of mechanical ventilation, and presence or absence of (1) fever (defined as a temperature of greater than 38.3°C [100.9°F] rectally), (2) leukocytosis (WBC greater than 10,000 per cubic millimeter), (3) leukopenia (WBC less than 5,000 per cubic millimeter), (4) pathogenic bacteria in pulmonary secretions or

pulmonary wedge specimens, (5) response to antibiotic therapy, and (6) abnormalities in chest roentgenograms. At autopsy the diagnosis of bronchopneumonia was based on focuses of consolidation with intense polymorphonuclear leukocyte accumulations in bronchioles and adjacent alveoli scattered through several lung sections.

A total of 24 patients met the criteria for analysis; 14 (58 percent) had histologic pneumonia, while 10 (42 percent) had only diffuse alveolar damage (Table 26-4). The features of fever, leukocytosis, and presence of bacterial pathogens even on specimens obtained through the flexible bronchoscope (the protected specimen brush catheter was not used in this study) did not allow differentiation. Improvement on antibiotic therapy also was not a useful indicator of the presence or absence of bacterial pneumonia. The occurrence of localized areas of consolidation on chest roentgenogram was most useful. Overall the accuracy of the clinical diagnosis of pneumonia in the ARDS patient was only 64 percent. Observations such as these indicate the need for clinical-pathologic correlations and improved diagnostic measures, and the difficulty in assessing preventive interventions and outcome measures.

Suprainfection of a previously existing respiratory infection may result in a new nosocomial infection when a new pathogen is cultured from sputum and clinical or radiologic evidence indicates that the new organism is associated with deterioration in the patient's condition.

While more stringent criteria may suggest a higher degree of specificity in diagnosis and enable greater assurance in distinguishing between suprainfection and supracolonization, they may result concomitantly in lower selectivity, especially when even the more stringent criteria have only moderate specificity. For this reason and because the largest data base from

TABLE 26-4. Correlation of clinical findings with histologic evidence of pneumonia

| Clinical feature | Pneumonia (no.) | (n = 14) (%) | Nonpneumonia (no.) | (n = 10) (%) |
|---|---|---|---|---|
| Fever | 14 | (100) | 8 | (80) |
| Leukocytosis or leukopenia | 14 | (100) | 8 | (80) |
| Pathogens in sputum | 12 | (86) | 7 | (70) |
| Pathogens on wedged catheter specimen | 5/5 | (100) | 3/4 | (75) |
| Localized consolidation on roentgenogram | 8 | (57) | 3 | (30) |
| Response to antibiotics | | | | |
| Worsened | 7/13 | (54) | 5/9 | (56) |
| Improved | 2/13 | (15) | 3/9 | (33) |
| Accuracy of clinical diagnosis | 9 | (64) | 8 | (80) |

Source: Andrews, C. P. et al. *Chest* 80:254, 1981.

which comparisons and trends can be developed is that of the CDC, it would seem that their definition should be employed unless there are specific justifications in a study for not doing so. Under the latter circumstances, it is essential that the diagnostic criteria used be defined.

*Microbiologic Criteria*

Although expectorated sputum is usually the most readily available material for microbiologic examination, it is not the most satisfactory material for examination in patients with complicated pneumonia or in debilitated patients who are at risk for developing nosocomial pneumonia. Expectorated sputum is contaminated by oropharyngeal flora, which may not be representative of the cause of the pneumonia. Attempts have been made to reduce the error in diagnosis introduced by the oropharyngeal flora by means of repeated washing of expectorated sputum. This procedure, however, does not absolutely ensure that the bacteria isolated from the washed sputum originated in the lower respiratory tract. In addition, the procedure places a great burden on the bacteriology laboratory. It has also been suggested that the true bacterial cause of the pneumonia can be identified by quantitative culture techniques. Our group and others have found, however, that this procedure does not necessarily identify the cause of the lung infection (Fig. 26-1).

Organisms isolated from blood, pleural fluid, lung, bronchial washings, or transtracheal aspirates in patients with clinical evidence of pneumonia should be reported as pathogens.

Transtracheal aspiration (TTA) has been used as a means of avoiding direct pharyngeal contamination in obtaining material for Gram stain and culture [4]. The clinical courses of patients with pneumonia have been correlated with the results of Gram staining and culture of both expectorated sputum and sputum obtained by TTA, and it has been demonstrated that the latter procedure is more likely to yield specimens that indicate the correct bacterial cause of the pneumonia. TTA allows for the identification of anaerobic bacteria; this is not possible with expectorated sputum, because anaerobes are normal inhabitants of the oropharyngeal cavity. Even with TTA, however, more than one bacterial species is usually isolated, and based on data obtained from direct lung puncture, most pneumonias (at least community-acquired pneumonias) are monomicrobial. The problem with interpretation of TTA results is shown in Table 26-5. In a canine model of *Streptococcus pneumoniae* pneumonia, TTA was found to have a 30 percent false-positive contamination rate and a specificity of only

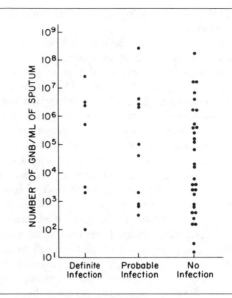

FIG. 26-1. The count of gram-negative bacilli (*GNB*) per milliliter of sputum. Specimens were obtained from 22 of 26 patients with definite or probable infection at the time of diagnosis; 17 specimens contained gram-negative bacilli. These results are compared with those from specimens of 31 patients who had no clinical signs of infection. (From Johanson, W. G., et al. *Ann. Intern. Med.* 77:701, 1972.)

10 to 20 percent [55]. TTA cannot be used in intubated patients.

Although the incidence of serious complications is low, the procedure carries some risk. It is contraindicated in patients with thrombocytopenia or other clotting disorders. Because the antipseudomonal penicillins (carbenicillin, ticarcillin, piperacillin, mezlocillin, and azlocillin) and third-generation cephalosporins (especially moxalactam) may interfere with

TABLE 26-5. Correlation of aerobic and anaerobic isolates among paired specimens obtained by telescoping plugged catheter (TPC) and transtracheal aspiration (TTA) from patients with suspected anaerobic infections

| Results | Anaerobic isolates | Aerobic isolates (potential pathogens) |
|---|---|---|
| Complete agreement | 7 | 9 |
| Partial agreement | 3 | 0 |
| No agreement | 3[a] | 4[b] |

[a]*Bacteriodes* species isolated from two TTA with no growth on TPC; no growth on 1 TTA with *Bacteriodes* species isolated from TPC.
[b]*Escherichia coli, Klebsiella pneumoniae, Steptococcus pneumoniae,* and *Hemophilus influenzae* isolated from TTA but not isolated on TPC.
Source: Bordelon, J. Y., et al. *Am. Rev. Respir. Dis.* 128:465, 1983.

platelet function, required therapy may interpose a contraindication.

Although transtracheal aspiration has been the "gold standard," more recent studies have better defined its limitations. Concurrently, alternative techniques have been developed and evaluated. Use of these more invasive techniques generally has been restricted to the patient with persistent pulmonary infiltrates or immunocompromised patients with progressive pulmonary infiltrates. These alternative techniques include flexible fiberoptic bronchoscopy with use of the protected specimen brush (telescoping plugged catheter), bronchial washings, or transbronchial biopsy; transthoracic direct needle aspiration of the lung; and open lung biopsy (Table 26-6). Winterbauer and colleagues [100] have reported that none of 60 control patients had greater than 4000 cfu per brush on quantitative culture, while in 29 of 33 episodes of clinically defined lower respiratory infections there were more than 4000 cfu per brush. Additionally, only 1 of 60 control patients had antibody-coated (AC) bacteria in their lower respiratory secretions, but AC bacteria were demonstrated in 24 of 33 episodes of infection. While such modifications may be helpful, the recently developed telescoping plugged catheter (TPC) or protected specimen brush (BFW Brush, Medi-Tech), which is introduced through the flexible fiberoptic bronchoscope, appears to provide comparable information without additional laboratory procedures. In both animal models and humans the TPC provides a high degree of sensitivity and specificity with the morbidity of bronchoscopy (Table 26-5)[6,38].

Comparison of the value of transbronchial biopsy with that of open lung biopsy in the immunocompromised patient is more controversial. Fiberoptic bronchoscopy with brush and wash specimens and transbronchial biopsy compares well with open lung biopsy for *Pneumocystis carinii* [10] but has failed to

identify cytomegalovirus in the bone marrow transplant patient [84]. In clinical circumstances in which a fulminant course is likely, open lung biopsy remains the procedure of choice. Where there is less urgency, transbronchial biopsy provides a reasonable alternative for the diagnosis of *P. carinii* pneumonia (PCP). A negative biopsy does not exclude PCP, however, and a subsequent open lung biopsy needs to be considered.

Blood cultures should be obtained from all patients with nosocomial pneumonia. Bacteremia occurs in one-fourth to one-half of the patients. Procedures such as counterimmunoelectrophoresis (CIEP) and coagglutination to detect antigens in sputum or urine are being developed and appear very promising [30].

Although the value of bacteriologic study of sputum remains in serious doubt, it is likely that expectorated sputum specimens will continue to be submitted to clinical bacteriology laboratories for culture because of reticence on the part of physicians and patients to use invasive procedures and medical contraindications to fiberoptic bronchoscopy or transtracheal aspiration. Therefore, a simple screening procedure to ascertain the degree of oropharyngeal contamination in expectorated sputum would be helpful. If contamination were present to a significant degree, cultures would yield a large number of different species that not only would complicate and prolong the bacteriologic procedures but also could overgrow the true causative agent. The effects of culturing oropharyngeal flora can hardly be regarded as a meaningful exercise for either the laboratory or the physician.

Bartlett [3] has proposed an objective system for evaluating the quality of lower respiratory tract secretions (see Chapter 7). Gram stains are examined under $\times$ 100 magnification after oil is placed on the slide to improve clarity. The slide is examined for

TABLE 26-6. Comparison of procedures for obtaining microbiologic specimens for diagnosis of nosocomial pneumonias

| Procedure | Sensitivity | Specificity | Morbidity |
|---|---|---|---|
| Expectorated sputum | High | Almost nil | Nil |
| Transtracheal aspiration | High | Low | Low |
| Fiberoptic bronchoscopy | | | |
|   Standard catheter brush | High | Low[a] | Low |
|   Washings | Moderate | Low | Low |
| Protected specimen brush[b] | High | High | Low |
|   Transbronchial biopsy | Moderate | High | Moderate |
| Transthoracic needle aspiration | Low | High | High |
| Open lung biopsy | High | High | High |

[a]Use of quantitative cultures and antibody coating of bacteria may increase sensitivity (Winterbauer, R. H., et al. *Am. Rev. Respir. Dis.* 128:98, 1983).
[b]Also called *telescoping plugged catheter*.

the presence of neutrophils, mucus, and squamous epithelial cells. A rough quantitative estimate is made by applying a scoring system (Table 26-7). If the total score is zero or less, a report of "oropharyngeal contamination, please repeat" is rendered. Specimens with scores of +1 to +3 are cultured. Complete speciation and susceptibility testing are performed only if the number of potential pathogens isolated does not exceed the score. A score of +3, for example, signifies the absence of oropharyngeal material and the presence of mucus and abundant neutrophils.

Using a similar system, Murray and Washington [57] attempted to provide bacteriologic evidence, including comparison with transtracheal aspirates, to support the criteria of Bartlett. These investigators found (Table 26-8) that specimens with more than ten epithelial cells per low-power (× 100) field (groups 1 through 4) yielded similar numbers of species (4.2 to 4.4), in contrast to the smaller number of different isolates recovered from specimens showing less than ten epithelial cells (group 5) and transtracheal aspirate specimens (2.7 and 2.4, respectively). The number of leukocytes bore no relationship to the number of isolates. It is of particular note that at the time of this study, 75 percent of the sputum samples received in the laboratory were contaminated with more than ten epithelial cells per field and were judged to be unsatisfactory for culture. It is important to reserve such a screening criterion (i.e., less than ten squamous epithelial cells per field at × 100 magnification) for sputum bacteriology only. In patients with suspected mycoplasmal, viral, fungal, or mycobacterial illness, the degree of oropharyngeal contamination is relatively less important.

In the event that the clinical illness does not indicate the need for, or there are contraindications to, transtracheal aspiration, microscopic examination of sputum employing the criteria of Murray and Washington appears to be of value in determining the

TABLE 26-7. Criteria for scoring the quality of specimens of lower respiratory tract secretions

| Observation* | Score |
| --- | --- |
| More than 25 neutrophils per field | +2 |
| 10 to 25 neutrophils per field | +1 |
| Mucus | +1 |
| 10 to 25 squamous cells per field | −1 |
| More than 25 squamous cells per field | −2 |

*Field examined under oil at × 100 magnification (× 10 objective).
Source: Bartlett, R. C. *Medical Microbiology: Quality, Cost, and Clinical Relevance.* New York: Wiley, 1974.

TABLE 26-8. Relationship between specimen group and mean number of bacterial species isolated

| Group | Cellular composition (no./field)* Epithelial | Leuko-cytes | Speci-mens (no.) | Mean number of species isolated |
| --- | --- | --- | --- | --- |
| 1 | >25 | <10 | 54 | 4.2 |
| 2 | >25 | 10–25 | 42 | 4.2 |
| 3 | >25 | >25 | 119 | 4.4 |
| 4 | 10–25 | >25 | 68 | 4.2 |
| 5 | <10 | >25 | 99 | 2.7 |
| TTA | — | — | 47 | 2.4 |

TTA = transtracheal aspirate.
*Field examined at × 100 magnification (× 10 objective).
Source: Murray, P. R., and Washington, J. A. *Mayo Clin. Proc.* 50:339, 1975.

acceptability of a specimen for bacterial culture. The use of such techniques should greatly sharpen the accuracy of defining causation in patients with nosocomial lower respiratory tract infections.

## GENERAL FACTORS AFFECTING SUSCEPTIBILITY

The normal human respiratory tract is provided with a variety of mechanisms that act to protect the lungs from infection. The lower respiratory tract is protected by the glottis and larynx, and material passing these barriers stimulates the expulsive cough reflex. Removal of small particles impinging on the walls of the trachea and bronchi is facilitated by their mucociliary lining, and the growth of bacteria reaching normal alveoli is inhibited by their relative dryness and by a dual phagocytic system that involves both granulocytes and alveolar macrophages (95). Any anatomic or physiologic derangement of these coordinated defenses tends to augment the susceptibility of the lungs to infection. Anesthesia, alcoholic intoxication, convulsions, and disturbed innervation of the larynx depress the cough reflex and may permit aspiration of infected material. Alterations in the tracheobronchial tree leading to anatomic changes in the epithelial lining or to localized obstruction increase the vulnerability of the lungs to infection. Local or generalized pulmonary edema resulting from viral infection, inhalation of irritant gases, cardiac failure, or contusion of the chest wall provides a fluid menstruum in the alveoli for the growth of bacteria and their spread to adjacent areas of the lung. Viral infection of the respiratory epithelium with concomitant disruption of its component cells interferes significantly with the clearance of bacteria from the lungs.

## SOURCES AND MODES OF ACQUISITION

Microorganisms may invade the alveolar level of the lung in sufficient density to produce pneumonia by one of three routes: (1) aspiration from the oropharynx, (2) suspension in inhaled gas, or (3) lymphohematogenous spread (by way of the vasculature).

### Bronchogenous Spread by Aspiration of Oropharyngeal Bacteria

MECHANISMS  Most bacterial pneumonia is due to microorganisms that make up the flora of the oropharynx, and aspiration of such organisms is probably the principal mechanism underlying nosocomial pneumonia. Indirect evidence supports this hypothesis. Pneumococci instilled into the nose of unanesthetized rabbits have been noted to appear in the lung within minutes. When the bronchi of dogs were occluded with sterile cotton plugs and atelectasis was allowed to occur, pharyngeal organisms were recovered distal to the occlusion. Culture of specimens from human lungs at autopsy has revealed bacterial species similar to those cultured from the pharynx. It has been suggested that these findings are due to agonal or postmortem invasion of the tracheobronchial tree. The findings, however, are also compatible with the terminal failure of clearance mechanisms that had suppressed bacterial growth in the lungs during life. The aspiration into the lung of radiopaque material instilled into the oropharynx of normal sleeping adults was demonstrated by Amberson [1] in 1937. A recent study using a radioisotope tracer showed that 45 percent of healthy young adults aspirated from the nasopharynx into the lung during sleep [39]. Persons with abnormal swallowing, decreased gag reflex, or decreased cough are more likely to aspirate and to aspirate larger inocula. Experimentally, inoculum size is an important determinant of pulmonary bacterial clearance [91]. It is of note that in some organisms, larger inocula are more effectively cleared than smaller inocula.

OROPHARYNGEAL COLONIZATION OF NORMAL PERSONS  The oropharynx of a normal person apparently does not provide a suitable environment for the growth of aerobic gram-negative bacilli; only about 2 percent of normal persons harbor more than occasional aerobic gram-negative bacilli at any given time. When multiple culture determinations are performed on normal persons, the cumulative percentage of subjects with at least one positive culture result increases, but previously positive persons usually are negative. This indicates that colonization is transient in normal persons, although the length of colonization has not been defined. Using more sensitive broth culture media that were selective for aerobic gram-negative bacilli, Rosenthal and Tager (71) detected small numbers of Enterobacteriaceae or *Pseudomonas aeruginosa* in 18 percent of normal persons. Furthermore, massive exposure of normal persons to these organisms does not result in colonization of the upper respiratory tract. Thus normal persons are only at slight risk (perhaps 2 percent are at risk) for developing gram-negative bacillary pneumonia by aspiration of oropharyngeal flora.

FACTORS PREDISPOSING TO COLONIZATION  Alcoholic, diabetic, and chronically or severely ill patients lose effective colonization immunity. Colonization of the oropharynx with gram-negative bacilli is associated with adherance of these organisms to buccal epithelial cells. Woods and associates [101] have shown that the host alterations associated with increased susceptibility to adherence by *P. aeruginosa* is the loss of fibronectin from the cell surface. Colonization of the upper respiratory tract by gram-negative bacilli precedes the development of nosocomial pneumonia in most patients. Exposure to such organisms from an exogenous source is common but not necessary, because it has been found [40] that approximately 20 percent of patients sufficiently ill to be admitted to a medical intensive care unit were colonized at the time of admission. Although previous therapy with antimicrobial drugs facilitates colonization and possibly the occurrence of pneumonia, it is similarly not a prerequisite.

As anticipated from the concentration of chronically and severely ill patients in a hospital setting, gram-negative bacillary oropharyngeal colonization is especially prevalent among hospitalized patients. There is a rapid rise in the incidence of colonization for the first few hospital days, which suggests that there is a "susceptible pool" of patients who are particularly predisposed to colonization. The patients most prone to colonization are those with features reflecting severe illness, such as coma, hypotension, acidosis, azotemia, and alterations in the leukocyte count; in such patients, the incidence of colonization approaches 75 percent. An increased prevalence of colonization among patients with respiratory disease or endotracheal intubation suggests that factors impairing lung clearance may also promote colonization. Hospitalized patients who are not critically ill have a far lower prevalence of oropharyngeal colonization (approximately 30 to 40 percent).

SOURCES OF ORGANISMS  The occurrence of clusters of patients colonized with the same species of gram-negative bacilli suggests that, in part, the bacteria are transmitted from patient to patient within the hospital setting. The 20 percent incidence of colonization at the time of admission and the subsequent colonization of some patients with bacterial species not isolated from other patients in the same environment, however, suggest that many patients are colonized with organisms indigenous to each patient. The gastrointestinal tract is the most likely site from which the bacilli spread.

Ventilatory equipment may serve as a reservoir from which patients may become colonized with bacteria through several routes. Surface contamination of inhalation therapy equipment could serve as a source from which the patient's face, mouth, or nose could become colonized; such has not been demonstrated directly. Development of satisfactory methods for disposing of fluid that condenses in tubing is needed. The exhalation side of the circuit has received little attention; however, effluent may contaminate the patient's immediate surroundings such as bed linens. From the contaminated local environment, secondary transmission by the patient's own hands or by hospital personnel to the index patient or to other patients can occur. Of course, contamination of the internal parts of the equipment may also lead to oropharyngeal colonization. The relative importance of ventilatory equipment as a source of oropharyngeal bacteria probably varies widely among hospitals [15]. In one observation [41] on the occurrence of colonization of the oropharynx with aerobic gram-negative bacilli, inhalation therapy was not a factor that could be significantly correlated with colonization.

*Bronchogenous Spread by Airborne Organisms*
MECHANISMS  Infection may be transmitted at some distance by infected small particles, or aerosols, that are generated by coughs and sneezes. Such particles range in size from 1 $\mu$ to more than 20 $\mu$ in diameter, remain airborne for long periods, may disseminate widely in the local environment such as a hospital ward, and may potentially infect large numbers of persons.

The minimum infectious dose of a number of pathogenic bacteria is less if they are delivered in aerosols of a size capable of deposition beyond the level of the ciliated epithelium. It has been estimated that at least 50 percent of 1.0- to 2.0-$\mu$ particles,

when delivered to the mouth or nose of an individual, are capable of entering the bronchial tree distal to the terminal bronchioles (lowest level of ciliated epithelium), where host defense mechanisms may be overcome more easily.

The most important mechanism for the dissemination of bacteria by ventilatory equipment is the aerosolization of organisms into the stream of gas delivered by such equipment in particle sizes that are sufficiently small to be deposited in terminal lung units. Most types of nebulizers are designed to deliver aerosols in a size range of 1.0 to 2.0 $\mu$ to ensure humidification or the delivery of medications to the lower reaches of the tracheobronchial tree.

Except for tuberculosis and circumstances in which patients are receiving inhalation treatments, airborne transmission is probably of little importance in the epidemiology of nosocomial bacillary pneumonia. The bacterial density in the air, even in hospitals, is quite low.

AIRBORNE SPREAD FROM PERSONS  In controlled experiments, natural airborne transmission of coxsackie virus A21 has been demonstrated. Adenovirus type 4 has been found in droplets expelled in coughs and in the air of rooms occupied by military recruits ill with adenoviral pneumonia. These observations suggest that airborne transmission is important in the transmission of these two infections and may be important in other viral infections of the respiratory tract, such as influenza. Riley and associates [69] demonstrated the infectiousness of air on a tuberculosis ward, although they concluded that viable airborne tubercle bacilli are not very numerous and that the air of a room occupied by a tuberculous patient may not be very dangerous if it is breathed for only a short time.

ROLE OF NEBULIZATION EQUIPMENT  Since gases such as oxygen or compressed air are essentially free of water vapor, their administration without humidification results in desiccation of the upper airways and may significantly predispose the patient to infection. Hence, a method for increasing the water vapor content of administered gases is essential, even though it results in the concomitant, increased risk of bacterial contamination of the moisture source. There are two markedly differing principles used to increase the humidity of gases delivered to the tracheobronchial tree. The first of these involves humidification; the second, nebulization (Fig. 26-2). Definition of these terms becomes essential, because differences in terminology with resultant confusion exist in the literature.

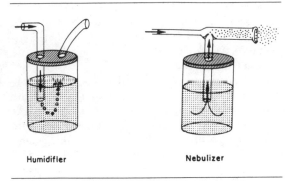

Humidifier                    Nebulizer

FIG. 26-2. Differences in principles of operation of humidifiers and nebulizers. (From Sanford, J. P., and Pierce, A. K. In Brachman, P. S., and Eickhoff, T. C. [Eds.], *Proceedings of the International Conference on Nosocomial Infections.* Chicago: American Hospital Association, 1971. Reprinted with permission.)

Humidifiers are devices that saturate gas with water vapor; they do not aerosolize droplet water. Most clinical humidifiers cause the stream of gas to bubble through water, although some humidifiers used in pediatric services cause the stream of gas to be blown across the surface of water.

In contrast, nebulizers not only saturate the gas with water vapor, but also disperse an aerosol of droplets. Most clinical nebulizers are gas driven and operate on the venturi principle. Venturi-type nebulizers may be of small volume (5 to 30 ml) for dispensing specific medication, or they may contain a large reservoir (approximately 500 ml) for the administration of moisture. The large-volume nebulizers may be operated at room temperature or they may be heated, usually to temperatures of 55°C (131°F). The temperature of the air delivered to the patient decreases to 33°C to 35°C (91.4°F to 95°F). Aerosols also may be produced by dropping liquid onto the surface of a rapidly spinning disc; such nebulizers, which are infrequently used in adult medicine, also incorporate large-volume reservoirs. A third means of creating aerosols is by ultrasonic nebulizers, in which droplets are produced by a rapidly oscillating crystal.

Disinfection of each type of equipment and even different devices employing the same design principle must be evaluated independently.

In our initial observations, we demonstrated that the reservoir nebulizer was the major site that became contaminated and from which bacterial dissemination occurred. The survival and multiplication of some bacterial species in the reservoir nebulizer fluid provide an effective amplification mechanism whereby even small numbers of initially contaminating bacteria ultimately may be delivered in large quantities to a patient.

There are multiple potential routes by which the fluid-containing reservoir initially may become contaminated. The relative importance of one route over another cannot be determined from the available data. The sources to be considered include at least the following (Fig. 26-3): the oxygen, compressed air, or other gas that is administered to the patient and that often drives the nebulizer may be contaminated; room air, which usually is added through the dilutor ports to decrease the concentration of inspired oxygen, may provide another source; personnel may contaminate the inside of the reservoir container during cleaning or replenishing of the fluid in the reservoir. (We even have had personnel contaminate the reservoir by attempting to be more cautious than called for in cleansing procedures; they washed the jars with 3% hexachlorophene-containing soaps that were unfortunately contaminated.) The water or other fluid placed in the reservoir must be sterile. Numerous outbreaks of pulmonary colonization and infection have been traced to the nebulization of contaminated medications. Organisms present in secretions from the patient's nose or mouth may contaminate the fluid that tends to condense in the plastic delivery tubing connecting the nebulizer to the face mask. Bacteria have been shown to survive for considerable time in such fluid. Massive contamination may result from emptying the condensate that collects in the delivery tubing back into the reservoir. Morris [54], however, detected contamination of the condensate in only one of 96 specimens. In a recent study Christopher and associates [9] found that retrograde contamination from tubing to a heated cascade humidifier did not occur since bacteria were inhibited at the 55°C (131°F) temperature. Failure to disinfect portions of the nebulizer, such as the nebulizer jet, may occur because of entrapment of air that prevents contact with liquids if liquid disinfectants are being used. Under these circumstances, the nebulizer jet serves as a nidus from which reinoculation of the reservoir may occur.

Whichever primary mechanisms are operative, even reservoir nebulizers that are initially sterile and used by only one individual very frequently become contaminated within 24 hours of clinical use. The bacterial multiplication that then occurs results in an amplification of organisms, which can be delivered in larger numbers and in a particle size that can be delivered to the lower reaches of the tracheobronchial tree.

Potential Means By Which Reservoir May Become Contaminated

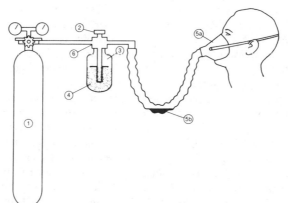

FIG. 26-3. Potential means by which reservoir of nebulizer may become contaminated. Key to figure: (1) Oxygen, compressed air, or other gas source; (2) room air via dilutor parts; (3) hand contact with inside of jar during refilling; (4) contaminated water used to fill reservoir; (5) organisms from patient's nose or mouth (5a), contaminated condensate (5b), which may then reflux into reservoir; (6) failure to sterilize nebulizer jet.

### Lymphohematogenous Spread

Invasion of the lung through the pulmonary vasculature is possible when there is a peripheral site of infection that is causing bacteremia, such as staphylococcal pneumonia secondary to septic thrombophlebitis associated with an indwelling venous catheter, *Escherichia coli* pneumonia as a complication of pyelonephritis, and *P. aeruginosa* pneumonia in the burned patient. In the majority of patients with nosocomial bacillary pneumonia, however, no distant locus can be identified.

### Control Measures*

The patients most likely to develop nosocomial bacterial pneumonia are those who (1) have had a recent surgical operation; (2) have conditions that make aspiration likely; (3) are exposed to contaminated respiratory therapy equipment, receive improper respiratory care, or have instrumentation of the respiratory tract; (4) are colonized in the oropharynx with aerobic gram-negative bacilli; or (5) have impaired immunologic function. Efforts to prevent nosocomial bacterial pneumonia have, therefore, emphasized (1) pre-

*From Simmons, B. P., and Wong, E. S. CDC Guidelines for the prevention of nosocomial pneumonia. *Am J. Infect Control* 11:230, 1983.

venting postoperative cases of pneumonia by giving therapy and instruction to high-risk patients, (2) preventing aspiration, (3) keeping respiratory therapy equipment clean and using proper techniques with patients whose respiratory tract is instrumented, and (4) preventing colonization.

Because the risk of pneumonia is not the same for all surgical patients and may be negligible for some, it is important to identify those patients scheduled for an operation who are at high risk of developing pneumonia [26]. These patients include those who are older (more than 70 years), are obese, have chronic obstructive pulmonary disease or a history of smoking, have abnormal pulmonary function tests (especially decreased maximum expiratory flow rate), have a tracheostomy or will be intubated for a prolonged time, or will have abdominal (especially upper abdominal) or thoracic operations. These patients may benefit from interventions designed to reduce their risk of pneumonia, especially therapies designed to expand the lung and prevent atelectasis after an operation.

Most patients can expand their lungs adequately after an operation by taking deep breaths periodically. However, patients may not take such deep breaths unless they are encouraged to do so. Patients can be encouraged to breathe deeply and expand their lungs by use of routine "stir-up" regimens that involve efforts to stimulate coughing, turning in bed, and walking. A device, the incentive spirometer, also appears to encourage periodic, voluntary expansion of the lung. The intermittent positive pressure breathing (IPPB) machine may be useful to assist lung expansion in high-risk patients who are cooperative but too weak to take deep breaths voluntarily. High airway pressures are often necessary to expand the lung with IPPB; such pressures may harm some patients, for example, by allowing gas to enter the esophagus and thus markedly elevating esophageal and gastric pressures. Such complications may be prevented by terminating IPPB before high pressures are reached. Unfortunately, such pressure-oriented treatments do not adequately expand the lung and do not decrease postoperative pulmonary complications. Thus the role of IPPB in preventing post operative pneumonia has not been determined [48]. Using blow bottles does not appear to decrease postoperative pulmonary complications and may in fact reduce lung volumes unless a deep breath is taken before blowing begins. If patients are not able to cough adequately, secretions may remain in the airways and interfere with pulmonary function and efforts to expand the lung. If a patient is having trouble with retained secretions that are not removed by coughing, chest physical therapy (breathing exercises, postural drainage and percussion, and efforts to stimulate coughing) is useful to help patients expectorate sputum [49]. Data on two modalities used to maintain lung expansion, positive end-expiratory pressure (PEEP) and continuous positive airway pressure (CPAP) by face mask, are too sparse to permit drawing definite conclusions concerning their efficacy.

The humidity of the anesthetic gases given during the operation may also be important in determining the risk of pneumonia. Prolonged breathing of dry gases, especially inadequately humidified oxygen ($O_2$) and nitrous oxide ($N_2O$), desiccates the respiratory mucosa, hampers ciliary function, and thus impairs respiratory defense mechanisms.

Patients who aspirate frequently or in large amounts or who aspirate gastric contents are at high risk of developing pneumonia. These patients usually have one or more of the following risk factors: (1) a depressed level of consciousness, (2) dysphagia due to neurologic or esophageal disorders, or (3) a nasogastric tube in place [50]. Prevention of pneumonia in such patients may be difficult, but patients with depressed consciousness who are likely to regurgitate can be intubated or fed by methods that make regurgitation unlikely, for example, by intravenous hyperalimentation or a feeding jejunostomy.

## DISINFECTION AND STERILIZATION OF VENTILATORY EQUIPMENT

Several methods have been suggested for the sterilization of inhalation therapy equipment. Based on surface-culturing techniques, the mechanical ventilator, rather than the reservoir nebulizer, is frequently the focus of major concern. Although ventilators, like other hospital equipment, should receive reasonable hygienic care, they are not a major source of bacterial contamination of inspired gas. The use of bacterial filters in various positions in the stream of gas flow in ventilators also has been suggested. A filter on the driving gas of the ventilator or nebulizer eliminates only one source of potential contamination, and hence filters do not ensure sterility of the effluent gas from the nebulizer. Filters interposed between the nebulizer and patient are not practical, because they would not permit the passage of the therapeutic aerosol. Primary attention must be directed to disinfection of the reservoir nebulizer (see Chapter 14).

### Definitions
In the published material on inhalation therapy equipment, varied terminology has been employed to describe the processes used to prevent transmission of disease. We have used the term "decontamination" for many of the procedures; however, according to common usage, this is inappropriate, and the term should be reserved for the process that renders contaminated items safe to handle with reasonable care. *Disinfection,* the more correct term, may be defined as the virtual elimination of all harmful microorganisms, except spores, in an attempt to prevent transmission of disease. *Sterilization* is the complete destruction or removal of all organisms (see Chapter 14). Objects that contact skin or mucous membranes, such as respiratory therapy equipment other than the apparatus itself, should receive at least a high level of disinfection and ideally should be sterilized before assignment to patients.

### Sterilization Methods
There are three methods potentially available for the sterilization of inhalation therapy equipment: steam autoclaving, cold soaking with activated glutaraldehyde germicidal solution, and ethylene oxide gas. (See the CDC *Guideline for Hospital Environmental Control:Cleaning, Disinfection, and Sterilization of Hospital Equipment* [80].)

AUTOCLAVING Steam autoclaving is usually not practical because of the sensitivity of the equipment to heat. We have used this procedure successfully, however, for older types of nebulizers that were constructed of cast aluminum.

GLUTARALDEHYDE Immersion in a germicidal solution may be used either to disinfect or to sterilize equipment, but ten hours of submersion in activated glutaraldehyde is required for sterilization; submersion for less time results in disinfection. The greatest limitation to liquid sterilization (or disinfection) is its unreliable penetration. To sterilize an item, the active chemical must contact all bacteria-laden surfaces. Entrapment of air often prevents adequate liquid contact during treatment, which is a particular problem with inhalation therapy equipment, because nebulizer jets are usually encased in hollow areas.

ETHYLENE OXIDE Since gases are completely miscible with air, the ideal chemical sterilant is a gas such as ethylene oxide. Ethylene oxide denatures bacterial proteins through a process of alkylation. Moisture is essential to this reaction. Raising the temperature also hastens the reaction; sterilization is achieved six to eight times faster at 54°C (130°F) than at 21°C (70°F). Ethylene oxide is absorbed into various plastics and must be allowed to diffuse out before the plastic is used in prolonged contact with tissues to avoid its local irritant effect; this process is termed *aeration.* Aeration periods depend on several factors: the duration of exposure to ethylene oxide, the aeration environment, the type of plastic, and the intended use of the item. Although aeration may often require 24 to 48 hours, units are available to reduce all aeration periods to 8 hours. The major problem of ethylene oxide sterilization is the expense of the equipment required to ensure safe, prompt, effective sterilization and aeration. This technique, however, appears to be the most satisfactory, provided it is remembered that under in-use conditions, recontamination can occur within 24 hours, even if a piece of equipment is used by only one patient.

*Disinfection Methods*
Many hospitals do not have the capability to sterilize all their inhalation therapy equipment with ethylene oxide. Also, it is not feasible to aerosolize the most effective liquid chemical sterilant, activated glutaraldehyde, to ensure that the nebulizer jets are sterilized. Thus various other disinfecting procedures have been employed and shown to be effective if rigorously applied and monitored [77]. With these procedures, it is important to cleanse the equipment mechanically. Exudates should not be allowed to dry. Equipment should be rinsed initially with cold water to avoid coagulation of protein and then washed using mechanical cleansing and detergent.

PASTEURIZATION Heating to 75°C (167°F) for ten minutes will kill vegetative forms of bacteria, and even washing at 60°C (140°F) for two minutes destroys most bacteria. The use of hot-water "pasteurization" has been successfully employed by several groups. Roberts and associates [70] immersed equipment for a period of 15 minutes at 80°C to 85°C (176°F to 185°F), whereas Nelson and Ryan [59] processed equipment for 30 minutes at 70°C (158°F). Nelson and Ryan were concerned that jets in equipment might not be disinfected by this method, because it is questionable whether the water enters the tiny orifices. All items with small orifices or jets were disassembled and disinfected with activated glutaraldehyde (immersion for ten minutes), rinsed in a solution of one ounce of sodium bisulfite per gallon of water, and then pasteurized and air-dried by blowing air at 38°C (100°F) over the equipment.

OTHER DISINFECTANTS Disinfectant solutions with greater antimicrobial activity than acetic acid, such as chlorhexidine diacetate and formaldehyde, can also be nebulized. However, the potential toxicities of chlorhexidine and similar agents, when nebulized into patient areas or inadvertently into patients, have not be sufficiently defined to allow their use without considerable study.

COPPER SPONGES It has been reported [17] that the placing of a copper sponge in the reservoir jars of venturi nebulizers results in the nebulizer contents remaining sterile. The institution of this method of cleaning in an intensive care unit resulted in an apparent reduction in the incidence of pulmonary infections. Although these investigators concluded that the sterility of reservoir nebulizers could be maintained for 48 hours or longer, they noted that in practice, the nebulizers and all parts distal to them were changed every 24 hours, a procedure that should have greatly improved the chances for sterility. Our own experience with this method has been limited to observations on the ability of the copper sponge to sterilize nebulizer solutions following intentional inoculation of bacteria into the nebulizer contents. We have been disappointed by the erratic ability of copper sponges to maintain sterility.

OTHER PROCEDURES Grieble and coworkers [28] have found that the daily use of phenolic disinfectants or dilute acetic acid did not sterilize spinning-disc nebulizers. It was found that daily sterilization with ethylene oxide was necessary to prevent contamination. Since this procedure was considered impractical in their clinical setting, the use of spinning-disc nebulizers was discontinued in their hospital.

Rhoades and associates [68] have found that ultrasonic nebulizers were not sterilized either by soaking in a disinfectant solution or by the nebulization of 0.25% acetic acid for 30 minutes. However, 2% acetic acid nebulization for 30 minutes successfully removed bacteria from a nebulizer. It has also been found that 7.5% hydrogen peroxide nebulization for 20 minutes may be an effective disinfecting procedure for ultrasonic nebulizers; it is suggested that such equipment be treated at least once every 24 hours.

One of the early regimens for controlling microbial contamination of reservoir, venturi-type nebulizers involved initial sterilization of the equipment with either ethylene oxide or steam autoclaving, or immersion in a disinfectant solution (e.g., glutaraldehyde or a phenolic disinfectant) in the inhalation therapy department. Daily nebulization with 0.25% acetic acid was then employed after the equipment had been assigned to a patient [66]. Dilute acetic acid was chosen because it is relatively nontoxic, which enabled the procedure to be performed at the patient's bedside. While acetic acid is bactericidal for only about one-third of gram-negative bacilli and gram-positive cocci, significant microbiologic failure of the regimen was not encountered. When properly used, acetic acid treatment renders the effluent gas from most venturi nebulizers virtually sterile. It is of note, however, that when the acetic acid method was transferred from laboratory procedure into routine hospital use, the results were disappointing. It was found subsequently that the failure to achieve disinfection of the effluent gas from nebulizers resulted from personnel error or faulty nebulizer jets. A continuous monitoring program and the replacement of pitted nebulizer jets resulted in the effluent gas being contaminated less than 10 percent of the time while in use.

It is not possible to control contamination of all types of reservoir venturi nebulizers safely by the described regimen. Some nebulizers used in pediatric tents have been demonstrated to be resistant to this method. It has been found that such nebulizers must be sterilized at least every 48 hours; either autoclaving or ethylene oxide may be used, and acetic acid nebulization is carried out on alternate days.

During the period immediately preceding the institution of a program of culturing the effluent from inhalation therapy equipment and of disinfection employing acetic acid nebulization, the prevalence of necrotizing pneumonia was 7.9 percent [66]. Under the epidemiologic circumstances of the hospitalized patient, the histologic appearance of necrotizing pneumonia has been found to be specific enough to serve as an index of the frequency of all pneumonia due to aerobic gram-negative bacilli. The prevalence of this lesion increased from 1.8 percent of all autopsies in 1957 to 7.9 percent of autopsies in 1963. This increase was significantly correlated with the use of reservoir nebulization treatments. With a program of surveillance and disinfection, and in the face of a 9 percent increase in the use of reservoir nebulization treatments, the incidence of necrotizing pneumonia in 1966 and 1967 decreased to 2.2 and 2.1 percent of autopsies. This accompanied a decrease in the frequency of contamination of reservoir nebulizers from 84 percent to less than 10 percent. Subsequently, in a totally independent study of the occurrence of colonization of the oropharynx and the development of pneumonia in patients in a medical intensive care unit, inhalation treatments were not significantly associated with the acquisition of aerobic gram-negative bacilli [41].

## USE OF DISPOSABLE AND INTERCHANGE OF REUSABLE EQUIPMENT

Most hospitals have found that it is easier to replace solutions and critical equipment at established intervals than to establish "in-use" disinfection programs. Many using the replacement approach recommend that reservoirs be completely emptied and refilled with sterile solutions every 8 to 24 hours and breathing circuits changed every 24 hours. Most of these recommendations have been empirical and not subjected to in-use validation. Lareau and coworkers [46] failed to demonstrate any difference between the incidence of pneumonia in patients whose ventilator circuits were changed at 8 hours and those for whom they were changed every 24 hours. In a hospital in which respirator tubing and nebulizer fluids were routinely changed at 24 hours, none of 68 cultures of nebulizer fluid taken after 24 hours of use was positive [15]. In an extension of observations on tubing change at 24- and 48-hour intervals, Craven and colleagues [13] found only low levels of contamination of inspiratory-phase gas and lack of a significant increase in colonization of tubing between 24 and 48 hours. They suggest that changing respirator tubing at 48 hours rather than 24 hours poses no increased risk to the patient, yet results in significant savings.

Results of several studies also suggest that in-use microbiologic sampling of respiratory therapy equipment is unwarranted in the absence of high endemic rates of nosocomial pneumonia or epidemics.

## CARE OF THE PATIENT WITH AN ENDOTRACHEAL TUBE OR TRACHEOSTOMY

Patients with endotracheal tubes or tracheostomies were recognized early to be at high risk for the development of nosocomial pneumonias. Despite early recognition, infection control practices have been less successful than in many other areas. Most recommendations are directed at preventing cross-contamination by use of sterile equipment and aseptic technique. Tracheal suction should be performed only when clinically indicated, rather than on a routine basis. To avoid or at least minimize damage to the trachea requires training in the use of the tracheal suction catheter. It is essential to avoid withdrawing the catheter up the trachea with suction applied in a manner analogous to vacuum-cleaning a rug. When suction is applied, the catheter should not be withdrawn.

Despite meticulous care, colonization of tracheostomy sites occurs regularly. Because of this inevitability, antibiotic administration via the endotracheal tube has been evaluated [43]. Although the procedure is of short-term benefit, over intervals resistant bacteria have been selected and the end result has been modification rather than elimination of the microbial flora.

## CDC GUIDELINES FOR PREVENTION OF NOSOCOMIAL PNEUMONIA*

The Centers for Disease Control has developed consensus guidelines for the prevention of nosocomial pneumonia. The procedure is a modification of the Delphi technique. A draft of recommendations is prepared and widely circulated to knowledgeable individuals, who are requested to categorize each statement or recommendation (Table 26-9). A multidisciplinary group made up of persons who have worked in the area is convened to discuss and reach a consensus on the draft of specific recommendations. Because the guidelines are based on consensus, there are specific recommendations, especially in categories II and III, with which persons in the working group and others may disagree.

*From Simmons, B. P., and Wong, E. S. CDC Guidelines for the prevention of nosocomial pneumonia. *Am J. Infect Control* 11:230, 1983.

TABLE 26-9. Ranking scheme for recommendations

Category I. Strongly recommended for adoption:*
Measures in category I are strongly supported by well-designed and controlled clinical studies that show effectiveness in reducing the risk of nosocomial infections or are viewed as useful by the majority of experts in the field. Measures in this category are judged to be applicable to the majority of hospitals regardless of size, patient population, or endemic nosocomial infection rate and are considered practical to implement.

Category II. Moderately recommended for adoption:
Measures in category II are supported by highly suggestive clinical studies or by definitive studies in institutions that might not be representative of other hospitals. Measures that have not been adequately studied but have a strong theoretical rationale indicating that they might be very effective are included in this category. Category II measures are judged to be practical to implement. They are not to be considered a standard of practice for every hospital.

Category III. Weakly recommended for adoption:
Measures in category III have been proposed by some investigators, authorities, or organizations, but to date lack both supporting data and a strong theoretical rationale. Thus they might be considered important issues that require additional evaluation; they might be considered by some hospitals for implementation, especially if such hospitals have specific nosocomial infection problems or sufficient resources.

*Recommendations that advise against the adoption of certain measures can be found in the guidelines that follow. These negative recommendations are also ranked into one of the three categories depending on the strength of the scientific backing or opinions of the members of the working group. A negative recommendation in category I means that scientific data or prevailing opinion strongly indicates that the measure not be adopted. A negative recommendation in category III means that, given the available information, the measure under consideration should probably not be adopted; such a measure, however, requires additional evaluation.
Source: Simons, B. P., and Wong, E. S. CDC guidelines for the prevention and control of nosocomial pneumonia. *J. Infect. Control* 11:230, 1983.

*Recommendations*

1. Perioperative measures for prevention of postoperative pneumonia
   a. Patients who will receive anesthesia and will have an abdominal or thoracic operation or who have substantial pulmonary dysfunction, such as patients with chronic obstructive lung disease, a musculoskeletal abnormality of the chest, or abnormal pulmonary function tests, should receive preoperative and postoperative

therapy and instruction designed to prevent postoperative pulmonary complications such as pneumonia. The therapy and instruction, which are recommended below in *1b* through *1g*, should be given by a person trained to administer them. *Category I*

b. Whenever appropriate, preoperative therapy should include treatment and resolution of pulmonary infections, efforts to facilitate removal of respiratory secretions (for example, by use of bronchodilators and postural drainage and percussion), and discontinuance of smoking by the patient. *Category I*

c. Preoperative instruction should include discussions of the importance in the postoperative period of frequent coughing, taking deep breaths, and ambulating (as soon as medically indicated). During the discussions, the patient should demonstrate and practice adequate coughing and deep breathing *Category I*

d. An incentive spirometer should be used for preoperative instruction in deep breathing and for postoperative care. *Category III*

e. Postoperative therapy and instructions should be designed to encourage frequent coughing, deep breathing, and, unless medically contraindicated, moving about in the bed and ambulating. *Category I*

f. If conservative measures (mentioned in *1e* above) do not remove retained pulmonary secretions, postural drainage and percussion should be done to assist the patient in expectorating sputum. *Category II*

g. Pain that interferes with coughing and deep breathing should be controlled, for example, by use of analgesics, appropriate wound support for abdominal wounds (such as placing a pillow tightly across the abdomen), and regional nerve blocks. *Category I* (Caution: narcotics may reduce the urge to cough and breathe deeply.)

h. Systemic antibiotics should not be routinely used to prevent postoperative pneumonia. *Category I*

2. Handwashing
Hands should be washed after contact with respiratory secretions, whether or not gloves are worn. Hands should be washed before and after contact with a patient who is intubated or has had a recent tracheostomy. (See *Guideline for Hospital Environmental Control: Antiseptics, Handwashing, and Handwashing Facilities*.) *Category I*

3. Fluids and medications
a. (1) Only sterile fluids should be nebulized or used in a humidifier. These fluids should be dispensed aseptically; that is, contaminated equipment should not be allowed to enter or touch the fluid while it is being dispensed. *Category I*

(2) After a large container (bottle) of fluid intended for use in a nebulizer or humidifier has been opened, unused fluid should be discarded within 24 hours. *Category II*

b. Either single-dose or multi-dose vials can be used for respiratory therapy. If multi-dose vials are used, they should be stored (refrigerated or at room temperature) according to directions on the vial label or package insert. Vials should be used no longer than the expiration date given on the label. *Category II*

4. Maintenance of in-use respiratory therapy equipment
a. (1) Fluid reservoirs should be filled immediately before—but not far in advance of—use. Fluid should not be added to replenish partially filled reservoirs; that is, if fluid is to be added, the residual fluid should first be discarded. *Category II*

(2) Water that has condensed in tubing should be discarded and not allowed to drain back into the reservoir. *Category I*

b. (1) Venturi wall nebulizers and their reservoirs should be routinely changed and replaced with sterilized or disinfected ones every 24 hours. *Category I*

(2) Other nebulizers (including medication nebulizers) and their reservoirs and cascade (high volume) humidifiers and their reservoirs should be changed and replaced with sterilized or disinfected ones every 24 hours. *Category II*

(3) Room air humidifiers that create droplets to humidify (and thus are really nebulizers) should not be used. *Category I*

c. Reusable humidifier reservoirs for use with wall oxygen outlets should be cleaned, rinsed out, and then dried daily. *Category II* (Disposable reservoirs for use with wall oxygen outlets may be safe for long periods, and it is not known whether these need to be routinely changed before they are empty.

d. The tubing (including any nasal prongs) and any mask used to deliver oxygen from a wall outlet should be changed between patients. *Category I*

e. Breathing circuits (including tubing and exhalation valve) should be routinely changed and replaced with sterilized or disinfected ones every 24 hours. *Category II*

f. When a respiratory therapy machine is used to treat multiple patients, the breathing circuit should be changed between patients and replaced with a sterilized or disinfected one. *Category II*

5. Disposable equipment

No pieces of respiratory therapy equipment that are designed for single use (disposable) should be reused. *Category I*

6. Processing reusable equipment*

a. All equipment to be sterilized or disinfected should be thoroughly cleaned to remove all blood, tissue, food, or other residue. It should be decontaminated before or during cleaning if it is marked "contaminated" and received from patients in certain types of isolation. *Category I*

b. Respiratory therapy equipment that touches mucous membranes should be sterilized before use on other patients; if this is not feasible, it should receive high-level disinfection. *Category I*

c. Breathing circuits (including tubing and exhalation valves), medication nebulizers and their reservoirs, venturi wall nebulizers and their reservoirs, and cascade humidifiers and their reservoirs should be sterilized or receive high-level disinfection. *Category I*

d. Since coolant chambers for ultrasonic nebulizers are difficult to disinfect adequately, these chambers should be gas-sterilized (ethylene oxide) or have at least 30 minutes of contact time with a high-level disinfectant. *Category I*

e. The internal machinery of ventilators and breathing machines should not be routinely sterilized or disinfected between patients. *Category I* (Disinfection or sterilization may be necessary only after a machine is potentially contaminated by extremely dangerous agents, such as Lassa fever virus.)

f. Respirometers and other equipment used to monitor several patients in succession should not directly touch parts of the breathing circuit. Rather, extension pieces should be used between the equipment and breathing circuit and should be changed between patients. If no extension piece is used and such monitoring equipment is directly connected to contami-

nated equipment, the monitoring equipment should be sterilized or receive high-level disinfection before use on other patients. *Category II*

g. Once they have been used for one patient, hand-powered resuscitation bags (for example, Ambu† bags) should be sterilized or receive high-level disinfection before use on other patients. *Category I* (There are no data to suggest that these bags need to be changed routinely during use on 1 patient.)

7. Microbiologic monitoring

a. In the absence of an epidemic or high endemic rate of nosocomial pulmonary infections, the disinfection process for respiratory therapy equipment should not be monitored by cultures; that is, routine sampling of such equipment should not be done. *Category I* (This recommendation differs slightly from a previous CDC recommendation. See text of this guideline for a discussion of this recommendation.

b. Because of the difficulty in interpreting results, routine microbiologic sampling of respiratory therapy equipment while it is being used by a patient is not recommended. *Category I*

8. Patients with tracheostomy

a. Tracheostomy should be performed under aseptic conditions in an operating room, except when strong clinical indications for emergency or bedside operation intervene. *Category I*

b. Until a recent tracheostomy wound has had time to heal or form granulation tissue around the tube, "no-touch" technique should be used or sterile gloves should be worn on both hands for all manipulations at the tracheostomy site. *Category II*

c. (1) When a tracheostomy tube requires changing, a sterile tube or one that has received high-level disinfection should be used. *Category I*

(2) Aseptic technique, including the use of sterile gloves and drapes, should be used when a tube is changed. *Category II*

9. Suctioning of respiratory tract

a. Risk of cross-contamination and excessive trauma increases with frequent suctioning. Thus suctioning should not be done routinely but only when needed to reduce substantial secre-

---

*See also *Guideline for Hospital Environmental Control: Cleaning, Disinfection, and Sterilization of Hospital Equipment.*

†Use of trade names is for identification only and does not constitute endorsement by the Public Health Service, U.S. Department of Health and Human Services.

tions, which may be indicated by increased respiratory difficulties or easily audible "gurgling" breathing sounds. *Category I*

b. Suctioning should be performed using "no-touch" technique or gloves on both hands. *Category I* (Although fresh gloves should be used for each suctioning, sterile gloves are not needed.)

c. A sterile catheter should be used for each series of suctioning (defined as a single suctioning or repeated suctioning done with only brief periods intervening to clear or flush the catheter). *Category I*

d. If tenacious mucus is a problem and flushing of the catheter is required, sterile fluid should be used to remove secretions from it; fluid that becomes contaminated during use for one series of suctioning should then be discarded. *Category I*

e. (1) Suction collection tubing (up to the canister) should always be changed between patients. *Category I*

(2) Suction collection canisters when used on one patient need not be routinely changed or emptied. *Category III*

(3) Unless used in short-term care units (recovery or emergency rooms), suction collection canisters should be changed between use on different patients. *Category II*

(4) If used in short term care units, suction collection canisters need not be changed between patients but should be changed daily. *Category III*

(5) Once they are changed, reusable suction collection canisters should be sterilized or receive high-level disinfection. *Category II*

f. With portable suction devices, which may discharge contaminated aerosols, high-efficiency bacterial filters should be used between the collection bottle and vacuum source. *Category III* (When used with wall suction units, such filters have not been shown to be useful for infection control.)

10. Protection of patients from other infected patients or staff

a. Patients with potentially transmissible respiratory infections should be isolated according to the current edition of *Isolation Techniques for Use in Hospitals*. (This recommendation is not categorized. A new edition of the isolation manual is being developed.)*

b. Personnel with respiratory infections should

---

*The new edition is now available (see Chapter 9).

not be assigned to the direct care of high-risk patients, for example, neonates, young infants, patients with chronic obstructive lung disease, or immunocompromised patients. *Category II*

c. If an influenza epidemic is anticipated, a prevention program should be started for all patient-care personnel and high-risk patients. This program could include use of influenza vaccine and antiviral chemoprophylaxis. *Category I*

## *STAPHYLOCOCCUS AUREUS* INFECTIONS

### *General Aspects*

TRANSMISSIBILITY   The distribution of staphylococci in nature has probably been studied more fully than any comparable bacteriologic problem. For all practical purposes, *S. aureus* has no significant reservoir outside of humans or animals. There is general agreement that the main reservoir in humans is the nose, specifically the squamous epithelium of the vestibule. Skin surfaces harboring staphylococci become colonized from the nose. To remain endemic, staphylococci have to pass from one person to another; their main asset in achieving this is their ability to withstand drying. Based on prevalence studies in normal adults residing in urban areas, the average nasal-carrier rate for staphylococci is 50 percent. In sequential studies on hospital personnel, it was found that 15 percent were consistently negative, while 36 percent were persistent carriers. The persistent carriers had higher numbers of organisms, based on quantitative studies, than the transient carriers (see Chapter 31).

The development of staphylococcal lower respiratory tract infection may be either bronchogenous or secondary to lymphohematogenous dissemination from peripheral sites to the lung. In the former instance (which is the more common), the acquisition of staphylococci appears to be primarily through contact transmission rather than by aerosols. Once staphylococci have been established on the mucosa, spread to the tracheobronchial tree can occur through aspiration, and provided the inoculum is sufficient, the bronchopulmonary antimicrobial defenses are compromised, or both, lower respiratory infection can ensue.

PREDISPOSING FACTORS   Staphylococcal pneumonia in infants usually occurs as a primary infection of the respiratory tract, but it may also derive by lymphohematogenous spread from the skin or from other infections. It may also occur as a complication of measles, chickenpox, influenza, or cystic fibrosis. The highest incidence occurs among infants.

Staphylococcal pneumonia in adults is usually associated with a previous viral respiratory tract infection, such as influenza. It may also occur as a complication of acute bacterial endocarditis or septic thrombophlebitis; septic emboli may involve the lungs.

Five to fifteen percent of all nosocomial pneumonia is caused by *S. aureus* (see Tables 26-2 and 26-3).

CLINICAL FEATURES  The illness usually begins as an upper respiratory tract infection with fever, nasal obstruction or discharge, and cough associated with irritability and anorexia. The symptoms may progress rapidly or gradually to increasing cough, tachypnea, dyspnea, and subcostal retractions. Severe infections in young infants may be manifested by increasing respiratory distress, abdominal distention, pallor, cyanosis, prostration, and possibly, death.

The physical findings vary with the type of pulmonary involvement. Staphylococcal infection of the lung may be followed by consolidation, abscess formation, pneumatoceles, empyema, pneumothorax, or pyopneumothorax, either singly or in combination. In children, the roentgenographic lesion is apt to appear as multiple cysts because of the characteristic pneumatocele formation. In adults, the pulmonary lesions appear as confluent areas of consolidation with rapid progression to abscess formation and cavitation.

Pneumatocele formation is a hallmark of staphylococcal pneumonia. It is thought to be an emphysematous bleb within the pulmonary interstitial tissue and is presumably produced as follows: the staphylococci invade the bronchial wall and peribronchiolar tissues, producing inflammation and abscess formation. The perforation of the bronchial wall by the abscess enables air to pass into the interstitial space. A ball-valve effect traps the air, thereby producing a cyst or pneumatocele. Thus the bleb is a secondary manifestation of the bronchial and peribronchial infection. Pneumatoceles usually clear spontaneously within a variable period of four weeks to four months.

Pneumothorax results from the rupture of a pneumatocele. Sudden onset of severe dyspnea, cyanosis, prostration, and shock may indicate tension pneumothorax. Empyema occurs as the result of rupture of an abscess into the pleural cavity. Pyopneumothorax develops if the abscess connects with a bronchus.

The blood picture characteristically reveals an increase in the number of polymorphonuclear leukocytes. Occasionally, however, the white blood cell count is normal or low. The roentgenographic findings may reveal rapidly changing infiltrations, pneumatoceles, pneumothorax, empyema, or pyopneumothorax.

THERAPY  Since the early 1940s, the prevalence of penicillin-resistant strains of staphylococci detected in hospitalized patients has risen from between 0 and 12 percent to at least 80 percent (see Chapter 11). The occurrence of staphylococcal pneumonia represents a medical emergency, because rapid progression is typical and the rates are high for morbidity and mortality, which ensue without therapy or with ineffective antimicrobial therapy. Initial empirical treatment should include the parenteral administration of a penicillinase-resistant semisynthetic penicillin, such as nafcillin. In the patient who is allergic to penicillin, alternatives include parenteral vancomycin or a first-generation cephalosporin. If methicillin-resistant *S. aureus* strains are prevalent in the epidemiologic setting in which the patient has acquired staphylococcal pneumonia, empirical therapy should be vancomycin intravenously (not a cephalosporin). Additional therapy directed at maintenance of adequate oxygenation, drainage of loculated infection, and correction and prevention of fluid and electrolyte imbalance is essential, and in many patients, it is as critical as the antimicrobial therapy, especially with the development of pneumatoceles and pyopneumothorax.

*Prevention of Endemic Infections*
The ubiquity of staphylococci, their ready adaptability, and the nature of the parasite-host relationship make it difficult to control human staphylococcal infections.

Since there is little evidence that healthy persons carrying staphylococci in the nose are primarily responsible for transmitting infection even to premature and newly born infants (potentially the most susceptible recipients), masks are not recommended. Washing one's hands with an antibacterial detergent (e.g., an iodophor) before and after handling patients is recommended. The routine use of hexachlorophene-containing detergents is probably safe for personnel, although evidence of absorption can be demonstrated. If these detergents are present in work areas, however, they are likely to be used on newborns or in other than epidemic circumstances, in which their use should be avoided.

The detection and treatment of asymptomatic nasal staphylococcal carriers is not indicated. However, the chronic nasal carrier who is plagued with recurrent boils or styes or has been shown to have an excessive rate of postoperative surgical wound infections should be treated. Short-term systemic antimicrobial therapy has been ineffective in more than temporary suppression of nasal carriage. One of two approaches can be taken. Prolonged use of a regimen of applying a topical antistaphylococcal ointment such as 0.1% neomycin in neobase, gentamicin, or bacitracin to the nasal vestibule three to four times daily may decrease the number of staphylococci carried [7]. A more recently reported regimen of rifampin (300 mg orally twice daily) and cloxacillin or dicloxacillin (500 mg orally four times daily) for 10 days resulted in eradication of nasal staphylococcal carriage in a high proportion of carriers [98].

It is most important to exclude all persons with active staphylococcal infections of the skin or mucous membranes, who may be shedding particularly virulent staphylococci, from patient-care areas. The prophylactic use of antimicrobial agents for contacts of pneumonia cases is not recommended. Proper isolation of patients with staphylococcal pneumonia is important and will reduce risks of cross-infection by contact and airborne spread (see Chapter 9).

### Epidemic Infections

INCIDENCE   Epidemics of staphylococcal lower respiratory tract infections were particularly common in the mid-1950s and early 1960s in association with outbreaks of staphylococcal skin infections in premature and newborn infants (these were associated with strains lysed by bacteriophages 80/81), and in adults following the influenza A2 ($H_2N_2$ [Asian] and $H_3N_2$ [Hong Kong]) pandemics of 1957–58 and 1968–70. During the 1957–58 influenzal pandemic, although the occurrence of *Streptococcus pneumoniae* predominated in many series of patients, Hers and associates [37] demonstrated staphylococci in 69 of 103 (67 percent), Martin and coworkers [50] in 11 of 17 (65 percent), and Petersdorf and coworkers [63] in 5 of 11 (45 percent) fatal cases of pneumonia.

HIGH-RISK AREAS   The areas of highest risk are the premature and newborn nursery areas and patient-care areas in which patients with respiratory problems may be congregated, for example, respiratory intensive care units.

SOURCES OF INFECTION   The sources and modes of spread are the same as those for endemic infections. In newborn nursery areas, transmission via the hands of personnel is the most important route. Transmission via aerosols or fomites is less important.

CONTROL OF OUTBREAKS   The prevention and control of outbreaks of nosocomial staphylococcal pneumonia mainly depend on the interruption of the transmission of *S. aureus* in newborn nurseries. The prompt control of epidemics of staphylococcal skin infections is especially important, because pneumonia as a result of lymphohematogenous spread may complicate such infections. The control of staphylococcal skin infections in neonates is described in depth in Chapter 31 of this text.

## PNEUMOCOCCAL PNEUMONIA

### General Aspects

TRANSMISSIBILITY   *Streptococcus pneumoniae* organisms are normal inhabitants of the human upper respiratory tract in 5 to 60 percent of the population, depending on the season. Most cases of pneumonia probably derive from aspiration of organisms from the oropharynx. Pneumococcal infection occurs predominantly during the winter and early spring. Morbidity and mortality rates are higher for blacks than for whites. Person-to-person transmission by droplets is undoubtedly common, but true epidemics of pneumococcal pneumonia are rare, even in closed populations. *S. pneumoniae* is responsible for 5 to 10 percent of all nosocomial pneumonias (see Tables 26-2 and 26-3). Patients with pneumococcal infections caused by penicillin-sensitive strains need not be isolated, because the risk of cross-infection is relatively small. Taking proper precautions in handling the respiratory secretions of such patients is adequate.

PREDISPOSING FACTORS   Invasion of the tissues of the nasopharynx rarely, if ever, occurs, and "pneumococcal pharyngitis" is a doubtful entity. Viral respiratory infections predispose to pneumococcal pneumonia. There is generally a high incidence of pneumococcal pneumonia during epidemics of viral influenza, and a frequent clinical association is seen with sporadic viral respiratory infections.

CLINICAL FEATURES   Pneumococcal pneumonia is often preceded for a few days by coryza or some other form of common respiratory disease. The onset is usually so abrupt that patients frequently can state the exact hour that the illness began. There is a sudden shaking chill in more than 80 percent of cases, a rapid rise in temperature, and a corresponding tachycardia.

About 75 percent of patients develop severe pleuritic pain and cough and produce pinkish or "rusty" mucinoid sputum within a few hours. The chest pain is agonizing, and respirations become rapid, shallow, and grunting as the patient tries to splint the affected side. Patients appear acutely ill; nausea, headache, and malaise are not prominent, however, and most individuals are alert. Pleuritic pain and dyspnea are the dominant complaints.

This "classic" clinical presentation occurs with lobar pneumococcal pneumonia; however, a recent analysis of pneumococcal pneumonia in hospitalized patients demonstrated that lobar pneumonia developed in only one-third of patients and bronchopneumonia in two-thirds [61]. Underlying disease (e.g., alcoholism, chronic pulmonary disease) was common in both groups. Symptoms and signs in the bronchopneumonic group consisted most commonly of fever (92 percent), cough (33 percent), and cough productive of purulent sputum (49 percent). Other features such as chills, pleuritic chest pain, nausea, and vomiting occurred in less than 15 percent of patients.

In the untreated disease, there is sustained fever of 39.2°C to 40.6°C (102.5°F to 105°F), continued pleuritic pain, cough, and expectoration; abdominal distention is frequent. Herpes febrilis (labialis) is a common complication.

Physical examination of the patient with lobar pneumonia reveals restricted motion of the affected hemithorax. Tactile fremitus may be decreased during the initial day of illness but is usually increased when consolidation is fully established. The percussion note is dull. Early in the course of infection, breath sounds are diminished, but as the lesion evolves, they become tubular or bronchial in quality, and bronchophony and whispered pectoriloquy can be elicited. These findings are accompanied by fine, crepitant rales.

THERAPY   In the United States, resistance of *S. pneumoniae* strains to benzylpenicillin (penicillin G) occurs with great rarity (see Chapter 11). Before 1965 the great majority of pneumococci were inhibited by penicillin concentrations of 0.04 μg/ml or less [16]. This situation could change; in May 1977, strains of *S. pneumoniae* that were highly resistant to penicillin G, methicillin, cephalosporin, tetracycline, erythromycin, clindamycin, chloramphenicol, trimethoprim-sulfamethoxazole, and all the aminoglycosides were isolated from patients and carriers in several locations in the Republic of South Africa. These multiply drug-resistant strains were initially susceptible to rifampin, vancomycin, bacitracin, and fusidic acid. Resistance to rifampin, however, is known to occur readily, and resistant strains have already been encountered in patients treated with rifampin and fusidic acid. Subsequently, several single, highly resistant strains (MIC for penicillin G ≥ 4 μg/ml) have been isolated in

the United Kingdom, New Guinea, Australia, and the United States (Minnesota, Colorado). Isolates belong to a limited number of serotypes: 6A, 6B, 14, and 19A. However, these strains have not spread. These rare "penicillin-resistant" strains should not be confused with strains that are "relatively" penicillin-resistant (MICs of 0.1 to 1.0 μg/ml), which represent 3 percent of U.S. isolates [16]. Strains that are resistant to the tetracyclines and, to a lesser extent, to erythromycin are clinically significant and are observed in the United States.

The antimicrobial agent of choice is benzylpenicillin (penicillin G). Optimal results have been achieved with dosages of 80,000 units (10,000 units every three hours) of aqueous crystalline penicillin G per day. The usual recommended dose of 600,000 units of aqueous procaine penicillin G intramuscularly twice daily provides a wide margin of safety; it also minimizes the influence on the normal microbial flora and the possibility of supracolonization and suprainfection. In the patient who is allergic to penicillin, alternative agents include erythromycin (the prevalence of resistant strains is less than 1 percent), the cephalosporins, and clindamycin. It should be emphasized that the aminoglycosidic antibiotics (gentamicin, tobramycin, amikacin, and netilmicin) are not effective against pneumococci in the usually recommended safe doses.

Pneumococcal pneumonia usually improves promptly when an appropriate antimicrobial drug is given. Within 12 to 36 hours after initiation of treatment with penicillin, the temperature, pulse, and respiration begin to fall and may reach normal values, the pleuritic pain subsides, and the spread of the inflammatory process is halted. In approximately half the patients, however, the temperature requires four days or longer to become normal, and a failure of the patient's temperature to reach normal in 24 to 48 hours should not prompt a change in antibacterial therapy in the absence of other indications.

Roentgenographic resolution often requires six to eight weeks. In a comparison of community-acquired (26 patients) with nosocomial (36 patients) pneumococcal bacteremia, more of the patients with nosocomial disease had ultimately fatal underlying diseases, and these patients had undergone more manipulation of the respiratory tract. The mortality in the community-acquired group was 18 percent compared with 67 percent in the nosocomial group [58]. Of the 36 patients with nosocomial bacteremia, 35 were either seen in the clinic or hospitalized for more than two weeks. Pneumococcal vaccine could have been administered to these patients.

*Prevention of Endemic Infections*

Despite 83 pneumococcal serotypes, most of the serious infections are caused by a limited number; organisms of capsular types 1 through 8 account for 60 percent of such infections in adults. The efficacy of prophylactic vaccination with 50 μg each of the capsular polysaccharides of pneumococcal types 1, 2, 5, and 7 was demonstrated convincingly by MacLeod and coworkers [48] in 1945, and the properties of hexavalent vaccines were studied later by Heidelberger, MacLeod, and DiLopi [35]. Most individuals receiving such vaccines showed an antibody response to all six antigens, and half-maximal levels of antibody persisted for five to eight years following a single injection of vaccine. Preparations of pneumococcal vaccines were available commercially for a short period, but they were removed from the market because their use was considered unnecessary by most physicians. Despite these attitudes, pneumococcal pneumonia with bacteremia remained a major infectious cause of death in the United States. This view has been challenged by more recent clinical and epidemiologic studies, and vaccines of capsular types 1 through 9 and types 12, 14, 18, 19, and 23 are especially indicated for those at high risk of infection and death. Of patients with pneumococcal bacteremia who die despite treatment with penicillin or tetracycline, approximately 60 percent die within five days of onset of illness. In light of observations such as these, new polyvalent pneumococcal vaccines have been relicensed. One vaccine consists of capsular polysaccharides from the 14 most prevalent pneumococcal types accounting for at least 80 percent of pneumococcal disease, while a more recent vaccine contains antigens from the 18 most prevalent types. A cost-effectiveness analysis has provided evidence supportive of the recommendation for immunizing all persons aged 65 years or older and persons with high-risk conditions aged 45 to 65 years [99]. Nevertheless, pneumococcal immunization programs have not received wide-scale acceptance. In recent studies it has been shown that 55 to 75 percent of adults aged 20 to 64 with high-risk conditions or 65 or greater without high-risk conditions who were hospitalized with pneumococcal bacteremia had one or more instances of hospitalization within the five years up to but not including the three weeks previous to development of pneumococcal bacteremia [22,23,44]. Based on these observations, a more targeted pneumococcal prevention program is both feasible and highly appropriate. Under such a program, at the time of discharge from the hospital, regardless of reason for admission, all previously unimmunized high-risk patients aged 45 years or older and all patients aged 65 years or older regardless of risk would be offered polyvalent pneumococcal vaccine.

*Epidemic Infections*

Epidemics of nosocomial pneumococcal pneumonia have rarely been reported. The above mentioned multiply drug-resistant strain of pneumococcus in the Republic of South Africa caused outbreaks in children hospitalized in several different hospitals [5]. Measles and previous antibiotic therapy appeared to be important conditions predisposing to pneumonia. Control of these outbreaks was achieved by cohorting infected and colonized patients, vancomycin treatment of cases and carriers, closing hospital wards housing carriers, placing carriers in isolation wards or an isolation hospital, and culturing new admissions and transferring carriers to the isolation hospital.

## *STREPTOCOCCUS PYOGENES* PNEUMONIA

*General Aspects*

TRANSMISSIBILITY  Soon after birth, α-hemolytic streptococci appear in the upper part of the respiratory tract and may be isolated therefrom throughout life. Streptococci of Lancefield groups C and G and, more rarely, organisms of groups other than A may be isolated from the oropharynx of 5 percent or more of the normal population.

In general, at least 5 percent of the people of any community harbor group-A streptococci in their oropharynx. The prevalence varies and depends on the culture methods used as well as on environmental, host, and bacterial factors. Persons under 20 years of age are most likely to harbor group-A streptococci, especially if the tonsils are present.

Following either apparent or inapparent infection, the carrier state usually persists for several months and occasionally for longer periods. As the carrier state progresses, the streptococci lose their ability to produce M protein, so that by the eleventh week, about 40 percent of strains cannot be typed.

Ability to spread disease appears to be an attribute of individuals who have been infected recently. Whether such persons harbor more numerous streptococci in the nose and throat or whether the organisms are especially capable of spreading to other persons cannot be determined from the available evidence. It is established that nasal carriers of group-A streptococci are likely to spread disease. The spread of streptococci in any population group is related to the degree of exposure, and, during the winter months when people are confined to enclosed areas and are under crowded conditions, dissemination of bacteria is especially likely to occur.

Group-A streptococci naturally deposited in dust and on blankets will not produce respiratory infections in humans. The evidence implicates the direct mode of transfer as being primarily responsible for the dissemination of such infections.

PREDISPOSING FACTORS Pneumonia caused by "aerobic" streptococci accounts for less than 5 percent of all cases of nosocomial pneumonia. Except in the newborn—in whom group-B streptococci are a major cause of neonatal sepsis that may include pneumonia—pneumonia is almost invariably caused by group-A streptococci and may arise secondarily to an infection of the upper part of the respiratory tract. Epidemics have been observed following influenza and measles.

CLINICAL FEATURES Primary group-A streptococcal pneumonia is rare in the absence of influenza. The onset of pneumonia tends to be abrupt, with symptoms of chills, fever, anorexia, and vomiting. Cough, sputum that is pink and thin, and chest pain are characteristic. The temperature is usually high 40°C (104°F), and fever is intermittent. Examination reveals scattered, fine rales, but signs of lobar consolidation are rare.

A characteristic feature of group-A streptococcal pneumonia is the early development (within four days of onset of illness) of an empyema (metapneumonic).

THERAPY All strains of *Streptococcus pyogenes* remain susceptible to benzylpenicillin (penicillin G). Strains that are resistant in vitro to the tetracyclines have been reported.

The antimicrobial agent of choice is benzylpenicillin. A dose of 600,000 units of aqueous procaine penicillin G administered intramuscularly twice daily provides an adequate margin of safety and minimizes the influence on the normal microbial flora as well as the possibility of supracolonization and suprainfection. Alternative agents for treating the patient who is allergic to penicillins include erythromycin, the cephalosporins, and clindamycin. As is the case with pneumococci (see previous section), the aminoglycosidic antibiotics (gentamicin, tobramycin, amikacin, and netilmicin) are not effective as single agents against group-A streptococci in the usually recommended safe doses.

*Control of Infections*
There are no specifically recommended measures for the prevention of group-A streptococcal pneumonia per se. However, proper control of infections in other sites (see Chapters 27, 30, and 31) will reduce the chances of nosocomial acquisition of these organisms.

There are no reports of nosocomial epidemics of group-A streptococcal pneumonia.

## PNEUMONIA CAUSED BY ENDOGENOUS, AEROBIC, GRAM-NEGATIVE BACILLI

*General Aspects*
TRANSMISSIBILITY *Klebsiella pneumoniae, Enterobacter aerogenes, Escherichia coli,* and *Proteus* species are aerobic, gram-negative bacilli that are commonly found among the endogenous flora of the gastrointestinal tract of hospitalized patients. Collectively, they are responsible for about one-quarter to one-third of all cases of nosocomial pneumonia (see Tables 26-2 and 26-3). In normal subjects, pharyngeal acquisition of these aerobic gram-negative bacilli is infrequent. In contrast, chronically or severely ill persons lose the ability to resist colonization of the oropharynx with this group of microorganisms [40]. Nosocomial pneumonia caused by these organisms may then occur following bronchogenous spread of the oropharyngeal organisms. This mechanism of acquisition of pneumonia is generally more common for these agents than is spread through aerosols, which may also occur.

Selden and associates [78], in the study of an endemic of nosocomial infections caused by a multiply drug-resistant strain of *K. pneumoniae* type 30, cultured this strain from stool specimens of 34 of 138 (25 percent) patients on acute-care wards, whereas only 6 of the 138 patients (4 percent) were found to be pharyngeal carriers. None of 22 psychiatric patients was an intestinal carrier, and only one of 54 physicians and nurses cultured was a carrier. All isolates from an inanimate environmental survey were obtained from patient areas. Procedures that were significantly associated with intestinal colonization were urinary catheterization, inhalation therapy, general anesthesia, and treatment with certain antimicrobial agents (ampicillin, cephalothin, and sulfonamides). How the *Klebsiella* organisms were introduced into the patients' intestinal tract was not defined, but it is assumed to be through contact with personnel who transiently picked up strains on their hands (the hands of two of eight nursing personnel on the intensive-therapy unit yielded positive cultures). In personnel intestinal colonization did not follow the transient acquisition of *Klebsiella* on their hands, probably because they were not receiving antibiotics. Similarly, Story [86] observed that 76 percent of

TABLE 26-10. Variables associated with colonization of the respiratory tract with gram-negative bacilli (GNB) in 213 patients admitted to a medical intensive care unit

| | GNB Colonization | | |
| Variable | Present (no.) | Absent (no.) | Significance level |
|---|---|---|---|
| Sex | | | |
| Men | 57 | 66 | |
| Women | 38 | 52 | NS |
| Smoker | | | |
| Yes | 56 | 67 | |
| No | 39 | 51 | NS |
| Coma[a] | | | |
| Yes | 35 | 26 | |
| No | 60 | 92 | $p < .05$ |
| Hypotension[b] | | | |
| Yes | 19 | 6 | |
| No | 76 | 112 | $p < .01$ |
| Sputum present | | | |
| Yes | 71 | 46 | |
| No | 24 | 72 | $p < .001$ |
| Tracheal intubation | | | |
| Yes | 36 | 20 | |
| No | 59 | 98 | $p < .001$ |
| Inhalation therapy | | | |
| Yes | 88 | 98 | |
| No | 7 | 20 | NS |
| Antimicrobial drugs | | | |
| Yes | 38 | 12 | |
| No | 57 | 106 | $p < .001$ |
| Arterial pH $\leq$ 7.31 | | | |
| Yes | 33 | 16 | |
| No | 62 | 102 | $p < .001$ |
| Blood urea nitrogen $\geq$ 50 mg/ml | | | |
| Yes | 10 | 2 | |
| No | 85 | 116 | $p < .05$ |
| White blood cell count > 15,000 or < 4,000 | | | |
| Yes | 37 | 18 | |
| No | 58 | 100 | $p < .001$ |
| Hemoglobin < 8 gm/100 ml | | | |
| Yes | 2 | 1 | |
| No | 93 | 117 | NS |

NS = not significant; $p$ = probability.
[a]Defined as loss of consciousness with no response to commands, but there may be response to painful stimuli.
[b]Systolic blood pressure less than 80 mm Hg or requiring vasopressors for more than four hours.
Source: Johanson, W. G., et al. Ann. Intern. Med. 77:701, 1972.

patients with nosocomial *Proteus* infections were intestinal carriers of the *Proteus* organisms.

In a previous study [41], we noted that the prevalence of colonization increased as the severity of illness increased. Indicators of the severity of illness associated with colonization in this study were coma, hypotension, acidosis, azotemia, and either marked leukocytosis or leukopenia (Table 26-10). The increased frequency of colonization among patients with respiratory disease, sputum production, or endotracheal intubation suggests that conditions that impair lung clearance may also promote colonization. In contrast to our earlier findings, neither colonization nor infection was related to the use of inhalatin therapy, because reservoir nebulizers had been recognized as potential sources of infection and an effective equipment-care regimen had been instituted. Although antimicrobial therapy may have played a role in some patients, our data indicate that most instances of colonization occurred independently of such therapy. Kaslow and colleagues [42] have reported cross-colonization by *Proteus* species with the occurrence of systemic infections, and they identified the catheterized urinary tract as an intermediate reservoir.

Colonization of the respiratory tract with aerobic gram-negative bacilli plays a major role in the pathogenesis of nosocomial lower respiratory tract infections [65]. In the study of Johanson and associates [41], 22 of 95 patients (23 percent) who were colonized developed infections, compared to 4 of 118 patients (3.4 percent) in whom colonization was not shown. Tillotson and Finland [88] observed that 25 percent of their colonized patients developed nosocomial infections, and Klick and coworkers [45] reported that 11 of 69 patients (16 percent) who were colonized with aerobic gram-negative organisms developed pneumonia.

From these observations, it seems reasonable to conclude that the transmission of aerobic gram-negative bacilli, especially *K. pneumoniae* and *Proteus* species, from the gastrointestinal tract of one patient to another can occur, especially if the patients are taking oral antimicrobial agents. The spread between patients is probably through the hands. In the susceptible host colonization of the oropharynx occurs, which is followed by the development of pneumonia in 15 to 25 percent of such patients.

CLINICAL FEATURES The "classic" clinical pattern is that of acute primary *Klebsiella* pneumonia. As with pneumococcal pneumonia, the onset is usually sudden (90 percent) and associated with cough productive of sputum (90 percent), pleuritic chest pain (80 percent), and true rigors (60 percent). Early prostration is a usual feature. Occasionally the acute onset is preceded by an undifferentiated upper respiratory infection and cough. Rarely, epigastric pain and vomiting are the initial symptoms. The characteristic sputum has been described as a nonputrid, homogeneous, thick mixture of blood and mucus, often brick-red, that is sufficiently thick to be expectorated with difficulty. This typical sputum is seen in one-quarter to three-quarters of patients. In some patients, the sputum is thin, resembling currant jelly, although in most it is either blood-tinged or rusty. Frank hemoptysis may occur. On examination, patients appear acutely ill, febrile, dyspneic, and often cyanotic. Although temperatures are often said to be less than those observed with pneumococcal pneumonia, two-thirds of the patients have temperatures between 39°C and 40°C (102°F and 104°F). Tachycardia coincides with the fever. Chest examination typically reveals signs of pulmonary consolidation; there may be loss of lung volume as manifested by decreased size, expansion of the involved hemithorax, and diaphragmatic elevation. Auscultation may reveal suppressed breath sounds with few rales, even when advanced consolidation has occurred. Involvement of more than one lobe is frequent (occurring in two-thirds of patients), and there is a predilection for the upper lobes.

The clinical features of pneumonia due to aerobic gram-negative bacilli other than *K. pneumoniae* are generally similar to those observed in patients with *Klebsiella* pneumonia, except that hemoptysis is unusual.

*E. coli* pneumonia tends to present as a bronchopneumonic process in the lower lobes. The pulse is proportional to the temperature. Early findings include rales without consolidation. Empyema formation is less common than in infection with *Klebsiella* or *Pseudomonas*.

*Proteus* species also produce a clinical picture similar to that of *Klebsiella* infection: fever, chills, dyspnea, pleuritic chest pain, and cough productive of purulent sputum. Signs of consolidation are usual. Roentgenograms reveal dense infiltrates in the posterior segment of an upper lobe or superior segment of the right lower lobe. Progression to lung abscess formation or empyema is common.

THERAPY Empirical treatment is usually initiated while results of sputum cultures and antibiotic sensitivity studies are awaited. Treatment must take into consideration any microbiologic feature that is unique to the specific care area or the hospital and must be based on a knowledge of the susceptibility patterns of organisms within the area or hospital. An essential element of infection control programs is the regular tabulation and reporting of such data. For Enterobacteriaceae and Pseudomonadaceae in the critically ill patient, especially if immunocompromised, combination drug therapy with a $\beta$-lactam and an aminoglycoside antibiotic is indicated. The choice of aminoglycoside (gentamicin, tobramycin, amikacin, or netilmicin) varies, depending on the specific organisms that make up the endemic bacterial flora of the area and their resistance-susceptibility patterns. When the results of cultures and subsequent sensitivity studies are available, empirical regimens should be modified by discontinuing unneeded or ineffective drugs and using the least toxic effective drugs. Duration of therapy should be based on clinical response and should be continued until the patient has been afebrile approximately seven days. Radiographic resolution usually takes much longer. The use of aerosolized antibiotics has been recommended by some. The evidence that they have therapeutic benefit is controversial. Meticulous measures directed at supportive care, the maintenance of clear airways, adequate but not excessive ventilation and oxygenation, adequate fluid and electrolyte replacement, and often, the control of delirium tremens, are essential. Intermittent positive pressure breathing and chest physiotherapy have not been shown to hasten the rate of resolution [27].

*Prevention of Infections*
Because the most important mode of spread between patients appears to be through contact via the hands, the implementation of rigorous hand-washing procedures should be of major importance in minimizing the colonization of susceptible patients who are introduced into high-risk areas such as intensive care units. In addition, restriction of antimicrobial agents may minimize the ability of resistant strains to colonize the intestinal tract. These recommendations appear rational, but are not of proven efficacy.

Using a more positive approach, Klastersky, Hedley-Whyte, and colleagues [24,43,45] have attempted to suppress the colonization of the oropharynx and tracheobronchial tree by repeated atomization, instillation, or both, of antimicrobial agents. In their initial studies [24,45], the use of aerosolized polymyxin B was shown to decrease the frequency of colonization of the oropharynx with sensitive strains, especially *P. aeruginosa,* and to prevent the occurrence of pneumonia. With prolonged use, however, polymyxin B—resistant strains of *Flavobacterium meningosepticum* were found, and these were associated with higher mortality rates than those observed with other organisms. Similarly, Klastersky and associates [43] instilled gentamicin into endotracheal tubes, a procedure that was effective until gentamicin-resistant strains of *Providencia* species, *Pseudomonas* species, and *Klebsiella* species emerged. Subsequently, this group has used aminosidine (paromomycin) and polymyxin B with clinical effectiveness; however, the ultimate appearance of resistant strains, such as *Pseudomonas cepacia*, seems most likely. Regimens such as these should be considered investigational and may be hazardous.

## PNEUMONIA CAUSED BY EXOGENOUS, AEROBIC, GRAM-NEGATIVE BACILLI

### General Aspects

TRANSMISSIBILITY Microorganisms that can survive and multiply in fluids can be readily disseminated as potentially infectious aerosols by certain types of ventilation equipment. *Pseudomonas aeruginosa, Pseudomonas maltophilia, P. cepacia, Achromobacter* species, *Serratia marcescens, Flavobacterium meningosepticum,* and *Acinetobacter calcoaceticus* are the most common organisms found in nebulizer fluid and aerosols, and bronchogenous spread through inhalation of aerosols should be suspected when nosocomial pneumonia produced by these agents occurs. In addition, such contaminated aerosols may also result in oropharyngeal colonization. Pneumonia produced by this group of agents is more likely to derive from the acquisition of exogenous organisms than from the endogenous gastrointestinal flora of patients. These organisms collectively are responsible for about one-tenth to one-fifth of all nosocomial pneumonias.

The bacterial species isolated in our initial studies of nebulizer fluid and aerosols are tabulated in Table 26-11. Multiple species of organisms were isolated more commonly than a single species. In no samples were gram-positive organisms recovered. This general pattern has held in subsequent studies that are based on aerosol samples, although Nelson and Ryan [59] isolated gram-positive organisms from aerosol samples from 8 of 27 patients (*Staphylococcus epidermidis,* five isolates; *S. aureus,* three isolates; viridans streptococci, two isolates; and hemolytic streptococci, one isolate).

Because of the failure to detect gram-positive cocci in our initial studies and because several patients had staphylococcal pneumonia at the time inhalation therapy was instituted, Reinarz and colleagues [67] studied the persistence of *S. aureus* strain 502A following massive contamination of a reservoir nebulizer. The reservoir nebulizer jars of three intermittent positive-pressure breathing (IPPB) machines were filled with cultures of viable *S. aureus* strain 502A. The number of organisms varied from $1.3 \times 10^9$ to $2.5 \times 10^9$ viable units per milliliter. After flushing with sterile distilled water, viable staphylococci in the aerosols exceeded 10,000 cfu per cubic foot of air. After eight hours, species of aerobic gram-negative bacilli were isolated from the aerosols generated by each of the machines. Furthermore, the number of staphylococci was less than 500 cfu per cubic foot. By 24 hours, staphylococci were no longer isolated, but, in contrast, large numbers of aerobic gram-negative bacilli (*Acinetobacter calcoaceticus* var. *anitratus* and *Achromobacter* species) were isolated. This lack of persistence of staphylococci should not have been unanticipated, because McDade and Hall [51] had shown in 1963 that the survival of strains of *S. aureus* was diminished at high relative humidity.

The ability of various microorganisms to proliferate in the fluid in the reservoir nebulizer is important in determining the organisms that predominate. Maki and Martin [49] have shown that organisms of the tribe Klebsielleae (*Klebsiella, Enterobacter,* and *Serratia*) can multiply in 5% dextrose in water, whereas pseudomonads do not. Favero and associates [21] found that "naturally occurring" strains of pseudomonads—that is, strains inoculated directly from water sources in the hospital—multiply rapidly in distilled water. Interestingly, strains precultured in broth before inoculation grew poorly. Although Sanders and coworkers [72] observed that the strains of *S. marcescens,* serotype 014:H4, that were isolated in an outbreak of infection due to contaminated inhalation therapy medications (especially Alevaire) would multiply in such products, intensive study of the growth characteristics of the many bacterial species associated with inhalation therapy has not been reported.

CLINICAL FEATURES In patients with *Pseudomonas* pneumonia, apprehension, toxicity, confusion, and progressive cyanosis are characteristic. Relative bradycardia may occur. Alteration in diurnal temperature patterns, with the peak temperature occurring in early morning, was noted by Crane and Lerner [12]. The physical signs over the thorax are not characteristic. The development of empyema is common and occurs in 22 to 80 percent of cases. Roentgenograms reveal bilateral bronchopneumonic infiltrates, usually in the lower lobe, which often are nodular and may undergo necrosis, and abscesses, which may be small but are often greater than 1 cm in diameter. A pattern of interstitial infiltration may be seen.

*Serratia* infections have been associated with the clinical oddity "pseudohemoptysis"; this results from the red pigment, prodigiosin, produced by some strains of *S. marcescens.* Other features may include abscess formation, empyema, or both.

TABLE 26-11. Results of bacterial cultures of inhalation therapy equipment at various hospitals

| Hospital | Source of cultures | Number of positive cultures | Bacterial species (number of isolates) | | | | | | | | Prevalent organism |
|---|---|---|---|---|---|---|---|---|---|---|---|
| | | | Pseudomonas species | Flavobacterium meningosepticum | Acinetobacter calcoaceticus var. anitratus | Alcaligenes faecalis | Achromobacter species | Acinetobacter calcoaceticus var. lwoffi | Serratia marcescens | Enterobacter aerogenes | |
| A | Aerosol | 62 | 32 | 12 | 20 | 27 | 15 | 3 | 3 | 4 | Pseudomonas aeruginosa |
| | Nebulizer fluid | 44 | 21 | 7 | 5 | 22 | 5 | 3 | 3 | 4 | |
| B | Aerosol | 20 | 4 | 15 | 2 | 9 | 4 | 1 | 0 | 0 | Flavobacterium meningosepticum |
| | Nebulizer fluid | 22 | 9 | 12 | 0 | 5 | 1 | 2 | 0 | 0 | |
| C | Aerosol | 6 | 3 | 2 | 0 | 1 | 1 | 0 | 0 | 0 | Pseudomonas aeruginosa |
| | Nebulizer fluid | 7 | 4 | 2 | 0 | 2 | 1 | 1 | 0 | 0 | |
| D | Aerosol | 13 | 3 | 2 | 11 | 1 | 2 | 3 | 0 | 0 | Acinetobacter calcoaceticus var. anitratus (Herellea) |
| | Nebulizer fluid | 9 | 1 | 2 | 8 | 1 | 1 | 0 | 0 | 0 | |
| E | Aerosol | 20 | 18* | 5 | 0 | 2 | 0 | 1 | 0 | 0 | Pseudomonas species* |
| | Nebulizer fluid | 19 | 18* | 1 | 0 | 0 | 0 | 0 | 0 | 0 | |

*Isolates studied at Centers for Disease Control and reported as Pseudomonas species. Isolates studied by Dr. S. G. Carey at Walter Reed Army Institute of Research were considered to resemble closely Cytophaga johnsonae.

Clinical experience with the other bacterial genera, such as *Hafnia* and *Flavobacterium,* is limited, but other characteristics suggest that the clinical features of their infections are similar to those of *Klebsiella* infections.

THERAPY Mortality rates in the range of 80 percent are not uncommon with *Pseudomonas* pneumonia, whereas they may be lower with infections due to the other gram-negative orgranisms.

The antimicrobial regimen of choice may be selected according to the antimicrobial susceptibilities anticipated in a given community, but they must be confirmed by tests on the organisms infecting the individual patient. In general, *P. aeruginosa* is most susceptible to the newer penicillins (carbenicillin, ticarcillin, piperacillin, azlocillin, and mezlocillin), some of the third-generation cephalosporins (cefoperazone, ceftazidime, and cefsulodin), imipenem, and the newer aminoglycosides (gentamicin, tobramycin, amikacin, and netilmicin). In contrast, *P. cepacia* may be susceptible only to chloramphenicol and trimethoprim-sulfamethoxazole. *E. coli* is susceptible to the same agents as *P. aeruginosa,* and in addition, most strains are susceptible to cephalothin or cefazolin. *S. marcescens* and the indole-positive *Proteus* species are most susceptible to the aminoglycosides. As with *Klebsiella* pneumonia, meticulous attention to supportive care is as important as the antimicrobial therapy in treating pneumonias caused by these other gram-negative bacilli.

### Prevention of Infections

A proper disinfection and sterilization program for respiratory equipment is the major means of preventing endemic infection (see previous section, Disinfection and Sterilization of Ventilatory Equipment). Inadequate disinfection of such equipment is also the major cause of nosocomial pneumonia outbreaks, and a careful review of procedures is mandatory when an outbreak caused by these organisms is identified. In addition, the possibility of a contaminated common vehicle added directly to the nebulizers, such as a contaminated multidose medication vial, should be carefully investigated. Given the infection risks associated with use of ventilatory equipment with reservoir nebulizers, the use of such apparatus should be restricted to clinical situations in which it is clearly indicated.

## PULMONARY TUBERCULOSIS

### Risk of Infection

Airborne spread of *Mycobacterium tuberculosis* is a recognized occupational hazard for persons working in hospitals, but the risk has lessened with the development of effective preventive programs and with the secular decrease in morbidity from tuberculosis [92]. Although Riley and associates [69] demonstrated the infectiousness of air on a tuberculosis ward, the average concentration of infectious particles was one per 11,000 cubic feet. Infectious particles were added at a rate of 25 to 30 particles per day. Moreover, the initiation of treatment, the presence of resistant organisms, or both, were associated with less relative infectivity; for example, if the relative infectivity of drug-susceptible organisms for an untreated patient is 100, susceptible strains from treated patients have a relative infectivity of 4, while resistant organisms from untreated patients have a relative infectivity of 28 and those from treated patients, a relative infectivity of 10. These authors observed one patient with laryngeal tuberculosis, however, who produced one infectious particle per 200 cubic feet of air. From these observations, they concluded that viable airborne tubercle bacilli normally were not very numerous and that the air of a room occupied by a tuberculous patient may not be very dangerous to breathe for a short time.

Annual skin-test conversion rates are reported to be 1.6 percent and 2.3 percent in general hospital employees but may be considerably higher. Ehrenkranz and Kicklighter [19] reported tuberculin skin-test conversion in 23 employees of a general hospital that was attributed to exposure to a patient with undetected tuberculous bronchopneumonia. In an air-conditioned ward on which the patient spent 57 hours, where high-efficiency filters were not present in the ventilatory systems and where air from patients' rooms was recycled to employee areas, 21 of 60 tuberculin-negative personnel (35 percent) converted their skin tests, and two converters had evidence of active infection.

Even the smear-negative patient may pose a risk. Catanzaro [8] observed that 10 of 13 (77 percent) susceptible hospital staff members present at the time of bronchoscopy of a smear-negative, culture-positive patient in a respiratory intensive care unit converted their purified protein derivative (PPD) skin tests. Rough calculations suggested that during bronchoscopy and intubation, the index case produced at least 249 infectious units per hour.

### Prevention of Microbial Contamination of the Air

CHEMOTHERAPY This is the most effective means of preventing microbial contamination of the air, since it reduces coughing due to tuberculosis (which produces droplet nuclei), the amount of sputum, and the number of organisms in the sputum. Therapy should be started at the time a presumptive diagnosis of tuberculosis is made, and it is the most important continuing means of infection control.

COVERING THE NOSE AND MOUTH    This procedure decreases the likelihood of atomized secretions becoming airborne.

MASKS    Patients may also reduce the addition of bacilli to the air by wearing masks; however, patients should generally not be required to wear masks in their rooms. To be effective, masks must filter out particles as small as 1 $\mu$, cover the nose and mouth, fit snugly, and be discarded or sterilized after each use. Masking a coughing patient when someone enters his room may reduce the addition of bacilli to the air but will not completely eliminate the hazard of transmission, since the room air would already be contaminated if the patient had been coughing previously without covering his or her mouth.

### Removal of Airborne Organisms

Air control is necessary in rooms of known or suspected transmitters and in places where persons with untreated tuberculosis might contaminate the air, for example, intensive care units, emergency rooms, admitting areas, outpatient waiting rooms, hallways, and x-ray departments (see Chapters 14 and 18).

Any room with proper air control can be used for patients with tuberculosis. Rooms do not have to be set aside for the exclusive use of tuberculosis patients.

Mechanical ventilation and ultraviolet irradiation are methods of air control. Either method or a combination of both may be used, depending on structural and engineering factors.

MECHANICAL VENTILATION    The patient's room should have fresh air introduced through a central or window unit and air exhausted to the outside through an individual room exhaust fan or a central exhaust system, usually through a lavatory exhaust. Preferably such air is not recirculated, but when necessary it should be passed through a high-efficiency filter or irradiated with ultraviolet light.

ULTRAVIOLET LIGHTS    Upper-room ultraviolet irradiation kills bacteria in the air, thus providing the equivalent of air changes, and when properly installed and maintained, supplements the ventilation system.

### Employee Surveillance Program

Every hospital should have an employee tuberculosis surveillance program; the specific details will vary

according to the dimension of the tuberculosis problem (see Chapter 2).

INITIAL EXAMINATION    A tuberculin skin test (purified protein derivative, 5 tuberculin units) should be provided to all employees at the time of hiring, and a chest roentgenogram should be obtained on those who have a positive reaction to the skin test. The CDC has examined the impact of the "booster" phenomenon on tuberculosis screening programs for hospital personnel. McGowen [52] found "boosting" occurred in 5.7 percent of persons who received a second test one week after the first. Retesting at one year showed that 13 of the 24 employees whose skin test exhibited boosting continued to have a reading of 10 mm or more. Based on these observations, the CDC guidelines recommend that new employees whose reactions are less than 10 mm receive a second test, at least one week but no more than three weeks after the first. Subsequently, Valenti and associates [93] have followed these guidelines and found no "boosting" effect in 416 new hospital employees. These researchers recommend that hospitals contemplating adoption of the two-step method perform a pilot study to assess the frequency of the "booster" phenomenon. If it is less than 1 percent, two-step testing is likely to be cost-ineffective.

PREVENTIVE TREATMENT    Preventive treatment should be given to infected employees, unless specifically contraindicated, to prevent them from developing disease and infecting others. New infections among employees should be reported to the local health department so family contacts may be given skin tests, roentgenograms, or both.

REPEAT TUBERCULIN SKIN TESTS    Policies for repeating skin tests should be determined by the risk of acquiring a new infection. The following factors should be considered:

1. The number and location of tuberculosis patients admitted to the hospital indicate the relative risks of different types of employees being exposed (Table 26-12).
2. The number and location of tuberculosis patients in the community will assist in determining the risk of employee exposure in the community.
3. The number of employees already infected should be determined, so employees at risk of developing disease and infecting others can be identified.
4. The number of employees who become infected will reflect the risk of becoming infected in the hospital and in the community.

TABLE 26-12. Relative hazard of multiple exposures to initially unsuspected tuberculosis by occupational category

| Occupation | Percentage of total occupational category with more than two exposures |
|---|---|
| X-ray technicians | 38.2 |
| Licensed practical nurses | 12.7 |
| Registered nurses* | 9.2 |
| Attendants | 5.1 |
| Medical students | 4.8 |
| Physicians | 4.5 |
| Student nurses | 1.2 |

*Emergency-room registered nurses were at highest risk of multiple exposures.
Source: Craven, R. B., et al. *Ann. Intern. Med.* 82:628, 1975.

5. The flow of air throughout the hospital should be assessed to determine the possibility of airborne transmission of infection from one area to another (e.g., from patient areas to service areas, or vice versa).

If the risk of exposure to tuberculosis is small or infrequent, it is not necessary to repeat skin tests on a routine basis. If certain areas of the hospital and certain categories of workers have either greater exposure to diagnosed and undiagnosed cases or higher rates of new infections, however, regular tests should be repeated every six months.

Periodic chest roentgenograms of employees who have completed an adequate course of treatment or preventive treatment should be discontinued. They should be instructed to report immediately if they have any symptoms that may be due to tuberculosis.

Depending on their risk of developing disease, persons who are infected and who are unable to take preventive treatment should have a chest roentgenogram every six to twelve months. They, too, should be encouraged to report promptly any respiratory symptoms that may be due to tuberculosis. Special surveillance of these employees should be provided if they work in areas of the hospital in which patients with immune deficiencies are treated, or they may be transferred to other parts of the hospital.

INVESTIGATION OF CASE CONTACTS   Careful investigations should be conducted when there is an inadvertent exposure to a "potential transmitter." Tuberculin skin tests should be immediately provided to exposed persons who previously had a negative reaction to the skin test. Those who are still negative should be retested ten weeks from the time of exposure. Preventive therapy may be necessary for some negative reactors with heavy exposure, because they may be infected even though their skin tests have not yet converted.

RECORDS   Accurate records should be kept on each employee to monitor infection rates and determine risks. The record should include the date of each tuberculin skin test and the method and specific antigen used; measurement of the skin-test reaction in millimeters; the date of any known exposure to infectious tuberculosis, the date and result of chest roentgenograms of positive skin-test reactors; the dates of initiation and completion of preventive treatment; and the dates of diagnosis, initiation, and completion of treatment if disease occurs.

EVALUATION   Data should be analyzed at periodic intervals to determine and revise policies. The best index of the effectiveness of the infection control program will be the absence of new infections in employees.

## LEGIONELLA PNEUMONIA

### General Aspects
Since the identification in January 1977 of the organism that caused legionnaires' disease in Philadelphia the year before, at least 23 *Legionella* species have been recognized, with 10 serogroups of *Legionella pneumophila*. The importance of *L. pneumophila* and other *Legionella* species as causes of focal outbreaks of nosocomial pneumonia was recognized early [36,56]. Subsequently, when appropriate diagnostic methods have been used, Legionellaceae have been incriminated as commonly as other aerobic gram-negative bacilli in endemic nosocomial pneumonia (see Table 26-2).

TRANSMISSIBILITY   Legionellaceae are ubiquitous in water. Isolation has been reported from the hot springs at Yellowstone Park, the rain forests in Puerto Rico, numerous lakes, irrigation sprinklers in Israel, industrial coolant fluids, and circulating potable water in buildings such as hotels and hospitals. Blue-green algae (Cyanobacteria) appear to facilitate the multiplication of *L. pneumophila* [89]. Inhalation of aerosols (less than 5 $\mu$ mean diameter) containing *L. pneumophila* seems the most likely mode of acquisition. The rubber washers in showers and taps can partially inactivate residual chlorine and hence facilitate growth. Tobin and colleagues [90] made 42 isolates of *L. pneumophila* from 31 hospitals or hotels; 6 of the institutions were associated with cases of legionnaires' disease, but in 25 there was no known association with disease. In areas in which disease has occurred and studies initiated, attack rates have been relatively low (e.g., 2 per 100).

PREDISPOSING FACTORS  Overall, the male to female ratio of cases has been 3:1, although in some outbreaks there have been no significant differences in attack rates between men and women. Attack rates increase progressively with increasing age. Other risk factors that have been incriminated include history of smoking, presence of lung disease, diabetes mellitus, cancer, renal disease, and exposure to the potable water system (e.g., use of showers).

CLINICAL FEATURES  Initial impressions were that legionnaires' disease presented as a pulmonary infection with major extrapulmonary—central nervous system, hepatic, gastrointestinal, and renal—manifestations [75]. It is now recognized that the clinical spectrum of legionellosis varies from asymptomatic or mild flu-like illness to a devastating fulminant pneumonia. In Philadelphia in 1976, the case fatality ratio was 16 percent. There are no distinctive clinical or radiographic features; diagnosis is based on laboratory findings. Optimal detection depends on use of direct fluorescent antibody (DFA) staining of secretions or tissues, culture, and serologic testing. Specimens for DFA staining should be obtained to minimize the presence of oropharyngeal flora (see Table 26-6). Culture of the organism has the advantage of high specificity. Sensitivity has been improved by use of buffered charcoal yeast extract agar supplemented with α-ketoglutarate. Pretreatment with acid or heat and added antibiotics facilitates the selection of Legionellaceae. Detection of antibodies by the indirect fluorescent antibody (IFA) test remains the mainstay of diagnosis. Use of polyvalent antigen pools is advisable for full screening. Based on IFA tests, a "confirmed" diagnosis depends on at least a fourfold rise in antibody titer between acute and convalescent-phase serums, with the final titer being at least 1:128. A "presumptive" diagnosis is usually based on the occurrence of a compatible illness and a single convalescent-phase serum titer of at least 1:256.

THERAPY  Assessment of treatment is still hampered by lack of properly controlled clinical trials. Because Legionellaceae are facultative intracellular organisms replicating particularly in pulmonary macrophages, in vitro antibiotic susceptibilities have limited clinical relevance. Erythromycin and rifampin remain the recommended antibiotics for L. pneumophila. Rifampin should not be given as a sole agent because of

rapid development of resistance. Treatment should be for several weeks. Relapse after a two-week course of erythromycin therapy is not uncommon. Such relapses appear not to be due to the development of resistance and response to reinstitution of erythromycin. Therapy for Legionella species other than L. pneumophila is even more difficult to assess. Erythromycin is recommended. L. micdadei may respond to trimethoprim-sulfamethoxazole; L. gormanii is relatively resistant in vitro to erythromycin.

### Control of Infections

ENVIRONMENTAL SOURCES  Selective media suitable for recovery of L. pneumophila directly from environmental sites are commercially available. In the presence of disease, treatment of contaminated water systems should be undertaken. Procedures that have been used include cleaning, chlorination, and heating—usually a combination of all three. "Shock" chlorination of the system for intervals such as 12 hours at levels in excess of 15 ppm free chlorine has been used. Following such chlorination it often is necessary to maintain residual chlorine levels of 3 to 15 ppm for prolonged intervals. The temperature of the central hot water supply can be raised from the usual 43°C–46°C to 77°C (110°F–115°F to 170°F) for an interval—often 72 hours. (Joint Commission on Accreditation of Hospitals regulations stipulate that under ordinary circumstances the hot water temperature in hospitals should not exceed 54°C [130°F].) If higher temperatures are used, it is mandatory to post warning signs to avoid scalding. With these interventions, Legionella has been eliminated or the frequency of isolation greatly decreased.

What should be done with the finding of Legionella in water systems in the absence of disease? There is a difference of opinion. If the contamination involves hospital areas housing immunosuppressed patients, treatment would seem reasonable; for other areas, however, current consensus suggests no special measures be undertaken.

COMMUNICABILITY  In the Philadelphia epidemic of 1976, a striking feature was the absence of human-to-human transmission. Subsequent extensive study has not modified this conclusion.

## VIRAL, CHLAMYDIAL, AND RICKETTSIAL INFECTIONS

### Nosocomial Viral Respiratory Infection: Influenza and Respiratory Syncytial Viruses

GENERAL ASPECTS  Although nosocomial infections caused by most viral agents have been recognized, relatively little attention has been directed toward such infections that affect the lower respiratory tract. Chapters 35 and 37 discuss varicella, cytomegalovirus, and other viruses that may sometimes produce lower respiratory tract infections.

During the 1957–58 influenza pandemic (Influenza "Asian" $H_2N_2$), a study was implemented at the Veterans Administration Hospital, Livermore, California, to determine whether the ultraviolet disinfection of droplet nuclei in the air would block the transmission of influenza to a susceptible population during an epidemic (Table 26-13) [53]. These observations indicated a reduction in seroconversions among patients in rooms that received ultraviolet irradiation. The attack rates among hospitalized patients whose rooms were not irradiated with ultraviolet light, however, are comparable to those in the community (as judged by experience in hospital personnel). More recent reports have confirmed similar attack rates for hospitalized and nonhospitalized infants and adults.

In a study that involved a pediatric ward in Great Britain [25], cross-infections from patients admitted with infections caused by respiratory syncytial virus, influenza A, and parainfluenza virus were documented (Table 26-14). The relative hazard of cross-infection was greatest for influenza A virus (nearly one cross-infection took place for each four admissions) and least with respiratory syncytial virus (one cross-infection for about 15 admissions).

PREVENTION OF EPIDEMIC INFECTION   Protection against influenza A can be provided both by immunization and by the chemoprophylactic agent, amantadine or its congeners. The protection provided by amantadine, which is effective only against influenza A virus, is comparable to that afforded by an effective vaccine. Disadvantages include the necessity for twice-daily medication throughout an outbreak

TABLE 26-13. "Aerial isolation" through disinfection of droplet nuclei by ultraviolet radiation

|  | Initially negative | Fourfold rise in influenza titer | |
|---|---|---|---|
|  |  | Number | Percentage |
| Patients |  |  |  |
| Radiated | 209 | 4 | 2 |
| Nonradiated | 396 | 75 | 19 |
| Personnel | 511 | 92 | 18 |

Source: McLean, R. D. *Am. Rev. Respir. Dis.* 83:36, 1961.

and the occurrence of minimal, amphetamine-like side effects in 4 to 27 percent of recipients. However, when patients at high risk of complications (such as those with underlying heart disease or chronic pulmonary disease and older patients [74] have not been immunized and are hospitalized during an epidemic, chemoprophylaxis with amantadine hydrochloride should be strongly considered. Although isolation of patients with such infections has not been deemed necessary, precautions in handling their respiratory secretions are indicated to reduce the possibility of nosocomial transmission.

RESPIRATORY SYNCYTIAL VIRUS   Respiratory syncytial virus (RSV), a common nosocomial pathogen, is the most important cause of lower respiratory disease in children less than two years of age (see Chapter 35). Generally it occurs in annual epidemics of two to three months' duration, often beginning in late December. Hall [31] demonstrated that patients infected with RSV shed large amounts of virus in respiratory secretions for a mean duration of one week. RSV can be recovered from gowns, tissues, or table tops for up to seven hours, from which they can be transferred to hands [32]. The primary mode of transmission appears to be direct person-to-person contact. Infant-to-infant transmission is almost never demonstrated, hence personnel are primarily involved. Control measures include careful hand-washing and change of gowns between patients. Masks do not appear necessary. During periods of RSV prevalence, infants with respiratory illness who are admitted to the hospital should be placed in single rooms or cohorted with other infants with RSV illness. There is no vaccine against RSV.

PARAINFLUENZA AND RHINOVIRUS   Nosocomial transmission of parainfluenza types 1, 3, and 4A on pediatric services and in adult renal transplant patients has been documented [18]. Nosocomial transmission of rhinoviruses (common colds) is well recognized although less well documented. For both parainfluenza and rhinoviruses, the primary mode of transmission is direct person-to-person contact. The same control measures used for RSV apply.

*Chlamydial and Rickettsial Infections*
*Chlamydia psittaci,* the causative agent of psittacosis, can be spread from person to person. Outbreaks involving nosocomial spread to nurses are known. In the 1943 epidemic in Louisiana, there were 8 deaths among 19 recognized infections in nursing attendants, which emphasizes the potential importance of nosocomial transmission of this respiratory infection.

TABLE 26-14. Cross-infections related to admissions with virus infections

| Virus type | No. of admissions | No. of cross-infections | Ratio of admissions to cross-infections |
|---|---|---|---|
| Respiratory syncytial virus | 219 | 15 | 14.6:1 |
| Influenza A | 61 | 16 | 3.8:1 |
| Parainfluenza, type 1 | 55 | 5 | 11.0:1 |
| Parainfluenza, type 2 | 9 | 0 | — |
| Parainfluenza, type 3 | 56 | 13 | 4.3:1 |
| Parainfluenza, type 4A | 7 | 1 | 7.0:1 |
| Parainfluenza, type 4B | 7 | 0 | — |
| *Totals* | 414 | 50 | 8.3:1 |

Source: Gardner, P. S., et al. *Br. Med. J.* 2:571, 1973.

*Q* fever, caused by *Coxiella burnetii,* may also be mentioned, because it is often associated with respiratory symptoms and signs, and instances of its spread to hospital personnel have been recorded.

## PNEUMOCYSTIS CARINII PNEUMONIA

### General Aspects

*Pneumocystis carinii* pneumonia (PCP) outside of the United States has usually been associated with endemic or epidemic focuses in nurseries for premature infants or in foundling homes. It appears as a plasma-cell pneumonia during the first year of life; symptoms appear between the sixth and the twelfth week. Predisposing factors are prematurity, marasmus, and malnourishment.

PREDISPOSING FACTORS  In the United States, the disease occurs sporadically in patients of various ages who invariably either are suffering from a chronic disease, malignancy, or immunologic disorder or have a history of immunosuppressive therapy (see Chapter 37). Since 1980 the occurrence of *Pneumocystis carinii* pneumonia has been a major feature of the acquired immunodeficiency syndrome (AIDS). The first large outbreak of PCP in the United States occurred at St. Jude's Children's Research Hospital in Memphis, Tennessee, where 17 cases were documented during 1968 and 1969 [62]. Subsequently, a cluster of 11 cases occurred in a three-month period in 1973 at Memorial Sloan-Kettering Cancer Center, New York [82].

TRANSMISSIBILITY  The mode of transmission and natural habitat of *P. carinii* are unknown. A few case reports with circumstantial evidence of person-to-person transmission plus the epidemic pattern in nursing homes justify the isolation of active cases from other patients who are at risk. Nevertheless, the occurrence of person-to-person transmission has not been proved.

CLINICAL FEATURES  The clinical characteristics of premature and newborn infants with *P. carinii* pneumonia include an average age at onset of 3.4 months and an average age at death of 4.2 months. The usual duration of illness is three to five weeks. Presenting symptoms include dyspnea in most infants (90 percent) and anorexia, cough, tachypnea, and cyanosis, each present in about one-half of the infants. Clinical signs include dyspnea, cyanosis, and tachypnea in over 90 percent of infants, and cough, fever, and rales are each demonstrated in approximately one-quarter of infants. Radiographic findings include diffuse bilateral infiltrates in all cases, with the presence of adventitious air in about one-fifth of the patients.

THERAPY  Both pentamidine isethionate and trimethoprim and sulfamethoxazole (TMP-SMX) have proved effective in treating *P. carinii* pneumonia. For patients with AIDS whose PCP progresses during TMP-SMX therapy, pentamidine is recommended. TMP-SMX has been successful in preventing the infection. Many oncologists recommend that all patients receive prophylactic TMP-SMX at the initiation of induction chemotherapy. In centers in which the occurrence of PCP has been uncommon, routine prophylactic chemotherapy is usually not recommended. When malnutrition is the cause of susceptibility, special diets are prophylactic.

Patients need carefully monitored oxygen therapy, but oxygen toxicity must be avoided. In severe cases, ventilatory assistance with a continuous negative-pressure system, as used in treating the respiratory distress syndrome of newborns, has been successful.

## PULMONARY ASPERGILLOSIS

*General Aspects*

*Aspergillus* infection is a frequent complication of acute leukemia [73]. In recent years, the frequency of fungal infections has increased; they are reported as the cause of death in 14 percent of a large series of leukemic patients. In the series reported by Bodey [5] from the National Cancer Institute, during a ten-and-one-half-year period major fungal infections were observed in 24 of 100 fatalities with acute leukemia, candidiasis occurred in 29 of 100 fatalities, and *Aspergillus* was incriminated in 8 of 100 fatalities. The lung was involved in 92 of 98 patients with aspergillosis (see Chapter 37).

SOURCES  The differences in the prevalence of aspergillosis in patients with acute leukemia treated with similar chemotherapeutic regimens in different institutions suggest that major differences in environmental contamination exist that make aspergillosis a major problem in some centers and not in others. This hypothesis is supported by the observation that with the moving of patients into a new hospital at Woods Veterans Administration Center in Wisconsin, the aspergillosis that had been common almost disappeared. Organisms are probably acquired mainly from environmental sources by airborne spread.

CLINICAL FEATURES  In 60 of 92 patients with pulmonary aspergillosis, the lung was the only site of infection. The pattern of pulmonary aspergillosis is unusual in the patient with acute leukemia. The two commonly reported primary forms—mycetoma (fungus ball) and allergic bronchopulmonary aspergillosis—were essentially absent. The most common manifestation was necrotizing bronchopneumonia. All but three of the patients with necrotizing bronchopneumonia had symptoms, usually dyspnea, fever, and tachycardia. Cough commonly was nonproductive. Only three patients of 30 with necrotizing pneumonia (10 percent) had hemoptysis, and six (20 percent) had pleuritic chest pain. Roentgenographic evidence was varied; five patients (17 percent) had no x-ray evidence of pneumonia, even shortly before death.

In patients with postive chest roentgenograms, patchy pneumonitis often was first noticed in the last week of life. Hemorrhagic pulmonary infarction was found in 29 of the 92 cases with pulmonary aspergillosis (32 percent); at necropsy, each of these 29 patients had prominent vascular invasion by mycelial elements, with occlusion and thrombosis of pulmonary vessels. In this group of 29 patients, pleuritic chest pain occurred in 61 percent and was often associated with a pleural friction rub.

Fifteen patients had pulmonary lesions characterized primarily by abscess formation, and eight patients had lobar pneumonia caused by *Aspergillus* organisms. The clinical and roentgenographic findings of dense, lobar consolidation suggested the presence of specific bacterial agents, such as *Klebsiella* and pneumococci.

LABORATORY DIAGNOSIS  The diagnosis of aspergillosis in patients with acute leukemia is difficult. In the National Cancer Institute series reported by Young and associates [103], 82 percent of the patients had antemortem fungal cultures, but only 34 percent had one antemortem culture positive for *Aspergillus*, and only 9 percent had more than one positive culture. In another study, Young and Bennett [102] subjeted serum specimens to a battery of serologic tests; the specimens were obtained within the last three weeks of life from 15 patients with invasive aspergillosis. Using the techniques of double diffusion in agar gel, complement fixation, immunoelectrophoresis, and indirect fluorescent-antibody determinations, no antibodies to *Aspergillus fumigatus* were detected despite subsequent histologic and cultural evidence of widespread invasive aspergillosis.

THERAPY  In view of the difficulties in reaching a definite diagnosis, initiation of treatment is often delayed. The treatment of choice is the parenteral administration of amphotericin B, which is not of proved value. Responses seem more closely related to the induction of remission in the underlying process, usually acute leukemia.

## MISCELLANEOUS CAUSES

Organisms other than those mentioned may sometimes produce nosocomial pneumonia, especially in immunosuppressed patients (see Chapter 37).

## REFERENCES

1. Amberson, J. B. Aspiration bronchopneumonia. *Int. Clin.* 3:126, 1937.
2. Andrews, C. P., Coalson, J. J., Smith, J. D., and Johanson, W. G., Jr. Diagnosis of nosocomial bacterial pneumonia in acute diffuse lung injury. *Chest* 80:254, 1981.
3. Bartlett, R. C. *Medical Microbiology: Quality, Cost, and Clinical Relevance.* New York: Wiley, 1974.
4. Berk, S. L., Holtsclaw, S. A., Kahn, A., and Smith, J. K. Transtracheal aspiration in the se-

verely ill elderly patient with bacterial pneumonia. *J. Am. Geriatr. Soc.* 29:228, 1981.

5. Bodey, G. P. Fungal infections complicating acute leukemia. *J. Chronic Dis.* 19:667, 1966.

6. Bordelon, J. Y., Legrand, P., Gewin, W. C., and Sanders, C. V. Telescoping plugged catheter in suspected anaerobic infections. *Am. Rev. Respir. Dis.* 128:465, 1983.

7. Byran, C. S., Wilson, R. S., Meade, P., and Sill, L. G. Topical antibiotic ointments for staphylococcal nasal carriers: Survey of current practices and comparison of bacitracin and vancomycin ointments. *Infect. Control* 1:153, 1980.

8. Catanzaro, A. Nosocomial tuberculosis. *Am. Rev. Respir. Dis.* 125:559, 1982.

9. Christopher, K. L., Saravolatz, L. D., Bush, T. L., and Conway, W. A. Potential role of respiratory therapy equipment in cross-infection: A study using a canine model for pneumonia. *Am. Rev. Respir. Dis.* 128:271, 1983.

10. Coleman, D. L., Dodek, P. M., Luce, J. M., Golden, J. A., Gold, W. M., and Murray, J. F. Diagnostic utility of fiberoptic bronchoscopy in patients with *Pneumocystis carinii* pneumonia and the acquired immunodeficiency syndrome. *Am. Rev. Respir. Dis.* 128:795, 1983

11. Conwill, D. E., Werner, S. B., Dritz, S. K., Bissett, M., Coffey, E., Nygaard, G., Bradford, L., Morrison, F. R., and Knight, M. W. Legionellosis: The 1980 San Francisco outbreak. *Am. Rev. Respir. Dis.* 126:666, 1982.

12. Crane, L. R., and Lerner, A. M. Gram-negative pneumonia in hospitalized patients. *Postgrad. Med.* 58:85, 1975.

13. Craven, D. E., Connolly, M. G., Jr., Lichtenberg, D. A., Primeau, P. J., and McCabe, W. R. Contamination of mechanical ventilators with tubing changes every 24 or 48 hours. *N. Engl. J. Med.* 306:1505, 1982.

14. Craven, R. B., Wenzel, R. P., and Atuk, N. O. Minimizing tuberculosis risk to hospital personnel and students exposed to unexpected disease. *Ann. Intern. Med.* 82:628, 1975.

15. Cross, A. S., and Roup, B. Role of respiratory assistance devices in endemic nosocomial pneumonia. *Am. J. Med.* 70:681, 1981.

16. Dajani, A. S. Antibiotic-resistant pneumococci. *Pediatr. Infect. Dis.* 1:143, 1982.

17. Deane, R. S., Mills, E. L., and Hamel, A. J. Antibacterial action of copper in respiratory therapy apparatus. *Chest* 58:313, 1970.

18. DeFabritus, A. M., Riggio, R. R., David, D. S., et al. Parainfluenza type 3 in a transplant unit. *J.A.M.A.* 241:384, 1979.

19. Ehrenkranz, N. J., and Kicklighter, J. L. Tuberculosis outbreak in a general hospital: Evidence of airborne spread of infection. *Ann. Intern. Med.* 77:377, 1972.

20. Eickhoff, T. C., Brachman, P. S., Bennett, J. V., and Brown, J. F. Surveillance of nosocomial infections in community hospitals. I. Surveillance methods, effectiveness, and initial results. *J. Infect. Dis.* 120:305, 1969.

21. Favero, M. S., Carson, L. A., Bond, W. G., and Petersen, N. J. *Pseudomonas aeruginosa*: Growth in distilled water from hospitals. *Science* 173:836, 1971.

22. Fedson, D. S., and Baldwin, J. A. Previous hospital care as a risk factor for pneumonia: Implications for immunization with pneumococcal vaccine. *J.A.M.A.* 248:1989, 1982.

23. Fedson, D. S., and Chiarello, L. A. Previous hospital care and pneumococcal bacteremia: Importance for pneumococcal immunization. *Arch. Intern. Med.* 143:885, 1983.

24. Feeley, T. W., duMoulin, G. C., Hedley-Whyte, J., Bushnell, L. S., Gilbert, J. P., and Feingold, D. S. Aerosol polymyxin and pneumonia in seriously ill patients. *N. Engl. J. Med.* 293:471, 1975.

25. Gardner, P. S., Court, S. D. M., Brocklebank, J. T., Downham, M. A. P. S., and Weightman, D. Virus cross-infection in paediatric wards. *Br. Med. J.* 2:571, 1973.

26. Garibaldi, R. A., Britt, M. R., Coleman, M. L., Reading, J. C., and Pace, N. L. Risk factors for postoperative pneumonia. *Am. J. Med.* 70:677, 1981.

27. Graham, W. G. B., and Bradley, D. A. Efficacy of chest physiotherapy and intermittent positive-pressure breathing in the resolution of pneumonia. *N. Engl. J. Med.* 299:624, 1978.

28. Grieble, H. G., Colton, F. R., Bird, T. J., Torgo, A., and Griffith, U. G. Fine-particle humidifiers: Source of *Pseudomonas aeruginosa* infections in a respiratory-disease unit. *N. Engl. J. Med.* 282:531, 1970.

29. Gross, P. A., Neu, H. C., Aswapokee, P., Van Antwerpen, C., and Aswapokee, N. Deaths from nosocomial infection: Experience in a university hosital and community hospital. *Am. J. Med.* 68:219, 1980.

30. Guzzetta, P., Toews, G. B., Robertson, K. J., and Pierce, A. K. Rapid diagnosis of community-acquired bacterial pneumonia. *Am. Rev. Respir. Dis.* 128:461, 1983.

31. Hall, C. B. Shedding and spreading of respiratory syncytial virus. *Pediatr. Res.* 11:236, 1977.

32. Hall, C. B., Douglas, R. G., Jr., and Geiman, J. M. Possible transmission by fomites of respiratory syncytial virus. *J. Infect. Dis.* 141:98, 1980.

33. Hall, C. B., Douglas, R. G., Jr., Geiman, J. M., and Messner, M. K. Nosocomial respiratory syncytial virus infections. *N. Engl. J. Med.* 293:1343, 1975.

34. Hedemark, L. L., Kronenberg, R. S., Rasp, F. L., Simmons, R. L., and Peterson, P. K. Value of bronchoscopy in establishing the etiology of pneumonia in renal transplant recipients. *Am. Rev. Respir. Dis.* 126:981, 1982.

35. Heidelberger, M., MacLeod, C. M., and DiLopi, M. M. Human antibody response to simultaneous injection of six specific polysaccharides of pneumococcus. *J. Exp. Med.* 88:369, 1948.

36. Helms, C. M., Massanari, R. M., Zeitler, R., Streed, S., Gilchrist, J. R., Hall, N., Hausler, W. J., Sywassink, J., Johnson, W., Wintermeyer, L., and Hierholzer, W. J., Jr. Legionnaires' disease associated with a hospital water system: A cluster of 24 nosocomial cases. *Ann. Intern. Med.* 99:172, 1983.

37. Hers, J. F. Ph., Masurel, N., and Mulder, J. Bacteriology and histopathology of the respiratory tract and lungs in fatal Asian influenza. *Lancet* 2:1141, 1958.

38. Higuchi, J. H., Coalson, J. J., and Johanson, W. G., Jr. Bacteriologic diagnosis of nosocomial pneumonia in primates: Usefulness of the protected specimen brush. *Am. Rev. Respir. Dis.* 125:53, 1982.

39. Huxley, E. J., Viroslav, J., Gray, W. R., and Pierce, A. K. Pharyngeal aspiration in normal adults and patients with depressed consciousness. *Am. J. Med.* 64:565, 1978.

40. Johanson, W. G., Pierce, A. K., and Sanford, J. P. Changing pharyngeal bacterial flora of hospitalized patients: Emergence of gram-negative bacilli. *N. Engl. J. Med.* 281:1137, 1969.

41. Johanson, W. G., Pierce, A. K., Sanford, J. P., and Thomas, G. D. Nosocomial respiratory infections with gram-negative bacilli: The significance of colonization of the respiratory tract. *Ann. Intern. Med.* 77:701, 1972.

42. Kaslow, R. A., Lindsey, J. O., Bisno, A. L., and Price, A. Nosocomial infection with highly resistant *Proteus rettgeri*. *Am J. Epidemiol.* 104:278, 1976.

43. Klastersky, J., Hensgens, C., Noterman, J., Monawad, E., and Mennier-Carpentier, F. Endotracheal antibiotics for the prevention of tracheobronchial infections in tracheotomized unconscious patients. *Chest* 68:302, 1975.

44. Klein, R. S., and Adachi, N. Pneumococcal vaccine in the hospital: Improved use and implications for high risk patients. *Arch. Intern. Med.* 143:1878, 1983.

45. Klick, J. M., duMoulin, G. C., Hedley-Whyte, J., Teres, D., Bushnell, L. S., and Feingold, D. S. Prevention of gram-negative bacillary pneumonia using polymyxin aerosol as prophylaxis. II. Effect on the incidence of pneumonia in seriously ill patients. *J. Clin. Invest.* 55:514, 1975.

46. Lareau, S. C., Ryan, K. J. and Diener, C. F. Relationship between frequency of ventilator circuit changes and infectious hazard. *Am. Rev. Respir. Dis.* 118:493, 1978.

47. Mackowiak, P. A., Martin, R. M., and Smith, J. W. Role of bacterial interference in the increased prevalence of oropharyngeal gram-negative bacilli among alcoholics and diabetics. *Am. Rev. Respir. Dis.* 120:589, 1979.

48. MacLeod, C. M., Hodges, R. G., Heidelberger, M., and Bernhard, W. G. Prevention of pneumococcal pneumonia by immunization with specific capsular polysaccharides. *J. Exp. Med.* 82:445, 1945.

49. Maki, D. G., and Martin, W. T. Nationwide epidemic of septicemia caused by contaminated infusion products. IV. Growth of microbial pathogens in fluids for intravenous infusion. *J. Infect. Dis.* 131:267, 1975.

50. Martin, C. M., Kunin, C. M., Gottlieb, L. S., and Finland, M. Asian influenza A in Boston 1957–1958. II. Severe staphylococcal pneumonia complicating influenza. *Arch. Intern. Med.* 103:532, 1959.

51. McDade, J. J., and Hall, L. B. An experimental method to measure the influence of environmental factors on the viability and pathogenicity of *Staphylococcus aureus*. *Am. J. Hyg.* 77:98, 1963.

52. McGowan, J. E., Jr. The booster effect: A problem for surveillance of tuberculosis in hospital employees. *Infect. Control.* 1:147, 1980.

53. McLean, R. D., Discussion in international conference on Asian influenza. *Am. Rev. Respir. Dis.* 83:36, 1961 (Part 2).

54. Morris, A. H. Nebulizer contamination in a burn unit. *Am. Rev. Respir. Dis.* 107:802, 1973.

55. Moser, K. M., Maurer, J., Jassy, L., Kremsdorf, R., Konopka, R., Shure, D., and Harrell, J. H., Sensitivity, specificity, and risk of diagnostic procedures in a canine model of *Streptococcus pneu-*

*moniae* pneumonia. *Am. Rev. Respir. Dis.* 125:436, 1982.

56. Muder, R. R., Yu, V. L., McClure, J. K., Kroboth, F. J., Kominos, S. D., and Lumish, R. M. Nosocomial legionnaires' disease uncovered in a prospective pneumonia study. *J.A.M.A.* 249:3184, 1983.

57. Murray, P. R., and Washington, J. A. Microscopic and bacteriologic analysis of expectorated sputum. *Mayo Clin. Proc.* 50:339, 1975.

58. Mylotte, J. M., and Beam, T. R., Jr. Comparison of community-acquired and nosocomial pneumococcal pneumonia. *Am. Rev. Respir. Dis.* 123:265, 1981.

59. Nelson, E. J., and Ryan, K. J. A new use of pasteurization: Disinfection of inhalation therapy equipment. *Respir. Care* 16:97, 1971.

60. Noone, M. R., Pitt, T. L., Bedder, M., Hewlett, A. M., and Rogers, K. B. *Pseudomonas aeruginosa* colonization in an intensive therapy unit: Role of cross-infection and host factors. *Br. Med. J.* 286:341, 1983.

61. Ort, S., Ryan, J. L., Borden, G., D'Esopo, N. Pneumococcal pneumonia in hospitalized patients. *J.A.M.A.* 249:214, 1983.

62. Perera, D. R., Western, K. A., Johnson, H. D., Johnson, W. W., Schultz, M. G., and Akers, P. V. *Pneumocystis carinii* pneumonia in a hospital for children. *J.A.M.A.* 214:1074, 1970.

63. Petersdorf, R. G., Fusco, J. J., Harter, D. H., and Albrink, W. S. Pulmonary infections complicating Asian influenza. *Arch. Intern. Med.* 103:262, 1959.

64. Peterson, P. K., Ferguson, R., Fryd, D. S., Balfour, H. H., Jr., Rynasiewicz, J., and Simmons, R. L. Infectious diseases in hospitalized renal transplant recipients: A prospective study of a complex and evolving problem. *Medicine* 61:360, 1982.

65. Pierce, A. K., and Sanford, J. P. Aerobic gram-negative bacillary pneumonias. *Am. Rev. Respir. Dis.* 110:647, 1974.

66. Pierce, A. K., Sanford, J. P., Thomas, G. D., and Leonard, J. S. Long-term evaluation of decontamination of inhalation therapy equipment and the occurrence of necrotizing pneumonia. *N. Engl. J. Med.* 282:528, 1970.

67. Reinarz, J. A., Pierce, A. K., Mays, B. B., and Sanford, J. P. The potential role of inhalation therapy equipment in nosocomial pulmonary infections. *J. Clin. Invest.* 44:831, 1965.

68. Rhoades, E. R., Ringrose, R., Mohr, J. A., Brooks, L., McKown, B. A., and Felton, F.

Contamination of ultrasonic nebulization equipment with gram-negative bacteria. *Arch. Intern. Med.* 127:228, 1971.

69. Riley, R. L., Mills,, C. C., O'Grady, F., Sultan, L. U., Wittstadt, F., and Shivpuri, D. N. Infectiousness of air from a tuberculosis ward. *Am. Rev. Respir. Dis.* 85:511, 1962.

70. Roberts, F. J., Cockcroft, W. H., and Johnson, H. E. A hot water disinfection method for inhalation therapy equipment. *Can. Med. Assoc. J.* 101:30, 1969.

71. Rosenthal, S., and Tager, I. B. Prevalence of gram-negative rods in the normal pharyngeal flora. *Ann. Intern. Med.* 83:355, 1975.

72. Sanders, C. V., Luby, J. P., Johanson, W. G., Barnett, J. A., and Sanford, J. P. *Serratia marcescens* infections from inhalation therapy medications: Nosocomial outbreak. *Ann. Intern. Med.* 73:15, 1970.

73. Sanford, J. P. Aspergillosis. In Tice, F. (Ed.), *Practice of Medicine*, vol. III. Hagerstown, Md.: Harper & Row, 1975.

74. Sanford, J. P. Influenza: Consideration of pandemics. *Adv. Intern. Med.* 15:419, 1969.

75. Sanford, J. P. Legionnaires' disease: One person's perspective. *Ann. Intern. Med.* 90:699, 1979.

76. Sanford, J. P., and Pierce, A. K. Current Infection Problems—Respiratory. In Brachman, P. S., and Eickhoff, T. C. (Eds.), *Proceedings of the International Conference on Nosocomial Infections.* Chicago: American Hospital Association, 1971.

77. Sanford, J. P., and Pierce, A. K. Inhalation Therapy Equipment. In DeLouvois, J. (Ed.), *Selected Topics in Clinical Bacteriology.* London: Bailliere-Tindall, 1976.

78. Selden, R., Lee, S., Wong, W. L. L., Bennett, J. V., and Eickhoff, T. C. Nosocomial *Klebsiella* infections: Intestinal colonization as a reservoir. *Ann. Intern. Med.* 74:657, 1971.

79. Selwyn, S., McCabe, A. F., and Gould, J. C. Hospital infection in perspective: The importance of the gram-negative bacilli. *Scott. Med. J.* 9:409, 1964.

80. Simmons, B. P. CDC guidelines for the prevention and control of nosocomial infections: Guidelines for hospital environmental control. *Am. J. Infect. Control* 11:97, 1983.

81. Simmons, B. P., and Wong, E. S., CDC guidelines for the prevention and control of nosocomial infections: Guidelines for the prevention of nosocomial pneumonia. *Am. J. Infect. Control* 11:230, 1983.

82. Singer, C., Armstrong, D., Rosen, P. P., and

Schottenfeld, D. *Pneumocystis carinii* pneumonia: A cluster of eleven cases. *Ann. Intern. Med.* 82:772, 1975.

83. Singer, C., Armstrong, D., Rosen, P. P., Walzer, P. D., and Yu, B. Diffuse pulmonary infiltrates in immunocompromised patients. *Am. J. Med.* 66:110, 1979.

84. Springmeyer, S. C., Silvestri, R. C., Sale, G. E., Peterson, D. L., Weems, C. E., Huseby, J. S., Hudson, L. D., and Thomas, E. D. Role of transbronchial biopsy for the diagnosis of diffuse pneumonias in immunocompromised marrow transplant recipients. *Am. Rev. Respir. Dis.* 126:763,765, 1982.

85. Stevens, R. M., Teres, D., Skillman, J. J., and Feingold, D. S. Pneumonia in an intensive care unit. *Arch. Intern. Med.* 134:106, 1974.

86. Story, P. *Proteus* infections in hospital. *J. Pathol.* 68:55, 1954.

87. Thoburn, R., Fekety, R. F., Cluff, L. E., and Melvin, V. B. Infections acquired by hospitalized patients. *Arch. Intern. Med.* 121:1, 1968.

88. Tillotson, J. R., and Finland, M. Bacterial colonization and clinical superinfection of the respiratory tract complicating antibiotic treatment of pneumonia. *J. Infect. Dis.* 119:597, 1969.

89. Tison, D. L., Pope, D. H., Cherry, W. B., and Fliermans, C. B. Growth of *Legionella pneumophila* in association with blue-green algae (Cyanobacteria). *Appl. Environ. Microbiol.* 39:456, 1980.

90. Tobin, J. O'H., Swann, R. A., and Bartlett, C. L. R. Isolation of *Legionella pneumophila* from water systems: Methods and preliminary results. *Br. Med. J.* 282:515, 1981.

91. Toews, G. B., Gross, G. N., and Pierce, A. K. Relationship of inoculum size to lung bacterial clearance and phagocytic cell response in mice. *Am. Rev. Respir. Dis.* 120:559, 1979.

92. U.S. Dept. of Health, Education, and Welfare. *Guidelines for the Prevention of TB Transmission in Hospitals.* Atlanta, Ga: Center for Disease Control, 1974.

93. Valenti, W. M., Andrews, B. A., Presley, B. A., and Reifler, C. B. Absence of the booster phenomenon in serial tuberculin testing. *Am. Rev. Respir. Dis.* 125:323, 1982.

94. Valenti, W. M., Betts, R. F., Hall, C. B., Hruska, J. F., and Douglas, R. G., Jr. Nosocomial viral infections. II. Guidelines for prevention and control of respiratory viruses, herpes viruses, and hepatitis viruses. *Infect. Control* 1:165, 1980.

95. Vial, W. C., Toews, G. B., and Pierce, A. K. Early pulmonary granulocyte recruitment in response to *Streptococcus pneumoniae. Am Rev. Respir. Dis.* 129:87, 1984.

96. Voris, L. P. V., Belshe, R. B., and Shaffer, J. L. Nosocomial influenza B virus infection in the elderly. *Ann. Intern. Med.* 96:153, 1982.

97. Wenzel, R. P., Osterman, C. A., Hunting, K. J., and Gwaltney, J. M. Hospital-acquired infections. I. Surveillance in a university hospital. *Am. J. Epidemiol.* 103:251, 1976.

98. Wheat, L. J., Kohler, R. B., Luft, F. C., and White A. Long-term studies of the effect of rifampin on nasal carriage of coagulase-positive staphylococci. *Rev. Infect. Dis.* 5:S459, 1983.

99. Willems, J. S., Sanders, C. R., Riddiough, M. A., and Bell, J. C. Cost-effectiveness of vaccination against pneumococcal pneumonia. *N. Engl. J. Med.* 303:553, 1980.

100. Winterbauer, R. H., Hutchinson, J. F., Reinhardt, G. N., Sumida, S. E., Deardon, B., Thomas, C. A., Schneider, P. W., Pardee, N. E., Morgan, E. H., and Little, J. W. Use of quantitative cultures and antibody coating of bacteria to diagnose bacterial pneumonia by fiberoptic bronchoscopy. *Am. Rev. Respir. Dis.* 128:98, 1983.

101. Woods, D. E., Straus, D. C., Johanson, W. G., Jr., and Bass, J. A. Role of fibronectin in the prevention of adherence of *Pseudomonas aeruginosa* to buccal cells. *J. Infect. Dis.* 143:784, 1981.

102. Young, R. C., and Bennett, J. E. Invasive aspergillosis: Absence of detectable antibody response. *Am. Rev. Respir. Dis.* 104:710, 1971.

103. Young, R. C., Bennett, J. E., Vogel, C. L., Carbone, P. P., and DeVita, V. T. Aspergillosis: The spectrum of disease in 98 patients. *Medicine* (Baltimore) 49:147, 1970.

After urinary tract infection, surgical wound infection is the commonest nosocomial infection; it is responsible for increasing the cost, disability, and mortality related to surgery. Meticulous preoperative and intraoperative care by the surgeon are the two mainstays in reducing the incidence of wound infection. To these tenets should be added a third—wound surveillance—to be described in this chapter.

## HISTORY

In 1861 Louis Pasteur showed bacteria to be responsible for the putrefaction of meat. Four years later Joseph Lister applied the concept to the prevention of "wound putrefaction" by the use of carbolic acid. This discovery, far more than the development of anesthesia, was the turning point for the rapid progression of surgery. The Listerian concept of antisepsis was not instantly accepted; in the Franco-Prussian War of 1870, for example, von Nussbaum still had a 100 percent mortality in the performance of 34 through-the-knee amputations. Indeed, as late as 1874 Erichsen, professor of surgery at University College Hospital in London, stated, "The abdomen, the chest, and the brain would be forever closed to the intrusion of a wise and humane surgeon" [13]. It is ironic that Lister, who was Erichsen's intern in 1852, was responsible for disproving this prophecy.

In the 1880s von Bergmann introduced autoclaves and aseptic surgery, and Kocher, of Berne, Switzerland, perfected meticulous, bloodless surgery. Kocher's achievement was an unobtrusive but remarkable advance, and by 1899 he was able to report a 2.3 percent infection rate in his thyroid surgery.

## INCIDENCE AND COST

Different authors have reported overall wound infection rates varying from 4.7 to 17.0 percent (Table 27-1). This chapter concentrates on the findings of two large studies: the National Research Council (NRC) five-hospital study to determine the influence of ultraviolet light [23], and the Foothills Hospital wound study [7,8].

A consideration often overlooked in infection studies is the monetary cost of a wound infection. In the

This chapter is dedicated to the memory of Dr. William Altemeier, a pioneer in surgical infection. His untimely death prevented plans to collaborate in preparing the second edition of this chapter.

TABLE 27-1. Comparison of wound sepsis rates in present-day studies

| Author | Country | No. of operations | Sepsis rate (%) |
|---|---|---|---|
| Clarke | England | 382 | 13.6 |
| Robertson | Canada | 1,917 | 9.3 |
| Williams, et al. | England | 722 | 4.7 |
| Public Health Laboratory Service | England | 3,276 | 9.4 |
| Rountree, et al. | Australia | 198 | 14.0 |
| Myburgh | South Africa | Not noted | 17.0 |
| National Research Council | United States | 15,613 | 7.5 |
| Cruse and Foord | Canada | 62,939 | 4.7 |

Foothills Hospital, a wound infection prolongs the patient's hospital stay by 10.1 days. A bed-day now amounts to about $400, and a wound infection therefore costs about $4000 for hospitalization alone. To this figure must be added the sums representing wages lost, decreased productivity, and payments from medical insurance plans. In the University of Virginia, Swartz (as quoted by Altemeier) [3], in 1968–69, calculated the cost of wound infection in 48 patients on the basis of salary lost, hospital costs, and surgeon's charges as $6700 to $9500 per patient. It must be kept in mind that hospital costs have risen three or fourfold since 1969.

## THE FOOTHILLS HOSPITAL WOUND STUDY

In 1965 we decided to use wound infection as the common denominator for surgical infection surveillance in our hospital, and two years later we embarked on a ten-year prospective study of all surgical wounds at the Foothills Hospital, with four aims in mind: (1) to obtain an accurate record of the monthly and yearly wound infection rates; (2) to complete a ten-year bank of statistics against which future variables could be compared; (3) to assess the relative importance of the various factors that influence the infection rate; and (4) to reduce the infection rate.

The ten-year goal was achieved in 1977 with the study of 62,939 wounds. The discussion in this chapter draws chiefly on information from this ten-year data bank. The study has proved of such quality-control value to our hospital that it is being continued, and we now compare our yearly statistics with the data bank to single out changes in etiologic factors.

*Method*
A surgical research nurse in charge of wound surveillance has been employed full-time. She personally observes all wounds during each patient's hospital stay and after discharge by telephoning surgeons' offices.

The 80 bits of information collected for each patient are recorded on a protocol sheet, coded into numerals, and transferred to the hospital computer, which is programmed to provide monthly and yearly infection reports (see Chapter 4). The computer also compiles an annual report for each surgeon, showing them their own clean infection rates compared to the average clean rate of their division peers.

*Definitions*
The definitions used in the 1964 NRC study [23] were used. For the purposes of the study, a wound is defined as infected if pus discharges from it. A wound showing any of the Celsian signs of inflammation or a serous discharge is observed on a daily basis until it resolves (uninfected) or pus discharges (infected).

*Wound Categories*
At the time of the operation the circulating nurse allocates all wounds to one of four categories of contamination. At Foothills Hospital we combined the NRC categories of "refined clean" and "other clean" into the single category of "clean wounds":

1. Clean. Wounds in which the gastrointestinal or respiratory tract was not entered, no apparent inflammation was encountered, and no break in aseptic technique occurred. Cholecystectomy, appendectomy in passing, and hysterectomy were included in this category if no acute inflammation was present.

2. Clean contaminated. Clean operations in which the gastrointestinal or respiratory tract was entered but there was no significant spillage.
3. Contaminated. Operations in which acute inflammation without pus formation was encountered or in which gross spillage from a hollow viscus occurred. Fresh traumatic wounds and operations in which a major break in aseptic technique occurred were included in this category.
4. Dirty. Operations in which pus was encountered or in which a perforated viscus was found. "Old" traumatic wounds were also included in this group.

Excluded from this study were oral, rectal, and vaginal operations, burns, and circumcisions.

*Results*

The overall wound infection rate in 62,939 wounds was 4.7 percent (Table 27-2). Ten percent of infected wounds only become evident after the patient is discharged from the hospital, an aspect of infection surveillance commonly overlooked in surveys.

The overall wound infection rate is not of use in epidemiology unless the contamination categories are known. Table 27-2 shows the infection rates in the four wound categories, varying from 1.5 percent in clean wounds to 40 percent in dirty wounds. This serves as a ready reminder that contamination at the time of the operation is the single most important factor in the production of succeeding wound infection.

The clean infection rate, which has proved to be our most useful measure for surveillance and research, is one of the most valuable reflections of surgical care in any hospital. Endogenous contamination is minimized in these wounds, and the influence of other factors such as exogenous contamination (e.g., skin preparations, hand scrubs) or patient resistance (e.g., age, malnutrition) can be more accurately evaluated. The clean wound infection rate also allows for comparison among hospitals, among hospital depart-

ments, and among the divisions of surgery, as well as among individual surgeons (see Fig. 27-1 for divisional rates and Fig. 27-2 for the surgeons' clean infection rates).

A number of surgeons at the Foothills Hospital, over a period of ten years, achieved a clean wound infection rate of less than 1 percent (Fig. 27-2). Since surgeons in each discipline do the same operations on similar patients and use the same operating rooms and wards, the variation in the clean wound infection rate must be ascribed to differences in operating technique. The surgeons with these low infection rates pride themselves on this achievement; they take pains with their preoperative workup and use fastidious operative technique.

An additional conclusion can be drawn from the surgeons' infection rates with regard to care on the surgical wards. The clean wound infection rate did not differ among the four wards in which eight general surgeons admitted patients. Because the same dressing and isolation techniques were used, we concluded that the surgeon was responsible for his or her infection rate, and that postoperative ward care did not play a significant role in the variation in development of wound infections. This finding led to a change in ward regulations: nurses do not wear gloves or masks during the performance of dressings, and clean wounds are exposed after 48 hours. The septic wound isolation technique has been simplified to the extent that patients whose wound discharge can be contained in dressings are allowed to roam, without restriction, throughout the ward and hospital. These steps have saved much effort and expense.

*Monthly Review*

We have come to consider the clean infection rate our most useful measure in infection and quality control: 0 to 1 percent is ideal, 1 to 2 percent is acceptable, and more than 2 percent is a cause for concern and investigation. The monthly clean infection rate is displayed and discussed in the surgical

TABLE 27-2. Analysis of infection rates related to wound types in the Foothills Hospital study

|  | Total number | Number infected | Percentage |
|---|---|---|---|
| Clean | 47,054 | 732 | 1.5 |
| Clean contaminated | 9,370 | 720 | 7.7 |
| Contaminated | 442 | 676 | 15.2 |
| Dirty | 2,093 | 832 | 40.0 |
| Overall | 62,939 | 2,960 | 4.7 |

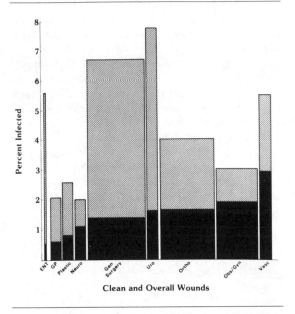

FIG. 27-1. The rate of infection of clean wounds (solid area) and overall wounds (cross-hatched area) observed in the various departments of Foothills Hospital from 1967 to 1977.

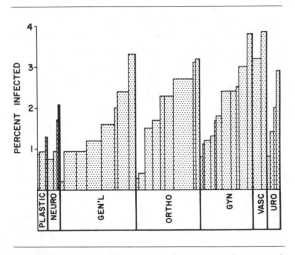

FIG. 27-2. The rate of infection of clean wounds achieved by surgeons in the various departments of Foothills Hospital over the 10-year period 1967–77.

business meetings and at the Infection Control Committee meeting. A monthly review of the infection rate keeps everyone aware of the hazard of infection. This method of surveillance and feedback of information produced a 50 percent reduction in both the overall and clean infection rates, when the first and second six-month periods were compared (see Chapter 3).

## FACTORS INFLUENCING THE INFECTION RATE

Two major factors determine whether a wound will become infected: the dose of bacterial contamination and the resistance of the patient.

### Contamination
Contamination of the wound can occur from extraneous sources (exogenous contamination) or from the patients own bacteria (endogenous contamination) (see Chapter 1).

SURGEONS' HANDS   In 1847 Semmelweis indicated the hands of surgeons and students as the carriers of infection in puerperal sepsis, although he did not appreciate that bacteria were being transferred. He introduced hand-washing with hypochlorite solution and reduced the mortality. Lister soaked his hands in 5% carbolic solution and developed cracks in his skin and nails. He said he could always identify a fellow Listerian on shaking hands because the skin was hard and cracked and the nails brittle. Halsted developed the surgical glove because his operating-room nurse developed an allergy to the bichloride of mercury used during operations. Factors that influence contamination of the surgeon's hands are the skin antiseptic, the length of surgical scrub, and the significance of glove punctures and are discussed in the next sections.

*Skin antiseptic.*   Price [28] showed years ago that although transient bacteria are reduced by soap and water, they rapidly regenerate inside the glove, making an antiseptic essential for hand-scrubbing. Several skin disinfectants are popular. Hexachlorophene (pHisoHex) is effective against gram-positive organisms only and is slow-acting but long-lasting. However, hexachlorophene became unpopular when Butcher and coworkers [4] showed that it was absorbed and detectable in the blood after three hand scrubs.

Povidone-iodine (Betadine) acts more rapidly than hexachlorophene, is effective against gram-positive and gram-negative organisms, but does not have a prolonged intraglove action.

Chlorhexidine (Hibitane) has been shown to be very effective by Lowbury and Lilly [19]. It can be used as a scrub solution with rapid action against gram-positive and gram-negative organisms, and it has a prolonged action inside the glove.

*Length of scrub.* Dineen [11] made bacterial counts of surgeons' hands at the end of two-hour operations and found no difference between five- and ten-minute scrubs, provided an antiseptic was used. Galle and colleagues [14] reported that a ten-minute scrub under running water requires a surprising 50 gallons of water. Most surgeons at our hospital now use brush scrubs for only three to five minutes at the beginning of an operating list and for two to three minutes between cases when they often use a sponge. This practice has not been associated with an increase in the clean wound infection rate, allows obvious savings, and reduces hand excoriation.

*Gloves.* In 1958, Penikett and Gorrill [27] conceived of an ingenious device to detect glove punctures. One pole of a battery is connected to the scrub basin and the other to a terminal that the surgeon can touch with his or her forehead. A hole in the glove completes the circuit and triggers an alarm. The electronics department in our institution constructed a glove tester based on this principle. We tested 1209 pairs of gloves before and after surgery and found 142 (11.6 percent) were punctured at the end of the procedure.

Somewhat to our surprise, not a single wound infection occurred in these 142 patients. The likely explanation is that after an antiseptic hand scrub, insufficient viable organisms escape from a glove puncture to produce an infection. There is probably little risk in operating without gloves—except perhaps hepatitis to the surgeon!

THE PATIENT'S SKIN *Length of preoperative hospital stay.* The longer a patient stays in the hospital before an operation, the greater is the likelihood of a subsequent wound infection (Fig. 27-3). With a one-day preoperative stay the clean wound infection rate is 1.2 percent, with a one-week preoperative stay it is 2.1 percent, and if he or she stays in for more than two weeks, it becomes 3.4 percent. The likelihood is that the patient's skin becomes increasingly contaminated with hospital organisms.

*Preoperative shower.* A preoperative shower using hexachlorophene for washing has value in reducing wound infection. The clean wound infection rate was 2.3 percent if the patient did not shower, 2.1 percent if a shower with soap was used, and 1.3 percent if hexachlorophene was used. The present policy at the Foothills Hospital is to provide patients with chlorhexidine solution to use in the shower.

*Shaving the operative site.* In the Foothills Hospital study the clean wound infection rate was 2.3 percent in patients shaved with a sharp razor before their operation, 1.4 percent in patients who had hair re-

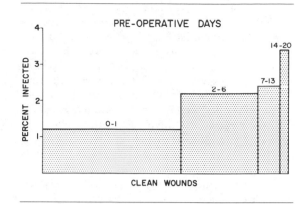

FIG. 27-3. Relationship of length of hospital stay to wound infection. The longer a patient is in the hospital before an operation, the more susceptible he or she is to infection of the wound.

moved with an electric razor, and 0.9 percent in those who had no form of hair removal. Seropian and Reynolds [29] report a clean wound infection rate of 5.6 percent in patients after razor shaving compared to 0.6 percent after depilatory hair removal. Hamilton and colleagues [15] demonstrated with electron microscopy the skin damage of shaving compared to the benign effect of a depilatory. They postulate bacterial growth in the razor nicks. At Foothills Hospital we have not found the depilatory creams to be universally efficacious in removing body hair at the site of operation, and we content ourselves with minimum shaving, preferably with an electric shaver.

*Preparation of the patient's skin.* Lowbury and Lilly [19] have found that 1% iodine in 70% alcohol and 0.5% chlorhexidine in 70% alcohol are the two most effective skin antiseptics. During the first four years of the Foothills study, skin preparation consisted of a vigorous ten-minute wash with green soap followed by an alcohol rinse. The clean wound infection rate was 2 percent. During the last three years the preoperative routine was changed: a few hours before surgery the area of the operation was washed with an iodophor sponge on the ward followed by a three-minute preparation of 0.5% chlorhexidine in 70% alcohol in the operating theatre. With this method of preparation, the clean wound infection rate is 1.6 percent. We still use this method with one modification: chlorhexidine scrub solution (Hibiscrub) is used on the ward instead of iodophor because of its longer action.

*Draping.* Three materials are currently in use to isolate the area of the incision: (1) conventional cotton drapes, (2) disposable prefabricated drapes, and (3) plastic adhesive drapes.

The problem with cotton drapes is bacterial strike-through whenever the cotton becomes wet, for example, through depositing of wet instruments on the patient's knee area. This problem is overcome at our institution by placing a thin sheet of sterile plastic over the "instrument area" before applying the cotton drapes. We believe this simple maneuver is one of the reasons for the low clean wound infection rate with the use of cotton drapes at Foothills Hospital. Some of the disposable drapes have excellent water-repellent qualities and do not require the sheet of plastic. If disposable drapes are used, it is important to check whether they are water-repellent; otherwise, the choice between cotton and disposable drapes can be made entirely on an economic basis.

Adhesive plastic drapes introduced to cover the exposed skin beside the wound, appeared an attractive concept. However, reports by Paskin and Lerner [26] have shown an increased infection rate with adhesive drapes because bacteria proliferate with the sweating beneath these drapes. At Foothills Hospital the use of cotton drapes in clean wounds was associated with a 1.5 percent infection rate (405 out of 26,303), while the addition of adhesive plastic drapes was associated with a clean wound infection rate of 2.3 percent (214 out of 9,252). As a consequence, adhesive plastic drapes are not used routinely at our institution, resulting also in money saved.

THEATRES, ANESTHETISTS AND AIR-HANDLING At Foothills Hospital there was no difference in the clean wound infection rate among the various operating theatres. Similarly, there has been no difference in the clean wound infection rate for different anesthetists. Carriers of infection are rare, fortunately, but will be detected quickly with a meticulous wound surveillance program. Personnel with upper respiratory infections do not constitute a hazard, but anyone with a staphylococcal infection should be excluded from the operating room.

*Air-handling.* Lister originally felt that air contamination was the main hazard in infection and employed a carbolic spray. Once he appreciated that contact spread was more important, the air spray was abolished. A resurgence of interest in air sterility occurred in the last 15 years because of two developments: (1) National Aeronautics and Space Administration projects showed air-handling techniques to be important in the assembly of electronic components for spacecraft and (2) Sir John Charnley reduced the infection rate of total hip replacement operations from 9 percent to 1 percent by using elaborate air-handling techniques. There has been much argument regarding whether the installation and maintenance of high-efficiency particulate air (HEPA) filtration and unidirectional airflow equipment are worthwhile (see Chapter 20). The controversy appeared to be settled in North America when surgeons reported infection rates of less than 1 percent for hip replacement operations performed in conventional operating rooms. At Foothills Hospital the clean wound infection rate for hip replacement operations is 1.9 percent (7 out of 373); however, a recent study by Lidwell and colleagues [18] has disturbed our complacency. They reported a significant reduction in the postoperative wound infection rate among patients operated on in rooms with ultraclean air as compared to a comparison group.

Our present policy in joint replacement operations is to mark the theatre door "closed" to restrict traffic; anyone with a skin infection is excluded, and movement and talking are kept to a minimum.

ENDOGENOUS CONTAMINATION  The overriding importance of endogenous contamination is clear from the analysis of wound categories (Table 27-2). Endogenous contamination is the main risk because of the large dose of organisms available from the bowel or other hollow muscular systems. Krizek and Robson [17] found that traumatic wounds were likely to become infected if they contained more than 500,000 organisms per gram of tissue; no wounds became infected if the bacterial count was less than $10^5$. Methods to reduce the dose of endogenous contamination in large bowel surgery are mechanical bowel preparation and use of oral antibiotics.

*Mechanical bowel preparation.* The conventional mechanical bowel preparation consists of laxatives, a low-residue diet, and repeated enemas for three days. Whole gut lavage (WHOGULA) provides better mechanical cleansing with less discomfort in nonobstructed patients [5,9]. The technique is simple: a small nasogastric tube is passed and Ringer's lactate is infused at the rate of 3 L per hour. Defecation commences after approximately half an hour. The infusion is continued until such time as the effluent is clear, which usually takes about three hours. Patients who have had the classic bowel preparation at one time and WHOGULA at another much prefer the latter method.

*Oral antibiotics.* The erythromycin-neomycin regime described by Nichols and associates [24] is the one most commonly used after mechanical bowel preparation. Erythromycin base 1 gm and neomycin 1 gm are administered by mouth at 1300, 1400, and 2300 hours for operations booked at 0800 hours the following day. In patients cleansed with WHOGULA, the antibiotic can be added to the last liter of infusion.

PROPHYLACTIC ANTIBIOTICS   The broad indications for prophylactic antibiotics include operations in which contamination is expected and operations in which infection could be catastrophic (e.g., implantation of vascular or orthopedic prostheses).

Prophylactic antibiotics must be given preoperatively. Miles and coworkers [21] demonstrated that for antibiotics to be effective they have to be present in the tissue fluids within three hours of bacterial contamination. Alexander and coworkers [2] noted in addition the pharmacologic differences in tissue penetration of antibiotics. Ampicillin, for example, reached zenith within one hour, cephalosporins between one and two hours, and clindamycin after two hours.

*Resistance of the Patient*
Culbertson and associates [10] have stated that the risk of wound infection varies according to the following equation:

$$\frac{\text{Dose of bacterial contamination} \times \text{virulence}}{\text{Resistance of the host}}$$

This equation explains the heavily contaminated wound healing without infection in the patient with superb host defense mechanisms. Because all wounds are contaminated to some extent, it also explains the high infection rate in the immunocompromised patient. The concept of improving the resistance of the patient is as old as Hippocrates, whose essential credo in patient management was to assist the *vis medicatrix naturae* (the healing power of nature). Host resistance can be classified into general and local factors.

GENERAL FACTORS   Most studies reveal an increase in the wound infection rate in association with advancing age [23]. The Foothills statistics regarding age are illustrated in Figure 27-4.

Diabetes, obesity, and malnutrition are also associated with an increase in the wound infection rate. Among malnourished surgical patients undergoing clean surgical procedures at the Foothills Hospital, 16 percent developed postoperative wound infections [6]. Statistics of the Glasgow Royal Infirmary during the last century showed that in 1860 the average income improved and that with better nutrition there was an associated reduction in typhus and ulcers of scurvy. His hypothesis is that the reduction in the

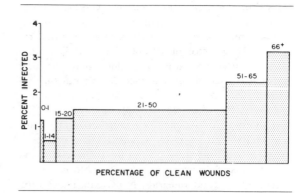

FIG. 27-4. Relationship of age to wound infection. Older patients are more likely to develop infection of clean wounds than are younger patients.

surgical infection rate at that institution was as much due to better nourishment as to the application of carbolic acid in 1865! This theory regarding the improvement of the general resistance of the patient by means of nutrition would vindicate some opponents of Lister who claimed as good wound results with simple cleanliness in operating on well-to-do patients. It also reinforces the well-known concept in elective operations of preoperative stabilization of diabetes (Foothills Hospital, clean wound infection rate, 7.8 percent), weight reduction in the obese (Foothills Hospital, clean wound infection rate, 6.9 percent), and correction of malnutrition by means of total parenteral nutrition.

LOCAL FACTORS   The local resistance of the wound is much more important than the general resistance of the patient. In 1536, Ambroise Paré rediscovered the gentle Hippocratic handling of wounds when he found that war wounds healed better when "mismanaged" with bland irrigation rather than treated with boiling oil. In the 1890s Kocher demonstrated statistically the low wound infection rate achievable by meticulous hemostasis. Halsted visited Kocher in Berne, adopted his technique, and promulgated the principles of wound care: complete hemostasis, adequate blood supply, removal of all devitalized tissue, obliteration of dead space, use of fine nonabsorbable sutures, and wound closure without tension.

*Foreign bodies in wounds.*   In 1957 Elek and Conen [12] quantified these observations by injecting the forearms of British medical students at St. George's Hospital with measured numbers of staphylococci. They found that 6.5 million *Staphylococcus aureus* organisms were required to produce a subcuticular abscess, but that only 100 organisms were necessary if they were injected into the area of a subcutaneous silk suture. The foreign body reduced the local resistance by a factor of 10,000. Howe and Marston [16] produced an additional reduction in the local resistance when tissue was included within the ligature.

*Blood supply of the wound.*   Miles and Niven [22] first showed that shocked experimental animals with impaired wound perfusion required 10,000-fold fewer organisms to initiate a wound infection. Sonneland [30] showed a direct relation between blood loss and succeeding wound infection in patients undergoing colonic gastric operations. Securing complete hemostasis and preventing wound hematoma remain the first dicta of wound management. Hemostasis can be obtained by means of electrocoagulation. Provided only the bleeding vessel is seized with the finest pair of nontoothed forceps (McIndoe) for coagulation, thus leaving a minimal amount of dead tissue, there is no difference in the clean wound infection rate with or without use of the electrocoagulation unit.

*Sutures and staples.*   Because of the finding of Elek and Conen [12], subcutaneous sutures are not used at the Foothills Hospital. The recent advent of skin staples also appears to be an advantage because staples do not transgress the subcutaneous tissues and are nonreactive. The horizontal part of the staple does not impinge against the skin, and cross-hatching of the wound is thus avoided.

*Drains.*   The introduction of closed wound suction drains has been a great advance, especially in the prevention of hematoma formation. Alexander and coworkers [1] showed that a hematoma rapidly becomes deficient in opsonins. A closed wound suction drain removes the stagnant wound fluid, allowing ingress of fresh opsonin-laden fluid. At Foothills Hospital we have found clean wound suction drainage of value in wounds in which hematoma formation is likely, such as spinal fusions. McIlrath and colleagues [20] have shown the benefit of subcutaneous hemovacs in abdominal operations. Indeed, a subcutaneous clean wound suction drain enhances the resistance of the wound so much that we rarely have to resort to delayed primary closure in contaminated wounds.

There is little to be said for the use of Penrose drains. Nora [25] has shown that these drains allow bacteria entry down to the tip of the drain, and it is not surprising that the wound infection rate is increased when the Penrose drain is brought out through the wound.

Furthermore, a Penrose drain is uncomfortable and requires extra nursing time. We timed student nurses attending to closed wound suction drains and Penrose drains. It took them five minutes to empty and measure the clean wound suction drain, compared to 35 minutes to redress the effluent from an abdominal Penrose drain.

*Delayed primary closure.*   Hunter first advocated delayed primary closure in his management of gunshot wounds in the Belle Isle Campaign of 1761, and this technique has had to be rediscovered in every war since that time, including the recent Falkland Islands conflict. Primary closure of gunshot wounds by Argentine surgeons had disastrous consequences. Delayed primary closure is essential for gunshot wounds and traumatic wounds with tissue destruction, and remains the standby for any heavily contaminated incisional wounds.

## COMMON TYPES OF WOUND INFECTIONS

### Staphylococcal Wound Infections

Staphylococcal infections usually have an incubation period of four to six days and tend to be localized; there is an initial area of erythema and subsequent swelling, pain, and central necrosis with the formation of an abscess containing thick, creamy, odorless, and usually yellow pus. Lymphadenitis may rarely occur, but septicemia is common. In closed incisional wounds, the symptoms and signs of staphylococcal infection include redness about the margins, swelling, and increasing local pain; the pain is throbbing in character and often synchronized with the pulse beat. Fever and leukocytosis are usually present. When invasive regional or systemic infection occurs, malaise, higher fever, lymphangitis, lymphadenitis, chills, and sweats usually develop. In open wounds, a purulent discharge is the principal sign of infection. The responsible organism in the majority of instances is coagulase-positive *S. aureus.* Many of these strains are β-hemolytic, liquefy fibrin and gelatin, and produce yellow pigment in cultures.

The treatment of staphylococcal wound sepsis depends primarily on early recognition, antibiotic therapy, and surgical opening of the whole infected wound. Other methods of treatment include the established principles of rest, heat, elevation, and general support. Each patient with a staphylococcal infection should be considered individually and treated according to the nature of the infection and associated diseases.

Infected sutured wounds should first be reopened with a hemostat at the point of maximum pain, swelling, or fluctuation, and the opening enlarged to the size of the cavity. The cavity is then gently irrigated with saline solution and loosely packed open with fine mesh gauze. If pus and necrotic material are present, their removal is important. Antibiotics should be administered before any wound manipulation.

The antibiotics recommended for treatment of patients with staphylococcal wound sepsis depend on the antibiotic sensitivities and any hypersensitivity of the patient to the available antibiotics. A penicillinase-resistant penicillin or a cephalosporin is the agent of choice in most hospitals, since the majority of strains are usually resistant to penicillin. Alternative drugs for patients with hypersensitivity to the penicillins include erythromycin, clindamycin, and vancomycin.

It should be kept in mind that antibiotic therapy alone in the presence of infected wounds with pus formation is inadequate and incomplete; it should be supplemented by incision and drainage as indicated previously. Antibiotic therapy should be started before surgical drainage, however, to produce bacteriostatic or bactericidal concentrations of the drug in the blood and tissues that will inhibit the growth of any bacteria disseminated by the operative procedure. In the presence of staphylococcal wound infection and invasion of the bloodstream, adequate therapy usually results in clearance of the organisms from the bloodstream within 36 to 72 hours in association with a decrease in the signs of local invasiveness. The presence of devitalized tissue, prostheses such as metal pins and plates, or other foreign bodies often limits the effect of the antibiotic therapy until such material is removed (see Chapter 29).

EPIDEMIOLOGIC CONSIDERATIONS Sources. The majority of S. aureus strains that cause endemic postoperative incisional wound infections are derived from strains colonizing the patient, whereas outbreaks occasionally derive from a member of the operating-room staff who has active clinical staphylococcal disease or is an asymptomatic disseminating carrier.

Prevention and control. The risk of S. aureus infection is several times higher in colonized patients, which suggests that attempts should be made to prevent such colonization in the preoperative period. Limiting the preoperative stay of patients to the minimum is recommended, because colonization rates increase with increasing duration of hospitalization, and strains acquired in the hospital may have enhanced virulence and a greater spectrum of resistance to antibiotics.

A surveillance system allows for the instant recognition of an outbreak of infection and of the personnel who attended the operations of the involved patients (see Chapter 4). Usually no single culprit is identified. A formal investigation of the infection and discussion with the surgeons invariably produce an instant reduction in the infection rate. Although epidemics associated with asymptomatic disseminating carriers are described, they have not been found to be a problem in our institution during the last 20 years.

### S. Epidermidis Wound Infections

Staphylococcus epidermidis is a normal member of the cutaneous bacterial flora; however, it is increasingly being implicated in wound infection, especially in operations employing prosthetic devices (see Chapter 29).

### Gram-Negative Bacillary Wound Infections

Wound infections caused by aerobic gram-negative bacilli have become more frequent and of increasing importance in recent years. Following the discovery and general use of penicillin, secondary or superimposed infections by various gram-negative bacilli have developed during treatment and have become a serious and increasing threat in modern surgical practice. This phenomenon is related to the rapid extension of new and complex surgical operations and diagnostic procedures to elderly and other poor-risk patients whose resistance is decreased by debilitating trauma, associated chronic diseases, and leukocyte-suppression therapy.

The genera and species most frequently identified in aerobic gram-negative bacterial infections are *Escherichia coli*, *Enterobacter*, *Proteus*, and *Pseudomonas aeruginosa*. These organisms are commonly associated with the anaerobic bacterium *Bacteroides fragilis* and anaerobic streptococci because these infections result from contamination with gut contents.

Wound infections caused by these gram-negative bacilli have a longer incubation period than staphylococcal or streptococcal infections, and a period of 7 to 14 days is not unusual. Furthermore, the local signs of inflammation are less marked than in staphylococcal wound infection, and patients may present instead with signs of systemic sepsis.

MANAGEMENT The treatment of purely gram-negative bacillary infections of postoperative incisional wounds includes adequate drainage, antibiotic therapy with the appropriate agents given systemically, and elevation and rest of the involved areas. The removal by sharp dissection of all necrotic tissue from these lesions is recommended.

Failure to drain obscure abscesses or similar focuses that are contributing to the septicemia usually results in death. However, the diagnosis of deep-seated or obscure abscesses can be made quite difficult by the masking effect of antibiotic or steroid therapy.

If mixed gram-negative and gram-positive organisms are found in the pus, the patient should be treated with an aminoglycoside and either clindamycin or metronidazole.

Contact isolation is recommended for patients with major wound infections and drainage/secretion precautions for minor or limited wound infections (see Chapter 9).

### Aerobic Streptococcal Infections

GROUP-A STREPTOCOCCAL INFECTIONS  The majority of invasive streptococcal infections in wounds are caused by aerobic, $\beta$-hemolytic, group-A streptococci. Such infections run a relatively rapid and fulminant course. The local process is one of diffusing cellulitis, lymphangitis, and lymphadenitis, with a large blood-filled local bleb at its primary focus. There is little tendency to form abscesses, but local breakdown, gangrene, or necrotizing fasciitis can occur. The infection is thus characterized by the development of thin, watery pus. Streptococcal invasion of the bloodstream is frequent and relatively early.

The systemic manifestations include chills, fever, tachycardia, sweats, prostration, and other signs of toxemia. Frequent examinations should be made to detect metastatic infectious complications as early as possible. Each is treated according to its individual location and characteristics.

*Surgical scarlet fever* may occur rarely as a postoperative infection in a postoperative wound, and the hemolytic streptococci are associated with this lesion. The condition is characterized by spreading cellulitis with redness, swelling, and frequently, bullous formation in and about the margins of the wound, as well as by a typical scarlatiniform eruption that starts at the wound and spreads peripherally over the body. The rash usually develops two to four days postoperatively.

Erysipelas, another type of cellulitis caused by a hemolytic strain of *Streptococcus*, may occur infrequently in lacerated wounds, particularly those about the face, after an incubation period of one to three days. Ushered in by chills, high fever, rapid pulse, and severe toxemia, it usually runs its course in a period of four to nine days. It is characterized by an area of advancing cellulitis with sharply demarcated, irregular, elevated, and indurated margins. The appearance of the infected skin is striking and immediately suggests the diagnosis.

Acute hemolytic streptococcal gangrene is characterized by subcutaneous gangrene, thrombosis of the nutrient vessels, and resultant patchy slough of the overlying skin. It usually develops in the extremities, although the perineum, face, and other parts of the body may be involved.

Aerobic streptococcal infections caused by organisms other than group-A streptococci tend to be much less invasive. Group-D streptococci are encountered in clean-contaminated and contaminated wounds of the gastrointestinal tract.

*Management.*  The treatment of aerobic hemolytic streptococcal infections consists primarily in the control of their invasive characteristics by antibiotics, rest, elevation, and warm compresses. Penicillin is the antibiotic of choice, and erythromycin, clindamycin, and cefamandole are alternatives. Enterococcal strains (such as *Streptococcus faecalis* and other group-D streptococci) are far less invasive than group-A streptococci and should be treated with ampicillin or a combination of ampicillin and an aminoglycoside.

*Epidemiologic Considerations.*  Streptococcal infections of incisional wounds are usually secondary to contamination from endogenous sources such as the upper respiratory tract, draining infected sinuses, other infected wounds, or contaminated instruments or dressings. Several outbreaks have been traced to asymptomatic disseminators of group-A streptococci who worked in the operating room. Interestingly, the majority of these persons have been anesthetists, and rectal, rather than pharyngeal, colonization has been the source from which organisms were dispersed. There are no reports of outbreaks resulting from streptococcal pharyngitis of surgical team members.

Outbreaks should be investigated as indicated in the preceding section on staphylococcal infections; the objectives of such an investigation are to identify and treat disseminating carriers.

### Microaerophilic and Anaerobic Streptococcal Infections

MICROAEROPHILIC STREPTOCOCCAL INFECTIONS Microaerophilic streptococcal infections usually occur and act in synergism with *S. aureus* or *Proteus* species. Meleney's chronic progressive cutaneous gangrene is rare nowadays but most commonly follows operations for purulent infections of the chest or peritoneal cavity. The condition is caused by the synergistic action of a microaerophilic nonhemolytic *Streptococcus* strain and an aerobic *S. aureus*. The incubation period is 10 to 14 days after the operation. The wound and surrounding skin become tender, red, and edematous, particularly around stay sutures. A carbuncular infection develops within a few days around the wound margins or stay suture holes, and the central area assumes a purplish or purplish-black color. A wide area of bright red cellulitis develops around the central purplish area, and central ulceration follows. This results in the characteristic appearance of the lesion, which consists of a central, enlarging area of ulceration bordered by a purplish-black, narrow margin of gangrenous skin and a large area of spreading cellulitis. Pain and tenderness are usually striking features, particularly in the region of the purplish-black margin.

*Management.* This infection is slowly progressive and may ultimately cause death unless specific treatment is instituted. Local excision of gangrenous margins or other conservative methods usually fail to check this process. Radical excision of the lesion with knife or cautery and general antibiotic therapy with penicillinase-resistant penicillin or a cephalosporin will promptly arrest the infection and permit early skin grafting and healing. Zinc peroxide cream or ointment was used in the past and may be of value.

ANAEROBIC STREPTOCOCCAL INFECTIONS Peptostreptococci may produce a variety of severe postoperative infections with or without bacteremia, particularly after operative procedures on the genital, intestinal, or respiratory tracts. The microorganism is difficult to grow bacteriologically, and routine cultures are frequently inadequate for detecting its presence. Careful bacteriologic studies, however, show that it is a frequent bacterial component of many infections seen in incisional wounds and deep abscesses. The pus produced by peptostreptococcal infection characteristically is thick and grayish and has a fetid anaerobic odor.

*Management.* The treatment of infections produced by *Peptostreptococcus* includes surgical drainage of abscesses; the antibiotic of first choice is penicillin G; tetracycline and erythromycin are alternative agents.

*Other Types of Wound Infections*
SURGICAL DIPHTHERIA Postoperative wounds very rarely become infected by the Klebs-Löffler bacillus (*Corynebacterium diphtheriae*), and the resultant infection usually is characterized by an acute ulceration and cellulitis with infiltration of the skin and subcutaneous tissues around the wound. A chronic, indolent ulceration of an open wound that fails to heal is another clinical type. The diagnosis is suggested by the development on the lesion of a pseudomembrane that bleeds readily when its removal is attempted. The diagnosis is proved by recovering the organism in special cultures from the wound. Testing for toxin should also be done, either in vitro or in vivo (by inoculation of guinea pigs).

*Management.* The treatment consists of contact isolation of the patient, the administration of diphtheria antitoxin, and the systemic administration of penicillin.

MIXED OR SYNERGISTIC INFECTIONS A large group of wound infections that complicate surgical operations or trauma are caused by a mixed bacterial flora. This group has a polymicrobic causation; the bacterial mixture may consist of aerobic, anaerobic, gram-negative, and gram-positive microorganisms whose origin most often is a lesion or perforation of the gastrointestinal, respiratory, or genitourinary tract. The aerobic and anaerobic bacteria often relate to each other in symbiosis, and their synergistic action determines the characteristic nature of these septic processes. The process spreads, producing abscess formation, thrombosis of neighboring vessels, and extending necrosis, particularly of the areolar tissue. Crepitation of the infected tissue may develop as a result of the bacterial action of the clostridia, anaerobic streptococci, or associated aerogenic or aerobic bacilli.

Successful treatment depends on early diagnosis and adequate surgical drainage of the infected wound if it is closed. X-rays for soft-tissue detail may be helpful in showing the presence of progressive gaseous infiltration and may aid in the diagnosis of associated crepitant cellulitis or abscess. Bacterial necrosis of tissue may be excessive, particularly in postoperative abdominal wounds. Antibiotic therapy with penicillin G and an appropriate broad-spectrum antibiotic is recommended. Gentamicin, tobramycin, tetracycline, cefamandole, and clindamycin are agents to consider for this purpose. The associated impairments of wound healing and intestinal ileus may lead to wound dehiscence. Septicemia with one or more bacteria may occur during the progress of this lesion.

GAS GANGRENE AND CLOSTRIDIAL WOUND INFECTIONS Clostridial infections occasionally occur in clean wounds but are most likely in the presence of extensive damage to muscle masses, impairments of regional blood supply, gross contamination by dirt and other foreign bodies, and significant delay in adequate surgical treatment. Amputation of a gangrenous lower limb is the most common elective operation to be complicated by gas gangrene. The onset of the infection is usually spectacular and the mortality high.

The microorganisms that cause such infection are anaerobic; the most frequent type is *Clostridium perfringens*. Other clostridia, such as *C. novyi*, *C. sporogenes*, *C. septicum*, *C. histolyticum*, and *C. sordellii*, may occur alone or in combination with *C. perfringens*.

Clinical forms of infection other than gas gangrene include cellulitis, synergistic infections, tetanus, and wound botulism. Only gas gangrene will be considered here.

*Manifestations of gas gangrene.* Gas gangrene is a spreading clostridial myositis, which may be crepitant, edematous and noncrepitant, mixed, or profoundly toxemic. It is primarily an infection of the muscles that spreads rapidly and involves to a lesser degree the neighboring connective tissues. The accumulation of edema and gas in the fascial compartments produces an expanding pressure that aids in the lateral and longitudinal spread of the infection and contributes to additional necrosis of the muscles. In this manner, groups of muscles, an entire limb, or large areas of the body may become successively involved.

The muscles become hemorrhagic and friable during the early stages of the process and noncontractile later, and they exude a brown, watery, foul discharge that frequently contains bubbles of gas.

The most effective way of preventing gas gangrene and other clostridial infections is early and adequate surgery of wounds with removal of contaminated foreign bodies and devitalized tissues. Most experimental and clinical evidence indicates that antibiotic therapy alone cannot be relied on to prevent the occurrence of clostridial infections. Prophylactic administration of gas gangrene antitoxin has been of little or no practical value in the prevention of gas gangrene. Hyperbaric oxygen treatment is supportive and of equivocal value.

In the treatment of established gas gangrene, success depends on early diagnosis and the institution of prompt emergency operative treatment that includes multiple incisions and fasciotomy for decompression and drainage of the fascial compartments, excision of the involved muscles, and open amputation when necessary. Early and adequate surgery is the most reliable and effective primary treatment. Antibiotic therapy with penicillin in large doses intravenously has been effective. Erythromycin is an alternative agent. Antibiotic therapy has been most effective when used as an adjunct to the operative procedure.

Polyvalent gas gangrene antitoxin administered pre- and postoperatively is also of equivocal value in treating established gangrene, and many surgeons doubt its efficacy. Other supportive treatment, such as the administration of plasma, electrolytes and steroids, is essential.

TUBERCULOUS INFECTIONS OF WOUNDS    Postoperative wounds may occasionally become infected by the tubercle bacilli, particularly following operations on known or unknown tuberculous lesions. This complication should rarely occur in modern surgical practice if antituberculosis agents are used. The infection may be apparent as a cold abscess, an indolent ulceration, one or more chronically draining sinuses, or a granulomatous lesion with ulceration. The diagnosis should be proved by biopsy or demonstration of the organism. Treatment consists of the usual therapy for tuberculosis, including two or more antituberculosis chemotherapeutic agents.

ACTINOMYCOTIC INFECTIONS    Actinomycotic infections are usually caused by *Actinomyces israelii* and may develop in wounds made in the presence of deep-seated actinomycosis, such as ileocecal or thoracic lesions. This fungal infection is characterized by the development of a chronic, stony-hard, granulomatous mass, usually in the cervicofacial, thoracic, or abdominal area. It subsequently breaks down to form central abscesses and multiple sinuses, which discharge a peculiar seropurulent fluid containing "sulfur" granules. There is adherence of the mass to the overlying skin, which then assumes a bronze or purplish-red color. The diagnosis is suggested by the appearance of the lesion and is proved by demonstration of the ray fungus in the pus or biopsied material by microscopic examination of the culture.

The lesion may be resistant to therapy, but antibiotic therapy over a prolonged period of several months may produce excellent results. Penicillin is the antibiotic of choice.

OTHER MYCOTIC INFECTIONS    It is impossible to give a description of all types of mycotic infections that may occur in incisional wounds. Numerous causative agents other than *Actinomyces* may cause infections of various types of wounds, including *Candida, Blastomyces, Coccidioides, Sporotrichum, Mucor, Aspergillus, Fusarium*, and *Nocardia*.

The *Candida* organisms have become serious problems; they are the mycotic agents found most frequently in infected wounds, particularly in burn patients, patients undergoing intensive antibiotic therapy, and those undergoing immunosuppressive therapy. Long-term infusion or hyperalimentation has been incriminated as a factor leading to the development of yeast infections in a wide variety of surgical conditions. When the organism is identified in wounds, it has often been discounted or considered to be of little clinical significance. Disseminated candidiasis may easily be missed because the organism may be poorly stained. For active established *Candida* infections, treatment with the intravenous administration of amphotericin B is recommended.

VIRAL INFECTIONS  Herpesvirus, varicella, poxvirus, and cytomegalovirus are rare causes of incisional wound infections.

## REFERENCES

1. Alexander, J. W., Korelitz, J., and Alexander, N. S. Prevention of wound infections: A case for closed suction drainage to remove wound fluids deficient in opsonic proteins. *Am. J. Surg.* 132:59, 1976.
2. Alexander, J. W., Sykes, N. S., Mitchell, M. M., and Fisher, M. W. Concentration of selected intravenously administered antibiotics in experimental surgical wounds. *J. Trauma* 13:423, 1973.
3. Altemeier, W. A., Burke, J. F. Pruitt, B. A., Jr., and Sandusky, W. R. (Eds.) Incidence and Cost of Infection. *Manual on Control of Infection in Surgical Patients.* Philadelphia: Lippincott, 1976, p. 11.
4. Butcher, H. R., Ballinger, W. F., Gravens, D. L., Dewar, N. E., Ledlie, E. F., and Barthel, W. F. Hexachlorophene concentrations in the blood of operating room personnel. *Arch. Surg.* 107:70, 1973.
5. Crapp, A. R., Powis, S. J. A., Tillotson, P., Cooke, W. T., and Alexander-Williams, J. Preparation of the bowel by whole-gut irrigation. *Lancet* 2:1239, 1975.
6. Cruse, P. J. E. Surgical wound sepsis. *C. M. A. Journal* 102:251, 1970.
7. Cruse, P. J. E., and Foord, R. A five-year prospective study of 23,649 surgical wounds. *Arch. Surg.* 107:206, 1973.
8. Cruse, P. J. E., and Foord, R. The epidemiology of wound infection: A 10-year prospective study of 62,939 wounds. *Surg. Clin. North Am.* 60:1, 1980.
9. Cruse, P. J. E., and McPhedran, N. T. Complications of surgery. In Beahrs, O. (Ed.), *General Surgery.* New York: Houghton Mifflin, 1978, pp. 1–24.
10. Culbertson, W. R., et al. Studies on the epidemiology of postoperative infection of clean operative wounds. *Ann. Surg.* 154:599, 1961.
11. Dineen, P. An evaluation of the duration of the surgical scrub. *Surg. Gynecol. Obstet.* 129:1181, 1969.
12. Elek, S. D., and Conen, P. E. The virulence of

*Staphylococcus pyogenes* for man: A study of the problems of wound infection. *Br. J. Exp. Pathol.* 38:573, 1957.
13. Erichsen, J. E. *On Hospitalism and the Causes of Death after Operations.* London: Longmans, Green, 1874.
14. Galle, P. C., Homesley, H. D., and Rhyne, A. L. Reassessment of the surgical scrub. *Surg. Gynecol. Obstet.* 147:214, 1978.
15. Hamilton, H. W., Hamilton, K. R., and Lone, F. J. Preoperative hair removal. *Can. J. Surg.* 20:269, 1977.
16. Howe, C. W., and Marston, A. T. A study on sources of postoperative staphylococcal infection. *Surg. Gynecol. Obstet.* 115:266, 1962.
17. Krizek, T. J., and Robson, M. C. Biology of surgical infection. *Surg. Clin. North Am.* 55:1261, 1975.
18. Lidwell, O. M., Lowbury, E. J. L., Whyte, W., Blowers, R., Stanley, S. J., and Lowe, D. Effect of ultraclean air in operating rooms on deep sepsis in the joint after total hip or knee replacement: A randomized study. *Br. Med. J.* 285:10, 1982.
19. Lowbury, E. J. L., and Lilly, H. A. Disinfection of the hands of surgeons and nurses. *Br. Med. J.* 1:1445, 1960.
20. McIlrath, D. C., Van Heerden, J., and Edis, A. J. Closure of abdominal incisions with subcutaneous catheters. *Surgery* 4:4112, 1976.
21. Miles, A. A., Miles, E. M., and Burke, J. The value and duration of defense reactions of the skin to the primary lodgement of bacteria. *Br. J. Exp. Pathol.* 38:79, 1957.
22. Miles, A. A., and Niven, J. S. F. The enhancement of infection during shock produced by bacterial toxins and other agents. *Br. J. Exp. Pathol.* 31:73, 1950.
23. National Research Council Division of Medical Sciences, Ad Hoc Committee of the Committee of Trauma. Postoperative wound infections: The influence of ultraviolet irradiation of the operating room and various other factors. *Ann. Surg.* 160 (Suppl. 2):1, 1964.
24. Nichols, R. L., Condon, R. E., Gorbach, S. L., and Nyhus, L. M. Efficacy of preoperative antimicrobial preparations of the bowel. *Ann. Surg.* 176:227, 1972.
25. Nora, P. In discussion of Cruse, P. J. E., and Foord, R. A five-year prospective study of 23,649 wounds. *Arch. Srug.* 107:206, 1973.
26. Paskin, D. L., and Lerner, H. J. A prospective study of wound infections. *Am. Surg.* 35:627, 1969.

27. Penikett, E. J. K., and Gorrill, R. H. The integrity of surgeons' gloves tested during use. *Lancet* 2:1042, 1958.

28. Price, P. B. The bacteriology of normal skin: A new quantitative test applied to a study of the bacterial flora and the disinfectant action of me-chanical cleansing. *J. Infect. Dis.* 63:301, 1938.

29. Seropian R., and Reynolds, B. M. Wound infections after preoperative depilatory versus razor preparation. *Am. J. Surg.* 121:251, 1971.

30. Sonneland, J. Postoperative infection. II. Etiological factors. *Pacific Med. Surg.* 74:165, 1966.

# 28 INFECTIONS OF CARDIAC AND VASCULAR PROSTHESES

John P. Burke

The development of synthetic materials that are chemically inert and durable enough to retain their geometric and other physical properties over many years has made possible the wide application of reconstructive operations on the heart and blood vessels. Devices that are commonly implanted in the cardiovascular system include cardiac total-valve prostheses, patches for repairing congenital heart defects, arterial grafts, permanent cardiac pacemakers, and arteriovenous shunts for performing hemodialysis. Ventriculoatrial shunts for treating hydrocephalus are discussed in Chapter 34 and will not be specifically addressed in this chapter.

All prosthetic devices have the propensity to fail because of mechanical, thromboembolic, or infectious complications. The risk of these complications continues throughout the "life" of the prosthesis. Operations to implant prostheses, therefore, should be viewed as palliative rather than curative. Fortunately, failure of the prosthesis need not be catastrophic because replacement is often feasible.

More than 25 varieties of cardiac valve substitutes are now available, and all yield comparable results in terms of survival [41,57]. Current heart valve prostheses may be classified as either mechanical or tissue valves. The caged-ball and tilting disc valves are the two principal types of mechanical prostheses. Tissue valves may be of either human or animal origin. Human homografts are now seldom used. The various types of porcine xenografts that have been widely implanted in the past decade are constructed of an aortic valve removed from a pig, treated with glutaraldehyde for sterilization and tanning, and mounted on a prosthetic support. Bovine pericardial xenografts are similar to the porcine valves and have been increasingly used in recent years. The long-term durability of xenografts is not yet well-established [2,13,51].

## NATURE OF INFECTIONS

### Incidence

Patients who receive cardiovascular implants are predisposed to a variety of nosocomial infections. The overall frequency of infections following open-heart operations, for example, has ranged from 8 to 44 percent [15,53]. The highest rates of infection have been found when special efforts have been made to identify minor and asymptomatic infections. The most common infections are of the respiratory tract, of the surgical wound, and bacteremia. Maki [46] has pointed out that the incidence of bacteremia in this population rivals that reported in acute leukemia.

The frequencies of intracardiac and other infections that occur in tissues adjacent to the different prostheses vary widely and, in some instances, are lower in more recent studies than in earlier ones [48,64]. Table 28-1 shows the approximate ranges of these rates for each of the major groups of prostheses. It is not possible to give an accurate incidence of infection for each device because the duration of follow-up in most reports is either variable or unspecified. The highest rates of infection are associated with appliances such as external arteriovenous cannulas that are continuously exposed to skin flora. Endocarditis has occurred more often with aortic than with mitral prostheses, although this has not been true in all series [58] or in more recent periods [2,64]. The risk does appear greater after multiple valve implantations than after single valve implantation. Similarly, the risk of infection appears greater with a prosthetic cardiac valve than with a patch repair of a congenital heart defect.

Infections at the site of a prosthetic implant account for a minuscule proportion of the entire spectrum of nosocomial infections. Nonetheless, the cost of these infections is high compared to that of many other types of nosocomial infection, and for patients with infected cardiac valve prostheses, the mean case-fatality rate was 54.6 percent in eight studies reported recently [48].

The small numbers of reported cases, the anecdotal nature of many reports, and the lack of a centrally coordinated national surveillance of patients who receive prosthetic implants are each responsible for important gaps in epidemiologic information. Collaborative multicenter studies and computer-assisted reporting systems for the long-term follow-up of patients with prostheses are beginning to appear and may help to establish baseline levels of endemic infections associated with these prostheses [35,45]. One

TABLE 28-1. Frequencies of cardiovascular prosthesis–associated infections

| Type of prosthesis [reference] | Percentage of patients with infections |
|---|---|
| Cardiac | |
|   Valve prosthesis [48] | 1.4–6.3 |
|   Patch repair [59] | 0.1–2.7 |
| Vascular | |
|   Arterial graft [42] | 0.25–6.0 |
|   Permanent pacemaker [11] | 0.13–12.6 |
|   Arteriovenous cannulas [38] | 2.5–26.6* |

*Rate per 100 patient-months.

example of the benefits to a community hospital of surveillance of selected clean cardiac and vascular surgical procedures has been reported in which modest increases in wound infection rates led to the uncovering of possible problems in the cleaning of sternal saws and in the inappropriate timing of "on-call" prophylactic antibiotics [32].

Epidemics in cardiovascular surgery units have generally been recognized by the occurrence of infections due to an unusual pathogen, rather than from an analysis of the overall infection rate. An "outbreak" of four cases of *Aspergillus* infections associated with cardiac prostheses that occurred in a three-year period in one hospital and two cases of *Penicillium* endocarditis in another hospital, for example, were traced to environmental contamination [25,26]. Organisms of the *Mycobacterium fortuitum* complex, including *Mycobacterium chelonei*, have been recognized as an intrinsic contaminant of porcine-valve prostheses, a cause of epidemic sternal wound infections following cardiac surgery, and a cause of prosthetic-valve endocarditis. While modifications of the glutaraldehyde disinfection regimen used by a company to prepare porcine bioprostheses appear to have reduced the risk of such intrinsic contamination, the possible source of contamination in several outbreaks is still unidentified [31]. Nonsterile ice water used for cooling the cardioplegic solution was the possible environmental source in one outbreak [40].

A few experiences have raised the disturbing possibilities that outbreaks due to common organisms may also be insidious and protracted. Clustering of cases of prosthetic-valve endocarditis caused by *Staphylococcus epidermidis* has been observed and was associated with an attack rate of 10 percent over a 32-month period in one hospital [20,27]. In one outbreak, methicillin-resistant *S. epidermidis* sternal wound infections were linked to a chronic carrier of the epidemic strain [47].

Other recent investigations have identified previously unsuspected sources and pathways of infection. *Pseudomonas cepacia* and *Pseudomonas maltophilia* bacteremias after open-heart surgery have been linked to contaminated transducers used with intraarterial pressure-monitoring systems that became contaminated even though disposable transducer domes were used [24,65]. An outbreak of bacteremia with *Enterobacter cloacae* among aortic-valve surgery patients was associated with nonsterile manometers used to measure the pressure of cardioplegia solution injected into the coronary arteries [9].

Finally, outbreaks associated with the injudicious use of quaternary ammonium compounds as disinfectants have been a recurring problem in cardiovascular surgery units (see Chapter 14). In the early years of open-heart surgery, improper cleaning of cardiopulmonary bypass equipment with these agents was responsible for bacteremic infections. Recently, contaminated disinfectants used on various surfaces in the operating room were also associated with contamination of blood in extracorporeal circulators and with subsequent cases of sternal wound infection and endocarditis due to *Serratia marcescens* [22].

*Pathogens*
A wide variety of bacterial, mycobacterial, fungal, and rickettsial species have been identified from infections associated with cardiovascular prostheses. Although gram-negative bacilli are the most frequent isolates in many nosocomial infections, this has not been true of cardiac and vascular prosthesis–associated infections (Table 28-2). Gram-negative bacilli are especially common in retroperitoneal vascular prostheses contaminated from the gastrointestinal or genitourinary tract. Multiple organisms are often isolated in mixed culture from infections associated with cardiac pacemakers and arterial grafts. *Staphylococcus aureus* and *Pseudomonas* species are the pathogens most frequently responsible for infections of vascular access sites for hemodialysis. Recent reports have documented shunt site infections due to unusual causes such as *Legionella pneumophila* and *Cephalosporium* [34,50].

Organisms that have been judged to be of low virulence are often recovered from these infections and cannot be easily dismissed as contaminants in blood cultures. Staphylococci, especially *S. epidermidis*, are involved most often in prosthetic-valve endocarditis. Streptococci (both α-hemolytic and group-D), a variety of enteric gram-negative bacilli, diphtheroids, *Candida*, and *Aspergillus* are also commonly found. The relative frequencies of the different pathogens may vary in different centers; for example, *S. epidermidis* was found in only 2 of 45 cases at the Mayo Clinic [67]. The patterns of microbial species reported from infections associated with patch repairs for congenital heart defects are similar to those from prosthetic valve infections, although staphylococci may be more frequent with prosthetic valve endocarditis [35].

*Classification of Infections*
Existing Centers for Disease Control (CDC) guidelines for determining the presence of infection and for classifying it can be applied to nosocomial infections related to intravascular prostheses [10]. In many instances, however, these definitions are not entirely satisfactory and require additional interpretation. A diagnosis of prosthesis-associated infection requires confirmation by the attending physician because some patients may have bacteremia or fungemia from a focal infection without involvement of the prosthesis [55] and others with prosthesis-associated infection may not have positive blood cultures [62].

Infections related to prosthetic cardiac valves have been classified according to the time of onset of symptoms as either *early* (less than 60 days after the operation) or *late* (more than 60 days after) [18]. Patients

TABLE 28-2. Causative agents of infections associated with cardiac and arterial prostheses

| | No. (%) of cases | |
| --- | --- | --- |
| Etiologic agent | Cardiac prosthesis[a] | Arterial prosthesis[b] |
| *Staphylococcus epidermidis* | 130 (28.1) | 6 (3.7) |
| *Staphylococcus aureus* | 65 (14.1) | 82 (50.9) |
| Gram-negative bacilli | 69 (14.9) | 52 (32.3) |
| *Streptococcus pneumoniae* | 5 (1.1) | |
| Group-D streptococci | 32 (6.9) | 3 (1.9) |
| Other streptococci | 79 (17.1) | 14 (8.7) |
| *Micrococcus* | 6 (1.3) | 3 (1.9) |
| Diphtheroids | 30 (6.5) | 1 (0.6) |
| *Neisseria* | 1 (0.2) | |
| *Listeria monocytogenes* | 2 (0.4) | |
| *Candida* | 30 (6.5) | |
| *Aspergillus* | 12 (2.6) | |
| Other fungi | 1 (0.2) | |
| Total | 462 (100.0) | 161 (100.0) |

[a]From Mayer, K. H., and Schoenbaum, S. C. *Prog. Cardiovasc. Dis.* 25:43, 1982.
[b]Multiple organisms reported in 21 cases. From Liekweg, W. G., Jr., and Greenfield, L. J. *Surgery* 81:335, 1977.

in these two groups differ from each other in their epidemiologic and clinical features; early infections are considered to arise most commonly from intraoperative contamination, and late cases from bacteremias such as those associated with dental, urinary, or other medical procedures. Infections associated with vascular prostheses may also be classified as either early or late in onset by the same (60-day) criterion [43].

The clinical onset of infection related to an intracardiac prosthesis may be delayed until weeks or months after the operative procedure and discharge from the hospital. The incubation period of postoperative infections related to prosthetic materials is often uncertain and probably varies within broad limits, perhaps depending on such factors as the virulence of the organism, size of the inoculum, prophylactic use of antibiotics, and host resistance.

Infections that become apparent within 60 days after placement of a cardiovascular prosthesis should be classified as nosocomial. In addition, intravascular infections that are secondary to nosocomial infections in other sites, such as the urinary or respiratory tract, should be considered separate nosocomial infections, even though their onset may occur more than 60 days postoperatively. A patient who enters the hospital with an intravascular infection for which he or she receives a vascular graft or prosthesis and who later develops postoperative infection with a new and different organism involving the implanted material should also be considered to have a nosocomial infection.

The majority of late infections should be considered community-acquired, however, because the causative agents recovered from them are often those seen in classic infective endocarditis in patients without prosthetic devices. It is unknown which, if any, of these late infections may originate from operative contamination or bacteremia while the patient is hospitalized. It is noteworthy, however, that in two clusters of prosthetic valve endocarditis due to S. epidermidis, 12 of 17 cases were late-onset [20,27]. In an outbreak of infections due to organisms of the M. fortuitum complex associated with cardiac surgery, 3 of 6 cases had late onsets [40]. Fungal endocarditis with manifestations occurring months after cardiac surgery and after documented fungemia also suggests that late cases of fungal endocarditis may be nosocomial [49].

### Diagnostic Criteria

The sudden appearance of a regurgitant murmur or cardiac failure, the disappearance of the distinct click of a mechanical prosthetic valve, or an abnormal tilting motion of the valve demonstrated fluoroscopically are each virtually diagnostic of endocarditis in patients with prosthetic cardiac valves and sustained bacteremia. Furthermore, bacteremia that is persistent after extracardiac sources of infection have been eliminated strongly supports a diagnosis of endocarditis. Criteria have been presented to categorize the diagnosis of endocarditis as "definite," "probable," or "possible" [63]. Varying combinations of findings that support a diagnosis of endocarditis in the presence of any type of intracardiac prosthesis have also been discussed [17].

Positive blood cultures are not as frequent in patients with vascular graft infections as in those with prosthetic valve endocarditis. Bleeding, clotting, or other evidence of malfunction of the graft are diagnostic of infection in the presence of purulent wound drainage, exteriorization of the graft, or systemic sepsis.

In the presence of clinical findings of infection, the discovery of microorganisms by microscopy or culture in vegetations or pus removed from completely intravascular prostheses at either repeat operation or autopsy is evidence of active infection. A positive culture from a removed arteriovenous cannula or an extruded cardiac pacemaker in conjunction with the recovery of the same organism from a blood culture obtained from a different site is also evidence of intravascular infection. In most other instances, the diagnosis of infection at the site of a cardiovascular prosthesis is indirect and is based on the presence of either typical clinical findings or repeated positive blood cultures, or both.

### Predisposing Factors

Postoperative endocarditis occurs more often following open-heart surgery that requires the implantation of foreign material than following other open-heart procedures. Foreign bodies may potentiate infection both by reducing the inoculum of bacteria required to induce inflammation and by promoting sequestration of bacteria in areas inaccessible to host defenses [19] (see Chapter 27). Bacterial adherence to the prosthetic device may also be important in the genesis of foreign-body-associated infections.

The risk of infection has generally been thought to be greater in procedures involving the placement of a prosthesis in a high pressure system with turbulent blood flow, which might explain, in part, the higher infection rates with prosthetic valve implantations than with patch repairs of congenital heart defects. The relative risks of infection cannot be given for all the various models of the available cardiac valve prostheses. Two of the most common types of prostheses currently employed—the Hancock porcine xenograft and various models of the Starr-Edwards plastic and metal valves—have been shown to have similar rates of infection [54].

Cardiopulmonary bypass itself appears to reduce the defense mechanisms of patients as well as to increase the opportunities for operative contamination. Concomitant infection in other sites, such as the urinary or lower respiratory tract, the surgical wound, and venous and arterial catheters, provides a source for direct contamination during the operative procedure and also predisposes to bacteremia with seeding of the prosthetic device. The risk of infection at the site of a femoral-popliteal arterial graft is increased by open, infected lesions on the legs at the time of the operation [29].

The most important single factor shaping the character of postoperative endocarditis and other infections related to cardiovascular prostheses is the use of antimicrobial agents before, during, and after operative procedures. The extensive preoperative use of antibiotics may increase the risk of postoperative endocarditis when an intracardiac prosthesis is implanted [44]. The reasons for this are not clear, but they may be related to the replacement of "normal flora" by antibiotic-resistant species and the overgrowth of certain microbial flora of the skin, mucous membrances, or gastrointestinal tract. The use of prophylactic antimicrobial agents during and after operations has been responsible for shifting the patterns of infecting agents to a more antibiotic-resistant group of pathogens including *S. epidermidis*, the diphtheroids, and various fungi [4].

The overall risk of infection is probably greater with longer than with shorter courses of chemotherapy, both pre- and postoperatively. When a major break in aseptic technique occurs during the operation, however, prophylaxis merges with early treatment, and a prolonged course of high-dose chemotherapy may be desirable.

Certain patients have other risk factors that are commonly associated with nosocomial infections. Serious underlying illnesses (e.g., congestive heart failure, rheumatoid arthritis, and diabetes mellitus) and the use of medications (e.g., steroids and indomethacin) are associated with decreased host resistance and often with defective inflammatory or immune responses, which thereby increases the risks of both prosthesis-associated infection and other focal infections. Recently, a high carriage rate of *S. aureus* in asymptomatic patients receiving hemodialysis has been suggested to be related to an increased incidence of shunt infections and bacteremia [39]. This is consistent with the observation that the risk of staphylococcal infections of incisional wounds in general is increased in patients who carry *S. aureus* in the anterior nares (see Chapter 27).

## SPECIMENS

### Collection

Isolation of the pathogen from blood cultures is the essential laboratory procedure for the diagnosis and effective treatment of intravascular infections. The techniques for obtaining specimens are far more important than the use of special media or the ability of the laboratory to isolate unusual microbial species (see Chapter 7).

The bacteremias accompanying prosthetic valve endocarditis have not been studied with quantitative blood cultures during the untreated course of the disease, as were those of native valve endocarditis in the preantibiotic era. In one report, blood cultures were not as uniformly positive in prosthesis cases as in nonprosthesis cases of endocarditis [63]. Nonetheless, as in other intravascular infections bacteremia is probably continuous, and timing of blood cultures should not be critical. Blood cultures should be obtained at various intervals, however, to document the *persistence* as well as the *presence* of bacteremia. It seems reasonable to recommend that at least three blood samples be obtained with separate venipunctures. More than six blood cultures are rarely necessary. In urgent clinical circumstances in which there is a need to begin antibiotic therapy promptly, these samples might be collected at hourly, or even more frequent intervals.

In adults a total blood sample of 50 to 60 ml should be sufficient to allow detection of low-density bacteremia. The blood from each sample is distributed between aerobic and anaerobic culture bottles at the time of collection. The sample obtained from a single venipuncture, however, should not be divided among more than one "set" of culture bottles since potential contaminants introduced during blood collection may be assigned clinical importance if all the cultures are positive. The yield from additional blood cultures is small when five or six samples taken at different times are negative.

The microorganisms that are the most common contaminants in blood cultures (e.g., *S. epidermidis* and diphtheroids) are also often responsible for infections associated with cardiac and vascular prostheses.

The rate of false-positive cultures depends on the aseptic precautions used in obtaining specimens; calculation of this rate in one's own hospital is helpful for interpreting reports of cultures and for stimulating efforts to improve the techniques of collection. The chance that a single blood culture is falsely positive should not be more than 2 or 3 percent [5].

Use of alcohol (70% to 95% isopropanol or 70% ethanol) for skin cleansing followed by tincture of iodine (2%) is preferred for preparing the skin for venipuncture. Solutions of benzalkonium chloride and other quaternary ammonium compounds should not be used for skin disinfection because these agents are relatively inactive against gram-negative bacilli and may become contaminated with such organisms. Outbreaks of pseudobacteremia caused by contaminated blood-drawing equipment [21] and collection tubes [30], benzalkonium chloride [37], and povidone-iodine [7] have been reported.

The disinfecting agent should be allowed to act for about one minute, and the venipuncture site should not be probed with a finger unless it has been decontaminated or unless surgical gloves are worn.

In adults the smallest amount of blood taken for culture on each occasion should be 10 ml; 1- to 2-ml samples are often taken from infants. The sample is then inoculated into a liquid culture medium that is at least tenfold greater in volume to dilute the antibacterial substances of the whole blood. Organisms from the deeper layers of the skin may adhere to the outside of the needle used for venipuncture; therefore, the needle must be removed and replaced with a sterile needle before the blood is inoculated from a syringe into the culture bottles. The diaphragm top of the bottle should be wiped with alcohol or tincture of iodine before the needle is inserted. Alcohol may be used to remove residual iodine on the skin after the blood culture is collected.

If the patient has been receiving a penicillin or cephalosporin, penicillinase may be added to the medium to block the antibiotic effect. When this is done, however, a sample of penicillinase should be cultured as a control to detect any contamination of the enzyme preparation. A commercial device for the removal of antibiotics from blood using an adsorbent resin has been introduced recently; the clinical usefulness of this device has not yet been established [60].

Direct communication between the physician and laboratory personnel is necessary for evaluating these serious infections. The physician should be responsible for ensuring that a colony of any microorganism recovered is placed in a holding medium and not discarded by the laboratory as a "contaminant." A separate colony from each positive culture should be preserved for later typing by either biochemical reactions, antibiotic sensitivity patterns (antibiograms), phage typing, or serologic methods when these results may be useful for determining whether the organisms are pathogens or contaminants (see Chapter 7). If the isolates are clearly different, their probable clinical significance is reduced. Specimens of the isolated microorganism will also be necessary for tests to estimate the effectiveness of antibiotic treatment.

When the clinical findings suggest intravascular infection and the conventional blood cultures are negative, special procedures should be employed to recover potential pathogens. Nutritionally variant streptococci may fail to grow in routine culture media unless they are supplemented with pyridoxal hydrochloride. In special instances, incubation of the cultures should be continued for two to three weeks so that organisms such as *Candida*, fastidious gram-negative rods, *Hemophilus*, and *Cardiobacterium* might be isolated. Special procedures for recognizing cell wall–defective bacterial variants (L-forms) may be performed in research laboratories. The techniques of lysis filtration and lysis centrifugation may permit greater sensitivity for detecting bacteremia [60], and the use of biphasic media improves the yield of fungi.

Negative blood cultures may be found in patients with intravascular infections due to *Chlamydia, Rickettsia, Aspergillus, Candida*, and certain other fungi. If embolism to a major artery occurs, the embolus should be removed and later examined and cultured to detect the presence of fungi. *Candida* and *Aspergillus* may be isolated more often from arterial blood than from venous blood [60]. Blood cultures are also occasionally negative when bacterial infection involves the right side of the heart.

*Transport of Specimens*

Because antibacterial substances and antibodies in whole blood may interfere with bacterial growth, blood for culture must be inoculated into the medium at the bedside. Many commercially available blood culture media also contain substances (e.g., sodium polyanetholsulfonate) that inhibit such antibacterial activity. No special precautions are necessary for the transport of the culture bottle, which may be kept at room temperature. Refrigeration of the culture bottle will delay bacterial growth.

Specimens of the prosthetic apparatus or tissues obtained from operations and autopsies should be immediately delivered to the laboratory in sterile containers rather than in formaldehyde solutions.

# CLINICAL ASPECTS OF INTRAVASCULAR INFECTIONS

## Manifestations

GENERAL FEATURES  The symptoms and signs of intravascular infection related to prosthetic materials are similar to those of classic infective endocarditis, with some important differences. The intravascular location is the feature that all these infections have in common and that is responsible for their protean manifestations. The specific clinical features are determined by the type and location of the prosthesis, nature of the responsible microbial agent, and presence of underlying chronic illness, especially uremia.

The most common symptoms are nonspecific, such as fever, malaise, and weakness. Indeed, a surprisingly high proportion of patients appear entirely well at the time of the first positive blood culture. Fever and other signs of infection may be suppressed by injudicious antibiotic treatment, or they may not occur in the presence of chronic illness such as uremia. In patients whose illness begins early in the postoperative period, the dominant symptoms may be of associated infection, such as pneumonia and wound infection.

VALVULAR PROSTHESES  In patients with prosthetic cardiac valves, the occurrence of regurgitant murmurs and severe cardiac failure as a result of separation of sutures from the valvular annulus is highly suggestive of endocarditis. These infections are frequently accompanied by embolic phenomena and sometimes produce aortic aneurysms and myocardial abscesses. The valve itself may become occluded by a thrombus. Other findings usually associated with endocarditis— such as anemia, hematuria (macroscopic or microscopic), Roth's spots, subungual hemorrhages, conjunctival petechiae, and enlargement of the spleen— help to direct attention to the possibility of intravascular infection. However, more than 50 percent of patients subjected to open-heart surgery with cardiopulmonary bypass develop conjunctival petechiae postoperatively that are unrelated to infection [66].

Prediction of the tempo of the clinical course cannot be based reliably on knowledge of the responsible microbial species. Rapid destruction of the valvular annulus may occur in prosthetic-valve infections due to organisms such as S. epidermidis that have been judged to be of low virulence as well as in infections due to S. aureus.

Fungal endocarditis with unusually large and friable vegetations is often complicated by embolic occlusion of the large arteries, especially those in the lower extremities. The complications of uveitis or endophthalmitis are especially suggestive of infection due to Candida species.

OTHER VASCULAR PROSTHESES  In endocarditis following polytef (Teflon) patch repair of a congenital heart defect (e.g., ventricular septal defect), the only evidence of infection may be fever, either low-grade or spiking. Separation of the patch with or without subsequent embolism may occur.

Inflammation at the operative site may be found in patients with infected arterial grafts, subcutaneous cardiac pacemakers, and arteriovenous shunts. Common signs of infections related to arterial grafts are bleeding, clotting of the prosthesis, localized abscess, chronic draining sinus, and peripheral septic emboli with secondary abscesses. Arteriovenous shunts may also show instability of the polytef cannula, oozing of blood, repeated clotting, or local abscess.

## Management

INITIAL TREATMENT  The management of infections associated with intravascular prostheses requires the use of high doses of microbicidal agents intravenously and a consideration of the removal and possible replacement of the prosthesis. The principles of antimicrobial therapy are similar to those for the treatment of infective endocarditis with native heart valves [16]. Full bacteriologic study of the sensitivity of the pathogen is necessary for optimal treatment of these intravascular infections. Nonetheless, chemotherapy must begin before the results of sensitivity tests become available. The selection of antimicrobial agents at that time is based on consideration of the usual sensitivities of the specific pathogen and the antimicrobial agents previously used for that patient. The pathogen should be assumed to be resistant to the prophylactic antibiotics used for open-heart surgery. Postoperative infections commonly occur, however, with organisms that are fully sensitive to the prophylactic antibiotics, especially in prosthetic-valve endocarditis due to S. epidermidis.

If because of fulminant illness it is necessary to begin treatment before the responsible pathogen is isolated, the selection of specific antimicrobials should be influenced by consideration of the types and sensitivities of pathogens isolated from similar patients in that hospital. Even in such urgent circumstances, however, it is possible to obtain five or six blood cultures before treatment is begun. Either a penicillinase-resistant penicillin, a cephalosporin, or vancomycin should be included in the antibiotic regimen to "cover" the possibility of staphylococcal infection.

TREATMENT FOR SPECIFIC PATHOGENS Specific drugs of choice cannot be listed for many pathogens, in part because of the changing and unique patterns of antibiotic resistance in different hospitals. However, guidelines for the selection of antimicrobial agents with activity against important pathogens can be given.

A penicillinase-resistant penicillin is used for infections due to *S. aureus*, although penicillin G can be used if the MIC of the organism is less than 0.1 $\mu$g/ml. Some experts believe that the combination of gentamicin and a penicillinase-resistant penicillin affords more rapid killing of *S. aureus*.

Methicillin-resistant *S. epidermidis* strains usually contain subpopulations that are resistant to cephalosporins even though susceptibility tests may indicate the isolates are sensitive. The optimum treatment regimen for *S. epidermidis* endocarditis may require vancomycin plus rifampin or an aminoglycoside [36]. Vancomycin is also indicated for methicillin-resistant *S. aureus*. Special care is required when disc sensitivity tests are used to detect resistance to penicillinase-resistant penicillins (see Chapter 11). Apparent resistance of staphylococci should be confirmed by tube-dilution tests.

Most patients who are allergic to penicillin can be safely treated with cephalosporins, although some patients are allergic to both. A cephalosporin can be used if the reaction to penicillin is mild or the history is vague. Vancomycin is a suitable alternative for patients with a history of a life-threatening reaction to either a penicillin or a cephalosporin.

Every effort should be made to use a penicillin or cephalosporin because they are the most effective antimicrobials in treating intravascular infections due to susceptible organisms. Skin tests are useful for predicting more severe penicillin reactions, and guidelines have been suggested for management of penicillin allergy in patients with bacterial endocarditis [23]. Hyposensitization to penicillin may be attempted for selected patients who are skin test positive.

Intravascular infections due to viridans streptococci, enterococci, or diphtheroids may be treated with combined penicillin G and gentamicin. The addition of gentamicin, while not strictly necessary for infections due to viridans streptococci, may provide a more rapid bactericidal effect. Some strains of diphtheroids are resistant to this combination, and other strains may be difficult to test for sensitivity because of their slow growth. Vancomycin with or without an aminoglycoside appears to be an effective alternative.

Infections due to gram-negative bacilli nearly always require early operative intervention. Failure of treatment with antibiotics is a major problem, in part because the antimicrobial agents that are most active against gram-negative bacilli have either prohibitive toxicity for the high-dose therapy needed, poor diffusibility in tissues, or bacteriostatic properties only. Initial therapy must always include at least two antimicrobial agents that are likely to be effective against recent nosocomial isolates of that species in the hospital in which the patient was most likely infected. At the present time, gentamicin, tobramycin, netilmicin, and amikacin are likely to possess the widest spectrum of activity against gram-negative bacilli from nosocomial infections. One of the antibiotics selected should be either a broad-spectrum penicillin (ampicillin, carbenicillin, ticarcillin, piperacillin, azlocillin, or mezlocillin) or a cephalosporin.

*Pseudomonas* infections associated with intracardiac prostheses are a special problem. The results of antimicrobial therapy are dismal—even with in vitro demonstration of the sensitivity of the organism to the antimicrobial agents used—and removal and replacement of the prosthesis may be life-saving.

Yeast and fungal infections, which are usually due to either *Candida* or *Aspergillus* species, require removal of the prosthesis and systemic treatment with amphotericin B.

The effectiveness of chemotherapy is generally monitored by determining the antibacterial activity of the patient's serum against the organism recovered from the blood (or from the prosthesis itself) with a serial, twofold dilution test. Numerous problems have been associated with such tests, including determining the most appropriate time for collection of the blood specimen (peak vs. trough antibiotic levels), lack of standardized methods for performing the tests, and lack of evidence that the results are of prognostic value [14].

Antibiotic assays are a suitable substitute for serial, twofold dilution tests of the patient's serum when the infecting organism is known to be sensitive, and such assays can assist in preventing toxicity from excessive drug levels. Serum concentrations should be maintained within acceptable therapeutic ranges. Assays are probably preferable in monitoring therapy with antibiotics that are highly protein-bound or very sensitive to pH changes, since erratic results sometimes occur with the serum dilution method.

The optimal duration of antibacterial treatment has not been determined. Therapy should generally be continued for at least four weeks. Most experts recommend longer treatment for cardiac prosthesis–associated infection than for native-valve endocarditis.

REMOVAL OF PROSTHESES Vigorous antibiotic therapy will cure some intravascular prosthesis infections; in others, antibiotics may suppress the systemic signs and symptoms while the infection persists at the site of the prosthesis. Antibiotic therapy of prosthetic-valve endocarditis fails more often in cases with an early postoperative onset than in those with a late onset. To detect antibiotic failure at the earliest possible time, it is useful to obtain blood for culture periodically during treatment and, especially, in the weeks and months after the completion of treatment, irrespective of the lack of fever or other signs of infection.

Removal of an intracardiac prosthesis is necessary when antibiotic therapy has failed to clear the bacteremia. Other indications for the removal of a prosthetic valve, in addition to uncontrolled infection or resistance of the organism to available bactericidal chemotherapeutic agents, include dysfunction of the valve (manifested by a regurgitant murmur, abnormal angulation of a partially detached valve seen on roentgenogram or fluoroscopy, or severe cardiac failure), major systemic embolism, and suspected yeast or fungal infection.

Furthermore, it seems advisable to recommend removal of the prosthesis early in the course of prosthetic-valve endocarditis complicated by factors associated with an unfavorable outcome [6]. Such factors include infection caused by organisms not easily treated by antibiotics (e.g., staphylococci, gram-negative bacilli, and fungi). In the presence of indications for the removal of the prosthesis, temporizing for more than a few days with antibiotic therapy does not appear to reduce the risk of relapse. The presence of active infection is not a contraindication to cardiac surgery in these patients. It is unknown how long antibiotics should be continued postoperatively, and recommended schedules vary from two to six weeks.

Dysfunction of the prosthetic valve or systemic embolism will often be the only evidence of involvement of the prosthesis when blood cultures are negative. Fungi are responsible for many of these infections, and removal of the prosthesis is necessary for cure.

## EPIDEMIOLOGIC CONSIDERATIONS

### Sources and Prevention

In general, nosocomial infections at the site of a prosthetic implant may arise either from direct contamination at the time of the operation or from bacteremic seeding of the prosthesis secondary to another focal infection. Appropriate preoperative care and aseptic surgical technique may lessen the risk of the former circumstance; practices described elsewhere in this book related to the prevention of urinary, respiratory, wound, and vascular-access-device-related infections will assist in the control of the latter situation (see Chapters 25, 26, 27, and 36).

PATIENT-CARE PRACTICES Many operative procedures to implant cardiac or vascular prostheses are semielective, thereby allowing for meticulous preoperative care. In one review, nearly one-half of the patients with prosthetic-valve endocarditis had clinical evidence of an extracardiac infection at the time of surgery [52]. Special attention should be given to the preoperative diagnosis and treatment of focal infections, especially periodontal, prostate, and urinary infections.

Some surgeons recommend washing the patient's skin daily with a 3% hexachlorophene emulsion for one to two days before the operation [12]. Preoperative shaving is associated with increased infection rates; clipping immediately before the operation is the preferred method for hair removal [1] (see Chapter 27).

Many procedures to implant a cardiovascular prosthesis are so complex and lengthy that eventual breaks in aseptic technique are almost inevitable. Punctured gloves, for example, occur with nearly every sternotomy. Considering the many opportunities for contamination of the operative field, the low infection rates observed suggest that infections may be caused by either uncommonly massive contamination, unusually virulent microorganisms, or especially dangerous personnel shedders. Nonetheless, firm discipline in the operating room, avoidance of unnecessary traffic and talking, and exclusion of personnel with overt skin infections should assist in the control of infection.

The development and maintenance of the professional skills of the nursing and technical staff are especially important. The Inter-Society Commission for Heart Disease Resources has recommended guidelines for the clinical and physical environment in which cardiac surgery may be performed most effectively [56].

Measures for the prevention of arteriovenous shunt–associated infections are similar to those for the prevention of intravenous catheter–associated infections (see Chapter 36). Because the cannula is exposed on the surface of an extremity, the site is continually subject to microbial contamination from the patient's own flora as well as from external sources, including dialysis fluid and equipment. The surgically created subcutaneous arteriovenous fistula is used more often than external cannulas in most hemodialysis centers, in part because there is a lower risk of infection with the internal fistula.

A topical antimicrobial agent, such as neomycin–polymyxin B–bacitracin, and a dry sterile gauze dressing may be placed over the external shunt, which is then covered with an occlusive bandage. The dressing should not be disturbed between dialysis periods. Aseptic technique during dialysis should be used in the care of the external shunt. Personnel who handle the shunt should wear gloves, and both patient and nurse should wear face masks whenever the dressing is removed.

ENVIRONMENTAL FACTORS  The majority of nosocomial infections associated with cardiovascular prostheses are thought to occur as a result of direct contamination of the prosthesis in the operating room. Blood in the heart-lung bypass machine appears to be an important source for this contamination. The fact that the most common microbial species recovered from blood cultures obtained from various sites during bypass are the most common pathogens found in cases of postoperative prosthetic-valve endocarditis has been cited as evidence of the role of contamination of the bypass machine. Indeed, positive cultures of pump-oxygenator blood are associated with an increased risk of later infection [3]. Furthermore, the predominance of gram-positive organisms recovered from these cultures is cited to justify prophylactic treatment of the patient with a penicillinase-resistant penicillin or a cephalosporin.

Blood in the operative field is returned by suction tubing to the pump oxygenator for recirculation. These suction lines have been found to yield the highest frequency of positive blood cultures when samples are obtained from several different sites during heart-lung bypass procedures. Nearly 25% of blood cultures from this site may be positive. Direct contamination from operating-room air at the site of the turbulent blood-air interface is, of course, suspected. One possible means of partially reducing this source of contamination is clamping the suction tubing when it is not in use.

The instruments and equipment for bypass procedures should be thoroughly cleaned of debris, autoclaved, and assembled under aseptic conditions before use. The use of disposable membrane and bubble oxygenators has done much to simplify the problems of sterilization. Many centers use a bacterial filter in the oxygen supply line because the oxygen itself and the junction between the nonsterile oxygen tank and the oxygenator may be sources of potential contamination.

The operating-room air should have a slight positive pressure in relation to the surrounding areas, and the doors must be kept closed. U.S. Public Health Service standards require at least 20 complete changes of operating room air per hour [61]. The development of clean-room technology and laminar (or unidirectional) airflow systems that are capable of reducing the microbial concentration to less than one organism per cubic foot has provided a research tool for the investigation of the relation of airborne bacteria to wound infection (see Chapters 27 and 29). Conventional air-conditioning systems, however, are capable of reducing the microbial concentration in operating-room air to between one and three organisms per cubic foot. Nonetheless, it seems advisable to protect prostheses from prolonged exposure to operating-room air before their insertion in the patient.

A variety of other unproven measures have been recommended to reduce environmental contamination in operating rooms. A few—such as regular cleaning of the operating-room floor with a phenolic disinfectant and the use of disposable, waterproof, paper draping materials and surgical gowns—are reasonable and in widespread use; others—such as changing shoe covers at the entrance to the operating room and passing all traffic over disinfectant-soaked blankets—appear irrational and useless. All such measures should be secondary to attention to proper aseptic techniques, hand-scrubbing, and minimizing number of personnel and traffic within the operating room (see Chapter 20).

Inadequate sterilization of the prosthesis before insertion has also been suspected as a cause of subsequent infection. Prosthetic materials that cannot be autoclaved are frequently sterilized by ethylene oxide. Intrinsic contamination is more likely for materials treated with ethylene oxide. Neither of these techniques is used for porcine valves, which are treated with glutaraldehyde. When sterilization is undertaken by a hospital, the process should be monitored with bacterial spore strips. Many surgeons have resorted to soaking the device in an antibiotic-containing solution just before insertion, with the hope of killing any surviving organisms in the interstices of the fabric of the prosthesis. Contamination of the prosthesis could occur from soaking in a nonsterile antibiotic solution, however, and patients who are allergic to the antibiotics used may be inadvertently exposed to serious reactions by this practice.

PROPHYLACTIC ANTIBIOTICS  The benefits of antibiotic prophylaxis in cardiac valve replacement remain uncertain, but it has become standard practice to use such prophylaxis [28] (see Chapter 11). No placebo-controlled studies have been performed in the past decade, and there is almost no available information on infection rates in patients not receiving antibiotics. One study, however—a large randomized, double-blind evaluation of cefazolin versus placebo during arterial reconstructive operations—supports the use of antibiotic prophylaxis for surgery involving the abdominal aorta and lower extremities [33].

Antibiotic prophylaxis directed at specific pathogens known to be sensitive to the drug will probably be effective. Thus prophylactic treatment with penicillinase-resistant penicillins or cephalosporins probably reduces the incidence of postoperative infection with *S. aureus* and other sensitive pyogenic cocci. This use of antibiotics is well established and will not change unless infections with antibiotic-resistant microorganisms become recognized with increasing frequency. The task of the hospital epidemiologist is to document and analyze the occurrences of infection so that obsolete or inappropriate prophylaxis may be recognized at the earliest possible time.

Prophylactic antibiotics should be started no earlier than a few hours before the operation. The optimal duration of prophylactic treatment has not been established, but several studies have failed to show any justification for prolonging their use beyond two days. Many surgeons insist on continuing them, however, until all possible sources of contamination, such as arterial catheters, have been removed.

## Management of Outbreaks

METHODS OF INVESTIGATION  To apply control measures for an outbreak, it is necessary to identify the source and mode of spread of the pathogen. The first step is to prepare a line-listing of the cases. Although only a few cases may have occurred, a detailed listing of the clinical and epidemiologic circumstances of each case is made, and each feature shared by two or more cases is expressed as a ratio. The listing should include the dates of onset and the outcome of the infections. Additional factors might include the ages and sexes of the patients, underlying diseases that predispose to such infections, duration of preoperative hospitalization, dates of operations, types and suppliers of the prostheses, methods of sterilization and handling of prostheses before insertion, locations of the operating rooms, names of surgeons and other members of the surgical teams, results of cultures and antibiograms of isolates, prophylactic antimicrobial agents used, duration of anesthesia and pump time, proportion of emergency and nighttime procedures and of emergency reoperations, proportion who experienced intraoperative problems such as bleeding

and difficulty in weaning from the pump, and presence of other focal infections [8]. These data should also be collected from a group of patients who underwent comparable surgical procedures during the same time period but who did not develop infections associated with their prostheses. Analysis of these data may suggest factors associated with the cases that will set directions for the investigation (see Chapter 5).

Recent operating-room records should be reviewed to determine the total number of operative procedures of a similar nature that have been performed. These procedures should be tabulated separately for periods before and during the epidemic for use in determining changes in the infection rate. At the same time that these data are being collected and analyzed, a review of aseptic techniques, methods for disinfecting equipment, and the mechanics of the ventilating system in the operating room may reveal a productive area for special bacteriologic study.

The pathogen recovered from each case should be saved, whenever possible, both for serum inhibition tests to be used in evaluating treatment and for later laboratory study to characterize the "epidemic strain." Review of the susceptibilities to antimicrobial agents of the pathogens will help to determine whether a single strain or multiple strains are involved, and such susceptibility data may lead the epidemiologist to recommend changes in prophylactic antibiotic use (see Chapter 7).

While the investigation is proceeding, the epidemiologist should recommend a protocol for collecting prospective data from new patients. For example, culture of blood from the bypass machine after each operation will help to establish the frequency of contamination from this source. If such cultures have been routinely performed, an immediate review of the results from preepidemic and epidemic periods is useful. Prospective cultures of prostheses just before insertion might also be undertaken, especially when the epidemic strain is an organism that is more likely than others to resist sterilization or the prostheses are subjected to disinfecting rather than sterilizing procedures. Diphtheroids, staphylococci, and spore-forming bacilli, for example, are more difficult to sterilize than gram-negative bacilli, and mycobacterial species appear to be relatively resistant to certain disinfectants. The temptation to obtain nasopharyngeal or other swabs for culture from personnel and environmental cultures from the operating room should be resisted until the foregoing tasks have been completed. Because the pathogens from these infections are ubiquitous, positive cultures from such human and environmental sites have limited meaning and may be misleading. Cultures from these sites should only be obtained when epidemiologic data suggest that one of these sites may be relevant to the outbreak, and isolates of appropriate identity should then be fully characterized and compared with isolates of the "epidemic strain" from cases.

CONTROL  The measures taken to control an epidemic are determined by the epidemiologic findings and the urgency of the problem. In an outbreak with a high attack rate that is recognized as a grave threat to the safe conduct of such operations, it may be necessary to close the operating room temporarily and suspend procedures. In less urgent circumstances—usually when the outbreak is insidious and protracted—thoughtful investigation may precede the application of control measures. Appropriate control measures should not be withheld pending completion of the investigation if there is a reasonable chance that additional cases will be prevented by their institution (see Chapter 5).

Available data should be reported to local and federal health authorities. Pooled data from multiple institutions may be necessary to establish conclusively low-frequency, intrinsic contamination of commercially distributed prosthetic materials.

If the investigation fails to uncover the source of the outbreak, the operating room should be temporarily closed and thoroughly cleaned. The importance of hand-washing and aseptic technique should be stressed to personnel. In some circumstances, discontinuation of the use of ineffective prophylactic antibiotics alone may control the outbreak, even if the source is not found. Prompt removal or elimination of a possible source suggested by the epidemiologic investigation, even when the data are inconclusive, will allow the epidemiologist to evaluate a hypothesis through well-planned, continuing surveillance. Regardless of the solution to the problem, surveillance of patients on the involved services should continue with the purpose of either evaluating the control-prevention measures or providing additional data that may help define the cause (see Chapter 4).

# REFERENCES

1. Alexander, J. W., Fischer, J. E., Boyajian, M., Palmquist, J., and Morris, M. J. The influence of hair-removal methods on wound infections. *Arch. Surg.* 118:347, 1983.

2. Angell, W. W., Angell, J. D., and Kosek, J. C. Twelve-year experience with glutaraldehyde-preserved porcine xenografts. *J. Thorac. Cardiovasc. Surg.* 83:493, 1982.

3. Ankeney, J. L., and Parker, R. F. Staphylococcal Endocarditis Following Open Heart Surgery Related to Positive Intraoperative Blood Cultures. In Brewer, L. A., III (Ed.), *Prosthetic Heart Valves.* Springfield, Ill.: Charles C Thomas, 1969, pp. 719–728.

4. Archer, G. L., and Armstrong, B. C. Alteration of staphylococcal flora in cardiac surgery patients receiving antibiotic prophylaxis. *J. Infect. Dis.* 147:642, 1983.

5. Bartlett, R. C., Ellner, P. D., and Washington, J. A., II. *Cumitech 1: Blood Cultures.* Washington, D.C.: American Society for Microbiology, 1974.

6. Baumgartner, W. A., Miller, D. C., Reitz, B. A., Oyer, P. E., Jamieson, S. W., Stinson, E. B., and Shumway, N. E. Surgical treatment of prosthetic valve endocarditis. *Ann. Thorac. Surg.* 35:87, 1983.

7. Berkelman, R. L., Lewin, S., Allen, J. R., Anderson, R. L., Budnick, L. D., Shapiro, S., Friedman, S. M., Nicholas, P., Holzman, R. S., and Haley, R. W. Pseudobacteremia attributed to contamination of povidone-iodine with *Pseudomonas cepacia. Ann. Intern. Med.* 95:32, 1981.

8. Bor, D. H., Rose, R. M., Modlin, J. F., Weintraub, R., and Friedland, G. H. Mediastinitis after cardiovascular surgery. *Rev. Infect. Dis.* 5:885, 1983.

9. Centers for Disease Control. Bacteremia among aortic-valve surgery patients—Boston. *Morbid. Mortal. Weekly Rep.* 31:88, 1982.

10. Centers for Disease Control. *Outline for Surveillance and Control of Nosocomial Infections. Appendix II. Guidelines for Determining Presence and Classification of Infection,* May 1970.

11. Choo, M. H., Holmes, D. R., Jr., Gersh, B. J., Maloney, J. D., Merideth, J., Pluth, J. R., and Trusty, J. Permanent pacemaker infections: Characterization and management. *Am. J. Cardiol.* 48:559, 1981.

12. Clark, R. E., Amos, W. C., Higgins, V., Bemberg, K. F., and Weldon, C. S. Infection control in cardiac surgery. *Surgery* 79:89, 1976.

13. Cohn, L. H., Mudge, G. H., Pratter, F., and Collins, J. J., Jr. Five- to eight-year follow-up of patients undergoing porcine heart-valve replacement. *N. Engl. J. Med.* 304:258, 1981.

14. Coleman, D. L., Horwitz, R. I., and Andriole, V. T. Association between serum inhibitory and bactericidal concentrations and therapeutic outcome in bacterial endocarditis. *Am. J. Med.* 73:260, 1982.

15. Conte, J. E., Jr., Cohen, S. N., Roe, B. B.,

and Elashoff, R. M. Antibiotic prophylaxis and cardiac surgery: A prospective double-blind comparison of single-dose versus multiple-dose regimens. *Ann. Intern. Med.* 76:943, 1972.

16. Dismukes, W. E. Prosthetic Valve Endocarditis: Factors Influencing Outcome and Recommendations for Therapy. In Bisno, A. L. (Ed.), *Treatment of Infective Endocarditis.* New York: Grune & Stratton, 1981, pp. 167–191.

17. Dismukes, W. E., and Karchmer, A. W. The Diagnosis of Infected Prosthetic Heart Valves: Bacteremia Versus Endocarditis. In Duma, R. J. (Ed.), *Infections of Prosthetic Heart Valves and Vascular Grafts: Prevention, Diagnosis, and Treatment.* Baltimore: University Park Press, 1977, pp. 61–78.

18. Dismukes, W. E., Karchmer, A. W., Buckley, M. J., Austen, W. G., and Swartz, M. N. Prosthetic valve endocarditis: Analysis of 38 cases. *Circulation* 48:365, 1973.

19. Dougherty, S. H., and Simmons, R. L. Infections in bionic man: The pathobiology of infections in prosthetic devices. Part I. *Curr. Probl. Surg.* 29:217, 1982.

20. Downham, W. H., and Rhoades, E. R. Endocarditis associated with porcine valve xenografts. *Arch. Intern. Med.* 139:1350, 1979.

21. DuClos, T. W., Hodges, G. R., and Killian, J. E. Bacterial contamination of blood-drawing equipment: A cause of false-positive blood cultures. *Am. J. Med. Sci.* 266:459, 1974.

22. Ehrenkranz, N. J., Bolyard, E. A., and Wiener, M. Antibiotic-sensitive *Serratia marcescens* infections complicating cardiopulmonary operations: Contaminated disinfectant as a reservoir. *Lancet* 2:1289, 1980.

23. Erffmeyer, J. E., and Lieberman, P. Management of Penicillin Allergy in Patients with Bacterial Endocarditis. In Bisno, A. L. (Ed.), *Treatment of Infective Endocarditis.* New York: Grune & Stratton, 1981, pp. 209–233.

24. Fisher, M. C., Long, S. S., Roberts, E. M., Dunn, J. M., and Balsara, R. K. *Pseudomonas maltophilia* bacteremia in children undergoing open heart surgery. *J.A.M.A.* 246:1571, 1981.

25. Gage, A. A., Dean, D. C., Schimert, G., and Minsley, N. *Aspergillus* infection after cardiac surgery. *Arch. Surg.* 101:384, 1970.

26. Hall, W. J., III. *Penicillium* endocarditis following open heart surgery and prosthetic valve insertion. *Am. Heart J.* 87:501, 1974.

27. Hammond, G. W., and Stiver, H. G. Combination antibiotic therapy in an outbreak of prosthetic endocarditis caused by *Staphylococcus epidermidis. Can. Med. Assoc. J.* 118:524, 1978.

28. Hirschmann, J. V., and Inui, T. S. Antimicrobial prophylaxis: A critique of recent trials. *Rev. Infect. Dis.* 2:1, 1980.

29. Hoffert, P. W., Gensler, S., and Haimovici, H. Infection complicating arterial grafts: Personal experience with 12 cases and review of the literature. *Arch. Surg.* 90:427, 1965.

30. Hoffman, P. C., Arnow, P. M., Goldmann, D. A., Parrott, P. L., Stamm, W. E., and McGowan, J. E., Jr. False-positive blood cultures: Association with nonsterile blood collection tubes. *J.A.M.A.* 236:2073, 1976.

31. Hoffman, P. C., Fraser, D. W., Robicsek, F., O'Bar, P. R., and Maundy, C. U. Two outbreaks of sternal wound infections due to organisms of the *Mycobacterium fortuitum* complex. *J. Infect. Dis.* 143:533, 1981.

32. Kaiser, A. B. Effective and creative surveillance and reporting of surgical wound infections. *Infect. Control* 3:41, 1982.

33. Kaiser, A. B., Clayson, K. R., Mulherin, J. L., Jr., Roach, A. C., Allen, T. R., Edwards, W. H., and Dale, W. A. Antibiotic prophylaxis in vascular surgery. *Ann. Surg.* 188:283, 1978.

34. Kalweit, W. H., Winn, W. C., Jr., Rocco, T. A., Jr., and Girod, J. C. Hemodialysis fistula infections caused by *Legionella pneumophila. Ann. Intern. Med.* 96:173, 1982.

35. Kaplan, E. L., Rich, H., Gersony, W., and Manning, J. A collaborative study of infective endocarditis in the 1970s: Emphasis on infections in patients who have undergone cardiovascular surgery. *Circulation* 59:327, 1979.

36. Karchmer, A. W., Archer, G. L., and Dismukes, W. E. *Staphylococcus epidermidis* causing prosthetic valve endocarditis: Microbiologic and clinical observations as guides to therapy. *Ann. Intern. Med.* 98:447, 1983.

37. Kaslow, R. A., Mackel, D. C., and Mallison, G. F. Noscomial pseudobacteremia: Positive blood cultures due to contaminated benzalkonium antiseptic. *J.A.M.A.* 236:2407, 1976.

38. Kaslow, R. A., and Zellner, S. R. Infection in patients on maintenance hemodialysis. *Lancet* 2:117, 1972.

39. Kirmani, N., Tuazon, C. U., Murray, H. W., Parrish, A. E., and Sheagren, J. N. *Staphylococcus aureus* carriage rate of patients receiving long-term hemodialysis. *Arch. Intern. Med.* 138:1657, 1978.

40. Kuritsky, J. N., Bullen, M. G., Broome, C. V., Silcox, V. A., Good, R. C., and Wallace,

R. J., Jr. Sternal wound infections and endocarditis due to organisms of the *Mycobacterium fortuitum* complex. *Ann. Intern. Med.* 98:938, 1983.

41. Lefrak, E. A., and Starr A. *Cardiac Valve Prostheses.* New York: Appleton-Century-Crofts, 1979.

42. Liekweg, W. G., Jr., and Greenfield, L. J. Vascular prosthetic infections: Collected experience and results of treatment. *Surgery* 81:335, 1977.

43. Liekweg, W. G., Jr., Levinson, S. A., and Greenfield, L. J. Infections of Vascular Grafts: Incidence, Anatomic Location, Etiologic Agents, Morbidity, and Mortality. In Duma, R. J. (Ed.), *Infections of Prosthetic Heart Valves and Vascular Grafts: Prevention, Diagnosis, and Treatment.* Baltimore: University Park Press, 1977, pp. 239–250.

44. Lord, J. W., Jr., Imperato, A. M., Hackel, A., and Doyle, E. F. Endocarditis complicating open-heart surgery. *Circulation* 23:489, 1961.

45. MacGregor, D. C., Covvey, H. D., Wilson, G. J., Schwartz, L., Scully, H. E., and Wigle, E. D. Computer-assisted reporting system for the follow-up of patients with prosthetic heart valves. *Am. J. Cardiol.* 42:444, 1978.

46. Maki, D. G. Epidemic Nosocomial Bacteremias. In Wenzel, R. P. (Ed.), *CRC Handbook of Hospital Acquired Infections.* Boca Raton, Fl.: CRC Press, 1981, pp. 462–464.

47. Maki, D., Zilz, M., Alvarado, C., Robbins, J., and Parisi, J. Methicillin-Resistant *Staph. epidermidis* Surgical Wound Infections Linked to a Chronic Carrier. In *Program and Abstracts of the Twenty-Second Interscience Conference on Antimicrobial Agents and Chemotherapy.* Washington, D.C.: American Society for Microbiology, 1982, Abstract no. 566.

48. Mayer, K. H., and Schoenbaum, S. C. Evaluation and management of prosthetic valve endocarditis. *Prog. Cardiovasc. Dis.* 25:43, 1982.

49. McLeod, R., and Remington, J. S. Postoperative Fungal Endocarditis. In Duma, R. J., (Ed.), *Infections of Prosthetic Heart Valves and Vascular Grafts: Prevention, Diagnosis, and Treatment.* Baltimore: University Park Press, 1977, pp. 163–234.

50. Onorato, I. M., Axelrod, J. L., Lorch, J. A., Brensilver, J. M., and Bokkenheuser, V. Fungal infections of dialysis fistulae. *Ann. Intern. Med.* 91:50, 1979.

51. Oyer, P. E., Miller, D. C., Stinson, E. B., Retiz, B. A., Moreno-Cabral, R. J., and Shumway, N. E. Clinical durability of the Hancock porcine bioprosthetic valve. *J. Thorac. Cardiovasc. Surg.* 80:824, 1980.

52. Quenzer, R. W., Edwards, L. D., and Levin, S. A comparative study of 48 host valve and 24 prosthetic valve endocarditis cases. *Am. Heart J.* 92:15, 1976.

53. Rosendorf, L. J., Daicoff, G., and Baer, H. Sources of gram-negative infection after open-heart surgery. *J. Thorac. Cardiovasc. Surg.* 67:195, 1974.

54. Rossiter, S. J., Stinson, E. B., Oyer, P. E., Miller, D. C., Schapira, J. N., Martin, R. P., and Shumway, N. E. Prosthetic valve endocarditis. *J. Thorac. Cardiovasc. Surg.* 76:795, 1978.

55. Sande, M. A., Johnson, W. D., Jr., Hook, E. W., and Kaye, D. Sustained bacteremia in patients with prosthetic cardiac valves. *N. Engl. J. Med.* 286:1067, 1972.

56. Scannel, J. G. (Chairman). Report of the Inter-Society Commission for Heart Disease Resources. Optimal resources for cardiac surgery: Guidelines for program planning and evaluation. *Circulation* 52:A-23, 1975.

57. Silverman, N. A., and Levitsky, S. Current choices for prosthetic valve replacement. *Mod. Concepts Cardiovasc. Dis.* 52:35, 1983.

58. Slaughter, L., Morris, J. F., and Starr, A. Prosthetic valvular endocarditis: A 12-year review. *Circulation* 47:1319, 1973.

59. Stanton, R. E., Lindesmith, G. G., and Meyer, B. W. *Escherichia coli* endocarditis after repair of ventricular septal defects. *N. Engl. J. Med.* 279:737, 1968.

60. Tilton, R. C. The laboratory approach to the detection of bacteremia. *Annu. Rev. Microbiol.* 36:467, 1982.

61. U.S. Dept. of Health and Human Services, Health Resources Administration, Hyattsville, Md. *Minimum Requirements of Construction and Equipment for Hospitals and Medical Facilities,* 1982.

62. Van Scoy, R. E. Culture-negative endocarditis. *Mayo Clin. Proc.* 57:149, 1982.

63. Von Reyn, C. F., Levy, B. S., Arbeit, R. D., Friedland, G., and Crumpacker, C. S. Infective endocarditis: An analysis based on strict case definitions. *Ann. Intern. Med.* 94(Part I):505, 1981.

64. Watanakunakorn, C. Prosthetic valve infective endocarditis. *Prog. Cardiovasc. Dis.* 22:181, 1979.

65. Weinstein, R. A., Emori, T. G., Anderson, R. L., and Stamm, W. E. Pressure transducers as a source of bacteremia after open heart surgery: Report of an outbreak and guidelines for prevention. *Chest* 69:338, 1976.

66. Willerson, J. T., Moellering, R. C., Jr., Buckley, M. J., and Austen, W. G. Conjunctival
petechiae after open-heart surgery. *N. Engl. J.
Med.* 284:539, 1971.

67. Wilson, W. R. Prosthetic Valve Endocarditis:
Incidence, Anatomic Location, Cause, Morbid-
ity, and Mortality. In Duma, R. J. (Ed.), *Infec-
tions of Prosthetic Heart Valves and Vascular Grafts:
Prevention, Diagnosis, and Treatment.* Baltimore:
University Park Press, 1977, pp. 3–13.

# 29  INFECTIONS OF SKELETAL PROSTHESES

William Petty
Jorge Franco
William F. Enneking

Plastic and metal skeletal prostheses have been used by orthopedic surgeons in the treatment of many clinical problems—principally fracture repair and partial joint replacement—for several decades. In the past decade, prostheses for replacing the hip, knee, and finger joints have been used increasingly, while surgeons and engineers continue to develop total replacement prostheses for other joints [6, 14]. Patients who have been in constant pain and unable to walk or take care of themselves can now be successfully rehabilitated by the insertion of such prosthetic devices. Unfortunately, not all these efforts are successful. The most common complication following total joint replacement is loosening of the prosthetic components. Although infection is less common than loosening, it is much more likely to lead to permanent failure of the procedure. These infection lead to compromise or loss of function of the prosthesis and occasionally have led to the death of the patient.

Since total hip replacement (THR) has been studied more extensively from the standpoint of infection than operations involving any other skeletal prosthesis, the ensuing discussion centers around this procedure and device. The principles enumerated, however, pertain to all implantable skeletal devices.

## CLASSIFICATION OF INFECTIONS

### Early (Acute) Infections
Early infections are defined as those that occur during the first postoperative month. As a general rule, all such infections should be considered to be nosocomial. Early infections are subdivided according to whether they are superficial or deep to the fascia lata.

*Suprafascial (superficial) infections,* the most common of all surgical infections in THR, possess the characteristics of incisional wound infections (see Chapter 27). Since superficial infections have a good prognosis compared to deep infections, they are omitted in the majority of reports dealing with THR complications.

*Deep wound infections* include all infections extending deep to the fascia lata. In large series, these acute infections are much less common than the late, deep infections. This difference appears to be related to increasing awareness by surgeons resulting in stricter aseptic discipline in the operating room.

### Late Infections
Late infections present after the patient has resumed painless function. Such infections are deep wound

infections that are noted months or even years after apparently successful THR, and they represent a mixture of nosocomial and community-acquired infections; information is nearly always insufficient to permit reliable differentiation.

## INCIDENCE

The incidence of surgical wound infections involving the use of skeletal prostheses varies widely in different reports. Infection rates range from approximately 6 percent in prosthetic knee replacement [9] and correction of scoliosis with Harrington instrumentation [11] to less than 1 percent in prosthetic hip replacement (Table 29-1). This variation in infection rate is not completely understood but could be related to factors such as anatomic site, selection of patients, immunologic status of the patient, experience and technique of the surgeon, and characteristics of the implant.

The rate of deep infections following total hip replacements varies among institutions, but it is recognized that the usual expected wound infection rate varies from less than 1 percent to 3 percent. Table 29-1 displays the major series of deep wound infections associated with THR reported in the literature; the composite mean wound infection rate for the entire series of published reports is 2.1 percent.

## PATHOGENS

The principle pathogenic organisms reported in a composite of publications on deep wound infections following THR are listed in Table 29-2. In practice, isolation of suspected microorganisms from an infected prosthetic hip is not always easy. In some large series of THR, the microbial cause of deep wound infection is not documented in at least 12 percent of cases [3]. Because of this problem, surgeons tend to consider the isolation of any organisms from deep tissue as conclusive evidence of infection. This situation is compounded by the fact that a normally saprophytic organism, *Staphylococcus epidermidis,* is one of the leading causes of wound infection in THR.

### Staphylococcus aureus
Coagulase-positive *S. aureus* causes about one-half of all deep infections following THR (Table 29-2). This species is seen more frequently in early than in late infections. For additional microbiologic, clinical, and epidemiologic features, the reader should refer to Chapters 27 and 31.

### Staphylococcus epidermidis
The term *coagulase-negative staphylococci* is used by most clinical laboratories to encompass all members of the family Micrococcaceae other than *S. aureus.* The majority of clinical microbiology laboratories do not dis-

TABLE 29-1. Rates of deep wound infection in total hip replacement surgery

| Authors | Country | Number of operations | Deep wound infection rate | Duration of follow-up |
|---|---|---|---|---|
| Bentley and Duthie | England | 229 | 2.3% | 1 to 4 years |
| Bergstrom, et al.[a] | Sweden | 283 | 4.9% | |
| Buchholtz and Noack | W. Germany | 3205 | 2.3% | 1 to 5 years |
| Chapchal, et al. | Netherlands | 340 | 0 | 3 months to 4 years |
| Charnley[b] | England | 5600 | 1.6% | >2 to 10 years |
| Eftekhar and Stinchfield | U.S.A. | 700 | 0.4% | 6 months to 3.5 years |
| Fitzgerald, et al. | U.S.A. | 658 | 1.1% | >18 months |
| Freeman, et al. | Scotland | 360 | 3.6% | 6 months to 6 years |
| Johnston | U.S.A. | 360 | 3.6% | — |
| Lazanski | U.S.A. | 501 | 0.8% | 6 months to 5 years |
| Leinbach and Barlow | U.S.A. | 700 | 1.0% | 6 months to 4 years |
| Moczyuski, et al.[a] | U.S.A. | 237 | 9.7% | — |
| Murray | U.S.A. | 808 | 1.5% | 3 months to 4 years |
| Nicholson | New Zealand | 1666 | 2.5% | 1 to 2 years |
| Ring | England | 887 | 0.7% | 1 to 8 years |
| Wilson, et al.[c] | U.S.A. | 436 | 9.8% | — |
| Total | | 16,970 | 2.1% | |

[a]Authors have reported a decrease in infection rate to less than 2.5 percent in their latest cases.
[b]Author has reported a decrease in infection rate to less than 1 percent in later cases.
[c]Superficial infections and deep infections were not separated.

TABLE 29-2. Bacterial etiology of deep wound infections following 17,170 total hip replacement operations

| Organism | Early infections (%) | Late infections (%) | Total (%) |
|---|---|---|---|
| Staphylococcus aureus | 58 | 39 | 50 |
| Staphylococcus epidermidis | 21 | 41 | 29 |
| Gram-negative rods | 17 | 10 | 14 |
| Others* | 4 | 5 | 7 |
| Overall | 60 | 40 | 100 |

*Includes group-D streptococci, group-A streptococci, Peptococcus, group-B streptococci, Peptostreptococcus, and anaerobic Corynebacterium.

tinguish S. epidermidis from other Micrococcaceae species; hence the relative frequency of these two groups of organisms in reported infections is not known, and potentially important clinical and epidemiologic differences remain undisclosed. We will refer to coagulase-negative staphylococci as S. epidermidis.

S. epidermidis has assumed the role of a major pathogen in implant surgery; it causes approximately 29 percent of all infections following THR (see Table 29-2), including approximately 21 percent of early acute infections, and approximately 41 percent of late infections. The true incidence of infection due to S. epidermidis is very difficult to calculate. There has been a tendency to consider its mere presence as indicating infection; therefore, the infection rate of 29 percent due to these organisms may be somewhat inflated, especially in early infections. Undoubtedly, S. epidermidis is a bona fide pathogen in late infections after THR operations; when these organisms are cultured from deep tissue, especially when cultured from several specimens, they should be considered causative agents of the infection.

### Aerobic Gram-Negative Rods
These organisms are responsible for a much smaller proportion of THR infections than other surgical wound infections (see Chapters 24 and 27). Gram-negative rods are isolated from about one-fifth of early, deep THR wound infections and from only about one-tenth of late infections (see Table 29-2).

### Anaerobes
Although anaerobic surgical wound infections are receiving increasing attention, they have seldom been reported in THR patients, and anaerobes have been infrequently recovered from wounds at the time of surgery. Evidence is increasing that the lack of reported infections with anaerobic organisms is due to a lack of proper anaerobic culture techniques; many infections previously considered "sterile" may be caused by anaerobic organisms.

## MICROBIOLOGIC DIAGNOSIS

Microbiologic findings can only be considered as supportive evidence in the diagnosis of hip infections. Clinical diagnosis clearly is of primary importance, but the identification of the pathogenic organisms involved is highly valuable, especially for choosing the appropriate antimicrobial therapy. The following points should be kept in mind when collecting specimens or interpreting the results of cultures.

### Swabs and Liquid Specimens
A superficial (skin) swab of the wound is not a suitable specimen, because in most cases it is impossible to determine whether the isolates are members of the normal skin flora or the causative agents of the infection. These swab specimens also are not adequate for the recovery of anaerobic organisms (see Chapter 7).

When pus is present, it should be aspirated with a needle and immediately taken to the laboratory. This is the best specimen (short of a tissue biopsy) for recovering both anaerobic and aerobic organisms. If possible, such a specimen should be collected before antibiotic therapy is started.

### Biopsy Specimens
When tissue from biopsy is sent to the laboratory for culture, deep tissue should be used to minimize contamination; the specimens should be handled as cautiously as possible to avoid contamination of the tissue with gloves, gown, and the like. The presence of one or two colonies in a tissue specimen must be interpreted with caution. S. epidermidis, diphtheroids, micrococci, and some streptococci are ubiquitous organisms in the surgical theatre, and airborne contamination of biopsy specimens with these organisms is a possibility.

A negative Gram stain of a tissue section is not to be interpreted as indicating the absence of infection, but it must be kept in mind that the occurrence of some granulomatous tissue may be directly related to the presence of the acrylic cement, the prosthesis itself, or both. As a part of exploratory surgery in a clinically suspected, infected hip without microbiologic evidence of infection, multiple specimens should be submitted to the laboratory, including pieces of deep tissue, cement, pseudocapsule, and so on. Recovery of the same organisms from several areas is important because such data should rule out specimen contamination.

### Specimens for Anaerobes

For the best recovery of anaerobic organisms, the laboratory must be provided with a proper specimen. All liquid specimens should be collected in syringes to maintain anaerobic conditions. Transport tubes for tissue or swabs must be oxygen-free; these tubes are commercially available under a variety of brand names. Finally, the laboratory must have appropriate anaerobic isolation and identification equipment (see Chapter 7).

## PREDISPOSING FACTORS

### Operative Factors

It has long been recognized that bacteria produce necrosis of the bone, when an infection occurs, by destroying the tenuous blood supply in the marrow spaces or haversian canals. Bacteria in this environment are relatively inaccessible to host defense mechanisms and antibiotics. Thus the presence of necrotizing organisms in bone leads to persistent infection until the necrotic sequestrated bone is spontaneously extruded or removed.

The insertion of a prosthetic device compromises the blood supply of the microenvironment around the implant. Bleeding from bone cannot be controlled in the usual surgical fashion; therefore, all skeletal implants are surrounded by a hematoma. The fact that both early and late infections of total joint replacements are often caused by organisms of low virulence has suggested that the implant materials, used because of either their chemistry or their structure, may inhibit the host ability to deal effectively with contaminating organisms. There is both in vitro and in vivo experimental data suggesting that some implant materials are more likely than others to be associated with infection because of inhibition of normal immune mechanisms [7]. The bone cement, polymethylmethacrylate, has been most strongly incriminated in this respect. The bone necrosis surrounding a total joint replacement implant is probably caused by a combination of surgical insult, heat of polymerization, and toxicity of methylmethacrylate monomer. Other implant materials, particularly the ions of some metallic alloys, may also be toxic to mammalian tissues; this may become increasingly important due to the increased surface area present in implants designed for biologic fixation (bone in-

growth) [9]. The presence of necrosis and hematoma provides favorable growth conditions for microorganisms.

THR surgery is associated with the implantation of two large foreign bodies. It has been established experimentally that fewer *S. aureus* organisms are needed to establish an infection in the presence of a foreign body (see Chapter 27).

Finally, a large wound may be exposed to contamination for a relatively long period of time (two or three hours) in technically difficult cases or in the hands of inexperienced operators.

These factors conspire to produce a high risk of infection. This risk, coupled with the serious disability from infected implants, has led to major efforts to prevent postoperative sepsis associated with these procedures [8].

### Previous Hip Surgery

A substantial portion of THR patients with infection have had previous hip operations. It is well known that the incidence of infection in refined, clean cases is lower than that in those operated on previously [13]. Approximately one-third of THR operations are now being done after the failure of other types of implants. These "idiopathic" painful hips may be due to occult infection. Despite negative preoperative cultures, the incidence of infection in THR is twice as high in such cases compared to the incidence in previously unoperated hips. Under circumstances in which the surgeon strongly suspects infection, it may be preferable to remove the device, carefully obtain culture and biopsy specimens from the wound, and close it. If subsequent studies indicate that occult infection is not present and if the wound is well healed, subsequent THR might be contemplated with relative safety. Others prefer to rely on Gram-stained smears, frozen sections, and gross inspection to reach an intraoperative decision; the validity of these methods in determining whether or not infection is present has not been firmly established.

When clinically obvious, occult deep infection compromises a previous implant, the safest management is implant removal, wound drainage or suction irrigation, appropriate antibiotic treatment, and a delay of a few weeks to many months with no signs of inflammation before undertaking a repeat THR. Some advocate implant excision, radical debridement, antibiotic lavage, and THR with massive antibiotic treatment. THR after a short delay or immediate exchange of infected implant for a replacement implant is more likely to be successful with gram-positive organisms. Immediate or early THR following the diagnosis of infection with gram-negative organisms has a high likelihood of failure, and even after a significant period of apparent quiescence of infection, infections with gram-negative organisms are more likely to be associated with recurrent infection when a new prosthesis is implanted.

### Other Factors

Another factor that may contribute to infection is obesity. Conclusive data are not available, but circumstantial evidence points out that obese patients are more prone than nonobese patients to development of superficial wound infections. This difference appears to be related to the heavy retraction required on the subcutaneous tissue, which leads to necrosis and difficulty in closing the subcutaneous space in obese patients.

A large number of patients receive steroid therapy for rheumatoid arthritis. It has been shown by Charnley [3] as well as others that these patients are at a higher risk of infection than other candidates for total joint replacement.

## GENERAL CONTROL MEASURES

Orthopedic surgeons involved in THR operations have gone to great lengths in an attempt to control surgical wound infections. The pioneers in THR experienced an initial infection rate of 8 to 10 percent. As noted in Table 29-1, the infection rate has decreased in the last decade to approximately 2 percent. Although some surgeons have emphasized antibiotic prophylaxis, others are advocates of "clean-room" surgery employing either a unidirectional airflow system (UAFS) or the use of ultraviolet (UV) lights. In all the series reported in Table 29-1, prophylactic systemic antibiotics, clean-air rooms, or both were used except in those of Chapchal and associates [10], Nicholson [21], and Bucholtz and Noack [21]. The last authors used gentamicin mixed with the methylmethacrylate.

### Surgical Techniques

An awareness of the infection problem in THR has led to the "rediscovery" of strict discipline in the operating room, with emphasis on meticulous aseptic surgery, double gloving, double masking, and the use of hoods and body-exhaust systems that employ relatively impermeable gowns. Such techniques have been accepted as routine procedure in THR surgery. Preparation of the skin before surgery is done meticulously because of the closeness of the surgical area to the perineum. Proper draping of the incision is

important to avoid endogenous contamination. The use of self-sealing plastic drapes about the perineum has been of particular help in decreasing wound contamination with perineal flora.

### Clean-Air Room System

The "clean-air" room has become popular among orthopedic surgeons, mainly because of the enthusiastic support of Charnley [3], Nelson [15], and others. The clean-air room usually has a unidirectional airflow system installed in a plexiglass or glass enclosure to which only the surgical personnel are allowed access. In many clean-air systems, the surgeons and supportive personnel inside the enclosure also wear body-exhaust suits. Airflow systems of two major types are available: horizontal and vertical. When horizontal airflow systems are used, great care must be taken in setting up the operating room to avoid having bacteria forced into the area of the wound when personnel or other obstructions get between the source of airflow and the operative site. It was demonstrated in one study that the infection rate is increased with the use of horizontal airflow systems if this principle is ignored [20]. For similar reasons, body-exhaust suits must be used with vertical airflow systems.

UAFS equipment is capable of delivering a high volume of unidirectional air that has been filtered by high-efficiency particulate air (HEPA) filters capable of removing more than 99 percent of particles greater than $3\mu$ in size. This equipment provides an air volume sufficient to exchange the air of a room at a rate of up to 300 changes of room air per hour (Fig. 29-1).

Body-exhaust suits consist of a helmet attached to a vacuum pump that is capable of sucking out all the expired air of the surgeon, thus controlling the microbial fallout from the head, neck, and other body surfaces of the surgeon.

The surgical enclosure unit usually consists of a series of transparent panels with dimensions of up to 10 by 20 feet. In addition to providing particulate-free air, the enclosure ensures restriction of traffic around the operating table. Furthermore, the body-exhaust suits impose both discipline and close surgical teamwork. Many consider these side benefits as significant as the "clean" air, but feel they can be achieved without the inconvenience and expense of the system. The efficacy of such systems in reducing airborne particulate and microbial contamination at the periphery of the wound has been established in many studies. There is now strong evidence in a well-controlled study that this reduction in contamination

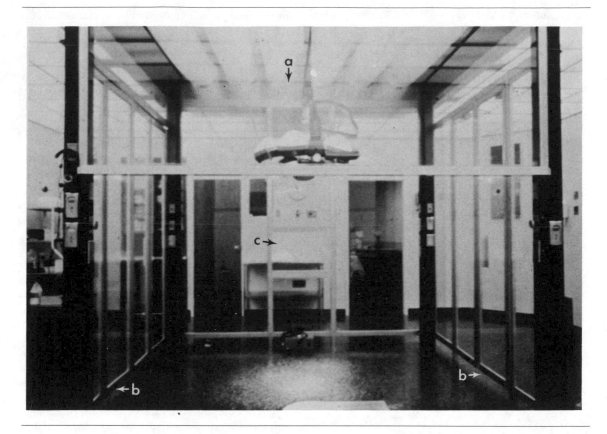

FIG. 29-1. A vertical unidirectional airflow system. Air enters from the ceiling of the enclosure through HEPA filters and flows downward (a) to exit beneath the enclosing walls (b). A pass-through window (c) serves for instrument exchange. The opening for the patient in the foreground is sealed by a plastic drape that leaves the patient's head and neck and anesthesia personnel outside the enclosure.

results in a significant reduction of wound infection rate in total joint replacement operative procedures [10].

The question of whether or not a clean-air system is really a necessity in controlling sepsis in THR cannot be answered in absolute terms. It would appear that the wound infection rates under optimal conventional surgical conditions with thoughtful antibiotic therapy and proper patient selection are approximately the same as they are when the surgical conditions are modestly improved with clean-air systems without antibiotics. Whether to use a clean room seems to require a judgment based on local conditions, rather than a decision based on a universal rule.

*Prophylactic Antibiotic Therapy*

A national survey showed that 87 percent of orthopedic surgeons used antibiotic prophylaxis in total joint replacements [16]. This figure is not surprising, because the use of prophylactic antibiotics in THR has been widely advocated. Numerous studies strongly suggest a decrease in deep infection rates with ap-

propriate use of perioperative antibiotics. Such antibiotic use is especially important when "clean-air" systems are not available or cannot be used to maximum efficiency. The literature abounds with reports of undesirable side effects following the use of prophylactic antibiotics, the emergence of antibiotic-resistant organisms, alteration of the normal flora, allergic side effects, and so on, and the surgeon must be aware that the routine use of prophylactic antibiotics in the absence of a "real" indication may be more dangerous to the patient than beneficial (see Chapter 11). These disadvantages of the use of prophylactic antibiotics may be largely obviated by avoiding extended administration of the antibiotic.

The timing of the dosage is critical. It has been

established both clinically and experimentally that if optimal results are to be expected from prophylactic antibiotics, the antibiotic concentration in the tissues must be high at the time of surgery (when inoculation with organisms occurs) or very shortly thereafter. Prophylactic antibiotics should be administered parenterally, at the time of anesthetic induction. In patients who are allergic to penicillins and/or cephalosporins, vancomycin is an excellent choice. There is no clinical evidence supporting the use of prolonged prophylactic antibiotics in THR, however, and experimental evidence indicates that prolonged treatment is unnecessary [1, 3]. Most authorities agree that under most circumstances administration of prophylactic antibiotics beyond 48 to 72 hours postoperatively is probably neither necessary nor beneficial.

As previously mentioned, *S. aureus* is the leading cause of infection in THR surgery. If prophylactic antibiotics are to be used to prevent *S. aureus* infection, a semisynthetic, penicillinase-resistant penicillin (e.g., methicillin) or cephalosporin should be given. Cephalosporins have been used increasingly for prophylaxis in total joint replacement surgery; cefazolin should be considered the agent of choice. Although the second- and third-generation cephalosporin agents are often used, their efficacy against the staphylococci that most commonly cause infections after total joint replacement is not as good as that of the first-generation cephalosporin agents.

## EARLY DEEP WOUND INFECTIONS

### Clinical Features

MANIFESTATIONS AND MANAGEMENT  The prompt clinical diagnosis of postoperative wound infections following THR surgery is very important because the earlier the treatment is started, the better the chances are of salvaging the prosthesis.

Acute deep infections present two to five days following surgery and are associated with fever, leukocytosis, and red-hot inflammation. Frequently, pus drains from the wound. Such infected patients should initially be treated vigorously with high doses of the appropriate antibiotics and incision and drainage of the wound. In most instances, subsequent removal of the device is required to achieve closure of the draining sinuses. As long as such preliminary steps contain the infection, the removal of the prosthesis should be delayed until it is certain that removal is inevitable. This state is manifested by recurrent dislocation, gross loosening of the device, or continued

drainage. Once it is clearly established that an early acute infection is superficial in the fascia lata, it must be decompressed to prevent deep extension. These infections cause little systemic toxicity, and when evacuated show no deep communication with the device. Should drainage persist an unusual length of time, communication must be sought by fluoroscopy and contrast roentgenographic study.

ANTIBIOTIC THERAPY  Therapy should be directed toward the organisms involved and should be based on the antibiogram of the pathogenic organisms. If an infection is suspected and the culture results are not available, antibiotic treatment should be started immediately to prevent the involvement of the prosthesis. *S. aureus* is responsible for about 60 percent of these infections (see Table 29-2); therefore, an antistaphylococcal drug such as methicillin or a cephalosporin is the antibiotic of choice. *S. epidermidis* causes about 20 percent of acute deep infections, and methicillin will effectively treat sensitive strains. Resistance of *S. epidermidis* to methicillin and similar penicillins is frequently found in some hospitals, however, and a cephalosporin antibiotic, rather than methicillin, might be chosen for initial therapy in these circumstances (see Chapter 28). An aminoglycoside antibiotic should be given in addition, because about 17 percent of acute infections are caused by gram-negative organisms (see Table 29-2). As soon as the laboratory results are available, the antibiotic therapy should be adjusted according to the type of organisms found. Serum bactericidal levels against the specific organism causing the infection may be helpful, especially when dealing with infections caused by gram-negative organisms.

In most hospitals in the United States, methicillin-resistant strains of *S. aureus* are uncommon. In England and Germany, however, there are increasing problems with methicillin-resistant *S. aureus,* which points out the importance of performing adequate antibiotic susceptibility tests (see Chapter 11). If an antibiotic must be chosen in the absence of susceptibility testing, the physician should use antibiotics that are most effective against the organisms that have been isolated from acute deep infections in the hospital. Updated information regarding susceptibility patterns of organisms in the hospital should be routinely available through the clinical microbiology laboratory or the hospital epidemiologist (see Chapter 7).

### Sources and Modes of Acquisition

The sources and modes of acquisition of organisms that produce surgical wound infections are systematically described in Chapter 27. Only features especially pertinent to infected THR prostheses are described in the following section.

GLOVE PUNCTURES   Direct contact spread by hands of personnel may play a role. Puncture holes in the surgical gloves at the time of surgery are a common finding, especially in orthopedic surgery, in which surgeons handle hammers, saws, power tools, sharp wires, and the like (see Chapter 27). It has been shown by Wise and colleagues [23] that up to 1.8 $\times$ 10$^5$ organisms can be cultured from inside the gloves after a surgical procedure. Ninety-eight percent of the gloves cultured were positive for microorganisms, and fourteen percent of them were positive for S. aureus; the implication of this study is simply that when gloves are punctured during surgery by a surgeon who is a heavy carrier of S. aureus, the wound may be inoculated with a sufficiently large number of organisms to cause wound infection.

POSTOPERATIVE HAND TRANSMISSION   Transmission from the hands of personnel after surgery (e.g., in wards or intensive care units) is a more controversial subject. It is doubtful that it plays a significant role in THR patients because the wound is covered at the time of surgery and the dressings are not usually removed for several days, allowing sufficient time for the skin to seal. The opportunity for infection to enter from the "outside" appears to be remote.

STAPHYLOCOCCUS AUREUS SHEDDERS   S. aureus resides in the skin as well as in the anterior nares of many of the surgical personnel and patients. Desquamated skin loaded with S. aureus is released in the air and can settle into the open wound. It is conceivable that these organisms may cause a wound infection in this type of high-risk procedure. It has been our experience that when personnel demonstrated to be "shedders" are present on a surgical team that is using clean-room techniques, S. aureus has not been recovered from the air, and no S. aureus infections attributable to such shedders have developed.

AIRBORNE SPREAD   Airborne spread from sources other than the patient and surgical personnel that leads to wound contamination and infection does not appear to be an important component in the epidemiology of early deep surgical wound infections. Filtration of the air and improved air-conditioning systems have controlled the spread of organisms from the outside as well as from adjacent wards.

ENDOGENOUS SOURCES   These are clearly a source of infection in many surgical wounds, and skeletal implants are no exception. The number of infections of endogenous origin, compared to other sources of contamination, has not been clearly established. It is highly probable that some of the acute implant infections and a larger proportion of the late infections are endogenous.

### Prevention

CLEAN-ROOM SYSTEM   Clearly, an institution with a high acute infection rate, in which surgical conditions are less than optimal and drug-resistant organisms are prevalent, would do well to consider seriously the use of a "clean room." The system does not make up for poor surgical technique any more than antibiotics do. Of necessity, however, it does impose a discipline on personnel who, in many hospitals, are not within the direct control of the surgeon. If a clean room is unavailable, infection rates can be reduced by the use of strict operating-room and surgical techniques; this may be combined with appropriately selected and administered prophylactic antibiotics.

INVESTIGATION AND ATTACK OF CAUSES   When the infection rate is above the expected range of 1 to 3 percent, the situation deserves a thoughtful approach. A blind rush to institute control measures should be avoided. Rather, attempts first should be made to find out why the infection rate is high. The first steps are to review the surgical techniques and conduct epidemiologic studies of the infections (see Chapters 5 and 27).

Carriers (i.e., shedders) that disseminate S. aureus into the environment may be responsible for surgical infections, but a carrier on the surgical team should not necessarily be considered a dangerous source of staphylococcal infections. If staphylococcal strains from a carrier have the same characteristics, including antibiograms, as those recovered from infected wounds, however, this should be sufficient to incriminate the carrier presumptively as a dangerous shedder (see Chapters 1 and 31). Epidemiologic incrimination of such a carrier requires the demonstration of a significantly higher risk of infection with the "epidemic strain" among patients whose THR operations are attended by the carrier than among patients whose THR procedures are not attended by the carrier. Such carriers should be managed as indicated in Chapter 27.

If surgical personnel are the sources of sporadic S. aureus infections, special efforts—such as the use of

UAFS, body-exhaust suits, and impermeable gowns—may be employed to minimize shedding. If the strains are usually traced to the patients (i.e., are endogenous), the method of preparation of the surgical area before surgery should be reviewed, and antibiotic prophylaxis should be considered.

## LATE DEEP WOUND INFECTIONS

### Clinical Features

MANIFESTATIONS It is necessary to emphasize the importance of the supplementary use of acrylics in implant fixation and its relation to late deep wound infections. The acrylic is used as a "cement" to fix the prosthesis to the bone. Loosening of the prosthesis is one of the universal symptoms of late infections. A few bacteria causing bone resorption at the interface between the bone and the acrylic are sufficient to cause surgical failure. S. epidermidis is of special importance in this respect, since it is a very frequent contaminant in surgical wounds. Even though these organisms are considered to be of relatively low virulence, they are capable of causing bone resorption with subsequent loosening of the prosthesis. S. epidermidis is about twice as frequent in late infections as in early infections, and it slightly surpasses S. aureus as a cause of late deep infections (41 percent versus 39 percent, respectively; see Table 29-2). Gram-negative bacilli are less commonly associated with late infections.

Late deep wound infections present months or years after surgery. Due to their usually insidious nature, a high index of suspicion is necessary to establish the diagnosis at the earliest possible time. Early warnings are continuous pain in the hip area and a slightly elevated erythrocyte sedimentation rate (ESR). Fever and leukocytosis are usually absent. The first sign suggestive of the presence of late infections is loosening of the prosthesis, which is usually detected roentgenographically. Periosteal new bone formation about the femoral stem–acrylic complex is usually associated with loosening, and this may be the initial sign of deep occult infection. Mechanical loosening of the prosthesis can also occur as a late complication in the absence of infection, and its appearance on roentgenograms is similar to that of "infective" loosening.

All late infections are not insidious, and some present with the typical characteristics of acute deep wound infections, that is, fever, leukocytosis, abscess formation with or without sinus tracts, inflammation, and so on.

MANAGEMENT In general, late deep wound infections resolve only after the prosthesis is removed. In a few instances, hip function may be salvaged by the removal of the loose device, debridement of the surrounding infected tissue, suction, irrigation, and the administration of antibiotics. Led by Bucholtz [21] in West Germany, many surgeons recommend the insertion of a new prosthesis using antibiotics (e.g., gentamicin) mixed with the methylmethacrylate. There are insufficient data at the present time to determine the true efficacy of this approach. Experimental studies [22] have shown that the activity of gentamicin incorporated in methylmethacrylate is detectable for .more than 70 weeks. Additional research in this area is needed to determine the usefulness of such an approach for the treatment and prevention of infection following THR surgery.

ANTIBIOTIC THERAPY Antibiotic treatment in patients with infections of insidious onset can be postponed until the identification of the microorganisms and their antibiotic sensitivity patterns are established. This postponement is possible because by the time the infection is diagnosed, extensive involvement is present. When the culture reports are negative and a clinical diagnosis of infection is strongly suspected, the following factors should be taken into consideration in choosing an antibiotic: late infections are almost always (about 80 percent) due to staphylococci, either S. aureus or S. epidermidis; negative culture results may be obtained because of a failure to isolate strict anaerobic organisms; Gram stains have been known to be positive, and wound cultures, negative. In such cases, guidance in choosing appropriate antibiotics may be provided by the morphology and staining characteristics of the organisms.

In summary, an antistaphylococcal agent will usually be the drug of choice; preferably, one may be used that will be adequate for coagulase-negative staphylococci (see earlier comments about therapy of early infections). When anaerobes are suspected, clindamycin seems to be a good choice, and S. aureus and S. epidermidis may also be susceptible to this drug. The choice of therapy for S. epidermidis infection should depend, whenever possible, on the antibiogram of the isolated pathogen. Choosing an antibiotic in the absence of laboratory results is difficult, because S. epidermidis strains vary greatly in terms of their antibiotic susceptibility patterns.

### Diagnostic Considerations

The following systematic approach is useful in evaluating the presence of latent deep infection about a skeletal prosthesis in a patient with a history of continuous pain accompanied by an elevated ESR.

ROENTGENOGRAPHY Roentgenograms should be evaluated to determine whether or not the following indications of infection are present. Loosening of the prosthesis is a common sign, but it is not diagnostic of infection. This diagnosis may require both fluoroscopy and arthrography. The arthrograms are performed to find out whether or not the injected dye can be seen in the interface between the acrylic cement and the bone; this test is sometimes positive even when the roentgenograms show no apparent loosening (Fig. 29-2). Arthrograms are also valuable to visualize abscess cavities and to determine whether sinus tracts communicate with the prosthesis. Periosteal reactive bone formation is another common finding in infection. Bone resorption about the cement, if present, will facilitate the diagnosis of osteomyelitis, and it is the most reliable roentgenographic sign of infection about a prosthesis (see Fig. 29-2).

JOINT ASPIRATION The aspiration of a prosthetic hip joint to obtain material for microbiologic examination is technically difficult but is of critical importance in evaluation of the patient with suspected infection associated with total joint replacement. Because the pseudocapsule must be entered with the needle, an arthrogram may be needed to determine the position of the needle.

RADIONUCLIDE SCINTIMETRY The use of this technique has been suggested in the diagnosis of hip infections. Scintimetric results may be positive in the absence of positive roentgenographic findings. Scintimetry may also occasionally sharply delineate whether the acetabular component, the femoral component, or both are involved. Care should be taken in the interpretation of bone scintimetric results, however, because high scintimetric values may be due to periarticular bone formation rather than infection. Loosening of the prosthetic components, which is much more common than infection, will also be associated with increased uptake of radionuclides. Several investigators have suggested that the gallium scan can be effectively used in differentiating septic from aseptic component loosening. However, the efficacy of this technique has recently been questioned [4]. An even newer technique being used experimentally that may show more promise in differentiating between septic and aseptic loosening of components is radionuclide scanning of indium-labeled white blood cells [12].

BIOPSY OF THE CAPSULE Frequently the definitive diagnosis of infection requires examination of a biopsy specimen from the capsule. Biopsy specimens are usually obtained as part of the surgical procedure to remove the prosthetic device when it must be removed because of loosening. The material obtained should be from the deep tissue or bone to minimize contamination. The material should be sent for microbiologic culture and histologic examination (see previous section Microbiologic Diagnosis). It is important to realize that chronic granulation of tissue may normally be found about the prosthesis. This lining tissue is covered by a fibrinous membrane, and by itself is not a diagnostic sign of an infective process.

### Sources and Modes of Acquisition

The sources of organisms that cause late infections are puzzling. It was felt previously that they were acquired at the time of surgery and remained dormant until the infection was detected. Alternatively, the organisms may be seeded into the area via the bloodstream from distant focuses; for example, brushing the teeth may cause transient bacteremias.

Charnley [3] and Ericson and associates [4] have shown a reduction in the incidence of late infections when control measures were instituted in the surgical theatre. Their results suggest that at least a portion of the late infections are acquired at the time of surgery. Additional evidence against a principal role for endogenous sources of late infections may be provided by the profile of causative agents, since this profile differs markedly from that of naturally occurring bacterial endocarditis (mainly viridans streptococci), and the latter infections clearly derive from bacteremic "seeding."

There are convincing reports in the literature of infections of total joint replacements following infection elsewhere in the body. These may be infections with either gram-positive or gram-negative organisms; several deep gram-negative infections have been reported following infections of the urinary tract with the same organism. There is not enough evidence at this time to determine whether late infections are due most often to surgical contamination or to late hematogenous spread. It seems clear, however, that endogenous sources and acquisition by direct and indirect contact at the time of surgery are each responsible for some infections.

Regarding endogenous infection, it is worth pointing out that many patients become colonized with *S. aureus* after admission. This colonization may be the source of a subsequent "endogenous" infection. Persistent colonization may be important because a

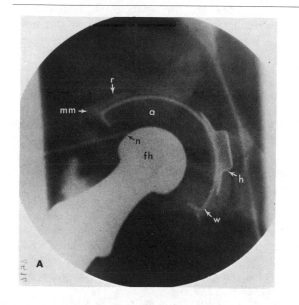
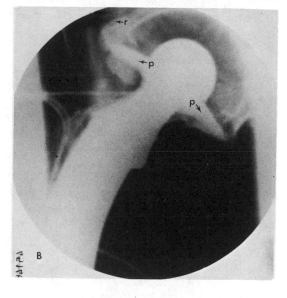

FIG. 29-2. Arthrogram of 67-year-old patient who had pain for 2 months following 14 months of pain-free function. After THR, there were no systemic or laboratory manifestations of infection. Cultures obtained during the procedure showed no growth.

A. An AP view of the prosthesis. The tip of the needle (*n*) is in the articulation of the metallic prosthetic femoral head (*fh*) and the radiolucent polyethylene acetabular component (*a*). The methylmethacrylate used to bond the polyethylene socket to the adjacent bone is made radiodense by adding barium to it (*mm*). The circular wire (*w*) marks the junction between the plastic socket and the bonding methylmethacrylate. The wire "hat" (*h*) restrains methylmethacrylate from entering the pelvis. There is a distinct line of bone resorption (*r*) between the bone-methylmethacrylate interface that suggests loosening.

B. After aspiration, an injection of opaque dye outlines the cavity about the prosthetic joint (*p*). Dye can be seen in the zone of resorption (*r*), which positively indicates loosening of the prosthesis and is highly suggestive of indolent infection. Culture of the aspirant yielded coagulase-negative staphylococci.

number of THR patients require bilateral hip replacements involving one or two periods of hospitalization.

### Prevention

Prevention of infections with *S. epidermidis,* the most common cause of late infections, appears to be a very difficult task because of the large numbers of *S. epidermidis* organisms in the environment. The number of *S. epidermidis* organisms needed to establish a wound infection in a system including acrylics, polyethylene, metal, and bone is not known. If a large inoculum is needed to initiate an infection (more than 100 organisms), then preventive measures such as clean-air systems (e.g., UAFS) may be helpful in reducing the number of organisms settling in the wound during THR operations (with UAFS, it is calculated that less than five microorganisms per hour settle in a wound).

The use of prophylactic antibiotics to reduce the likelihood of endogenous contamination may be important if there is a significantly large number of endogenous infections. Prophylactic antibiotic administration for THR patients undergoing procedures likely to result in transient bacteremia might well be justified, and a controlled study of the effectiveness of this approach might provide additional insights into the relative importance of endogenous sources.

For infections that are acquired at the time of surgery, remain dormant, and subsequently cause late wound infection, all the preventive measures described previously for the prevention of early infections should be used. "Clean" rooms, prophylactic antibiotics, or both at the time of surgery should be useful in the prevention of such infections.

### REFERENCES

1. Bowers, W. H., Wilson, F. C., and Green, W. B. Antibiotic prophylaxis in experimental bone infections. *J. Bone Joint Surg. (Am.)* 55:795, 1973.

2. Burke, J. F. The effective period of preventative antibiotic action in experimental incision and dermal lesions. *Surgery* 50:161, 1961.
3. Charnley, J. Postoperative infections after total hip replacement with special reference to air contamination in the operating room. *Clin. Orthop.* 87:162, 1972.
4. Collie, L. P., Fitzgerald, R. H., and Brown, M. L. *In Vivo Localization of Technetium and Gallium Radionuclides in Infected Bone.* Transactions of the Twenty-Ninth Annual Meeting of the Orthopedic Research Society, 1983, p. 301.
5. Ericson, C., Lidgren, L., and Lindberg, L. Cloxacillin in the prophylaxis of postoperative infections of the hip. *J. Bone Joint Surg. (Am.)* 55:808, 1973.
6. Ewald, F. C., Scheinberg, R. D., Pow, R., Thomas, W. H., Scott, R. D., and Sledge, C. B. Capitellocondylar total elbow arthroplasty. *J. Bone Joint Surg.* 62-A:1259, 1980.
7. Fitzgerald, R. H., Jr., Peterson, I. F. A., Washington, J. A., II, Van Scoy, R. E., and Coventry, M. C. Bacterial colonization of wounds and sepsis in total hip arthroplasties. *J. Bone Joint Surg. (Am.)* 55:1242, 1973.
8. Hill, C., Flamant, L., Mazar, F., and Evrard, J. Prophylactic cefazolin versus placebo in total hip replacement: Report of a multicenter double-blind randomized trial. *Lancet* 1:795, 1981.
9. Kettlekamp, D. B., and Leach, R. B. Total knee replacement. *Clin. Orthop.* 94:2, 1973.
10. Lidwell, O. M., Lowbury, E. J. L., Whyte, W., Blowers, R., Stanley, S. J., and Lowe, D. Effect of ultraclean air in operating rooms on deep sepsis in the joint after total hip or knee replacement: A randomized study. *Br. Med. J.* 285:10, 1982.
11. Lonstein, J., Winter, R., Moe, J., and Gaines, D. Wound infection with Harrington instrumentation and spine fusion for scoliosis. *Clin. Orthop.* 96:222, 1973.
12. Merkel, K. D., Fitzgerald, R. H., Jr., Brown, M. L., and Dewanjel, M. K. *Comparison of Indium-WBC and Sequential Technetium-Gallium Imaging in Suspected Low-Grade Osteomyelitis.* Transactions of the Twenty-Ninth Annual Meeting of the Orthopedic Research Society, 1983, p. 204.
13. National Academy of Sciences, National Research Council. Postoperative wound infections: The influence of ultraviolet irradiation of the operating room and of various other factors. *Ann. Surg.* 160(Suppl.):1, 1964.
14. Neer, C. S., II, Watson, K. C., and Stanton, F. J. Recent experience in total shoulder replacement. *J. Bone Joint Surg.* 64-A:319, 1982.
15. Nelson, J. P. The operating room environment and its influence on deep wound infections. In *The Hip: Proceedings of The Fifth Open Scientific Meeting of The Hip Society.* St. Louis: Mosby, 1977, p. 129.
16. Operating-Room Survey. Operating-room survey finds most orthopaedic surgeons use antibiotics regularly. *Orthop. Rev.* 3:156, 1974.
17. Petty, R. W. The effect of methylmethacrylate on phagocytosis and bacterial killing by human polymorphonuclear leucocytes. *J. Bone Joint Surg.* 60-A:752, 1978.
18. Petty, R. W., and Goldsmith, S. Resection arthroplasty following infected total hip arthroplasty. *J. Bone Joint Surg.* 62-A:889, 1980.
19. Petty, R. W., Spanier, S., and Silverthorne, C. *Influence of Skeletal Implant Materials on Infection.* Transactions of the Twenty-Ninth Annual Meeting of the Orthopedic Research Society, 1983, p. 137.
20. Salvati, E. A., Robinson, R. P., Zeno, S. M., Koslin, B. L., Brown, B. D., and Wilson, P. D., Jr. Infection rates after 3175 total hip and total knee replacements performed with and without a horizontal unidirectional filtered airflow system. *J. Bone Joint Surg.* 64-A:525, 1982.
21. Stinchfield, F. E. Statistics on total hip replacement. *Clin. Orthop.* 95:2, 1973.
22. Wahlig, H., Hameister, W., and Grieben, A. Uber die freisetzung von gentamycin aus polymethylmethacrylat. I. Experimentelle untersuchungen in vitro. *Langenbecks Arth. Chir.* 331:169, 1972.
23. Wise, R. I., Sweeney, F. J., Jr., Haupt, G. J., and Waddell, M. A. The environmental distribution of *Staphylococcus aureus* in an operation suite. *Ann. Surg.* 149:30, 1958.

# 30 INFECTIONS OF BURN WOUNDS

Bruce G. MacMillan
Ian Alan Holder
J. Wesley Alexander

Nosocomial infections have been more prevalent following major burns than perhaps any other condition in medicine. From the earliest recordings concerning this type of injury, infection has been the leading cause of death. Even now, the development of life-threatening nosocomial infection remains the major obstacle to successful therapy, despite recent improvements in care that have led to opportunity for survival for some patients with 90 percent burns or even greater.

## NATURE OF INFECTIONS

It is sometimes difficult to determine the presence and degree of infection in burn wounds, since they are invariably contaminated with microbes. This problem has led to the establishment of several guidelines for more exacting evaluation, but all fall short of their intended goal. To compound the problem, multiple organisms are often involved in infections of the burn wound, and it is not rare to find two or more organisms associated with septicemia or other types of invasive infection.

### Incidence

The incidence of serious infections in the burned patient varies with the size of the burn. With current methods of topical chemotherapy, serious infections are not expected in otherwise healthy patients with burns involving less than 30 percent of the total body surface area. A progressive increase in the incidence of serious infection, however, is seen as the size of the burn increases, necessitating constant vigilance and repeated evaluation. The extent of the problem is shown in Figure 30-1, which is constructed from admission data from the University of Cincinnati Hospital Burn and Trauma Unit and the Cincinnati Shriners Hospital during the period 1964 to 1982. These admissions are broken into one four-year and three five-year periods to emphasize the improvement in prevention of infectious complications during this period. The data shown involve only patients with 30 to 90 percent burns who survived for at least five days after admission. Overall mortality caused by infection in these patients dropped from 26 percent in the 1964–67 period to 12 percent in the 1978–82 period, and the rate of nonseptic deaths dropped from 15 percent in the earlier period to 6 percent in the

Supported in part by the Cincinnati Shriners Burns Institute and USPHS Grant 5-P01-GM 15428-06.

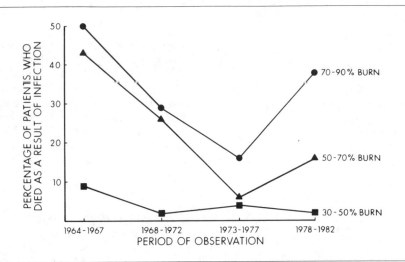

FIG. 30-1. Deaths caused by infection in a major burn unit. There is a clear association with the size of the burn injury (see text).

later period. The rates of change for these two sets of patients are almost equal (56 and 60 percent, respectively). Of all the patients who died between 1964 and 1967 with burns of greater than 30 percent, 64 percent died of infections, while in the period 1978 to 1982, 66 percent died with infection. The fact that nearly two-thirds of all patients with burns of greater than 30 percent who die following burn injury die as a result of infection underscores the complexity and seriousness of the continuing problem.

Septic problems were even worse in the preceding decade. In a review of 1049 patients treated at the U. S. Army Surgical Research Unit between January 1953 and December 1962, there were 228 deaths that occurred after the first five days following admission, and 184 (80.7 percent) were caused by septicemia [20].

The important relationship of the age of the patient and the size of the burn to the risk of infection has been emphasized by many authors and was especially well documented by Thomsen [29]. Suffice it to say that the incidence of infection increases with age (dramatically so in patients over the age of 60) and with size of burn (infection affects nearly all patients with more than 40 percent burns).

*Pathogens*

Nowhere in medicine and surgery has the changing parade of pathogens been more evident than in burns (Fig. 30-2). Before the availability of penicillin and the sulfonamides, hemolytic *Streptococcus pyogenes* was the pathogen most frequently recognized. The clinical course of such infections was often dramatic; an invasive streptococcal cellulitis would spread rapidly to become a fulminating infection with generalized toxicity, and early death of the patient would ensue. In 1933, Aldrich [1] reported that all severe burns at the Johns Hopkins Hospital were colonized with streptococci within the first day. In 1935, Cruickshank [8] noted that two-thirds of patients in a hospital in Glasgow had hemolytic streptococci on their wounds three to six days after admission and in 1941, from the same institution, an incidence of 83 percent acquisition of hemolytic streptococci was found within a few days of admission. By 1945, however, Colebrook and Lond [7] noted that significant group-A streptococcal infections had been almost eliminated by the use of penicillin.

By 1943 both *Staphylococcus aureus* and gram-negative bacteria were coming into prominence as causes of burn-wound infection, when Meleney [18] reported bacteriologic studies from 347 burns associated with military injuries early in World War II. Hemolytic streptococci were very frequent in the wounds, but he noted that staphylococci were the most numerous of the pathogens in persistent infections, and the gram-negative aerobic bacilli were close behind. Many of those patients were treated with local or systemic sulfonamides. During the 1950s *S. aureus* emerged as the predominant organism, and in the study of Moncrief and Teplitz [20] *S. aureus* was recovered from the blood in 75 percent of patients who died of septicemia in 1954. By the early 1960s, however, *Pseudomonas aeruginosa* had surpassed *S. aureus* in frequency. Many advances in the control of *P. aeruginosa* resulted in a sharp decline in the rate of

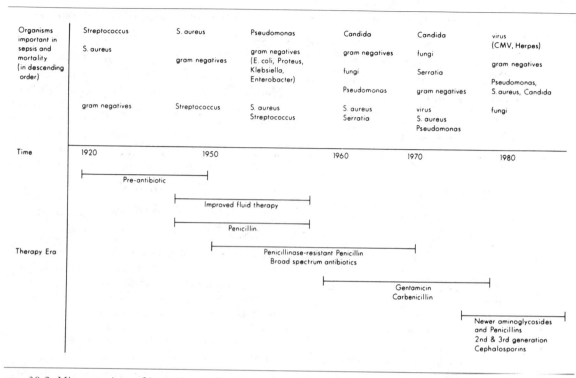

FIG. 30-2. Microorganisms of importance in burn infections: changing patterns with time.

fatal infections, but it still continues to be an important pathogen.

Data collected by the National Nosocomial Infection Study for the years 1980–82 reveal that gram-negative microorganisms are recovered from burns most frequently, with gram-positive microorganisms a close second (Table 30-1). Fungi and anaerobes constitute only a small percentage of total microorganisms isolated. The breakdown of these organisms by genera is presented in Table 30-2. *S. aureus* and *P. aeruginosa* are the most frequently isolated gram-positive and gram-negative organisms. Enterococci constitute another major group of gram-positive isolates, while gram-negative microorganisms—*Escherichia coli, Enterobacter cloacae, Serratia marcescens,* and *Klebsiella* species—are also important in burn infections. *Candida albicans,* other *Candida* species, and other fungi account for a small percentage of potentially dangerous burn infections. Of more recent concern has been an increase in the number of infections resulting from a variety of viruses. Currently it would seem that virtually any organism can become a lethal pathogen in the seriously burned patient.

The changing pattern of flora in the burn wound often reflects changing methods of therapy more than any other factor, and although the ecology of the burn-wound flora can be altered by therapy, the burn wound cannot be sterilized. All too often, the administration of antimicrobial agents merely provides an environmental pressure for a change in the burn-wound flora to more resistant organisms. To complicate the picture additionally, there is ample evidence that depression of numerous immune resistance factors in seriously burned patients contributes in a major way to both proliferation of microbes on the burn wound and their systemic invasion.

The incidence of recovery of significant pathogens at the Cincinnati Shriners Burns Institute from 1978–82 is shown in Figures 30-3 and 30-4. The relative incidence of pathogens may vary remarkably among institutions because of differences in therapy and institutional microbial ecology, which are often

TABLE 30-1. Distribution of groups of microorganisms recovered from infected burns

| Group | Percentage of total |
|---|---|
| Gram-negative organisms | 51.8 |
| Gram-positive organisms | 42.6 |
| Fungi | 4.4 |
| Anaerobes | 1.0 |

From the National Nosocomial Infection Study, 1980–82.

TABLE 30-2. Distribution of 648 microorganisms recovered from infected burns

| Organisms | Number recovered | Percentage of total |
|---|---|---|
| *Staphylococcus aureus* | 157 | 24.2 |
| *Pseudomonas aeruginosa* | 135 | 20.8 |
| Enterococci | 76 | 11.7 |
| *Escherichia coli* | 50 | 7.7 |
| *Enterobacter cloacae* | 50 | 7.7 |
| *Serratia marcescens* | 39 | 6.0 |
| *Klebsiella* species | 22 | 3.4 |
| *Staphylococcus epidermidis* | 19 | 2.9 |
| *Candida albicans* | 14 | 2.3 |
| *Proteus* species | 12 | 1.9 |
| Non-*Enterococcus* streptococci | 12 | 1.9 |
| *Pseudomonas* species | 6 | 0.9 |
| Anaerobes | 6 | 0.9 |
| *Acinetobacter* species | 5 | 0.8 |
| *Aspergillus* species | 4 | 0.6 |
| *Candida* (non-albicans) | 3 | 0.5 |
| *Providencia* species | 2 | 0.3 |
| Other bacteria | 28 | 4.3 |
| Other fungi | 8 | 1.2 |

Source: National Nosocomial Infection Study, 1980–82.

brought about by pressures related to antibiotic therapy.

*Community-Acquired versus Nosocomial Infections*
Infections of burn wounds or skin grafts placed at a burn site should be considered nosocomial if the onset of the infection occurs during hospitalization. Infection of burn wounds on initial admission should be classified as community-acquired; these are most likely to be encountered among persons with minor burns whose injury did not initially require hospital care.

## CLINICAL AND MICROBIOLOGIC CLASSIFICATION

Unfortunately, infections of the burn wound often fail to segregate into neat categories that facilitate accurate classification. Several factors contribute to the problem; for example, the wounds themselves differ considerably in extent and depth. Occasionally, burns on one portion of the body may become massively infected, while other areas remain relatively unaffected. To complicate matters additionally, wounds that appear to be uninfected sometimes heal poorly, whereas others that have a heavy purulent discharge

FIG. 30-3. Percent recovery of gram-negative organisms in burn wounds of 558 acute patients. GNR = gram-negative rods.

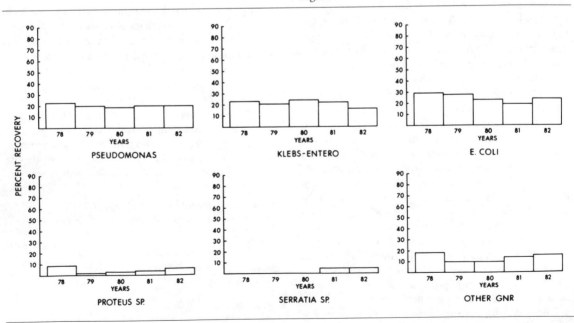

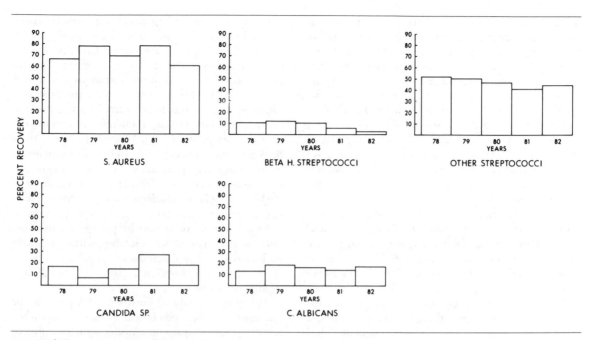

FIG. 30-4. Percent recovery of gram-positive organisms and *Candida* in burn wounds of 558 acute patients.

may heal without incident. There are often associated infections of the urinary tract or respiratory tract, and infections may occur as a complication of the use of intravenous lines or other instrumentation. These conditions are considered elsewhere in Part II of this text and will not be discussed in this chapter except to emphasize their relatively high frequency in the burn patient.

Unfortunately, there is no universal agreement regarding definitions of infection associated with burn injury. The complex physiologic derangements associated with the burn, the necessity for intensive therapeutic manipulation, and the marked overlapping between microbial infections and microbial contamination all contribute to the numerous exceptions that invalidate any inflexible rule. We feel that it is nevertheless useful to categorize infections of burn wounds (excluding specific complicating infections of secondary sites) into three admittedly overlapping divisions: (1) noninvasive infections of the burn wound, (2) invasive infections without bacteremia, and (3) invasive infections with bacteremia. To facilitate consistent surveillance of nosocomial burn infections, noninvasive infections with heavy exudation of purulent material and all invasive burn infections should be reported. All burns with large numbers of organisms in the eschar, however, represent potentially important sources of cross-infections, and these must not be ignored in epidemiologic investigations of infection problems.

### Noninvasive Infections

Infection occurs to some extent in virtually all burn wounds, and colonization with one microorganism or a mixture of microorganisms is universal. Usually, when careful cultures are made of the wound, there is a predominant organism with other bacteria and fungi occurring in lesser numbers. The numbers of bacteria in the exudate or in the dead eschar vary from as few as 10 to up to $10^{10}$ organisms per gram without evidence of invasive infection. Heavy colonization of the wound is unusual within the first few hours, but it is seen more regularly after several days have passed. When surface proliferation reaches a critical number for the interaction between the particular microbe and the immune system of the host, it is followed by invasive infection.

During the second and third weeks after the burn, a layer of granulation tissue develops at the interface between the viable and the nonviable tissue of the burn wound. Associated with the increased vascularity and reactivity of this layer of granulation tissue, resistance to invasion by microorganisms increases progressively. Healthy granulation tissue can resist invasion by extraordinary numbers of bacteria placed on its surface. The dead eschar begins to separate during this same time, the separation resulting in part from enzymes associated with the granulation layer and partly from degradative enzymes produced by microbes in the eschar. Being a dead tissue that is exposed to varying degrees of external contamination, the eschar is an excellent pabulum for microbial proliferation. Control of this proliferation is the basis for successful treatment of significant burn injury. When there are large numbers of bacteria in the eschar, hydrolysis occurs at a more rapid rate, and microbial products that are capable of causing systemic responses in the patient also diffuse across the granulation barrier.

The clinical criteria for noninvasive infection of the burn wound vary somewhat with the age, size, and depth of the wound. In general, the clinical picture of noninvasive infection is characterized by the rapid separation of the eschar and an increased or heavy exudation of purulent material from the burn wound.

Cultures of the eschar or drainage usually show $10^6$ organisms or more per gram of material. Incisive biopsies into healthy tissues, however, usually reveal less than $10^5$ organisms per gram of tissue and, on frozen section, do not show bacteria invading normal tissue. Systemic manifestations of infection are mild to moderate and include a low-grade but spiking fever and a mild-to-moderate leukocytosis without a marked shift to immature forms of granulocytes. The patient remains alert and responsive. One of the great benefits of recognizing noninvasive infection of the burn wound is to prevent its progression to invasive infection.

*Invasive Infections without Bacteremia*
Such infections occur more commonly with some organisms (e.g., *Streptococcus pyogenes*) than with others (e.g., *Candida albicans*). In the host with marked depression of immune resistance, however, all microbes seemingly can become pathogens. The lack of quantitative measurements in clinical observation has led to the performance of quantitative bacteriology to establish and confirm the extent of colonization and invasion. In general, quantitative cultures of specimens from incisional biopsies into viable tissues of the burn wound that yield counts of $10^5$ or more organisms per gram of tissue are considered to represent invasive infection [25]. Counts of $10^{10}$ or $10^{11}$ organisms per gram of tissue are often found with invasive infections. Correlation between such counts and the clinical status of the patient varies considerably with individual strains of organisms as well as with their genus and species.

In invasive infections of the burn wound, the once-healthy appearance of the granulation bed deteriorates with the invasion of organisms into viable tissue. Invaded tissues become edematous and pale and do not bleed briskly from abraded surfaces. As the infection progresses, the surface may become dry and crusty, and in very advanced infections the wound may become frankly necrotic. Unless the process is halted very early, invasion of a partial-thickness wound can quickly convert it into a full-thickness injury that later requires grafting [23]. "Conversion" of partial-thickness injuries occurs not only because of damage to the vestiges of epithelial structures by the organisms, but also because of progressive thrombosis of the blood supply of the affected wound, which results in extension of necrosis into the subcutaneous tissues.

Frozen sections of incisive biopsy specimens of the burn wound may show microbes within formerly healthy tissue. The diagnosis of fungal infection by the identification of hyphae is particularly facilitated by this technique.

The onset of invasive burn wound sepsis may be rather sudden, but the clinical picture is more often superimposed in a patient who already has a purulent drainage, spiking temperatures, and leukocytosis. Early and moderately severe cases usually show an augmentation of the fever, an additional elevation in the white blood cell count, and a decrease in the ratio of segmented to nonsegmented neutrophils. In more severe cases of burn wound sepsis, the temperature may fall to subnormal levels, and the peripheral white blood cell count may be depressed. However, there is nearly always a moderate-to-marked decrease in the ratio of segmented to nonsegmented neutrophils. The cheerful and alert patient usually becomes less responsive, and his or her condition may progress to coma in very severe cases. In some patients, such a picture can be present in the absence of bacteriologic confirmation of septicemia; this was originally pointed out by Moncrief and Teplitz [20], who noted toxemia and death in their patients from *P. aeruginosa* infection without confirmed bacteriologic proof of septicemia. The diffusion of toxins from certain bacteria through the burn eschar to the systemic circulation seems to play an important role. It is much more frequent, however, for bloodstream invasion to occur as a concomitant complication of invasive burn wound infection.

The occurrence of burn-wound sepsis always requires vigorous treatment for a successful outcome.

*Invasive Infections with Bacteremia*
Both colonizing and invading bacteria may enter the lymphatics and traverse into the systemic circulation, and direct invasion of bacteria into blood vesels can

also occur. Thus when repeated blood-culture specimens are taken on a routine basis in patients with large burns, it is not unusual to recover organisms. Recovery of organisms by blood culture in a burn patient sometimes occurs without clinical evidence of systemic infection, and as mentioned before, septic death can occur without septicemia. Furthermore, bacteremia and septicemia in burn patients may derive from other sites of infection, and these may be caused by the same organisms as those isolated from the burn wound. Because of this, some burn centers have placed decreasing emphasis on monitoring burn sepsis by repeated blood cultures. Although it is true that both false-negative and false-positive blood cultures can be obtained, there is nevertheless a very good correlation between clinical evidence of septicemia and the presence of positive blood cultures. It is our strong feeling that differentiation among bacteremia, septicemia, and burn-wound sepsis should not be too rigid, and that the entire clinical and bacteriologic picture must be taken into account in the frequent and critical reevaluation of infections in these patients.

It is apparent that the clinical manifestations of invasive infection of the burn wound associated with septicemia and bacteremia are really not much different from those that occur without bacteremia. The former deserve separate classification, however, because of the objective nature of the diagnosis. In cases of invasive burn wound sepsis with septicemia and bacteremia, it is not unusual to recover more than one organism from the blood culture, which indicates that such patients have a generalized lack of resistance to infection. In our experience, the large majority of patients with burn wound sepsis also have associated bacteremia.

## MICROBIOLOGIC SPECIMENS

Routine bacteriologic monitoring is an essential component of any well-run burn unit. There are considerable differences in the techniques and practices used, however, based on economic consideration and individual preferences. Practices vary from taking occasional culture specimens of the burn wound with a moist swab, to regular, almost daily, incisive biopsies of the burn wound under local anesthesia for quantitative cultures [25]. There is almost universal agreement that methods to quantitate the number of bacteria on the surface of the wound do not accurately reflect the degree of invasion into normal tissue. Routine qualitative cultures of the burn wound provide information concerning the types of bacteria on the wound and their antibiotic sensitivity patterns. Coupled with careful clinical monitoring, surface cultures can provide a useful guide for the choice of antimicrobial agents in patients who require treatment on a clinical basis. It is the practice in our unit to culture wounds after cleansing, either at the time of dressing change and debridement or following hydrotherapy. It is advisable to culture more than one area.

We have found that the most practical technique for routine use in our unit is to sample a wound area using a moist sterile swab; the swab is immediately placed into a transport medium and promptly processed. It has not been helpful to perform routine quantitative culturing on the burn surface, and quantitative incisive biopsies have been too expensive for routine monitoring. Incisive biopsies, however, may be extremely helpful in the evaluation of selected patients, particularly in the diagnosis of invasive fungal infection. The presence of mycelia on frozen sections of biopsy specimens from viable tissue is diagnostic of invasive fungal infection.

## DEFECTS IN IMMUNE RESPONSE

Virtually every measurement of immune response has been found to be abnormal at some time following burn injury [2]; these include depression of circulating immunoglobulin G (IgG) and complement levels, especially in association with hemodilution and protein loss during the first week following injury; abnormalities of complement function; depressed response of circulating antibody to certain antigens, especially in large burns after the fifth day following the burn; a decrease in chemotactic activity of leukocytes; lymphoid depletion in both primary and secondary lymphoid organs, especially in relation to the T-cell population of lymphocytes; altered T-cell function; abnormal response to antigens that cause delayed hypersensitivity reactions (e.g., tuberculin, streptokinase, and the like); prolongation of allografts; depressed response to nonspecific stimuli; and abnormalities of the antibacterial function of neutrophils. Undoubtedly, any of these could contribute in a significant way to the development of nosocomial infections in burn patients. Clinical and laboratory correlative studies from our unit, however, have suggested that abnormalities of neutrophil function and of the opsonic proteins are foremost among the factors that predispose to infection in burn patients. We do not believe that abnormalities of lymphoid function are of primary concern in seriously burned patients.

## GENERAL CONTROL MEASURES

### Patient-Care Practices

Perhaps nowhere else in medicine are patient-care practices more important in controlling infection. Of most importance is the principle emphasized by Aldrich in 1933: "It must be stressed that there is no way to heal a burn and adequately care for the patient without constant supervision and interest" [1].

DEBRIDEMENT  Since the burn wound is a nonviable tissue that is continuously exposed to the external environment, common sense has dictated that the removal of this dead tissue should decrease infection by limiting bacterial growth in the eschar. When the portal of entry is closed by autograft or suitable biologic dressings, an additional advantage can be achieved.

Progressive debridement of all nonviable tissue as it begins to separate from the viable interface followed by autografting is the time-honored method of treatment. Debridement should be vigorous, and the burn wound should be continually monitored for the development of infection. Daily care is required for successful management. The use of enzymatic debridement has received repeated evaluation during the past several years, but at the present time it appears that its potential for harm exceeds its usefulness [11].

Surgical excision is another means of early removal of the burn eschar. Full-thickness excision by either cold knife, electrocautery, or laser has been quite helpful in the management of both small and large burns. Another technique, tangential excision, also has considerable value in both second- and third-degree injuries. One of the reasons for improved survival in patients with very large burns during recent years is the introduction of the technique of excision of large areas of third-degree burns on admission with immediate autografting; this procedure can modify the injury to one of lesser severity.

NUTRITION  With the pain, inanition, marked fluid loss, interruption of daily routine by therapeutic measures and physical therapy, and repeated trips to the operating theatre, the patient is apt to become deficient in caloric intake. In addition, losses from the burn wound and the marked increase in the catabolic rate (which can be almost double that of normal persons) magnify the problem and can precipitate a marked nutritional deficit. In patients with large burns, this nutritional deficit cannot be managed by regular dietary regimens. In the past, it was not uncommon to see loss of body weight of 20 percent or more following a large burn. Sepsis was a frequent acompanying factor. To correct these deficiencies, regimens of intravenous hyperalimentation were begun, but even when the caloric intake was improved to meet metabolic demands, the incidence of septic complications was not diminished [24]. Because of the central intravenous catheter problems (see Chapter 36) associated with parenteral hyperalimentation, a program of oral hyperalimentation was instituted at the Cincinnati Shriners Burns Institute in 1971. Concurrent with this program was an associated improvement in patient mortality and a marked decrease in deaths related to septicemia. The effect of oral hyperalimentation is confounded by the simultaneous change in other variables; nonetheless, it appeared to be an important factor. An analysis of the variables that might have contributed to this abrupt and outstanding improvement in our septic problem showed that the patients who received oral hyperalimentation regimens had a marked improvement in neutrophil function compared to previously studied patients who did not receive oral hyperalimentation. Since a direct correlation exists between the ability of circulating neutrophils from burn patients to kill bacteria in vitro and the incidence of septic complications in such patients [4], this improvement seems critically important. From analysis of the data it would appear that either alimentation by the oral route with improved hepatic metabolism or the added administration of vitamins and minerals was the more important contributing factor [13].

### Environmental Control

BURN UNITS  Before the advent of burn-unit care, the transfer of invasive organisms from adjacent patients was a crucial problem. Even within modern, controlled burn units, the vital importance of regulating environmental factors to control nosocomial infections needs to be repeatedly emphasized. New burn units should be planned and constructed to permit patient care to be delivered in a protected environment with reduced microbial contamination within the area of patient care. Access to the patient-care area should be limited to personnel concerned with the care and support of the patients. Any visitors to the unit should comply with the rigid rules followed by personnel, including the wearing of caps, masks, shoe covers, and operating-room attire. The no-touch technique using a mask, gloves, and a gown or apron should be used on all patients with exposed wounds, with strict attention to mandatory handwashing and the use of disposable materials whenever possible. Dirty areas should be contained. At our institution, color-coding techniques greatly assist in containment. Conventional air-handling equipment can be used, and laminar-flow units and patient-care isolators are not essential. Special attention should be given to measures for control of fomites and the care of supporting equipment such as respirators and nebulizers. Additional environmental control may be necessary for certain patients, such as those harboring group-A streptococci, who usually should be placed in strict isolation (see Chapter 9).

MacMillan [16] has emphasized that in a rigidly controlled burn-care unit, the most common nosocomial reservoirs, in order of decreasing importance, were found to be the patients themselves, personnel, sinks, floors, food, soaps, respirators, warming and cooling equipment, and hydrotherapy equipment. The most common organisms recovered from these areas have been *P. aeruginosa* and saprophytic gram-positive and gram-negative organisms. *Staphylococcus aureus,* α-hemolytic streptococci, *Proteus,* and *Candida albicans* were less frequently isolated. The strains of *Pseudomonas aeruginosa* isolated from environmental sources were invariably rough strains, whereas those isolated from patient sources were invariably smooth strains.

In a highly controlled burn unit, environmental factors contributing to the development of nosocomial infections in burned patients can be minimized, but without control such variables may assume major significance. The techniques necessary for general environmental control are discussed in Chapter 14 and elsewhere in this book.

HYDROTHERAPY EQUIPMENT Conventional hydrotherapy equipment poses a significant risk of transmitting organisms from patient to patient. Such equipment, however, can be modified by removing the agitator and using disposable plastic liners in which tubes are incorporated for compressed air. When such tubes are punctured in appropriate areas, the compressed air leaving the vents agitates the water and helps in the debridement of the burn wound. When physical-therapy personnel protect themselves with plastic gloves and plastic aprons, burn patients can be treated in these facilities without running the risk of becoming contaminated from the burn wounds of other patients who have used the same area [17].

*Antibiotic Therapy*
Prophylactic and therapeutic antimicrobial regimens have played an important role in the control of infection in burn patients.

TOPICAL THERAPY Topical therapy was tried intermittently after the introduction of antimicrobial agents, but it was not very successful until 1964 [19]. It is now a routine component in the management of any serious burn injury. Topical agents merely control the numbers of bacteria sufficiently to prevent invasive infection. With any antimicrobial drug, resistant strains may arise, and it is for this reason that the burn wound must be carefully monitored and the topical agent changed if infection becomes obvious. Ointments as a vehicle for the application of topical drugs have largely been replaced by water-soluble creams or solutions. A variety of topical agents are available and in clinical use today. The major agents used are gentamicin sulfate, mafenide acetate, silver sulfadiazine, and nitrofurazone, but silver nitrate solution and povidone-iodine are also used. However, a variety of potential problems have been reported in using each of these drugs. Silver sulfadiazine, although a useful agent, has been associated with leukopenia, and more recently, resistant strains have emerged.

Mafenide acetate is an extremely useful agent, but it has the disadvantage of aggravating metabolic disorders and pulmonary complications in many patients with burns exceeding 50 percent. It also has the disadvantage of causing significant burning on application, particularly over second-degree injuries. While silver nitrate does not penetrate into the burn wound, it is an effective topical agent, has a low cost, and is currently in use at this and some other institutions. Povidone-iodine ointment and gentamicin ointment should generally be reserved as secondary agents; an iodofor is particularly useful to control overgrowth of *Candida* in the burn wound, and gentamicin will control overgrowth of *Pseudomonas* or *Staphylococcus.* Gentamicin should not be used as a primary agent, because of the emergence of resistant pathogens. In fact, no one agent is uniformly effective against all microorganisms colonizing burn wounds. Routine sequential testing for the effectiveness of topical agents permits early change of the agent when resistant organisms arise.

SYSTEMIC CHEMOPROPHYLAXIS For several decades, penicillin has been used prophylactically to prevent the occurrence of acute, invasive streptococcal infections of the burn wound (see Chapter 11). With the extensive use of topical antimicrobial agents, however, streptococcal infection in burns is now a rare event. Penicillin causes the emergence of resistant organisms and a deleterious change in the ecology of the burn-wound flora [16]. Thus we recommend careful monitoring of the burn wound and nasopharyngeal flora for beginning signs of infection or colonization and delaying specific therapy until there is clinical or bacteriologic evidence of streptococcal infection or colonization. Other prophylactic systemic antibiotics clearly encourage the emergence of antibiotic-resistant pathogens in the nosocomial environment and should not be used in burn patients.

## GROUP-A *STREPTOCOCCUS PYOGENES*

### General Aspects

TRANSMISSIBILITY  Group-A *Streptococcus pyogenes* is a highly transmissible organism that can cause rapidly lethal infections in the burn patient.

CLINICAL COURSE  The clinical course is characterized by an abrupt deterioration in the wound that is associated with an increase in wound pain, redness, induration, and swelling. Redness extending from the margin of the burn wound is perhaps the most significant sign of streptococcal infections, which characteristically invade into normal tissues. Within hours of the onset of the more fulminant infections, systemic symptoms occur, characterized by a high, spiking fever, rapid tachycardia, and flushing of the face. Untreated, the condition can progress rapidly to death. Leukocytosis with a marked shift to the left is characteristic. Shock usually does not occur until the condition is terminal. Most streptococcal infections are seen within the first week following burn injury, and invasive infection of healthy granulation tissue by *Streptococcus* rarely occurs. It is for this reason that penicillin has been used so extensively for prophylaxis during the early burn period.

The freshly grafted wound and fresh donor site are other sites that frequently become infected with group-A *Streptococcus pyogenes*. The clinical course is usually less abrupt, and of more concern is the loss of grafts from infection or the conversion of a donor site to a full-thickness injury.

PREDISPOSING HOST FACTORS  These are not different from those of other types of bacterial infection in burn patients, but from the available data it would appear that a decrease in serum opsonic activity during the first 10 to 15 days after injury is especially important. Perhaps of more significance as a predisposing factor is carriage of the organism by the patient, because those who carry streptococci in oropharyngeal sites are at a much higher risk.

THERAPY  Fortunately, group-A *Streptococcus* infection almost always responds to penicillin therapy. For those individuals allergic to penicillin, alternative drugs include erythromycin, vancomycin, and the cephalosporins. Patients wtih penicillin allergy tend to be sensitive to cephalosporin as well, and cephalosporins should probably not be used in those with a history of severe penicillin reactions. Streptococci are exquisitely sensitive to vancomycin, and this is the drug of choice in treating serious life-threatening infection in a patient with penicillin allergy. It is well to remember that although gentamicin has a broad spectrum of activity against most staphylococcal organisms, it is relatively ineffective against streptococcal infections.

### Endemic Infections

INCIDENCE  Despite the high transmissibility, endemic infections are much more common than epidemic infections in well-run burn units. Positive cultures from burn wounds for group-A *Streptococcus* are found in 5 to 10 percent of all admissions to the Cincinnati Shriners Burns Institute. Clinical infections became evident in only a few of these individuals, however, and such infections are relatively minor. Only one life-threatening infection with group-A *Streptococcus* has occurred during the last decade, and this was in a patient undergoing a reconstructive orthopedic procedure.

SOURCES  The major source of the group-A streptococci that cause endemic infection is the nasopharynx of the patient. The patient's wounds can also be an important source, however, particularly the small, chronically draining wounds in ulcerated burn scars or burn sites that are slow to heal. Fomites and other environmental sources do not seem to play a prominent role in endemic infections.

MODES OF SPREAD  Spread is usually within the patient, either from the nasopharynx or from open areas to recently grafted sites. Less common but very important is spread by nursing and supporting personnel from one patient to another by contaminated hands or possibly by colonization in the nares and dissemination to susceptible patients.

PREVENTION  Prevention of endemic infections by group-A streptococci is best accomplished by bacteriologic monitoring of the patient and his wound. Every patient should have a nasopharyngeal culture as well as cultures of all wounds on admission to a burn unit. Such cultures should be repeated on a routine, periodic basis during the hospital stay. Patients who have or develop a positive culture for group-A *Streptococcus* should be isolated immediately and treated with systemic penicillin therapy until the cultures are negative. Any patient with positive cultures in the recent past that required an operation or debridement should be given prophylactic penicillin therapy to protect against invasive infection by hemolytic *Streptococcus*. We feel that it is not indicated to give penicillin prophylactically to patients for most reconstructive procedures or for debridement or grafting in patients with negative cultures. We also feel that the routine administration of penicillin during the first five days after the burn injury is not necessary in well-controlled burn units. While it has been claimed that penicillin does little harm, data from our unit would suggest that the microbial flora of the wound can be adversely shifted to a more resistant population in patients who have received prophylactic penicillin on a routine basis [16].

### Epidemic Infections

INCIDENCE With good environmental control and bacteriologic monitoring, epidemic infections should be exceedingly rare. However, most older, experienced burn surgeons have observed the devastating consequences of such outbreaks in the prepenicillin era. In our unit, such an outbreak has not occurred in over 20 years.

HIGH-RISK AREAS Both open wards and intensive care units can pose high risks in hospitals that treat burns in such areas. The enhanced risk is related mostly to a high density of patients with susceptible wounds, which in turn results in inadequate protective isolation of the burn patient.

SOURCES In epidemic infections, nursing and supporting personnel must be highly suspected, but initial infections may come from the patients or visitors (see Chapters 27 and 31).

MODES OF SPREAD In contrast to endemic infections, spread is usually by contact from carriers or from personnel who transmit the infection from patient to patient.

CONTROL OF OUTBREAKS Strict isolation procedures should be used to control any acute group-A β-hemolytic streptococcal burn infection. All patient-care personnel and patients should have cultures of the nares, oropharynx, and wounds, and epidemiologic studies should be undertaken to identify potential disseminating carriers (see Chapters 5, 27, and 31). Patients with positive cultures should be isolated and treated with penicillin (see Chapter 9). Personnel with positive cultures must be removed from patient-care duties until either they are treated and have negative cultures or their strains are shown to be different

from the epidemic strain on the basis of M and T typing. Strict attention to "no-touch" technique is essential to the control and prevention of outbreaks, and gloves and masks should be worn anytime there is contact with the wound. One important aspect of the prevention of such outbreaks is to prohibit visitation by persons with upper respiratory tract infections.

### STAPHYLOCOCCUS AUREUS

### General Aspects

TRANSMISSIBILITY *S. aureus* is an organism of moderate virulence that is easily transmitted. The extremely large numbers of organisms that may colonize or infect burns are accompanied by significant risks of transmission by contact and airborne routes. Because they survive even in the dried state, staphylococci can become airborne on dust particles and desquamated epithelial cells, but contact is by far the most important mode of their transmission in burn patients.

CLINICAL FEATURES Patients who develop invasive infections of the burn wound with *S. aureus* have an insidious course; two to five days often elapse between the earliest symptoms and the full-blown infection. These patients have early dissolution of granulation tissue in the burn wound, become hyperpyretic with a leukocytosis, develop disorientation that is often severe, and often develop a prominent gastrointestinal ileus. Shock is not infrequent and is often accompanied by renal failure.

PREDISPOSING HOST FACTORS The most important host factor that predisposes to staphylococcal infections appears to be an abnormality of the antibacterial function of the neutrophils. Serum factors seem to be less important in the control of this microorganism than they are in other infections.

THERAPY Fortunately, many antimicrobial agents are effective against *S. aureus*. Although penicillin is effective against some strains, the high incidence of penicillin resistance makes it mandatory that other antibiotics be chosen as a primary agent. In our unit, systemic nafcillin has proved to be a valuable drug. The occasional strains that have been nafcillin-resistant have been uniformly susceptible to vancomycin. Antibiotics should only be administered when there is evidence of invasive infection of the burn wound. Because of the problem of superinfection, therapy should be restricted to relatively short time intervals.

To reverse a tendency to administer the antistaphylococcal drugs for too long a time, we recommend a thorough reassessment of the need for their continuation after each five days of therapy. Generally, *S. aureus* cannot be eradicated completely from a burn wound until the wound is covered by graft.

### Endemic Infections

INCIDENCE *Staphylococcus aureus* is one of the most important organisms causing infection in burn patients [30]. Approximately 60 percent of all patients become colonized with *S. aureus* on their burns, and it is the leading cause of septicemia in our burn unit at the present time. With the availability of effective antimicrobial agents for the treatment of systemic infections, however, mortality from staphylococcal infection in our unit is rare.

SOURCES Environmental sources are probably much more important for *S. aureus* than for most of the organisms encountered in the burn unit. Indeed, the organism is almost ubiquitous. Furthermore, patients colonized in the anterior nares may spread the organisms to their burns. The greatest source of endemic spread is the nosocomial reservoir. For this reason, it is extremely important to develop rigid environmental control techniques, as mentioned previously.

MODES OF SPREAD Staphylococcal carriers among personnel can be an important source, but the most important mode of spread is usually via personnel from patient to patient in an environment that is not closely controlled. Fomites and even food are occasionally implicated.

PREVENTION Evironmental control is of utmost importance in preventing endemic infection by *S. aureus*; these measures have already been outlined. In addition, the restrictive use of systemic antibiotics favors easier control of this infection. Among the topical agents, povidone-iodine and mafenide acetate appear to give reasonably good control for *S. aureus* infection, and our strains have been uniformly susceptible to nitrofurazone.

### Epidemic Infections

Epidemic infections with *S. aureus* occur at a low incidence, even in high patient-density areas such as intensive care units. When they do occur, epidemiologic studies and bacteriologic surveys of personnel for carriers should be performed. If carriers are epidemiologically associated with the outbreak, they should be temporarily excused from duty, and attempts should be made to eradicate the colonizing strain (see Chapters 27 and 31).

## PSEUDOMONAS AERUGINOSA

### General Aspects

TRANSMISSIBILITY *P. aeruginosa* is an organism of low pathogenicity that rarely causes infections in immunologically normal individuals. However, it grows well in moist environments, especially in open wounds; it is resistant to most commonly used antibiotics; and it invades frequently in immunodepressed individuals.

CLINICAL FEATURES Invasion of the burn wound by *P. aeruginosa* may occur either abruptly or slowly. In a typical case, the burn wound develops a heavy, green-pigmented, foul-smelling discharge over a period of two or three days. In rapidly advancing and invasive infections, the eschar may become dry, and previously healthy granulation tissues develop a shaggy, green exudate and later progress to form patchy, black areas of necrosis. In certain cases, however, the granulation tissue may not show necrotic areas and may not have a greenish exudate. Gangrene in nonburned areas (ecthyma gangrenosum) is often seen before death in patients with septicemia. Patients usually become hypothermic and have a depressed white cell count and clinical ileus, but they are usually not disoriented until the disease is terminal.

PREDISPOSING HOST FACTORS Predisposing host factors are extremely important in the development of infections with *P. aeruginosa*. In burn patients, these factors are related both to abnormalities of the antibacterial function of neutrophils and to deficiencies in serum opsonins, that is, specific natural or immune antibody and components of the complement system. With heavy colonization of the burn wound, a selective consumption of specific antibody can occur that renders the patient increasingly susceptible to the organism on the burn wound.

VIRULENCE FACTORS In addition to host factors that predispose patients to *P. aeruginosa*, research in recent years has defined several virulence-associated factors for this microorganism. These include elastase, alkaline protease, and exotoxin production and motility. Several additional factors have also been defined. It is the activity of these virulence-associated factors, alone or in concert, taken together with the predisposing host factors, that makes *P. aeruginosa* infections in burn patients the most devastating of the gram-negative infections.

THERAPY In the treatment of established septicemia in the burn patient, polymyxin B and colistin are relatively toxic and almost totally ineffective. In recent years, certain aminoglycoside antibiotics—especially gentamicin, tobramycin, and amikacin—have been the antibiotics of choice in the treatment of *Pseudomonas* septicemia. Simultaneous administration of carbenicillin has been useful in selected cases, especially in overwhelming infections. One alarming observation has been a marked increase in the numbers of bacteria in some hospitals that have been found to be resistant to gentamicin, carbenicillin, and even the newer aminoglycosides.

Some newer penicillins—piperacillin and azlocillin—show significant antipseudomonal activity in vitro, but resistance develops rapidly in patients when they are used alone. Newer third-generation cephalosporin antibiotics hold some promise based on in vitro test results, but the clinical experience using these drugs is too limited for any assessment to be made.

MONITORING SERUM AMINOGLYCOSIDE LEVELS Gram-negative infections, particularly those due to *P. aeruginosa*, *Klebsiella pneumoniae*, and *Enterobacter* species, are frequently the cause of death of patients suffering from major burns. Septicemia and burn-wound sepsis resulting from these pathogens have in the past produced an alarmingly high mortality rate. Because of the favorable antibacterial spectrum of gentamicin and other aminoglycosides, these agents have become widely used in the treatment of burn sepsis. Optimal treatment with these agents requires the careful establishment of dosage schedules.

In 1976 Zaske and coworkers [32], using a digital computer program nonlinear regression analysis of postinfusion serum concentration versus time analysis, calculated the estimated half-lives of gentamicin in burn patients. They found that the recommended dosage of 5 mg/kg/day resulted in shorter half-lives in burned compared to nonburned persons, and that this shortened half-life in burned patients led to extended periods of subtherapeutic serum antibiotic concentrations. Furthermore, it was determined that among adult burn patients, there was a wide variability of gentamicin half-lives and that younger burn patients eliminated gentamicin even more rapidly than older burn patients. By establishing clearance curves on individual patients and calculating drug half-lives, the clinician can adjust both the dosage and the frequency of treatment to maintain serum antibiotic levels in the therapeutic range over the whole treatment period.

Shortly after it was established that gentamicin was cleared more rapidly in burned patients, we established individualized dosage schedules for our patients using the procedures just described. Clearance curves were determined for each patient after a standard gentamicin dosage of 5 mg/kg/day. Serum gentamicin concentrations were determined using an enzyme-multiplied immunoassay technique. We have found that serum for these assays can be obtained by venipuncture or from finger-stick samples. Gentamicin levels obtained by the two methods showed a strong correlation. These data were used in a digital computer program nonlinear regression analysis that provided estimates of gentamicin half-lives in the individual patients. From these analyses it was determined that the gentamicin half-lives ranged from 50 to 90 minutes in our patients. Younger patients and patients with larger burns had half-lives closer to 50 minutes than to 90 minutes. With the half-life determined in each patient for the standard dosage, the computer can be asked to determine what dose would be necessary to achieve desired therapeutic levels in each patient. In our institution, we feel that the desired therapeutic dosage would be one in which the peak level is 12 mg/ml or slightly less and the trough level is 1 mg/ml or less. Using these values as our desired therapeutic gentamicin levels, we had to adjust our dosage of gentamicin upward. Dosages of 8 mg/kg/day to 20 mg/kg/day have been used in our patients, and each dosage is individualized to the specific patient based on data obtained from the initial clearance rate of the standard dosage.

While it is not entirely clear why burn patients clear gentamicin more rapidly than nonburn patients, Goodwin and colleagues [9] report that the size of the kidneys in burn patients exceeds their normal size two- or threefold. The more rapid perfusion that takes place in these kidneys may explain why gentamicin and other aminoglycoside antibiotics, which are excreted exclusively by the kidneys, are cleared more rapidly. Under these circumstances, optimal aminoglycoside therapy can be ensured only by monitoring serum levels and appropriately adjusting dosage and frequency of treatment.

The established dosage schedule should be checked at intervals of seven to ten days in the early course of the aminoglycoside therapy to ensure that levels are being adequately maintained and that half-lives are not changing during this time. This technique probably represents one of the major therapeutic advancements in delivering and assessing systemic antibiotic therapy.

*Endemic Infections*

INCIDENCE  As indicated before, it is difficult to establish the incidence of infection by any one organism in burn patients because of the spectrum between colonization and frank sepsis. In surveys in the Cincinnati Shriners Burns Institute, from 1974 to 1982 between 20 and 30 percent of all admitted patients became colonized with *P. aeruginosa* on their burns during their hospital stay (Fig. 30-5).

SOURCES  A survey in our intensive care unit demonstrated that the major source of *P. aeruginosa* on a patient's burn wound was the patient himself, predominantly via the gastrointestinal tract [17]. This observation has been emphasized by others [10, 28]. Nosocomial acquisition of *P. aeruginosa* in the gastrointestinal tract is common among seriously ill hospitalized patients. *P. aeruginosa* was found in a number of environmental areas, but these were not felt to be reservoirs for pathogenic organisms, since the organisms were invariably of the rough, nonpathogenic type not found on patients. Other reports relating to *Pseudomonas* in hospital environments, however, have indicated that fomites (including mop buckets, sink traps, faucet aerators, respirators, nebulizers, hospital food, contaminated oral medications, and flowers) may be reservoirs for *P. aeruginosa* [14, 15]. The first two items are probably of little or no importance as proximate sources of infective organisms.

MODES OF SPREAD  The predominant mode of spread within burn units is transference by personnel who have direct patient contact. Another important mode of spread in some burn units is via whirlpool and Hubbard tank units, especially when extensive decontamination and aseptic procedures are not followed properly.

PREVENTION  Colonization of the burn patient by *P. aeruginosa* is extremely difficult to prevent. General control measures are important in preventing the spread of this organism, and topical therapy has been beneficial in limiting its growth in colonized patients. Increases in antibiotic resistance patterns emphasize the need for an immunologic approach to therapy. A variety of immunologic approaches to *Pseudomonas* prophylaxis have been tried. Vaccines prepared against lipopolysaccharides, polysaccharides, ribosomes, exoproducts, outer membranes, and flagella have been tried in experimental animals, and in some cases, clinical trials. While some of these preparations appear to have some merit, continued research is necessary before widespread use of antipseudomonal vaccines can occur. Passive immunization using IgG fractionated from the serum of volunteers immunized with *Pseudomonas* antigens appears to be a practical approach to immunotherapy and is closer to being available for clinical use than is active immunization [3].

*Epidemic Infections*

Epidemic infections with *P. aeruginosa* are practically nonexistent in a well-controlled environment. Outbreaks traced to contaminated hydrotherapy and respiratory equipment have occurred, and these sources should be carefully evaluated if an outbreak develops.

## OTHER ORGANISMS CAUSING BURN INFECTIONS

### *Candida albicans*

CLINICAL COURSE  Invasive infection caused by *Candida albicans* is not frequently seen; it occurs commonly only in patients who have extensive and debilitating burn injuries. Such patients have usually received broad-spectrum antibiotics for relatively long periods of time for the treatment of other infectious complications. Clinically, the granulating wound usually becomes dry and flat with a yellow or orange color. There is a gradual downhill course, during which the patient's temperature and white blood cell count usually remain unchanged.

PREDISPOSING HOST FACTORS  The mechanisms for defense against *Candida* infections are essentially the same as those for bacterial infections, although delayed hypersensitivity mechanisms seem to be more

FIG. 30-5. Colonization rate with *Pseudomonas aeruginosa* at the Cincinnati Shriners Burns Institute.

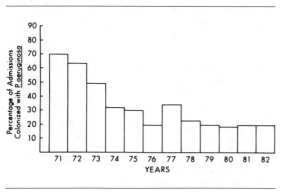

important and antibody-mediated immune reactions less important for ridding the host of these pathogens. Such agents infrequently cause primary infections, but they are troublesome opportunistic invaders in patients with abnormalities of host resistance such as occur in some immunologic deficiency diseases or during immunosuppressive therapy. An improvement in the survival rate for the extensively burned patient has contributed to the rise in the incidence of serious yeast and fungal infections. *Candida* often becomes the predominant organism of mucosal surfaces and burn wounds when the usual bacterial flora have been destroyed by antibiotic therapy, and superinfections not infrequently follow successful treatment for systemic bacterial sepsis. Among mycotic agents, *Candida albicans* is the most frequent cause of both local and systemic infections as a secondary invader, probably because of its normal occurrence in the gastrointestinal tract. At one time, it was believed that only *C. albicans* among the *Candida* species caused infections in burn patients. We now know that other *Candida* species, especially *C. tropicalis* and *C. parapsilosis*, cause severe, often fatal infections in burn patients. A report of any *Candida* species in the wounds and/or body fluids of a burned patient should be viewed with concern.

While the presence of *Candida* on the burn wound only is of little clinical significance in the majority of cases, colonization may precede invasion, which can herald the occurrence of *Candida* septicemia and systemic mycosis. In this instance biopsies of the burn wound can be of great help, because the demonstration of pseudohyphae deep in viable subcutaneous tissue by wound biopsy can alert the clinician to the danger of possible *Candida* septicemia and systemic candidiasis [22]. Systemic candidiasis can also be suspected by the demonstration of *Candida* organisms in the urine. Krause and coworkers [12] have demonstrated candiduria in a human promptly after swallowing a pure culture of *Candida albicans*, and they have shown that invasion from the gastrointestinal tract can be effectively controlled by the use of oral nystatin (Mycostatin).

Colonization of the burn wound depends on several predisposing factors, including antibiotic therapy. Nash and associates [21] have shown a tenfold increase in the occurrence of fungi on burn wounds following the use of mafenide acetate cream as a topical antibacterial agent at the U.S. Army's Institute of Surgical Research. Seelig [27] has noted the development of candidiasis in patients receiving multiple systemic broad-spectrum antibiotics. Williams and colleagues [31] have noted an increase in the incidence of can-

didiasis in association with certain therapeutic measures, that is, the use of blood transfusions, central venous pressure lines, and intravenous hyperalimentation therapy.

THERAPY  Local colonization of *Candida* in the burn wound can be controlled by the incorporation of nystatin (Mycostatin) in the appropriate topical antibacterial agent. Systemic spread from the gastrointestinal tract can be effectively controlled by the use of oral nystatin. Early invasive candidiasis should be treated by the discontinuation of systemic antibiotic therapy whenever possible, the removal of intravenous and urinary catheters, and the intravenous administration of amphotericin B.

ENDEMIC AND EPIDEMIC INFECTIONS  Colonization of burn wounds by *C. albicans* in patients treated at the Cincinnati Shriners Burns Institute has increased from 30 to 50 percent during the early 1970s. This increase paralleled a steady rise in the incidence of disseminated candidiasis, and systemic candidiasis became the major cause of septic deaths in this unit for a short while. Endemic colonization on the wounds of burn patients can be minimized by the limited and selective use of antibiotic therapy, including, whenever possible, the avoidance of broad-spectrum agents such as tetracycline, nutritional support by the oral route, the use of intravenous hyperalimentation only in patients who are suffering from a superior mesenteric artery syndrome, and the administration of intravenous fluids for short periods through butterfly (scalp vein) needles. Consideration might also be given to the prophylactic use of oral nystatin in units experiencing high rates of *Candida* infection. Putting the above practices into use at our institution has reduced the recovery of *C. albicans* to below 20 percent of all burn patients over the past five years.

Epidemic infections of candidal organisms are rarely seen in well-controlled burn units. The major source of cross-infection with fungal organisms in the burn unit has been the inappropriate use of hydrotherapy equipment. This mode of dissemination can be eliminated by the use of protective liners on hydrotherapy equipment.

*Other Mycotic Infections*
GENERAL ASPECTS  With improved control of burn-wound sepsis caused by gram-negative and gram-positive bacteria, increasing numbers of mycotic infections of the burn wound have been reported. One study from the Institute of Surgical Research reported 30 cases of invasive infection with fungi of the Phy-

comycetes or *Aspergillus* species [5]. Of the 30 patients, 9 died from invasive fungal infections, and 6 from bacterial sepsis. Of 15 surviving patients, 7 required amputation to eradicate their disease. Phycomycetes or *Aspergillus* was recovered in culture from only nine patients. Fungi of the Phycomycetes class were identified histologically as the offending organisms in 22 cases and an *Aspergillus* in eight cases. Of the 22 cases of invasive Phycomycoses identified histologically, two were further identified as *Rhizopus* and the remaining 19 were probably *Mucor*. The incidence of clinically significant fungal burn wound infections was approximately 3 percent of patients treated for thermal injury. Other fungal organisms recovered from burn wounds included isolated species of *Geotrichum*, *Rhodotorula*, *Cephalosporium*, *Penicillium*, *Trichosporon*, *Trichophyton*, *Fusarium*, and *Fonsecaea* [6], but these did not seem to invade. Little is known about their transmissibility, sources, and modes of spread within burn units.

CLINICAL OBSERVATIONS   The mycotic infections cited above were most frequently seen between days nine and 15 after the burn, and the majority of patients had burns of greater than 30 percent. Clinical signs included fever, swelling, and conversion of the burn wound. The most frequent manifestations were ulceration, induration, edema, tenderness, early separation of the eschar, and muscle necrosis. Hyphal invasion of viable tissue is diagnostic of fungal burn wound infection. Invasion may be identified by microscopic examination of frozen sections from incisional biopsy specimens.

Hyphal invasion of viable tissue very often extends laterally to involve unburned subcutaneous tissues beneath unburned skin, and hyphae often invade through the fascia and into skeletal muscle. Thrombosis and vascular necrosis of the tissue are common because of invasion of the blood vessel walls. The vascular invasion is also responsible for dissemination of organisms into the abdominal and thoracic organs and the central nervous system. At the Cincinnati Shriners Burns Institute, we have had only one death caused by these agents (a disseminated *Mucor* infection). In this patient, there was rapid invasion of normal tissue followed by general dissemination and death within a short time after the diagnosis.

PREDISPOSING HOST FACTORS   Little is known about the host factors that predispose to invasive fungal infections of this type in burned patients. Such infections, however, have been seen with increasing incidence in other disorders associated with decreased host resistance, particularly in patients with malig-

nancies of the lymphoid and reticuloendothelial systems and in those with diabetes mellitus, especially when acidosis is present.

THERAPY   Effective therapy of invasive fungal infections in burn patients must be instituted promptly. Therapy consists primarily of radical excision of the involved area [5]. Immediate histologic examination of the excisional margins is a helpful adjunct to excisional therapy to document complete removal. Following surgical excision, frequent examination of the remaining wound to detect areas of incomplete excision is necessary. Amputation may be necessary to eradicate the disease. Early aggressive therapy with Amphotericin B has been found effective in reducing mortality from *Candida* sepsis and has also been successful in treating *C. tropicalis* and *C. parapsilosis* sepsis.

*Other Aerobic Gram-Negative Bacteria*
PATHOGENIC AGENTS   Gram-negative enteric bacteria other than *Pseudomonas aeruginosa* have become increasingly important in infections occurring in burn patients. These organisms include *Escherichia*, *Klebsiella*, *Proteus*, *Enterobacter*, *Providencia*, *Acinetobacter*, and *Alcaligenes*. *Salmonella* and *Shigella* species do not seem to cause infections of the burn wound. The gram-negative organisms generally appear on a burn wound as a consequence of contamination from the endogenous flora of the patient or the environment, but the most important factor in their becoming pathogenic is the selective elimination of competing gram-positive organisms from the burn wound by antibiotic therapy. Another problem of special importance is that these organisms can be controlled on the burn wound, but they can rarely be eliminated by antibiotic therapy. When antibiotic-resistant strains begin to appear, the transfer of resistance (R) factors to nonresistant strains occurs (frequently even to different genera), which leads to the accumulation and proliferation of antibiotic-resistant organisms within the nosocomial environment of the burn unit [26] (see Chapters 11 and 12).

TRANSMISSIBILITY   Most of the gram-negative bacteria of enteric origin have low pathogenicity, and most infections occur because the host is immunologically compromised. Cross-colonization of the gastrointestinal tract of hospitalized patients is facilitated by the use of antibiotics to which prevalent nosocomial strains are resistant.

CLINICAL FEATURES   Invasive infections may show deterioration of healthy granulation tissue, which becomes edematous and pale. Classic ecthyma gangrenosum is rare with gram-negative organisms other than *Pseudomonas*, but progressive thrombosis of vessels extensively invaded can occur and result in conversion of partial-thickness injuries to full-thickness injuries. The clinical picture of systemic infections with these gram-negative organisms in burn patients is similar to that of gram-negative septicemia in other patients. Systemic infection is usually heralded by an initial elevation in temperature, which may be followed by hypothermia in later stages. Hypotension is not uncommon. Either leukocytosis or leukopenia may be present, but there is usually a marked shift in the differential count to immature forms.

PREDISPOSING HOST FACTORS Abnormalities of complement, natural antibody, and neutrophil antibacterial function have all been shown to be important in the development of systemic invasion with these organisms.

THERAPY Systemic gentamicin has been our drug of choice for initial treatment of gram-negative sepsis before specific antibiotic-sensitivity patterns are established, but therapy should be altered if so indicated by specific sensitivities. Topical therapy is determined based on the results obtained using an agar well diffusion topical antimicrobial test assay.

PREVENTION Most infections caused by gram-negative bacteria are endemic, and there is a relatively high incidence of superinfections following therapy for infections with gram-positive organisms. The usual source of the gram-negative agents is the gastrointestinal tract of the patients themselves. Hyperendemic disease caused by one or more of the pathogens may occur from time to time within particular burn units, and it probably results from the establishment of a large reservoir of a particular strain. Such strains are usually multiply-drug-resistant and are selected by the continuous use of particular popular antibiotic regimens. They are usually found in the patients and environment of the burn unit, and continual cross-colonization and infection of new admissions take place. Parenteral antibiotic therapy in burn patients should thus be restricted to situations with clear indications, and periodic shifts in popular drug regimens, when possible, might also be considered. Hands of personnel and contact with contaminated hydrotherapy units can spread these organisms. The prevention of such infections depends on excellent care of the burn wound and strict attention to the general control measures mentioned earlier in this chapter.

*Anaerobic Bacterial Infections*
Anaerobic infections following burn injury are surprisingly infrequent, possibly because of the aerobic environment of the burn wound in most instances. However, early contamination with clostridial species, including *Clostridium perfringens* and *Clostridium tetani*, is relatively common. In very deep burns, such as can occur with electrical injuries in which muscle necrosis is often associated, prevention of gas gangrene and tetanus should be of great concern, and early debridement or excision of dead tissue is advisable. Tetanus in the burn patient is a potential hazard in almost every case, but it can be easily prevented by current active and passive immunization procedures. In present practice, both gas gangrene and tetanus are exceedingly rare. Other types of anaerobic infections, such as those caused by *Bacteroides* species, are also very uncommon and cause no particular problem.

*Viral infections*
Viral infections have increasingly been reported in burn patients. Herpesvirus and cytomegalovirus are the agents most frequently found, either by serologic tests or by direct culture. The clinical significance of these findings is not clear at the present time.

## REFERENCES

1. Aldrich, R. H. The role of infection in burns: The theory and treatment with special reference to gentian violet. *N. Engl. J. Med.* 208:299, 1933.
2. Alexander, J. W. Infections in the patient with severe burns. In Nahmis, H. J., and O'Reilly, R. J. (Eds.), *Immunology of Human Infections*, vol. I. New York: Plenum Publishing. (In press.)
3. Alexander, J. W., and Fisher, M. W. Immunization against *Pseudomonas* in infection after thermal injury. *J. Infect. Dis.* 130:S152, 1974.
4. Alexander, J. W., and Meakins, J. L. A physiological basis for the development of opportunistic infections. *Ann. Surg.* 176:273, 1972.
5. Bruck, H. M., Nash, G., and Pruitt, B. S., Jr. Opportunistic fungal infection of the burn wound with phycomycetes and *Aspergillus*. *Arch. Surg.* 102:476, 1971.
6. Bruck, H. M., Nash, G., Stein, J. M., and Lindberg, R. B. Studies on the occurrence and significance of yeasts and fungi in the burn wound. *Ann. Surg.* 176:108, 1972.
7. Colebrook, L., and Lond, M. B. The control of infection in burns. *Lancet* 1:6511, 1948.

8. Cruickshank, R. The bacterial infection of burns. *J. Pathol. Bacteriol.* 31:367, 1935.

9. Goodwin, C. W., Aulick, L. H., Becker, R. A., and Wilmore, D. W. Increased renal perfusion and kidney size in convalescent burn patients. *J.A.M.A.* 244:1588, 1980.

10. Haynes, B. W., Jr., and Hench, M. E. Hospital isolation system for preventing cross-contamination by staphylococcal and pseudomonas organisms in burn wounds. *Ann. Surg.* 162:641, 1965.

11. Hummel, R. P., Kautz, P. D., MacMillan, B. G., and Altemeier, W. A. The continuing problem of sepsis following enzymatic debridement of burns. *J. Trauma* 14:572, 1974.

12. Krause, W., Matheis, K., and Wulf, K. Fungemia and funguria after oral administration of *Candida albicans*. *Lancet* 1:598, 1969.

13. Lennard, E. S., Alexander, J. W., Craycraft, T. K., and MacMillan, B. G. Association in burn patients of improved antibacterial defense with nutritional support by the oral route. *Burns* 1:95, 1975.

14. Lowbury, E. J. L. Infection of burns. *Br. Med. J.* 1:994, 1960.

15. Lowbury, E. J. L., and Fox, J. The epidemiology of infection with *Pseudomonas pyocyanea* in a burns unit. *J. Hyg.* (Camb.) 52:403, 1954.

16. MacMillan, B. G. Burn wound sepsis: A ten-year experience. *Burns* 2:1, 1975.

17. MacMillan, B. G., Edmonds, P., Hummel, R. P., and Maley, M. P. Epidemiology of *Pseudomonas* in a burn intensive care unit. *J. Trauma* 13:627, 1973.

18. Meleney, F. L. The study of the prevention of infection in contaminated accidental wounds, compound fractures, and burns. *Ann. Surg.* 118:171, 1943.

19. Moncrief, J. A. The development of topical therapy. *J. Trauma* 11:906, 1971.

20. Moncrief, J. A., and Teplitz, C. Changing concepts in burn sepsis. *J. Trauma* 4:233, 1964.

21. Nash, G., Foley, F. D., Goodwin, M. N., Bruck, H. M., Greenwald, K. A., and Pruitt, B. A., Jr. Fungal burn wound infection. *J.A.M.A.* 215:1664, 1971.

22. Nash, G., Foley, F. D., and Pruitt, B. A., Jr. *Candida* burn-wound invasion: A cause of systemic candidiasis. *Arch. Pathol.* 90:75, 1970.

23. Order, S. E., Mason, A. D., Jr., Walker, H. L., Lindberg, R. F., Switzer, W. E., and Moncrief, J. A. The pathogenesis of second- and third-degree burns and conversion to full-thickness injury. *Surg. Gynecol. Obstet.* 120:983, 1965.

24. Popp, M., Law, E., and MacMillan, B. G. Parenteral nutrition in the burn child: A study of 26 patients. *Ann. Surg.* 179:219, 1974.

25. Pruitt, B. A., Jr., and Foley, F. D. The use of biopsies in burn patient care. *Surgery* 73:887, 1973.

26. Roe, E., and Jones, R. J. Effects of topical chemoprophylaxis on transferable antibiotic resistance in burns. *Lancet* 1:109, 1972.

27. Seelig, M. The role of antibiotics in the pathogenesis of *Candida* infections. *Am. J. Med.* 40:887, 1966.

28. Shooter, R. A., Walker, K. A., Williams, V. R., Horgan, G. M., Parker, M. T., Asheshov, E. H., and Bullimore, J. F. Fecal carriage of *Pseudomonas aeruginosa* in hospital patients: Possible spread from patient to patient. *Lancet* 2:1331, 1966.

29. Thomsen, M. The burns unit in Copenhagen. VI. Infection rates. *Scand. J. Plast. Reconstr. Surg.* 4:53, 1970.

30. Thomsen, M. The burns unit in Copenhagen. VIII. Bacteriology. *Scand. J. Plast. Reconstr. Surg.* 4:126, 1970.

31. Williams, R., Chandler, J., and Orloff, J. J. *Candida* septicemia. *Arch. Surg.* 103:8, 1971.

32. Zaske, D. E., Sawchuk, R. J., Gerding, D. N., and Strate, R. G. Increased dosage requirements of gentamicin in burn patients. *J. Trauma* 16:284, 1976.

# 31 EPIDEMIOLOGY OF *STAPHYLOCOCCUS AUREUS* AND GROUP-A STREPTOCOCCI

Donald A. Goldmann

## HISTORICAL CONTEXT

A review of staphylococcal and streptococcal epidemiology leads directly to the historical roots of infection control. Epidemics of puerperal sepsis first suggested that hospital-acquired infections could be a major cause of morbidity and mortality and might require an organized approach to control. Modern-day hospital infection control programs have developed largely in response to outbreaks of staphylococcal disease in the 1950s and 1960s. Thus it is not surprising that the early infection control literature was dominated by studies concerning the epidemiology of streptococcal and staphylococcal infection, and a rich and varied literature it is. More recently other pathogens, particularly gram-negative bacilli, appeared to be supplanting gram-positive cocci on hospital wards, and the emphasis of the infection control literature changed accordingly. In the last few years, however, the field has come full circle as the emergence of methicillin-resistant *Staphylococcus aureus* has rekindled interest in staphylococcal epidemiology.

## EPIDEMIOLOGY OF GROUP-A STREPTOCOCCAL INFECTIONS

### Transmission

Although streptococci have been a scourge of obstetric wards and surgical services for centuries, group-A streptococcal nosocomial infection is relatively rare today. Group-A streptococci are recovered from less than 1 percent of all surgical wound infections in hospitals participating in the National Nosocomial Infections Study. Thus the occurrence of even one group-A streptococcal infection is reason for concern, and two or more cases in a short period of time should alert the infection control team that a full-scale epidemic investigation is warranted to determine the source of the outbreak.

Perhaps because streptococcal epidemics occur sporadically and unpredictably in hospitals, much of what we know about the transmission of group-A streptococci comes from a series of remarkably careful studies in military populations performed by Rammelkamp and Wannamaker and their colleagues [20,21, 25,34]. It had already been demonstrated that streptococcal infections could be spread by contact with infected cutaneous lesions. Furthermore, it had been established that streptococcal disease could be trans-

483

mitted to susceptible volunteers by inoculating the pharynx with secretions from patients with streptococcal pharyngitis. Thus it was known that transmission could occur by direct contact with the skin or secretions of infected individuals. The military studies were designed to answer two pivotal questions: (1) could streptococci be transmitted by droplet nuclei generated from the respiratory tract of infected or colonized individuals? and (2) could dust and other environmental fomites serve as reservoirs for the airborne spread of streptococci? These studies therefore addressed one of the fundamental issues in infection control—the relative importance of airborne and contact transmission of infection.

To obtain a rough assessment of the relative significance of airborne transmission via dust or droplet nuclei versus direct contact spread via large droplets or respiratory secretions, Rammelkamp's group studied the incidence of streptococcal disease among susceptible soldiers as a function of the distance of their bunks from the beds of colonized or infected recruits. If the risk of infection were increased only among soldiers whose bunks were very close to those of the index cases, the direct contact theory would be supported. On the other hand, if the incidence of infection were independent of location in the barracks, airborne spread would be the most likely explanation. In fact the risk of a recruit acquiring group-A streptococcal disease turned out to be inversely proportional to the distance between his bunk and that of a carrier (Fig. 31-1). At a distance of 30 feet, the acquisition rate was no higher than the background incidence of streptococcal infection among recruits in a control population. If the beds were located right next to each other, the risk more than tripled.

Although this study suggested that most streptococcal disease is transmitted by direct contact with large droplets, the possibility remained that some infections could be spread by contaminated dust or other environmental reservoirs. It seemed particularly important to rule out airborne transmission, since it was known that soldiers who carry streptococci in their throat or nose expel a prodigious number of bacteria onto their clothes, blankets, and other personal articles. Moreover, dust collected from barracks housing colonized or infected soldiers routinely yields enormous numbers of streptococci, and streptococci can remain viable in the environment for days. To find out whether contaminated dust or blankets could spread group-A streptococcal infections among susceptible individuals, the following experiments were performed.

The initial studies were made possible by a bizarre but routine military procedure. Each new recruit was

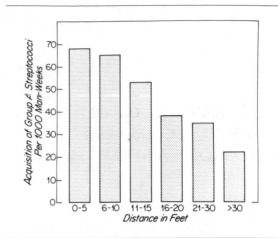

FIG. 31-1. Acquisition rates for group-A streptococci according to bed distance from the nearest carrier. (From Rammelkamp, C. H., Mortimer, E. A., Jr., and Wolinsky, E. Transmission of streptococcal and staphylococcal infections. *Ann. Intern. Med.* 60:756, 1964.)

issued a set of wool blankets that he used until he was transferred to another unit or was admitted to a hospital. Unless these blankets were grossly soiled, they were reissued to a new recruit without cleaning. Thus it was common practice to issue blankets heavily contaminated with streptococci to susceptible soldiers. In the clinical study, blankets were donated by 83 colonized soldiers, including 15 who had just been hospitalized because of streptococcal disease. The blankets were stored for either 24 hours or 6 days and then reissued. Recipients were followed closely for acquisition of streptococci and clinical disease. A control group received laundered blankets that were shown not to harbor streptococci. Acquisition rates turned out to be slightly lower in soldiers issued the contaminated blankets (Fig. 31-2), although this difference was not statistically significant. Six recruits who received a contaminated blanket did develop streptococcal disease, but in only two cases did the serotype isolated from the throat of the soldier match the serotype from the contaminated blanket.

In the next experiment, five volunteers were placed in a small enclosure while approximately 50 to 100 gm of contaminated dust were blown in. The soldiers were asked to sweep the floor for 10 minutes and to rest in a chair for 10 additional minutes. Air samples taken during the study period contained 100 to 1600 streptococci per cubic foot. It was obvious that the volunteers had inhaled a considerable amount of contaminated dust since dust could be seen easily in

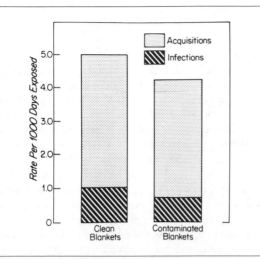

FIG. 31-2. Acquisition and infection rates with eight types of streptococci of men with clean or contaminated blankets. (From Perry, W. D., Siegel, A. C., Rammelkamp, C. H., et al. Transmission of group-A streptococci. I. The role of contaminated bedding. *Am. J. Epidemiol.* 66:89, 1957.)

mucus expelled by coughing or nose blowing for as long as six hours after exposure. No infections were observed, even though none of the volunteers had antibody to the streptococcal serotypes found in the dust.

To document additionally the inability of contaminated dust to transmit streptococcal infections, dust was sprinkled on the pharynx of 13 volunteers. Six other volunteers had dust containing 1,800 to 42,000 streptococci blown into the mouth. Streptococci could be recovered from the pharynx only transiently, and there were no infections.

Finally, 37 airmen were placed in a barracks while 50 to 150 gm of contaminated dust were blown into the room. The airmen lived in the barracks for 18 to 24 hours before sweeping it clean. No infections occurred.

These experiments suggest that airborne streptococci are not very infectious and rarely if ever produce pharyngitis in susceptible persons. Rather, it appears tha close contact with respiratory secretions or droplets from colonized or infected patients is critical for transmission to occur.

Although airborne streptococci seem to be virtually incapable of producing pharyngitis, it does not necessarily follow that streptococci falling into a wound from contaminated air would be unable to initiate a streptococcal wound infection. Only a few streptococcal surgical wound infection outbreaks have been

reported in the modern nosocomial infection literature, so data concerning the transmission of these infections are scarce. It is worth noting that the literature is virtually devoid of descriptions of outbreaks traced to a nasopharyngeal carrier on the medical or nursing staff. Rather, the reported epidemics have been attributed to vaginal or anal carriers among operating personnel. It is possible that this reflects a reporting bias: anal or vaginal carriers may be perceived as unusual and therefore worthy of documentation, whereas epidemics caused by nasopharyngeal carriers may be seen as too mundane to warrant publication. Regardless, the reported outbreaks provide reasonably strong evidence that streptococci may reach operative wounds via the air [1,26,27,31].

Streptococci have been recovered from settling plates placed in operating rooms occupied by carriers who were linked epidemiologically to the surgical wound infections, and it has been suggested that streptococci are aerosolized by flatus or shed during exercise. As emphasized previously, mere dissemination of bacteria into the environment does not prove that these organisms actually were responsible for the observed infections. However, the carriers in some of the reported outbreaks had no direct contact with the infected patients. It is not known why airborne streptococci disseminated by carriers apparently can cause wound infections but not pharyngitis. Perhaps the open surgical wound is much more susceptible than the pharynx to airborne streptococci.

### Epidemic Investigation

As soon as an outbreak of group-A streptococcal nosocomial infection is recognized, the infection control team should immediately initiate a search for a carrier on the hospital staff (see Chapter 5). Of course the possibility of person-to-person transmission via the hands of personnel cannot be ignored, particularly in the newborn nursery and on other nonsurgical services, but streptococcal operative wound infections are generally inoculated in the operating room and can virtually always be traced to a carrier. As noted above, the recent literature suggests that the carrier is more likely to be colonized with streptococci in the anus or vagina than in the throat, but the prudent epidemiologist will not begin an investigation by indiscriminately culturing a particular anatomic site. Rather, a formal epidemiologic investigation should be undertaken to ascertain whether infected patients had a significantly greater exposure to individual members of the staff. Personnel identified by the epidemiologic investigation should be questioned closely about recent sore throats, skin infections, or vaginal or anal symptomatology. Although perineal disseminators may be totally asymptomatic, most of the carriers reported in the literature have had mild symptoms that could easily be missed by a casual investigation. For example, the surgeon responsible for the outbreak reported by Richman and colleagues [26] suffered from external hemorrhoids to which he applied corticosteroid ointment daily. The circulating nurse implicated in the epidemic described by Berkelman and associates [1] had chronic bouts of diarrhea complicated by shallow perineal ulcers.

Isolation of streptococci from anal or vaginal cultures taken from someone who has been linked epidemiologically to an outbreak is strong evidence pointing to the source of the problem, particularly since group-A streptococci are rarely found at these sites in healthy adults. However, it is usually desirable to obtain additional laboratory data to prove that the carrier is colonized or infected with the same strain of group-A streptococci that was recovered from the nosocomial infections. First, serogrouping should be performed to confirm that the organism is indeed group A, since streptococci of groups B, C, and G can also be both $\beta$-hemolytic and bacitracin-susceptible. Serogrouping occasionally yields surprises. Goldmann and Breton [9] found that the $\beta$-hemolytic streptococci recovered from a small cluster of orthopedic infections were of group C, and group-C streptococci were subsequently isolated from the anus of a member of the surgical staff. If additional microbiologic confirmation is required, group-A streptococci can be classified by reference laboratories according to their M and T antigens and by their serum opacity reaction [18]. Occasionally the symptom complex caused by the streptococci is so distinctive that it is clear that all the cases are associated with the same strain. For example, Richman and coworkers [26] recognized their outbreak when two cases of scarlet fever occurred on the orthopedic service within a short period of time.

Nasopharyngeal carriers of group-A streptococci can usually be treated successfully with penicillin or erythromycin, but vaginal and anal carriers pose a greater challenge. Oral penicillin may fail to eradicate anal carriage. Oral vancomycin, which is not absorbed from the bowel, has been advocated as a supplement to penicillin therapy. Other regimens may have to be tried empirically. Even if it appears that anal or vaginal carriage has been eliminated, vigilance should be maintained. In one outbreak [1] vaginal carriage recurred with a different strain of *Streptococcus*, leading to a renewed outbreak of streptococcal disease that received considerable attention in the national press.

## EPIDEMIOLOGY OF *STAPHYLOCOCCUS AUREUS* NOSOCOMIAL INFECTIONS

### Transmission

Group-A streptococcal nosocomial infections gave the advocates of airborne and direct contact theories of transmission an excuse to have a skirmish; the epidemics of *S. aureus* infection in the 1950s and 1960s provided an opportunity to start a war. British investigators performed a vast number of detailed microbiologic studies to demonstrate how carriers of staphylococci could heavily contaminate the air. This extensive literature is not well known in the United States, and Americans with an interest in staphylococcal epidemiology have largely ignored the careful work of Hare, Ridley, Shooter, Nobel, Davies, Blowers, Lidwell, and many other British colleagues. Indeed, with the exception of Walter and Kundsin [35], who elaborated on the principles developed by Wells [37], the concept of airborne transmission of staphylococci has had few advocates in the United States. Among the many investigators who have sought to put airborne spread in perspective are Rammelkamp in the United States [25] and Williams in Great Britain [41]. The issues have been summarized succinctly by Williams, who wrote in 1966: "It is a characteristic of the airborne route of infection. . . . that whenever there is the possibility of aerial transfer there is almost always the possibility of transfer by other routes. This is perhaps especially true of the forms of staphylococcal infection that have been most extensively studied, namely, those occurring in hospitals" [41]. This debate between proponents of airborne and contact spread is of more than historical interest; those who enthusiastically promote the performance of surgery in laminar airflow operating rooms [16] or under ultraviolet lights [23] are merely reflecting their continued belief in the importance of airborne spread of staphylococci and other bacteria.

Since most of the outbreaks of staphylococcal disease in the 1950s and 1960s were caused by a single phage type (often referred to as 80/81, although these strains were generally also lysed by other phages), early British investigators naturally concentrated on identifying carriers who might be disseminating the epidemic strain on wards and in the operating room. Had they been faced with the kinds of outbreaks that we tend to see today, which generally are caused by more than one phage type, it is possible that their research would have focused on the role of the patient's endogenous staphylococcal flora and the importance of transmission of staphylococci on the hands of personnel. Instead, they doggedly pursued staphylococcal carriers and shedders.

The principal site of staphylococcal colonization is the anterior nares. If repeated cultures are performed, up to 80 percent of adults are found to harbor *S. aureus* in the nose at one time or another [38]. In most persons the carrier state is transient, but 20 to 40 percent of adults remain colonized for months or even years. Often the same strain remains in residence for prolonged periods of time, and if it is eradicated a new strain of *Staphylococcus* tends to take its place. The factors that predispose to stable colonization are unknown. Hospital personnel and patients tend to have higher colonization rates than persons outside the hospital environment, particularly during nosocomial staphylococcal outbreaks.

When it was recognized that hospital personnel could be carriers of staphylococci, some hospitals required routine nasal cultures of personnel so that they could be treated before they transmitted their staphylococci to patients. This practice never gained widespread acceptance for a number of reasons: (1) staphylococci are most efficiently liberated directly from the nose of a healthy carrier when air is forcefully expelled, creating a loud snorting sound [11]; (2) many carriers may be present on hospital wards without any infections occurring in patients; (3) even if there is an outbreak of staphylococcal infection on a ward, personnel who become nasal carriers may be innocent bystanders rather than the cause of the problem; (4) routine nasal cultures are expensive, and the resulting reams of data are generally uninterpretable; and (5) eradication of the nasal carrier state is difficult at best.

Although the nose itself probably is not important in the direct dispersal of staphylococci, shedding is more likely to occur in nasal carriers who have a heavy growth of staphylococci on nasal swab cultures [4]. Moreover, the nose is the site that supports colonization of the entire skin surface of most carriers. Eradication of staphylococci from the nose is generally accompanied by elimination of *S. aureus* from the entire body. In some staphylococcal carriers, however, the perineum is the primary site of colonization, and staphylococci may not be found on repeated cultures of the nose [38].

Both nasal and perineal carriers continually shed staphylococci on skin squames—aptly called "rafts" by British investigators. Because of their size, shape, and weight, these contaminated squames may be carried along on currents of air in the hospital, resulting in airborne dispersal of staphylococci (see Chapter 1). Fortunately, most colonized hospital personnel shed modest numbers of squames, and the relatively small number of staphylococci dispersed into the environment are quickly diluted by conventional air-han-

dling systems and washed away by standard housekeeping practices. A small percentage of colonized persons disperse much larger numbers of staphylococci into their immediate environment, however, and are referred to as "heavy shedders." High concentrations of airborne staphylococci may result, and staphylococci contaminating the environment may remain viable for long periods of time. Dermatologic disorders, such as eczema and psoriasis, clearly predispose to skin scaling and shedding, but in most cases the reason for heavy shedding is not readily apparent. Carriers who have a heavy growth of staphylococci on culture of the anterior nares tend to colonize body sites more readily than carriers with scant nasal colonization [40], but this observation does not explain the phenomenon of heavy shedding per se.

Some insight into staphylococcal shedding patterns has been gained by studying the dispersion of staphylococci from volunteers confined to a small enclosure. The test chamber may be either quite rudimentary or very elaborate (Fig. 31-3), but the basic principle involves collecting and quantitatively culturing the air in the chamber for staphylococci while the subject wears various types of clothing and moves about as instructed. Using this experimental technique, it has been demonstrated repeatedly that men are more likely than women to be heavy shedders [2, 12]. If a male heavy shedder is placed in a chamber clothed only in polyethylene or tightly woven cloth underpants, dispersal of staphylococci is practically eliminated, indicating that most bacteria are shed from the perineum of carriers [12]. However, subsequent studies demonstrated that there was little value in subjecting carriers to the discomfort of wearing plastic underwear since staphylococcus-bearing skin squames were liberated from other body sites when the shedder was fully clothed, presumably due to the friction of fabric against the skin [19]. Skin staphylococci readily escaped from street clothing and standard operating-room garb [30], but dispersion could be reduced somewhat by clothing made of tightly woven fabric [3]. Taken to the extreme, efforts to eliminate shedding in the operating room have led to the development of total body suits with individual ventilation and exhaust systems. Although these suits are a logical extension of the staphylococcal shedding experiments just mentioned, it is important to emphasize that such radical and costly measures should rarely be necessary since very few hospital personnel actually shed significant numbers of staphylococci. Nosocomial outbreaks of staphylococcal infection, whether in the operating room or on the wards, have seldom been traced to a shedder on the hospital staff or to environmental contamination. For this reason,

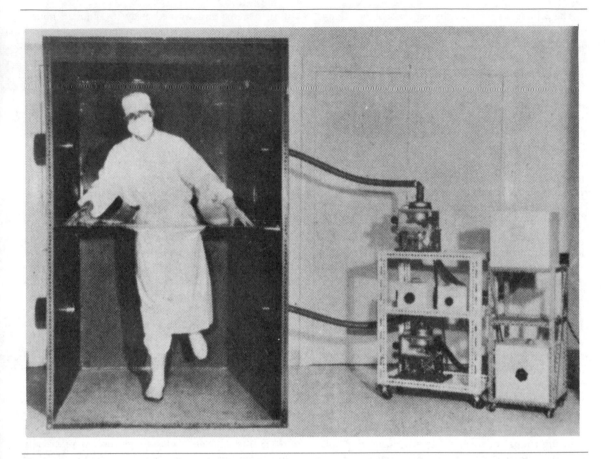

FIG. 31-3. Test chamber with door removed showing waistline division, air-inlet filters, and air-sampling equipment. (From Bethuen, D. W., et al. *Lancet* 27:4, 1965.)

most hospital epidemiologists discourage extreme measures to eliminate shedding and concentrate instead on good aseptic surgical technique, careful handwashing, and other measures designed to reduce direct contact transmission.

*Epidemic Investigation*
The key to detecting the presence of a staphylococcal shedder lies not in surveillance cultures, but in careful surveillance for nosocomial staphylococcal infections (see Chapter 4). If an increasing incidence of infection is noted, phage typing is requested to determine whether a single epidemic strain is responsible (see Chapter 7). Occasionally antibiotic resistance profiles may be helpful, particularly if the strains are resistant to methicillin or specific aminoglycosides. Aminoglycoside-resistant strains can be additionally characterized by plasmid analysis (see Chapter 12). When an epidemic strain is identified, personnel should not be cultured indiscriminately. Rather, the microbiologic investigation should focus on persons who ap-

pear to be associated epidemiologically with infected patients. These persons should be inspected carefully for signs of infection and questioned regarding recent infections or skin problems. Cultures of the nose, perineum, and sites of possible skin infection or dermatitis should be obtained, and any resulting *S. aureus* isolates should be phage-typed. Of course it is difficult to know whether a staff member is colonized because of his or her contact with infected patients or vice versa. Formal shedding studies are cumbersome unless the infection control team happens to be in possession of a shedding chamber, but a rough measure of the intensity of shedding can be obtained by quantitatively culturing the carrier's clothing, or by asking the carrier to exercise in a small, poorly ventilated room in which settling plates have been placed.

Staphylococcal epidemics caused by heavy shedders

definitely are the exception rather than the rule, and most hospital epidemiologists probably will never be confronted by such an outbreak. At some point in the workup of almost all staphylococcal outbreaks, however, the infection control team will be forced at least to consider the possibility that a carrier is at the heart of the problem. Understandably, staff members tend to become apprehensive as the investigation proceeds, particularly if the investigators seem to be interested in their contact with the infected patients. Thus it is extremely important to proceed in a frank and forthright manner, to eschew premature conclusions based on incomplete data, and to avoid capricious culturing forays (see Chapter 5). If the epidemiologic study clearly implicates one person, the infection control team must expect to encounter guilt and fear. A surgeon, for example, may have justifiable anxiety about possible litigation and damage to his or her career. Depending on the tact and skill of the investigators, the implicated staff member may be fully cooperative or may display the hostility and defensiveness of someone accused. It is essential for the infection control team to speak with one voice and to follow a rational plan of action that has been discussed fully with the directors of the appropriate services.

If the epidemiologic evidence is very strong, it is prudent to remove the presumed carrier from patient-care activities while cultures are obtained. If staphylococci are recovered on culture, treatment is generally begun before phage typing results are available, since reference laboratories may be unwilling to perform typing on an urgent basis. Since the carrier will usually want to return to work as soon as possible, the infection control team will be under considerable pressure to expedite treatment and issue work clearance. Unfortunately, there are no universally accepted criteria for determining when it is safe to send a carrier back to the wards. Certainly work should not be permitted until cultures of at least the nose and perineum are negative, although it must be realized that negative cultures while still undergoing therapy may indicate that the carrier state is suppressed but not eradicated. When treatment is concluded, therefore, the carrier should again be removed from work until follow-up cultures are performed and the results are available. Alternatively, some infection control teams may elect to take a more conservative approach and to suspend patient-care activities for the entire period of treatment until follow-up cultures are negative. In either case, careful surveillance should be carried out after the carrier returns to work, since the carrier state and shedding may recur. Some authorities advocate placing settling plates in the immediate

work environment for a period of several months as an additional, but untested, security measure.

A staggering array of systemic and topical antimicrobial regimens has been used in an effort to eradicate nasal carriage of staphylococci [38]. Systemic agents have included cephalosporins, semisynthetic penicillins, erythromycin, tetracycline, and fusidic acid. All these agents temporarily suppress the carrier state during therapy, but when adequate follow-up cultures are performed, staphylococci reappear in the majority of persons. Rifampin, given in combination with another systemic agent to retard emergence of rifampin resistance, is a promising alternative to previously available regimens [39] but requires additional testing. If the staphylococci acquire resistance to the antibiotic being administered, staphylococcal shedding may actually increase, perhaps reflecting suppression of competing nasal flora. Topical antimicrobials, including lysostaphin, gentamicin, neomycin, chlorhexidine, vancomycin, and bacitracin, have been equally unsuccessful in eradicating the carrier state.

In addition to administering antibiotics and applying antimicrobial ointments to the nose, the infection control team may try other strategies that have not been tested systematically in staphylococcal carriers. Although suppression of nasal staphylococci eventually leads to elimination of staphylococci from other sites, it seems logical to try to hasten this process along by prescribing daily hexachlorophene showers during the treatment period. This approach is especially appealing in carriers who have colonization of the perineum or other sites in the absence of nasal colonization. Since other members of the carrier's family may also be colonized with the outbreak strain, thus providing a reservoir for recolonization of the shedder, it seems reasonable to treat them if nasal cultures yield staphylococci. In refractory cases, it may be advisable to recommend laundering of clothing and bedding as well as a thorough housecleaning to reduce the burden of staphylococci in the household.

Rarely, persistent or recurrent shedding of staphylococci may jeopardize a health professional's career. When all else fails, it is reasonable to consider trying bacterial interference. In the 1960s Shinefield and coworkers [28] discovered that implantation of *S. aureus* strain 502A in the umbilicus and nose of neonates could prevent—or interfere with—colonization and infection with more virulent staphylococcal strains, such as phage type 80/81 (see discussion following). Bacterial interference with strain 502A was subsequently tried in adults suffering from recurrent furunculosis; it showed considerable success provided the carrier state was first suppressed with antibiotics [32]. Although the implantation of strain 502A in neonates occasionally resulted in 502A infections, this complication has not been noted in adults and presumably would not cause problems for otherwise healthy carriers. Of course it is unknown whether successfully recolonized carriers would become heavy shedders of 502A, which might then produce infections in susceptible patients.

The vast literature concerning staphylococcal carriers and shedders tends to obscure the fact that the patients themselves frequently serve as reservoirs for staphylococci, and that staphylococci are transmitted from patient to patient on the hands of personnel. Thus prompt isolation of patients with documented staphylococcal infections is extremely important. Drainage-secretion precautions (gown and gloves when touching infective material) recommended by the Centers for Disease Control [6] suffice for most infections (see Chapter 9). However, contact precautions (single room and mask when close to the patient, as well as gown and gloves) are often recommended for extensive cutaneous infections, such as infected burns and staphylococcal pneumonia. Fear of airborne transmission is at the root of the single-room recommendation—transmission by skin squames in the case of cutaneous infections and by droplet nuclei in the case of pneumonia. Indeed the rooms of these patients quickly become contaminated with large numbers of staphylococci, so a single room may be reasonable in spite of the apparent rarity of airborne spread. Masks are recommended to protect personnel from colonization with nosocomial staphylococcal strains. Again this may be logical, but even if a member of the attending staff is colonized it is exceedingly unlikely that he or she will become a heavy shedder.

### Staphylococcal Disease in the Nursery
Over the years the nursery has provided numerous opportunities to study the acquisition and transmission of *S. aureus*. Newborns seldom acquire staphylococci from their mothers at the time of birth but rapidly become colonized if they are admitted to a nursery where many babies are already colonized. The umbilicus is usually the initial site of colonization [13], but staphylococci quickly spread to the nose and other skin sites. Spread from infant to infant undoubtedly occurs via the hands of the doctors and nurses who care for colonized babies; airborne transmission almost never occurs. These principles, which are widely accepted today, were hotly disputed before Rammelkamp and his colleagues performed their classic

studies of nursery staphylococcal epidemiology in the 1950s [25].

Rammelkamp's studies were carried out in a small ward containing seven bassinets (Fig. 31-4). A baby known to be colonized with staphylococci was placed in one of these beds. Newborns were then admitted directly to the ward and placed either right next to the index baby or 4.5 or 11 feet away. The three nurses who cared for the noncolonized newborns wore double masks and washed their hands with hexachlorophene after each patient contact; the index patient was cared for by separate personnel. Nasal cultures were obtained from the babies every other day. Of the 91 newborns brought onto this special ward, only 3 became colonized with the index baby's staphylococcal strain. During two weeks of this study, one of the nurses, who was colonized with *S. aureus*, sat for eight hours per day in the chair between the two bassinets in position 1 (Fig. 31-4). Although she did not wear a mask, none of the babies in the room acquired her strain of *Staphylococcus*. This is hardly surprising since the probability that she was a heavy shedder was very small. More interesting results were obtained by allowing this nurse and another colonized nurse to handle the noncolonized babies in a routine fashion. Approximately 20 percent of the babies cared

FIG. 31-4. Results of exposure of infants to carriers of staphylococci. (From Rammelkamp, C. H., Mortimer, E. A., Jr., and Wolinsky, E. Transmission of streptococcal and staphylococcal infections. *Ann. Intern. Med.* 60:756, 1964.)

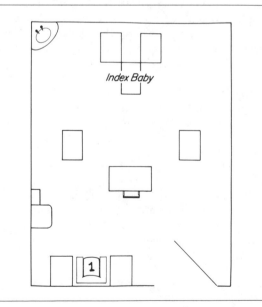

*Index Baby*

1

for by these nurses acquired their caretakers' staphylococcal strains.

A subsequent study revealed that these staphylococci were transferred to the babies by direct contact with organisms on the nurses' hands. In this study, the same two nurses and a third carrier handled 37 infants for ten minutes each through the ports of an Isolette incubator. Fifty-four percent of these babies acquired staphylococci from their nurse, as determined by phage typing of organisms recovered from cultures of the nose and umbilicus. This study demonstrated that so-called Isolettes do not effectively shield newborns from the most important route of staphylococcal cross-infection in the nursery—transmission via the hands.

Even in spacious, well-staffed nurseries, spread of staphylococci may be difficult to control (see Chapter 19). Transmission occurs much more readily in crowded, hectic nurseries. Staffing appears to be a particularly critical factor. Haley and Bregman [10] were able to demonstrate that clusters of staphylococcal infections occur significantly more frequently when patient-staff ratios are highest.

Control of nursery staphylococcal outbreaks is facilitated by prompt recognition, but detection is not always easy. Most well babies spend only two or three days in the nursery, so hospital-acquired staphylococcal infections may not become manifest clinically until the baby is at home. Moreover, the majority of infections are quite mild and do not require readmission to the hospital. Therefore, community pediatricians must be encouraged to report all staphylococcal infections to the infection control office. Seemingly trivial infections, such as pustulosis, omphalitis, circumcision wound infection, and conjunctivitis, have just as much epidemiologic significance as infant mastitis, septic arthritis, or osteomyelitis. Community obstetricians should also participate in the reporting process, since a single case of maternal mastitis may be the initial sign of a nursery problem.

In an effort to predict when a staphylococcal outbreak is imminent, some nurseries routinely monitor staphylococcal colonization rates by culturing the umbilicus and nose when babies are discharged. Such surveillance cultures are expensive and rarely helpful. Although there is a rough correlation between the number of babies colonized with staphylococci and the incidence of staphylococcal infections [8], many nurseries routinely find high colonization rates without experiencing an outbreak. Surveillance cultures may be more informative when performed to determine the impact of specific control measures on transmission of staphylococci in the nursery or to verify that a particular epidemic strain has been eradicated.

The severe outbreaks of staphylococcal disease that struck nurseries in the 1950s and 1960s led to the introduction of a variety of infection control measures. Perhaps the simplest and most effective was routine bathing of neonates with 3% hexachlorophene [7]. Hexachlorophene, with its excellent and persistent activity against gram-positive bacteria, drastically reduced staphylococcal colonization and subsequent infection. By eliminating the normal gram-positive cutaneous flora along with the *S. aureus*, hexachlorophene paved the way for colonization by nosocomial gram-negative bacilli such as *Pseudomonas* [17], but this appeared to be a minor disadvantage at the time since the importance of neonatal gram-negative infections had not yet been recognized. Of greater concern were reports of hexachlorophene toxicity. Patients with burns or extensive dermatitis who were bathed with large amounts of hexachlorophene developed a convulsive disorder associated with cystic degenerative changes in the white matter. Similar neuropathologic changes were seen in infant animal models treated with topical hexachlorophene [15], as well as in human neonates, particularly premature infants [24,29]. The human studies were retrospective, and there has been no convincing evidence that bathing full-term infants with hexachlorophene is hazardous. Nonetheless, in 1972 the Food and Drug Administration recommended against routine use of hexachlorophene in nurseries. This recommendation resulted in a sharp decline in hexachlorophene bathing and a significant increase in the number of outbreaks of nursery staphylococcal disease in the United States [14]. Balancing the potential risks and benefits of hexachlorophene use, it seems reasonable to avoid routine bathing of newborns. However, hexachlorophene may be a valuable adjunct to other control measures during a staphylococcal outbreak. As an added measure of safety, some investigators suggest diluting the hexachlorophene 1:4 or 1:5 and omitting baths for premature infants, although it is possible that these compromises could reduce efficacy.

Since the umbilicus is one of the initial sites of staphylococcal colonization in the neonate, a variety of topical antiseptics have been applied to it in an effort to abort colonization without washing the entire body surface. The basic validity of this approach has been demonstrated by studies using triple dye, an aqueous mixture of brilliant green, proflavine hemisulfate, and crystal violet [22], but the safety of this agent has not been evaluated extensively. Other topical antiseptics such as bacitracin, alcohol, and iodophors may be as effective as triple dye and more acceptable aesthetically, but none has been studied adequately.

When topical antiseptics and conventional infection control measures failed to halt epidemics of severe staphylococcal disease in the 1960s, Shinefield and colleagues [28] tried the more radical approach of bacterial interference (see previous discussion). In general, implantation of S. aureus 502A in the nose and umbilicus was highly successful in preventing colonization by nosocomial staphylococcal strains. Although this strategy fell into disfavor when epidemics of staphylococcal disease abated and reports of occasional serious disease due to 502A appeared, bacterial interference remains a possible approach in difficult-to-control nursery epidemics.

The emphasis in the medical literature on topical antiseptics and bacterial interference tends to obscure the fact that adherence to standard infection control routines is of primary importance in limiting the transmission of staphylococci in the nursery. Thorough hand-washing after contact with infants is imperative (see Chapter 9). Hexachlorophene may be used for routine hand-washing when a staphylococcal problem is recognized in the nursery but probably should be avoided at other times because its use may encourage transmission of gram-negative bacilli on the hands. Infants with staphylococcal infections should be placed on drainage-secretion precautions [6]. Consideration should be given to placing babies with intercurrent viral respiratory infections on full contact precautions (mask when close to the patient and single room required), because such babies tend to aerosolize large numbers of staphylococci into the environment—the so-called cloud baby phenomenon described by Eichenwald and colleagues [5]. Colonized babies may be segregated with infected babies in a separate part of the nursery and, if possible, assigned separate nursing staff (see Chapter 19). Some nursery staffs have elected to use a cohort admissions system to reduce the opportunity for person-to-person spread. In a typical system, all infants admitted in a 48-hour period are placed in a single room, and traffic of personnel from this room to other rooms is minimized or avoided altogether. After 48 hours, the room is closed to additional admissions and not reopened until the entire cohort has been discharged and the room cleaned thoroughly. Clearly the success of cohorting depends on the availability of separate nursery areas and sufficient personnel. In nurseries with inadequate facilities and insufficient staff, elegant cohorting and isolation arrangements may be

impossible, and the only way to cope with an escalating rate of staphylococcal infection is to close the units temporarily to new admissions (see Chap. 35).

Outbreaks of nursery staphylococcal disease frequently are caused by multiple phage types and presumably result from lapses in technique rather than the presence of a carrier on the obstetrical or neonatal staff. Unfortunately, as noted previously phage typing results are seldom available immediately, and pressure may mount to treat all nasal carriers. This is understandable and perhaps unavoidable since there may be few epidemiologic clues in a busy nursery in which most of the staff have contact with most of the infants. Since few nursery staphylococcal outbreaks have been shown to be caused by shedders on the staff, however, it may be more prudent to stress good aseptic technique and other standard infection control measures than to jump immediately to wholesale treatment of nasal carriers.

### Methicillin-Resistant S. Aureus

The emergence of methicillin-resistant S. aureus as a major nosocomial pathogen in recent years (see Chapter 10) has resulted in increased interest in staphylococcal epidemiology. Indeed, it is interesting to watch a new crop of epidemiologists reaffirming the observations made by their mentors two decades ago. In general, studies performed to date have yielded few surprises, but there is increasing evidence that methicillin-resistant staphylococci have a few epidemiologic idiosyncrasies [33]. Efforts to eradicate methicillin-resistant staphylococci from infected or colonized patients have been remarkably unsuccessful, particularly if the patient has a smoldering source, such as a colonized decubitus ulcer or chronic pulmonary infection. Once colonized or infected, patients may become lasting reservoirs for resistant strains. When these patients are readmitted to the hospital or transferred to other institutions, their staphylococci may be transmitted to other patients via the hands of personnel who are unaware of the dangerous organisms in their midst. Interinstitutional spread of methicillin-resistant staphylococci has been well documented, and transfer of colonized patients without proper warnings is inexcusable.

Although methicillin-resistant staphylococci appear to survive well on the skin, it is interesting to note that nasal colonization of hospital personnel has been quite uncommon [33]. In most studies, fewer than 2 percent of personnel who have been in contact with colonized or infected patients have developed nasal colonization. In one interhospital outbreak, however, transmission of infection was attributed to a rotating member of the surgical house staff who developed nasal colonization following a paronychia [36].

Once introduced into a hospital, methicillin-resistant staphylococci generally become endemic nosocomial pathogens. Very few institutions have been able to eradicate resistant organisms once they have become established. Not surprisingly, infection control programs have seen the methicillin-resistant staphylococcus as a major threat and have insisted on isolating infected or colonized patients. The Centers for Disease Control (CDC) revised *Guidelines for Isolation Precautions in Hospitals* [6] recommend contact isolation for patients colonized or infected with methicillin-resistant staphylococci at any site. This category of isolation is quite stringent, requiring a single room and a mask for those coming close to the patient, as well as gown and gloves on contact. Since some patients with methicillin-resistant staphylococci heavily contaminate their environment, these precautions seem reasonable. Alternatively, precautions can be tailored to fit the needs of individual patients, based on an estimation of the degree of staphylococcal shedding into the environment. For example, a single room and mask precautions may not be necessary for patients who are colonized only in the nose and on the skin, particularly if there is no dermatitis or wound and if settle plates or air-sampling reveal no airborne methicillin-resistant staphylococci. Some clinicians attempt to eradicate staphylococcal carriage in such patients if long-term hospitalization or transfer to a chronic-care facility is anticipated. Rifampin, usually given in combination with another antibiotic such as trimethoprim, may be effective in patients with straightforward nose and skin colonization with methicillin-resistant staphylococci (see p. 489).

## REFERENCES

1. Berkelman, R. L., Martin, D., Graham, D. R., Mowry, J., Freisem, R., Weber, J. A., Ho, J. L., and Allen, J. R. Streptococcal wound infections caused by a vaginal carrier. *J.A.M.A.* 247:2680, 1982.

2. Bethune, D. W., Blowers, R., Parker, M., and Pask, E. A. Dispersal of *Staphylococcus aureus* by patients and surgical staff. *Lancet* 1:480, 1965.

3. Blowers, R., and McCluskey, M. Design of operating room dress for surgeons. *Lancet* 2:681, 1965.

4. Ehrenkranz, N. J. Person-to-person transmission of *Staphylococcus aureus:* Quantitative characterization of nasal carriers spreading infection. *N. Engl. J. Med.* 271:225, 1964.

5. Eichenwald, H. F., Kotsevalov, O., and Fasco, L. A. The "cloud baby": An example of bacterial viral interactions. *Am. J. Dis. Child.* 100:161, 1960.

6. Garner, J. S., and Simmons, B. P. Guidelines for isolation precautions in hospitals. *Infect. Control* 4:247, 1983.

7. Gezon, H. M., Thompson, D. J., Rogers, K. D., Hatch, T. F., and Taylor, P. M. Hexachlorophene bathing in early infancy: Effect on staphylococcal disease and infection. *N. Engl. J. Med.* 270:379, 1964.

8. Gillespie, W. A., Simpson, K., and Tozer, R. C. Staphylococcal infection in maternity hospital: Epidemiology and control. *Lancet* 2:1075, 1958.

9. Goldmann, D. A., and Breton, S. J. Group-C streptococcal surgical wound infections transmitted by an anorectal and nasal carrier. *Pediatrics* 61:235, 1978.

10. Haley, R. W., and Bregman, D. A. The role of understaffing and overcrowding in recurrent outbreaks of staphylococcal infection in a neonatal special care unit. *J. Infect. Dis.* 145:875, 1982.

11. Hare, R., and Thomas, C. G. A. The transmission of *Staphylococcus aureus*. *Br. Med. J.* 2:840, 1956.

12. Hill, J., Howell, A., and Blowers, R. Effect of clothing on dispersal of *Staphylococcus aureus* by males and females. *Lancet* 2:1131, 1974.

13. Jellard, J. Umbilical cord as reservoir of infection in maternity hospital. *Br. Med. J.* 1:925, 1957.

14. Kaslow, R. A., Dixon, R. E., Martin, S. M., Mallison, G. F., Goldmann, D. A., Lindsey, J. D., II, Rhame, F. S., and Bennett, J. V. Staphylococcal disease related to hospital nursery bathing practices: A nationwide epidemiologic investigation. *Pediatrics* 51(Suppl.):418, 1973.

15. Kimbrough, R. D., and Gaines, T. B. Hexachlorophene effects on the rat brain: Study of high doses by light and electron microscopy. *Arch. Environ. Health* 23:114, 1971.

16. Lidwell, O. M., Lowbury, E. J. L., Whyte, W., Blowers, R., Stanley, S. J., and Lowe, D. Effect of ultraclean air in operating rooms on deep sepsis in the joint after total hip or knee replacement: A randomized study. *Br. Med. J.* 285:10, 1982.

17. Light, I. J., Sutherland, J. M., Cochran, M. L., and Scitorius, J. Ecological relationship between *Staphylococcus aureus* and *Pseudomonas* in a nursery population. *N. Engl. J. Med.* 278:1243, 1968.

18. Maxted, W. R., and Widdowson, J. P. The Protein Antigens of Group-A Streptococci. In Wannamaker, L. W., and Matsen, S. M. (Eds.), *Streptococci and Streptococcal Diseases.* New York: Academic, 1972, p. 251.

19. Mitchell, N. J., and Gamble, D. R. Clothing design for operating-room personnel. *Lancet* 2:1133, 1974.

20. Perry, W. D., Siegel, A. C., and Rammelkamp, C. H., Jr. Transmission of group-A streptococci. II. The role of contaminated dust. *Am. J. Hyg.* 66:96, 1957.

21. Perry, W. D., Siegel, A. C., Rammelkamp, C. H., Jr., Wannamaker, L. W., and Marple, E. C. Transmission of group-A streptococci. I. The role of contaminated bedding. *Am. J. Hyg.* 66:85, 1957.

22. Pildes, R. S., Ramamurthy, R. S., and Vidyasagar, D. Effect of triple dye on staphylococcal colonization in the newborn infant. *J. Pediatr.* 82:907, 1973.

23. Postoperative wound infections: The influence of ultraviolet irradiation of the operating room and of various other factors. *Ann. Surg.* 160(Suppl.):1, 1964.

24. Powell, H., Swarner, O., Gluck, L., and Lampert, P. Hexachlorophene myelinopathy in premature infants. *J. Pediatr.* 82:976, 1973.

25. Rammelkamp, C. H., Jr., Mortimer, E. A. Jr., and Wolinsky, E. Transmission of streptococcal and staphylococcal infections. *Ann. Intern. Med.* 60:753, 1964.

26. Richman, D. D., Breton, S. J., and Goldmann, D. A. Scarlet fever and group-A streptococcal surgical wound infection traced to an anal carrier. *J. Pediatr.* 90:387, 1977.

27. Schaffner, W., Lefkowitz, L. B., and Goodman, J. S. Hospital outbreak of infections with group-A streptococci traced to an asymptomatic anal carrier. *N. Engl. J. Med.* 280:1224, 1969.

28. Shinefield, H. R., Ribble, J. C., and Boris, M. Bacterial interference between strains of *Staphylococcus aureus,* 1960–1970. *Am. J. Dis. Child.* 121:148, 1971.

29. Shuman, R. M., Leech, R. W., and Alvord, E. C. Neurotoxicity of hexachlorophene in the human. I. A clinicopathologic study of 248 children. *Pediatrics* 54:689, 1974.

30. Speers, R., Jr., Bernard, H., O'Grady, F., and Shooter, R. A. Increased dispersal of skin bacteria into the air after shower baths. *Lancet* 1:478, 1965.

31. Stamm, W. E., Feeley, J. C., and Facklam, R. R. Wound infections due to group-A *Streptococcus* traced to a vaginal carrier. *J. Infect. Dis.* 138:287, 1978.

32. Steele, R. W. Recurrent staphylococcal infection in families. *Arch. Dermatol.* 116:189, 1980.

33. Thompson, R. L., Cabezudo, I., and Wenzel, R. P. Epidemiology of nosocomial infections caused by methicillin-resistant *Staphylococcus aureus. Ann. Intern. Med.* 97:309, 1982.

34. Wannamaker, L. W. The Epidemiology of Streptococcal Infections. In McCarthy, M. (Ed.), *Streptococcal Infections.* New York: Columbia University Press, 1954, p. 157.

35. Walter, C. W., and Kundsin, R. B. The airborne component of wound contamination and infection. *Arch. Surg.* 107:588, 1973.

36. Ward, T. T., Winn, R. E., Hartstein, A. I., and Sewell, D. L. Observations relating to an interhospital outbreak of methicillin-resistant *Staphylococcus aureus:* Role of antimicrobial therapy in infection control. *Infect. Control* 2:453, 1981.

37. Wells, W. F. *Airborne Contagion and Air Hygiene.* Cambridge, Mass.: Harvard University Press, 1955.

38. Wheat, L. J., Kohler, R. B., and White, A. Treatment of Nasal Carriers of Coagulase-Positive Staphylococci. In Maibach, H. I., and Aly, R. (Eds.), *Skin Microbiology: Relevance to Clinical Infection.* New York: Springer, 1981, pp. 50–58.

39. Wheat, L. J., Kohler, R. B., White, A. L., and White, A. Effect of rifampin on nasal carriers of staphylococci. *J. Infect. Dis.* 144:177, 1981.

40. White, A. Relation between quantitative nasal cultures and dissemination of staphylococci *J. Lab. Clin. Med.* 58:273, 1961.

41. Williams, R. E. O. Epidemiology of airborne staphylococcal infection. *Bacteriol. Rev.* 30:660, 1966.

# 32 INFECTIOUS GASTROENTERITIS

Herbert L. DuPont
Bruce S. Ribner

Microorganisms that cause outbreaks of foodborne illness in the community also have the potential for causing similar events in hospitalized patients. However, certain forms of gastroenteritis—such as that caused by foodborne toxins of *Clostridium perfringens*, *Clostridium botulinum*, *Staphylococcus aureus*, and *Bacillus cereus*, as well as that produced by the ingestion of food contaminated with group-A streptococci and *Vibrio parahaemolyticus*—have not been recognized to be transmissible from person to person within the hospital. The control of these diseases in the hospital depends on safe food-handling practices as discussed in Chapter 16, and such forms of gastroenteritis are not considered additionally in this chapter.

Infectious or communicable gastroenteritis caused by *Salmonella* other than *S. typhi*, *Escherichia coli*, *Shigella*, and rotavirus receive primary attention in this chapter. In addition, the chapter separately addresses *Clostridium difficile* (an agent with a high degree of communicability that causes antibiotic-associated colitis), *Yersinia enterocolitica* (an agent that has produced communicable nosocomial infections involving the gastrointestinal tract), staphylococcal enterocolitis (a noncommunicable form of nosocomial gastroenteritis), and necrotizing enterocolitis (a disease of uncertain, possibly infectious cause). Nosocomial transmission of *Vibrio cholerae* has produced nosocomial infectious gastroenteritis in areas endemic for this disease, but the agent will not be discussed here because of the rarity of endemic cases in the United States.

Infectious gastroenteritis differs from most other hospital-associated infections, which characteristically result from endogenous organisms in persons with markedly altered resistance. Enteric infections caused by the agents just mentioned are nearly always exogenously acquired, often occur in clusters or epidemics, and are usually due to the introduction of a virulent organism through the ingestion of contaminated foods or medications, through short-term carriers among patients and hospital staff, or through patient-to-patient transmission on the hands of personnel. Although host factors such as age and debility are important, healthy patients and hospital personnel also are frequently involved in outbreaks of these infections.

## INCIDENCE

The true incidence of nosocomial infectious gastroenteritis is not known. Such enteric infections are markedly underreported in the United States because of the common occurrence of noninfectious diarrhea among hospital patients and personnel with its attendant complacency, and because laboratory techniques are significantly limited in delineating some bacterial and viral pathogens. The absence of well-defined criteria for the diagnosis of nosocomial gastrointestinal infection has contributed additionally to the underreporting of this condition. It has also resulted in variation in the criteria used by different infection control practitioners, with subsequent disparities in the rates reported by different institutions.

The National Nosocomial Infections Study (see Chapter 24) for the period January 1980 through December 1982 found enteric nosocomial infections to represent only the twelfth most frequent nosocomial infection reported. Of all patients discharged from the 82 reporting hospitals, only 371, or 0.01 percent, experienced nosocomial gastrointestinal infections. This represented only 0.3 percent of all nosocomial infections detected. Of these 371 patients with gastrointestinal infections, 99 did not have a pathogen isolated and 82 had no diagnostic tests performed. Of the remaining 190 patients, 40 had *C. difficile* identified as the causative pathogen, while 35 had nontyphoidal *Salmonella* species, 11 had *E. coli,* 5 had rotaviruses, and 2 had *Shigella* isolated. An additional 97 isolates were contained within 39 categories of pathogens, including fungal, bacterial, and viral agents.

There were marked differences among services in the rate of nosocomial enteric infections. The highest rates were found on pediatric (0.04 percent) and newborn (0.03 percent) services, reflecting the underlying susceptibility of the hosts and the inherent difficulty in controlling diseases spread primarily through the fecal-oral route in the younger age groups. Medical and surgical services had intermediate rates (0.008 percent) of infection, and obstetric and gynecologic services had the lowest rates of enteric nosocomial infection (0.002 percent).

Causative pathogens also tended to differ by service. Among newborn patients *Salmonella* species were the most frequently identified pathogen. On pediatric services viral pathogens tended to be most common. Medical patients were primarily infected by *C. difficile* and *Salmonella* species. Surgical patients were far more likely to have *C. difficile* isolated than any other pathogen.

## DIAGNOSTIC CRITERIA

### Clinical and Microbiologic Criteria
There is wide variation in the clinical symptoms experienced by patients with these enteric infections.

Some patients become asymptomatic excreters of a potential pathogen, while others show varying forms of diarrheal disease. Organisms that invade the intestinal epithelial lining usually elicit a febrile response in addition to causing diarrhea. In infections with pathogens that invade the colonic mucosa primarily, symptoms of colitis occur, including urgency, tenesmus, and bloody, mucoid stools (dysentery). Diarrhea or loose stools in a patient with unexplained fever should be diagnosed as infectious gastroenteritis, regardless of culture results for bacterial pathogens. When diarrhea or loose stools occur in an afebrile patient or in a febrile patient whose fever has other likely causes, the identification of a recognized pathogen in stools or by serologic testing is necessary for this diagnosis.

Diarrhea of noninfectious origin—such as that caused by cathartics, inflammatory diseases of the gastrointestinal tract, and surgical resections and anastomoses—should be carefully differentiated from the diarrhea of infectious gastroenteritis. Alterations in the gastrointestinal flora because of antibiotic administration are commonly associated with diarrhea; such cases of diarrhea should not be reported as gastroenteritis unless enterocolitis occurs, in which event they should be reported as noninfectious gastroenteritis.

### Classification of Infections
Diarrhea with onset after admission that is associated with a positive culture for organisms recognized as causative of infectious gastroenteritis should be regarded as a nosocomial infection. The interval between the time of admission and the onset of clinical symptoms must be greater than the known incubation period for that agent (see subsequent sections) unless there are associated cases among other hospital patients or personnel. Alternatively, nosocomial infections may be diagnosed if a stool culture obtained shortly before or just after admission is negative for the pathogen in question and the pathogen is subsequently cultured from the patient.

## PREDISPOSING HOST FACTORS

### Defective Gastric Defenses
There is evidence to indicate that gastric acid plays an important role in the defense against ingested organisms. The bactericidal action of stomach acid greatly reduces or eradicates ingested organisms and thus reduces the inoculum of organisms that subsequently reaches the intestine. Physiologic or pathologic achlorhydria, which is most common in premature infants and elderly patients, may underlie the increased risks of certain enteric infections seen in

these groups. Although unstudied, variations in gastric acidity may also partly determine which person becomes ill following the ingestion of a contaminated common vehicle. Antacid use has been shown to greatly facilitate colonization of the intestine with vaccine strains of *Shigella* and to increase the frequency of gastrointestinal acquisition of nosocomial strains of aerobic gram-negative rods. It is probable that anticholinergic medications act similarly. Persons with histories of gastric resection and vagotomy are known to be at higher risk of acquiring cholera than normal persons.

The time during which ingested substances are in contact with gastric acid may be important. Water without food tends to traverse the stomach more rapidly than solid food, reaching the neutralizing secretions of the duodenum more rapidly. The inoculum of organisms required to produce infection is probably reduced when transmitted by water. Waterborne outbreaks of salmonellosis have occurred when low concentrations of the organism are present, whereas large numbers are usually required for foodborne transmission of these organisms.

### Antibiotic Therapy

The oral or systemic administration of antibiotics to which an epidemic strain is resistant greatly facilitates cross-colonization and infection (see Chapter 11). These effects presumably occur because of a reduction in the competitive interference of normal, sensitive flora against the ingested strains, which in effect reduces the inoculum required for establishment of the pathogen. The continued administration of the drug following acquisition of the pathogen may permit the selective outgrowth of the pathogen and result in much greater concentrations of the organism in the feces than might otherwise occur. The chances of transmission and risk of disease are thereby increased.

Antibiotic administration may also predispose certain patients to diarrhea by enteric pathogens sensitive to the antibiotic. This may occur during therapy or shortly after termination of the antibiotic. In such cases, the pathogen is able to replicate more rapidly than the suppressed normal flora, reaching concentrations not normally achievable when the normal flora is at pretherapy levels. These elevated concentrations may lead to enteritis and increase the risk of cross-infection in a manner similar to that of resistant pathogens.

### Crowding and Staffing Factors

A ratio of staff to patients that is insufficient encourages infractions in hand-washing and isolation techniques, especially in critical-care areas. Even careful hand-washing, however, is sometimes ineffective in removing gram-negative rods from the hands, and a slight but definite risk of transmitting organisms by direct contact with successive patients exists even after hand-washing. Thus inordinately low staff-to-patient ratios may lead to increased risk of cross-colonization and infection. Crowding of patients also increases the risk of cross-infection. While crowding of patients is often accompanied by insufficiencies in staff, it may be independently important in that it increases the risk of indirect contact spread through environmental sources, especially in nurseries.

## GENERAL CONTROL MEASURES

In controlling the spread of enteric infections within the hospital environment, a number of general measures can be taken regardless of the specific pathogen responsible. The most important mode of cross-infection for enteric bacterial pathogens in the hospital is usually the fecal-oral route, where indirect contact spread of organisms occurs from patient to patient on the hands of personnel. Outbreaks may also result from the ingestion of contaminated food, medication, or test materials.

### Hand-washing

Since the most important means of spread of enteric bacterial pathogens is via hand transfer, effective hand-washing is among the most important measures to prevent disease transmission. Although it is unlikely that all potentially pathogenic microorganisms can be removed by hand-washing, the level of contamination can be reduced, in most cases, below that necessary for disease transmission among healthy children and adults. Among debilitated patients or newborn infants, the required dose of enteropathogens needed to produce disease probably is substantially lower. In areas housing such patients, additional measures for the prevention of cross-infection may be required.

### Surveillance

It is necessary to have an alert hospital surveillance program that continually reviews clinical patterns of infection in the hospital and evaluates bacteriologic reports from the diagnostic microbiology laboratory. Such a program is often instrumental in defining the extent of an outbreak before it has reached serious proportions and represents the foundation of an effective infection control program (see Chapter 4).

Surveillance must include hospital personnel, particularly food handlers, as well as patients. One important means of minimizing nosocomial diarrheal disease is to establish an effective personnel health service. Food handlers, nurses, and ancillary staff having direct contact with patients should be encouraged to communicate with the personnel health service when an episode of acute gastroenteritis occurs among themselves. Stool cultures should be performed, and the ill person removed from work until culture results and the clinical course of the disease can be evaluated (see Chapter 2).

All personnel with an acute diarrheal illness should be removed from food handling and direct patient contact until the diarrhea has resolved. If stool cultures reveal the presence of an infectious pathogen, the employees should not return to food handling and should not care for patients in high-risk areas (e.g., intensive care units, newborn nurseries, transplant services) until two stool specimens obtained a minimum of 24 hours apart are negative for the pathogen. Employees from whom an enteric pathogen is isolated may care for patients in low-risk areas on resolution of diarrhea and before elimination of the infectious pathogen from the stool. However, such employees must be instructed to pay careful attention to thorough hand-washing after use of toilet facilities.

No infant born of a mother with diarrhea or with stool cultures positive for an enteric pathogen should be admitted to the nursery ward. Any infant with loose, watery, or bloody diarrhea should be handled with enteric precautions until a noninfectious cause for the diarrhea has been identified.

Similarly, patients of all ages admitted to the hospital with unexplained diarrhea, or developing diarrhea while in the hospital, should be placed in enteric isolation until an infectious etiology has been ruled out. Historically such patients have led to well-documented outbreaks of nosocomial gastroenteritis by both bacterial and viral agents.

### Use of Antispasmodic Drugs

Treatment of acute gastroenteritis with drugs to decrease the motility of the gut and produce symptomatic relief of diarrhea may have undesirable side-effects in select patients. In persons with severe illness due to invasive pathogens (*Shigella, Salmonella*, and *Campylobacter*), worsening of clinical illness may result. Drugs such as diphenoxylate hydrochloride and atropine (Lomotil) should be avoided in the treatment of nosocomial gastroenteritis when patients have significant fever or are passing bloody mucoid stools.

### Prompt Investigation of Cases

The occurrence of two or more cases of nosocomial infectious gastroenteritis caused by the same organism within a few weeks should prompt a review of the exposures common to these cases (see Chapter 5). Case-control investigations are less likely to establish the source of infections conclusively when the number of cases is small, and microbiologic sampling of foods, medications, or equipment common to cases may be of special value in this circumstance. Culture surveys of other patients hospitalized in the same patient-care areas as those with cases of disease and of employees working in these areas may identify asymptomatically infected persons, and such persons should be included with symptomatic patients for purposes of epidemiologically establishing possible sources.

Hospital outbreaks of enteric disease may be caused by patients or hospital personnel who are short-term carriers of a specific pathogen. Comparison of the exposures of cases and controls to specific personnel (see Chapter 5) and culture surveys of hospital personnel and asymptomatic patients may help to identify the carriers responsible for such outbreaks. Occasionally environmental factors—such as air, dust, bedside tables, thermometers, and mattresses—are important in contact spread. If a common vehicle such as food, contaminated equipment, or contaminated oral medication or test solution can be identified, its removal or disinfection may assist in terminating the outbreak.

Secondary cases often occur following disease outbreaks caused by contaminated vehicles, and the chance of epidemiologically identifying responsible sources may be improved in such situations by focusing attention on early cases and on patients whose illnesses seem unlikely to have derived from person-to-person spread.

On occasion epidemiologic studies may indicate that the central kitchen is responsible for the dissemination of a bacterial pathogen. Removal of food handlers with recent diarrheal disease or kitchen personnel with positive cultures on culture surveys may result in termination of the epidemic. In the vast majority of instances, however, foodborne outbreaks of nosocomial gastroenteritis derive from inadequate handling of products from food-producing animals, rather than from contamination of the food by food handlers.

### Outbreak Management

During an epidemic it is usually helpful to isolate patients with asymptomatic as well as symptomatic infections in separate rooms with separate lavatory facilities. Enteric precautions are necessary in which glove-gown-stool precautions should be undertaken.

In nurseries in which enteric isolation of individual cases is not possible, cohort systems (see Chapter 19) should be employed during an epidemic to minimize the risk of cross-infection. Successful control of outbreaks sometimes requires repeated culture surveys coupled with a special type of cohorting. Infants who are ill or colonized with the epidemic organism can sometimes be grouped together into a cohort that is physically separated from noninfected infants. Personnel caring for these infants must not care for noninfected infants, and no equipment should be shared between the two groups. Only milk packaged in sterile containers should be used, common equipment shared among babies should be removed, and infants should be confined to their own bassinets or Isolettes. To prevent additional spread of infection, infants born outside the hospital should not enter the nursery during an epidemic of diarrhea. Unnecessary contact with babies by hospital personnel or contact between infants should be eliminated during epidemics. An adequate sized nursing and hospital staff is especially important in the management of nursery epidemics.

Not only is it important to isolate patients with active disease as long as indicated (see Chapter 9), but infected patients should be discharged from the hospital as soon as their condition allows them to be managed at home. Uninfected patients should also be discharged as soon as possible from hospital areas experiencing an outbreak of nosocomial gastroenteritis.

## SALMONELLA INFECTIONS

### General Aspects

CLINICAL AND MICROBIOLOGIC FEATURES In salmonellosis fever, nausea, and vomiting develop and are followed shortly thereafter by abdominal pain and watery diarrhea. Frequently mucous strands can be found in stool specimens, while gross blood is found in slightly less than 10 percent of cases. In shigellosis and *Campylobacter* enteritis, stools are bloody in approximately 50 percent of cases.

Newborns have a predisposition to disease. Approximately 50 percent of exposed infants develop illness once a case is introduced into a nursery. *Salmonella* infections in infants may result in septicemia or disseminated focal disease such as meningitis, abscesses, or osteomyelitis. They may also result in asymptomatic intestinal colonization. Some neonates become persistent intestinal carriers of salmonellae, and their cultures may remain positive for over a year.

Others who are at high risk are the aged and the debilitated. Patients with malignant disease have an unexplained predisposition to the development of sal-

monellosis, and the frequency of bloodstream invasion in such patients is quite high. Persons housed in nursing homes represent another segment of hospitalized patients in whom explosive outbreaks may occur with high fatality rates.

In a patient with acute gastroenteritis, the isolation of *Salmonella* from a stool culture is generally sufficient to establish the cause of the disease. This is true because of the relatively high degree of pathogenicity of these enteric bacteria, plus the fact that long-term carriers are unusual.

THERAPY Antimicrobial therapy has been shown in numerous studies to prolong the intestinal excretion of salmonellae. Most of these studies have involved oral therapy, and recent data with ampicillin suggest that parenteral administration may be more effective. Mild, uncomplicated *Salmonella* gastroenteritis should not be treated. However, in patients in whom bloodstream invasion occurs—most commonly newborn or extremely debilitated patients, particularly those with malignant disease—antimicrobials often are instrumental in recovery from infection and may be lifesaving. In general ampicillin, chloramphenicol, and trimethoprim-sulfamethoxazole provide the most effective therapy.

In addition to prolonging the period of excretion of the infecting strains, the administration of antimicrobial agents may, on occasion, make the clinical infection more severe or cause clinical relapse of infection when the drug administered is one to which the infecting strain is resistant. Antimicrobial therapy also increases the chance of the infecting organism acquiring additional resistances (see Chapter 11).

### Epidemiologic Considerations

CLASSIFICATION OF INFECTIONS Incubation periods for salmonellosis vary from 6 to 72 hours. The incubation period varies inversely with the size of the infecting dose. Patients with positive cultures and an onset of gastroenteritis 72 hours or more after admission should be considered to have nosocomial infections. Persons with onsets within 6 to 72 hours of admission should be considered to have nosocomial infections only when epidemiologic evidence makes nosocomial acquisition likely. Isolation of salmonellae from a patient's stool in the absence of clinical symptoms of gastroenteritis should be reported as a nosocomial infection only if previous stool cultures during hospitalization were negative.

TRANSMISSIBILITY While person-to-person transmission of *Salmonella* strains is unusual among healthy persons outside of the hospital environment, these organisms can be transmitted on the hands of health-care workers or by person-to-person spread among the aged, debilitated, or newborn patients in the hospital setting. Communicability of this organism from patients to hospital personnel or to community contacts is uncommon because larger doses are necessary to infect healthy persons and the precautions routinely used by hospitals in managing patients with gastroenteritis.

INCIDENCE  About 50 percent of infections occur on the newborn service or pediatric floor. The remaining cases occur mainly among patients on the surgical or medical services.

Since 1963 the Centers for Disease Control has maintained nationwide surveillance of salmonellosis. Between 1963 and 1972, 112, or 28 percent, of the total reported outbreaks occurred in institutions (hospitals, nursing homes, and custodial institutions) [1]. Approximately 3500 cases were reported in these outbreaks among institutionalized populations, which represented 13 percent of the total reported cases. In 1979, 13 percent of reported outbreaks in the United States occurred in institutions. These outbreaks accounted for only 1.4 percent of all the cases occurring in outbreaks that year. The average institutional outbreak involved 6 patients, contrasting with the average noninstitutional outbreak, which involved 69 cases.

SOURCES AND MODES OF ACQUISITION  The nosocomial salmonellosis that occurs in the pediatric population, especially in newborns, is characteristically spread from person to person. The organism is typically introduced into the nursery by an infant who acquired the infection from its mother at delivery, but it can also be introduced by a carrier among the personnel or, more rarely, through foods and medications. Spread from infant to infant within the nursery then occurs on the hands of personnel. Fomites may be important in cross-infections, and persistence of the organism in dust and other environmental sites is sometimes responsible for perpetuating an outbreak. Epidemics have been traced to contaminated delivery-room resuscitation equipment and the water baths used for heating infant formula [28]. A commercially distributed, special nutritional formula that contained contaminated egg albumin has caused *Salmonella infantis* outbreaks when administered orally or by tube feeding. Outbreaks of *S. kotthus,* a serotype that has a tendency to be excreted from infected bovine mammary glands, have been traced to contamination of human breast milk collected to feed premature infants. Although it is unclear whether the

breast milk was primarily or secondarily contaminated, inadequate storage and handling of the milk following collection allowed the organisms to proliferate to significant levels.

Outbreaks in nurseries are generally smaller than those commonly seen in nosocomial *Salmonella* infections in adults [1]. In adult infections, a common source can usually be incriminated. The common source may be previously contaminated, raw or undercooked meats or other products of food-producing animals (e.g., eggs or milk products), or food that has become contaminated after cooking because of organisms on equipment or surfaces in the kitchen [14,19]. Food contaminated by a short-term *Salmonella* carrier working in the kitchen is much less commonly responsible. On occasion a medication contaminated by *Salmonella* serves as a vehicle, especially medications containing enzymes and hormones of animal origin (e.g., pepsin, bile salts, vitamins, and endocrine gland extracts). Sporadic cases caused by intermittent exposure to infrequently used medications can produce a puzzling epidemiologic problem that requires a careful case-control approach for its solution (see Chapter 5).

In homes for the aged, epidemics often are initiated by the ingestion of contaminated food, and the epidemic may be perpetuated by cross-infection among debilitated patients by means of health-care workers.

Less frequent sources of *Salmonella* infections include yeast, dried coconut, carmine dye, and inadequately disinfected equipment used on successive patients (e.g., Gomco suction and endoscopy equipment).

The specific serotype of *Salmonella* may provide a clue to the source. Some serotypes commonly infecting humans such as *S. typhimurium* derive from a variety of sources, but some have strong associations with particular sources that may suggest likely sources of human infection: *S. choleraesuis* is associated with porcine sources; *S. cubana,* with cochineal insects used to prepare carmine dye; *S. dublin,* with bovines; *S. pullorum,* with poultry sources; and so on. Many additional correlations exist between serotypes and sources among the 2000 or so serotypes of *Salmonella.* Establishing that several different cases were caused by the same serotype may also be of value in suggesting a common source of infection. This is especially true when cases have occurred sporadically in different hospital areas. For this reason, all *Salmonella* isolated from nosocomial infections should be serotyped.

CONTROL  Safe food-handling practices as outlined in Chapter 16 are especially important in the prevention of nosocomial salmonellosis. In addition to the prompt epidemiologic identification and removal of common sources and implementation of the measures mentioned earlier in this chapter concerning outbreak management, thorough cleaning and disinfection of fomites and environmental surfaces in a nursery after discharge of infected infants is also important (see Chapter 19). Prophylactic antibiotics are contraindicated as a control measure.

## ESCHERICHIA COLI INFECTIONS

### General Aspects

CLINICAL AND MICROBIOLOGIC FEATURES  *Escherichia coli* can produce gastroenteritis in children and adults by several different mechanisms. Strains that produce keratoconjunctivitis in the guinea pig eye (the Sereny test) tend to produce an invasive *Shigella*-like illness. Disease caused by such strains appears rare in the United States, although a large common-source outbreak caused by contaminated imported French cheese has been documented. Loose, watery diarrhea, usually mild but sometimes severe and resembling that of cholera, is associated with certain strains of *E. coli* that produce enterotoxin. Both heat-labile and heat-stable toxins have been identified. Disease can be produced by either type of enterotoxin, although both are frequently produced by the same strain. Enterotoxin-producing strains appear to be major causes of travelers' diarrhea and are frequent causes of gastroenteritis in developing countries. Enterotoxigenic *E. coli* occasionally causes outbreaks of diarrhea in the United States, characteristically traced to contaminated food or water. One large hospital nursery outbreak has been reported [26].

E. coli belonging to the classic enteropathogenic serotypes (EPEC) appears to produce disease by mechanisms not yet fully understood, since disease caused by such strains cannot be explained on the basis of the previously described mechanisms [9]. In more recent studies, a high percentage of EPEC strains have been enteroadherent, as seen in HEp-2 tissue culture cells [3]. EPEC has previously been considered a common cause of nursery outbreaks, which sometimes were explosive with high attack rates and fulminating clinical courses [29]. Reports of such outbreaks are almost unheard of in the United States in recent years. Undoubtedly this relates at least in part to the decreasing availability of serotyping procedures in hospital diagnostic laboratories over the past ten years. During any hospital outbreak of diarrhea, particularly when it has occurred in the newborn nursery, EPEC should be considered in the differential diagnosis.

The clinical expression of EPEC infections varies considerably—probably as a result of differences in pathogenic mechanisms—from minimal, watery diarrhea to fulminating disease with septicemia. There appears to be a great deal of unexplained variability even among strains with the same serotype, and occasional outbreaks occur in newborn nurseries in which attack rates exceed 50 percent and mortality rates are high. EPEC outbreaks are almost totally confined to newborn nurseries, and infants and young children, especially those less than two years of age, appear to be primarily at risk. The association of EPEC disease with the very young may not be totally correct, because such strains are generally considered to occur only in children less than four years of age with diarrhea and appropriate laboratory tests are only performed in this age group.

Clinicians should be aware that the laboratory procedures used to determine the serogroup of isolates have certain deficiencies. Non-EPEC serotypes that cross-react with EPEC serotypes can agglutinate in pooled test sera to give a false-positive test result that can be identified only by complete serotyping. Also, *E. coli* implicated in cases of diarrhea not belonging to EPEC serotypes and not producing the conventional heat-labile or heat-stable toxins of enterotoxigenic *E. coli* may be enteroadherent in HEp-2 cells.

THERAPY  Disease caused by enterotoxin-producing strains of *E. coli* was shown to respond favorably to antibiotics to which the organisms are sensitive in studies conducted in Mexico, an area where such disease has a high endemic frequency. The duration and severity of diarrhea are reduced by such therapy. Although controlled trials have not been conducted, antibiotic therapy would appear to be indicated on clinical grounds for *Shigella*-like disease caused by invasive strains, and responses comparable to those seen in treatment of shigellosis (see *Shigella* Infections below) might be anticipated.

The value of antimicrobial therapy for EPEC disease is presently controversial, and part of this controversy doubtlessly derives from the difficulty in ensuring that the EPEC was the cause of the gastroenteritis. In some instances, a lack of response to antibiotics may have occurred because EPEC isolated from cases was an incidental finding in disease caused by other agents, especially rotaviruses. When gastroenteritis occurs in a premature or full-term nursery and a causative role can be ascribed to EPEC, uncontrolled trials suggest that orally administered gentamicin, colistin, or neomycin for a one-week course of treatment may be of value. Systemic antibiotics should also be given to all such patients if sepsis occurs in one or more affected infants. Since the isolation of EPEC in a sporadic case of gastroenteritis is presently of uncertain value in establishing the cause, such laboratory findings offer little or no guidance to the clinician; the clinical severity of the illness is the only factor useful in deciding whether to institute treatment.

### Epidemiologic Considerations

CLASSIFICATION OF INFECTIONS    Incubation periods for EPEC disease are commonly 24 to 48 hours, but they may occasionally be much longer. Children with onset of gastroenteritis 48 hours or longer after admission should be considered to have nosocomial infections, as well as all infants who develop EPEC disease at any time during hospitalization following birth in the hospital. Isolation of an enteropathogenic serotype of E. coli from a stool culture in the absence of clinical symptoms of gastroenteritis should not be reported as an infection. For consistency in surveillance, an infection should be reported when an EPEC strain is isolated from a patient with gastroenteritis in whom no other recognized pathogen is identified.

TRANSMISSIBILITY    The only known population at risk to develop nosocomial enteric infections due to E. coli strains are newborn infants and young children. When an enteropathogenic E. coli strain is introduced into a nursery, hospital personnel and community contacts may become asymptomatic carriers of the organism, especially during an episode of infantile diarrhea, and may serve as an important epidemiologic link in the transmission of the disease to the newborns [24]. Enteric disease caused by enterotoxigenic E. coli is only very rarely transmitted from person to person.

INCIDENCE    EPEC is third to Clostridium difficile and Salmonella as a reported cause of infectious nosocomial diarrheal disease caused by bacteria in the NNIS data. At the present time, these organisms are identified by serotype analysis. Outbreaks ascribed to EPEC have become much less common over the last decade. Only five outbreaks caused by such strains were investigated by the CDC since 1970 (see Chapter 24). Only a few outbreaks of nosocomial disease caused by enterotoxin-producing E. coli have been reported [26].

SOURCES AND MODES OF ACQUISITION    The most common source of EPEC infections is an infected child admitted to a newborn nursery or readmitted to a pediatric ward. The infant may have acquired the infection at the time of delivery or may have acquired the organism during hospitalization and had an onset of enteric disease in the early days after discharge from the hospital. Secondary spread of the infecting strain to other infants occurs on the hands of hospital personnel or from articles in the nursery that have been contaminated with the strain during an epidemic. Pharyngeal colonization of infants is common during epidemics, and although unproved, may be an important intermediate step in producing disease in some cases. Proliferation of organisms at this site might produce an inoculum that is capable of establishing infection in the lower gastrointestinal tract.

Epidemics of infantile EPEC diarrhea have occurred at times when the organism can be detected in the dust and fomites within the hospital environment. Asymptomatic carriers are probably important as a cause of epidemics among susceptible infants and include antepartum mothers, hospital staff, or other children without disease. During periods of infantile diarrhea outbreaks, approximately 5 percent of pediatric patients without intestinal infection and up to one-third of antepartum women have been shown to harbor EPEC organisms in their stool. Outbreaks in the nursery usually follow the introduction of a new serotype of EPEC by a newly admitted, infected child or by colonized hospital personnel. The infecting strain is transmitted among children, generally on the hands of attendants or through articles and equipment in communal use.

A single large, protracted nosocomial outbreak caused by a strain of E. coli that produced heat-stable enterotoxin and did not belong to a recognized enteropathogenic serotype has been reported [26]. The disease appears to have been transmitted by means of cross-contamination of oral feedings. The epidemic strain did not colonize or produce disease in adults despite its presence in multiple environmental sites. Illness was mild and characterized by three to five days of watery diarrhea without pus or blood in the stools. Prophylactic oral colistin, to which the multiply drug-resistant strain was sensitive, was ineffective in preventing acquisition. Antibiotic resistance and enterotoxin production were co-linked on a transmissible plasmid of the epidemic strain [31].

CONTROL    Control measures mentioned earlier in this chapter and elsewhere [12] can be helpful in curtailing an EPEC outbreak. Such measures are not indicated, however, unless a causative role can be ascribed to an EPEC strain on the basis of the previously outlined criteria. Colonization of infants with an EPEC strain in the absence of enteric disease attributable to the strain is not an indication for control measures.

Enterotoxigenic E. coli strains are thought to be

transmitted mainly by food and water, and prevention of disease from these sources can be accomplished by proper food handling and chlorination of water supplies.

## SHIGELLA INFECTIONS

### General Aspects

CLINICAL AND MICROBIOLOGIC FEATURES Shigellosis, or bacillary dysentery, often represents a distinct clinical entity. Fever develops in 50 percent of the patients, and mucus with or without blood can be documented in the stool within one or two days after the onset of diarrhea. Patients are usually more toxic and symptoms more severe with this form of enteric infection than with others.

When newborns are infected by a *Shigella* strain, the mortality rate is higher, and complications (e.g., intestinal perforation and septicemia) develop with a higher frequency than in other common bacterial causes of gastroenteritis [11,32]. Although there is some evidence that breast-fed infants show an increased resistance to *Shigella*, nearly all hosts are extremely susceptible to these organisms.

*Shigella sonnei* and *S. flexneri* are the species principally responsible for disease in the United States. *S. sonnei* strains can be differentiated from each other by colicin typing, and *S. flexneri* strains by serotyping. Clinicians should be aware that *Salmonella-Shigella* agar, a popular medium for stool cultures in many clinical laboratories, is toxic to many *S. flexneri* strains. For optimal recovery of strains, specimens should not be placed in holding or transport media but should be plated directly onto blood or xylose, lysine, and deoxycholate (XLD) agar as soon as possible after collection.

THERAPY In bacillary dysentery, appropriate antimicrobial agents are clearly beneficial in decreasing the excretion of the pathogenic shigellae and improving clinical symptoms. Trimethoprim-sulfamethoxazole (TMP/SMX) is the treatment of choice for all cases of shigellosis when susceptibility testing is not available. A 3- to 5-day course is generally adequate. The dose for children is TMP 10 mg/kg/day plus SMX 50 mg/kg/day in two divided doses; for adults it is TMP 160 mg and SMX 800 mg twice a day. When strains are known to be susceptible, ampicillin can be used in children (100 mg/kg/day, in divided doses, IV or PO), and tetracycline (2.5 gm in a single oral dose) can be given to adults. Antibiotic therapy is associated with the emergence of multiple drug resistance in originally sensitive strains, which is presumably caused by R-factor transfer from endogenous gastrointestinal flora. Thus patients should remain in enteric isolation until posttreatment cultures are negative.

### Epidemiologic Considerations

CLASSIFICATION OF INFECTIONS Incubation periods for shigellosis vary from one to six days. Patients with positive cultures and an onset of gastroenteritis 24 hours or more after admission should be considered to have nosocomial infections unless epidemiologic evidence of community-acquired infection is found (e.g., occurrence of shigellosis in family contacts before the onset of the patient's illness). Isolation of shigellae from a patient's stool in the absence of clinical symptoms of gastroenteritis should be reported as a nosocomial infection only if previous stool cultures during hospitalization were negative or isolation occurs during a documented hospital outbreak due to the recovered strain.

TRANSMISSIBILITY While *Shigella* strains represent the most potentially communicable of the bacterial pathogens, the striking clinical disease often helps the physician spot the illness early and promptly institute effective therapy and control measures. Such early detection partly explains the usual, surprising lack of spread within the normal hospital environment. Other patients, hospital personnel, and community contacts appear to be at risk of developing bacillary dysentery when exposed to an infected patient because of the very low dose of organisms (less than $10^3$) necessary to produce disease.

INCIDENCE Although any hospitalized patient is at risk of developing nosocomial shigellosis when a case is admitted, only rarely do outbreaks occur [27]. The only population at high risk is that of persons housed in residential institutions for the mentally retarded, where crowded living conditions, poor personal hygiene, and overworked nursing personnel all appear to be important causes of serious outbreaks.

Shigellosis was reported in only two of the 371 patients with nosocomial enteric infections during the 1980–82 period in NNIS data. How many of the 10,000 to 13,000 cases of shigellosis reported each year in the United States come from hospitals is unknown. Between 10 and 20 percent of the cases of shigellosis reported each year, however, come from residential institutions for the retarded.

SOURCES AND MODES OF ACQUISITION The usual sources are short-term carriers of the disease who are either ill or in the convalescent stages of their disease.

In custodial institutions, a few long-term carriers may be present and may serve as an important reservoir. Long-term carriage, however, is rare. On occasion, shigellosis develops when contaminated food is ingested that was prepared by a person who was carrying the organism following an episode of disease. The vast majority of cases, however, are secondary to person-to-person spread of infection. Infections are rarely acquired by indirect-contact spread from inanimate environmental sources, since these organisms are only able to survive for short periods in the environment.

CONTROL   Antibiotics are effective in eradicating sensitive strains of *Shigella* from the gastrointestinal tract, but as noted earlier, infecting strains have a propensity to develop multiple drug resistance in response to therapy. Thus treatment of culture-positive patients should be coupled with individual enteric isolation procedures for each patient to prevent the potential emergence and continued spread of a strain that has acquired additional antibiotic resistances (see Chapter 9).

Streptomycin-dependent vaccine strains of *Shigella* have been tested as a control measure in mental institutions with high endemic rates of shigellosis. The duration of protection is short, however, as it is with the natural disease. Furthermore, multiple oral doses of vaccine must be given, vaccine strains can be transmitted to nonimmunized patients, and there is a potential risk of reversion of such strains to streptomycin-independent virulent organisms.

## VIRAL GASTROENTERITIS

Recent studies have spotlighted the major role of rotaviruses as a cause of gastroenteritis [6,25]. Nosocomial transmission of rotavirus [4,8,25], hepatitis A virus [10], and adenoviruses [8] has been documented. Nosocomial adenoviral gastroenteritis, which appears to be much less frequent than rotaviral infections and produces milder clinical illness, will not be discussed in this section.

While the transmission of hepatitis A infection is rare in the hospital setting, it is mentioned here because of the occasional presentation of patients with unexplained diarrhea caused by hepatitis A (see Chapter 35). The diarrhea may antedate the onset of clinical jaundice by several days, or jaundice may not occur. The high titers of infectious virus in the stool during the preicteric phase make these patients excellent sources of hepatitis A nosocomial infection in settings in which good hand-washing practices are not followed.

### Rotavirus Infections

INCIDENCE   Rotaviruses are probably the most frequent enteric pathogens found in persons less than five years of age in the United States (see Chapter 35). Prospective studies of hospital nurseries have shown nosocomial infection rates of 33 to 49 percent, with 8 to 28 percent of the infected babies experiencing clinical diarrheal disease [2,22]. Infection rates tend to follow the seasonal pattern observed in the general community, with peak incidence in the winter and lowest incidence in the summer. An outbreak of rotavirus infection has also been reported in hospitalized geriatric patients [20].

CLINICAL ASPECTS   Illness begins with the sudden onset of fever and vomiting and continues with moderate or severe watery diarrhea that generally lasts about five days. Dehydration severe enough to require hospitalization is frequent among patients with community-acquired illness. The causative agent can be identified either by the direct demonstration of virus by electron microscopy in stool or rectal swabs of patients or by serologic means. A commercially available kit for accurate and rapid identification of rotavirus is currently available (Rotazyme test). It makes use of a modified enzyme-linked immunoadsorbent assay. Nosocomial rotavirus gastroenteritis should be strongly suspected in a child one year of age or younger who develops nonbacterial gastroenteritis 72 hours or more after admission.

SOURCES AND MODES OF ACQUISITION   Rotavirus disease appears to be highly infectious, and it can be spread from patients with disease to susceptible persons by direct contact. The peak incidence in winter suggests that droplet spread from the upper respiratory tract may play a role in transmission, since respiratory spread is a common feature of most illnesses with seasonal peaks in the winter. Nosocomial transmission probably occurs indirectly from patient to patient on the hands of hospital personnel as well as by person-to-person spread from patients with disease to susceptible persons when such patients are inadequately isolated. Hospital personnel are generally immune and do not carry the virus.

PREVENTION AND CONTROL   Rotaviruses are highly immunogenic, and serologic studies indicate a high level of acquired immunity in persons over five years of age. These findings raise the possibility of ultimate control of the disease by vaccine. Children with nosocomial nonbacterial gastroenteritis should be placed on enteric precautions; although not currently recommended in Centers for Disease Control (CDC) guidelines, consideration should be given to the use of masks on older children to prevent potential droplet transmission when they are transported out of the isolation area.

## OTHER GASTROINTESTINAL DISEASES

### Clostridium difficile colitis

It is now known that *C. difficile* is the major cause of antibiotic-associated colitis. The organism is rapidly and efficiently transmitted to hospital staff and patients unless strict enteric precautions are carried out.

INCIDENCE Of the 371 nosocomial gastrointestinal infections reported by NNIS hospitals in 1980–82, *C. difficile* was the most common agent identified, occurring in 40 patients. Considering the difficulty in diagnosing *C. difficile* colitis, this incidence undoubtedly reflects only a portion of the cases that occurred.

CLINICAL ASPECTS Characteristically, *C. difficile* produces profuse diarrhea and fever that are temporally related to a course of antimicrobial therapy. Stools often contain mucus and blood. The major antibiotics associated with the disease are clindamycin, cephalosporins, and ampicillin. Nearly all commonly used antibiotics have been implicated in the process. Diagnosis is based on the clinical setting (diarrhea in a patient receiving an antibiotic) plus the use of other diagnostic tests and procedures. Sigmoidoscopy reveals the characteristic white or yellow plaques of pseudomembranous colitis. The toxin of *C. difficile* is demonstrated by documenting a histotoxic effect in tissue culture cells that is inhibited by clostridial antitoxin.

Therapy includes stopping the antibiotic, administering fluids and electrolytes, and instituting chemotherapy. For mild cases cholestyramine 1 gm qid is given PO until diarrhea is controlled, while moderate-to-severe cases are treated with vancomycin 125 mg qid PO for 10 to 14 days. Relapses occur in as many as 20 percent of cases. Vancomycin should be used again in such patients. For patients too ill to be given an oral drug, metronidazole can be given intravenously.

SOURCES AND MODES OF ACQUISITION *C. difficile* can be cultured from the vagina of many women and from the intestine of most newborns. About 4 percent of adults harbor the organism in the lower intestinal tract. When persons receive an antibiotic to which *C. difficile* is resistant, the organism is encouraged to proliferate. Pseudomembranous enterocolitis results when the *C. difficile* grows to certain levels and produces high concentrations of toxin. The organism is highly communicable and can be transmitted from those affected to others despite its previous absence in the gut. Spread by cross-contamination occurs in the hospital among patients of all ages when cases of antibiotic-associated colitis occur [16,17,21]. The environment becomes contaminated and toxigenic *C. difficile* spores may remain viable on environmental surfaces for periods of up to five months [16].

PREVENTION AND CONTROL In addition to therapy, affected patients should be placed under enteric precautions (see Chapter 9). Because of spore formation, the environment should be considered contaminated. Careful cleansing of the room and environmental objects should be undertaken after discharge of the patient. Sigmoidoscopes and colonoscopes need to be carefully sterilized. It is not known whether special methods of environmental cleaning need to be developed for the causative organism.

### Staphylococcal Enterocolitis

In contrast to *C. difficile* colitis, staphylococcal enterocolitis is not transmissible from person to person; however, the disease may be an important source from which nosocomial strains of *Staphylococcus aureus* can be transmitted.

INCIDENCE The true incidence of such infections is unknown. Since the appreciation of *C. difficile* as the common cause of pseudomembranous colitis, the reported incidence of staphylococcal enterocolitis has dropped sharply. Only nine cases were reported in the NNIS reporting period of 1980–82. The proportion of such cases in which *S. aureus* was truly the causative agent of gastroenteritis is uncertain. Staphylococcal enterocolitis occurs sporadically, and epidemics have not been reported.

CLINICAL ASPECTS In certain hosts in whom there is impaired resistance due to surgery, antimicrobial therapy, alcoholism, or diabetes mellitus, staphylococci may grow to large numbers in the intestinal tract and be responsible for morphologic damage to the intestinal mucosa that results in diarrhea and fever of varying severity. Intestinal involvement varies widely from minimal and self-limiting "enteritis" to fulminating "pseudomembranous enterocolitis" [5]. Patients with enteritis have diarrhea of a variable nature, often mild and watery, and may have low-grade fever, but they are not extremely toxic. Pseudomembranous enterocolitis frequently presents with fulminating and dehydrating diarrhea; bloody, mucoid stools; fever; leukocytosis; and toxemia. The entire colon may be involved with the disease, and there may be some involvement of the small intestine. Mortality rates in such patients are high and range from 10 to 50 percent.

The diagnosis is established by documenting abundant polymorphonuclear leukocytes and sheets of gram-positive cocci in stool specimens, which on subsequent culture grow large numbers of *S. aureus*. Proctologic examination shows a white membrane that reflects areas of mucosal necrosis in those with pseudomembranous enterocolitis.

Patients should receive replacement fluid and electrolytes. Both oral vancomycin [15] and fecal retention enemas containing stool flora from a healthy person (the latter may have only historical significance) have been shown to be of value in treating patients with serious forms of the disease. Parenteral semisynthetic penicillinase-resistant penicillin treatment is advised for very toxic patients.

SOURCES AND MODES OF ACQUISITION    *S. aureus* can be cultured from the stool of about 10 percent of normal adults, but it is normally present in small numbers. Intestinal carriage of these organisms is twice as common in hospitalized patients as in persons outside the hospital environment. Most strains that cause staphylococcal enterocolitis are multiply drug resistant, and some have been shown to produce an enterotoxin in laboratory tests. Pathogenic strains are probably acquired mainly from nosocomial sources, and they proliferate to displace normal flora when antibiotics to which they are resistant are administered. Staphylococcal enterotoxin is probably not important in the pathogenesis of the disease, since otherwise clinically identical pseudomembranous enterocolitis occurs following infection with nonenterotoxigenic strains. Destruction or replacement of normal endogenous flora is probably the principal inciting factor.

PREVENTION AND CONTROL    Prompt cessation of previously administered antibiotics and administration of oral vancomycin to patients with more serious staphylococcal enteritis may prevent the disease from progressing to pseudomembranous enterocolitis. Large numbers of *S. aureus* are often disseminated from patients with these diseases, and strict, rather than enteric, isolation procedures should be considered (see Chapter 9).

*Neonatal Necrotizing Enterocolitis*

Neonatal necrotizing enterocolitis (NEC) is a frequently fatal disease that usually affects sick premature infants. The disease is characterized by ischemic necrosis of the gastrointestinal tract and intramural gas (pneumatosis intestinalis), and it frequently results in intestinal perforation, peritonitis, and septicemia. NEC frequently occurs in epidemics within nurseries, which suggests an infectious cause. Three pathogenetic factors underlie the occurrence of disease: injury to the intestinal mucosa, due to relative ischemia from stress in newborns or other causes; the presence of intraluminal enteric bacteria; and enteral feedings that provide a metabolic substrate for the bacteria.

Most reports of NEC have not incriminated a particular bacterium as a cause of the disease, perhaps indicating that many strains of gram-negative bacteria may be involved in its pathogenesis. However, a particular strain of bacteria prevalent in the nursery has occasionally been linked with an epidemic of NEC [13]. The prophylactic use of systemic antibiotics does not prevent colonization of an infant's gastrointestinal tract with gram-negative bacteria, and most studies have shown no efficacy of such drugs in preventing NEC. The prophylactic use of oral kanamycin, however, appeared effective in one study [7].

Additional studies of sporadic and epidemic NEC cases, including careful aerobic and anaerobic culture studies of cases and controls, should assist in determining the role of microorganisms in this disease.

*Yersinia enterocolitica Infections*

Nosocomial transmission of infections caused by *Yersinia enterocolitica* has rarely been reported, but it probably occurs far more commonly than reports indicate. The organism, a gram-negative rod, can easily be misidentified, and sometimes prolonged cold enrichment is required for its optimal recovery from stool specimens. Early symptoms are usually those of fever and acute enterocolitis, and the abdominal pains are frequently so similar to those of appendicitis that appendectomies are performed. Mesenteric adenitis or ileitis is generally discovered. A wide variety of other features can be seen, including arthritis and erythema nodosum. Although the reservoir of the organism is in animals, person-to-person transmission also occurs, and nosocomial transmission has sometimes involved personnel [30].

A more deliberate search for this organism in otherwise unexplained nosocomial gastroenteritis outbreaks should be encouraged when clinical features suggest it is a possible causative agent. In addition to culture studies, serologic tests may be helpful in establishing the diagnosis of infection with this organism.

*Other Pathogens*

In addition to the enteropathogens discussed, outbreaks of nosocomial gastroenteritis have been caused by *Citrobacter freundii* [23], *Listeria monocytogenes* [18], and a variety of other agents. Although *Campylobacter jejuni* was encountered only rarely in the NNIS survey, it will undoubtedly prove to be an important cause of nosocomial gastroenteritis now that the organism can be readily identified in hospital laboratories. The ability of pathogens other than those normally associated with gastrointestinal disease to produce gastroenteritis must be remembered when evaluating an outbreak. One should be cautious not to dismiss lightly unusual pathogens recovered from stool cultures during the investigation of nosocomial enterocolitis.

# REFERENCES

1. Baine, W. B., Gangarosa, E. J., Bennett, J. V., and Barker, W. H., Jr. Institutional salmonellosis. *J. Infect. Dis.* 128:357, 1973.
2. Chrystie, I. L., Albrey, M. B., and Crewe, E. B. Rotavirus infections of neonates. *Lancet* 2:1149, 1977.
3. Cravioto, A., Gross, R. J., Scotland, S. M., and Rowe, B. An adhesive factor found in strains of *Escherichia coli* belonging to the traditional infantile enteropathogenic serotypes. *Curr. Microbiol.* 3:95, 1979.
4. Davidson, G. P., Bishop, R. F., Townley, R. R. W., Holmes, I. H., and Ruck, B. J. Importance of a new virus in acute sporadic enteritis in children. *Lancet* 1:242, 1975.
5. Dearing, W. H., Baggenstoss, A. H., and Weed, L. A. Studies on the relationship of *Staphylococcus aureus* to pseudomembranous enterocolitis and to postantibiotic enteritis. *Gastroenterology* 38:441, 1960.
6. Echeverria, P., Blacklow, N. R., and Smith, D. H. Role of heat-labile toxigenic *Escherichia coli* and reovirus-like agent in diarrhea in Boston children. *Lancet* 2:1113, 1975.
7. Egan, E. A., Mantilla, G., Nelson, R. M., and Eitzman, D. V. A prospective controlled trial of oral kanamycin in the prevention of neonatal necrotizing enterocolitis. *J. Pediatr.* 89:467, 1976.
8. Flewett, T. H., Boyden, A. S., and Davies, H.

Epidemic viral enteritis in a long-stay children's ward. *Lancet* 1:4, 1975.
9. Goldschmidt, M. C., and DuPont, H. L. Enteropathogenic *Escherichia coli:* Lack of correlation of serotype with pathogenicity. *J. Infect. Dis.* 133:153, 1976.
10. Goodman, R. A., Carder, C. C., Allen, J. R., Orenstein, W. A., and Finton, R. J. Nosocomial hepatitis A transmission by an adult patient with diarrhea. *Am. J. Med.* 73:220, 1982.
11. Haltalin, K. C. Neonatal shigellosis: Report of 16 cases and review of the literature. *Am. J. Dis. Child.* 114:603, 1967.
12. Harris, A. H., Yankauer, A., Greene, D. C., Coleman, M. B., and Phaneuf, M. Y. Control of epidemic diarrhea of the newborn in hospital nurseries and pediatric wards. *Ann. N.Y. Acad. Sci.* 66:118, 1956.
13. Hill, H. R., Hunt, C. E., and Matsen, J. M. Nosocomial colonization with *Klebsiella,* type 26, in a neonatal intensive care unit associated with an outbreak of sepsis, meningitis, and necrotizing enterocolitis. *J. Pediatr.* 85:415, 1974.
14. Hirsch, W., Sapiro-Hirsch, R., Berger, A., Winter, S. T., Mayer, G., and Merzbach, D. *Salmonella edinburg* infection in children: A protracted hospital epidemic due to a multiple drug resistant strain. *Lancet* 2:828, 1965.
15. Khan, M. Y., and Hall, W. H. Staphylococcal enterocolitis: Treatment with oral vancomycin. *Ann. Intern. Med.* 65:1, 1966.
16. Kim, K.-H., Fekety, R., Batta, D. H., Brown, D., Cudmore, M., Silva, J., Jr., and Waters, D. Isolation of *Clostridium difficile* from the environment and contacts of patients with antibiotic-associated colitis. *J. Infect. Dis.* 143:42, 1981.
17. Larson, H. E., Barclay, F. E., Honour, P., and Hill, I. D. Epidemiology of *Clostridium difficile* in infants. *J. Infect. Dis.* 146:727, 1982.
18. Larsson, S., Cederberg, A., Ivarsson, S., Svanberg, L., and Cronberg, S. *Listeria monocytogenes* causing hospital-acquired enterocolitis and meningitis in newborn infants. *Br. Med. J.* 2:473, 1978.
19. Mackerras, I. M., and Mackerras, M. J. An epidemic of infantile gastro-enteritis in Queensland caused by *Salmonella bovis-morbificans* (Basenau). *J. Hyg.* (Camb.) 47:166, 1949.
20. Marrie, T. J., Lee, S. H., Faulkner, R. S., Ethier, J., and Young, C. H. Rotavirus infection in a geriatric population. *Arch. Intern. Med.* 142:313, 1982.

21. Mulligan, M. E., George, W. L., Rolfe, R. D., and Finegold, S. M. Epidemiological aspects of *Clostridium difficile*–induced diarrhea and colitis. *Am. J. Clin. Nutr.* 33:2533, 1980.

22. Murphy, A. M., Albrey, M. B., and Crewe, E. B. Rotavirus infections of neonates. *Lancet* 2:1149, 1978.

23. Parida, S. N., Verma, I. C., Deb, M., and Bhujwala, R. A. An outbreak of diarrhea due to *Citrobacter freundii* in a neonatal special care nursery. *Indian J. Pediatr.* 47, 81, 1980.

24. Rogers, K. B. The spread of infantile gastroenteritis in a cubicled ward. *J. Hyg.* (Lond.) 49:40, 1951.

25. Ryder, R. W., McGowan, J. E., Hatch, M. H., and Palmer, E. L. Reovirus-like agent as a cause of nosocomial diarrhea in infants. *J. Pediatr.* 90:698, 1977.

26. Ryder, R. W., Wachsmuth, I. K., Buxton, A. E., Evans, D. G., DuPont, H. L., Mason, E., and Barrett, F. F. Infantile diarrhea produced by heat-stable enterotoxigenic *Escherichia coli*. *N. Engl.*

J. Med. 295:849, 1976.

27. Salzman, T. C., Scher, C. D., and Moss, R. Shigellae with transferable drug resistance: Outbreak in a nursery for premature infants. *J. Pediatr.* 71:21, 1967.

28. Schroeder, S. A., Aserkoff, R., and Brachman, P. S. Epidemic salmonellosis in hospitals and institutions: A five-year review. *N. Engl. J. Med.* 279:674, 1968.

29. Taylor, J. Infectious infantile enteritis, yesterday and today. *Proc. R. Soc. Med.* 63:1297, 1970.

30. Toivanen, P., Toivanen, A., Olkkonen, L., and Aantaa, S. Hospital outbreak of *Yersinia enterocolitica* infection. *Lancet* 1:801, 1973.

31. Wachsmuth, I. K., Falkow, S., and Ryder, R. W. Plasmid-mediated properties of a heat-stable enterotoxin-producing *Escherichia coli* associated with infantile diarrhea. *Infect. Immun.* 14:403, 1976.

32. Whitfield, C., and Humphries, J. M. Meningitis and septicemia due to *Shigellae* in a newborn infant. *J. Pediatr.* 70:805, 1967.

# 33  PUERPERAL ENDOMETRITIS

William J. Ledger

## NATURE OF INFECTIONS

### Incidence

There is good evidence that the incidence of puerperal endometritis reported from individual hospitals with active surveillance of these infections (1 to 4 percent) is probably unchanged from the most accurate figures available from the preantibiotic decade of the 1920s. This statement should not be construed as an apology for modern obstetrics, for the status of puerperal endometritis and sepsis has dramatically changed in that same time interval. The most severe infections—those resulting in maternal death from sepsis—have virtually been eliminated from modern obstetrics.

The reported incidence is higher than that noted in the National Nosocomial Infections Study (NNIS) (see Chapter 24), in which an incidence of less than 1 percent was found. Possible reasons for this lower incidence are noted in the following sections.

### Deficiencies in Reporting Infections

Obstetricians, who are surgically oriented physicians, tend to underestimate the incidence of nosocomial infections, including postpartum endometritis. This phenomenon of individual physician inaccuracy in assessing the frequency of infections reflects commonly observed patterns of clinical practice. Most patients with the early symptoms of a postpartum endometritis, such as temperature elevation, are first discovered at night and not during the traditional early-morning rounds of physicians (Fig. 33-1). In the majority of occasions, these patients are placed on systemic antibiotics without prior culture studies. A nationwide evaluation of over 12,000 women undergoing hysterectomy who were cared for by obstetrician-gynecologists revealed that over 50 percent had received systemic antibiotics without prior culture tests [6]. A rapid response of the patient to the administered antibiotics with a quick return of temperature levels to normal may cause the attending physician to disregard the case as "true" morbidity. In this context, the reader must be aware that any nationwide survey will detect only a portion of all cases of endometritis during any study interval. Despite the fact that some cases are inevitably missed by surveillance systems such as that of the NNIS, pooled microbiologic data from cases that are reported do provide a good assessment of the major pathogens involved in postpartum endometritis.

Underestimates of the incidence of endometritis in modern obstetrics are also based on continued dependence on a preantibiotic-era definition of morbid-

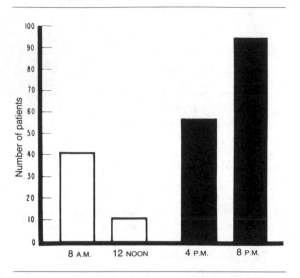

FIG. 33-1. The first temperature elevation of obstetric patients with postpartum morbidity. The majority of patients had initial rises in the late afternoon or evening hours.

ity based on temperature elevations. This definition was established by American obstetrician-gynecologists between the first and second World Wars, and it is based on four separate oral temperature recordings each postpartum day; *morbidity* is defined as an oral temperature of 38°C (100.4°F) or greater on any two of the first 10 postpartum days, excluding the first 24 hours after delivery. This definition successfully excluded from consideration patients with one temperature elevation shortly after delivery as well as those who had a single temperature elevation later but no evidence of a postpartum pelvic infection. On a statistical basis, nearly all the women from the preantibiotic era who met these temperature criteria for morbidity had a pelvic infection, whether uterine or urinary tract. Appropriate microbiologic studies could be performed, and such patients could be isolated from other obstetric patients.

The great setback for a clear understanding of infectious disease in antibiotic-era obstetrics has been the maintenance of this formerly valid standard in the face of antibiotic use. Employment of powerful systemic antibiotics in postpartum patients with the first elevation of temperature may yield an immediate clinical response with rapid and persistent defervescence of fever. If the obstetric service adheres to the old temperature-defined morbidity standards, the patient is not counted in morbidity statistics. This accounts in part for the frequent discrepancy between the low recorded morbidity figures and the high systemic antibiotic use in obstetric units.

*Community-Acquired Versus Nosocomial Infections*
All postpartum endometritis should be considered a nosocomial infection, unless the amniotic fluid is infected at the time of admission or the patient was admitted 48 hours or more following rupture of the membranes. Some infections in the latter group are nosocomial, however, and available microbiologic, clinical, and epidemiologic data should be carefully reviewed to determine whether the infection is community-acquired or nosocomial.

*Mechanisms of Infection*
The uterus has excellent local defense mechanisms to protect itself against invasion by contaminating organisms from the lower genital tract. These defenses are present in the nonpregnant state, as is demonstrated by the rapid clearance of the lower genital tract bacteria that are carried into the endometrial cavity during the insertion of an intrauterine device [14]. During pregnancy, Galask and associates [5] have demonstrated inhibition of bacterial growth by the amniotic fluid. The stress of labor and delivery probably results commonly in uterine acquisition of organisms from the nonsterile lower genital tract, but most postpartum patients remain free of symptoms as the uterus rapidly clears itself of the potentially pathogenic bacteria introduced from the vagina.

Postpartum endometritis occurs when these efficient uterine defense mechanisms are overcome by a combination of too many bacteria, the introduction of especially virulent bacterial strains, or local alterations (e.g., soft tissue damage or the incomplete removal of the placenta) that provide a nidus for the development of a postpartum infection.

Postpartum pelvic infection follows a pattern of progression (Fig. 33-2) with ascension of the organisms into the endometrial cavity, invasion of the myometrium, extension into parametrial areas beyond the uterus, and bloodstream invasion in some instances [1]. If this progression is unchecked by the appropriate use of systemic antibiotics and anticoagulants when indicated, then myometrial, parametrial, or adnexal abscesses can occur with suppurative involvement of the pelvic veins, septic pelvic thrombophlebitis, and even distant septic metastases to the liver and lung. In addition to the appropriate use of systemic medical agents, adequate uterine drainage must be ensured, and operative intervention for the drainage or removal of a pelvic abscess may be necessary for cure.

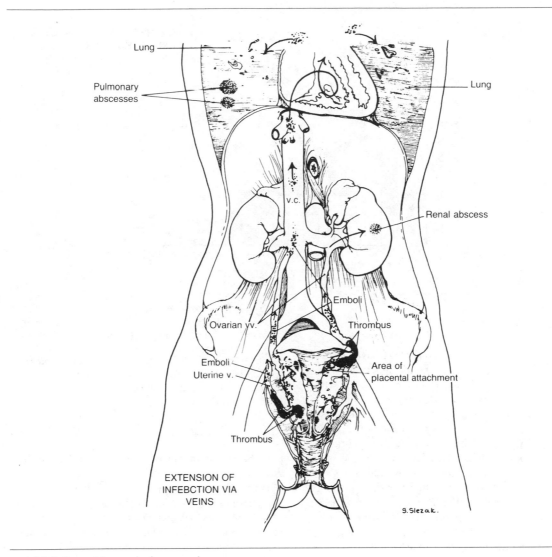

Lung

Pulmonary
abscesses

Lung

V.C.

Renal abscess

Emboli

Ovarian vv.

Thrombus

Emboli

Uterine v.

Area of
placental attachment

Thrombus

EXTENSION OF
INFEBCTION VIA
VEINS

9. Slezak.

FIG. 33-2. Potential spread of untreated postpartum
endometritis.

## PREDISPOSING HOST FACTORS

### Host Susceptibility

The well-nourished pregnant patient is far less likely
to have infectious problems than her poorly nour-
ished, anemic counterpart. In addition, risk of infection increases with prolonged rupture of the fetal
membranes before delivery, with increasing length
of labor, and with retention of fetal membranes or
placental fragments after delivery.

### Transvaginal Monitoring

In addition to reducing mortality rates, the availability of antibiotics has dramatically changed the
practice of obstetrics-gynecology. Prolonged transvaginal monitoring of maternal intraamniotic pressures and transvaginal attachment of a fetal scalp
electrode for electrocardiograph readings could not
have been considered if antibiotics were not available
for postpartum use by obstetricians and neonatolo-
gists. However, these advances have been accompanied by enhanced infection risks. Among obstetric
patients, the incidence of endometritis is relatively
high in monitored patients as compared to unmon-
itored patients [6]. In a clinic population, where there
is a moderately high level of background infection,
this difference is less apparent [2] (see Figs. 33-3 and
33-4).

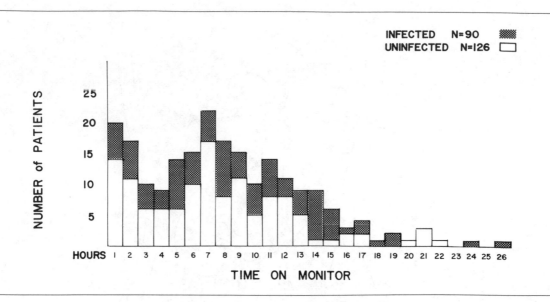

FIG. 33-3. The length of time of internal monitoring and the number of women with and without infection who delivered vaginally. Each bar represents the total number of women monitored for that time interval. (From Gassner, C. B., and Ledger, W. J. The relationship of hospital-acquired maternal infection to invasive intrapartum monitoring techniques. *Am. J. Obstet. Gynecol.* 126:33, 1976.)

### Cesarean Section

Advances in the science of neonatology have increased fetal survival and increased the incidence of cesarean section for fetal indications in situations in which maternal risk of postpartum infection is increased. The frequency of infection following a cesarean section is ten times greater than that following vaginal delivery. The obstetric service at the New York Hospital–Cornell Medical Center is now doing cesarean sections for infants estimated to weigh 700 gm or more, instead of 1000 gm, the limit that previously existed. The result of this new criterion has been a dramatic reduction in perinatal mortality rates [15], but these results have been achieved by judgments that increase the maternal risk of infection; our own assessment would be that the benefits to the fetus of this new obstetric philosophy outweigh the risks to the mother.

## DIAGNOSTIC CRITERIA

### Clinical

The clinical diagnosis of postpartum endometritis is based on a number of findings, but the most significant factor is fever. Generally, these women have an oral temperature elevation to about 38°C (100.4°F) and a tachycardia consistent with this rise. Patients usually have uterine tenderness and often have tenderness beyond the uterus in the parametrial and adnexal regions. A decrease in the normal postpartum uterine lochial flow is often noted 6 to 12 hours preceding the temperature elevation, and the lochial flow may be foul smelling.

If the physician makes a clinical diagnosis of endometritis and begins administration of systemic antibiotics with or without positive culture results, the patient should be included in all infection surveillance and postpartum morbidity statistics.

Attempts to assess the presence of a postpartum endometritis through evaluation of commonly employed, indirect hematologic measures of infection have not been successful. The phenomena of labor and delivery are accompanied by changes in the commonly employed parameters to measure the presence or absence of a bacterial infection. Thus a normal patient in labor or postpartum who has no clinical evidence of an active bacterial infection may have an elevated white blood cell count (even above 20,000) with an increase in the percentage of immature leukocytes, an elevated sedimentation rate, and a striking increase in the percentage of white cells that have engulfed and reduced nitroblue tetrazolium during incubation. With these facts in mind, there should be no enthusiasm for dependence on such laboratory tests to determine the diagnosis of infection.

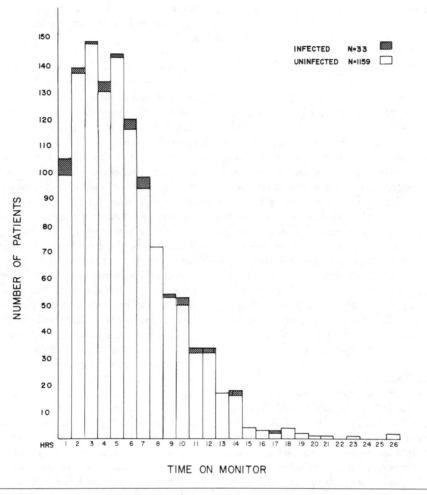

FIG. 33-4. The length of time of internal monitoring and the number of women with and without infection who delivered by cesarean section. Each bar represents the total number of women monitored for that time interval. (From Gassner, C. B., and Ledger, W. J. The relationship of hospital-acquired maternal infection to invasive intrapartum monitoring techniques. *Am. J. Obstet. Gynecol.* 126:33, 1976.)

*Microbiologic*

Bacterial isolations in the clinical microbiology laboratory usually do not establish the diagnosis of a postpartum endometritis. The sole exception is the discovery of a group-A β-hemolytic *Streptococcus,* which should trigger specific physician responses for treatment, isolation, and investigation. The reasons for the usual lack of useful diagnostic, but not therapeutic, information from the microbiologic laboratory are manifold. Most culture techniques for sampling the postpartum endometrial cavity include a transcervical approach, which of necessity involves contamination by the abundant bacterial flora normally present in the endocervical canal of asymptomatic women. Also, the organisms recovered from the endometrial cavity of endometritis patients are usually the same as those normally inhabiting the vagina and endocervix of sexually active women.

The above considerations do not mean that the laboratory will not be helpful, for it may indirectly contribute to the diagnosis or lack of diagnosis and give therapeutic guidance for treating postpartum endometritis. Assistance in excluding the diagnosis of postpartum endometritis may be provided, for example, in the febrile postpartum patient with no localizing uterine signs of infection when a significant bacterial colony count is obtained from a properly collected urine sample, and the fever resolves successfully following therapy with an antibacterial agent (e.g., a nitrofurantoin) with limited action outside of the urinary tract.

## SPECIMEN COLLECTION AND TRANSPORT

### Transvaginal Specimens

The greatest difficulty facing clinicians in their attempts to sample the postpartum endometrial cavity microbiologically is in obtaining specimens that are free of vaginal and cervical contamination. To date, most techniques have stressed the transvaginal and transcervical approach to the endometrial cavity. Various techniques have been tried to decrease contamination from endocervical canal organisms, including the use of plastic or metal tubing through which specimens can be collected. There has been little physician enthusiasm for these more complicated diagnostic procedures. Also, there have been no reports of attempts to quantitate the recovery of bacteria, similar to the methods of the colony counts of urine specimens, which might separate vaginal and endocervical contaminants from the more numerous pathogens from the site of infection.

### Transabdominal Specimens

An alternative microbiologic method to the transcervical technique is the transabdominal approach. We have attempted this approach in a limited number of patients and have had no serious complications with the method. More significant has been the greater frequency of recovery of microorganisms with this approach than with a blood culture. The importance of this technique in future microbiologic sampling remains to be established by more extensive study.

## PERITONEAL CULTURES

Transvaginal cul-de-sac aspirations have been tried in women with a clinical diagnosis of postpartum endomyometritis. The yield of positive cultures was much higher than with the transabdominal approach, but the impact of surface vaginal contamination on the results is not known.

### Use of Blood Cultures

The most useful microbiologic technique, when it is positive, is the blood culture. A positive result focuses the clinician's attention on the most significant microorganisms in the infectious process. Those that invade the bloodstream are critical for the physician's

therapeutic consideration. This diagnostic technique is positive in as many as 60 percent of febrile patients who deliver by cesarean section.

### Transport

Significant changes in microbiologic sampling and the transportation of specimens have been brought about by the growing physician awareness of the importance of anaerobic microorganisms in postpartum infections. The recovery of anaerobes is crucially dependent on the clinician's efforts to reduce exposure of the specimens to atmospheric oxygen. Time is a critical factor, because exposure of a swab of the infection site to atmospheric oxygen for a few minutes or less will reduce or eliminate certain anaerobic organisms. A number of alternative laboratory systems have been proposed to eliminate such exposure. Transport media have been used, either liquid for primary culture or semisolid for transport to the laboratory and primary plating there. Alternatively, gassed tubes, free of oxygen, have been used for transport to a laboratory where primary plating and anaerobic incubation can be performed (see Chapter 7).

There is a major weakness in all these clinical schemes for the obstetrician-gynecologist. Figure 33-1 documents the first temperature elevation of obstetric patients with postpartum morbidity, which is the logical time for initial patient evaluation [10]. It is clear that the majority of microbiologic samples will be obtained late in the afternoon or in the early evening, when laboratory coverage, particularly by technicians with familiarity in anaerobic methods, will usually be inadequate. An alternative to this scheme involves bringing the laboratory to the patient's bedside. This can be accomplished with anaerobic or prereduced blood agar plates, prereduced blood agar plates with vancomycin and kanamycin added, and thioglycolate broth. Inoculated medium is placed in an anaerobic chamber containing the Gas-Pak and is then placed into an ordinary incubator in the hospital. The laboratory can then work with the specimen during the daylight hours. This technique has allowed recovery of anaerobic organisms from over 70 percent of submitted specimens.

## GENERAL CONTROL MEASURES

### Patient-Care Practices

PRENATAL CARE   The emphasis on the preventive aspects in patient care has been heavily weighted toward patient management during pregnancy, labor, and delivery. For the patient in labor, most obstetricians believe that the results of prenatal care culminating in delivery largely determine the frequency and severity of postpartum endometritis.

RECTAL AND VAGINAL EXAMINATIONS One of the great changes in practice patterns in obstetrics in the past several years has been the virtual abandonment of the rectal examination during labor. Rectal examination was firmly established in the preantibiotic era and was predicated on the belief that it would avoid the introduction of exogenous organisms into the vagina. Since the most feared bacterial pathogens—the group-A $\beta$-hemolytic streptococci—were often introduced into the vagina from personnel sources, prohibition of vaginal examination was undoubtedly beneficial. A number of studies demonstrated no differences in the postpartum endometritis rate when patients undergoing vaginal examination during labor were compared to those having rectal examination. These results probably reflect the low frequency of involvement of exogenous organisms such as group-A $\beta$-hemolytic streptococci in postpartum endometritis. Both rectal and vaginal examinations, however, can result in the displacement of organisms from the lower genital tract to the uterus, and these manipulations, as well as other manipulations with similar risks (e.g., intrauterine placement of forceps or the physician's hand at delivery), should be limited to as few as necessary for good management of the patient.

PROPHYLACTIC ANTIBIOTICS Recently interest has grown in the use of prophylactic antibiotics for the patient in labor who needs a cesarean section (see Chapter 11). Most studies to date have shown diminished postpartum morbidity. The timing of the dosage for prophylaxis is in question. Preoperative administration delivers a therapeutic level of antibiotic to the fetus and can make evaluation for neonatal sepsis more difficult. A more popular method is administration after clamping of the cord. Recently there has been increasing use of antibiotic solution lavage in the operating room.

HAND-WASHING AND GLOVES In the nineteenth century, Semmelweis recognized the importance of hand transfer of organisms from the postmortem room and the autopsy in the production of endometritis; physicians carried the bacterial pathogens from the autopsy room on their hands and clothing to the vagina and endocervix of the patient in labor, which led to the subsequent development of infection. Semmelweis' great achievement was to require hand-bathing in an antiseptc solution by physicians before the next patient was seen to break the chain of bacterial contamination and infection. Hand-washing and the use of sterile gloves for vaginal examinations remain important general control measures.

*Environmental Factors*
Environmental factors are infrequently involved in the development of postpartum endometritis. Indeed, the studies of the effect of ultraviolet irradiation on the rate of all postoperative wound infections [3] suggest that this would be the case in the delivery room, because they showed that there was little impact on clinical results despite reductions in the bacterial contamination of air (see Chapter 20). The lack of importance of the environment would be especially anticipated in the case of endometritis, because most of these infections derive from the patients' endogenous bacterial flora.

*Therapy*
The cornerstones of therapy in patients with a postpartum endometritis are adequate uterine drainage and the use of appropriate antimicrobials. Uterine drainage must be ensured, and the maneuver of removing membranes provides the patient undergoing clinical examination the added benefit of an assessment of the extent of infection; a microbiologic specimen may also be obtained at this time.

Antibiotics are frequently used for cure. They usually are prescribed before the results of culture susceptibility tests are known, and the initial choices reflect the individual physician's philosophy of antibiotic use, which should be based on past experiences with similar patients. At LAC-USC Medical Center, they will frequently use a single antibiotic like ampicillin or a cephalosporin to treat the patient who is not allergic to penicillin and who has had a vaginal delivery. This course usually results in cure, even in the patient with a concomitant bacteremia, because these agents provide coverage against most of the commonly recovered organisms. In patients who have had a cesarean section, our antibiotic coverage includes a combination of clindamycin and an aminoglycoside, usually gentamicin. This combination of antibiotics provides coverage against most of the commonly recovered aerobes and anaerobes and has shown superior results to the previously employed combination of penicillin and an aminoglycoside. Alternatively, a second- or third-generation cephalosporin such as cefoxitin or one of the newer broad-spectrum penicillins such as mezlocillin can be used alone.

## ENDOGENOUS INFECTIONS FROM LOWER GENITAL TRACT FLORA

The microorganisms mainly responsible for postpartum endometritis are nearly always endogenous to the patient; that is, they normally reside in the gastrointestinal and lower genital tracts (vagina and endocervix) of asymptomatic, sexually active, pregnant women. The stress of labor and delivery, rupture of the membranes, frequent vaginal examinations by the medical team caring for the patient, use of monitoring devices, and delivery by the intrauterine placement of forceps or physicians' hands all introduce opportunities for uterine acquisition of lower genital tract flora. After introduction, they may find a suitable uterine environment where they can survive and invade.

The endogenous organisms that most frequently become pathogenic and result in an endometritis include certain aerobic streptococci ($\alpha$-hemolytic streptococci, the group-B $\beta$-hemolytic streptococci, and the enterococci); anaerobic cocci (*Peptostreptococcus* and *Peptococcus*); gram-negative enteric aerobes (*Escherichia coli, Proteus mirabilis,* and *Klebsiella* species); and finally, gram-negative anaerobic rods, *Bacteroides fragilis, B. bivius,* and *B. disiens.* There is evidence that nearly all of the patients with endometritis, particularly those with severe infections, have a mixed infection with more than one organism involved. The implications of such microbiologic findings for multiple antibiotic use have not been settled by prospective study.

Epidemics of endometritis caused by these organisms have not been recognized, and their control depends on avoiding predisposing factors, when possible, and adherence to general control measures.

### Gram-Negative Aerobic Bacterial Infections
INCIDENCE   The National Nosocomial Infections Study (NNIS) data indicate that gram-negative aerobes were the most commonly recovered pathogens (see Chapter 24). From 2692 patients with endometritis, *E. coli* was recovered in 732, *Klebsiella* in 179, and *P. mirabilis* in 154. This frequent recovery of *E. coli* matches our own surveillance data on endometritis and postpartum bacteria; this has consistently been the most common organism recovered. On many obstetric services, gram-positive anaerobic cocci are the most frequently isolated pathogens.

CLINICAL FEATURES   A patient with postpartum endometritis due to a gram-negative aerobe can be seriously ill. This is particularly true in the patient

with an associated bacteremia. There are no distinctive clinical signs, however, to alert the clinician to the possibility that these organisms are involved.

THERAPY   The low frequency of antimicrobial-resistant organisms is a major advantage to the clinician treating women with endometritis due to a gram-negative aerobe. Most postpartum obstetric patients have intact host defense mechanisms and usually have not had prolonged exposure to systemic antimicrobial therapy before labor and delivery or prolonged hospitalization before delivery. Effective first-line drugs include the aminoglycosides, gentamicin, and tobramycin. Since there are a few resistant gram-negative aerobic organisms seen in these patients, we usually rely on gentamicin as our most frequently used aminoglycoside, with amikacin reserved for the patient who is suspected of having gram-negative aerobic bacterial sepsis or who had repeated exposure to antibiotics for urinary tract infections during pregnancy. The cephalosporins are highly effective against such gram-negative aerobes, and these are an acceptable alternative to aminoglycosides. Chloramphenicol has shown effectiveness in the laboratory against gram-negative aerobes, but I do not prescribe it in these patients because of my concern about bone-marrow toxicity.

### Bacteroides fragilis Infections
INCIDENCE   The NNIS data indicate that *Bacteroides* species were the most common anaerobes isolated from patients with postpartum endometritis. Undoubtedly, the majority of these isolates are *B. bivius* or *B. disiens.*

CLINICAL FEATURES   Patients wtih postpartum endometritis due to *B. fragilis, B. bivius*, or *B. disiens* can be seriously ill, and they frequently have lochia with a fecal ordor. A hallmark of established postpartum pelvic infections due to this organism is their chronicity, even in the face of appropriate antibiotic coverage. This is indirectly reflected in a number of patient assessments. Such patients may require many days of antibiotic therapy and operative intervention (Fig. 33-5) before they become afebrile [8]. In addition to this clinical assessment, the urinary mucopolysaccharide/creatinine index, a measure of ground-substance turnover that is elevated in patients with a pelvic infection, remains elevated for a longer period of time in women with *B. fragilis* infection [11]. Pelvic abscess formation is not uncommon, and operative drainage or removal may be necessary for cure, despite the use of appropriate antibiotics in adequate

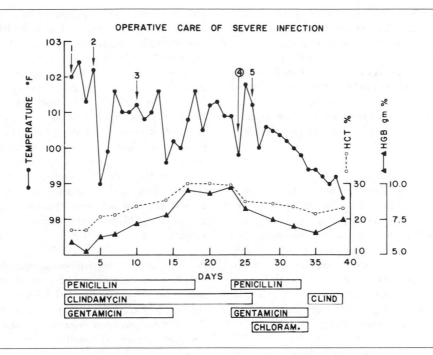

FIG. 33-5. The complicated postpartum course of a patient with an endometritis. This septic Jehovah's Witness was admitted to our hospital (point 1 on the graph) following a cesarean section and the development of postpartum sepsis in another hospital. Hyperalimentation was begun at point 2 and continued until point 3. At point 4, a hysterectomy and bilateral salpingooophorectomy were performed. Postoperatively (point 5), chloramphenicol was started. The *Bacteroides fragilis* organisms recovered from the excised tissue were susceptible in the laboratory to both clindamycin and chloramphenicol.

dosages. Septic thrombophlebitis with septic emboli may also follow infections with this organism.

THERAPY Pospartum endometritis due to *B. fragilis, B. bivius*, or *B. disiens* requires specific antibiotic strategies. The current first-line drugs of choice are clindamycin and metronidazole. Clindamycin has been associated with pseudomembranous enterocolitis, a serious clinical entity that affects more than one in 25,000 treated patients (see Chapters 11 and 32). Alternative drugs include the newer cephalosporins and broad-spectrum penicillins.

Operative removal and drainage of pelvic abscesses, treatment of septic pelvic thrombophlebitis with intravenous heparin therapy, and continued use of appropriate antibiotics may result in a rapid defervescence of fever in a patient with previously persisting temperature spikes.

*Peptostreptococcus and Peptococcus Infections*
INCIDENCE The NNIS report does not include anaerobic gram-positive cocci among the frequently recovered organisms in patients with endometritis. This undoubtedly reflects shortcomings in anaerobic microbiologic techniques in the initial culture study of patients with endometritis. Microbiologic studies of patients with postpartum endometritis in the preantibiotic era showed *Peptostreptococcus* to be the most commonly isolated organism [16], and this is true on some services today. In surveillance studies of obstetric infections with proper anaerobic culture techniques, however, *Peptostreptococcus* and *Peptococcus* are each recovered from the endometrium and bloodstream of patients with endometritis in numbers equivalent to those of *Bacteroides* species, and if combined in the category of gram-positive anaerobic cocci, they are numerically more common than *Bacteroides*.

CLINICAL FEATURES A postpartum endometritis due to gram-positive anaerobic cocci can be suspected in a patient whose lochia has a putrid, fecal odor. Pelvic abscess formation can occur, and operative drainage or removal may be necessary for cure, despite the use of appropriate antibiotics as judged by in vitro antibiotic susceptibility testing. The postpartum retention of fetal membranes or placental fragments has frequently been observed with these infections.

THERAPY   *Peptostreptococcus* and *Peptococcus* are both quite susceptible to clindamycin in dosage levels that are easily exceeded in the serum by frequently administered therapeutic doses of this agent. Other alternative antibiotics include the newer cephalosporins and penicillins.

### Aerobic Streptococcal Infections

INCIDENCE   The NNIS report noted that groups B and D streptococci and $\alpha$-hemolytic streptococci occurred more frequently in endometritis than the group-A $\beta$-hemolytic streptococci but less frequently than any of the previously mentioned gram-negative aerobes. This frequency pattern varies from our own surveillance data on postpartum endometritis. In our patients with endometritis or an associated bacteremia, these aerobic streptococci were more frequently recovered than any organism except *E. coli*.

CLINICAL FEATURES   Postpartum endometritis due to aerobic streptococci has no characteristic clinical findings that distinguish it from endometritis due to other organisms.

THERAPY   The group-B $\beta$-hemolytic streptococci and $\alpha$-hemolytic streptococci are susceptible to penicillin and clindamycin. The group-D $\beta$-hemolytic streptococci have unique antibiotic susceptibility patterns. In the laboratory, the organism is frequently not susceptible to penicillin or an aminoglycoside alone, but when both antibiotics are used together or when ampicillin is substituted for penicillin, there is both laboratory and clinical evidence of a response. In the penicillin-allergic patient with enterococcal endometritis, erythromycin is the antibiotic of choice, since the cephalosporins and clindamycin have little effectiveness against this group of organisms.

## GROUP-A $\beta$-HEMOLYTIC STREPTOCOCCAL INFECTIONS

In contrast to the preceding category of infections, endometritis caused by group-A streptococci commonly derives from exogenous sources, is highly invasive and transmissible, and has produced outbreaks requiring special measures for control.

### General Aspects

TRANSMISSIBILITY   The group-A $\beta$-hemolytic streptococci are highly contagious agents (see Chapter 31).

For this reason, obstetricians justifiably fear the introduction of this organism into the labor-room environment lest it will be transmitted to patients in labor and result in serious cases of postpartum endometritis. A patient with an active *Streptococcus pyogenes* infection can transmit these organisms to patients or medical personnel, resulting in colonization. Hospital personnel can be asymptomatic carriers of group-A streptococci and transmit the organisms to patients in labor. Community contacts may be important in the transmission of this organism, particularly in the modern obstetric setting that so frequently allows husband and wife to be together during all of labor and delivery. This practice can be dangerous if the husband is a carrier of group-A streptococci.

INCIDENCE   The importance of group-A $\beta$-hemolytic streptococcal infections is not based on a high frequency of infections but rather on the clinical invasiveness and epidemiologic virulence of such strains. The low frequency of isolation matches our surveillance experience with endometritis and the bacteremia associated with it.

SOURCES AND MODES OF ACQUISITION   Endogenous sources are probably mainly responsible for specific cases. The vagina of such patients is often asymptomatically colonized with group-A streptococci when the patient is admitted to the delivery room, but patients may also have an upper respiratory tract infection or skin lesion that harbors such organisms.

The most common method of spread of exogenous organisms involves direct transmission of the organism from personnel who are asymptomatic carriers to the patient. Clinically infected personnel may also be responsible (see Chapters 27, 30, and 31). Personnel may become colonized after providing care to a patient with postpartum endometritis; they may then transmit these organisms to patients in labor.

### Clinical Considerations

MANIFESTATIONS   There are a number of distinctive clinical features seen in the patient with group-A $\beta$ hemolytic streptococcal endometritis. Historically, this entity has been called "puerperal fever," "puerperal sepsis," and "childbed fever." The most striking feature is the early onset of high spiking fevers (Fig. 33-6) in the postpartum patient [9]. Patients appear critically ill, but abdominal and pelvic examinations reveal diffuse tenderness with no localizing signs. The cervical discharge is usually clear and watery, is not purulent, and contains many gram-positive cocci when the exudate is Gram stained.

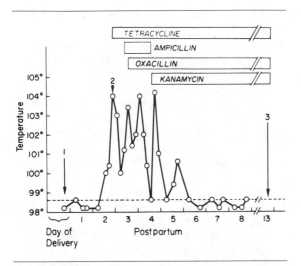

FIG. 33-6. The early onset of a high, spiking temperature pattern in a postpartum patient with group-A β-hemolytic streptococcal endometritis. Despite the use of penicillin analogs (ampicillin and oxacillin), the patient required several days to become completely afebrile. The patient delivered at point 1 on the chart, was started on antibiotic treatment at point 2, and was discharged at point 3.

Although this organism is very susceptible to penicillin and clindamycin, patients with endometritis frequently do not become afebrile for 48 hours or more (see Fig. 33-4).

THERAPY  The drug of choice for treating group-A β-hemolytic streptococcal endometritis remains penicillin G; clindamycin is also effective against this organism. Tetracycline is not an acceptable alternative for treating patients with this infection because of the frequency of resistant strains.

### Epidemic Infections

REPORTED OUTBREAKS  In recent years, sporadic outbreaks of group-A β-hemolytic streptococcal endometritis epidemics have been reported in New York City [13] and Boston [4]. In the New York City outbreak, there were 9 confirmed cases, while in Boston there were 20 women with this diagnosis.

SOURCES  In the New York City outbreak, the source of the bacteria that were disseminated around the hospital was colonized, asymptomatic newborn infants. In Boston, a common source was the cutaneous lesions of an anesthesiologist [4]. A preantibiotic era study of this problem found many personnel colonized with such streptococci [17]. Colonization of medical personnel and subsequent transmission to

patients in labor seem to be the crucial ingredients in the maintenance of an epidemic. Another outbreak of group-A streptococcal infections affecting obstetric-gynecologic patients was ultimately traced to an anesthesiologist who was an asymptomatic rectal carrier of the organism [12]. Thus operating-room sources of this type should be suspected in endometritis outbreaks that exclusively or primarily involve patients with cesarean sections.

### Prevention and Control

PREVENTION  Infections due to this organism are so serious that the discovery of one case of puerperal sepsis should be considered an epidemic. The patient needs to be placed in wound and skin isolation, and hospital personnel should gown and glove before providing personal care (see Chapter 9). All labor and delivery room personnel on duty during this patient's labor and delivery should be screened for possible infections by history and physical examination, and cultures should be obtained on their nose, throat, any suspected skin lesion, and rectum. Lochial culture specimens should be obtained from postpartum patients who had been in the delivery room at the same time as the infected patient, and appropriate antibiotics should be given to those whose cultures are positive for group-A streptococci. Personnel whose cultures are positive for the same strain as the one isolated from the infected patient (which is established by M and T typing) should be relieved of patient-care responsibilities until appropriate antibiotic therapy has resulted in negative cultures. All culture-positive personnel should be treated if the typing of strains cannot be done expeditiously.

CONTROL OF OUTBREAKS  There were a number of significant differences between the preantibiotic era epidemics and those recently reported. The preantibiotic era study reported maternal deaths, and the outbreak was controlled only by closing the maternity service of the hospital until all infected patients had been discharged [17]. The recent epidemics have been controlled by the use of appropriate antibiotics, isolation of infected patients, epidemiologic identification of disseminating carriers, and eradication of carried strains by proper treatment of colonized or infected hospital personnel. If initial nose and throat cultures of personnel epidemiologically associated with the outbreak are negative, multiple culture specimens should be obtained, including ones from rectal and vaginal sites. In Boston, all admissions to the service in the midst of the epidemic were treated with penicillin or penicillin-like antibiotics [4]. Such broad-scale prophylaxis may be especially indicated at the time an outbreak is first recognized, because it may permit a maternity unit to remain open while epidemiologic and microbiologic investigations are undertaken. If such investigations are successful in identifying the sources and modes of spread, then attention focused on these areas should obviate the need for continued chemoprophylaxis of patients. Outbreaks should be promptly reported to local health authorities.

# REFERENCES

1. Eastman, N. J., and Hellman, L. M. In Williams, L. W. (Ed.), *Obstetrics* (13th ed.). New York: Appleton-Century-Crofts, 1966.
2. Gassner, C. B., and Ledger, W. J. The relationship of hospital-acquired maternal infections to invasive intrapartum monitoring techniques. *Am. J. Obstet. Gynecol.* 126:33, 1976.
3. Howard, J. M., Barker, W. F., Culbertson, W. R., Grotzinger, P. T., Jovine, V. M., Keehn, R. J., and Ravdin, R. G. Postoperative wound infections: The influence of ultraviolet irradiation of the operating room and of various other factors. *Ann. Surg.* 160(Suppl.):1, 1964.
4. Jewett, J. F., Reid, D. E., Safon, L. E., and Easterday, C. L. Childbed fever—a continuing entity. *J.A.M.A.* 206:344, 1968.
5. Larsen, B., Snyder, I. S., and Galask, R. P. Bacterial growth inhibition by amniotic fluid. *Am. J. Obstet. Gynecol.* 119:492, 1974.
6. Larsen, J. W., Goldkrand, J. W., Hanson, T. M., and Miller, C. R. Intrauterine infection on an obstetric service. *Obstet. Gynecol.* 43:838, 1974.
7. Ledger, W. J., and Child, M. The hospital care

8. Ledger, W. J., Gassner, C. B., and Gee, C. Operative care of infections in obstetrics-gynecology. *J. Reprod. Med.* 13:128, 1974.
9. Ledger, W. J., and Headington, J. T. The group A beta-hemolytic streptococcus. *Obstet. Gynecol.* 39:474, 1972.
10. Ledger, W. J., Reite, A. M., and Headington, J. T. A system for infectious disease surveillance on an obstetric service. *Obstet. Gynecol.* 37:769, 1971.
11. Ledger, W. J., Thompson, G. R., and deVries, L. The influence of infection in obstetric and gynecologic patients upon increased uinary mucopolysaccharide excretion. *Am. J. Obstet. Gynecol.* 120:407, 1974.
12. McIntyre, D. M. An epidemic of *Streptococcus pyogenes* puerperal and postoperative sepsis with an unusual carrier site—the anus. *Am. J. Obstet. Gynecol.* 101:308, 1968.
13. Mead, P. B., Ribble, J. C., and Dillon, T. F. Group A streptococcal puerperal infection. *Obstet. Gynecol.* 32:460, 1968.
14. Mishell, D. R., Bell, J. H., Good, R. G., and Moyer, D. L. The intrauterine device: A bacteriologic study of the endometrial cavity. *Am. J. Obstet. Gynecol.* 96:119, 1966.
15. Paul, R. H., and Hon, E. H. Clinical fetal monitoring v. Effect on perinatal outcome. *Am. J. Obstet. Gynecol.* 118:529, 1974.
16. Schwarz, O. H., and Dieckman, W. J. Puerperal infection due to anaerobic streptococci. *Am. J. Obstet. Gynecol.* 13:467, 1927.
17. Watson, B. P. An outbreak of puerperal sepsis in New York City. *Am. J. Obstet. Gynecol.* 16:157, 1928.

# 34 NOSOCOMIAL CENTRAL NERVOUS SYSTEM INFECTIONS

Arthur L. Reingold
Claire V. Broome

Central nervous system (CNS) infections, including meningitis, ventricular shunt infections, ventriculitis, infected subdural hematomas, and intracranial abscesses, are among the least common but most serious hospital-acquired infections. CNS infections accounted for only 0.4 percent of the nosocomial infections reported through the National Nosocomial Infections Study (NNIS) during the time period 1980–82. Due to a variety of factors, however, including the age of patients at highest risk, organisms frequently involved, and difficulty of achieving adequate concentrations of effective antimicrobials in the cerebrospinal fluid (CSF), nosocomial CNS infections are associated with a high mortality rate, as well as severe neurologic impairment among many survivors. Consequently, prevention of such infections assumes greater importance than might seem warranted by their incidence.

As in other infection sites, it is sometimes difficult to determine whether a CNS infection in a hospitalized patient began in the hospital or in the community. Part of the difficulty arises from uncertainty about the incubation period between antecedent head trauma and subsequent development of meningitis; this incubation period can range from a day to many weeks. There is also uncertainty regarding how long a period between the implantation of a device such as a ventricular shunt and the development of a shunt infection is consistent with nosocomial acquisition of infection. Infections in patients with ventricular shunts are considered nosocomial in origin if onset occurs within 60 days of implantation, revision, or manipulation of a shunt. With the exception of patients with ventricular shunts, most patients with meningitis following neurosurgery have onset of symptoms within three weeks of the procedure, and approximately 50 percent of patients develop symptoms within one week of surgery [38]. As a general rule, all infections that occur during the first postoperative month should be considered nosocomial.

Patients who develop meningitis several days into their hospitalization, secondary to a community-acquired infection at another body site, also should have their meningitis classified as a nosocomial infection. The criteria employed by the NNIS categorize meningitis developing at least 48 hours after admission to the hospital as nosocomial in origin, even if there is a history of antecedent head trauma or if the meningitis is secondary to community-acquired bacteremia or infection at another site. Neonatal meningitis due to organisms acquired during passage through the birth canal is considered to be nosocomial when the baby is born in the hospital. However, the implications for hospital personnel may be quite different from those generated by other types of nosocomial meningitis.

These definitions, although necessary and useful for surveillance purposes, may result in the misidentification of the place of acquisition of infection in an individual patient. When multiple patients in the same institution develop meningitis and/or other infections due to the same organism, however, it usually becomes apparent that the infections are nosocomial in origin. Under these circumstances, rapid determination of the source of infection and mode of spread is vital to prevention of additional cases.

## PATIENTS AT RISK

While any hospitalized patient is at risk of acquiring a nosocomial CNS infection, three occasionally overlapping groups of patients are at greatest risk: neurosurgery patients, both with and without ventricular shunts; neonates, particularly those in neonatal intensive care units; and patients undergoing diagnostic or therapeutic procedures that involve penetrating the CNS. In NNIS hospitals, almost three-fourths of the nosocomial CNS infections reported in 1980–82 were from newborn nurseries and surgical services, with the highest rate of such infections seen in the newborn nursery (Table 34-1).

### Neurosurgery Patients
Patients undergoing neurosurgery are at risk of seeding of their CNS directly at the operative site at the time of surgery. In addition, they are at substantial risk of developing secondary CNS infections due to direct spread from an infected surgical wound or seeding of devitalized tissue during bacteremia caused by infection at another site, such as the urinary tract. Overall, the incidence of postoperative meningitis among approximately 7000 neurosurgery patients in one hospital-based study was 0.5 percent [38].

It has been suggested that the risk of postoperative CNS infection increases with increasing operative time and with increasing number of operative procedures, although the available evidence is not convincing. Prophylactic antimicrobials have not been demonstrated to decrease the risk of nosocomial CNS infections in neurosurgery patients in general [38], although randomized prospective studies are lacking. Furthermore, outbreaks of CNS infections in neurosurgical units caused by multiply resistant organisms have resulted from injudicious use of antimicrobials in such patients [51] (see Chapter 11).

### Ventricular Shunt Patients
Patients with ventricular shunts form a special subgroup of neurosurgery patients that merits separate discussion. The increased risk of CNS infections, both hospital- and community-acquired, among these patients has been recognized for many years, and factors related to that risk have been studied [2,44,61,62, 65]. Most investigators have reported that 10 to 20 percent of patients undergoing shunt insertion or revision develop shunt infections.

The fact that most shunt infections have onset within two months of surgery (70 percent in one large series) strongly suggests that the infecting organism is usually introduced during the perioperative period [61]. While it has been suggested that the risk of infection is a function of the number of previous procedures and the number of therapeutic or diagnostic entries into the CNS, a study of 289 shunt patients in one hospital has shown that the rate of infection is independent of the number of previous procedures and that multiple entries into the CNS need not be associated with an increased risk of CNS infection [61]. The same study failed to show any association between the rate of infection and underlying disease, type of shunt, presence or absence of a valve, type of valve, or depth of the catheter in the right atrium. Other studies have shown that the rate of infection varies with the neurosurgeon [39], and in at least one cluster of shunt infections, with the use of shunt extension tubing [personal communication, J. L. Ho].

The role of prophylactic perioperative antimicrobials in ventricular shunt patients remains unsettled. While some authors have noted a lower rate of shunt infections among patients given prophylactic anti-

TABLE 34-1. Nosocomial CNS infections in NNIS hospitals by hospital service, 1980–82

| Service | Number of cases (%) | Infection rate/100,000 discharges |
|---|---|---|
| Surgery | 216 (43) | 18.0 |
| Newborn nursery | 151 (30) | 42.0 |
| Medicine | 83 (17) | 7.0 |
| Pediatrics | 44 ( 9) | 20.0 |
| Obstetrics | 2 (<1) | 0.5 |
| Invalid | 2 (<1) | — |
| Total | 498 | |

microbials [57,61], others have not [44,64]. All of these studies have biases and/or include very small numbers of patients. A large, randomized, prospective controlled clinical trial of the efficacy of prophylactic antimicrobials in this setting is needed.

### Neonates

While neurosurgery patients are at increased risk of nosocomial CNS infections because of the disruption of the normal barriers against infection, neonates, in whom these barriers are in general not well developed, are at increased risk of developing secondary CNS infection whenever they become bacteremic. Thus the factors associated with an increased risk of nosocomial meningitis are the same as those associated with an increased risk of sepsis, and in outbreak settings the cases of nosocomial meningitis are usually only a subgroup of the affected infant population. Cases of nosocomial meningitis in neonates occur predominantly in neonatal intensive care units, presumably due to the fact that patients requiring care in such units are more premature and of lower birth weight, more likely to have invasive therapeutic and diagnostic procedures, more likely to be exposed to broad-spectrum antimicrobials, more likely to be exposed to potentially contaminated life-support systems, and more likely to have extended hospital stays. Other important factors thought to be associated with the development of nosocomial meningitis in such units include crowding, decreased nurse-to-infant ratio, and poor hand-washing practices.

### Other Patients

The last group of patients at increased risk of nosocomial meningitis includes persons undergoing diagnostic or therapeutic procedures that penetrate the CNS, such as lumbar puncture for removal of CSF or instillation of dyes or medications [19,34,46, 58], use of a CSF (Omaya) reservoir [54], and induction of spinal anesthesia [18]. While such infections are less common in the present-day era of presterilized, single-use needles, syringes, and other equipment, they do still occur.

## ETIOLOGIC AGENTS

Two-thirds of nosocomial CNS infections are caused by gram-negative bacilli and staphylococci, although the distribution by etiologic agent depends on the hospital service (Table 34-2). In contrast, *Hemophilus influenzae* and *Neisseria meningitidis*, the two most common causes of community-acquired bacterial meningitis, account for only 2 percent of reported nosocomial CNS infections.

### Neurosurgery Patients

There have not been many reports that systematically analyze the etiologic agents responsible for CNS in-

TABLE 34-2. Nosocomial CNS infections in NNIS Hospitals by etiologic agent and service, 1980–82

| Etiologic agent | Service | | | | |
| --- | --- | --- | --- | --- | --- |
| | Newborn nursery | Pediatrics | Surgery | Medicine | Total |
| Bacteria | | | | | |
| Gram-negative bacilli | 46 | 17 | 70 | 23 | 156 |
| *Staphylococcus aureus* | 12 | 6 | 26 | 13 | 57 |
| *Staphylococcus epidermidis* | 8 | 6 | 47 | 10 | 71 |
| Group-B streptococci | 42 | 4 | 1 | — | 47 |
| Other streptococci, excluding *Streptococcus pneumoniae* | 11 | 3 | 17 | 6 | 37 |
| *Listeria monocytogenes* | 4 | — | 1 | 4 | 9 |
| *Streptococcus pneumoniae* | 4 | — | 3 | 1 | 8 |
| *Hemophilus influenzae* | 2 | — | 3 | 2 | 7 |
| *Neisseria meningitidis* | 1 | — | — | 1 | 2 |
| Anaerobes | — | — | 2 | — | 2 |
| Other | — | — | 5 | — | 5 |
| Viruses | 2 | 1 | 1 | — | 4 |
| Fungi and yeast | 7 | 5 | 6 | 7 | 25 |
| Total | 139 | 42 | 182 | 67 | 430 |

fections in neurosurgery patients. In one large hospital series, however, investigators found that 69 percent of proven cases of meningitis in the postneurosurgical period were caused by gram-negative bacilli and an additional 19 percent by staphylococci [38] Of the cases of gram-negative bacillary meningitis, approximately 70 percent were caused by *Escherichia coli* and *Klebsiella pneumoniae*. While the data from NNIS hospitals in Table 34-2 show that only 70 (38 percent) of 182 nosocomial CNS infections on surgical services were due to gram-negative bacilli, it should be noted that the proportion of these cases that came from neurosurgical services is unknown, as is the number of ventricular shunt patients.

### Ventricular Shunt Patients

Unlike nosocomial CNS infections in other neurosurgical patients, infections in patients with ventricular shunts are primarily caused by staphylococci. *Staphylococcus aureus* and *Staphylococcus epidermidis* together accounted for 75 percent of shunt infections in one large series and 81 percent in a smaller series, with gram-negative bacilli causing most of the other infections [39,61]. Additional analysis of the data from one series, however, revealed that gram-negative enteric organisms caused 35 percent of the shunt infections in patients with ventriculoureteral shunts [61].

### Neonates

As shown in Table 34-2, no single organism or group of organisms accounts for a majority of the cases of neonatal meningitis, although gram-negative bacilli and group-B streptococci together were implicated in over 60 percent of cases. A similar pattern has been seen in another large series [38]. While cases of neonatal meningitis due to group-B *Streptococcus* and *Listeria monocytogenes* are usually thought to be the result of mother-to-infant spread of the causative organism during passage through the birth canal, well-documented instances of horizontal spread of these organisms within the hospital also have occurred [1,15,23,35,36,67].

### Outbreaks

Reported outbreaks or clusters of cases of meningitis in hospitalized neonates and/or neurosurgical patients have been caused predominantly by a wide variety of gram-negative genera, including *Escherichia, Klebsiella, Pseudomonas, Citrobacter, Serratia, Enterobacter, Acinetobacter, Proteus, Salmonella,* and *Flavobacterium* [4,7,9–10,12–13,25–29,32,41,48,50–53,56]. However, clusters of cases of nosocomial meningitis

caused by gram-positive organisms, including groups A and B *Streptococcus, S. aureus,* and *L. monocytogenes,* have been described [1,15,20,23,30,35,36,55,67], as have clusters of CNS infections caused by fungi and viruses [42,45,54].

Nosocomial spread of *H. influenzae* and *N. meningitidis* CNS infections appears to be quite rare. A single cluster of cases of *H. influenzae* infections, including meningitis, has been reported in a chronic-care hospital for children [24]. Also, secondary spread of *H. influenzae* in an acute-care hospital recently has been reported [6]. Whereas secondary spread of *N. meningitidis* among patients in the hospital may have been more common when the United States was still experiencing epidemic meningococcal disease, there is only one well-documented instance of such transmission in the recent medical literature [17].

## MODES OF SPREAD AND SOURCES OF INFECTION

The source of infection and mode of spread in cases of nosocomial meningitis are primarily a function of the organism involved and the affected patient population.

### Neurosurgery Patients

As mentioned earlier, neurosurgery patients are at risk of seeding of their CNS both during and after surgery, with either incompletely eradicated endogenous local flora or exogenous bacteria. In the former situation, bacteria found on the skin, such as *S. epidermidis* and *S. aureus,* are not completely killed by preoperative scrubbing and are thus able to enter the CNS via the surgical incision. Alternatively, staphylococci or gram-negative bacilli can be transmitted to patients by hospital personnel, during either surgery or postoperative wound care, or as a result of care unrelated to the neurosurgical procedure, such as manipulation of a urinary tract catheter or performance of respiratory therapy. In one cluster of cases of meningitis due to a *Klebsiella* species, for example, the neurosurgical patients were found to be colonized with the causative agent in the urinary and respiratory tracts also [52]. Furthermore, in one large series, 70 percent of neurosurgical patients with meningitis had the same organism isolated from another site before or at the same time as the initial isolation from the CSF [38].

During the investigation of several outbreaks of gram-negative bacillary meningitis in neurosurgical units, inanimate objects such as respirators [10] and a shaving brush used for preoperative preparation of the scalp [4] have been found to harbor the epidemic strain. While isolation of the epidemic strain from the environment in such settings has led to speculation about the role of fomites in transmission, a statistically significant association between exposure to the inanimate object and risk of infection has not been established.

### Ventricular Shunt Patients

Many ventricular shunt infections probably result from incomplete eradication of "normal" skin flora—particularly *S. epidermidis*—from the operative site before surgery. One study that examined this question in detail found that *S. epidermidis* was recovered from cultures of the operative site before closure in 58 of 100 operations to insert or revise shunts [8]. In 32 (55 percent) of these patients, the same organism (determined by colicin typing) was present in the nose or ear, on the scalp, or at the operative site before the operation. Of 9 patients whose shunts became infected, 7 had the infecting organism present at the operative site at the time of surgery. The finding in another study, however, that 35 percent of shunt infections in patients with ventriculoureteral shunts were due to gram-negative enteric organisms suggests that other sources of infection may be important in patients having this type of shunt procedure [61].

### Neonates

Clusters of cases of meningitis in neonates caused by gram-negative enteric organisms probably result from the introduction of the organism into the newborn nursery from the stool of an infant or mother, or from the stool, vagina, or hands of someone on the hospital staff, with subsequent spread between infants via the hands of hospital personnel and/or improperly sterilized equipment. Investigations in such settings frequently reveal that many more infants are colonized (particularly at the umbilical stump and in the stool) than are infected and that one or more members of the nursery staff carry the implicated organism on the hands or in the stool or vagina. In one such outbreak, continued carriage of the causative organism on the hands of a nurse was believed to be at least partially due to a chronic dermatitis of the hands [48].

The causative organism frequently can also be found on inanimate objects in the nursery. Equipment found to be contaminated in such outbreaks has included oxygen tubing, water bottles used to humidify inspired air, suctioning equipment, aspirator bottles, and Isolettes [7,9]. In one cluster of cases of *Flavobacterium* meningitis, contamination of the saline used

to rinse the eyes of newborn babies was suggested as the source of infection [50]. As in outbreaks in neurosurgical units, however, in none of these situations has exposure to the contaminated object or product been conclusively linked epidemiologically to the risk of developing meningitis.

Groups A and B streptococci, *S. aureus*, and *L. monocytogenes* are probably also introduced into nurseries by an infected infant, mother, or medical care provider and subsequently spread among infants via hospital personnel. As with gram-negative bacilli, the role of aerosols and fomites in the spread of these organisms remains unsettled.

### Other Patients

In any patient undergoing procedures that invade the CNS, contaminated medications and medical devices are a potential source of infection. Nosocomial meningitis has been linked to the use of contaminated amphotericin B suspensions given intrathecally [58] and to contaminated saline used during induction of spinal anesthesia [18]. In addition, five cases of streptococcal meningitis following myelography have been described, and the possibility that contaminated contrast medium may have been responsible has been suggested [46]. Finally, it is notable that cases of both community-acquired and nosocomial meningitis due to *L. monocytogenes* have been linked to consumption of raw vegetables [30,60].

## CLINICAL FINDINGS AND OUTCOME

Nosocomial meningitis does not differ clinically from meningitis acquired elsewhere. The clinical manifestations are largely a function of the patient's age and the presence of associated infections. Prompt recognition of nosocomial meningitis can be difficult, however, both in patients who have undergone recent neurosurgical procedures or invasion of the CNS and in neonates.

### Neurosurgery Patients

Meningitis following neurosurgery is characterized by fever, with 94 percent of patients having fever on the first day of illness [38]. Chills, headache, nausea and vomiting, irritability, malaise, cervical rigidity, coma, and a positive Kernig's sign are also common manifestations of postoperative meningitis. Many of these findings, however, are also present in uninfected neurosurgery patients during the postoperative period, due to the presence of blood and/or other foreign matter in the CNS and to the surgical trauma. Furthermore, changes in mental status in such patients can be difficult to assess.

The choice of antimicrobials for treatment is governed by the antimicrobial sensitivities of the infecting organism, while the route of administration (systemic and/or intrathecal) depends on the ability to achieve adequate levels of an effective antimicrobial in the CSF. The outcome for neurosurgical patients with meningitis is generally poor, but it is a function of the infecting organism and its antimicrobial sensitivities and of the underlying neurosurgical problem.

*Ventricular Shunt Patients*
Meningitis in patients with ventricular shunts is manifested by fever, nausea and vomiting, malaise, and meningeal signs [44,61]. Shunt infections per se can also be accompanied by local erythema over the shunt course, splenomegaly, anemia, and glomerulonephritis. CNS infections in shunt patients can become apparent within a day or two after surgery, or many months later [44,61,62]. The time interval between surgery and onset of illness is in large part a function of the infecting organism, with infections due to *S. aureus* usually becoming apparent early and infections due to *S. epidermidis* usually becoming apparent late [61]. Similarly, infections in patients with ventricular shunts can have an acute, rapidly progressive course (more common with *S. aureus* infections) or can be more indolent (more common with *S. epidermidis* infections).

There is substantial controversy about the role of antimicrobials (parenteral and/or intraventricular) alone in treating shunt infections, compared with antimicrobials plus removal of the shunt. Although antimicrobials alone have been reported to cure 36 to 41 percent of patients [40,59], many authors have reported poor results without the complete removal of the infected shunt [11,14,37,61,63]. Whether or not the infected shunt is removed, the outcome of meningitis in ventricular shunt patients tends to be better than in neonates and other neurosurgical patients.

*Neonates*
Meningitis in neonates is usually characterized by fever (although hypothermia also has been reported) and nonspecific findings such as poor feeding, decreased tone, lethargy, listlessness, a weak cry, irritability, dyspnea or apnea, and jaundice. Specific findings that point toward the CNS as the site of infection (e.g., bulging fontanelle, stiff neck) are frequently absent [47]. Since neonatal meningitis is usually associated with bacteremia, it is not surprising that the clinical findings are almost indistinguishable from those seen in neonatal sepsis without meningitis.

Onset of illness usually occurs four to eight days after birth, but can be as early as one day or as late as six weeks. Thus many cases of nosocomial meningitis in neonates do not become apparent until after discharge from the hospital. As in meningitis in neurosurgical patients, the choice of antimicrobials and the route of administration depend on the causative organism, its antimicrobial sensitivities, and the penetration of the antimicrobial agent into the CSF. The outcome of neonatal meningitis, while dependent on the causative organism, is generally poor; the fatality rate is 60 percent (approaching 100 percent in some outbreaks), and there is permanent neurologic damage in many survivors [47].

## LABORATORY FINDINGS

The laboratory findings in patients with nosocomial bacterial meningitis do not differ from those seen in other patients with bacterial meningitis. The opening pressure may be normal or increased; the CSF contains an elevated number of white blood cells, with a predominance of polymorphonuclear leukocytes; the CSF protein level is increased; the CSF glucose level is decreased; and bacteria may be visible on Gram stain. On rare occasions, the CSF may be entirely normal. Because the CSF protein level and leukocyte count may be elevated due to neurosurgery alone, however, and because organisms are not visible on Gram stain in approximately 50 percent of cases, a low CSF glucose concentration may be the only reliable indicator of meningitis in a neurosurgery patient until the CSF culture results are available [38]. While an elevated peripheral white blood cell count also is usually present in patients with meningitis, the frequent administration of corticosteroids to neurosurgery patients and the resultant leukocytosis can make these counts difficult to interpret.

## FACTITIOUS MENINGITIS
## AND PSEUDOOUTBREAKS

While CSF Gram-stain evidence of bacterial meningitis in several hospitalized patients over a short period of time is suggestive of a problem with nosocomial meningitis, it is worth keeping in mind that such findings can be spurious. False-positive CSF Gram stains can be caused by the presence of viable or nonviable organisms in the Gram-stain reagents, in transport media used for swabs, in the tubes used to centrifuge the CSF, and on improperly cleaned glass slides [21,31,43,49,66]. False-positive CSF Gram stains also have been attributed to the use of unoccluded needles in the performance of the lumbar puncture [33]. Problems such as these should be considered whenever CSF culture results fail to confirm positive CSF Gram-stain results; they can largely be avoided by proper cleaning of glass slides before use, filtration of staining reagents, and thorough rinsing of slides after staining.

## RISK TO HOSPITAL PERSONNEL

Hospital personnel in contact with infected patients are not thought to be at increased risk of developing meningitis except when the patient has meningitis or other invasive disease caused by N. meningitidis. Even when the patient has a meningococcal infection, the risk to hospital personnel is low and appears to be limited to those with unusually intimate contact with the patient's respiratory tract secretions (e.g., someone who has given the patient mouth-to-mouth resuscitation or suctioned the patient). The number of reported secondary meningococcal infections among medical personnel since the disappearance of epidemic meningococcal disease from the United States has been small [3,16,22], despite the fact that approximately 2500 patients with meningococcal meningitis and meningococcemia are admitted to U.S. hospitals each year [5].

Current recommendations for prevention of such cases seem to be adequate to protect hospital personnel. Recommendations include keeping patients with meningococcal infections in respiratory isolation (private room, with face masks worn by staff and visitors) until 24 hours after initiation of effective therapy and prompt use of chemoprophylaxis among hospital staff with unusually intimate exposure to respiratory secretions (see Chapter 9). Chemoprophylaxis of close community contacts of patients with meningitis caused by H. influenzae or N. meningitidis also is indicated. Such cases should be promptly reported to the appropriate state or local health department so that chemoprophylaxis can be given.

## SURVEILLANCE AND PREVENTION

The prevention of nosocomial meningitis does not differ fundamentally from the prevention of other nosocomial infections. An awareness of the problem and a surveillance system focused on high-risk areas such as neurosurgical wards and neonatal intensive care units are the keys to spotting cases early and preventing additional ones (see Chapter 5). Avoiding colonization of patients by impeccable surgical-wound and umbilical-stump care and scrupulous attention to hand-washing can probably prevent most cases of nosocomial meningitis.

The infection control nurse should carefully monitor the occurrence of cases of meningitis in neonates and neurosurgery patients. Given the generally poor outcome in cases of nosocomial meningitis, two or more cases due to a single organism, even if they are scattered in time, should be cause for additional investigation. In light of the sometimes prolonged incubation period, particularly in patients with ventricular shunts, such an investigation must include the following up of patients at risk who were not ill at the time of discharge. Culturing of the hospital environment and of hospital personnel, if undertaken at all, should follow and be guided by a thorough epidemiologic investigation.

## REFERENCES

1. Aber, R. C., Allen, N. Howell, J. T., Wilkinson, H. W., and Facklam, R. R., Nosocomial transmission of group-B streptococci. Pediatrics 58:346, 1976.
2. Anderson, F. M. Ventriculocardiac shunts. J. Pediatr. 82:222, 1973.
3. Artenstein, M. S., and Ellis, R. E. The risk of exposure to a patient with meningococcal meningitis. Military Med. 133:474, 1968.
4. Ayliffe, G. A. J., Lowbury, E. J. L., Hamilton, J. G., Small, J. M., Asheshov, E. A., and Parker, M.T. Hospital infection with Pseudomonas aeruginosa in neurosurgery. Lancet 2:365, 1965.
5. Band, J. D., Chamberland, M. E., Platt, T., Weaver, R. E., Thornsberry, C., and Fraser, D. W. Trends in meningococcal disease, United States 1975–1980, J. Infect. Dis. 148:754, 1983.
6. Barton, L. L., Granoff, D. M., Barenkamp, S. J. Nosocomial spread of Haemophilus influenzae type b infection documented by outer membrane protein subtype analysis. J. Pediatr. 102:820, 1983.
7. Bassett, D. C. J., Thompson, S. A. S., and Page, B. Neonatal infections with pseudomonas aeruginosa associated with contaminated resuscitation equipment. Lancet 1:781, 1965.
8. Bayston, R., and Lari, J. A study of the sources of infection in colonized shunts. Dev. Med. Child Neurol 16(Suppl. 32):16, 1974.
9. Becker, A. H. Infection due to Proteus mirabilis

in newborn nursery. *J. Dis. Child.* 104:69, 1962.

10. Berkowitz, F. E. Acinetobacter meningitis—a diagnostic pitfall: A report of 3 cases. *S. Afr. Med. J.* 61:448, 1982.

11. Bruce, A. M., Lorber, J., Shedden, W. I. H., and Zachary, R. B. Persistent bacteraemia following ventriculocaval shunt operations for hydrocephalus in infants. *Dev. Med. Child Neurol* 5:461, 1963.

12. Burke, J. P., Ingall, D., Klein, J. O., Gezon, H. M., Finland, M. *Proteus mirabilis* infections in a hospital nursery traced to a human carrier. *N. Engl. J. Med.* 284:115, 1971.

13. Cabrera, H. A., and Davis, G. H. Epidemic meningitis of the newborn caused by flavobacteria. *Am. J. Dis. Child.* 101:289, 1961.

14. Callaghan, R. P., Cohen, S. J., and Stewart, G. T. Septicaemia due to colonization of Spitz-Holter valves by staphylococci: Five cases treated with methicillin. *Br. Med. J.* 1:860, 1961.

15. Campbell, A. N., Sill, P. R., and Wardle, J. K. *Listeria* meningitis acquired by cross-infection in a delivery suite. *Lancet* 2:752, 1981.

16. Centers for Disease Control. Nosocomial meningococcemia—Wisconsin. *Morbid. Mortal. Weekly Rep.* 27:358, 1978.

17. Cohen, M. S., Steere, A. C., Baltimore, R., Graevenitz, A. V., Pantelick, E., Camp. B., and Root, R. K. Possible nosocomial transmission of group Y *Neisseria meningitidis* among oncology patients. *Ann. Intern. Med.* 91:7, 1979.

18. Corbett, J. J., and Rosenstein, B. J. *Pseudomonas* meningitis related to spinal anesthesia: Report of three cases with a common source of infection. *Neurology* 21:946, 1971.

19. Cutler, M., and Cutler, P. Iatrogenic meningitis. *J. Med. Soc. N. J.* 50:510, 1953.

20. Dillon, H. C. Group A type 12 streptococcal infection in a newborn nursery. *Am. J. Dis. Child.* 112:177, 1966.

21. Ericsson, C. D., Carmichael, M., Pickering, L. K., Mussett, R., and Kohl, S. Erroneous diagnosis of meningitis due to false-positive Gram stains. *South. Med. J.* 71:1524, 1978.

22. Feldman, H. A. Recent developments in the therapy and control of meningococcal infections. *DM* Feb. 1966, pp. 18–20.

23. Franciosi, R. A. Knostman, J. D., Zimmerman, R. A. Group-B streptococcal neonatal and infant infections. *J. Pediatr.* 82:707, 1973.

24. Glode, M. P., Schiffer, M. S., Robbins, J. B., Khan, W., Battle, C. U., and Armenta, E. An outbreak of *Hemophilus influenzae* type b meningitis in an enclosed hospital population. *J. Pe-*

*diatr.* 88:36, 1976.

25. Graham, D. R., Anderson, R. L., Ariel, F. E., Ehrenkranz, N. J., Rowe, B., Boer, H. R., and Dixon, R. E. Epidemic nosocomial meningitis due to *Citrobacter diversus* in neonates. *J. Infect. Dis* 144:203, 1981.

26. Gross, R. J., Rowe, B., and Easton, J. A. Neonatal meningitis caused by *Citrobacter koseri*. *J. Clin. Pathol.* 26:138, 1973.

27. Gwynn, C. M., and George, R. H. Neonatal *Citrobacter* meningitis. *Arch. Dis. Child.* 48:455, 1973.

28. Headings, D. L., and Overall, J. C., Jr. Outbreak of meningitis in a newborn intensive care unit caused by a single *Escherichia coli* Kl serotype. *J. Pediatr.* 90:99, 1977.

29. Hill, H. R., Hunt, C. E., and Matsen, J. M. Nosocomial colonization with *Klebsiella*, type 26, in a neonatal intensive-care unit associated with an outbreak of sepsis, meningitis, and necrotizing enterocolitis. *J. Pediatr.* 85:415, 1974.

30. Ho, J. L., Shands, K. N., Friedland, G., Eckind, P., and Fraser, D. W. A multihospital outbreak of type 4b *Listeria monocytogenes* infection. *ICAAC* Abstract, 1981, p. 632.

31. Hoke, C. H., Batt, J. M., Mirrett, S., Cox, R. L., and Reller, L. B. False-positive Gram-stained smears. *J.A.M.A.* 241:478, 1979.

32. Jentsch, H. J., Guggenbichler, J. P., and Waltl, H. Salmonella meningitis in the newborn. *Monatsschr. Kinderheilkd.* 127:415, 1979.

33. Joyner, R. W., Idriss, Z. H., and Wilfert, C. M. Misinterpretation of cerebrospinal fluid Gram stain. *Pediatrics* 54:360, 1974.

34. Kremer, M. Meningitis after spinal analgesia. *Br. Med. J.* 2:309, 1945.

35. Larsson, S., Cederberg, A., Ivarsson, S., Svanberg, I., and Cronberg, S. *Listeria monocytogenes* causing hospital-acquired enterocolitis and meningitis in newborn infants. *Br. Med. J.* 2:473, 1978.

36. Laugier, J., Borderon, J. C., Chantepie, A., Tabarly, J. L., and Gold, F. Meningite du nouveau-ne a *Listeria monocytogenes* et contamination en maternite. *Arch. Fr. Pediatr.* 35:168, 1978.

37. Luthardt, T. Bacterial infections in ventriculoauricular shunt systems. *Dev. Med. Child Neurol.* 22(Suppl.):105, 1970.

38. Mangi, R. J., Quintiliani, R., and Andriole, V. T. Gram-negative bacillary meningitis. *Am. J. Med.* 59:829, 1975.

39. McCarthy, M. F., Jr., and Wenzel, R. P. Postoperative spinal fluid infections after neurosurgical shunting procedures. *Pediatrics* 59:793, 1977.

40. McLaurin, R. L. Infected cerebrospinal fluid shunts. *Surg. Neurol.* 1:191, 1973.

41. Morgan, M. E. I., and Hart, C. A. Acinetobacter meningitis: Acquired infection in a neonatal intensive care unit. *Arch. Dis. Child.* 57:557, 1982.

42. Muschner, V. K., Dietzsch, H. J., Gottschalk, B., Liebscher, S., and Mank, H. Meningitisepidemid durch Coxsackievirus typ B 5 auf einer sauglingsstaion. *Kinderaerztl. Prax.* 7:290, 1972.

43. Musher, D. M., and Schell, R. F. False-positive Gram stains of cerebrospinal fluid. *Ann. Intern. Med.* 79:603, 1973.

44. Naito, H., Toya, S., Shizawa, H., Hisao, S., Hzaka, Y., and Tsukumo, D. High incidence of acute postoperative meningitis and septicemia in patients undergoing craniotomy with ventriculoatrial shunt. *Surg. Gynecol. Obstet.* 137:810, 1973.

45. Nardi, G., Grandi, D., Baroni, M., Bevilacqua, G., Tanzi, M. L., and Tedeschi, F. Epidemia da virus coxsackie di gruppo B in un reparto neonatale. *Ann. Sclavo* 18:793, 1976.

46. Noiby, N., Schneibel, J., and Sebbesen, O. Streptococcal meningitis after myelography. *Communicable Disease Report* Public Health Laboratory Service, Communicable Disease Surveillance Center, London, England, vol. 5, 1982.

47. Overall, J. C., Jr. Neonatal bacterial meningitis: Analysis of predisposing factors and outcome compared with matched control subjects. *J. Pediatr.* 76:499, 1970.

48. Parry, M. F., Hutchinson, J. H., Brown, N. A., Wu, C. H., and Estreller, L. Gram-negative sepsis in neonates: A nursery outbreak due to hand carriage of *Citrobacter diversus*. *Pediatrics* 65:1105, 1980.

49. Peterson, E., Thrupp, L., Uchiyama, N., Hawkins, B., Wolvin, B., and Greene, G. Factitious bacterial meningitis revisited. *J. Clin. Microbiol.* 16:758, 1982.

50. Plotkin, S. A., and McKitrick, J. C. Nosocomial meningitis of the newborn caused by a flavobacterium. *J.A.M.A.* 198:194, 1966.

51. Price, D. J. E., and Sleigh, J. D., Control of infection due to *Klebsiella aerogenes* in a neurosurgical unit by withdrawal of all antibiotics. *Lancet* 2:1213, 1970.

52. Price, D. J. E., and Sleigh, J. D. *Klebsiella* meningitis—report of nine cases. *J. Neurol. Neurosurg. Psychiatry.* 35:903, 1972.

53. Rance, C. P., Roy, T. E., Donohue, W. L., Sepp, A. Elder, R., and Finlayson, M. An epidemic of septicemia with meningitis and hemorrhagic encephalitis in premature infants. *J. Pediatr.* 61:24, 1962.

54. Ratcheson, R. A., and Ommaya, A. K. Experience with the subcutaneous cerebrospinal fluid reservoir: Preliminary report of 60 cases. *N. Engl. J. Med.* 279:1025, 1968.

55. Ravenholt, R. T., and LaVeck, G. D. Staphylococcal disease: An obstetric, pediatric, and community problem. *Am. J. Public Health* 46:1287, 1956.

56. Ribeiro, C. D., Davis, P., and Jones, D. M. *Citrobacter koseri* meningitis in a special care baby unit. *J. Clin. Pathol.* 29:1094, 1976.

57. Salmon, J. H. Adult hydrocephalus: Evaluation of shunt therapy in 80 patients. *J. Neurosurg.* 37:423, 1972.

58. Sarubbi, F. A., Jr., Wilson, M. B., Lee, M., and Brokopp, C. Nosocomial meningitis and bacteremia due to contaminated amphotericin B. *J.A.M.A.* 239:416, 1978.

59. Schimke, R. T., Black, P. H., Mark, V. H., and Swartz, M. N. Indolent *Staphylococcus albus* or *aureus* bacteremia after ventriculoatriostomy: Role of foreign body in its initiation and perpetuation. *N. Engl. J. Med.* 264:264, 1961.

60. Schlech, W. F., Lavigne, P. M., Bortolussi, R. A., et al. Epidemic listeriosis: Evidence for transmission by food. *N. Engl. J. Med.* 308:203, 1983.

61. Schoenbaum, S. C., Gardner, P., and Shillito, J. Infections of cerebrospinal fluid shunts: Epidemioloy, clinical manifestations, and therapy. *J. Infect. Dis.* 131:543, 1975.

62. Sells, C. J., Shurtleff, D. B., and Loeser, J. D. Gram-negative cerebrospinal fluid shunt—associated infections. *Pediatrics* 59:614, 1977.

63. Shurtleff, D. B., Foltz, E. L., Weeks, R. D., and Loeser, J. Therapy of *Staphylococcus epidermidis* infections associated with cerebrospinal fluid shunts. *Pediatrics* 53:55, 1974.

64. Tsingoglou, S., and Forrest, D. M. A technique for the insertion of Holter ventriculo-atrial shunt for infantile hydrocephalus. *Br. J. Surg.* 58:367, 1971.

65. Venes, J. L. Control of shunt infection: Report of 150 consecutive cases. *J. Neurosurg.* 45:311, 1976.

66. Weinstein, R. A, Bauer, F. W., Hoffman, R. D., Tyler, P. G., Anderson, R. L., and Stamm, W. E. Factitious meningitis: Diagnostic error due to nonviable bacteria in commercial lumbar puncture trays. *J.A.M.A.* 233:878, 1975.

67. Winterbauer, R. H., Fortuine, R., and Eickhoff, T. C. Unusual occurrence of neonatal meningitis due to group B beta-hemolytic streptococci. *Pediatrics* 38:661, 1966.

# 35 SELECTED VIRUSES OF NOSOCOMIAL IMPORTANCE

William M. Valenti
Paul F. Wehrle

Viral infections probably account for more nosocomial infections than previously realized; at least 5 percent of all nosocomial infections are due to viruses [146]. While much of the data on nosocomial viral infections comes from pediatric services [67,103,147], adults, especially the elderly and chronically ill, appear to be at risk as well [92,146,148].

The magnitude of nosocomial viral infections occurring in hospital employees has not been studied systematically. Except for anecdotal information regarding the acquisition of clinical disease (e.g., rubella), employee involvement in transmission of viral infections among patients can only be inferred. Health-care facilities bring together a great variety of workers of all ages with a wide range of educational and ethnic backgrounds, which complicates the implementation of infection control procedures. In addition, the numbers of pregnant women working in health-care facilities are probably greater than in any other work place, which adds to the complexities of protecting workers from developing infections. Medical facilities pose a serious challenge in terms of prevention of infection in both patients and personnel. Infection control personnel must be familiar with the potential for nosocomial transmission of viruses and must be aware of their modes of transmission and possible methods of control and prevention.

With the continued development of rapid viral diagnostic methods, new and improved vaccines, and antiviral chemotherapy, virology will become an increasingly important component of the infection control program in health-care facilities (see Chapter 37).

## RESPIRATORY VIRUSES

Transmission of respiratory viruses in health-care facilities is an annual event in temperate climates. Both patients and personnel are at special risk during the winter season, and large numbers of health-care personnel with acute respiratory illnesses become a major concern. In addition to pediatric patients [67], patients who seem to be at greatest risk of acquiring nosocomial viral respiratory disease are patients in closed or semiclosed populations such as psychiatric units [146] and patients in extended-care facilities [92].

The two major mechanisms of transmission of respiratory viruses are by means of droplet nuclei (small-particle aerosol) and droplets (large-particle spread). Droplet nuclei aerosols ($< 10\ \mu$ median diameter)

531

containing infectious virions are produced by coughing, sneezing, or talking and are capable of transmitting infectious virus over considerable distances (greater than 6 feet). Smallpox provided the classic example of this type of spread, but influenza virus and perhaps varicella and measles viruses also exhibit patterns of spread compatible with this mechanism. With droplet spread, other viral agents may be transmitted over shorter distances by mechanisms requiring close person-to-person contact, generally at a distance of less than 3 feet separating two persons. This method of transmission may occur when droplets produced by coughing or sneezing either directly infect the susceptible host (e.g., mucous membranes of the eye or nose) or contaminate the donor's hands or a fomite allowing infectious virus to be transferred indirectly to the skin or mucous membranes of a susceptible host. Infection in the susceptible host may also result from autoinoculation, with transfer of virus from hands to mucous membranes of the eye or nose. Rhinoviruses and respiratory syncytial virus exhibit patterns of spread compatible with close-contact transmission.

In the absence of viral diagnostic facilities, it may be possible to establish a presumptive viral diagnosis based on the predominant anatomic site of involvement in the respiratory tract, epidemiologic data such as season of the year, geographic location, type of patient population, and data from area surveillance activity.

### Influenza Virus

Influenza A and B viral infections are among the most communicable diseases of humans. They are characterized by explosive epidemics, and nosocomial transmission of influenza A [42,92] and B [148] has been well documented. Person-to-person transmission is thought to take place primarily by droplet nuclei. These aerosols may account for the explosive nature of influenza outbreaks, since, in a closed environment, one infected person can potentially infect large numbers of susceptible persons. During an outbreak of influenza A at the New York Hospital during the pandemic of 1957–58, 15 of 29 patients and 15 of 30 personnel on one hospital floor became infected, possibly from a single index case [42]. Influenza A viral infection may result in significant morbidity (e.g., primary influenza pneumonia, secondary bacterial pneumonia) and mortality. It may also pose a significant risk to elderly and/or chronically ill institutionalized patients [92], to patients in closed or semiclosed populations such as psychiatric patients [146], and to pediatric patients [63,146,155,156].

ISOLATION PRECAUTIONS Respiratory isolation with masks for hospital personnel, private room, and care in handling secretions and secretion-soiled articles would seem to be the most reasonable precautions for patients with proven or suspected influenza viral infection. However, the recently revised *Guidelines for Isolation Precautions in Hospitals* do not recommend these precautions (see Chapter 9), presumably due to the delay in diagnosis of influenza because diagnostic laboratories for viral isolation are not available to many health-care facilities. We still believe, however, that because influenza virus is transmitted by small-particle aerosols, patients who are admitted to the hospital with febrile respiratory illness at a time when influenza is prevalent in the community should be considered to have influenza until proved otherwise and should be placed on appropriate precautions including mask and private room. In hospital outbreaks involving large numbers of people, patients with influenza should be cohorted in the same room or on the same hospital floor [63]. Shedding of virus may persist for as long as five days after the onset of symptoms in adults [42], and for seven days or longer in children [63]. At the present time we maintain respiratory precautions for patients with influenza viral infection for seven days or the duration of clinical illness, whichever is longer.

IMMUNIZATION Vaccination in the fall of each year of patients with chronic underlying illnesses and persons over the age of 65 should result in 60 to 90 percent protection against influenza A and B infections for many hospitalized patients [19,21,114,115]. Additionally, vaccine appears to reduce mortality in those who acquire infection.

Although influenza viral infection in healthy, young hospital workers is often benign and self-limited, hospital staff who have contact with patients should be vaccinated because of their high degree of exposure to influenza and subsequent high risk of transmission of infection to hospitalized patients. Attempts at vaccinating hospital personnel are often unrewarding. Influenza vaccination programs directed at health-care workers should include an intensive educational effort; we have found that large numbers of hospital personnel are reluctant to be vaccinated because of misinformation regarding vaccine efficacy and its side effects, including Guillain-Barré syndrome [83]. While a significant association between A/New Jersey/swine influenza vaccines and Guillain-Barré syndrome was noted, similar association has not been noted with previous or subsequent vaccine formulations [77].

CHEMOPROPHYLAXIS O'Donoghue and colleagues [113] have shown that amantadine hydrochloride is 80 percent effective in preventing clinical nosocomial influenza A viral disease [113]. In addition, there is evidence to suggest that the effects of prophylactic amantadine plus vaccination are additive [107]. During periods of high prevalence of influenza viral infection in the hospital and/or community, amantadine may be used in unvaccinated hospital patients and personnel. Vaccination of susceptible persons should also be considered in the presence of an epidemic, in addition to amantadine administration, until an adequate serologic response to vaccine occurs— generally about two weeks after vaccination. The usual dose of amantadine is 200 mg per day in either a single or divided dose. If susceptible personnel are not vaccinated, amantadine must be continued for the duration of the outbreak. Amantadine is not effective prophylactically for influenza B infection. In view of the problems with compliance when large numbers of people are taking amantadine, vaccination against influenza remains the best preventive measure against the disease.

SPECIAL CONSIDERATIONS During documented influenza outbreaks, measures other than vaccination and amantadine chemoprophylaxis should be considered, depending on the severity of the outbreak: (1) curtailment or elimination of elective surgery and other elective admissions; (2) restriction of cardiovascular and pulmonary surgery; (3) restriction of hospital visitors, especially those with respiratory illnesses; and (4) work restriction for medical personnel with acute respiratory disease. Controlled studies to evaluate these measures have not been done. In addition, items 3 and 4 above, may be difficult to implement. It is often necessary to appeal to the common sense and good judgment of hospital personnel and visitors in restricting their contact in the hospital. If personnel recovering from influenza must work, it is advisable to assign them to areas of the hospital where influenza viral infections are prevalent.

### Respiratory Syncytial Virus

Respiratory syncytial virus (RSV) is the most frequent cause of lower respiratory tract disease in children less than two years of age [67]. In recent years RSV infections have accounted for approximately 45 percent of all admissions to the Strong Memorial Hospital for respiratory disease in children under two years of age [64]. It is also the most common nosocomial infection on our pediatric wards [65,146]. In addition, people in all age groups are potentially suscep-

tible to RSV infection, and because immunity is incomplete and not permanent, reinfections may occur throughout life [70]. RSV infections have also been documented in hospital personnel [65] and in elderly chronically ill patients [92]. Generally, RSV infections occur in annual epidemics of two to three months' duration, often beginning in late December. Early studies by Chanock and colleagues [29] showed that approximately 59 percent of children admitted to the hospital with nonviral diseases showed serologic conversion to RSV while hospitalized during periods of RSV prevalence in the community.

The primary mode of transmission of RSV appears to be by close person-to-person contact. Studies by Hall and coworkers [64,66] have elucidated the chain of transmission of RSV. These authors have also demonstrated that patients infected with RSV shed large amounts of virus in their respiratory secretions, with a mean duration of shedding of 6 to 7 days and a range of 1 to 21 days [64]. The virus can be recovered from the immediate environment of infected patients for prolonged periods of time. For example, RSV in nasal secretions from infected infants can be recovered for up to 30 minutes from contaminated skin, gowns, or paper tissues [66]. The virus appears to survive best on nonporous surfaces such as countertops and has been recovered for up to six hours from these surfaces [66]. Infectious virus can then be transferred from these environmental surfaces to hands and from hand to hand [66]. Studies in volunteers have also demonstrated that infection can be initiated by instillation of RSV-containing fluid into the mucous membranes of the eyes or nose but not the mouth. Therefore, spread by direct inoculation of drops or large particles or by self-inoculation after touching contaminated surfaces such as skin or fomites seems feasible. Spread by small-particle aerosols seems less likely since nosocomial outbreaks are not as explosive as those due to influenza virus, and studies in volunteers show that only persons cuddling infected infants and touching contaminated surfaces became infected with RSV. Persons did not become infected if kept more than 6 feet from an infected baby, suggesting that small-particle aerosol transmission is not a major route of transmission of RSV.

The risk of nosocomial RSV infection has been correlated with the duration of hospitalization; the risk increases with each subsequent week of hospitalization. In one study, RSV infection was acquired by 45 percent of contact infants hospitalized for one week or more. The rate of RSV acquisition increased with each subsequent week of hospitalization until all infants hospitalized four weeks or more became infected. The rate of infection was not related to underlying illness or age of the patient. In addition, the role of hospital personnel in the transmission of RSV is becoming increasingly important. Each year, approximately 50 percent of adult staff working on the pediatric service (nurses, house staff, and medical and nursing students) become infected with RSV. Conventional infection control measures such as hand washing, gowns, isolation or cohorting of infected infants, and cohorting of staff to infants have decreased the rate of nosocomial acquisition of RSV in patients but not in hospital personnel [65].

ISOLATION PRECAUTIONS During periods of increased RSV prevalence in the community, infants with respiratory illness who are admitted to the hospital should be placed in single rooms or cohorted with other infants with RSV illness (see Chapter 9). A clean gown should be worn for each contact with an infected infant, and the gown should be changed after each contact. To prevent cross-infection, hospital personnel caring for infected infants should not care for infants who don't have respiratory illness if at all possible. The need for a mask is not as clear, since the risk of droplet-nuclei aerosol transmission of RSV is small. However, masks probably assist in preventing droplet spread and thus may prevent transmission of RSV via close contact [28,29,67]. The importance of careful hand washing is evident.

IMMUNIZATION There is no effective vaccine for RSV.

SPECIAL CONSIDERATIONS Attempts to reduce nosocomial transmission of RSV should be directed toward hospital personnel. Education of patient-care staff should include special emphasis on both the mode of transmission of RSV and the role of personnel in the chain of infection.

Efforts should be made to curtail visits from family and friends who have respiratory illness, especially during periods of increased RSV prevalence in the community. In the absence of locally generated data on RSV prevalence, one can assume its occurrence during December through March in the United States and Europe. Children visiting pediatric services should be screened for present histories of respiratory illness of any kind and should be discouraged from visiting on the ward if there is any clinical respiratory disease.

### Parainfluenza Virus
Nosocomial transmission of parainfluenza types 1, 3, and 4a on pediatric services has been documented [106]. Mufson reports that 18 percent of infants who are well or infected with another respiratory pathogen at the time of admission to a children's hospital subsequently acquired nosocomial infections with parainfluenza type 3 [106]. Infections in hospitals have also been reported in adult renal transplant patients [38] and in elderly institutionalized patients [16]. Details of transmission of parainfluenza virus have not been fully elucidated, but transmission is believed to occur by contact spread, either direct (person-to-person) or indirect (person-to-fomite-to-person) [16]. Infections with parainfluenza types 1 and 2 are seasonal, with the greatest activity occurring during the fall months. Community epidemics with types 1 and 2 occur approximately every two years, while infections with parainfluenza virus type 3 tend to occur throughout each year.

ISOLATION PRECAUTIONS The importance of careful hand-washing cannot be overemphasized, especially in view of the proposed mechanism of transmission of parainfluenza virus. Precautions are similar to those used for RSV, with patients placed in a private room or cohorted together (see Chapter 9). Careful hand-washing and gown changes after each contact have been suggested as the most effective means of minimizing nosocomial transmission of parainfluenza viruses [16]. Precautions should be maintained for the duration of illness.

### Rhinovirus
Although rhinovirus infections are ubiquitous during the winter and spring months, they have not been recognized as important nosocomial pathogens [146,155,156]. Rhinovirus may be a cause of significant morbidity in premature infants. Recently, an outbreak of rhinovirus infection in premature infants in an intensive care nursery was documented [147]. The affected infants had significant respiratory distress related to rhinovirus infections, and one of them required intubation.

Large quantities of virus are present in nasal secretions and readily contaminate the hands of the infected person. Virus transmission appears to take place directly from hand to hand or indirectly via fomites. Virus may be inoculated from the recipient's hands via touching of the mucous membranes of the nose and eyes [72].

Careful hand-washing with soap and water appears to be the most effective way of minimizing transmission of rhinovirus. Dilute solutions containing 1% iodine have been shown to be effective skin antiseptics [71]. Since rhinoviruses are remarkably resistant to drying and survive for long periods of time on hard surfaces and plastic and synthetic fabrics [72], iodinated compounds may also be considered for use as disinfectants on surfaces contaminated with rhinovirus-containing secretions (see Chapter 14).

ISOLATION PRECAUTIONS Generally, precautions other than hand-washing are not recommended for patients with rhinovirus infection (see Chapter 9). However, cohorting of patients with rhinovirus infection in nurseries may sometimes be indicated.

*Adenovirus*

Adenovirus infections occur in the general population throughout the year. These viruses are quite stable and can be transmitted via a number of routes and cause a variety of illnesses. Adenoviruses are associated with conjunctivitis, keratoconjunctivitis, pharyngoconjunctival fever, pneumonia, and a pertussis-like syndrome. Respiratory transmission via aerosols occurs in all age groups [51], and volunteer studies have shown that inhalation of small doses of virus can initiate acute respiratory illness, including pneumonia [51]. Fecal-oral transmission occurs but probably is more important in children than in adults [51].

Hospital-acquired adenovirus infection has been reported in both patients and personnel [14,133,135]. Infections in neonates [47] and in pediatric patients [14,133,135] account for many of the reported cases of nosocomial adenovirus infections. Although adenovirus pneumonia has been reported more frequently in military recruits, adenovirus can be the cause of sporadic pneumonia in up to 10 percent of pediatric patients admitted with pneumonia [51]. Transmission of adenovirus from patients with pneumonia to hospital personnel has occurred in these situations, with personnel developing conjunctivitis and pharyngoconjunctival fever. Recently the role of adenovirus infections in immunocompromised hosts has led to speculation that adenoviruses, like herpesviruses, may be reactivated after primary infection [156]. Adenovirus has also been implicated as a cause of diffuse interstitial pneumonia in a renal transplant recipient [97] (see Chapter 37). All of these infections may have resulted from endogenous reactivation of adenovirus. Nosocomial transmission from staff with mild upper respiratory illness to immunocompromised patients may also have been involved.

An outbreak has been reported of epidemic keratoconjunctivitis due to adenovirus type 8, originating in a physician's office [37]. Of 98 persons subjected to ophthalmic procedures, 21 became infected. The physician's own eye infection probably served as a major source of virus with transmission to susceptible patients occurring by direct transfer of virus from the physician's hands and by indirect transfer of the virus

via a Schiötz tonometer. A similar outbreak of keratoconjunctivitis was associated with a contaminated ophthalmic solution in an industrial health clinic [130].

Recent evidence suggests that new types of adenovirus called noncultivable adenoviruses (NCAV) are a frequent cause of sporadic diarrhea in children [102]. Outbreaks of diarrhea among young children living at a Royal Air Force station in the United Kingdom and in a long-stay orthopedic ward suggest that these viruses can cause epidemic diarrhea and can act as nosocomial pathogens in addition to causing sporadic disease [118]. Adenovirus type 3 associated with diarrhea has also been transmitted in premature nurseries [47].

ISOLATION PRECAUTIONS Patients with adenovirus infection should be in private rooms if possible (see Chapter 9). Personnel should wear gowns and gloves when direct contact with skin and mucous membranes is anticipated. We also recommend a mask for personnel at all times; this is because available evidence suggests that airborne transmission of adenovirus takes place easily in closed populations and because of the apparent susceptibility of most adults to infection. Care must also be taken when handling secretions, contaminated articles, and contaminated linens. Because shedding of adenovirus may be quite variable and prolonged, it is not possible to determine for precisely how long a period these precautions should be maintained. For this reason it is recommended that these precautions be maintained for the duration of clinical illness.

IMMUNIZATION A live, attenuated trivalent vaccine containing adenovirus types 3, 4, and 7 has been used extensively in military personnel and has been found to be safe and reasonably effective. However, because of potency variations between lots of vaccine and the low incidence of serious disease resulting from adenovirus infection, routine use of this vaccine is not recommended.

SPECIAL CONSIDERATIONS Adenoviruses are quite stable and survive for long periods of time. Special care must be given to the decontamination and sterilization of contaminated instruments such as tonometers (see Chapter 14). Thorough cleaning followed by steam sterilization consisting of 15 psi for 15 minutes at 121°C (250°F), or 15 psi for 10 minutes at 126°C (259°F), or 29 psi for 3 minutes at 134°C (273°F) is recommended. The use of a disposable tonofilm to cover and preserve sterility of the tonometer has also been suggested [78]. Equipment now available for ocular pressure measurement without direct contact may be considered for use as well.

Once again scrupulous hand-washing between contacts cannot be overemphasized. Personnel with conjunctivitis present a hazard to patients; it is recommended that personnel with infectious conjunctivitis have no contact with patients in nurseries, obstetric units, or operating rooms until all drainage ceases.

## HERPESVIRUSES

The members of the family Herpesviridae include varicella-zoster virus (VZV), herpes simplex virus (HSV) types I and II, cytomegalovirus (CMV), and Epstein-Barr virus (EBV). Herpesvirus infections become latent or inactive after primary infection and can reactivate at a time remote from the primary infection. Infectious virus can be isolated in both primary and reactivated infections due to herpesviruses. Often primary infection is symptomatic, while reactivation infection often is asymptomatic [154]. In the United States most persons have come in contact with all the human herpesviruses (except herpesvirus II) by age 50 [154]. Thus nosocomial infection occurs relatively infrequently.

Transmission of the herpesviruses occurs primarily by direct-contact spread (person to person) and except for VZV requires close personal contact. Of the herpesviruses, VZV is the most capable of nosocomial involvement because of its direct-contact spread or airborne transmission. In addition because of particular underlying diseases or chemotherapy, many hospitalized patients are susceptible to reactivation of herpesvirus infections. When herpesviruses are transmitted in the hospital, however, nosocomial transmission may be difficult to establish since all but HSV I and II have prolonged incubation periods, and illness often develops after discharge.

In a 17-month period of careful viral surveillance, 20 cases of reactivation infection with herpesviruses were documented based on clinical criteria [146]. These infections were classified as endogenous nosocomial infections because signs and symptoms of infection were not apparent at the time of admission. During this same period, only one episode of primary CMV infection was detected; this was associated with virus from a transplanted kidney [146].

### Varicella-Zoster Virus

VZV, the most communicable of the herpesviruses, is the causative agent of chickenpox and herpes zoster (shingles). Nosocomial transmission of chickenpox is well recognized [61,87,101] and is a cause of mortality and serious morbidity in immunocompromised patients [101,104] (see Chapter 37). The primary mechanism of transmission of varicella is probably via direct contact with infectious lesions. However, nosocomial spread by the airborne route is also well documented [87]. Epidemiologic evidence suggests that patients may shed varicella virus in respiratory secretions as early as two days before the onset of rash [58], but this has never been proved by virus isolation.

Whenever possible, patients with uncomplicated chickenpox should not be admitted to the hospital because they present a hazard to susceptible patients and personnel. In addition, patients who develop chickenpox or are exposed to chickenpox while hospitalized should be discharged, if possible. Of course severely ill patients are exceptions to these rules.

ISOLATION PRECAUTIONS  Nonimmune patients exposed to chickenpox or patients with chickenpox should be isolated in a private room or cohorted (see Chapter 9). Precautions that prevent contact with both respiratory secretions and secretions from patients' vesicles are recommended. Although the duration of contagion is variable, the period of contagion of varicella virus from vesicles appears to decrease about five days after the onset of rash. Because this period is somewhat variable, isolation precautions should be continued until all skin lesions are completely dried and crusted.

The susceptible patient exposed to chickenpox who cannot be discharged from the hospital often presents a difficult problem regarding restriction of activity and isolation precautions. Because of the high degree of communicability of chickenpox, personnel and patients in the same unit as a patient with chickenpox should be considered exposed [69]. Furthermore, patients with negative or unknown histories of chickenpox should be considered susceptible and will require isolation precautions beginning 10 days after exposure and continuing until 21 days after the last exposure. Since communicability of disease before the onset of the rash is not accurately predictable, precautions or cohorting of exposed persons should be initiated on the tenth day after exposure. Unless immunity can be proved, these patients should remain isolated until discharged from the hospital or for 21 days, whichever occurs first.

Hospital workers exposed to persons with active varicella who have negative or unknown histories of previous varicella infection should not work with susceptible patients from the tenth to the twenty-first day after exposure [158]. If employee immunity to varicella can be proved, employees need not be sent home from work. If large numbers of employees are involved, these precautions may result in a significant expense to the hospital in time lost from work. In general, a history of previous chickenpox or herpes zoster in an adult or child is felt to be a reliable indication of immunity. In an attempt to control nosocomial transmission of chickenpox, the immune status in exposed persons with negative or unknown histories of chickenpox should be determined. While the complement fixation (CF) antibody test is inexpensive and easy to perform, this antibody does not persist indefinitely, and false-negative results may occur [57,161]. Newer tests, which are not as readily available as CF, include the fluorescent antibody to membrane antigen test (FAMA) and the immune adherence hemagglutination test (IAH); both tests are more reliable than CF since these antibodies are thought to persist indefinitely [161].

PROPHYLAXIS Varicella-zoster immune globulin (VZIG) is intended primarily for passive immunization of susceptible immunocompromised children after significant exposure to chickenpox or herpes zoster [23]. Available evidence suggests that if VZIG is administered within 96 hours of exposure, chickenpox can be prevented or modified in children with impaired immunity. VZIG has recently been licensed by the U.S. Food and Drug Administration and is available from 13 regional Red Cross Blood Centers [23]. The criteria for use of VZIG are shown in Tables 35-1 and 35-2. VZIG is not recommmended for susceptible workers who have been exposed to varicella-zoster virus.

### Herpes Zoster

Transmission of virus from patients with herpes zoster to produce chickenpox has occurred [4] but occurs less frequently than transmission of virus from patients with chickenpox. This may be due to the lower frequency of VZV in oral secretions of patients with herpes zoster than of patients with chickenpox.

ISOLATION PRECAUTIONS Localized herpes zoster requires secretion precautions to guard against acquisition of infection by direct contact with secretions from vesicles and from secretion-contaminated articles (see Chapter 9). A private room is desirable but not required.

Patients with disseminated herpes zoster should be cared for in the same way as patients with chickenpox. They require strict isolation precautions in a private room with negative air pressure.

TABLE 35-1. Indications for use of varicella-zoster immune globulin: patient factors

1. Susceptibility to varicella-zoster (see text)*
2. Significant exposure
3. Age of < 15 years, with administration to immunocompromised adolescents and adults and to other older patients on an individual basis (see text)
4. One of the following underlying illnesses or conditions:
   a. Leukemia or lymphoma
   b. Congenital or acquired immunodeficiency
   c. Immunosuppressive treatment
   d. Newborn of mother who had onset of chickenpox within 5 days before delivery or within 48 hours after delivery
   e. Premature infant (≥ 28 weeks' gestation) whose mother lacks a previous history of chickenpox
   f. Premature infants (< 28 weeks' gestation or ≤ 1000 gm) regardless of maternal history

*Patients should meet all four criteria.
Source: Centers for Disease Control. Recommendation of the immunization practice advisory committee (ACIP). Varicella-zoster immune globulin for the prevention of chickenpox. *Morbid. Mortal. Weekly Rep.* 33:84, 95, 1984.

TABLE 35-2. Indications for use of varicella-zoster immune globulin: exposure factors

1. One of the following types of exposure to persons with chickenpox or zoster:*
   a. Continuous household contact
   b. Playmate contact (generally > one hour of play indoors)
   c. Hospital contact (in same two- to four-bed room or adjacent beds in a large ward or prolonged face-to-face contact with an infectious staff member or patient)
   d. Newborn contact (newborn of mother who had onset of chickenpox five days or less before delivery or within 48 hours after delivery)
                        AND
2. Time elapsed after exposure is such that varicella-zoster immune globulin can be administered within 96 hours but preferably sooner

*Patients should meet both criteria.
Source: Centers for Disease Control. Recommendation of the immunization practice advisory committee (ACIP). Varicella-zoster immune globulin for the prevention of chickenpox. *Morbid. Mortal. Weekly Rep.* 33:84, 95, 1984.

Hospital personnel with negative or unknown histories of chickenpox should avoid contact with patients with either localized or disseminated herpes zoster.

Gershon [57] has shown that more than 95 percent of American-born women of childbearing age have detectable antibody to VZV. Ross [120] noted an 8 percent attack rate in historically susceptible adults with household exposure to chickenpox. A negative or unknown history of chickenpox in adults is often unreliable. These data suggest that the risk to hospital personnel for varicella acquisition from patients is small but measurable. The pool of susceptible persons, however small, represents a potential hazard for transmission of varicella to both susceptible patients and personnel.

Identification of persons with negative or unknown histories using reliable screening tests (FAMA or IAH) at the time of employment is an ideal infection control measure. Since these tests may not be readily available, selective screening should be done as quickly as possible after exposure to minimize the disruption of patient services.

### Herpes Simplex

Reactivation of HSV type I infection frequently occurs spontaneously in healthy patients or personnel as well as in immunocompromised hosts (see Chapter 37). Persons with reactivated HSV I infection rarely have intraoral lesions and often do not have labial lesions. Therefore, asymptomatic personnel potentially can transmit HSV I to susceptible patients. Recently, it has been shown that individuals with herpes simplex labialis (fever blisters) do not transmit virus efficiently in respiratory secretions [144]. However, the same investigators were able to recover virus from the hands of two-thirds of the patients with herpes labialis [144]. This transmission may explain the clusters of infections that have been described in burned patients [50] and in immunocompromised patients [110]. Transmission of infection from hospital patients to personnel is well documented. Direct inoculation of HSV I on fingers of personnel after contact with the infected patient's mouth can result in herpetic whitlow [59]. Herpetic whitlow can easily be mistaken for pyogenic paronychia and is often quite disabling to hospital personnel [59]. Available evidence suggests that herpetic whitlow can occur in immune or nonimmune persons [6]. In addition, primary herpes simplex stomatitis and pharyngitis can occur in hospital personnel [89]. A cluster of cases of primary HSV stomatitis and pharyngitis has occurred due to transmission of HSV I to patients in a dental office from a dental hygienist with herpetic whitlow [90].

HSV II and its potential for transmission from mother to newborn infant has long been a concern on obstetric and newborn services (see Chapter 19). When genital herpes is present in a mother at term, 40 to 60 percent of vaginally delivered infants will have clinically apparent infection with HSV II [109]. Approximately 50 percent of these infants will have severe or fatal illness. The risk of neonatal infection can be minimized, but not eliminated, if delivery is by cesarean section *and* membranes remain unruptured or have been ruptured for less than six hours [109]. The risk of infection at birth is also less if the mother's infection is reactivated rather than primary [109].

Although transmission of infection from mother to infant at the time of birth is well documented, evidence for transmission in the postpartum period is only indirect. Infection control policies under these circumstances are often ambiguous and confusing, and there is lack of uniformity from one institution to another [81,124]. It is generally agreed, however, that certain precautions may be indicated, depending on the clinical status of the mother.

ISOLATION PRECAUTIONS Infection control recommendations for mothers with known, suspected, or inactive herpes simplex have been described in detail [145] (see Chapter 9).

*Women with proven or clinically suspected genital herpes simplex at term.* Such women may transmit virus postnatally to their offspring as well as to other close contacts. Therefore, personnel should observe precautions, using gowns and gloves for direct contact with lesions containing virus. Perineal pads, dressings, and linen should be double-bagged. The mother may care for her baby, but she should be out of bed, wash hands thoroughly before contact with the baby, and wear a clean cover gown. The infant should be observed after birth for signs and symptoms of illness, and personnel should follow drainage-secretion precautions for direct contact with the infant. Currently, there are no data regarding use of the observation or isolation nursery for such infants after birth. The value of such a nursery for use in these cases is controversial, and nursery outbreaks of herpes simplex infection are uncommon. However, an observation nursery for these infants is recommended, and good technique including thorough hand-washing should be emphasized. These precautions do not restrict mother-baby contact yet offer some degree of protection for other infants in the nursery.

*Women with active nongenital herpes simplex at term.* Wound and skin precautions similar to those recommended for women with genital herpes simplex are reasonable for these women. A private room is not indicated. Mothers may care for their infants using the same precautions as noted for mothers with known or suspected genital herpes simplex with the addition of a mask or dressing to cover the lesions.

The infant may be kept in the general newborn nursery without isolation after birth if there has been no maternal contact. After the first contact with the mother, the infant should be placed in the suspect or isolation nursery, using precautions noted previously for babies born to mothers with active genital herpes simplex.

*Women with clinically inactive herpes simplex at term.* No special precautions are necessary for either the mother or infant.

SPECIAL CONSIDERATIONS  The issue of work restrictions for employees with herpes simplex infection is raised frequently. In determining such work restrictions, it is useful to distinguish between covered and uncovered active lesions of herpes simplex. Personnel who have uncovered or active lesions of herpes simplex should not work with newborn infants (term or preterm), burned patients, or immunocompromised hosts until all lesions have dried and crusted. Personnel with herpetic whitlow should be excluded from patient care until the lesions are dried and crusted. Wearing a glove on the involved hand has been suggested as an alternative, but it is not known if this is a truly effective barrier to disease transmission. Personnel who have active genital herpes simplex or covered lesions of herpes simplex are not restricted from patient contact, but strict hand-washing is required before and after patient contact.

Measures to prevent herpetic whitlow include wearing gloves on *both hands* if direct contact with oral or pharyngeal secretions is anticipated [59,145]. Gloves are especially important when suctioning patients and should be worn routinely during this procedure. Also, patients with proven or suspected herpes simplex labialis who require intensive nursing care should be placed on precautions that require the use of gloves whenever contact with these lesions is anticipated [59,145].

Recently, concern has arisen over the possibility of acquiring genital herpes simplex infections from inanimate surfaces, especially toilet seats. While the virus has been found to survive for short periods of time outside the human body, the geometric mean titer of virus on plastic and skin surfaces decreases rapidly during the first hour (Fig. 35-1) [144], although the falloff is not quite as rapid on cloth. Transmission of herpes simplex from inanimate surfaces such as plastic and cloth has not been documented. The general consensus of experts in the field of virology is that such transmission is rare or nonexistent and that herpes simplex virus is usually transmitted via direct contact with infectious lesions.

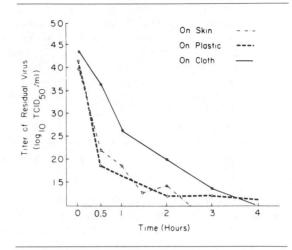

FIG. 35-1. Geometric mean titers of residual herpesvirus in saliva. TCID = tissue culture infective dose. (From Turner, R., Shehab, Z., Osborne, K., et al. Shedding and survival of herpes simplex virus from "fever blisters." *Pediatrics* 70:547, 1982, with permission.)

*Cytomegalovirus*

Cytomegalovirus, like other herpesviruses, requires direct contact for spread. There is increasing evidence to suggest that CMV infection may be a sexually transmitted disease. The virus is found in cervical and vaginal secretions and in semen. In addition, the prevalence of CMV antibody has been found to be greater in homosexual (96 percent) than in heterosexual (57 percent) men [44]. It has also been shown to increase with years of sexual activity and is higher in prostitutes than in nuns [153].

The potential for in-hospital transmission of CMV has long been a concern of hospital personnel because of its role in congenital malformations. Yeager [159] showed a slight excess of antibody conversion in pediatric nurses working with children who were shedding CMV compared to personnel without patient contact. These differences, however, were not statistically significant. In another setting, dialysis personnel failed to show any seroconversion after two years of follow-up [142]. More recently, it has been shown that pediatric health-care workers are not at increased risk of acquiring CMV infection compared to women in the community [46]. Case reports have also demonstrated lack of transmission of CMV from patients to health-care personnel by using restriction endonuclease techniques [157,160].

The risk of acquisition of CMV from blood transfusion has been established more clearly. This risk is reduced with leukocyte-poor blood and virtually eliminated if washed frozen red blood cells are used

[84]. It can also be eliminated by screening potential blood donors for antibody to CMV and by eliminating those with antibody. Patients undergoing renal transplantation are an important source of CMV [73] (see Chapter 37). The majority of such patients have reactivation of endogenous CMV as a result of the transplant process or from associated immunosuppressive therapy. We have classified these infections as endogenous nosocomial infections [146]. A small number of transplant patients acquire CMV exogenously from the transplanted kidneys or from circulating cells present in the transplanted kidney.

ISOLATION PRECAUTIONS   We suggest hand-washing as the only infection control precaution for patients with congenital or acquired CMV infection. Because the risk of transmission of CMV to hospital personnel appears low, hospital personnel are not screened for CMV antibody. Personnel should be educated regarding the mode of transmission of CMV, but pregnant personnel need not be discouraged from having contact with patients with known or suspected CMV infection nor is transfer to an alternative assignment necessary.

SPECIAL CONSIDERATIONS   At the present time routine screening for antibody to CMV of personnel on newborn, pediatric, or dialysis-transplant services is not recommended.

Patients undergoing renal transplantation and their donors or donor kidneys are tested for antibody to CMV before transplantation. Whenever possible, kidneys from antibody-negative donors are transplanted to antibody-negative recipients.

*Epstein-Barr Virus*
Epstein-Barr virus (EBV) is shed in high concentration from the oropharynx of infected patients. Although nosocomial transmission is relatively rare, infection has occurred through blood transfusion [143] and from blood contamination of dialysis equipment [33] (see Chapter 37). Since transmission of EBV from the respiratory tract has not been documented in hospitals, isolation precautions for patients with EBV infections are not indicated.

# HEPATITIS

*Hepatitis A*
Nosocomial hepatitis A has been known for many years to occur in institutions for the mentally retarded [91]. Crowded conditions and poor hygienic practices on the part of many patients in these institutions appear to be predisposing factors. Recently it has been shown that as many as 80 percent of susceptible institutionalized patients may develop hepatitis A virus (HAV) infection as measured by seroconversion of antibody to HAV within three years of admission [136]. This rate of seroconversion is considerably higher than the rate of seroconversion in noninstitutionalized adults or in child controls.

Transmission of HAV in general hospitals appears to be relatively uncommon. Nosocomial transmission from personnel to patient has not been reported and from patient to patient has rarely been reported. Transmission of HAV infection from patients to personnel has occurred infrequently [15]. Foodborne outbreaks have also occurred involving hospital workers primarily but also small numbers of patients [98].

ISOLATION PRECAUTIONS   Precautions for the care of patients with hepatitis have recently been reviewed and revised [46] (see Chapter 9). In general these recommendations avoid the "all-or-none" phenomenon of past guidelines, allowing for more flexibility based on known or anticipated contact with infectious material. Dienstag and colleagues [39] have shown that maximum fecal shedding of HAV occurs before the onset of symptoms [40]. Because of these data, some experts have recommended that no precautions be taken—once the symptomatic patient is admitted to the hospital, the time for maximal shedding should have passed. On the other hand, because viral shedding can be variable, isolation precautions should emphasize the importance of care and handling of feces, bedpans, and equipment or instruments contaminated with feces. Measures such as gowns, gloves, and masks are not required routinely but should be used whenever necessary to minimize contact with feces or material contaminated with feces. A private room is not required unless the patient is incontinent of feces.

PROPHYLAXIS   Immune serum globulin (IG) has been shown to be effective in preventing or modifying hepatitis A both before exposure and early in the incubation period. If given within two weeks of exposure, IG will prevent 80 to 90 percent of HAV infections.

*Hepatitis B*
Nosocomial transmission of hepatitis B is thought to occur most often by parenteral exposure to HBsAg-positive blood. Transmission can occur from an acutely ill patient, or more likely, from an asymptomatic person who is positive for HBsAg and is unaware of it. The HBsAg carrier state accounts for the pro-

longed period of potential HBV infectivity of some patients even after the acute infection has resolved. The infectivity of blood is best correlated with the presence of either DNA polymerase or hepatitis B "e" antigen (HBeAg). For infection control purposes, however, all blood positive for HBsAg should be considered infectious. Although HBsAg has been detected in all body fluids, the frequency with which fluids other than blood contribute to hospital infection is probably low. The mechanisms of transmission are listed below from the easiest to the hardest. [46].

1. *Overt parenteral.* Direct percutaneous inoculation by needles contaminated with serum or plasma (e.g., transfusion of contaminated blood or blood products, contaminated needle stick)
2. *Inapparent parenteral*
   a. Percutaneous inoculation of infective serum or plasma without overt needle puncture (e.g., contamination of cutaneous cuts, abrasions, or lacerations
   b. Contamination of mucosal surfaces by infected serum or plasma (e.g., pipetting accidents, accidental ingestion, other direct contact with mucous membranes of the eye or mouth)
   c. Contamination of mucosal surfaces by infective secretions other than serum or plasma (e.g., sexual activity)
   d. Transfer of infective material via fomites (e.g., toothbrushes, toys, drinking cups, horizontal surfaces in hospitals)

Clearly, ample opportunity exists for transmission of hepatitis B in the hospital to both patients and personnel.

Dienstag and Ryan [40] have reviewed the prevalence of hepatitis B markers in hospital personnel by job category [41]. Emergency-room nurses were found to have the highest prevalence of markers of previous HBV infection (30 percent). Other groups who appeared to be at high risk were surgical ICU nurses, phlebotomists, chemistry laboratory technicians, and surgical house officers. While this survey reflects the HBV status of employees in a large urban hospital, it also serves to underscore the fact that health-care workers are at higher risk of HBV infection than the general population. In a large survey reported by Denes and colleagues [38], evidence of previous HBV infection was higher among physicians practicing in urban communities, increased with the number of years in practice, and was highest among pathologists and surgeons [39]. Dentists and physicians have a similar overall rate of positivity [126].

The issue of work restrictions for the HBsAg-pos-itive worker is a controversial one (see Chapter 2). The CDC Guideline for Infection Control in Hospital Employees states that employees who are chronic carriers of HBsAg need not be restricted from patient contact unless they have been implicated in disease transmission [158]. While this recommendation may seem paradoxical, it points out the difficult and sensitive nature of the problem. All available evidence suggests that the greatest risk of nosocomial transmission of HBV takes place from patients to personnel [158]. Transmission of HBV from personnel to patients is not as clear. Epidemiologic data are available that show both transmission [54,119] and lack of transmission of hepatitis B [56,100] from HBsAg-positive personnel to their patients. Factors contributing to transmission of HBV from personnel to patients are probably the level and duration of antigenemia in the employee and the type of contact the employee has with the patient. From the available data, it appears that routine patient care that does not afford contact with blood of infected personnel does not present a risk to patients [56,100]. The physician surgeon or dental surgeon who is HBsAg-positive may present a different degree of risk to patients when performing surgical procedures. It is not possible to make general recommendations regarding restrictions for these personnel in the operating room as this type of evaluation should be made on an individual basis. Hopefully, as high risk personnel are vaccinated with the hepatitis B vaccine, the dilemma of the HBsAg-positive health care worker can be avoided.

ISOLATION PRECAUTIONS A private room is not required routinely for acute hepatitis B patients (see Chapter 9), although the patient who is incontinent of feces or is bleeding is managed best in a private room. While routine use of gowns, gloves, and masks is not required, any or all of these precautions should be used if patient contact may also involve contact with blood or other body fluids. Gloves should be used for direct contact with blood or blood-contaminated equipment such as intravenous catheters, drains, or soiled dressings. Precautions should also be taken to avoid contact with feces or that has been contaminated with blood (see Chapter 9).

PROPHYLAXIS *Preexposure prophylaxis.* The hepatitis B vaccine should be used as preexposure prophylaxis for hepatitis B in certain high-risk individuals. The vaccine is also recommended for certain health care workers such as dialysis workers, nurses in emergency rooms and ICUs and other personnel at high risk due to regular contact with blood [9,41,158] (see Chapter 2). The high-risk groups can be selected using a number of data sources from the facility including results of serologic screening done on an ongoing basis in some institutions, prevalence studies of hepatitis B markers in certain groups of employees, and records of needle punctures. Once the high-risk groups are identified in an institution, prevaccination screening for all vaccinated persons may not be necessary and will depend on the expected prevalence of hepatitis B markers and the cost of screening [9]. Groups of workers who are screened periodically due to the high risk of hepatitis B exposure (e.g., dialysis and laboratory workers) are automatically candidates for vaccination since it is implied that they are at high enough risk to require regular screening. In these cases, the vaccine is more cost-effective than routine screening because it offers the additional benefit of protection from hepatitis B and makes further screening unnecessary in those who respond with hepatitis B surface antibody (anti-HBs).

Other points for consideration when developing a hepatitis B vaccination program are:

1. Mandatory vaccination of high-risk employees as a condition of employment. This may be desirable but may be difficult to enforce especially for employees who are currently working. The legal ramifications of such a policy also need to be assessed.
2. Voluntary vaccination of high-risk individuals. This is a more practical approach to vaccination. This strategy then places the burden on the infection control team, department heads and supervisors, and hospital administration in terms of "marketing" the vaccine to employees.
3. Payment for the vaccine. This may be a critical factor in implementing a hepatitis B vaccine program. It would seem reasonable that once a facility designates a group of employees as high risk, the facility should also bear the cost of the program. The response to a program where the high-risk employee pays for the cost of the hepatitis B vaccine is generally poor. If the facility elects not to pay the entire cost of the vaccine, a more reasonable compromise is one in which the facility and the employee share the cost.
4. The decision not to offer the vaccine may be a viable alternative in some health care settings. This decision is best based on results of employee screening that show a low prevalence of HBV markers.
5. The vaccine has been shown to be immunogenic and effective in preventing hepatitis B [137]. Clinical trials in large numbers of homosexual men have shown that the vaccine is 100 percent effective in preventing hepatitis B infection in those who respond with hepatitis B surface antibody [137]. Although the response rate was 96 percent in field trials, the rates of seroconversion have not been as high in the experience of most hospital infection control programs. The site of injection has been suggested as one reason for variable response rates, and the deltoid muscle is now the recommended site of injection [26]. Even with response rates of 80 to 85 percent, however, vaccination clearly offers protection against hepatitis B in the majority of people who receive it and is a worthwhile infection control/employee health activity. The safety of the vaccine has been questioned by some as a result of the occurrence of the acquired immunodeficiency syndrome (AIDS) in certain high-risk groups whose serum may be used to manufacture the vaccine. The vaccine-manufacturing process has been shown to inactivate the human T-cell lymphotropic virus (HTLV-III) the cause of AIDS [9]. In addition, follow-up studies of vaccinees have failed to show an increased risk of AIDS when compared to unvaccinated controls [132].

*Postexposure prophylaxis.* Hepatitis B immune globulin (HBIG) and the hepatitis B vaccine are recommended for use as postexposure prophylaxis for hepatitis B. Current guidelines from the Immunization Practices Advisory Committee (ACIP) [20] state that these agents should be used together for the following types of contact: (1) parenteral inoculation of HBsAg-containing material, such as a needle stick or contamination of open skin with a large inoculum of HBsAg-positive blood; or (2) accidental ingestion of HBsAg-positive blood (e.g., pipetting accident); or (3) accidental splash of HBsAg-positive blood on the mucous membranes of the eye or mouth. Ideally, prophylaxis should be given as soon as possible but within seven days of exposure. HBIG is given once at a dose of 0.06 ml/kg at the same time as the first dose of hepatitis B vaccine. Additional doses of vaccine are given one and six months after the first dose. A second dose of HBIG is not given with this regimen. Workers who refuse the hepatitis B vaccine should be given two doses of HBIG (0.06 ml/kg each dose) one month apart (see Chapter 22).

One of the most difficult aspects of postexposure hepatitis B prophylaxis is to determine if the exposure was significant, that is, if it involved parenteral inoculation of HBsAg-positive material. It is also important that the HBsAg status of the source be determined as soon as possible. Infection control and employee health personnel should try to apply uniform and consistent criteria when evaluating the need for prophylaxis after a hepatitis B exposure. However, the final evaluation may need to be done on an individual basis in some cases.

Infants born to mothers who are HBsAg-positive at the time of delivery should also be given hepatitis B prophylaxis to prevent development of the HBsAg carrier state. Both HBIG and the hepatitis B vaccine should be given at the time of birth. One dose of HBIG (0.06 ml/kg) should be given along with the first dose of vaccine (0.5 ml). The additional doses of vaccine should be given one month and six months after the first [20].

SPECIAL CONSIDERATIONS One of the most important infection control measures for all forms of hepatitis involves the education of hospital personnel. Hospital staff must be aware of the modes of transmission of hepatitis viruses and the importance of appropriate precautions in the care of such patients. Obtaining blood from patients with HBsAg presents one of the greatest hazards to hospital personnel. In some cases, large numbers of personnel may be exposed to blood containing HBsAg before the patient is known to be HBsAg-positive. For this reason, and because patients may have detectable HBsAg before the onset of illness, blood from all patients should be considered infectious and handled appropriately. Special emphasis should be placed on avoiding contamination of skin and mucous membranes by blood spills from acutely ill patients who are HBsAg-positive. Since it is not possible to recommend specific precautions for each instance, employees should be encouraged to use precautions that will minimize contact with blood or blood-contaminated excretions and secretions at all times (see Chapter 22).

### Hepatitis B in Hemodialysis Units

Infection with HBV is an infection control hazard to both patients and personnel in many units [10] (see Chapters 17 and 37). Hepatitis B appears to be introduced into the dialysis unit by HBsAg-positive patients, who probably acquire their infection from transfusion of HBsAg-positive blood. Hemodialysis does not play a role in the spread of HAV infection [135]. In a study of 65 dialysis units conducted by the Centers for Disease Control (CDC) from 1967–70, 82 percent of the units surveyed had patients, staff, or both with hepatitis B [134]. In 1974 Szmuness and associates [134] reported overall rates of seropositivity (HBsAg- and anti-HBs-positive) in 15 U.S. dialysis units of 51 percent in patients and 34 percent in staff members. By 1980, the incidence of hepatitis B had decreased to one percent of patients and 0.7

percent of staff [1]. Once introduced into a dialysis unit, HBV infection can become endemic, with patients, personnel, and environmental surfaces acting as reservoirs of infection [127,128]. It should be noted that to date, transmission of HBV infection from hemodialysis personnel to patients has not been reported. Transmission to personnel from either HBsAg-positive patients or contaminated equipment or environmental surfaces, on the other hand, has been well documented [127]. The greatest risk in such instances has been shown to be contact with blood or blood-contaminated materials and instruments [127].

ISOLATION PROCEDURES Clearly, strictly enforced infection control precautions are required if hepatitis B transmission in dialysis units is to be contained [11] (see Chapter 9). A detailed discussion of these precautions is found in a CDC publication [10], and they are reviewed briefly here (see Chapter 17).

*Patients.* Ideally, patients who are HBsAg-positive should undergo dialysis in a separate room or another unit designated for hepatitis patients only. If this is not possible, the patient should undergo dialysis in an area removed from the mainstream of activity and should be separated from seronegative patients.

*Personnel.* Whenever possible, patients who are HBsAg-positive should be dialyzed by personnel who are also seropositive (positive for one or more markers: HBsAg, anti-HBs, anti-HBc) and who are thus immune to reinfection. Although not supported by controlled studies, it is recommended that a seropositive nurse perform the dialysis and that this nurse not work with any seronegative patients during the same shift to avoid accidental transmission of HBV to susceptible patients. Patients who are seropositive but have different markers may be cared for by the same staff member during the same shift regardless of the staff member's antigen status, since neither patient is susceptible to HBV infection.

The hemodialysis unit and infection control program should emphasize appropriate precautions in the care of patients and handling of blood and secretions. Dialysis equipment should not be shared by both HBsAg-positive and seronegative patients at any time. Routine preexposure prophylaxis with HBIG or IG is not recommended for either dialysis unit personnel or patients.

HEPATITIS SURVEILLANCE Regular hepatitis screening for dialysis patients and staff has been an important component of hepatitis B prevention programs in dialysis units for many years. However, this activity has only served to monitor the introduction and/or transmission of HBV in dialysis settings (see Chapters 2 and 17). Ideally all dialysis candidates should be screened for hepatitis B markers (HBsAg, anti-HBs and anti-HBc) prior to admission to the dialysis unit [10]. Similarly, all dialysis workers should be screened for hepatitis B markers prior to their employment in the unit. The use of the hepatitis B vaccine, however, should change the need for screening after admission or employment in dialysis centers. Vaccination can be a more cost effective activity than screening alone because it will obviate the need for hepatitis B screening in those who respond to the vaccine with protective levels of anti-HBs. Vaccination rather than screening offers the added advantage of providing immunity to infection rather than merely monitoring the introduction of hepatitis B into the hemodialysis unit [138].

Once dialysis patients and personnel have been vaccinated, those who respond with protective levels of anti-HBs can be screened less frequently (e.g., yearly) to check for persistence of antibody.

### Non-A, Non-B Hepatitis

Non-A, non-B hepatitis appears to be caused by more than one agent [105]. Available data suggest that transmission in the United States is primarily parenteral, through transfusions of blood or blood products [99]. Non-A, non-B hepatitis has become the most common form of posttransfusion hepatitis since the advent of routine screening of donor blood for HBsAg and elimination of HBsAg-positive donors. At the present time there are no commercially available diagnostic tests for non-A, non-B hepatitis.

ISOLATION PRECAUTIONS Isolation precautions for patients with non-A, non-B hepatitis are similar to those for patients with hepatitis B, with emphasis on precautions in handling blood or blood-contaminated articles.

PROPHYLAXIS Preliminary data suggest that IG may be useful in prophylaxis of non-A, non-B hepatitis [20], but additional study is required.

## RUBELLA

The introduction of rubella vaccine in 1969 has resulted in a marked decrease in the numbers of cases of rubella in school-aged children. The vaccine has not decreased the incidence of rubella in older age groups as dramatically, however [19,24]. From 1976

to 1979, over 70 percent of reported cases occurred in persons 15 years of age or older [24], and in 1980 46.6 percent of cases were over 15 years of age [73]. Overall seronegativity among hospital employees has been reported as high as 14 percent [44]. Outbreaks of rubella in hospitals have also been reported [94,116,117]. These outbreaks emphasize the potential for transmission of rubella in institutional settings and underscore the importance of immunity against rubella to protect patients and personnel. In general, efforts to vaccinate susceptible hospital personnel on a voluntary basis, especially physicians, have been disappointing [117].

ISOLATION PRECAUTIONS *Congenital rubella.* In congenitally acquired infection, virus may persist in pharyngeal secretions for many months after birth and may be shed for up to four years after birth [125]. In general these infants are not thought to be hazardous to others after about two to three years of age because little virus is present [68]. Infants with congenital rubella syndrome should be in private rooms and remain on precautions for the duration of hospitalization (see Chapter 9). Until additional data are available, we recommend that infants with congenital rubella who are less than two years of age be placed on precautions when readmitted to the hospital.

*Acquired rubella.* Patients with acquired rubella or susceptible patients who have been exposed to rubella should be isolated for 21 days after exposure and/or for five days after the onset of rash.

SCREENING AND IMMUNIZATION Regulations regarding screening and immunization for rubella in hospital personnel vary widely (see Chapter 2). The current rubella strategy in the United States involves elimination of the congenital rubella syndrome. The earlier narrower approach to rubella, which involved only vaccination of women of childbearing age, does not apply any longer. As a result of this broader approach, vaccination is recommended for all potentially susceptible persons, both males and females, in order to increase the pool of immune individuals [19]. The CDC Guideline for Infection Control in Hospital Employees recommends that health care workers who are likely to be in contact with patients with rubella or with pregnant women be immune to rubella [158]. Immunity to rubella is defined as laboratory evidence of a protective titer for rubella or evidence of vaccination with live rubella vaccine after 12 months of age [158]. Previous history of disease is not acceptable since many exanthematous diseases can be confused with rubella [19,158]. Also, the trivalent MMR vaccine should be used whenever possible. Available evidence suggests that vaccination with MMR of persons who are already immune to one of its components is not associated with significant adverse effects [19].

Schoenbaum [122] has outlined four possible strategies for rubella screening and immunization of hospital employees: (1) a voluntary program for screening and immunizing susceptible persons, (2) a mandatory program of screening and either voluntary or mandatory immunization of susceptible persons, (3) a voluntary or mandatory immunization program without prescreening, and (4) no program. It is advisable that hospitals develop obligatory rubella immunization program for susceptible personnel who may be in contact with pregnant patients. The epidemiology of rubella in hospitals certainly supports this action. The cost of such a program should be the responsibility of the hospital.

SPECIAL CONSIDERATIONS  Outbreak management. To prevent the transmission of rubella in outbreaks, those susceptible should be vaccinated promptly [19]. It is not recommended, however, that pregnant women be vaccinated [19]. McLaughlin and Gold [94] have outlined restrictions for use during outbreaks. Personnel with rubella should not work in any area of the hospital because of the risk of transmitting disease to susceptible persons. Immune or nonexposed staff should care for pregnant patients in their first trimester and, whenever possible, for all pregnant patients regardless of gestational stage [94]. Immune serum globulin may modify the disease in exposed persons, but its use is generally not recommended during pregnancy [94].

## MEASLES (RUBEOLA)

Large hospital outbreaks of measles were common in the past, but with the advent of measles vaccination programs, nosocomial infection has become rare.

ISOLATION PRECAUTIONS  A single room (or cohorting) is required and all personnel should observe respiratory precautions (see Chapter 9). We maintain precautions until seven days after onset of rash in known cases. When exposure to measles has occurred, the patient should be isolated from the fifth to the twenty-first day after exposure. If clinical disease occurs, isolation should continue for seven days after the appearance of the rash.

SPECIAL CONSIDERATIONS  *"Modified measles".* Measles modified by immune globulin (IG) may be overlooked or result in delays in diagnosis. Respiratory shedding of virus does occur in patients given IG, and the isolation precautions mentioned previously should be instituted and maintained.

*Atypical measles.* The syndrome occurs after exposure to wild measles virus in persons who have been vaccinated with the inactivated measles vaccination that was used before 1965 [108]. The illness is characterized by fever; an *unusual skin rash* that, like the measles rash, is maculopapular but is more likely to become petechial or hemorrhagic; and pulmonary manifestations; it appears to be caused by an altered immune response in a previously sensitized host [52]. The illness has also been recorded in persons vaccinated after 1965 with live attenuated vaccine [30]. Measles virus has not been isolated from patients with atypical measles. Because of this fact and the apparent pathogenesis of atypical measles, these patients are not thought to be infectious, and special isolation precautions are not recommended.

## MUMPS

Mumps virus is less communicable than either measles or varicella (chickenpox), and infections in compromised hosts have not been associated with the serious consequences that may follow measles or varicella [49]. Although nosocomial transmission has been documented [129], outbreaks are usually confined to families, schools, and military personnel.

ISOLATION PRECAUTIONS  Respiratory isolation and a private room are recommended; presently we maintain precautions until nine days after the onset of parotitis, at which time infectiousness appears to decrease (see Chapter 9).

## SLOW VIRUS INFECTION

### Creutzfeldt-Jakob Disease
Creutzfeldt-Jakob disease (CJD) is thought to be of viral origin with a long incubation period for 15 to 24 months. It is not "contagious" in the usual sense and does not appear to present excessive risks to hospital personnel. Sufficient concern dealing with the transmission of CJD in hospitals has arisen in the past few years, because the diagnosis has been proved or suspected in more patients. The disease has been reported to occur following corneal transplantation [45], as well as in two patients through contaminated

stereotactic electrodes used in previous neurosurgical procedures [5].

ISOLATION PRECAUTIONS  Precautions are recommended for patients with suspected CJD until the diagnosis has been ruled out [53,60] (see Chapter 9). If a diagnosis is established by brain biopsy, patients are maintained on precautions that emphasize care in handling of all body fluids and tissue, especially blood, cerebrospinal fluid, and brain tissue [53,60]. To facilitate understanding by hospital personnel, it should be stressed that these precautions are similar to those used for patients with hepatitis B. Once a diagnosis of CJD has been confirmed, precautions are maintained for the duration of hospitalization and for subsequent hospitalizations.

SPECIAL CONSIDERATIONS  A policy should be established to ensure additional precautions for specimens from CJD patients, equipment, and instruments used for patients with CJD [51]. The infection control nurse (ICN) should be notified of the admission of a CJD patient to the hospital. The ICN should then notify staff in other involved hospital departments and service areas, who should make the necessary arrangements for disposal and handling of specimens and sterilization of equipment and instruments. The details of such a policy have been described previously [53,60].

## GASTROENTERITIS VIRUSES

The two major causes of viral gastroenteritis were identified in the 1970s using immune electron-microscopic examination of stool and by electron-microscopic analysis of infected intestinal mucosa. The rotaviruses are a major cause of viral diarrhea in infants and children [140]. The calicivirus–like agents (Norwalk gastroenteritis–like agents) generally cause gastroenteritis in older children and adults [36].

### Rotavirus
The human rotavirus (HRV; human reovirus-like agent, or infantile gastroenteritis virus) is a major cause of gastroenteritis in infants and children during the winter in temperate climates [80] (see Chapter 32). Kapikian and coworkers [80] showed that approximately half of all children admitted to hospitals in the winter months because of gastroenteritis are afflicted with human rotavirus. Infants often are admitted to the hospital because of diarrhea and dehydration that may have been preceded by vomiting. Children 6 to 24 months of age are the most suscep-

tible to HRV infection, and serum antibodies are rapidly acquired during this period. The majority of adults have such antibodies. The presence of serum antibodies does not protect completely against reinfection, however, and natural and experimental infections in adults do occur [82,96]. Although adults may serve as a reservoir of infection despite the presence of preexisting antibody, the amount of virus shed is less than that shed by infectious children [82]. Approximately 55 percent of adult contacts of children with rotavirus infection develop serologic evidence of infection [82]. Asymptomatic shedding also occurs. Using electron-microscopy, Bolivar [7] showed that while 25 percent of symptomatic students had rotavirus in their stool, 12 percent of asymptomatic students also had rotavirus in their stool.

Transmission is by the fecal-oral route; although nosocomial infection affects newborn infants most frequently [82,131], infections in older children, adults, and hospital personnel also have been documented [35].

ISOLATION PRECAUTIONS  Isolation precautions should emphasize care in handling articles contaminated with feces (see Chapter 9). Patients with rotavirus are maintained on these precautions for the duration of hospitalization, because the duration of shedding can be quite variable.

SPECIAL CONSIDERATIONS  Rotaviruses are not readily isolated from tissue culture. The diagnosis is made by electron-microscopic examination of stool or by serologic methods (complement fixation [CF], enzyme-linked immunosorbent assay [ELISA], or counterimmunoelectrophoresis [CIE]). Because these tests may not be available in some institutions, the infection control nurse should be suspicious of rotavirus infection in infants who are admitted to the hospital for or become ill with vomiting, diarrhea, dehydration, and fever during the winter months.

It is recommended that all infants with diarrhea be maintained on isolation precautions pending the results of culture for bacterial pathogens and serologic study for rotavirus. When rotaviral and bacterial causes are ruled out, patients with presumed "nonbacterial gastroenteritis" are maintained on precautions for 48 hours after they become asymptomatic (see Special Considerations, following).

### Norwalk Gastroenteritis Virus and Related Agents
Included in this group are the Norwalk, Hawaii, W, and Montgomery County agents. These agents are major causes of viral gastroenteritis in children and adults and are associated with school, family, and

community outbreaks; they probably are transmitted by fecal-oral spread. Although nosocomial transmission has not been documented, it probably occurs in a manner similar to that of rotavirus.

ISOLATION PRECAUTIONS Precautions for Norwalk gastroenteritis–like agents should be the same as for rotavirus. Isolation in these cases, however, is maintained for 72 hours after symptoms have ceased, because the period of shedding appears to be somewhat shorter than that of rotavirus [141].

SPECIAL CONSIDERATIONS Like rotavirus, the Norwalk gastroenteritis–like agents cannot be isolated on viral culture. The only laboratory test presently available for identifying infected materials is immune electron-microscopy, which is tedious and not widely available. When rotavirus and nonbacterial pathogens have been ruled out, patients may be classified as having "nonbacterial gastroenteritis other than rotavirus." Other agents, such as coronavirus–like agents, astrovirus, and mini-reovirus agents, also may be involved.

## PICORNAVIRUSES

Of the three genera of the picornaviridae family (enterovirus, rhinovirus, and calicivirus), the enteroviruses are the most frequent causes of nosocomial infection. Included in the enterovirus group are coxsackieviruses A and B, echoviruses, polioviruses, and enterovirus types 68 to 71.

Enteroviruses cause sporadic disease throughout the year but are most prevalent in the community during the summer and fall in temperate climates [95,115,116]. Transmission of the virus is via the fecal-oral route, but droplet transmission has been described for coxsackie A21 and probably occurs with other enteroviruses as well [95]. Virus can be recovered easily from the oropharynx and rectum and may be shed for one month or more after infection. Transmission occurs in hosts with or without preexisting antibody [95].

### Nonpolio Enteroviruses
Infection is common in the general population, particularly among children, and results in a variety of illnesses. Patients may be asymptomatic or have mild illness with fever, rash, and upper respiratory and/or gastrointestinal symptoms. Symptomatic and severe disease occurs in newborn infants, particularly in full-term infants who may develop meningitis, encephalitis, myocarditis, and/or pericarditis in addition to

the other symptoms mentioned. In older children, infection often is asymptomatic or benign. For these reasons, most of the reported nosocomial enterovirus infections have been outbreaks in neonatal units [32,34,79,85,93], while nosocomial enterovirus acquisition among older children often is undetected.

Most nursery outbreaks involve the nonpolio enteroviruses. Often the virus is introduced into the nursery by an infected infant, and transmission occurs by indirect contact (i.e., from infant to infant via the hands of personnel). Infection also has been found in nursery personnel, suggesting that they may also serve as sources of infection [32].

The most consistent mode of acquisition of nonpolio enteroviruses in infants is transmission from the mother [32]. Transmission may take place before, during, or after delivery. In a study of 27 newborn infants with symptomatic infection, 30 percent had onset of symptoms within the first three days of life, and 60 percent of the mothers were symptomatic at the time of delivery [85]. In a prospective study done during enterovirus season, Cherry and colleagues [31] demonstrated that 2 of 55 women were shedding virus at the time of delivery, and one of these two transmitted virus to her child. Others have reported the endemic occurrence of enterovirus infection in nurseries [32]. Additional epidemiologic studies are needed, however, to determine the frequency with which infected infants are introduced into the nursery and the risk they pose to other babies and personnel.

ISOLATION PRECAUTIONS Because of the potentially serious consequences of enterovirus infection in newborn infants, precautions for the control of nosocomial enterovirus infection in the nursery are especially important. Infants with suspected or proven infection should be isolated in a private room or cohorted together (see Chapter 9). The cohort method of isolation may be useful in situations involving several infants and has proved to be an effective control measure in containing nursery outbreaks [34] (see Chapter 19). Enteric precautions for isolating infants, using gowns and gloves for direct contact, should be maintained. Gowns should be changed after each patient contact. The decision to close a nursery to new admissions is always difficult but may be necessary, especially with prolonged outbreaks, or if adequate cohort programs cannot be maintained. Rigorous and strict handwashing before and after each patient contact clearly is required, and its importance cannot be overemphasized.

Unless a particularly virulent enterovirus has been identified in the community (e.g., poliovirus or certain strains of enterovirus-71), such rigorous isolation precautions generally are not necessary for adults or for children beyond the neonatal period. Careful handling of feces and secretions, and soiled objects and instruments should be the rule for all patients with enterovirus infection.

PREVENTION   Often a thorough maternal history is the best way to identify the infant at risk during the enterovirus season, and a mild febrile illness in the mother during the summer may warn of infection in the infant. Any infant born to a mother who is known to have had a recent febrile illness should be placed in an observation nursery rather than the main nursery area (see Chapter 19).

In addition, nursery personnel should be aware of their potential for infecting the newborn. While it may not be possible or necessary to identify employees with these nonspecific illnesses, the importance of reporting febrile, respiratory, or diarrheal illnesses to the employee health service and the necessity for careful hand-washing as part of an inservice program for nursery personnel must be emphasized (see Chapter 2).

The attenuation of enterovirus disease by passive immunization has been suggested. Antibody does not protect against infection but appears to reduce the severity of disease and duration of virus shedding. The administration of immune serum globulin in the setting of a sudden and particularly virulent nursery outbreak has been suggested by Cherry [32].

*Polioviruses*
Poliovirus infection has become rare since the institution of widespread immunization programs, and nosocomial transmission of poliovirus is no longer a problem.

Virus shedding may follow vaccination with live oral polio vaccine (OPV) for a brief period of time. In general, paralytic poliovirus infection today is associated with the use of live oral polio vaccine, but this is rare [3,19,123]. Cases occur in recipients of live vaccine (recipient cases) or in their contacts (contact cases). The incidence of vaccine-induced paralysis in recipients is estimated to be 0.44 per million vaccinated [111], and in contacts, 1.5 per million vaccinated [111]. Several community outbreaks of paralytic polio among groups of nonimmunized persons were described recently [17], and serologic surveys have demonstrated that an unacceptably high proportion of the population remains at risk [112].

ISOLATION PRECAUTIONS   Children identified as having unspecified enterovirus infections should be isolated using precautions that minimize contact with secretions and excretions pending identification of the specific agent. Asymptomatic children subsequently found to be shedding poliovirus present a potential risk to certain high-risk patients, especially children with congenital immune deficiency diseases (e.g., agammaglobulinemia, hypogammaglobulinemia, combined immune deficiency states). It is recommended that, as a precaution, unimmunized children or children with congenital or acquired immune deficiency states not be placed in the same room as children who are known to be shedding poliovirus. However, routine screening of hospitalized children for poliovirus is not recommended.

IMMUNIZATION   Because of the persistence of wild and vaccine strains of poliovirus, adequate immunity against polioviruses is essential for both pediatric patients and hospital personnel. Routine vaccination of adults currently is not recommended [19].

SPECIAL CONSIDERATIONS   Enteroviruses are unusually stable and resist many commonly used disinfectants (e.g., 70% alcohol, 5% Lysol, and 1% quaternary ammonium compounds). The most effective virucidal agent is 5% sodium hypochlorite solution, which may be used for surface decontamination but is corrosive to metal, including stainless steel (see Chapter 14).

## RHABDOVIRUS

*Rabies*
Although nosocomial rabies is uncommon, two cases have been documented of human-to-human transmission of rabies from corneal transplantation [12,76]. Both donors had obscure neurologic illnesses, one resembling Guillain-Barré syndrome, and the other, flaccid paralysis. Because of this atypical presentation, the diagnosis of rabies was not suspected before the death of either donor, and their tissues were considered acceptable for transplantation.

Hospital personnel also are theoretically at risk when exposed to patients with rabies in whom the diagnosis may not be suspected before death [11]. In an investigation of hospital personnel exposed to one such patient, many employees were unable to recall the extent of exposure 15 to 43 days earlier. Because of this and because of the long duration of hospitalization of the index case, 198 of 371 hospital employees were thought to have had significant rabies exposure and advised to receive postexposure rabies prophylaxis [11].

Laboratory personnel working with bat colonies

and other potentially rabid animals also are at increased risk of this disease. Laboratory-associated rabies, presumably transmitted by aerosolization of laboratory virus strains, has been reported, [28], resulting in revised safety recommendations for laboratory personnel working with rabies virus [28].

ISOLATION PRECAUTIONS Strict isolation precautions are recommended for the duration of illness in patients with proven or suspected rabies (see Chapter 9).

IMMUNIZATION Human diploid cell rabies vaccine (HDCV), is recommended whenever available [18,22]. HDCV should be used in the following situations:

1. Individuals with documented rabies exposure
2. Individuals with probable or possible exposure
3. Laboratory workers working with bats or other potentially rabid animals, for preexposure prophylaxis

Postexposure prophylaxis of hospital personnel should be handled according to established recommendations [22]. In addition, local wounds should be cleansed with soap and water [2]. Preexposure prophylaxis of laboratory workers at high risk also should be undertaken. Personnel should not work with potentially rabid animals until a complete series of vaccine has been administered.

SPECIAL CONSIDERATIONS The potential for transmission of rabies in transplanted tissues presents serious problems in evaluating potential donors. The Infection Control Committee of the Strong Memorial Hospital and the Rochester Area Eye Bank have jointly agreed to the following policy: "Corneas from individuals who have died with a diagnosis of dementia, encephalopathy, undiagnosed neurological illness, multiple sclerosis, conjunctivitis, or other viral diseases including hepatitis B, rabies, or Creutzfeldt-Jakob disease should not be utilized for the purposes of corneal transplantation. Corneas in such cases may be accepted for research purposes if they are labeled 'Biohazard.' "

## ARENAVIRUSES

### Lymphocytic Choriomeningitis
Lymphocytic choriomeningitis (LCM) has been implicated as a cause of outbreaks of flu-like illness with aseptic meningitis in laboratory workers and other

hospital personnel [149]. It is not known to be transmitted from person to person in hospital settings other than after contact with laboratory animals.

ISOLATION PRECAUTIONS No special isolation precautions are required for patients with LCM infection.

## SMALLPOX

Before the elimination of smallpox by the World Health Organization's Smallpox Eradication Program, outbreaks were reported in both hospital personnel and patients [151].

The virus is quite stable and can survive in crusts, fluid, or dry material for very long periods of time [43]. Transmission of smallpox occurred by direct or indirect contact with infectious material. Infected patients were able to transmit the disease to others from the onset of the exanthem until the last crust was shed. Airborne transmission also occurred and appears to have caused the most recent laboratory-associated case, which occurred in a medical photographer working on the floor above a laboratory in which researchers were working with variola virus [13]. Airborne transmission via air currents was also the cause of a hospital outbreak of smallpox in Germany [19,27].

ISOLATION PRECAUTIONS Patients with suspected cases of smallpox should be isolated, using strict isolation precautions, until all crusts have been shed (see Chapter 9).

IMMUNIZATION At present smallpox vaccination is indicated only for laboratory workers who are using smallpox or related orthopox viruses (e.g., monkeypox, vaccinia) [19,27].

SPECIAL CONSIDERATIONS In May 1980 the World Health Organization (WHO) declared all countries free of smallpox. Nevertheless, stocks of smallpox virus remain in a few research and reference laboratories worldwide, presenting a small risk of smallpox in certain settings. Suspected cases must be reported immediately to local and state health authorities.

## ACQUIRED IMMUNODEFICIENCY SYNDROME

The acquired immunodeficiency syndrome (AIDS) appears to be a new disease entity that has emerged since 1979. The cause of this disease is a retrovirus named human T-cell lymphotropic virus (HTLV) type

III. This strain of retrovirus appears to be toxic to T4 helper lymphocytes.

The perplexing nature of the disease presents the greatest problems for infection control personnel. The disease is confined almost exclusively to several high-risk groups. Almost 75 percent of cases have occurred in homosexual or bisexual men, and 13 percent of cases occur in intravenous drug abusers. Smaller numbers of cases have occurred in hemophiliacs, transfusion recipients, and sexual or household contacts of high-risk individuals. To date, evidence suggests that close intimate contact is required for transmission of disease (e.g., sexual contact, shared needles). This evidence suggests that the disease is transmitted in a manner similar to hepatitis B. Unlike the situation with hepatitis B, however, hospital personnel do not seem to be at increased risk for disease [74]. Although cases of AIDS have been reported in hospital personnel who did not appear to belong to any other high-risk groups [8], histories in these cases may be incomplete, and they provide no new information regarding this disease in hospital personnel. Although numerous significant exposures from AIDS patients have occurred in hospital workers (e.g., needle sticks), none of the cases of AIDS reported to date have occurred in hospital workers who have had such accidents. The Hospital Infections Branch of the Centers for Disease Control is currently following persons prospectively who have had such accidents.

Currently there is no prophylaxis available for exposed persons. A screening test for antibodies to HTLV-III has been developed and is commercially available. Many persons in high-risk groups have antibodies to HTLV-III, and most of those with antibody have viremia. It should be remembered that the usual measures for hepatitis B prevention should be applied in employees who have significant exposures to patients with AIDS.

Infection control precautions should include care in handling blood, needles, and body fluids, similar to precautions used for hepatitis B. Masks, gowns, and gloves are not indicated for routine care but, as in hepatitis B, should be used if excess contamination with blood or body fluids is expected (e.g., patients who are bleeding or incontinent of feces). Central to the entire issue of infection control for this disease is education of hospital personnel. The epidemiology of AIDS does tell us how to deal with the disease and how to prevent it. These efforts will be enhanced in their effectiveness by use of current diagnostic tests for HTLV-III infections. The ultimate challenge for the infection control team may be to assist hospital personnel who care for patients with this perplexing disease.

## METHODS OF PREVENTING SPREAD OF VIRUSES

### Cohort Isolation Precautions

In hospital epidemiology, a cohort is a group of individuals kept together to minimize contact between members of the cohort and other patients or personnel to decrease opportunities for transmission of infectious agents.

Cohort isolation programs have proved effective in controlling some nursery outbreaks of *Staphylococcus aureus* [88] as well as those due to enteroviruses (see Chapter 19) [34]. Cohort isolation programs also have been used outside of nurseries during hospital outbreaks of influenza.

A program of cohort isolation generally consists of two groups of people, an *infected* group and an *uninfected* group, that are separated from one another. Occasionally a third group, an *exposed* group, is separated from the uninfected group and cared for separately from both of the other groups. This method of separation may involve the use of geographically distinct rooms or, if not available, physical separation in the same room. To ensure complete separation of cohorts, geographically separate rooms are preferable and should be used whenever possible. The separation of hospital staff often is overlooked, but this also is essential to a successful cohort program. Although it is not always possible to separate house staff and support personnel, the nursing staff caring for infected and noninfected cohorts should be separated as much as possible without disrupting services to patients. If possible, those caring for infected patients should be immune to the disease in question or receiving prophylactic treatment or vaccine. This immunity may be determined by previous infection or vaccination and may be identified by appropriate history of illness, vaccination, and/or antibody testing. In cohort programs for viral illness, especially respiratory viruses, the same groups of personnel ideally should care for the same cohort for the duration of isolation. This plan minimizes the risk of transmission of infection to the uninfected cohort. Personnel who have recently recovered from the viral illness under consideration also may care for the infected cohort. In other cohort programs (e.g., dialysis of HBsAg-positive patients or staphylococcal outbreaks in nurseries), personnel may work with different cohorts on different days but not during the same day. In many instances, groups of personnel such as house staff and support personnel cannot be restricted as easily. In these situations, personnel should see patients in the "clean" area first, then go to the "dirty" area.

It is also important to remember that separation of groups on the basis of symptoms alone will not guarantee that all members of the cohort have the same illness. It is desirable, therefore, to take appropriate steps to confirm the suspected diagnosis as quickly as possible to ensure proper cohorting of patients. More detailed guidelines for the use of cohort programs are presented in Table 35-3.

The cohort method of isolation may involve small numbers of patients and/or hospital staff, such as in the dialysis of HBsAg-positive patients in areas physically separate from main dialysis units [10]. Other uses of the cohort method may involve restriction of larger groups of patients and personnel; for example, outbreaks of respiratory viral infections, such as respiratory syncytial virus, are approached in this way [65].

In general, cohort programs using geographically separate areas of the same room are not recommended for the control of viral respiratory infections.

TABLE 35-3. General guidelines
for use of cohort isolation

1. Patients should be separated into cohorts of infected ("dirty") and noninfected ("clean") patients
2. Only persons with proven or suspected infection should be admitted to the infected cohort
3. All exposed (potentially infected) individuals should be included with the cohort of infected patients; in some instances, the potentially infected cohort may be separated into a third cohort
4. The infected cohort should be closed to new, uninfected admissions, and all new, uninfected admissions should be placed with the uninfected cohort
5. Personnel working with the infected cohort should be immune to the illness in question by either previous history of illness or vaccination *whenever possible*
6. Personnel should be assigned so that separate groups work with the infected and uninfected cohorts *whenever possible*; crossover between cohorts should be discouraged to minimize the risk of cross-infection of the uninfected cohort
7. Ideally, personnel should be separated for the duration of the cohort program, especially when viral illnesses are proved or suspected
8. When personnel must work in both areas, they should work in the "clean" area first, then work in the "dirty" area
9. The infected cohort area should be closed as patients are discharged from the hospital and may be used for new uninfected admissions after thorough cleaning of the area and its equipment

Source: Valenti, W. M., et al. *Infect. Control* 2:236, 1980, with permission.

*Communicable Disease Survey*

The purpose of the communicable disease survey (contagion check) is to screen pediatric patients and visitors quickly to determine whether they are currently infected or have been exposed to and are incubating any communicable diseases. The main concern of the survey is to prevent the introduction of varicella into the hospital, but other illnesses such as measles, mumps, and viral respiratory illnesses also should be considered. A "contagion check" should be done for every pediatric patient and child visitor, and is especially important during periods of peak virus activity in the community.

Before the admission of a pediatric patient to the hospital, information regarding the child's immunization history, susceptibility to chickenpox, and history of recent exposure to chickenpox should be obtained. Questions that may yield additional helpful information, shown in Table 35-4, may be included in the communicable disease survey, especially for child visitors. This survey is relatively uncomplicated and assists in screening patients who present potential hazards to susceptible patients and personnel. Susceptible pediatric patients who have been exposed to proven or suspected viral illnesses are placed on precautions as previously noted.

TABLE 35-4. Items to include in a
communicable disease survey

Essential components
  Immunization history
    Measles/mumps/rubella
    Polio
    Diphtheria/pertussis/tetanus
  Has the child had or recently been exposed to chickenpox?
Other considerations, especially for child visitors
  Has the child had or recently been exposed to the following?
    Measles
    Mumps
    German measles
    Hepatitis
  Does the child have any of the following now or has the child had any of the following recently?
    Streptococcal infection
    Cough, cold, or upper respiratory infection of any kind
    Diarrhea
    Vomiting
    Fever
    Rash
    Infection of any kind

Source: Valenti, W. M., et al. *Infect. Control* 2:236, 1980, with permission.

*Infection Control and the Pregnant Employee*

Employee health personnel and infection control personnel are often consulted by the pregnant employee regarding contact with patients who have various infectious diseases (see Chapter 2). In these situations, the concern is not only for the pregnant employee but also for the fetus, who may be at risk of developing infection in the perinatal period. To counsel patients effectively in these matters, employee health personnel should be familiar with the mode of transmission of the various infectious agents as well as their risk to the pregnant employee. The educational gain from these visits may be all that is required to resolve the employee's concerns.

The infectious processes that generate the most concern among pregnant employees include viral agents such as cytomegalovirus, herpes simplex, hepatitis B, rubella, and varicella zoster viruses.

*Work Restrictions for the Pregnant Employee*

It may sometimes be advisable to restrict particular types of contact between infected patients and pregnant personnel. However, the transfer of pregnant employees to other areas of the hospital or other positions is probably not necessary in most situations. A practical approach should be developed to deal with the issue of the pregnant health care worker in much the same way that the infection control practitioner deals with work restriction in other infection control problems, taking into consideration the rights of the employee as well as the protection of the patient.

It should be kept in mind that pregnancy by itself

TABLE 35-5. Recommendations for work restriction for pregnant employees

| | Restriction | | |
|---|---|---|---|
| Disease | No contact | Follow isolation precautions | Comment |
| AIDS | | X | No evidence of transmission to health-care workers. |
| Cytomegalovirus | | | |
| Congenital | | X | Risk of transmission very low in health-care settings |
| Acquired | | X | |
| Herpes simplex | | | |
| Genital | | X | |
| Other | | X | |
| Varicella-zoster | X* | If immune | If history of chickenpox is negative or unknown, employee should not have contact with patients with chickenpox or herpes zoster |
| Rubella | X* | If immune | Ideally, employee should be immune to rubella according to testing at employment or via vaccination |
| Hepatitis B | | | |
| Dialysis units | | X | Employees of hemodialysis units should be vaccinated against hepatitis B |
| Other areas | | X | |

*Until immunity is proved by serologic testing.

TABLE 35-6. Interaction of factors in nosocomial transmission of viruses

| Virus | Transmissibility | Susceptibility of staff or other patients | Resultant nosocomial risk |
|---|---|---|---|
| Respiratory viruses | | | |
| Influenza | High | Variable[a] | High |
| Respiratory syncytial | High | High | High |
| Rhinovirus | Moderate | Moderate[a] | Moderate |
| Other (e.g., adenovirus, coronavirus) | Moderate | Moderate[a] | Moderate |
| Hepatitis B | | | |
| Needle sticks | High | High | High |
| Other exposure | Low | High | Low |
| Herpes viruses | | | |
| Herpes simplex 1 | Low | Moderate[a] | Low |
| Herpes simplex 2 | Very low | Moderate[a] | Very low[b] |
| Varicella (chickenpox) or disseminated zoster | High | Very low[a] | Low[a] |
| Herpes-zoster (localized) | Moderate | Very low[a] | Very low |
| Epstein-Barr | Very low | Very low[a] | Very low |
| Cytomegalovirus | Low | Moderate[a] | Very low[c] |
| Rubella | High | Moderate[a] | High |

[a]High in pediatric age groups.
[b]Except to newborn during delivery or after rupture of membranes.
[c]Except for blood transfusion or organ transplantation.
Source: Valenti, W. M., et al. *Infect. Control* 2:236, 1980, with permission.

does not usually make an employee more susceptible to acquiring infectious diseases from patients. Transferring employees during pregnancy may not be realistic since the same infectious hazards may be present throughout the health-care facility. In addition, routine movement of personnel may create an unnecessary burden on the departments involved. Recommendations for work restriction for pregnant employees are noted in Table 35-5 and discussed in detail by Votra and colleagues [150].

*Special Considerations*
It is important to emphasize that some viral agents are more easily transmitted than others. Personnel may respond with extraordinary concern when caring for patients with cytomegalovirus infection, while influenza vaccination programs and precautions for other more highly contagious viruses are often overlooked. Table 35-6 reviews briefly the relative risk of transmission to hospital personnel and patients of commonly seen viruses.

The relationship of virology to infection control has only recently been appreciated; viral infections have traditionally been an enigma to infection control personnel. The health-care facility presents a unique challenge to virologists and infection control personnel as they attempt to develop comprehensive pro-grams for the control and prevention of nosocomial viral infections. Certainly the next few years should help clarify this relationship as additional developments in antiviral chemotherapy and rapid viral diagnostic techniques occur.

## REFERENCES

1. Alter, M. J., Favero, M. S., Peterson, N. J., et al. National surveillance of dialysis-associated hepatitis and other diseases 1976 and 1980. *Dialysis Transp.* 12:860, 1983.
2. Anderson, L. J., and Winkler, W. G. Aqueous quaternary ammonium compounds and rabies treatment. *J. Infect. Dis.* 139:494, 1979.
3. Basilico, F. C., and Bernat, J. Vaccine-associated poliomyelitis in a contact. *J.A.M.A.* 239:2275, 1978.
4. Berlin, B. S., and Campbell, T. Hospital-acquired herpes zoster following exposure to chickenpox. *J.A.M.A.* 211:1831, 1970.
5. Benoulli, C., Siegfried, J., Baumgartner, G., et al. Danger of accidental person-to-person transmission of Creutzfeldt-Jakob disease by surgery. *Lancet* 1:478, 1977.
6. Blank, H., and Haines, H. G. Experimental

reinfection with herpes simplex virus. *J. Invest. Dermatol.* 61:223, 1973.

7. Bolivar, R., Conklin, R. H., Vollett, J. J., Pickering, L. K., et al. Rotavirus in travelers' diarrhea: Study of an adult student population in Mexico. *J. Infect. Dis.* 137:324, 1978.

8. Centers for Disease Control. Prospective evaluation of health-care workers exposed via the parenteral or mucous-membrane route to blood or body fluids from patients with acquired immunodeficiency syndrome—United States. *Morbid. Mortal. Weekly Rep.* 34:101, 1983.

9. Centers for Disease Control. Hepatitis B vaccine: Evidence confirming lack of AIDS transmission. *Morbid. Mortal. Weekly Rep.*, 33:685, 1984.

10. Centers for Disease Control. *Hepatitis-Control Measures for Hepatitis B in Dialysis Centers.* Viral Hepatitis Investigations and Control Series, November 1977.

11. Centers for Disease Control. Human rabies—Pennsylvania. *Morbid. Mortal. Weekly Rep.* 28:75, 1979.

12. Centers for Disease Control. Human-to-human transmission of rabies via a corneal transplant. *Morbid. Mortal. Weekly Rep.* 29:25, 1980.

13. Centers for Disease Control. Laboratory-associated smallpox. *Morbid. Mortal. Weekly Rep.* 27:319, 1978.

14. Centers for Disease Control. Nosocomial outbreak of pharyngoconjunctival fever due to adenovirus, type 4—New York. *Morbid. Mortal. Weekly Rep.* 27:4, 1978.

15. Centers for Disease Control. Outbreak of viral hepatitis in the staff of a pediatrics ward—California. *Morbid. Mortal. Weekly Rep.* 26:77, 1977.

16. Centers for Disease Control. Parainfluenza outbreaks in extended-care facilities. *Morbid. Mortal. Weekly Rep.* 27:475, 1978.

17. Centers for Disease Control. Poliomyelitis—Pennsylvania, Maryland. *Morbid. Mortal. Weekly Rep.* 28:49, 1978.

18. Centers for Disease Control. Rabies prevention. *Morbid. Mortal. Weekly Rep.* 29:265, 1980.

19. Centers for Disease Control. Recommendation of the immunization practice advisory committee (ACIP). Adult immunization. *Morbid. Mortal. Weekly Rep.* 33: Supplement 1S, 1984.

20. Centers for Disease Control. Recommendation of the immunization practice advisory committee (ACIP). Postexposure prophylaxis of hepatitis B. *Morbid. Mortal. Weekly Rep.* 34:313, 1985.

21. Centers for Disease Control. Recommendation of the immunization practice advisory committee (ACIP). Prevention and control of influenza. *Morbid. Mortal. Weekly Rep.* 34:261, 273, 1985.

22. Centers for Disease Control. Recommendation of the immunization practice advisory committee (ACIP). Rabies prevention—United States, 1984. *Morbid. Mortal. Weekly Rep.* 33:393, 407, 1984.

23. Centers for Disease Control. Recommendation of the immunization practice advisory committee (ACIP). Varicella-zoster immune globulin for the prevention of chickenpox. *Morbid. Mortal. Weekly Rep.* 33:84, 95, 1984.

24. Centers for Disease Control. Rubella surveillance report. Jan. 1976–Dec. 1978. Issued May 1980.

25. Centers for Disease Control. Rubella in hospitals in California. *Morbid. Mortal. Weekly Rep.* 32:37, 1983.

26. Centers for Disease Control. Suboptimal response to hepatitis B vaccine given by injection into the buttock. *Morbid. Mortal. Weekly Rep.* 34:105, 110, 1985.

27. Centers for Disease Control. Smallpox vaccine. *Morbid. Mortal. Weekly Rep.* 34:341, 1985.

28. Centers for Disease Control. Veterinary Public Health Notes, July 1977.

29. Chanock, R. M., Kim, H. W., Vargosko, A. J., et al. Respiratory syncytial virus. I. Virus recovery and other observations during the 1960 outbreak of bronchiolitis, pneumonia, and respiratory diseases in children. *J.A.M.A.* 176:647, 1961.

30. Cherry, J. D., Feigin, R. D., Lobes, L. A., et al. Atypical measles in children previously immunized with attenuated measles virus vaccine. *Pediatrics* 50:712, 1973.

31. Cherry, J. D., Soriano, F., and Jahn, C. L. Search for perinatal virus infection: A prospective, clinical, virologic, and serologic study. *Am. J. Dis. Child.* 116:245, 1968.

32. Cherry, J. D. Non-polio enteroviruses. In Feigin, R. D., and Cherry, J. D. (Eds.), *Pediatric Infectious Diseases.* Philadelphia: Saunders, 1981, pp. 1316–1365.

33. Corey, L., Stamm, W. E., Feorino, P. M., et al. HBsAg-negative hepatitis in a hemodialysis unit: Relation to Epstein-Barr virus. *N. Engl. J. Med.* 293:1273, 1975.

34. Cramblatt, H. B., Haynes, R. D., Azimi, P. H., et al. Nosocomial infection with echovirus type 11 in handicapped and premature infants. *Pediatrics* 51:602, 1973.

35. Crystei, I. L., Totterdel, B., Baker, M. J., et al. Rotavirus infections in a maternity unit. *Lancet* 2:79, 1975.

36. Davidson, G. P. Importance of a new virus in acute sporadic enteritis in children. *Lancet* 1:242, 1975.

37. Dawson, C. R., and Darrel, R. Infections due to adenovirus type 8 in the United States. I. An outbreak of epidemic keratoconjunctivitis originating in a physician's office. *N. Engl. J. Med.* 268:1031, 1973.

38. DeFabritis, A. M., Riggio, R. R., David, D. S., et al. Parainfluenza type 3 in a transplant unit. *J.A.M.A.* 241:384, 1979.

39. Denes, A. E., Smith, J. L., Maynard, J. E., et al. Hepatitis B infection in physicians: Results of a nationwide seroepidemiologic survey. *J.A.M.A.* 239:210, 1978.

40. Dienstag, J. L., Feinstone, S. M., Kapikian, A. Z., et al. Fecal shedding of hepatitis A antigen. *Lancet* 1:765, 1975.

41. Dienstag, J. L., and Ryan, D. M. Occupational exposure to hepatitis B virus in hospital personnel: Infection or immunization? *Am. J. Epidemiol.* 115:26, 1982.

42. Douglas, R. G., Jr. Influenza in Man. In Kilbourne, E. D. (Ed.), *The Influenza Viruses and Influenza.* New York: Academic, 1975.

43. Downie, A. W. Poxvirus Group. In Horsfall, R. L., and Tamm, I. (Eds.), *Viral and Rickettsial Infections of Man* (4th ed.). Philadelphia: Lippincott, 1965, pp. 932–964.

44. Drew, W. L., Mintz, L., Miner, R. C., et al. Prevalence of cytomegalovirus infection in homosexual men. *J. Infect. Dis.* 143:188, 1981.

45. Duffy, P., Wolf, J., Collins, G., DeVoe, A. G., et al. Possible person-to-person transmission of Creutzfeldt-Jakob disease (letter). *N. Engl. J. Med.* 290:692, 1974.

46. Dworskey, M. E., Welch, K., Cassady, G., and Stagno, S. Occupational risk for primary cytomegalovirus infection among pediatric health care workers. *N. Engl. J. Med.* 309:950, 1983.

47. Eichewald, H. F., McCracken, G. H., and Kindberg, S. J. Virus infections of the newborn. *Prog. Med. Virol.* 9:35, 1967.

48. Favero, M. S., Maynard, J. E., Leger, R. T., et al. Guidelines for the care of patients hospitalized with viral hepatitis. *Ann. Intern. Med.* 91:872, 1979.

49. Feldman, H. A. Mumps. In Evans, A. S. (Ed.), *Viral Infections of Humans: Epidemiology and Control.* New York: Plenum, 1976, pp. 317–332.

50. Foley, F. D., Greenwald, K. A., Nash, M. C., and Pruitt, B. A. Herpes virus infection in burned patients. *N. Engl. J. Med.* 282:652, 1970.

51. Foy, H. M., and Grayston, J. T. Adenoviruses. In Evans, A. S. (Ed.), *Viral Infections of Humans: Epidemiology and Control.* New York: Plenum, 1976, pp. 53–69.

52. Fulginiti, V. A., and Arthur, J. M. Altered reactivity to measles virus: Skin test reactivity and antibody response to measles virus antigens in recipients of killed measles virus vaccine. *J. Pediatr.* 75:604, 1979.

53. Gadjusek, D. C., Gibbs, C. J., Asher, D. M., Brown, P., et al. Precautions in medical care of and in handling materials from patients with transmissable virus dementia (Creutzfeldt-Jakob disease). *N. Engl. J. Med.* 297:1253, 1977.

54. Garibaldi, R. A., Rasmussen, C. M., Holmes, A. W., et al. Hospital-acquired serum hepatitis: Report of an outbreak. *J.A.M.A.* 219:1577, 1972.

55. Garibaldi, R. A., Bryan, J. A., Forrest, J. N., et al. Hemodialysis-associated hepatitis. *J.A.M.A.* 225:384, 1973.

56. Gerber, M. A., Lewin, E. B., Gerety, M. D., et al. The lack of transmission of type B hepatitis in a special care nursery. *J. Pediatr.* 91:120, 1977.

57. Gershon, A. A., Kalter, Z. G., and Steinberg, S. Detection of antibody to varicella-zoster virus by immune adherence hemagglutination. *Proc. Soc. Exp. Biol. Med.* 151:762, 1976.

58. Gordon, J. E. Chickenpox: An epidemiological review. *Am. J. Med. Sci.* 244:362, 1962.

59. Greaves, W. L., Kaiser, A. B., Alford, R. H., et al. The problem of herpes whitlow among hospital personnel. *Infect. Control* 1:381, 1980.

60. Greenlee, J. E. Containment precautions in hospitals for cases of Creutzfeldt-Jakob disease. *Infect. Control* 3:222, 1982.

61. Gustafson, J. L. An outbreak of nosocomial airborne varicella. *Pediatrics* 70:550, 1982.

62. Gwaltney, J. M., Mosalski, P. B., and Hendley, J. O. Hand-to-hand transmission of rhinovirus. *Ann. Intern. Med.* 88:453, 1978.

63. Hall, C. B., and Douglas, R. G., Jr. Nosocomial influenza as a cause of intercurrent fever in infants. *Pediatrics* 55:673, 1975.

64. Hall, C. B. The shedding and spreading of respiratory syncytial virus. *Pediatr. Res.* 11:236, 1977.

65. Hall, C. B., Geiman, J. M., Douglas, R. G., Jr., and Meagher, M. P. Control of nosocomial respiratory syncytial virus infections. *Pediatrics* 62:728, 1978.

66. Hall, C. B., Douglas, R. G., Jr., and Geiman, J. M. Possible transmission by fomites of respiratory syncytial virus. *J. Infect. Dis.* 141:98,

1980.

67. Hall, C. B. Nosocomial viral respiratory infections: Perennial weeds on pediatric wards. *Am. J. Med.* 70:670, 1981.

68. Hanshaw, J. B., and Dudgeon, J. A. In Schaffer, A. J., and Markowitz, M. (Eds.), *Viral Diseases of the Fetus and Newborn.* Philadelphia: Saunders, 1978.

69. Hayden, C. F., Meyers, J. D., and Dixon, R. E. Nosocomial varicella. Part II. Suggested guidelines for management. *West. J. Med.* 130:300, 1979.

70. Henderson, F. W., Collier, A. M., Clyde, W. A., et al. Respiratory syncytial virus infections, reinfections, and immunity: A prospective longitudinal study in young children. *N. Engl. J. Med.* 300:530, 1979.

71. Hendley, J. O., Mika, L. A., and Swaltney, J. M. Evaluation of virucidal compounds for inactivation of rhinovirus on hands. *Antimicrob. Agents Chemother.* 14:690, 1978.

72. Hendley, J. P., Wenzel, R. P., and Gwaltney, J. M. Transmission of rhinovirus colds by self-inoculation. *N. Engl. J. Med.* 288:1362, 1973.

73. Hethcote, H. W. Measles and rubella in the United States. *Am. J. Epidemiol.* 117:2, 1983.

74. Hirsch, M. S., Wormser, G. P., Schooley, R. T., et al. Risk of nosocomial infection with human T-cell lymphotropic virus III (HTLV-III). *N. Engl. J. Med.* 312:14, 1985.

75. Ho, M., Suwansirikul, S., Dowling, J. N., Youngblood, L. A., et al. The transplanted kidney as a source of CMV infection. *N. Engl. J. Med.* 293:1109, 1975.

76. Houff, S. A., Burton, R. C., Wilson, R. W., Henson, T. E., et al. Human-to-human transmission of rabies virus by corneal transplant. *N. Engl. J. Med.* 300:603, 1979.

77. Hurwitz, E. S., Schonberger, L. B., Nelson, D. B., et al. Guillain-Barré syndrome and the 1978–79 influenza vaccine. *N. Engl. J. Med.* 304:1557, 1981.

78. Jawetz, E., Hanna, L., Sonne, M., et al. Laboratory infection with adenovirus type 8: Laboratory and epidemiologic observations. *Am. J. Hyg.* 69:13, 1979.

79. Jones, M. J., Kolb, M., Votava, H. F., et al. Intrauterine echovirus type 11 infections. *Mayo Clin. Proc.* 55:509, 1980.

80. Kapikian, A. Z., Kim, H. W., Wyatt, R. G., et al. Human reovirus-like agent as the major pathogen associated with "winter" gastroenteritis in hospitalized infants and young children. *N. Engl. J. Med.* 294:965, 1976.

81. Kibrick, S. Herpes simplex infection at term: What to do with mother, newborn, and nursery personnel. *J.A.M.A.* 243:157, 1980.

82. Kim, H. W., Brandt, C. D., Kapikian, A. Z., Wyatt, R. G., et al. Human reovirus-like agent infection occurrence in adult contacts of pediatric patients with gastroenteritis. *J.A.M.A.* 238:404, 1977.

83. Kuenz, J. C., and Valenti, W. M. An attitudinal study of an influenza vaccination program. Presented at the Eighth Educational Conference of the Association for Practitioners in Infection Control. Abstract #26, Atlanta, Ga., May 28, 1981.

84. Lang, D. J., Ebert, P. A., Rodgers, B. M., et al. Reduction of post-transfusion cytomegalovirus infections following use of leukocyte-depleted blood. *Transfusion* 17:391, 1977.

85. Lake, A. M., Lauer, B. A., and Clark, J. C. Enterovirus infections in neonates. *J. Pediatr.* 89:787, 1976.

86. Lawless, M. R., Abramson, J. S., and Harlan, J. E. Rubella susceptibility in sixth graders: Effectiveness of current immunization practice. *Pediatrics* 65:1086, 1980.

87. LeClair, J. M., Zaia, J. A., Levin, M. J., et al. Airborne transmission of chickenpox in a hospital. *N. Engl. J. Med.* 302:450, 1980.

88. Light, I. J., Brackvogel, M. S., Walton, R. L., and Sutherland, J. M. An epidemic of bullous impetigo arising from a central admission-observation nursery. *Pediatrics* 49:15, 1972.

89. Linneman, C. C., Jr., Buchman, T. G., Light, I. G., et al. Transmission of herpes simplex virus type I in a nursery for the newborn: Identification of viral isolates by DNA fingerprinting. *Lancet* 1:964, 1978.

90. Manzella, J., McConville, J., Valenti, W. M., et al. An outbreak of herpes simplex virus stomatitis in a dental practice. *J.A.M.A.* 252:2019, 1984.

91. Matthew, E. B., Sietzman, D. E., Madden, D. L., et al. A major epidemic of infectious hepatitis in an institution for the mentally retarded. *Am. J. Epidemiol.* 98:199, 1973.

92. Mathur, U., Bentley, D. W., and Hall, C. B. Concurrent respiratory syncytial virus and influenza A infections in the institutionalized elderly and chronically ill. *Ann. Intern. Med.* 93:49, 1980.

93. McDonald, L. L., St. Geme, J. W., and Arnold, B. H. Nosocomial infection with ECHO virus type 31 in neonatal intensive care unit. *Pediatrics* 47:995, 1971.

94. McLaughlin, M. C., and Gold, L. H. The New York rubella incident: A case for changing hos-

pital policy regarding rubella testing and immunization. *Am. J. Public Health* 69:287, 1979.

95. Melnick, J. L. Enteroviruses. In Evans, A. S. (Ed.), *Viral Infections in Humans: Epidemiology and Control.* New York: Plenum, 1976, pp. 163–201.

96. Meurman, O. H., and Laine, M. J. Rotavirus epidemic in adults. *N. Engl. J. Med.* 296:1289, 1977.

97. Meyerowitz, R. L., Stalder, H., Oxman, M. N., et al. Fatal disseminated adenovirus infection in a renal transplant recipient. *Am. J. Med.* 59:591, 1975.

98. Meyers, J. D., Romm, F. J., Then, W. S., and Bryan, J. A. Food-borne hepatitis A in a general hospital. *J.A.M.A.* 231:1049, 1975.

99. Meyers, J. D., Dienstag, J. L., Purcell, R. H., Thomas, E. D., and Holmes, K. K. Parenterally transmitted non-A, non-B hepatitis: An epidemic reassessed. Ann. Intern. Med. 87:57, 1977.

100. Meyers, J. D., Stamm, W. E., Kerr, M., et al. Lack of transmission of hepatitis B after surgical exposure. *J.A.M.A.* 240:1725, 1978.

101. Meyers, J. D., MacQuarrie, M. B., Merigan, T. C., and Jennison, M. H. Nosocomial varicella. Part 1: Outbreak in oncology patients at a children's hospital. *West J. Med.* 130:196, 1979.

102. Middleton, P. J., Azymanski, M. T., and Petric, P. J. Viruses associated with acute gastroenteritis in young children. *Am. J. Dis. Child.* 131:233, 1977.

103. Mintz, L., Ballard, R. A., Sniderman, S. H., Roth, R. S., et al. Nosocomial respiratory syncytial virus infections in an intensive care nursery: Rapid diagnosis by immunofluorescence. *Pediatrics* 64:149, 1979.

104. Morens, D. M., Bregman, D. J., West, C. M., et al. An outbreak of varicella-zoster virus infection among cancer patients. *Ann. Intern. Med.* 93:414, 1980.

105. Mosley, J. W., Redeker, A. G., Feinstone, S. M., et al. Multiple hepatitis viruses in multiple attacks of acute viral hepatitis. *N. Engl. J. Med.* 296:75, 1977.

106. Mufson, M. A., Mocega, H. E., and Krause, H. E. Acquisition of parainfluenza 3 virus infection by hospitalized children. I. Frequencies, rates, and temporal data. *J. Infect. Dis.* 128:141, 1973.

107. Muldoon, R. L., Stanley, E. D., and Jackson, G. G. Use and withdrawal of amantadine chemoprophylaxis during epidemic influenza A. *Am.*

*Rev. Resp. Dis.* 133:487, 1976.

108. Nadar, P. R., Horowitz, M. S., and Rousseau, J. Atypical exanthem following exposure to natural measles: Eleven cases in children previously inoculated with killed vaccine. *J. Pediatr.* 72:22, 1968.

109. Nahmias, A. N., Josey, W. E., Naib, Z. M., et al. Perinatal risk associated with maternal genital herpes simplex virus infection. *Am. J. Obstet. Gynecol.* 110:825, 1971.

110. Naragi, S., Jackson, G. G., and Jonasson, O. M. Viremia with herpes simplex type 1 in adults. *Ann. Int. Med.* 85:165, 1976.

111. Nathanson, N., and Martin, J. R. The epidemiology of poliomyelitis: Enigmas surrounding its appearance, epidemicity and disappearance. *Am. J. Epidemiol.* 110:672, 1976.

112. Nightingale, E. O. Recommendations for a national policy on poliomyelitis vaccination. *N. Engl. J. Med.* 297:249, 1977.

113. O'Donoghue, J. M., Ray, C. G., Terry, D. W., et al. Prevention of nosocomial influenza with Amantadine. *Am. J. Epidemiol.* 97:276, 1973.

114. Orenstein, W. A., Heseltine, P. N. R., LeGagnoux, S. J., and Portnoy, B. Rubella vaccine and susceptible hospital employees. *J.A.M.A.* 245:711, 1981.

115. Parkman, P. D., Galasso, G. H., Top, F. H., and Noble, G. R. Summary of clinical trials of influenza vaccines. *J. Infect. Dis.* 134:100, 1976.

116. Phillips, C. A., Aronson, M. D., Tomkow, J., et al. Enteroviruses in Vermont, 1969–1978: An important cause of illness throughout the year. *J. Infect. Dis.* 141:162, 1980.

117. Polk, B. F., White, J. A., DeGirolami, P. C., and Modlin, J. F. Outbreak of rubella among hospital personnel. *N. Engl. J. Med.* 303:541, 1980.

118. Richmond, S. J., Caul, E. O., Dunn, S. M., et al. An outbreak of gastroenteritis in young children caused by adenoviruses. *Lancet* 1:1178, 1979.

119. Rimland, D., Parkin, W. E., Miller, G. B., et al. Hepatitis B traced to an oral surgeon. *N. Engl. J. Med.* 296:953, 1977.

120. Ross, A. H. Modification of chickenpox in family contacts by administration of gamma globulin. *N. Engl. J. Med.* 267:369, 1962.

121. Ryder, R. W., McGowan, J. E., Hatch, M. H., and Palmer, E. L. Reovirus-like agent as a cause of nosocomial diarrhea in infants. *J. Pediatr.* 90:698, 1977.

122. Schoenbaum, S. C. Rubella policies for hospi-

tals and health workers (editorial). *Infect. Control* 2:366, 416, 1981.

123. Schonberger, L. B., McGowan, J. E., and Gregg, M. B. Vaccine-associated poliomyelitis in the United States, 1961–1972. *Am. J. Epidemiol.* 104:202, 1976.

124. Schreiner, R. L., Kleinman, M. B., and Gresham, E. L. Maternal oral herpes: Isolation policy. *Pediatrics* 63:247, 1979.

125. Shewmon, D. A., Cherry, J. D., and Kirby, S. E. Shedding of rubella virus in a 4½-year-old boy with congenital rubella. *Pediatr. Infect. Dis.* 1:342, 1982.

126. Smith, J. L., Maynard, J. E., Berquist, K. R., et al. Comparative risk of hepatitis B among physicians and dentists. *J. Infect. Dis.* 6:705, 1976.

127. Snydman, D. R., Bryan, J. A., Macon, E. J., and Gregg, M. B. Hemodialysis-associated hepatitis: Report of an epidemic with further evidence on mechanisms of transmission. *Am. J. Epidemiol.* 104:563, 1976.

128. Snydman, D. R., Bryan, J. A., London, W. T., et al. Transmission of hepatitis B associated with hemodialysis: Role of malfunction (blood leaks) in dialysis machines. *J. Infect. Dis.* 134:562, 1976.

129. Sparling, D. Transmission of mumps (letter). *N. Engl. J. Med.* 280:276, 1979.

130. Sprague, J. B., Hierholzer, J. C., Currier, R. W., et al. Epidemic keratoconjunctivitis. *N. Engl. J. Med.* 289:1341, 1977.

131. Steinhoff, M. C., and Gerber, M. A. Rotavirus infection of neonates. *Lancet* 1:775, 1978.

132. Stevens, C. E., et al. Increased incidence of AIDS in hepatitis B vaccine (letter). *N. Engl. J. Med.* 308:1163, 1983.

133. Straube, R. C., Thompson, M. A., Van Dyke, R. B., et al. Adenovirus type 7b in a children's hospital. *J. Infect. Dis.* 147:814, 1983.

134. Szmuness, W., Prince, A. M., Grady, G. F., et al. Hepatitis B infection: A point prevalence study in 15 U.S. hemodialysis centers. *J.A.M.A.* 227:901, 1974.

135. Szmuness, W., Dienstag, J. L., Purcell, R. H., et al. Hepatitis A and hemodialysis. *Ann. Intern. Med.* 87:8, 1977.

136. Szmuness, W., Purcell, R. H., Dienstag, J. L., and Stevens, C. E. Antibody to hepatitis A antigen in institutionalized mentally retarded patients. *J.A.M.A.* 237:1702, 1977.

137. Szmuness, W., Stevens, C. E., Harley, E. J., et al. Hepatitis B vaccine: Demonstration of efficacy in a controlled clinical trial in a high

risk population in the United States. *N. Engl. J. Med.* 303:833, 1980.

138. Szmuness, W., Stevens, C. E., Harley, E. J., et al. Hepatitis B vaccine in medical staff of hemodialysis units: Efficacy and subtype cross protection. *N. Engl. J. Med.* 307:4181, 1982.

139. Tada, H., Yanagida, M., Michina, J., Fujii, T., et al. Combined passive and active immunization for preventing perinatal transmission of hepatitis B virus carrier state. *Pediatrics* 70:613, 1982.

140. Tallett, S., MacKenzie, C., Middleton, P., et al. Clinical, laboratory and epidemiologic features of a viral gastroenteritis in infants and children. *Pediatrics* 60:217, 1977.

141. Thornhill, T. S., Kalika, A. R., Wyatt, R. G., et al. Pattern of shedding of Norwalk particle in stools during experimentally induced gastroenteritis in volunteers as determined by immune electronmicroscopy. *J. Infect. Dis.* 132:28, 1975.

142. Tolkoff-Rubin, N. E., Rubin, R. H., Keller, E. E., et al. Cytomegalovirus infection in dialysis patients and personnel. *Ann. Intern. Med.* 89:625, 1978.

143. Turner, A. R., MacDonald, R. N., and Cooper, B. A. Transmission of infectious mononucleosis by transfusion of pre-illness serum. *Ann. Intern. Med.* 77:751, 1972.

144. Turner, R., Shehab, Z., Osborne, K., et al. Shedding and survival of herpes simplex virus from "fever blisters." *Pediatrics* 70:547, 1982.

145. Valenti, W. M., Betts, R. F., Hall, C. B., et al. Nosocomial viral infections. II. Guidelines for prevention and control of respiratory viruses, herpesviruses, and hepatitis viruses. *Infect. Control* 1:165, 1980.

146. Valenti, W. M., Menegus, M. M., Hall, C. B., et al. Nosocomial viral infections. I. Epidemiology and significance. *Infect. Control* 1:33, 1980.

147. Valenti, W. M., Clarke, T. A., Hall, C. B., Menegus, M. A., et al. Concurrent outbreaks of rhinovirus and respiratory syncytial virus in an intensive care nursery: Epidemiology and associated risk factors. *J. Pediatr.* 100:722, 1982.

148. VanVoris, L. P., Belshe, R. B., and Shaffer, J. L. Nosocomial influenza B in the elderly. *Ann. Intern. Med.* 96:153, 1982.

149. VanZee, B. E., Douglas, R. G., Jr., Betts, R. F., Bauman, A. W., et al. Lymphocytic choriomeningitis in University Hospital personnel. *Am. J. Med.* 58:803, 1975.

150. Votra, E. M., Rutala, W. A., and Sarubbi, F.

A. Recommendations for pregnant employee interaction with patients having communicable infectious diseases. *Am. J. Infect. Control* 11:10, 1983.

151. Wehrle, P. F., Posch, J., Richter, K. H., and Henderson, D. A. An airborne outbreak of smallpox in a German hospital and its significance with respect to other recent outbreaks in Europe. *Bull. WHO* 43:669, 1970.

152. Weiss, K. E., Falvo, C. E., Buimovici-Klein, E., Magill, J. W., et al. Evaluation of an employee health service as a setting for a rubella screening and immunization program. *Am. J. Public Health* 69:281, 1979.

153. Weller, T. H. The cytomegaloviruses: Ubiquitous agents with protean manifestations. *N. Engl. J. Med.* 285:203, 267, 1971.

154. Wentworth, B. B., and Alexander, E. R. Seroepidemiology of infections due to members of the herpes virus group. *Am. J. Epidemiol.* 94:496, 1971.

155. Wenzel, R. P., Deal, E. C., and Hendley, J. O. Hospital-acquired viral respiratory illness on a pediatric ward. *Pediatrics* 60:367, 1977.

156. Wigger, H. F., and Blank, W. A. Fatal hepatic and bronchial necrosis in adenovirus infection with thymic alymphoplasia. *N. Engl. J. Med.* 275:870, 1977.

157. Wilfert, C. M., Huang, E., and Stagno, S. Restriction endonuclease analysis of cytomegalovirus deoxyribonucleic acid as an epidemiologic tool. *Pediatrics* 70:717, 1982.

158. Williams, W. W. *CDC Guidelines for Infection Control in Hospital Personnel.* Springfield, Va.: National Technical Information Service (NTIS), July 1983.

159. Yeager, A. S. Longitudinal serological study of cytomegalovirus in nurses and personnel without patient contact. *J. Clin. Microbiol.* 2:448, 1975.

160. Yow, M. D., Lakeman, A. D., Stagno, S., et al. Use of restriction enzymes to investigate the source of primary cytomegalovirus infection in a pediatric nurse. *Pediatrics* 70:713, 1982.

161. Zaia, J. A., and Oxman, M. N. Antibody to varicella-zoster-virus–induced membrane antigen: Immunofluorescence assay using monodisperse glutaraldehyde target cells. *J. Infect. Dis.* 136:519, 1977.

# 36 INFECTIONS DUE TO INFUSION THERAPY

Dennis G. Maki

## BACKGROUND AND MAGNITUDE OF THE PROBLEM

Each year over one-half of the 40 million patients hospitalized in the United States receive infusion therapy in some form for administration of fluid and electrolytes, blood products, drugs, or total parenteral nutrition, or, increasingly, for hemodynamic monitoring. Infusion therapy unfortunately has a substantial and generally underappreciated potential for producing iatrogenic disease, particularly "line sepsis," which is bacteremia originating either from the cannula used for vascular access or from contaminated infusate.

Fully one-third of all outbreaks of nosocomial bacteremia derive from infusion therapy in some form (Fig. 36-1). Also, up to one-third of all endemic nosocomial bacteremias, and the majority of candidemias, are infusion-related and derive mainly from vascular catheters.

Infusion-related sepsis is frequently unrecognized, most likely due to its relative infrequency. The percentage of infusions identified as producing sepsis—considerably less than 1 percent on the average—is sufficiently low that any single physician or nurse is unlikely to encounter more than an occasional case. But even such a low incidence of infection applied to the 20 million patients who receive infusion therapy in U.S. hospitals translates to many thousands of device-related septicemias nationwide each year. Neither the device nor fluid is cultured in many — possibly most—of these infections, and the infusion source thus remains undisclosed.

The premise that infusion-related sepsis is largely preventable forms the thesis for this chapter. The primary goal must not be simply to identify and treat these iatrogenic infections but rather to prevent them. By critically examining existing knowledge of the major reservoirs of nosocomial pathogens and their modes of transmission to infusions, rational and effective guidelines for prevention can be formulated.

The following sections present selected important events and findings related to infections deriving from infusion therapy rather than a comprehensive review of literature related to the topic. The reader is also referred to Chapter 38 in which some of the topics included in this chapter are discussed additionally.

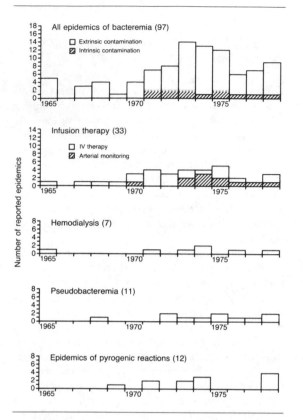

FIG. 36-1. Epidemics of nosocomial bacteremia and pyrogenic reactions by year, 1965 to 1978. (From published reports in English world literature; for epidemics of bacteremia, bacteremias constituted at least 25 percent of epidemic infections.)

## SOURCES OF INFUSION-RELATED INFECTION

There are two potential sources of bacteremic infection associated with any intravascular line: infection of the cannula* wound and contamination of the infusate administered through the cannula. Cannulas produce bacteremia far more frequently than does contaminated fluid. We cultured both the cannula and a sample of fluid at the time the infusion was discontinued in a prospective study of 790 in-use infusions [2]; contamination of infusate was identified only five times, and none of the patients involved had concomitant bacteremia. In contrast, five cannulas were shown to have produced septicemia in the

*Cannula is a general term that encompasses all devices used for temporary vascular access, including steel needles and plastic catheters of all types.

TABLE 36-1. Results of culturing infusate and cannula in 790 in-use infusions

| | Results on culture | |
|---|---|---|
| | Infusion fluid | Cannula |
| Total number cultured | 790 | 790 |
| Positive culture, number (%) | 5 (0.6) | 34 (4.3)[a] |
| Local infection, number (%) | 0 | 29 (3.7)[b] |
| Related septicemia, number (%) | 0 | 5 (0.6)[c] |

[a] $p < .001$ by Fisher's Exact test.
[b] Positive semiquantitative culture of the cannula.
[c] $p = .03$.
Source: Adapted from Band, J. D., and Maki, D. G. Ann. Intern. Med. 91:173, 1979.

absence of concomitantly contaminated fluid (Table 36-1).

## CLINICAL SYNDROMES

### Infusion Phlebitis

Local inflammation—pain, erythema, tenderness, or a palpable inflamed and thrombosed vein—is an extremely common complication of intravenous therapy, occurring with as many as 35 percent of peripheral intravenous infusions in some hospitals. Phlebitis is primarily a physiochemical phenomenon, deriving mainly from acidic and hypertonic fluids, irritating drugs (especially antibiotics and cytotoxic agents), and the mechanical effects of the cannula. Other factors that contribute to phlebitis may include particulate matter, the anatomic location of the cannula, the diameter and length of the cannula, the material of which it is made, and especially, the duration of cannulation.

Among this multitude of potential etiologic factors is infection, the exact contribution of which is not altogether clear. Only about one-half of patients with catheter-related septicemia display prodromal phlebitis. Using the semiquantitative culture method [21], however, which more clearly identifies local cannula-related infection, we estimate that about 20 percent of cases of infusion phlebitis are caused by infection of the cannula wound.

Phlebitis can also be produced by contaminated infusate. Patients with septicemia from intrinsically contaminated fluid in a large nationwide epidemic traced to the contaminated products of one manufacturer had a much higher incidence of phlebitis than patients receiving intravenous fluids who did not develop sepsis [20]. Most patients with infusion phlebitis do not develop cannula-related sepsis, but its presence connotes a substantially increased risk of infusion-related septicemia and indicates the need for immediate removal of the cannula.

### Suppurative Phlebitis

The most serious form of intravascular-line infection is septic or suppurative phlebitis resulting in septic thrombosis. This serious infection nearly always originates from plastic catheters that have been left in place for more than 48 hours. In suppurative phlebitis, the vein literally becomes an intravenous abscess, discharging myriads of organisms into the bloodstream. The clinical picture of refractory and, not uncommonly, overwhelming septicemia is typical. When this occurs, few patients survive unless the vein and its affected tributaries are excised surgically. However, suppurative phlebitis may be very insidious clinically. Local inflammation is present less than half the time, and the septic picture often occurs several days after the catheter is removed.

Suppurative phlebitis has been encountered most frequently in burn patients, and has often been first recognized at autopsy. Limited accessible peripheral veins for vascular access; failure to recognize the early signs of catheter-induced sepsis because fever, chills, and hypotension are attributed to the burn wound or other concomitant infections; an intrinsic hypercoagulable state; and the vast number of pathogenic organisms near the catheter wound create a milieu uniquely conducive to this infection. Suppurative phlebitis also occurs in nonburn patients, most commonly after prolonged venous catheterization, and may be more frequent with cannulation of veins of the leg. Venous cannulation of the lower extremity in adults is generally inadvisable.

Suppuration of the great central veins usually derives from catheters used for hyperalimentation in burn patients and has rarely been diagnosed during life. Patients typically die with refractory cryptogenic septicemia and septic pulmonary emboli.

The microorganisms most frequently implicated in suppurative phlebitis are the same organisms that cause uncomplicated cannula-related septicemia: *Staphylococcus aureus,* the nosocomial aerobic gram-negative bacilli (*Klebsiella, Enterobacter, Pseudomonas, Serratia,* and *Acinetobacter*), and *Candida.*

## DIAGNOSIS OF INFUSION-RELATED SEPSIS

Although stringent attention to asepsis will considerably reduce the incidence of intravascular-line sepsis, sporadic cases and even epidemics can be expected to occur occasionally because of human error, intrinsically contaminated products, or undue susceptibility to infection of patients. If affected patients are to survive, the causal relation between an infusion and a picture of sepsis must be recognized early.

The clinical features of infusion-related septicemia are indistinguishable from bloodstream infection arising from any other site, such as the urinary tract or an infected surgical wound, and do not appear to differ significantly on the basis of origin in the intravascular cannula or contaminated infusate. Line sepsis occurring in seriously ill patients can be particularly insidious. The bacteremia is often attributed to pneumonia or urinary tract or surgical wound infection or is simply accepted as "cryptogenic" and treated. About half of the outbreaks of infusion-related bacteremias have occurred in intensive care units, and most of the reported outbreaks of bacteremia from contamination of arterial pressure-monitoring systems have involved postcardiac surgery patients.

The following key observations should immediately bring to mind the possibility of sepsis arising from an infusion:

1. A patient receiving infusion therapy at the outset of septicemia
2. Inflammation at the cannula insertion site, especially with expressible purulence
3. Primary septicemia (i.e., no obvious local infection)
4. Patient unlikely candidate for septicemia (young or without underlying predisposing diseases)
5. Precipitous onset of overwhelming sepsis, often with shock (usually indicative of massively contaminated infusate or suppurative phlebitis)
6. Sepsis refractory to appropriate antimicrobial therapy until the culpable infusion is purposely or fortuitously removed

During a nationwide outbreak in 1970–71 due to intrinsic contamination of one manufacturer's products, patients treated with antibiotics to which the epidemic organisms were sensitive remained clinically septic, continued to have positive blood cultures after 24 hours or more of therapy, and did not improve clinically until their infusions were fortuitously or intentionally removed [20].

Focal retinal lesions—cotton-wool patches—may be present in patients with deep *Candida* infection deriving from hyperalimentation catheters, even in those without positive blood cultures. Careful ophthalmologic examination should be a routine part of the evaluation of patients receiving hyperalimentation who are suspected of having line sepsis. A confounding problem in studies of systemic candidiasis is whether the catheters themselves give rise to candidiasis or intravascular catheters "trap" blood-borne organisms originating from other sites. Septicemia from arterial catheters is frequently heralded by embolic lesions that manifest themselves as tender, erythematous papules, 5 to 10 mm in diameter, appearing in the distal distribution of the involved artery, usually in the palm or sole (Osler's nodes).

The microbiologic profile of septicemia (Table 36-2) can also strongly suggest an infusion-related cause. Certain microorganisms are so prevalent in line sepsis—*S. aureus* in cannula-related sepsis; *Enterobacter cloacae, Enterobacter agglomerans,* and *Pseudomonas cepacia* in sepsis from contaminated infusate; and *Candida* in hyperalimentation—that their recovery from blood cultures, even from only one patient, should prompt immediate search for an infusion-related cause. A cluster of cases should mandate a full-scale investigation, which may include culturing of in-use products and informing the local, state, and federal public health authorities. Such actions averted a second na-

TABLE 36-2. Microbial pathogens associated with infusion-related septicemia

| Source of septicemia | Major pathogens |
| --- | --- |
| Conventional infusion therapy<br>    Cannula | Coagulase-negative *Staphylococcus* (>50%)<br>*Staphylococcus aureus*<br>Enterococcus<br>*Klebsiella-Enterobacter*<br>*Serratia marcescens*<br>*Candida* species<br>*Pseudomonas aeruginosa*<br>*Pseudomonas cepacia*<br>*Corynebacterium* species (diphtheroids), JK-1 |
| Contaminated infusate | Tribe Klebsielleae (90%)<br>    *Klebsiella*<br>    Enterobacter*<br>    *Serratia*<br>*P. cepacia**<br>*Citrobacter freundii*<br>*Flavobacterium* |
| Hyperalimentation, Hickman-Broviac catheters<br>(most, catheter-related) | Coagulase-negative *Staphylococcus* (>50%)<br>*Candida* species, *Torulopsis glabrata*<br>*S. aureus*<br>*Klebsiella-Enterobacter*<br>Enterococcus |
| Contaminated blood products (contaminated infusate) | Pseudomonads other than *P. aeruginosa* (>50%)*<br>*S. marcescens*<br>*Achromobacter*<br>*Salmonella choleraesuis*<br>*Citrobacter*<br>*Flavobacterium* |
| Arterial pressure monitoring | *P. cepacia**<br>*Serratia*<br>*P. acidovorans*<br>*P. aeruginosa*<br>*Enterobacter*<br>*Flavobacterium*<br>*Candida* (very rare) |
| Regional intraarterial cancer chemotherapy (cather-related) | *S. aureus* |

*Septicemia caused by *E. cloacae, E. agglomerans,* or *P. cepacia,* in particular, should prompt investigations for contaminated infusate.
Source: Adapted from Maki, D. G. In Phillips, I., Meers, P. D., and D'Arcy, P. F. (Eds.), *Microbiological Hazards of Infusion Therapy.* Lancaster, England: MTP Press, 1976.

tionwide U.S. epidemic in 1973, when, prompted by five unexplained bacteremias in three hospitals, intrinsic contamination of one company's products was identified and a recall put into effect so rapidly that the outbreak was limited to the five initially recognized cases [8]. It must be emphasized that for surveillance of bacteremias to be maximally effective, all blood isolates must always be speciated completely [12]. Failure to do so during the 1970–71 nationwide epidemic resulted in major hospitals experiencing large numbers of cases that were recognized as infusion-related only in retrospect [20].

### Blood Cultures

When line sepsis is suspected, three blood cultures should be drawn, ideally from separate venipuncture sites. If antibiotics are being administered, blood cultures obtained immediately before a dose is due to be administered, when the blood antibiotic level is lowest, may produce a higher yield. Use of resin-containing media to adsorb and remove antibiotic present in the blood specimen may also increase the yield.

Deep *Candida* sepsis—systemic candidiasis—in contradistinction to bacterial septicemia, is frequently associated with negative blood cultures. Recovery of *Candida* may be considerably enhanced if blood culture bottles are transiently vented. Biphasic media (the Castaneda system), which incorporates both a liquid and a solid phase in the same tube, incubated aerobically at 30°C (86°F) considerably enhances the yield of *Candida* and other fungi from blood cultures.

The value of arterial or central venous blood cultures in the diagnosis of *Candida* sepsis and the pathophysiologic interpretation of positive specimens collected from catheters cannot be resolved until comparative studies are done with freshly inserted catheters or with in-use catheters that are carefully studied both histologically and microbiologically on removal.

It is common practice in many intensive care units to draw many of the routine blood cultures through central venous or arterial catheters, or in neonates, through umbilical catheters. Routine blood cultures obtained through central venous or arterial catheters in adults show reasonably good concordance with cultures drawn by conventional venipuncture, but rates of false-positive (contaminated) cultures are slightly higher with catheter-drawn specimens. In contrast, nearly half of all blood cultures drawn through umbilical catheters in neonates are contaminated, although cultures obtained immediately after insertion may have low rates of false positivity.

Quantitative blood cultures (using pour plates) drawn aseptically through hyperalimentation catheters provide an excellent method for diagnosis of catheter-related infection. Positive pour-plate blood cultures correlate well with positive semiquantitative cultures of catheter segments. Whereas this technique provides a possible method for earlier identification of infected catheters without having to remove the catheter first, it may misidentify infection due to contaminated infusate. Thus infusate should be cultured every time catheter-drawn blood cultures are performed.

The practice of drawing blood cultures through indwelling vascular catheters probably ought not be encouraged because of the risk of introducing contamination into the infusion with added manipulations. If, however, to preserve dwindling superficial veins it is considered necessary to use a vascular catheter to obtain blood cultures, an attempt should be made to use recently inserted catheters and to draw every other specimen by conventional percutaneous venipuncture. The use of the quantitative pour-plate techniques for processing catheter-drawn blood cultures deserves additional study.

### A Semiquantitative Technique for Culturing Cannulas

Many laboratories culture vascular catheters qualitatively, amputating the tip aseptically and immersing it in liquid medium. Unfortunately, a positive culture by this technique is diagnostically nonspecific, since a single organism acquired from the skin as the catheter is removed can yield a positive culture.

Most cannula-related septicemias derive from local infection of the transcutaneous cannula tract. Culture of the external surface of the withdrawn cannula should reflect the microbiologic status of the wound, and quantitative culture should more accurately distinguish infection from contamination. We have developed and standardized a semiquantitative method for culturing vascular cannulas on solid media [21]. The technique is as follows:

Before removing a cannula, the skin about the insertion site is first cleansed with an alcohol-impregnated pledget, mainly to reduce contaminating skin flora and remove any residual antimicrobial ointment. After the alcohol dries, the cannula is withdrawn, taking care to avoid contact with the surrounding skin. If pus can be expressed from the cannula wound, it is always Gram-stained and cultured separately. For short catheters and steel needles, the entire length of the cannula is amputated at the former skin surface-catheter junction (Fig. 36-2), using a sterile scissors for plastic catheters and snapping steel needles off with a sterile hemostat. For longer catheters, two 2-inch segments are cultured: the tip and the intracutaneous segment. The

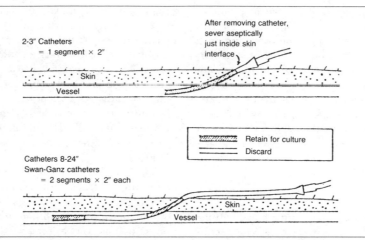

FIG. 36-2. Segments of vascular cannulas cultured semiquantitatively. (From Maki, D. G., et al. *J. Surg. Res.* 22:513, 1977, with permission.)

segments are transported to the laboratory in sterile transport tubes. The segment should be cultured as soon as possible after removal, ideally within 2 hours.

In the laboratory, using a flamed forceps, the segment is transferred onto the surface of a 100-mm 5% blood agar plate and is rolled back and forth at least four times across the agar surface. Plates are incubated aerobically at 37°C (98.6°F) for at least 72 hours. We do not believe it necessary to routinely culture cannulas anaerobically.

Colony counts on semiquantitative plates are bimodally distributed (Fig. 36-3), as they are on quantitative urine cultures; this method provides excellent discrimination between infection and insignificant contamination produced by catheters. Fifteen or more colonies growing on a semiquantitative plate is regarded as a positive culture, denoting local cannula-related infection. Based on experience with nearly 2000 cannulas, positive cultures found using this technique have a 15 to 40 percent association with concomitant bacteremias. Cannulas positive on semiquantitative culture are strongly associated with local inflammation, additionally affirming the validity of considering a positive semiquantitative culture ($\geq$ 15 colonies) to represent infection.

Culturing cannulas semiquantitatively accelerates the microbiologic identification of clinically significant isolates. The technique also shows promise in facilitating the diagnosis of suppurative phlebitis, which frequently is very difficult to diagnose clinically. The semiquantitative technique has excellent sensitivity and specificity in the diagnosis of cannula-related infection with peripheral and central venous catheters as well as umbilical catheters. The technique is clearly superior to culturing cannulas in broth.

Using this culture technique, we apply the following stringent criteria for defining a nosocomial bacteremia as cannula-related: (1) isolation of the same species in significant numbers on semiquantitative culture of the cannula and from blood cultures obtained by separate venipunctures with a negative culture of infusate, (2) clinical (or autopsy) and microbiologic data disclosing no other apparent source of septicemia, and (3) clinical features consistent with bloodstream infection.

The catheter segment can also be cultured by immersing and irrigating the catheter segment in broth and quantifying the number of eluted organisms by plating serial dilutions of the broth on surface plates [9]. Results are very similar to those obtained with the semiquantitative technique. This method produces excellent sensitivity in the diagnosis of device-related infection, excellent correlation between high counts ($> 10^3$ cfu) and device-related bacteremia, and a strong association between positive cannula cultures and local inflammation. This technique must be supplemented with cultures of infusate to differentiate between cannula-caused infection and a positive culture due to contaminated infusate.

## Method for Culturing Infusion Fluid

A variety of techniques are available for culturing parenteral admixtures and fluid medications. A relatively simple method, easily adaptable for use in the hospital when in-use fluids or parenteral medications are suspected of harboring contaminants, has been described previously [16]. Since there is no evidence that anaerobic bacteria can grow in parenteral admixtures or produce related septicemia, anaerobic culture techniques are not necessary unless blood or another biologic product is involved.

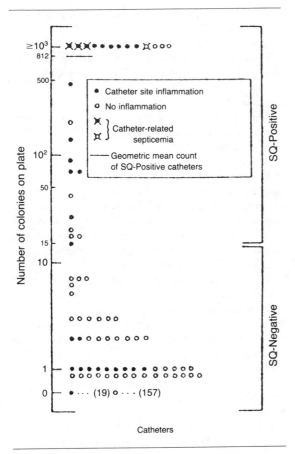

FIG. 36-3. Distribution of colony counts of 250 intravenous plastic catheters cultured by a semiquantitative technique. Note bimodal character of distribution. Presence of 15 or more colonies is regarded as a positive culture, denoting local infection of the catheter wound. (From Maki, D. G., et al. *N. Engl. J. Med.* 296:1305, 1977, with permission.)

## CANNULA-ASSOCIATED INFECTION

*Concepts of Pathogenesis and
Their Application to Prevention*

When a plastic catheter is inserted in a vessel, a loosely formed fibrin sheath forms around the intravascular portion of the device within 24 to 48 hours (Fig. 36-4), forming a nidus within which microorganisms can multiply and that shields them to an extent from host defenses and antibiotics. Thrombogenesis of cannula materials may play an important role in vulnerability to cannula-related infections. Continuous administration of low-dose heparin (1 unit per milliliter of hyperalimentation fluid) may reduce the rate of positive hyperalimentation catheter cultures and catheter-associated bacteremia.

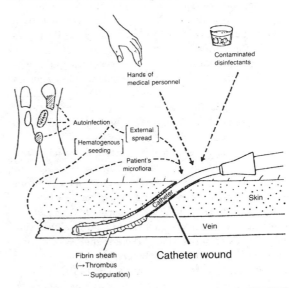

FIG. 36-4. Sources of vascular cannula-related infection. (Modified from Maki, D. G., In Phillips, I., Meers, P. D., and D'Arcy, P. F. [Eds.], *Microbiological Hazards of Infusion Therapy.* Lancaster, England: MTP Press, 1976, p. 106, with permission.)

A number of clinical observations and use of a semiquantitative technique for culturing cannulas indicate that most cannula-related septicemias begin as a local infection of the intradermal cannula wound. Aerobic bacteria, including *S. aureus, Staphylococcus epidermidis,* various gram-negative bacilli, diphtheroids, and enterococci, as well as *Candida* gain access to the cannula wound (and ultimately, the fibrin sheath) from external sources or colonize the cannula hematogenously. Anaerobic bacteria are very rare causes of device-related sepsis.

Most device-related septicemias are caused by the patient's own skin flora or by microorganisms transmitted from the hands of the person inserting the device. Presence of a preexistent infection, such as an infected surgical wound or a tracheostomy, contiguous to a subclavian or internal-jugular catheter conveys a greatly increased risk of infection of the cannula insertion site by the same species. Effective disinfection of the insertion site and meticulous attention to aseptic technique during the insertion, especially in heavily colonized or already infected patients, are clearly fundamental to prevention of device-related infection. Tincture of iodine (1% to 2% iodine in 70% alcohol) is inexpensive and well tolerated, and is probably the most effective disinfectant. Acceptable alternatives include an iodophor, tincture (not an aqueous solution) of 0.5% chlorhexidine, or 70% alcohol. Whatever disinfectant is used should be scrubbed on and left for at least 30 seconds before inserting the cannula.

Agents with unreliable activity against gram-negative bacilli, such as aqueous benzalkonium or aqueous chlorhexidine, should never be used. Many epidemics of intravascular-line sepsis have been traced to use of these agents, which had become heavily contaminated by *Pseudomonas* or *Enterobacter* species.

"Defatting" the skin with acetone is widely practiced as an adjunctive measure in the regimen for disinfecting catheter insertion sites, especially in intravenous hyperalimentation. However, our studies indicate that acetone defatting of catheter insertion sites has no effect on quantitative skin colonization contiguous to subclavian catheters, incidence of positive cultures of such catheters, or catheter-related septicemia (4 percent in both groups) [18].

Transient carriage of gram-negative pathogens on the hands of medical personnel assists in the spread of most types of bacterial infection; medical personnel commonly carry gram-negative bacilli on their hands, predominantly *Klebsiella* and *Enterobacter*. Carriage of gram-negative bacilli and *S. aureus* is usually transient, most often reflecting the presence of patients infected by the same species on a particular unit. Thus vigorous hand-washing must always precede insertion of a vascular cannula. With a high-risk cannula such as a hyperalimentation catheter or an arterial catheter or with a highly susceptible patient such as one with leukemia sterile gloves should be used.

Once inserted, the cannula should be firmly anchored and dressed with a sterile dressing. The relative merits and safety of conventional gauze and tape versus the transparent, occlusive, semipermeable adhesive plastic membranes (for example, Opsite) are as yet unresolved. Most total parenteral nutrition programs call for redressing the catheter every other day, first recleansing the site with disinfectant and reapplying a topical antimicrobial ointment. The optimal frequency and best regimen—disinfectants, occlusive versus nonocclusive dressing—for follow-up care of cannula sites remain to be determined by clinical study.

Whereas most device-related infections appear to be caused by microorganisms that migrate into the cannula tract from the exterior (see Fig. 36-4), increasing the distance between the skin surface and the vein by creating a subcutaneous tunnel has not been shown to reduce the incidence of catheter-related sepsis in hyperalimentation. However, incorporating a Dacron cuff on the subcutaneus portion of a Silastic catheter, seems to provide an element of protection against extrinsic infection of the tunnel and bloodstream. When implanted surgically, the cuff is rapidly ingrown by fibrous tissue that forms a potential biologic barrier against microbial invasion of the tract (the Hickman and Broviac catheters, described in subsequent sections).

Available data suggest that a topical antimicrobial agent applied to the catheter insertion site, especially a polyantibiotic ointment, confers some protection against device-related infection, but only marginally. If an ointment is to be used, a topical polyantibiotic preparation seems preferable for peripheral venous catheters, in which staphylococci are the predominant pathogens, and povidone-iodine ointment is best for central catheters used for hyperalimentation and for arterial catheters, in which *Candida* and resistant gram-negative bacilli are more frequent pathogens.

The cannula tip and its surrounding fibrin sheath can also, theoretically, become colonized hematogenously, but the true frequency with which this phenomenon occurs is unknown. Central venous and arterial catheters may be vulnerable. About 10 percent of arterial catheters exposed to bacteremias from distant unrelated sites of infection appear to have become colonized hematogenously and later gave rise to catheter-related septicemia caused by the same species. Such "rebound septicemias" are of special concern in vascular catheters used in burn patients. If a vascular catheter—especially a central venous or arterial catheter, or any vascular cannula in a burn patient—is exposed to high-grade bacteremia, it may be most prudent to replace it. Contaminants in the infusate administered through a device rarely colonize the cannula and its fibrin sheath.

### Incidence of Cannula-Related Infection

Every type of vascular cannula carries some risk of causing bacteremic infection, but the magnitude of risk *per cannula* varies greatly, depending on its type and the institution. In general, hazards appear greater with plastic catheters than small steel needles, long catheters than short catheters, and catheters inserted into the central circulation than peripheral venous catheters. Furthermore, catheters emplaced by surgical cutdown are considerably more hazardous than catheters inserted by percutaneous puncture. With virtually every type of cannula inserted in a peripheral vessel, the longer the device is left in place, the higher is the risk of related bacteremia. With reasonable care, few cannulas of any type produce septicemia until they have been in place for at least 48 hours. In most centers, plastic catheters left in for over 48 to 72 hours have been associated with rates of septicemia ranging between 2 and 5 percent. Unless there are extenuating circumstances, *peripheral* venous cannulas—irrespective of the type (short plastic catheters, long catheters used for hyperalimentation or pressure monitoring, or even small steel needles)—should be replaced no less frequently than every 72 hours [2]. Uniform compliance with this control measure would almost eliminate peripheral intravenous lines as a source of nosocomial bacteremia.

The lowest rates of line sepsis have been reported from institutions with established intravenous therapy teams that provide a uniform and high level of asepsis at the time of cannula insertion, maintain care thereafter, and carefully monitor all infusions at least daily, especially those used for hyperalimentation. However, the cost-effectiveness of using such teams for all infusion therapy has not been established by controlled clinical trial.

It must be pointed out that most of the published studies of device-related infection evaluated the older and larger polyethylene or polyvinylchloride catheters. The small polytef (Teflon) catheters now widely used appear to be less hazardous regarding infection, but there are no controlled comparative studies of these devices and of catheters made of other materials purported to cause less morbidity, such as Silastic.

*Infections Associated with Specific Cannulas*
STEEL NEEDLES  The lowest incidence of cannula-related infection has been reported with steel needles—especially the "scalp-vein" or "butterfly" needles used widely in pediatric patients. In studies of noncompromised patients given intravenous therapy through winged steel needles or heparin-lock needles, device-related septicemia has generally occurred in less than 0.2 percent. We found that even steel needles were associated with a significant incidence of septicemia, nearly 7 percent, in patients with hematologic malignancy, half of whom had severe granulocytopenia [1]. All septicemias occurred in granulocytopenic patients in whom needle placements exceeded 3 days ($p < 0.001$).

Plastic catheters are probably more hazardous than steel needles for routine intravenous therapy simply because they are more likely to remain in one location for prolonged periods. Tully and coworkers [31] reported the results of a large prospective study of 954 cases in which winged steel needles and small-bore plastic catheters were used in a noncompromised adult patient population. All devices were inserted and cared for by a nurse-intravenous therapy team, and most were removed within 48 hours, nearly all within 72 hours. No device-related septicemias occurred in either group, suggesting that if intravenous cannulas are inserted under conditions of scrupulous asepsis and removed without fail within 72 hours, plastic catheters probably pose no greater risk of bacteremia than steel needles.

CENTRAL CATHETERS FOR HYPERALIMENTATION
Providing nutritional support solely by the parenteral route—total parenteral nutrition or intravenous hyperalimentation—has become a widely used technique. Because the solutions used in parenteral alimentation are highly irritating to the vein, it is usually necessary to cannulate the central circulation, most often by percutaneous puncture of the subclavian or internal jugular vein. Catheters remain in the same location for prolonged periods, ranging from weeks to months, and patients requiring this form of therapy are typically debilitated and malnourished, and many already have active infections (see Chapter 37).

In the early years of this new application of infusion therapy, a number of centers experienced alarmingly high rates of complicating septicemia, reaching as high as 27 percent and averaging 7 percent. Organisms such as *S. aureus,* enterococci, and gram-negative bacilli, which commonly cause infections in conventional intravenous therapy, were often implicated, but the most common causes of septicemia were *Candida* species.

Most sepsis in hyperalimentation originates from the central catheter. There is little evidence that contaminated fluid accounts for many hyperalimentation-related infections. The basic admixture now used almost universally—crystalline amino acids in hypertonic glucose—is inhibitory to most organisms [13]. Hospitals with special hyperalimentation teams that stress stringent attention to aseptic technique during catheter insertion and in follow-up care of the catheter tend to experience rates of related sepsis of 2 percent or less. Home hyperalimentation programs that place maximal emphasis on instructing patients to take meticulous care of their own catheter and infusion consistently report rates of line sepsis of less than one case per five patient-years.

Hoshal [14] and Bottino and coworkers [4] have reported promising experiences with long *peripherally inserted* central venous silicone-elastomer catheters used for hyperalimentation. Only one case of catheter-related septicemia was identified among 116 patients treated for an average of 3 to 4 weeks; in Bottino's study, however, which was carried out in cancer patients, catheters were not removed routinely or cultured in most patients developing fever or other signs of sepsis, and the true incidence of catheter sepsis may have been considerably higher. Controlled comparative studies are needed to determine whether silicone catheters, allegedly less thrombogenic and phlebitogenic, are sufficiently safe to justify leaving them in a peripheral vein for many days longer than is considered safe with conventional intravenous catheters.

With consistent, excellent catheter care, there appears to be no need to replace subclavian or internal jugular hyperalimentation catheters routinely at prespecified intervals unless it was necessary to insert the catheter through a burn wound, in which event the catheter should be replaced every third day. The rate per day of catheter-related infection with central venous hyperalimentation catheters given optimal care is probably lower in many institutions than the rate per day with conventional infusion therapy through peripheral venous catheters because of the much greater distance between the skin surface and the bloodstream with subclavian or internal jugular catheters (measured in centimeters) compared to catheters in a peripheral vein (measured in millimeters). If a patient receiving hyperalimentation becomes septic without an obvious source or develops a persistent unexplained fever, however, the catheter should be removed and cultured. Interim nutritional support can be provided with 10% dextrose in water through a peripheral intravenous infusion.

Blackburn and coworkers [3] have developed an interesting approach to patients receiving hyperalimentation who develop unexplained fever. The central catheter is removed over a guide wire, using the Seldinger technique, and a new catheter is immediately inserted into the same tract. If the culture of the suspect catheter is positive, the new catheter (in the old, presumably infected, tract) is immediately removed. Conversely, if cultures are negative it is possible to examine objectively the suspect catheter microbiologically and exclude the device as a cause of infection without subjecting the patient to the risks of an entirely new subclavian or internal jugular catheter insertion.

It is difficult to find any rationale for the widespread practice of periodically and routinely replacing subclavian or internal jugular hyperalimentation (or other central venous) catheters by the Seldinger technique solely as a putative infection control measure. If the tract is yet uninfected, as it usually is, the extensive manipulation inherent in inserting a new catheter in the same tract may well increase the risk of infection. Conversely, if the tract is already infected at the time a new catheter is inserted, it remains infected, and there is no reason to believe the new catheter will reduce the risk of eventual systemic sepsis.

SPECIAL SURGICALLY IMPLANTED CENTRAL VENOUS CATHETERS Surgically implanted central venous catheters that incorporate a subcutaneous Dacron cuff, such as the Hickman or Broviac catheters, have gained widespread and enthusiastic use as all-purpose intravascular lifelines for patients who have undergone bone marrow transplantation, have leukemia or disorders requiring frequent vascular access, or are undergoing home hyperalimentation programs. Used for drawing all blood specimens as well as for administration of all parenteral fluids, drugs, and blood products, these devices are a major advance in terms of patient comfort; however, they have also been associated with device-related bacteremia. Their relative safety compared with peripherally inserted intravenous cannulas has not been established by comparative trials. Rates of septicemia (approximately one to two per patient-year), however, compare very favorably with historical controls from the same institutions and with sepsis rates originating from intravenous winged steel needles in leukemic patients.

ARTERIAL CATHETERS FOR HEMODYNAMIC MONITORING A form of infusion therapy with unique features that predispose to iatrogenic sepsis, especially of epidemic proportions, is the use of intraarterial infusions for hemodynamic monitoring and for obtaining arterial blood specimens (see Chapter 38). In large centers, most critically ill adults and newborns and all cardiovascular surgery patients are monitored routinely.

The incidence of endemic nosocomial bacteremia caused by intraarterial catheters is not as well established as that caused by venous catheters. Most reports of sepsis associated with arterial pressure monitoring involve epidemics related to contamination of the fluid used in these systems (discussed in a later section).

Catheters left in place for several days, especially those in place for five days or longer, and those inserted by cutdown rather than percutaneously are associated with greatly increased rates of infection. In contrast to most intravenous line sepsis, these infections are caused by enterococci, gram-negative bacilli, and *Candida,* very likely because most patients receiving such monitoring are likely to be receiving systematic antibiotics at the time.

Overall, about 10 percent of all nosocomial bacteremias occurring in high-risk patients subjected to prolonged monitoring originate from an arterial catheter. The percutaneous mode of placement is preferred. When prolonged arterial cannulation is required, the site should be rotated every four days.

Local pain or inflammation or clinical signs of sepsis without an obvious source should prompt removal and culture of the catheter.

PULMONARY ARTERY CATHETERS Flow-directed balloon-tipped Swan-Ganz catheters have been widely used to guide fluid therapy and monitor cardiac hemodynamics in postsurgical patients and patients with shock or cardiorespiratory failure.

Bacteremias occurring during subclavian Swan-Ganz catheter monitoring of a general intensive care unit population are infrequently (<2 percent) ascribed to the catheter.

Catheters inserted precutaneously by the Seldinger technique directly in the subclavian or internal jugular vein are probably less likely to cause device-related sepsis than catheters inserted in a peripheral vein and guided centrally, and they are more stable regarding position in the pulmonary circulation. Swan-Ganz catheters inserted in a peripheral vein should be considered peripheral venous catheters and ideally should be replaced every third day in patients requiring prolonged monitoring. It is less clear how frequently to replace catheters inserted directly into the central circulation by subclavian or internal jugular vein puncture using the Seldinger technique; such catheters should probably also be replaced every third day.

SUBCLAVIAN CATHETERS FOR HEMODIALYSIS Modified large-bore subclavian catheters designed to permit adequate access for emergency hemodialysis are associated with rates of catheter-related sepsis of approximately 3 percent per week; with an average 1- to 3-week course of dialysis through the device, approximately two septicemias occur per patient-year. This incidence is 6- to 15-fold higher than rates of bacteremia associated with surgically created subcutaneous fistulas (approximately 0.15 per patient-year) and external arteriovenous shunts (approximately 0.30 per patient-year).

Although some have advocated replacing the catheter routinely every week with a guide wire as an infection control measure, we eschew this practice. It seem preferable to promote hyperalimentation-quality aseptic catheter care while striving to obtain a safer and more permanent route for vascular access as quickly as possible, ideally within one to two weeks.

ARTERIAL CATHETERS FOR CANCER CHEMOTHERAPY Direct perfusion of tumor by selective intraarterial infusion of antineoplastic drugs is an established technique for the treatment of hepatic metastases and other nonresectable malignant tumor masses. We have examined the risks of infection associated with percutaneously inserted brachial artery catheters used for regional chemotherapy. About 1.5 percent of such catheters produce septicemia, nearly all caused by *S. aureus*. Difficult cannulations of the brachial artery and the need to reposition the catheter greatly increase the risk of infection. These infections produce a distinctive clinical syndrome, which facilitates identifying early catheter-related infection in a patient receiving intraarterial chemotherapy before bacteremia occurs. Typically, there are early localized pain, hemorrhage, and Osler's nodes distally, followed several days later by local inflammation, purulence, and signs of systemic sepsis.

UMBILICAL CATHETERS Umbilical catheters are used almost universally for vascular access in neonates. Prospective studies in some centers have documented a high incidence of positive catheter cultures and concomitant bacteremia (blood cultures obtained through separate venipunctures), ranging from 8 to 16 percent. High rates have been ascribed to the difficulty of maintaining asepsis in the luxuriant flora of the umbilical stump, which develops within 24 to 48 hours of birth. However, others have observed much lower rates of positive catheter cultures and essentially no related bacteremias. Reasons for such disparate observations are unclear. Prophylactic use of systemic antibiotics has not consistently reduced the incidence of umbilical catheter-related bacteremia. Catheterization of the umbilical artery rather than vein may be associated with fewer complications. Studies have not delineated a maximal upper limit of time for umbilical catheterization.

Umbilical catheters are sometimes identified as portals of bacteremia in nursery outbreaks. It is important to exclude infusion-related sepsis, unrecognized as such.

## SEPSIS FROM CONTAMINATED INFUSATE

It was many years after the introduction of intravascular catheters that they were ultimately recognized as an important source of serious iatrogenic infection. It required 35 years and the occurrence of epidemic bacteremias in hospitals across the United States in 1970 to 1971 [20] to bring about awareness that the fluid given in infusion (infusate) also was vulnerable to contamination. Epidemics of infusion-related bacteremia due to contaminated infusate are far more likely to be caused by organisms introduced during its preparation and administration in the hospital (extrinsic contamination) than by organisms introduced during its manufacture (intrinsic contamination).

We use the following criteria for defining a nosocomial bacteremia as caused by contaminated infusate: (1) recovery of the same species from cultures of infusate and from blood cultures obtained by separate venipuncture, with a negative semiquantitative culture of the cannula; (2) lack of another identifiable source of septicemia; and (3) clinical features consistent with bloodstream infection.

### Growth Properties of Organisms in Parenteral Fluids

We have evaluated the ability of 105 clinical isolates from human nosocomial infections—representing 9 genera and 13 species—to grow at room temperature (25°C [77°F]) in 5% dextrose in water, the most frequently used commercial parenteral solution [19]. Of 51 strains of the genera *Klebsiella, Enterobacter,* and *Serratia* in the family Enterobacteriaceae, 50 attained concentrations of 100,000 or more organisms per milliliter in 24 hours, beginning with washed organisms at an initial concentration of one organism per milliliter. In contrast only 1 of 54 strains of other bacteria—including staphylococci, *Escherichia coli, Pseudomonas aeruginosa,* and *Acinetobacter*—and of *Candida* displayed any growth in 5% dextrose in water. With most organisms, even with a level of contamination exceeding $10^6$ organisms per milliliter of fluid, evidence of microbial growth is usually not visible. Molds, usually introduced into the container through microscopic cracks, are most often responsible for cloudiness or filmy precipitates. Rapid multiplication in 5% dextrose in water appears limited mainly to certain members of the family Enterobacteriaceae and *Pseudomonas cepacia;* in distilled water, to *P. aeruginosa, P. cepacia, Acinetobacter,* and *Serratia;* and in lactated Ringer's solution, to *P. aeruginosa, Enterobacter,* and *Serratia.* Normal (0.9%) sodium chloride solution supports growth of most bacteria while supporting the growth of *Candida* rather poorly. *Candida* species do grow in synthetic amino acid—25% glucose solutions used in hyperalimentation—but only very slowly; most bacteria are greatly inhibited [13].

Most microorganisms, including *Candida,* are able to grow in commercial 10% lipid emulsion for infusion (Intralipid). Indeed, many of these grow almost as rapidly as in bacteriologic media. Accordingly, fat emulsions seem to possess considerable potential for producing epidemic nosocomial disease. However, sporadic septicemia clearly linked to in-use contamination of the product has been exceedingly rare. It is possible that the true frequency of septicemia caused by contaminated lipid emulsion is indeed very low because most users consistently re-

frigerate the product until use and administer it within four hours, as recommended by the manufacturer. Alternatively, the few reported cases of septicemia may also reflect lack of recognition.

The pathogens implicated in nearly 95 percent of all reported septicemias linked to contaminated fluid have been aerobic gram-negative bacilli able to proliferate rapidly at room temperature in the solution involved. It must be emphasized that microbial growth in most parenteral solutions—with the exception of fat emulsion—is rather limited. Thus the identity of an organism causing nosocomial septicemia can point toward contaminated fluid as a plausible source: *Enterobacter* species (particularly *Enterobacter agglomerans* or *E. cloacae*), *Flavobacterium* species, *P. cepacia,* or *Citrobacter* cultured from the blood of a patient receiving infusion therapy should prompt suspicion of contaminated infusate. Conversely, recovery of organisms such as *E. coli, P. aeruginosa, Acinetobacter, Proteus,* and staphylococci, all of which grow poorly if at all in parenteral admixtures, suggests that the septicemia is not due to contaminated infusate.

### Mechanisms of fluid contamination

Parenteral fluid can readily become contaminated during its administration in the hospital (Fig. 36-5). Culture surveys of intravenous fluids given in hospitals have revealed contamination rates that average about 5 percent. However, most organisms recovered from positive in-use cultures are common skin commensals that are generally considered of low virulence and grow poorly if at all in the fluid. The level of contamination is usually far too low (< one organism per milliliter) to produce clinical illness. When contamination occurs with gram-negative bacilli that are able to multiply in the product, however, the risk of sepsis increases greatly.

The risk of fluid becoming contaminated during use is closely related to the duration of uninterrupted infusion through the same administration set. Microorganisms capable of growth in the fluid, once introduced into a running infusion, can often persist in the administration set for many days despite multiple replacements of the bottle or bag and high rates of flow.

INTRAVENOUS FLUID    The incidence of nosocomial bacteremia caused by extrinsically contaminated intravenous fluid is not known but appears to be quite low, at least tenfold lower than the incidence of endemic cannula-related septicemia. Overall, it seems improbable that there is more than one case of septicemia from contaminated fluid for every 1000 infusions. However, infusate can be identified as a source

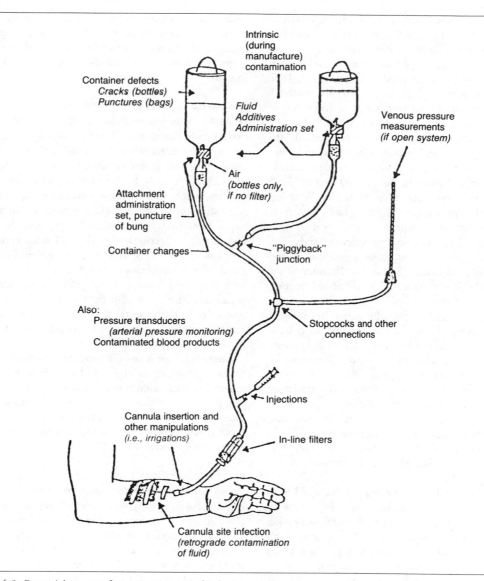

FIG. 36-5. Potential sources for contamination of infusion fluid. (Adapted from Maki, D. G. In Phillips, I., Meers, P. D., D'Arcy, P. F. [Eds.], *Microbiological Hazards of Infusion Therapy*. Lancaster, England: MTP Press, 1976, p. 120, with permission.)

of septicemia only if it is cultured. Because this rarely occurs in most hospitals, it is likely that the majority of sporadic (endemic) septicemias caused by contaminated fluid are unrecognized or attributed to the intravascular cannula.

During the 1971 nationwide epidemic due to the contaminated fluid of one manufacturer, we recommended, as an infection control measure, that the entire delivery system be routinely changed every 24

hours and that at every change of the cannula all equipment be totally replaced [12]. Several hospitals using the involved company's intrinsically contaminated products that instituted this control measure in early 1971 experienced a reduction in epidemic septicemias [20]. Since then, routinely replacing the delivery system every 24 hours has been practiced in most North American hospitals as the primary means of reducing the hazard of contaminated infusate.

Two independent studies have examined the safety and cost-effectiveness of using 48 hours as an interval for set change. Buxton and coworkers [6] randomized 600 intravenous infusions in a large municipal hospital to have the administration set changed at 24-

or 48-hour intervals. Sampling fluid from each infusion daily, they found 2.0 percent of systems that were changed every 24 hours and 2.3 percent changed every 48 hours became contaminated. None of their 13 contaminated systems produced septicemia. In a study of 790 in-use infusions, we also encountered no septicemias and found no significant difference in contamination rates of fluid in delivery systems changed at 24- or 48-hour intervals [2]. These studies indicate that changing delivery systems every 48 hours is justified in terms of safety and should result in considerable savings to hospitals. In our 500-bed hospital in 1977, the policy probably saved $160,000. Whether 72 hours, or even longer, might be an even more optimal interval for set replacement in terms of cost and safety requires additional prospective study.

We regard the following three situations as the only exceptions to using 48 hours as the interval for set change: (1) blood products are administered through the set, (2) intravenous lipid emulsion is administered, or (3) an epidemic of infusion-related septicemia is suspected. In these circumstances, we believe delivery systems should be changed routinely every 24 hours. Minute amounts of blood buffer acidic solutions, and blood and lipid emulsion also provide organic nutrients that greatly enhance the ability of many microorganisms to grow rapidly. If infusion-associated septicemias occur in epidemic numbers, especially those caused by gram-negative bacilli of such genera as *Enterobacter* or *Pseudomonas,* contaminated infusate of either extrinsic or intrinsic origin may be responsible.

The risks of sepsis due to contaminated fluid with routine set change every 48 hours are very low with all types of infusions, including hyperalimentation systems (which, as discussed, seem less prone than conventional intravenous infusions to produce sepsis from contaminated infusate), hemodynamic monitoring systems (we have found 48 hours to be a safe and cost-effective interval for replacement of the chamber dome and monitoring circuit), and infusions entered more than an arbitrary number of times per day.

Terminal, in-line, 0.22- or 0.44-$\mu$ membrane filters also hold promise as a means of reducing the hazard of contaminated infusate. However, filters do not consistently prevent passage of endotoxin, must be changed at frequent intervals, and periodically become blocked (often leading to added manipulations of the system, and paradoxically, greater potential for contamination). Furthermore, filters are expensive and have not consistently shown significant benefit in reduction of morbidity associated with infusion therapy. Until studies affirming benefit are

performed, changing the delivery system every 24 to 48 hours probably provides the best protection against infection from contaminated infusate. Filters may be of greatest value for removal of microparticulates from infusate.

CONTAMINATED FLUID IN ARTERIAL PRESSURE MONITORING  Whereas endemic bacteremias caused by extrinsically contaminated intravenous fluid are rare, arterial infusion appears to be considerably more likely to become contaminated during use and cause related septicemia, possibly because the infusion consists of a stagnant column of fluid subjected to frequent manipulations. In most outbreaks caused by contaminated intraarterial infusions used for hemodynamic monitoring, infections were derived from contaminated fluid within the transducer chamber dome located at the termination of the fluid column connected to the patient's bloodstream. Gram-negative organisms gain access during therapy from external reservoirs in the hospital and can be perpetuated if reusable chamber domes or the permanent transducers are not reliably sterilized.

Intraarterial infusions for pressure monitoring cause sporadic septicemias endemically derived from extrinsic contamination of the infusate. With prolonged monitoring, transducer chamber domes and continuous-flow devices should be replaced at periodic intervals, ideally with the administration set every 48 hours (see Chapter 38).

CONTAMINATED BLOOD PRODUCTS  Between less than 1 and 6 percent of blood units have been found to contain bacteria [15], yet endemic septicemias derived from transfusion of contaminated blood products have been rare, presumably because most blood products are routinely refrigerated, because contamination is low level, and because of universal awareness that blood products must be infused promptly after removal from refrigeration. Sepsis traced to contaminated whole blood has usually been associated with severe shock and high mortality because of the massive numbers of psychrophilic (cold-growing) organisms, such as *Serratia, Pseudomonas* other than *P. aeruginosa,* and other uncommon nonfermentative gram-negative bacilli, in the contaminated blood unit. In such circumstances, bacteria may be visible on a direct Gram-stained smear of the product.

Outbreaks of pyrogenic reactions and an epidemic of *Pseudomonas* species septicemia [30] have been traced to intrinsically contaminated normal serum albumin, and small epidemics of *E. cloacae* [15] and *Salmonella choleraesuis* [26] septicemia have been traced to organisms derived from contaminated platelet concentrates (which are maintained at 25°C [77°F] to enhance viability. Blood products should be infused promptly after they are removed from refrigeration. On completion of the transfusion, the entire delivery system should be replaced. If sepsis is suspected as being related to a contaminated blood product, the entire infusion should be removed. Aliquots of the remaining product should be cultured aerobically and anaerobically on solid medium, at both 35°C to 37°C (95°F to 99°F) and 16°C to 20°C (61°F to 68°F).

### Epidemic Infusion-Related Septicemia

Whereas approximately 8 percent of endemic nosocomial bacteremias in American hospitals are considered infusion-related, about one-third of all epidemics of hospital-acquired bacteremia derive from infusion therapy in some form (see Fig. 36-1).

EXTRINSIC CONTAMINATION  Even when commercially manufactured products are sterile on arrival in the hospital, circumstances of hospital use can compromise that initial sterility (see Figs. 36-4 and 36-5). Most sporadic infections related to infusion therapy, whether due to the cannula or contaminated infusate, are of extrinsic origin. Similarly, most reported epidemics have originated from exposure of multiple patients' infusions to a common source of contamination in the hospital.

Outbreaks of infusion-related bacteremia may be caused by unreliable chemical disinfectants such as aqueous benzalkonium in the United States and aqueous chlorhexidine in the United Kingdom used for cutaneous disinfection or, in recent years, for decontaminating transducer components used in hemodynamic monitoring (see Chapter 14).

Consecutive use of the same product also may result in outbreaks. In 1970 Sack [28] reported five cases of gram-negative septic shock in patients who had consecutively received an intraoperative infusion from a single bottle of succinylcholine in 5% dextrose in water. *Klebsiella pneumoniae* and *E. cloacae* were subsequently cultured from the fluid. Although the mechanism of contamination was not found in these cases, another case of *Klebsiella-Enterobacter* septicemia in the same hospital was attributed to a cracked bottle containing contaminated fluid. Entry of organisms through a minute crack was also postulated by Robertson [27] to be the cause of two cases of visible contamination of in-use fluid in one hospital in 1970; one case involved *Trichoderma* species and the other, *Penicillium*. One patient developed transient fungemia. A defect in a glass bottle, usually a crack, underlies fluid contamination with a fungus ball." Sepsis is uncommon following infusion of such fluid, but

fluid containers, bottles, or bags should always be examined before use and discarded if defects, cloudiness, or precipitates are present. Bottles lacking a vacuum should be discarded.

Multiply entered vials or containers used to compound intravenous medications or flush arterial monitoring systems are prone to contamination and may result in infusion-related septicemia, most commonly with gram-negative bacilli that thrive in aqueous solutions, such as *Flavobacterium*, *P. cepacia*, and *Serratia marcescens*.

Investigations in a number of outbreaks have documented contamination of in-use infusate or infection of cannula sites, most likely deriving from extrinsic contamination. The hospital reservoir of the epidemic pathogens, and often even the mode of transmission, have frequently eluded detection. Manipulations of the delivery system, especially the administration set, may have provided a means for access of microorganisms to the hands of medical attendants in some of these.

Compounding of admixtures is another important means by which contamination can be introduced. The greatest concern about this mode of contamination, especially if it occurs in a central pharmacy, is that a large number of patients may be exposed. Moreover, the delay between compounding and use provides opportunity for proliferation of introduced organisms. During a four-month period in 1975, 22 patients in a large university hospital developed *Candida parapsilosis* fungemia traced to contaminated solutions used for intravenous hyperalimentation. Plouffe and coworkers [25] discovered that a vacuum system in the hospital's pharmacy used to evacuate fluid from bottles before introducing other admixture components was heavily contaminated by the epidemic *Candida* strain. Presumably, organisms refluxed into bottles during compounding of the admixtures.

In March 1976 seven children in a pediatric hospital developed *Enterobacter aerogenes* septicemia traced to contaminated 5% dextrose in 0.2% sodium chloride solution to which potassium chloride had been added in the hospital's central pharmacy. A Centers for Disease Control (CDC) team [11] found that the pharmacist was using one syringeful of concentrated potassium chloride solution to add potassium to each of eight consecutive units of fluid. After compounding, bottles were permitted to stand at room temperature for up to 48 hours before use. The necessity for stringent attention to asepsis in central admixture programs cannot be overemphasized. Fluid admixtures should be used within six hours of admixing or be immediately refrigerated. No bottle or bag should hang for more than 24 hours.

ARTERIAL PRESSURE MONITORING   While the quantitative hemodynamic data derived from invasive hemodynamic monitoring is often of considerable value for the optimal management of critically ill patients, the potential for iatrogenic infective complications is also considerable. More than a dozen epidemics of nosocomial bacteremia deriving from intraarterial infusions used for hemodynamic monitoring have been reported in the world literature. In every outbreak, bacteremias were caused by extrinsically contaminated fluid, particularly within the transducer chamber dome (see Chapter 38). Nosocomial gram-negative microorganisms may gain access during therapy from external hospital sources, such as contaminated flush solutions or ice used to chill syringes, and can be perpetuated by failure to sterilize reusable chamber domes reliably.

The availability of disposable chamber domes would seem to have resolved the problem for hospitals of inadequate resterilization of these critical components. Outbreaks continue to occur, however, because of the failure to resterilize reliably the permanent transducer head between use with different patients. Donowitz and coworkers [10] have shown in simulation studies that organisms placed on the transducer head are readily transmitted to fluid in the monitoring circuit during manipulations of the system by medical personnel whose hands become contaminated. A potential risk of contamination may also be introduced by gas sterilization of disposable chamber domes, which sometimes produces cracks in the membrane.

All permanent or reusable transducer components should be cleansed and sterilized with ethylene oxide or glutaraldehyde between use with different patients, and disposable chamber domes should not be reused. Saline infusate should be used rather than glucose-containing solutions, which support growth of microorganisms.

With the ever-increasing number of hospital patients exposed to invasive hemodynamic monitoring, the increasing number of reports of infection may well reflect not only an increase in the number of procedures performed and greater general awareness, but a true increase in the incidence of infectious complications. Except during outbreaks, particularly those caused by rare pathogens such as *Flavobacterium* or *P. cepacia*, infusions of any type are rarely considered a cause of nosocomial bacteremia in most hospitals.

INTRINSIC CONTAMINATION   Since 1970 there have been several reported epidemics of infusion-related septicemia caused by intrinsically contaminated infusate, illustrating a variety of iatrogenic hazards of infusion therapy.

The first and largest epidemic had its onset in mid-1970 [7], when one U.S. manufacturer of large-volume parenterals began to distribute bottles of fluid with a new elastomer-lined screw cap closure. By early December 1970 the first cases of infusion-related septicemia caused by biologically characteristic strains of *E. cloacae* and *E. agglomerans* (formerly designated *Erwinia*) were reported to the CDC, although retrospective review subsequently showed that many hospitals had been experiencing epidemic bacteremias for several months. Although it was established very early, virtually at the outset of the investigation, that sepsis was associated with contaminated intravenous fluids, the ultimate source of contamination—*intrinsic* contamination of the new closures—was not conclusively established until March 1971. Between July 1970 and April 1971, 25 U.S. hospitals reported to the CDC nearly 400 cases of infusion-related septicemia [20]. More than 20 microbial species, including *E. agglomerans,* were isolated from closures of previously unopened bottles. Organisms could be dislodged from the cap liner and gain access to fluid when bottles were handled under conditions duplicating normal in-hospital use. The appearance of epidemic septicemias within individual hospitals parallelled the national distribution of the company's product with the new closures, and the epidemic was only terminated by a nationwide product recall.

During a six-month period in 1970 to 1971, seven patients with lymphoproliferative malignancy hospitalized in the Clinical Center of the National Institutes of Health developed cryptogenic *S. choleraesuis* septicemia. A meticulous epidemiologic investigation by Rhame and coworkers [26] ultimately linked the infections to one blood donor whose platelets had been given to every case. The donor was subsequently shown to have an asymptomatic focus of tibial osteomyelitis and was experiencing intermittent, very low-level bacteremia.

A third epidemic caused by intrinsically contaminated intravenous products was reported by Phillips and coworkers [24]. Between April 1971 and January 1972, 40 patients in a London, England hospital developed septicemia, urinary tract infection, or respiratory infection from softened, deionized distilled water manufactured in the pharmacy and used throughout the hospital. *P. cepacia* was recovered from infected patients and the water. When used for cooling bottles of parenteral fluid and other sterilized fluids in the hospital's rapid-cooling autoclave, this water often remained on the rubber stopper beneath the foil seal and presumably entered the bottle when the closure was punctured for clinical use. Water may also have entered some of the bottles directly during the cooling cycle.

In 1972 seven patients at a Plymouth, England, hospital developed profound shock after receiving 5% dextrose in water. Five patients died. Investigations by Meers and coworkers [22] showed that the fluid within approximately one-third of 155 bottles cultured from the implicated lot contained up to $10^7$ gram-negative bacilli per milliliter. Contamination was ultimately traced to faulty maintenance of autoclaving equipment at the manufacturer's plant.

In both of the aforementioned outbreaks in England, infusion products with rubber-stopper closures were implicated, emphasizing that no specific design can be assumed automatically to be safe.

A fifth outbreak, the third in this country, occurred in 1972, when a manufacturer increased pressure in his autoclaves, a move that would be expected to increase their efficiency. The exact mechanisms of contamination are uncertain. Apparently, however, this led to an increased pressure differential between the outside and inside of fluid-filled bottles, producing greater stress on the containers and their closures and possibly drawing contaminated cooling water into the partial vacuum inside the bottles. Between February and March 1973, five patients who received 5% dextrose in lactated Ringer's solution developed sepsis [8]. *Citrobacter freundii* was recovered from the blood of three patients, *E. cloacae* from one patient, and *E. cloacae* and *E. agglomerans* from the fifth. Low-level intrinsic contamination was demonstrated by careful cultures of previously unopened fluid.

Noncellular blood products such as normal serum albumin or plasma protein fraction are now produced commercially. Contamination of one lot can result in nosocomial disease involving patients in multiple, widely scattered hospitals. In 1973 11 patients at a Maryland hospital developed *Pseudomonas* septicemia, shown by Steere and coworkers [30] to be associated with receipt of 25% normal serum albumin made by a single manufacturer. Cultures of unused units showed contamination with *P. cepacia*. Because the product cannot be autoclaved, it is heated to 60°C (140°F) for 10 hours and then filtered. Contamination was thought to have been introduced in the manufacturing plant after the heat treatment, most likely during dispensing of the product into individual vials.

Sporadic pyrogenic reactions are very common with all types of blood products. It is likely that both normal serum albumin and plasma protein fractions frequently contain minute amounts of endotoxin—usually too little to produce human illness—because of the necessity of sterilizing these solutions by filtration rather than by autoclaving. Detection of epidemic pyrogenic reactions, especially those originating from contamination of commerical products or inadequately decontaminated and reprocessed reusable cardiac or angiographic catheters, is based on awareness of the phenomenon and careful epidemiologic investigations using case-control techniques.

In 1978 16 patients in two European hospitals developed *P. cepacia* bacteremia in the early postoperative period. The infections fortunately were very mild clinically. Investigations by Siboni and associates [29] disclosed that all of the affected patients had received intravenous fentanyl intraoperatively. The product was not routinely sterilized after preparation and dispensing, but a chemical preservative was added. Two lots of the product were found to be intrinsically contaminated with *P. cepacia*.

These epidemics illustrate how subtle and insidious the factors that influence sterility can be. In many instances, there was no documented failure of the sterilization process. Instead, seemingly minor alterations in the manufacturing process resulted in contamination of individual units in the manufacturing plant after the sterilization stage.

Although intrinsic contamination fortunately is exceedingly rare, its potential for harm is great because of the large numbers of patients in multiple hospitals who may be affected. Also, direct contamination of infusate at the manufacturing level gives contaminants an opportunity to proliferate to very high concentrations.

It is very likely that intrinsic contamination is a continuous source of infusion-related sepsis but of such low magnitude that the resulting sporadic septicemias are never identified as such. Only when infusion-associated septicemias are encountered in epidemic numbers is intrinsic causation likely to be recognized and proved. A substantial increase in the incidence of cryptogenic infusion-associated septicemia should prompt immediate studies to exclude intrinsic contamination.

There are no clinical clues to differentiate reliably between intrinsic and extrinsic contamination. Bacteremia from contaminated fluid has the same manifestations and signs as catheter-induced sepsis and other nosocomial septicemias. The few clues to infusion-related bacteremia—absence of an obvious source of infection, its common occurrence in patients without a predilection to systemic infection, and the dramatic clinical response to discontinuation of the infusion—do not differentiate between intrinsic and extrinsic sources of infection. The distinction must be made epidemiologically and microbiologically.

## MANAGEMENT AND PREVENTION OF INFUSION-RELATED INFECTIONS

### Management of Line Sepsis

Except for surgically implanted catheters, removing the entire infusion—the cannula as well as the entire delivery apparatus—is the single most important immediate therapeutic maneuver in the management of infusion-related septicemia. Failure to remove an infusion in its entirety may result in refractory chronic bacteremia, with a high risk of metastatic seeding and endocarditis. Both the cannula and a specimen of infusate should be cultured. The type and lot numbers of suspected products should be recorded, and all remaining samples should be retained for possible future investigation in the event that intrinsic contamination is suspected. Any data suggesting intrinsic contamination of a commercial product, especially if it may have produced human illness or simply has the potential to do so, should be immediately reported to local, state, and federal public health authorities.

The cannulation site should always be carefully examined for purulence. Milking the cannulated vein outward, toward the puncture wound, is a simple but helpful bedside maneuver. Extrusion of pus, which should be immediately Gram-stained and cultured, strongly suggests venous suppuration and should usually prompt surgical exploration of the vein, especially if the patient has unexplained fever or signs of sepsis. If milking the vein externally yields negative results but the patient has evidence of severe sepsis without an obvious source, an attempt may be made to aspirate the vein segment proximal to the cannular insertion site. If this maneuver also produces no purulent material, blind exploratory venotomy may be advisable. If sheets of polymorphonuclear leukocytes and microorganisms are seen microscopically in expressible pus or an aspirate or on exploration, the entire involved vein segment and its affected tributaries should be excised en bloc.

Suppuration (septic thrombosis) of a great central vein (the venae cavae or subclavian or iliofemoral veins) deriving from centrally placed catheters presents a far more difficult management problem. Angiographic studies showing the presence of great vein thrombosis in a patient with high-grade refractory septicemia strongly suggest this entity. We have found that heavier growth on semiquantitative culture of the tip of central catheters than of the proximal in-

tracutaneous segment, when associated with concomitant high-grade bacteremia persisting after removal of the catheter, is also very suggestive. If the patient is not gravely ill, septic thrombosis of the great central veins should be managed by adopting the therapeutic approach used in endocarditis, including high-dose, intravenous bactericidal antibiotics for four to six weeks, and possibly also including systemic anticoagulation. Surgical intervention is reserved for recurrent septic pulmonary emboli or refractory sepsis occurring despite optimal medical therapy. The affected iliofemoral or distal subclavian veins or inferior vena cava can be ligated, if necessary, and the clot removed surgically without resorting to cardiopulmonary bypass. When the proximal subclavian vein, the superior vena cava, or the proximal inferior vena cava are involved, therapy usually must be restricted to high-dose antibiotic therapy and anticoagulants alone. Surgical debridement of the infected clot might be considered as a last resort in an individual case.

A substantial number of device-related bacteremias with implanted Broviac or Hickman catheters can be successfully eradicated medically, without resorting to removal of the "lifeline" implanted catheters. These cases should also probably be treated as endovascular infections, with administration of high-dose bactericidal antibiotics, usually parenterally, for at least four weeks. The catheter should be removed if the bloodstream cannot be sterilized, the patient remains clinically septic after three to five days of intensive antimicrobial therapy, the tunnel is grossly infected at the outset, or septic pulmonary emboli occur.

Infusion-related sepsis often resolves itself without antimicrobial therapy following removal of an offending device and infusion. However, systemic antimicrobial therapy should be administered to patients who are clinically septic, patients whose wounds show expressible purulence, patients with suppurative phlebitis (even in the absence of documented bacteremia), and all patients with positive blood cultures—even with bacteremia that clears spontaneously on removal of the infusion. Drug selection may be guided by the results of previous blood cultures of Gram-stained smears of purulence. If these are unavailable, however, an initial microbial regimen effective against microorganisms known to be commonly associated with both catheter- and infusate-related infection is indicated. A combination of a penicillinase-resistant semisynthetic penicillin (e.g., methicillin, oxacillin, or nafcillin)—in penicillin-allergic patients, a cephalosporin, clindamycin, or vancomycin—and an aminoglycoside, such as tobramycin (or gentamicin or amikacin) will prove effective against most infusion-related bacterial pathogens. A seven- to ten-day course of systemic antimicrobial therapy is usually sufficient.

In general, empirical antifungal therapy in the initial regimen is rarely necessary or recommended. Objective evidence of systemic infection; positive blood cultures; presence of *Candida* or *Torulopsis* in pleural, ascitic, joint, or cerebrospinal fluid; histopathologic confirmation; ophthalmoscopic signs of retinitis; repeated recovery of yeasts from multiple anatomic sites; or possibly, positive serologic tests are usually recommended before initiating therapy with amphotericin B, 5-fluorocytosine, or miconazole.

Most device-related fungemias resolve spontaneously and rapidly after removal of the catheter, but there is a risk of metastatic infection becoming manifest at a later time without treatment, especially endophthalmitis or endocarditis. It may be most prudent to give a brief course of low-dose amphotericin B (approximately 200 to 300 mg total) even to patients with transient line-related fungemia, especially if the patient is immunosuppressed.

It is imperative to follow closely all patients who develop infusion-related bacteremia or fungemia, even if there has been a rapid and clear-cut favorable response to initial therapy. Latent focuses of deep infection such as endocarditis or endophthalmitis can become established even by transient bloodstream invasion, especially those with *S. aureus,* enterococcus, or *Candida. S. aureus* bacteremia deriving from a vascular cannula clearly can produce endocarditis. Similarly, there is a risk of *Candida* endophthalmitis and endocarditis not manifesting clinically until one or more months after a seemingly "self-limiting" cannula-related fungemia. In a prospective study, Montgomerie and Edwards [23] found that 5 of 23 patients receiving intravenous hyperalimentation developed *Candida* retinitis, which was usually silent; only 3 patients had positive blood cultures.

*Prevention of Line Sepsis*
All infusion systems, whether for simple intravenous therapy or for hemodynamic monitoring, must be recognized as potential portals for the entry of infection. Vigorous hand-washing before inserting a cannula, using sterile gloves for high-risk cannulas and in high-risk patients (e.g., those with leukemia), thoroughly disinfecting the site with a reliable germicide (e.g., tincture of iodine), and paying meticulous attention to aseptic technique throughout the insertion constitute the first line of defense against cannula-related infection. Thereafter, daily surveillance of all intravascular lines and limiting the duration of placement for hemodynamic monitoring to four days can greatly reduce the risk of cannula-related infection. Maximal care when compounding parenteral admixtures and handling infusions, and routinely replacing the entire delivery system at least every 48 hours are pivotal measures for reducing the risk of contaminated infusate. All apparatus used in association with an intravascular infusion, such as pressure transducer components, must be reliably sterile.

Additional research is needed to determine the value of in-line microbial filters, the relative risks of various intravascular devices and different catheter materials (such as Silastic), the relative safety of surgically implanted central venous catheters compared with peripheral intravenous cannulas in high-risk patients, the most effective regimen for cutaneous antisepsis, the optimal frequency for follow-up care of the infusion site in hyperalimentation, the cost-effectiveness of intravenous therapy teams to care for all infusions, and the best ways to educate physicians regarding the microbiologic hazards of infusion therapy and the need for stringent adherence to aseptic technique.

## REFERENCES

1. Band, J. D., Alvarado, C. J., and Maki, D. G. A semiquantitative culture technique for identifying infection due to steel needles used for intravenous therapy. *Am. J. Clin. Pathol.* 72:980, 1979.
2. Band, J. D., and Maki, D. G. Safety of changing delivery systems at longer than 24-hour intervals. *Ann. Intern. Med.* 91:173, 1979.
3. Blackburn, G. H., Bothe, A., and Lahey, M. A. Organization and administration of a nutrition support service. *Surg. Clin. North Am.* 61:709, 1981.
4. Bottino, J., McCredie, K. B., Groschel, D. H. M., and Lawson, M. Long-term intravenous therapy with peripherally inverted silicone elastomer central venous catheters in patients with malignant diseases. *Cancer* 43:1937, 1979.
5. Buckholtz, D. H., Young, V. M., Friedman, N. R., Reilly, J. A., and Mardinez, M. R. Bacterial proliferation in platelets stored at room temperature. *N. Engl. J. Med.* 285:429, 1971.
6. Buxton, A. E., Highsmith, A. K., Garner, J. S., West, M. C., Stamm, W. E., Dixon, R. E., and McGowan, J. E. Contamination of intravenous infusion fluid: Effects of changing administration sets. *Ann. Intern. Med.* 90:764, 1979.
7. Centers for Disease Control. Nosocomial bacter-

emias associated with intravenous fluid therapy—USA. *Morbid. Mortal. Weekly Rep.* 20(Suppl. 9):1971.

8. Centers for Disease Control. Septicemia associated with contaminated intravenous fluids. *Morbid. Mortal. Weekly Rep.* 22:99, 1973.

9. Cleri, D. J., Corrado, M. H., and Seligman, S. J. Quantitative culture of intravenous catheters and other intravascular inserts. *J. Infect. Dis.* 141:781, 1980.

10. Donowitz, L. G., Marsik, F. J., Hoyt, J. W., and Wenzel, R. P. *Serratia marcescens* bacteremia from contaminated pressure transducers. *J.A.M.A.* 242:1749, 1979.

11. Edwards, K. E., Allen, J. R., Miller, M. J., Yogev, R., Hoffman, P. C., Klotz, R., Marubio, S., Burkholder, E., Williams, T., and Davis, A. T. *Enterobacter aerogenes* primary bacteremia in pediatric patients. *Pediatrics* 62:304, 1978.

12. Goldmann, D. A., Maki, D. G., Rhame, F. S., Kaiser, A. B., Tenney, J. H., and Bennett, J. V. Guidelines for infection control in intravenous therapy. *Ann. Intern. Med.* 79:848, 1973.

13. Goldmann, D. A., Martin, W. T., and Worthington, J. W. Growth of bacteria and fungi in total parenteral nutrition solutions, *Am. J. Surg.* 126:314, 1973.

14. Hoshal, V. L. Total intravenous nutrition with peripherally inserted silicone elastomer central venous catheters. *Arch. Surg.* 110:644, 1975.

15. James, J. D. Bacterial contamination of preserved blood. *Vox. Sang.* 4:177, 1959.

16. Maki, D. G. Growth properties of microorganisms in infusion fluid and methods of detection. In Phillips, I., Meers, P. D., and D'Arcy, P. F. (Eds.), *Microbiological Hazards of Infusion Therapy.* Lancaster, England: MTP Press, 1976.

17. Maki, D. G., Jarrett, F., and Sarafin, H. W. A semiquantitative culture method for identification of catheter-related infection in the burn patient. *J. Surg. Res.* 22:513, 1977.

18. Maki, D. G., and MacCormick, K. N. Acetone "defatting" in cutaneous antisepsis. *Crit. Care Med.* 9:202, 1981.

19. Maki, D. G., and Martin, W. T. Nationwide epidemic of septicemia caused by contaminated infusion products. IV. Growth of microbial pathogens in fluids for intravenous infusion. *J. Infect. Dis.* 131:267, 1975.

20. Maki, D. G., Rhame, F. S., Mackel, D. C., and Bennett, J. V. Nationwide epidemic of septi-cemia caused by contaminated intravenous products. I. Epidemiologic and clinical features. *Am. J. Med.* 60:471, 1976.

21. Maki, D. G., Weise, C. E., and Sarafin, H. W. A semiquantitative culture method for identifying intravenous-catheter-related infection. *N. Engl. J. Med.* 296:1305, 1977.

22. Meers, P. D., Calder, M. W., Mazhar, M. M., and Laurie, G. M. Intravenous infusion of contaminated dextrose solution: The Davenport incident. *Lancet* 2:1189, 1973.

23. Montgomerie, J. Z., and Edwards, J. E. Association of infection due to *Candida albicans* with intravenous hyperalimentation. *J. Infect. Dis.* 137:197, 1978.

24. Phillips, I., Eykyn, S., and Laker, M. Outbreak of hospital infections caused by contaminated autoclaved fluids. *Lancet* 1:1258, 1972.

25. Plouffe, J. F., Brown, D. G., and Silva, J., Jr. Nosocomial outbreak of *Candida parapsilosis* fungemia related to intravenous infusions. *Arch. Intern. Med.* 137:1686, 1977.

26. Rhame, F. S., Root, R. K., MacLowry, J. D., Dadisman, T. A., and Bennett, J. V. *Salmonella* septicemia from platelet transfusions. *Ann. Intern. Med.* 78:633, 1973.

27. Robertson, M. H. Fungi in fluids: A hazard of intravenous therapy. *J. Med. Microbiol.* 3:99, 1970.

28. Sack, R. A. Epidemic of gram-negative organism septicemia subsequent to elective operation. *Am. J. Obstet. Gynecol.* 107:394, 1970.

29. Siboni, K., Olsen, H., Paun, E., Sogaard, P., Hjorth, A., Nielsen, K. N., Askgaard, K., Secher, B., Borghans, J., Khing-Ting, L., Joosten, H., Fredericksen, W., Jensen, K., Mortensen, N., and Sebbren, O. *Pseudomonas cepacia* in 16 nonfatal cases of postoperative bacteremia derived from intrinsic contamination of the anesthetic fentanyl: Clinical and epidemiologic observations in Denmark and Holland. *Scand. J. Infect. Dis.* 11:39, 1979.

30. Steere, A. C., Tenney, J. H., Mackel, D. C., Snyder, M. J., Polakavitz, S., Dunne, M. E., and Dixon, R. E. *Pseudomonas* species bacteremia caused by contaminated normal human serum albumin. *J. Infect. Dis.* 135:729, 1977.

31. Tully, J. L., Friedland, G. H., and Goldmann, D. A. Complications of intravenous therapy with steel needles and small-bore Teflon catheters. *Am. J. Med.* 70:702, 1981.

# 37 TRANSPLANT-RELATED INFECTIONS

Robert G. Brooks
Jack S. Remington

The increasing availability of human organ transplantation has expanded significantly the numbers of patients at risk for nosocomial infections. Although substantial improvements have been made in immunosuppressive regimens and surgical technique, infection still remains the most common cause of death in most transplant series [12,179,206,245]. It is therefore incumbent on physicians caring for organ transplant recipients to stay abreast of new information related to the special circumstances of infection in this unique population and the expanding number of opportunistic pathogens that cause infection in these patients.

In addition, an understanding is needed of the underlying host risk factors, surgical techniques, and immunosuppressive regimens unique to each transplant group, since these factors frequently determine the site and type of potential infections. Thus major determinants of infection may be viewed in light of the patient's underlying disease, the effect of the site of transplantation on local host resistance factors, and the type and duration of immunosuppressive therapy. For example, the patient with end-stage renal failure due to diabetes mellitus will continue to be at risk posttransplantation for infections seen more commonly with diabetes. Other host factors that may predispose to nosocomial infection, such as age, nutritional status, and incidence of pretransplant infections, vary markedly among different transplant groups.

Examples of infectious problems related to the specific type of allograft include (1) pneumonia, which is the most common site of infection in heart and lung transplant recipients (Table 37-1); (2) septicemia, which occurs more frequently in liver transplant and bone marrow transplant patients (Table 37-2); and the urinary tract, which is the site of infection most often observed in renal transplant patients [200]. These differences are often understandable in light of the surgical and postoperative factors that affect local host resistance. In the cardiac transplant patient, chronic cardiac failure with pulmonary edema, postoperative atelectasis, pleural fluid, and chest tubes combine with the patient's difficulty in coughing to compromise effectively the patient's defense against pulmonary pathogens. The high incidence of bacterial sepsis in the liver transplant recipient is related to the direct exposure of the biliary tract and graft to endogenous gastrointestinal flora [206,220]. In the renal transplant recipient, preoperative bacteriuria, urinary manipulation, and postoperative urinary catheters are the factors most often

TABLE 37-1. Infections in Stanford cardiac transplant patients treated with cyclosporine (Dec. 1980–Aug. 1983)

| Organism | Blood | Lung | Central nervous system | Gastro-intestinal tract | Urinary tract | Soft tissue | Dissem-inated | Other | Total isolates | Total patients |
|---|---|---|---|---|---|---|---|---|---|---|
| **Bacteria** | | | | | | | | | | |
| **Gram-negative** | | | | | | | | | | |
| Pseudomonas aeruginosa | 1 | 5 | | 3 | | | | | 9 | 8 |
| Escherichia coli | 1 | 3 | | 1 | 1 | | | 1 | 7 | 5 |
| Klebsiella pneumoniae | 2 | 2 | | 1 | 1 | | | | 6 | 4 |
| Serratia marcescens | 2 | 3 | 1 | | | 2 | | 2 | 10 | 6 |
| Enterobacter cloacae | 1 | | | 1 | | 1 | | 1 | 4 | 3 |
| Citrobacter freundii | 1 | 2 | | | 1 | | | | 4 | 2 |
| Proteus mirabilis | 1 | 1 | | | | | | | 2 | 1 |
| Acinetobacter linoffin | | | | 1 | | | | | 1 | 1 |
| Legionella pneumophila | | 5 | | | | | | | 5 | 5 |
| **Gram-positive** | | | | | | | | | | |
| Staphylococcus aureus | 2 | | | | 1 | 3 | | 3 | 9 | 5 |
| Staphylococcus, coagulase-negative | | | | | | 1 | | | 1 | 1 |
| Streptococcal species (other than enterococcus) | | 3 | | | | | | | 3 | 3 |
| Enterococcus | 5 | 5 | | 4 | 2 | 2 | | 2 | 20 | 14 |
| Listeria monocytogenes | | | 1 | | | | | | 1 | 1 |
| Mixed aerobic-anaerobic | | 2 | | 1 | | | | | 3 | 3 |
| Nocardia asteroides | | 2 | | | | 1 | | | 3 | 3 |
| **Fungi** | | | | | | | | | | |
| Aspergillus | 1 | 8 | | | | | 5 | | 14 | 8 |
| Candida | 1 | 1 | | | | 1 | | 1 | 4 | 2 |
| Cryptococcus | | 2 | | | | | | | 2 | 2 |
| **Protozoa** | | | | | | | | | | |
| Toxoplasma gondii | | | | | | | 1 | 1 | 2 | 2 |
| Pneumocystis carinii | | | | | | | | | 0 | |
| Total patients[a] | 11 | 29 | 1 | 5 | 5 | 7[b] | 6 | 11 | | |

[a]Patients may have multiple organisms infecting a single site.
[b]Includes five patients with mediastinitis, one with osteomyelitis, and one with subcutaneous nocardial infection.
Source: Stinson, E.B. Personal communication.

TABLE 37-2. Bacteria isolated from the bloodstream in selected organ transplant series

| Organism | Renal (Peterson et al. [179])[a] | Bone Marrow | | Heart (Stinson et al. [223])[b] | Liver (Schröter et al. [206])[b] |
| | | Meyers and Thomas [151][b] | Winston et al. [245][c] | | |
| --- | --- | --- | --- | --- | --- |
| Gram-negative | | | | | |
| Pseudomonas | 2 | 30 | 9 | 1 | 8 |
| Escherichia | 7 | 13 | 5 | 1 | 28 |
| Klebsiella | 1 | 13 | 7 | 2 | |
| Enterobacter | | 6 | 1 | 1 | |
| Proteus | 1 | 4 | | 1 | 6 |
| Serratia | | 3 | | 2 | 3 |
| Citrobacter | | | | 1 | 1 |
| Other aerobic gram-negative species | 1 | 1 | | | 4 |
| Total aerobic gram-negative organisms | 12 | 70 | 22 | 9 | 67 |
| Gram-positive | | | | | |
| Staphylococcus | | | | | |
| Coagulase-positive | 1 | 7 | 3 | 2 | 2 |
| Coagulase-negative | 2 | 5 | | | 2 |
| Enterococcus | 1 | | 1 | 5 | 15 |
| Streptococcal species | | 9 | 1 | | 6 |
| Propionibacterium | | 6 | | | |
| Corynebacterium | | 7 | | | |
| Other aerobic gram-positive species including Listeria | | 16 | | 1 | 4 |
| Total aerobic gram-positive organisms | 4 | 50 | 5 | 8 | 29 |
| Other | | | | | |
| Anaerobic only | 1 | 13 | 1 | | 20 |
| Mixed aerobic/anaerobic | 1 | | 3 | | 29 |
| Total | 18[a] | 133[b] | 31[c] | 17[b] | 145[b] |
| Patients at risk | 518 | Not given | 60 | 78 | 93 |
| Percent | 3.5 | | 52 | 22 | |

[a]Data expressed in number of patients.
[b]Data expressed in number of organisms.
[c]Data expressed in number of episodes.

cited as responsible for the increased incidence of posttransplantation urinary tract infections [15].

Suppression of cell-mediated immunity is necessary to circumvent rejection of grafts. Unfortunately, the profound deficits in immunologic status caused by immunosuppressive drugs have been associated with an untoward incidence of opportunistic infection. Traditional regimens have included corticosteroids, cytotoxic drugs such as cyclophosphamide and azathioprine, and antilymphocyte globulin. These regimens often produced marked deficits, not only in cell-mediated immunity, but in humoral immunity as well [29]. High doses of corticosteroids and antilymphocyte globulin were often needed for frequent rejection episodes, resulting in an increase in infections [140]. A recent addition to immunosup-

pressive drug regimens is cyclosporine, a cyclic polypeptide, which has been used in human transplant populations since 1978 [32]. The first partially selective immunosuppressive drug, it acts primarily on the helper arm of the T-lymphocyte population [241]. It has also been shown to block the development of cytotoxic effector cells [90] and interfere with the production of interleukins 1 and 2 [27]. Clinical experience has now accumulated with the use of this agent in renal [32], bone marrow [184], heart [173], and liver [55] allografts in humans, and it appears that not only is the incidence of graft loss decreased [60], but the overall incidence of infection has been reported to be reduced as well [55, 173].

This chapter focuses on infectious problems that are unique to the transplant population. Emphasis has been placed on cases and series published since 1978 to define recent trends in infections that are likely to shape the outlook for transplant patients in the coming years. No attempt is made to include references to all of the available literature but rather to focus on references that are most illustrative. Infections are discussed by both site and specific organism.

## INFECTION BY SITE

### Infection of the Bloodstream

RENAL TRANSPLANTS  Bacteremia has been a major problem in the renal transplant population, especially in patients with postoperative urinary tract infection. In 1971 McDonald and colleagues [143] at Tulane University reported 12 (24 percent) episodes of bacterial sepsis among 50 renal transplant recipients. Eleven of these infections were with enteric gram-negative bacilli. Nine of the ten patients who died had become bacteremic from their urinary tract. The authors reported that bilateral nephrectomy done before transplantation in 16 patients who had previous evidence of urinary tract infection caused a decrease in the incidence of posttransplant urinary tract infection and sepsis.

McHenry and coworkers [144] at the Cleveland Clinic reported 47 episodes of sepsis in 36 renal transplant patients. In 41 of the 47 episodes, renal impairment was present at the onset of sepsis, and 25 percent of the patients were leukopenic because of the necessity for increased immunosuppression due to rejection. Among the 47 episodes of sepsis, the major sites of origin were the urinary tract in 17 percent, the lung in 8 percent, and the wound in 7 percent. Mortality due to sepsis was 36 percent. Peterson and associates [179] in a more recent series from the University of Minnesota reported 18 (3.5 percent) episodes of bacteremia among 518 renal transplant patients who were followed for an average of 22 months posttransplantation. Gram-negative bacilli were responsible for ten of these episodes, and in seven of them the origin was the urinary tract. The markedly lower incidence of sepsis in this series may be due to several factors, including the use of cyclosporine as the standard immunosuppressive agent in some of the patients and the routine use of daily prophylactic oral trimethoprimsulfamethoxazole in an attempt to prevent infections due to *Nocardia* and *Pneumocystis*.

With improved perioperative urinary tract management [108] and prophylactic antibiotics [230] to decrease the incidence of the urinary tract as a site of sepsis, a larger proportion of bacteremias are now being reported to arise from the gastrointestinal tract [200]. In addition, *Listeria monocytogenes* has become a frequent cause of bacteremia in at least one major medical center [200].

BONE MARROW TRANSPLANTS  The transplant group most at risk for bacteremia is the bone marrow transplant group. In this population bacteremias are particularly likely to occur in the early posttransplantation period because of sustained granulocytopenia. Of 60 bone marrow transplant patients transplanted between 1973 and 1976 reviewed by Winston and colleagues [245] from the U.C.L.A. Bone Marrow Transplant Group, 32 (53 percent) had documented bacteremia with a median time to onset of nine days posttransplantation (Table 37-2 and Fig. 37-1). Patients with underlying acute leukemia, who received a more intensive pretransplantation regimen consisting of both multiple chemotherapeutic agents and radiation, had a higher incidence of posttransplantation bacteremia compared with patients transplanted for aplastic anemia. The lower gastrointestinal tract and oral cavity were considered to be the source of bacteremia in 66 percent of the patients. Overall mortality was 55 percent and did not differ by transplant group (acute leukemia or aplastic anemia). A mortality of 46 percent was seen among the 26 patients with infections due to gram-negative bacteria, whereas there was no mortality in the six patients who had bacteremia due to gram-positive organisms.

Data from the University of Washington in Seattle also document an early posttransplant peak in bacteremias in this group [151]. In comparison with the U.C.L.A. series, however, these authors reported that bacteremias occurred later. Twenty-six percent of the bacteremias occurred more than 50 days posttransplantation. The predominant pathogens in this series were also enteric gram-negative bacilli.

HEART TRANSPLANTS  Since 1980 78 heart transplant patients in whom cyclosporine was used have been followed at Stanford University Medical Center. As of August 1983, there have been 16 organisms isolated in 15 episodes of bacteremia among 11 of these patients (Tables 37-1 and 37-2) [223].

LIVER TRANSPLANTS  Bacteremia is a significant cause of transplant failure and patient morbidity in liver transplant recipients [206]. This is especially true when a functional loop of bowel is used for biliary

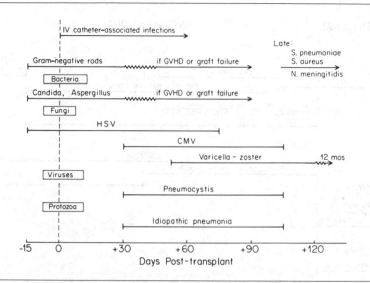

FIG. 37-1. Timetable for occurrence of infection in bone marrow transplant recipients. CMV = cytomegalovirus; GVHD = graft-versus-host disease; HSV = herpes simplex virus. (From Young, L. S. In *Proceedings of the Second International Symposium on the Compromised Host.* London, Academic, 1983, p. 27, with permission of the author.)

duct reconstruction [220]. This alteration allows direct bacterial contamination of the transplant itself. In a study of 77 liver transplant patients between 1963 and 1974 at the University of Colorado [206], there was a 69 percent incidence of bacteremia. In almost half of these episodes the bacteremia was due to more than one bacterial species. Twenty episodes of anaerobic bacteremia were reported, most often with *Bacteroides* or *Clostridium* species.

FUNGEMIA  Fungemia has also been a major problem, especially with bone marrow or liver transplantation. The U.C.L.A. Bone Marrow Transplant Group [245] reported 16 patients with fungemia—13 patients with *Candida* species, two with *Aspergillus,* and one with *Trichosporon*. Fungemia represented 33 percent of all bloodstream infections and had a mean time to onset of five days posttransplant. The mortality rate of 88 percent was significantly higher than that seen with bacteremias in this group. At the University of Washington [151], 40 (12 percent) of 330 total bloodstream isolates from bone marrow transplant recipients were due to *Candida* species. Although fungemia occurred throughout the posttransplantation period, a greater proportion of total bloodstream isolates were fungi (28 percent) after day

30 posttransplantation compared to the first month, when only 12 percent were fungi.

In a series of 100 consecutive liver transplants at the University of Colorado, Schröter and colleagues [205] reported eight (8 percent) cases of candidemia. *Candida albicans* was the most common cause of fungemia in this patient group.

*Infections of the Urinary Tract*
RENAL TRANSPLANTS  Infection of the urinary tract takes on special importance only in the renal transplant recipient. Urinary tract infection has been reported as the most common cause of bacterial infection in renal transplant series [111,156,187,200]. Major risk factors in these patients include pretransplantation urinary tract infections, prolonged catheterization of the urinary tract, and immunosuppressive therapy [197]. Urinary tract infection, especially in the first three months posttransplantation, is frequently associated with pyelonephritis, bacteremia, and a high rate of relapse when treated with the usual courses of antibiotics (Fig. 37-2) [200]. Conversely, infection that occurs more than six months after transplantation has been reported to be more benign and tends to be more responsive to conventional outpatient antibiotic regimens [79].

Of particular importance have been the complications of urinary tract infections in renal transplant patients. As discussed previously, urinary tract infections have played a significant role in bacteremic infection in the posttransplant period. Of additional concern is the role of urinary tract infection in the

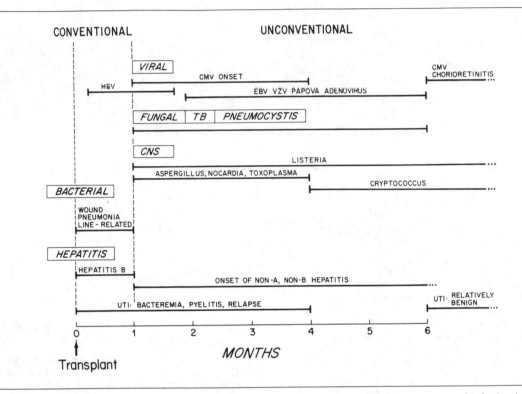

FIG. 37-2. Timetable for occurrence of infection in the renal transplant patient. HSV = herpes simplex virus; CMV = cytomegalovirus; EBV = Epstein-Barr virus; VZV = varicella-zoster virus; UTI = urinary tract infection. (From Rubin, R. H. In Rubin R. H., and Young, L. S. (Eds.), *Clinical Approach to Infection in the Compromised Host.* New York: Plenum, 1981, p. 553, with permission of the author.)

causation of graft rejection. Krieger and coworkers [112] studied 87 renal transplant patients transplanted in 1974 at the New York Hospital-Cornell Medical Center who were followed for at least 12 months. Urinary tract infection in the first month posttransplantation was associated with a particularly poor prognosis for graft survival. Of 22 patients with early urinary tract infection, 19 lost their graft. This relation of graft loss with early urinary tract infection was also observed in a series by Byrd and associates [30], in which a significant correlation existed between infection of the urinary tract with *Streptococcus faecalis* and subsequent graft failure at 1, 3, and 12 months posttransplant.

OTHER TRANSPLANTS  Urinary tract infections have not been a major problem in patients who received a bone marrow, liver, or heart transplant. Of 60 patients with bone marrow transplants studied by Winston and colleagues [245], only 3 had documented urinary tract infection, and at Stanford University Medical Center, 6 urinary tract infections have been observed in 5 of the 78 heart transplant patients receiving cyclosporine from December 1980 to August 1983 [223].

*Infection of the Lung*

Infections of the lung have been a major concern in all groups of transplant patients because of their frequency and morbidity (Table 37-3) [12,188,206,245]. Fever and pulmonary infiltrates in the transplant patient may be due to a variety of infectious agents. Because invasive procedures are often necessary to secure a diagnosis and begin appropriate therapy in these patients, a coherent approach to this problem must be formulated by each physician involved [243]. Following is an overview of this problem in each transplant group. Additional information on viral, fungal, and nocardial infections of the lung is provided under the individual sections concerning these agents.

RENAL TRANSPLANTS  Pneumonia has been reported to be the most common cause of death in renal transplant recipients [188,200]. Ramsey and colleagues

TABLE 37-3. Pneumonias in selected organ transplant series

| Type of infection | Renal (Ramsey et al. [188]) | Bone Marrow (Winston et al. [245]) | Heart (Stinson et al. [223]) | Liver (Schröter et al. [206]) |
|---|---|---|---|---|
| Viral | | | | |
|   Cytomegalovirus | 8 | 10 | 3 | 7 |
|   Herpes simplex | | | | 6 |
|   Other | 1 | 1 | | |
| Bacterial | | | | |
|   Gram-negative | | | | |
|     *Pseudomonas aeruginosa* | | 3 | 5 | 3 |
|     *Escherichia coli* | 1 | | 3 | 2 |
|     *Klebsiella-Enterobacter* group | 4 | | 2 | 5 |
|     *Serratia marcescens* | | | 3 | 4 |
|     *Proteus* species | | | | 2 |
|     Other gram-negative bacilli | 1 | | 6[a] | |
|   Gram-positive | | | | |
|     *Staphylococcus aureus* | 1 | 1 | | |
|     *Staphylococcus*, coagulase-negative | | | | |
|     *Streptococcus pneumoniae* | 4 | 1 | | |
|     Other stretococcal species | | | 2 | 3 |
|   Mixed aerobic infection | | | 4 | |
|   Anaerobic infection | 1 | | 2 | 1 |
| Nocardial | 8 | | 2 | 2 |
| Fungal | | | | |
|   *Aspergillus* species | 5 | 6 | 8 | 8 |
|   *Candida* species | | 3 | 1 | 6 |
|   Cryptococcal species | 1 | | 2 | |
|   Other | | 1 | | |
| Protozoal | | | | |
|   *Pneumocystis carinii* | 1 | 3 | | 10[c] |
|   *Toxoplasma gondii* | | | 1 | 1 |
| *Total* patients infected[b] | 36 | 29 | 33 | 39 |
| *Total* patients studied | 227 | 68 | 78 | 93 |
| Percent | 16 | 42 | 42 | 42 |

[a]Includes five patients with *Legionella pneumophila*.
[b]Several patients had more than one infection.
[c]Includes five patients listed as probable.

[188] studied 277 patients who received renal allografts at the Massachusetts General Hospital from October 1966 to March 1978 and noted 54 patients with fever and pulmonary infiltrates. In 36 patients (66 percent) the pneumonia was diagnosed as due to infection (20 bacterial, which included 8 nocardial, 9 viral, 6 fungal, and 1 protozoal infection due to *Pneumocystis carinii*). In addition, in 23 of these cases superinfection developed, often with a nosocomially-acquired pathogen of nosocomial origin such as *Pseudomonas aeruginosa,* other gram-negative bacilli, or *C. albicans*. A remarkable mortality of 96 percent was noted in this group with superinfection. In the first month posttransplantation, bacterial infection of the lung was of prime importance. In the period one to four months posttransplantation, viral, nocardial, and fungal pathogens predominated. More than four months posttransplantation, pulmonary infections were due to both conventional and opportunistic pathogens. Late bacterial infections appeared to take one of two forms: a community-acquired infection that occurred in patients with stable renal function, or a nosocomial infection with gram-negative bacilli in patients hospitalized for rejection episodes.

At the University of Pittsburgh, Ho and colleagues [96] compared 64 renal transplant patients taking cyclosporine, transplanted in 1981 or 1982, with 59 renal transplant patients who had received azathioprine and were transplanted between 1978 and 1980. Both groups received prednisone as well, and duration of follow-up was similar. They reported that 23 (39 percent) of the 59 azathioprine-treated patients, but only 5 (8 percent) of the 64 cyclosporine-treated patients had pulmonary infections. Before the routine institution of trimethoprimsulfamethoxazole prophylaxis in September of 1982, the incidence of infection with *P. carinii* was significantly higher (9 percent) in the cyclosporine-treated group compared to the azathioprine-treated group (3.4 percent) [84,96].

BONE MARROW TRANSPLANTS   Pneumonia has been a major cause of morbidity and mortality in the bone marrow transplant population [151,245]. The most common pneumonias in this group have been reported to be due to infection with demonstrable pathogens or to interstitial pneumonia of unknown cause.

Interstitial pneumonia of unknown cause is a syndrome rather than a distinct entity [151]. In the bone marrow transplant recipient, interstitial pneumonia may present as fever, cough (usually nonproductive), tachypnea, and generally, diffuse pulmonary infiltrates. Cytomegalovirus and *P. carinii* have been the agents most commonly isolated, but the majority of episodes have been of unknown cause even when lung tissue is examined histologically [150]. The period of highest risk is from one to four months posttransplantation [151]. The incidence of interstitial pneumonia has varied widely but has averaged 30 percent, and mortality has been approximately 75 percent [151,245]. Because of the high mortality, early attempts at diagnosis to rule out other treatable causes of this syndrome should be made. This usually requires an invasive procedure.

Infection with opportunistic pathogens has been the other main cause of pulmonary disease in bone marrow transplant recipients. In the U.C.L.A. series [245], 35 patients (51 percent) of 68 bone marrow transplants had pneumonia develop posttransplantation. Viral pneumonia was the most common demonstrable cause (26 percent), followed by fungal (23 percent), bacterial (12 percent), and *P. carinii* (7 percent) pneumonia. The median time posttransplantation of onset for viral pneumonia was day 74, compared to day 8 for fungal pneumonia and day 44 for bacterial pneumonia. Clinical symptoms or signs (e.g., fever, cough, sputum production) did not distinguish bacterial from nonbacterial pneumonias in this series. Sputum cultures were not helpful in defining bacterial or fungal pneumonias, and definitive diagnosis of bacterial pneumonia was made only at autopsy in four of five cases.

HEART TRANSPLANTS   Among the 78 cardiac transplant patients at Stanford University Medical Center who were treated with cyclosporine (December 1980 to August 1983), there have been 19 episodes of

bacterial pneumonia in 17 patients [223]. Five of these infections were due to *Legionella pneumophila*, and six were due to other gram-negative bacilli alone. *P. aeruginosa* was the most common isolate recovered (five), followed by *Serratia marcescens* and *Escherichia coli* (three each) and *Klebsiella, Citrobacter,* and *Enterobacter* species (two each). Four cases of pneumonia were due to mixed gram-negative and gram-positive organisms, and only two were due to gram-positive aerobic bacteria alone—one patient had pneumonia with enterococcus, and one had pulmonary infection due to another species of *Streptococcus*. In addition, two patients had mixed anaerobic infection. There have been 11 episodes of fungal pneumonia among these 78 patients. Eight were due to *Aspergillus,* two to *Cryptococcus,* and one to a *Candida* species. In addition, there were three cases of pneumonia due to cytomegalovirus, two to *Nocardia,* and one to *Toxoplasma gondii*. No cases of *P. carinii* pneumonia have been observed among the 78 patients treated with cyclosporine through August 1983. None of these patients received prophylaxis for *P. carinii*.

*Infection of the Wound*
RENAL TRANSPLANTS   Wound infections take on particular importance in the renal transplant population. Although different series vary widely with respect to incidence (less than 2 percent to greater than 50 percent), the potential for serious deep infection resulting in loss of graft or systemic infection has been recognized by numerous groups [114,200,208].

Kyriakides and colleagues [114] at the University of Minnesota reported an overall incidence of wound infection of 6.1 percent among 439 renal transplant recipients from August 1967 to July 1973. Unrelated cadaver kidneys, diabetes mellitus, urinary fistulas, and wound hematomas were all factors that predisposed to wound infection. Of 27 isolates *E. coli* was the most common (14), followed by enterococcus (12) and *C. albicans* (11). Superficial infection could be easily drained, but deep infections were much more serious. Loss of the kidney occurred in 12 (75 percent) of 16 patients with deep infections. Mycotic aneurysms of the renal artery occurred in 37.5 percent and septicemia in 62.5 percent of patients with deep wound infection. The authors stress the importance of the prevention of wound hematomas and urinary fistulas for the avoidance of wound infection.

HEART TRANSPLANTS   Among the 78 cardiac transplant patients treated with cyclosporine at Stanford University Medical Center since December 1980, eight episodes of sternotomy wound infections in five patients have been seen [223]. Three of these have been due to *Staphylococcus aureus*, two to *S. marcescens*, and one each to *Enterobacter*, *Streptococcus* (enterococcus), and *Candida* species. These infections are particularly difficult to treat, and long-term antibiotic therapy as well as surgical exploration and debridement may be necessary for cure.

LIVER TRANSPLANTS   Among the 93 liver transplant recipients studied by Schröter and associates [206] at the University of Colorado from March 1963 to November 1974, infection of the abdominal wound was common. Twenty-seven (30 percent) patients had a total of 38 bacterial and 23 fungal organisms isolated from their wounds. These infections were most often due to mixed flora; 13 contained both gram-negative enteric bacilli and *C. albicans*. Only four patients had an infection with a single bacterial species. In 8 of 23 patients whose cultures were positive for *C. albicans*, this was the only organism to grow. Twelve patients had sepsis with an organism that had also been isolated from the wound site.

*Infection of the Central Nervous System*
Infection of the central nervous system (see Chapter 34) is a major cause of morbidity and mortality in immunosuppressed populations [98]. The incidence of infection of the central nervous system in transplant patients has varied with the type of transplant and duration of follow-up (Table 37-4) [25,98,206, 227,245].

RENAL TRANSPLANTS   Two recent publications have reported on the incidence of central nervous system infection following renal transplantation (Table 37-4) [98,277]. Hooper and coworkers [98] at the Massachusetts General Hospital studied 300 renal transplant patients from 1969 to 1979. During this time, 20 patients (7 percent) developed central nervous system infection and nine (45 percent) of them died as a direct result of their infection. As observed in the cardiac transplant experience, *L. monocytogenes, Aspergillus fumigatus,* and *Cryptococcus neoformans* were the most common organisms isolated. The peak incidence of infection occurred one to four months posttransplantation. The infections due to *Cryptococcus* however, all occurred more than six months after transplantation in this group. The authors noted a strong association of leukopenia, azotemia, acute rejection, high daily dose of prednisone, and cytomegalovirus infection with the occurrence of central nervous system infection. Focal neurologic deficits were uncommon except with *Aspergillus* infection; three of the six patients had focal abnormalities.

Tilney and colleagues [227] from Brigham and Women's Hospital in Boston studied 678 renal allograft patients from March 1961 to January 1980

TABLE 37-4. Central nervous system infection in selected organ transplant series

| Organism | Renal | | Bone Marrow (Winston et al. [245]) | Heart (Britt et al. [25]) | Liver (Schröter et al. [206]) |
| | Hooper et al. [98] | Tilney et al. [227] | | | |
| --- | --- | --- | --- | --- | --- |
| *Aspergillus fumigatus* | 6 | 3[b] | 1 | 10 | 3 |
| *Cryptococcus neoformans* | 6 | 6 | | 5 | |
| *Listeria monocytogenes* | 7 | 8 | | 4 | |
| *Toxoplasma gondii* | 1 | | | 4 | 1 |
| Mucoraceae | 1 | | | 2 | |
| *Candida albicans* | | | | 1 | 2 |
| *Coccidioides immitis* | | 1 | | 1 | |
| Conventional bacteria | 1 | | 2 | 1 | 2 |
| *Nocardia asteroides* | | | | | 1 |
| *Total* patients infected | 20[a] | 18 | 3 | 27[c] | 8[c] |
| *Total* patients at risk | 300 | 678 | 60 | 182[d] | 93 |
| *Percent* with CNS infection | 7 | 2.7 | 5 | 13.6 | 8.6 |

[a]Two patients had two infections each.
[b]Two definite and one probable case.
[c]One patient had two infections.
[d]On whom 199 transplants were performed.

and found 18 cases (2.7 percent) of central nervous system infection. The causative agents in their cases were similar to those mentioned previously (Table 37-4). In this study, diabetes mellitus, use of high-dose corticosteroids, and coincident infections were all considered to be risk factors for central nervous system infection. In patients with fungal infection of the central nervous system, dissemination from a pulmonary site was the rule. The overall mortality rate was 44 percent in this series but was 20 percent when only patients diagnosed since 1974 were analyzed.

BONE MARROW TRANSPLANTS    Infections of the central nervous system have not been noted commonly in series of bone marrow transplant patients. In the U.C.L.A. Bone Marrow Transplant Series [245], three (5 percent) infections of the central nervous system were reported among 60 patients. The three cases, *S. aureus* brain abscess, *Klebsiella pneumoniae* meningitis, and encephalitis due to *A. fumigatus,* were each considered to be secondary to bloodborne dissemination. In a separate analysis of late infections that occurred in bone marrow transplant recipients, Atkinson and colleagues [7] from the University of Washington noted two cases of meningitis (cause not mentioned) and one case of herpes simplex encephalitis among 244 infectious episodes in 98 patients.

HEART TRANSPLANTS    At the Stanford University Medical Center, infection of the central nervous system has been a serious problem in heart transplant patients. Britt and coworkers [25], studying the first 199 transplants performed, reported 27 patients (13.6 percent) with intracranial infections (Table 37-4). *Aspergillus* species were responsible for ten cases of necrotizing meningoencephalitis, most of which occurred within the first three months posttransplantation. This disease most often presented with disorientation, obtundity, and multiple low-density lesions on computerized tomographic scanning. Although five patients were treated with systemic amphotericin B, none survived.

*T. gondii,* the next most common cause of an encephalitis-like picture, was often found in the setting of dissemination of this organism to multiple organs. Of the four patients in whom this diagnosis was made, it was made only at autopsy in three. *C. neoformans* (five cases) and *L. monocytogenes* (four cases) accounted for the vast majority of instances of central nervous system infections in which a meningitic picture predominated. Patients with *Cryptococcus* or *Listeria* meningeal infection most often presented with headache and lethargy; four patients had focal neurologic def-

icits. Examination of the cerebrospinal fluid was diagnostic in all cases of cryptococcal central nervous system infection. All four patients with *Listeria* meningitis had a negative Gram stain but were positive on culture. Two of the five patients with cryptococcal central nervous system infections died, whereas all of the patients with *Listeria* infection treated with penicillin survived.

LIVER TRANSPLANTS    In the study of liver transplant patients at the University of Colorado [206], 8 (8.6 percent) of 93 patients had central nervous system infection; *A. fumigatus* was the most common organism isolated (Table 37-4).

## SPECIFIC ORGANISMS CAUSING INFECTION IN TRANSPLANT PATIENTS

### Infection Due to Bacteria

Bacteria are the most common organisms that cause morbidity and mortality according to most transplant series [12,206,223,245]. This is particularly true in the early posttransplantation period when bacteremia, pneumonias, urinary tract infections, and wound infections are likely to occur. In a prospective study of infections in 518 renal transplant patients from 1977 to 1981, Peterson and coworkers [179] found 62 infectious episodes due to bacteria, which represented 30 percent of all infections. The mortality was 10 percent for all bacterial infections and increased to 22 percent when bacteremia was present. In addition, 20 patients had polymicrobic infections with bacteria, fungi, and/or viruses; in this group the mortality rate was 65 percent.

Bacterial infections in bone marrow transplant patients are of particular concern in the early posttransplantation period when the majority of patients are granulocytopenic. In the 60 bone marrow transplant patients reported by Winston and associates [245] from the U.C.L.A. Bone Marrow Transplant Group, bacterial infection accounted for 40 percent of all documented infection; the median time of onset of infection was 18 days posttransplantation.

According to a review of infectious complications after cardiac transplantation at Stanford University Medical Center from 1968 to 1978, 235 episodes of bacterial infection occurred in 94 patients. This accounted for 61 percent of all infections [12]. Of the 78 patients treated with cyclosporine since December 1980, bacteria have caused a total of 46 (40 percent) of the 116 infectious episodes that occurred in 58 patients [223].

GRAM-NEGATIVE BACILLI  The importance of gram-negative organisms as a significant cause of infection in hospitalized patients has been amplified by findings in the transplant patient population. Infections of the urinary tract, blood, wound, and lungs are more often due to gram-negative, usually enteric, bacilli, than to gram-positive organisms (Tables 37-2 and 37-3). *P. aeruginosa, E. coli* and members of the tribe Klebsielleae have been most commonly involved. These organisms may cause primary or secondary infections [188]. Substantiation of their etiologic involvement may be difficult because these bacterial species frequently colonize mucosal surfaces in hospitalized transplant patients [245]. Although the incidence of gram-negative infections (at least in the bone marrow transplant population) has declined in recent years, these organisms still remain a major cause of morbidity and mortality in this transplant group. Infection of transplant patients with gram-negative bacteria other than enteric gram-negative bacilli or *L. pneumophila* has been uncommon.

LEGIONELLA AND LEGIONELLA-LIKE ORGANISMS  Of growing concern have been the recent outbreaks of pneumonia due to *Legionella* in hospitalized transplant patients (see Chapter 26). Documented outbreaks have occurred in renal [65,80,82,137,138,228], bone marrow, [113] and heart transplant [131] patients.

*Renal transplants.*  Marshall and colleagues [138] identified 14 cases of legionnaires' disease in 92 renal transplant patients from 1972 to 1980 at the University of Vermont. The clinical syndrome did not appear to differ from that observed in other groups of patients with legionnaires' disease. The authors stress the importance of maintaining a high index of suspicion for *Legionella* in transplant patients with pulmonary infiltrates since erythromycin is not routinely administered for nosocomial pneumonia at most centers. Without proper therapy, the mortality of this disease is high [107,203].

From May 1977 to July 1978, 49 cases of legionnaires' disease were identified at Wadsworth Medical Center in Los Angeles. During this period, 6 of 12 renal homograft recipients acquired legionnaires' pneumonia, in contrast to 3 of 22 renal transplant patients during the preceding three years [82]. The high incidence in this group of patients resulted in the temporary discontinuation of renal transplantation at this center [82,107].

Renal transplant patients are reported to be at greater risk than the general population of acquiring infection with the Pittsburgh pneumonia agent *Legionella microdadei* [157,174,183,194]. Taylor and coworkers [226] from the University of Pittsburgh could find no clinical, laboratory, or radiographic manifestations that differentiated pneumonias due to the Pittsburgh pneumonia agent from those due to *L. pneumophila* or other bacteria. The 9 cases occurred among 77 patients who had renal transplantation performed from July 1977 through January 1980. The authors stress the importance of early diagnosis in the cure of this infection and have recommended the early use of open lung biopsy to obtain tissue for histologic examination and culture in any patient not diagnosed by noninvasive methods.

*Bone marrow transplants.*  Kugler and associates [113] from the University of Iowa reported five cases of *L. pneumophila* pneumonia after bone marrow transplantation for hematologic malignancies. *L. pneumophila* serogroup 1 was isolated from the hospital's hot water system. Retrospective serologic screening of 40 consecutive transplant recipients revealed the incidence of pneumonia due to *Legionella* to be 13 percent in this patient group—approximately four times higher than the incidence in the general population of Iowa [191]. This organism caused 23 percent of all pneumonias observed in this transplant group, and two of the five patients died despite treatment with erythromycin.

*Heart transplants.*  The first two cases of legionnaires' disease in cardiac transplant recipients were reported by Copeland and colleagues in 1981 [42]. These cases occurred three and nine weeks after cardiac transplantation. Both cases survived after therapy with intravenous erythromycin. Another case of legionnaires' disease in a cardiac transplant recipient was reported by Naot and coworkers [163]. This patient had pneumonia beginning ten weeks after transplantation. The diagnosis was substantiated by a positive Dieterle and fluorescent stain of a needle aspirate of lung as well as by seroconversion. Cavitation was observed in each of these three cases. Eight additional cases of legionnaires' disease have been seen in cardiac transplant recipients at Stanford University Medical Center from May 1982 through October 1983 [131]. In six of these cases diagnosis was made by positive smear or culture of lung tissue, and in three cases a retrospective diagnosis was made based on seroconversion. The majority of these cases occurred in the first month posttransplantation and had a rapid and pronounced rise in IgM titers against *L. pneumophila* by enzyme-linked immunosorbent assay (ELISA). In contrast, IgG responses as measured by ELISA were often minimal even when followed for months. All isolates were typed and found to be serotype 1. Water obtained from a water heater in the intensive care unit in which the cardiac transplant recipients were cared for also grew out *L. pneumophila* when first examined in October 1983.

GRAM-POSITIVE BACTERIA   Although gram-negative bacilli cause the majority of bacterial infections in transplant patients, gram-positive bacteria take on increased significance under certain conditions. Prolonged intravenous therapy and the use of indwelling central venous catheters have become increasingly common [128,244]. These lines subject the patient to increased risk of bloodstream infection (see Chapter 36). In one series [244], 20 of 22 bone marrow transplant patients with coagulase-negative staphylococcal bacteremia had indwelling central venous lines. Of the 22, 16 were also granulocytopenic. Previous colonization of mucocutaneous sites with coagulase-negative *Staphylococcus* occurred in all bacteremic patients before infection. In another study from Westminster Medical School in London [195], 12 of 33 bone marrow transplant patients had documented coagulase-negative staphylococcal bacteremia during a 15-month period (January 1981 to March 1982). Persistence of fever or complications (catheter exit-site infection [four], pneumonia [two], embolic skin lesions [one]), despite antibiotic therapy, necessitated premature removal of the catheter in nine patients.

Central venous lines have also been considered a risk factor for the development of *Corynebacterium* infection [166,177,218]. Stamm and coworkers [218] reported 32 (11 percent) cases of *Corynebacterium* bacteremia in 284 bone marrow transplant patients over a three-year period (1974 to 1977). Other risk factors appeared to be male sex, age greater than 16 years, immunosuppressive drugs, granulocytopenia, and previous colonization or local infection with this organism. This organism appeared to be of nosocomial origin in the majority of cases and to be best treated by specific antibiotic therapy and removal of the central venous line if present (see Chapter 36).

*Streptococcus pneumoniae* appears to play a role in posttransplantation infections in at least two specific patient populations. There is an increasing number of reports of pneumococcal bacteremia and sepsis in renal transplant patients who have received splenectomy pretransplantation. Linnemann and First [120] reported that within a six-year period 11 of 163 renal transplant patients with previous splenectomy had pneumococcal infection, compared with only one of 34 without splenectomy. Because of this increased risk, the authors recommend that pneumococcal vaccine be given to prospective renal transplant recipients before transplantation [120,121]. Bourgault and colleagues [22] reported five patients with pneumo-

coccal bacteremia, two of whom had fulminant sepsis, among 236 renal transplant patients with splenectomies, compared to no episodes in 57 renal transplant patients without previous splenectomy.

Long-term survivors of bone marrow transplantation also face an increased prospect of pneumococcal infection [238,247]. Winston and associates [247] documented 8 pneumococcal infections in 7 of 26 bone marrow transplant patients who had survived more than seven months posttransplantation. This represented an incidence of 27 percent. Six of the eight infections were bacteremias. Localized infection of the lung was the most common source (four patients). The source of bacteremia was reported to be the sinuses in two patients and the middle ear and meninges in one each. The authors suggest that abnormal opsonizing or complement activity may play a role in the predisposition to pneumococcal infection in this patient population.

LISTERIA   *Renal transplants.   L. monocytogenes* remains a major pathogen in organ transplantation patients. This is especially true of the renal transplant population. Nieman and Lorber [168], in a review of cases of listeriosis reported in the English literature from 1968 to 1978, noted that 22 percent of all cases of listeriosis in adults since 1968 were in renal transplant recipients. This figure probably underestimates the percentage of cases in renal transplant patients since several series [21,64,102] of listeriosis in renal transplant patients were not included because of insufficient details. *Listeria* caused meningitis, nonmeningitic central nervous system infection, or primary bacteremia in this series. Nieman and Lorber reported that among renal transplant patients 56 percent developed *Listeria* meningitis; this figure is similar to the 55 percent incidence of *Listeria* meningitis among all patients with listeriosis. Nonmeningitic central nervous system listeriosis, however, appeared to be more common in renal transplant recipients (17 percent vs. 6.5 percent). Mortality in both types of central nervous system *Listeria* infection was 30 percent. The incidence of primary bacteremia due to *Listeria* in renal transplant recipients (27 percent) was not different from that of all patients (24.5 percent). All 14 cases of *Listeria* endocarditis were in the nonrenal transplant group.

Stamm and associates [217] observed an outbreak of listeriosis in six renal transplant recipients in a tenweek period of 1979 at the University of Alabama. Investigation of the outbreak established that the first four cases were close contacts and all were infected by *L. monocytogenes* serotype 1b. Source of infection and route of spread were not identified. On the basis of their clinical experience, the authors recommended that individual renal transplant patients with listeriosis be cared for with secretion and excretion precautions and that they be treated with ampicillin and gentamicin. The same authors also reviewed the literature on listeriosis in renal transplant recipients from 1969 to 1980. Of the total of 102 cases, they found the major manifestation of disease was meningitis in 50 percent, parenchymal disease of the central nervous system in 10 percent, both meningitis and parenchymal disease of the central nervous system in 9 percent, and primary bacteremia in 30 percent. The overall mortality in renal transplant recipients was 26 percent. Pneumonia due to *L. monocytogenes* was present in seven patients (7 percent), five of whom died.

*Other transplants.* In the cardiac transplant patients who were taking cyclosporine between December 1980 and August 1983, there was only 1 case of *Listeria* central nervous system infection (Table 37-1). *Listeria* has not been reported as a frequent pathogen in recent series of bone marrow [245] or liver [206] transplant recipients.

MYCOBACTERIAL SPECIES *Renal transplants.* After renal transplantation, an incidence of mycobacteriosis from 0.65 to 1.7 percent has been reported [44,123,193]. Lloveras and coworkers [123] from the University of Minnesota found seven cases of mycobacterial infection during an 11-year period (1968 to 1980) among 1069 patients with renal allografts. Four of these cases were due to *Mycobacterium tuberculosis;* one presented as pulmonary disease and three as joint or subcutaneous tissue infection. An additional three patients had joint or subcutaneous infection with *Mycobacterium kansasii.* Six of the seven patients responded to antimycobacterial drugs.

Riska and Kuhlbäck [193] reported ten cases of mycobacterial disease, six of which were bacteriologically identified as *M. tuberculosis* among 584 patients who had received transplants at the University of Helsinki from 1964 to 1978. All ten patients had pulmonary tuberculosis with a time of onset from 1 to 32 months posttransplantation. The disease presented with fever in eight cases, cough or other respiratory symptoms in three, and pleural effusion in two. Treatment with isoniazid, rifampin, and either ethambutol or streptomycin was initiated in nine patients and resulted in clinical cure in all nine.

Spence and colleagues [214] from the University of Pennsylvania, reported five cases of mycobacterial infection among 565 renal transplant recipients during a 15-year period. Atypical mycobacteria were cultured from three of the five cases. There were two

cases of *M. kansasii* infection, both of which had soft-tissue involvement, and one case of combined *M. intracellularis* pulmonary disease and *M. tuberculosis* urinary tract involvement. The two cases of *M. tuberculosis* initially had only pulmonary involvement, but one patient relapsed after one year of treatment with isoniazid and ethambutol and died of disseminated mycobacterial disease. In four of the five patients, there were serious drug-related complications—hepatitis in one, myelosuppression in one, and neurologic symptoms in two.

Several other recent case reports have reemphasized the ability of atypical mycobacteria to infect the renal transplant population in extrapulmonary sites, especially skin and soft tissue [19,34,47,78,152,155].

The use of prophylaxis and optimum treatment of tuberculosis in the renal transplant group has not been agreed on [5,14,169,193,197]. Some authors suggest that the duration of therapy be longer than that used in nonimmunocompromised patients [11,123,214]. Based on their experience, Spence and colleagues [214] recommend screening and treating all prospective renal transplant patients with a history of tuberculosis exposure with multidrug therapy (i.e., isoniazid, ethambutol, and rifampin) for a minimum period of 18 months. If infection is documented posttransplantation, the authors suggest modifying immunosuppressive regimens (even if sacrifice of the allograft is necessary) and treating with the regimens listed previously for a minimum of 18 months. In the Massachusetts General Hospital Renal Transplant Program, routine isoniazid prophylaxis is not used [197]. However, one year of isoniazid prophylaxis is instituted in renal transplant patients who are recent tuberculin convertors, in those with a history of untreated or suboptimally treated tuberculosis in the past decade, and in patients with significant abnormalities on chest x-ray [197].

*Heart transplants.* Infection with atypical mycobacteria was found in 8 (5 percent) of the first 160 patients who had cardiac transplants performed at Stanford University Medical Center from January 1968 to December 1978 [212]. Of particular interest was the fact that five of these eight patients had previous documented infection with *Nocardia asteroides.* Four of these five infections were due to *M. kansasii* and one to *M. avium-intracellularis* complex. Three patients had lung involvement (all due to *M. kansasii*), one of which was also disseminated to skin. Two patients had subcutaneous involvement only (one due to *M. kansasii* and one to *M. avium-intracellularis*). The mean duration from transplantation to documentation of atypical mycobacteriosis was almost three years. The relative risk of developing atypical mycobacteriosis appeared to increase with time post-transplantation in this series. The significant risk (5 percent) of post-cardiac transplantation mycobacteriosis in this series of patients treated with traditional immunosuppressive regimens (i.e., azathioprine or cyclophosphamide plus corticosteroids with or without antithymocyte globulin) has not been seen in the recent experience with 78 cardiac transplant recipients who received cyclosporine plus corticosteroids. No cases of atypical mycobacteriosis have been reported in these 78 patients through August of 1983 [223].

*Other transplants.* No increase in incidence of mycobacterial infection has been recorded after bone marrow transplantation [245] or liver transplantation [206].

### Infection Due to Viruses

CYTOMEGALOVIRUS  Over the past several years, increasing numbers of reports have appeared attesting to the significance of cytomegalovirus infections in recipients of organ transplants [199]. (see Chapter 35). These infections have been most extensively studied in recipients of bone, kidney, and heart transplants; presumably some of the same features would be present in liver, pancreas, and lung allotransplant recipients, but data are not available to corroborate this presumption [16].

Before proceeding, a distinction must be made between cytomegalovirus infection and cytomegalovirus disease (see Chapter 1). As defined by Friedman [69], *cytomegalovirus infection* is a laboratory diagnosis that does not distinguish between symptomatic and subclinical infection. *Cytomegalovirus disease* combines clinical features with laboratory findings and indicates that in the opinion of the physician the virus detected by the laboratory offers the best explanation for the patient's clinical findings. Excretion of cytomegalovirus in urine or saliva, especially in immunocompromised patients, may be demonstrable for months or years after onset of infection [38,62]. Isolation of virus from these sources does not accurately predict the time of onset of infection. Isolation of cytomegalovirus from tissue or blood, demonstration of inclusion bodies or virus in histologic sections, or a fourfold or greater rise in antibody titer, however, provides stronger evidence that the infection is recently acquired [69]. Cytomegalovirus infection in transplant patients is of two types: *primary infection*, in which the transplant recipient has no evidence before transplantation of exposure to cytomegalovirus, and *secondary infection*, in which reactivation of latent virus occurs.

*Renal transplants.* At the time of transplantation, from 16 to 69 percent [76] of renal transplant recipients have no detectable antibodies to cytomegalovirus and are therefore susceptible to primary infection with this organism (see Chapter 35). The incidence of primary cytomegalovirus infection after transplantation varies widely (12 to 100 percent) [159,164] but averages 53 percent [76]. Although controversy still exists [13], it appears that the two most likely sources of cytomegalovirus infection in these patients are blood transfusion [50] or the transplanted kidney itself [18,95]. Strong circumstantial evidence exists to implicate transfusion of fresh blood as a risk factor for cytomegalovirus infection [3,87]; however, no correlation between the number of units transfused and the risk of cytomegalovirus infection has been substantiated. Serologic evidence implicating the donor kidney as a source of cytomegalovirus transmission appears stronger [18,95,162,229]. Betts and associates [18] reported that of 16 renal transplant patients who were seronegative for cytomegalovirus infection pretransplant and who received kidneys from seropositive donors, 13 (81 percent) had evidence of posttransplantation cytomegalovirus infection, compared with none of the 15 seronegative recipients who received a seronegative donor kidney. Numerous other series have documented this higher incidence of posttransplant cytomegalovirus infection in seronegative recipients of seropositive kidneys (Table 37-5).

From 31 to 84 percent of renal transplant patients are already seropositive for cytomegalovirus antibodies before transplantation and are therefore susceptible to reactivation (secondary infection) of latent cytomegalovirus [76] (Table 37-5). Surgery, anesthesia [213], or immunosuppressive therapy [53] may allow reactivation of cytomegalovirus infection in this group by interfering with immune responsiveness [122]. Renal transplant recipients who are seropositive for cytomegalovirus antibodies pretransplant have been reported to have a higher incidence of posttransplantation cytomegalovirus infection than recipients who were cytomegalovirus-seronegative, regardless of whether transplantation occurred with a kidney from a seropositive or a seronegative donor. In a review of 12 series from the literature, Glenn [76] found that 64 to 100 percent (mean 85 percent) of seropositive patients who had a renal transplant had posttransplantation cytomegalovirus infection compared with the 12 to 100 percent (mean 53 percent) incidence of cytomegalovirus infection in those who were seronegative.

Although cytomegalovirus has been reported to be the most common pathogen recognized in the first six months after renal transplantation [9], it is difficult to prove that any specific sign or symptom that

TABLE 37-5. Incidence of primary and reactivation cytomegalovirus infection after renal, bone marrow, liver, and cardiac transplantation

| Type of transplant (author, year, reference) | Total | | | Primary infections | | | Reactivation infections | | |
|---|---|---|---|---|---|---|---|---|---|
| | Inf[a] | N[b] | % | Inf | N | % | Inf | N | % |
| Renal transplants | | | | | | | | | |
| Spencer et al., 1974 [215] | 86 | 100 | 86 | 19 | 27 | 70 | 67 | 73 | 92 |
| Fiala et al., 1975 [62] | 24 | 26 | 92 | 9 | 11 | 81 | 15 | 15 | 100 |
| Ho et al., 1975 [95] | 21 | 32 | 66 | 13 | 22 | 59 | 8 | 10 | 80 |
| Nankervis et al., 1976 [162] | 34 | 50 | 68 | 14 | 22 | 64 | 20 | 38 | 71 |
| Armstrong et al., 1976 [4] | 10 | 23 | 43 | 3 | 12 | 25 | 7 | 11 | 64 |
| Balfour et al., 1977 [10] | 18 | 27 | 67 | 5 | 13 | 38 | 13 | 14 | 93 |
| Naraqi et al., 1977 [164] | 22 | 30 | 73 | 1 | 8 | 12 | 21 | 22 | 95 |
| Betts et al., 1977 [17] | 48 | 77 | 62 | 16 | 42 | 28 | 32 | 35 | 91 |
| Pass et al., 1978 [175] | 37 | 40 | 93 | 4 | 6 | 67 | 33 | 34 | 97 |
| Chatterjee et al., 1978 [35] | 32 | 35 | 91 | 4 | 6 | 67 | 28 | 29 | 97 |
| Light et al., 1979 [119] | 43 | 69 | 62 | 18 | 35 | 51 | 25 | 34 | 74 |
| Whelchel et al., 1979 [241] | 142 | 164 | 75 | 21 | 34 | 62 | 121 | 130 | 93 |
| Peterson et al., 1980 [178] | 20 | 78 | 25 | 4 | 21 | 19 | 16 | 57 | 25 |
| Marker et al., 1981 [135] | 181 | 320 | 57 | 59 | 169 | 35 | 122 | 151 | 81 |
| Walker et al., 1982 [237] | 31 | 84 | 37 | 11 | 40 | 28 | 20 | 44 | 46 |
| Gadler et al., 1982 [71] | 25 | 28 | 89 | 5 | 7 | 71 | 20 | 21 | 95 |
| Dummer et al., 1983 [55][c] | 13 | 17 | 76 | 3 | 4 | 75 | 10 | 13 | 77 |
| Dummer et al., 1983 [55][d] | 45 | 60 | 75 | 4 | 9 | 44 | 41 | 51 | 80 |
| *Total* renal transplants | 832 | 1260 | 66 | 213 | 488 | 44 | 619 | 782 | 79 |
| Bone marrow transplants | | | | | | | | | |
| Neiman et al., 1977 [167] | 37 | 80 | 46 | 10 | 44 | 23 | 27 | 36 | 75 |
| Liver Transplants | | | | | | | | | |
| Dummer et al., 1983 [54] | 12 | 18 | 66 | 5 | 8 | 62 | 7 | 10 | 70 |
| Heart transplants | | | | | | | | | |
| Pollard et al., 1982 [181] | 32 | 40 | 80 | 12 | 20 | 60 | 20 | 20 | 100 |
| Preiksaitis et al., 1983 [185] | 41 | 54 | 76 | 12 | 25 | 48 | 29 | 29 | 100 |
| Dummer et al., 1983 [54] | 13 | 13 | 100 | 2 | 2 | 100 | 11 | 11 | 100 |
| *Total* heart transplants | 86 | 107 | 80 | 26 | 47 | 55 | 60 | 60 | 100 |

[a]Number of patients infected.
[b]Number of patients at risk.
[c]Azathioprine-treated group.
[d]Cyclosporine-treated group.
Source: Adapted from Ho, M. Cytomegalovirus Infection in Transplant and Cancer Patients. In Remington, J. S., and Swartz, M. N. (Eds.), *Current Clinical Topics in Infectious Diseases.* New York: McGraw-Hill, 1980, p. 45.

appears after transplantation is associated with cytomegalovirus infection. However, the major manifestations of cytomegalovirus disease in the renal transplant patient have been divided into two major syndromes [199,211]. In the so-called benign or self-limited syndrome reported by Simmons and colleagues [211] at the University of Minnesota, fever; moderate leukopenia; and liver, pulmonary, and renal dysfunction were seen. These were often in association with an infiltrate on chest x-ray and typical findings of cellular rejection at kidney biopsy. This group, which had normal in vitro lymphocyte function, formed

antibody to the virus and generally had a spontaneous recovery from their illness. A second, smaller group had a so-called lethal syndrome. These patients had the same initial clinical findings (fever, leukopenia, pulmonary and renal dysfunction) but had no antibody response, no evidence of typical rejection on kidney biopsy, and depressed lymphocyte function, and they generally died with superimposed bacterial, fungal, or protozoal infection. Although several authors [215,225] have commented on the fact that patients with primary cytomegalovirus infection appear to have a higher incidence of symptoms compared to those with secondary disease, this more severe syndrome occurred in patients with both primary and reactivation disease.

Cytomegalovirus has been associated with a variety of disease states in the renal transplant patient in addition to the two mentioned above. Of particular importance are cytomegalovirus retinitis, which may progress to severe visual loss or blindness [176] and gastrointestinal ulceration and bleeding due to cytomegalovirus [66,67]. In addition, a distinct glomerulopathy associated with cytomegalovirus viremia has been reported [192].

Substantial controversy remains regarding the role of cytomegalovirus infection in allograft failure. Although many series [1,70,129,135] report an increased incidence of renal allograft rejection in patients with documented cytomegalovirus infection posttransplantation, this problem is compounded by the many variables reported to affect renal allograft survival, including HLA match, multiple blood transfusions [24], blood group [20], and the use of antithymocyte globulin (ATG) [43].

Opportunistic infections have been reported to be more common in renal transplant patients with cytomegalovirus infection [23,35]. In a series of 81 consecutive renal allografts in 78 recipients, Braun and Nankervis [23] reported that 11 of 12 transplantations complicated by bacteremia were also affected by nearly concurrent cytomegalovirus infection. Four of the eleven patients had primary cytomegalovirus infection and two of these patients had viremia. Chatterjee and coworkers [35] reported that among six patients seronegative for cytomegalovirus antibody pretransplant, four (66 percent) experienced active cytomegalovirus infection within two months, and four died of *Candida* or *Aspergillus* infection within six months after transplantation. Among the 22 patients who were seropositive to cytomegalovirus pretransplant, however, only one (4 percent) had a fungal infection.

Treatment of established cytomegalovirus disease in the renal transplant patient with antiviral agents [134] or hyperimmune plasma [49] has been attempted. Prophylaxis of cytomegalovirus infection in this group has also been examined. In the preliminary studies of vaccination of renal transplant patients preformed by Glazer and colleagues [75], vaccination (with the Towne 125 strain of cytomegalovirus) produced both humoral and cellular immunity, was not associated with significant morbidity, and did not result in reactivation of the vaccination strain with immunosuppression. Initial experience with a randomized trial of Towne-strain cytomegalovirus

versus placebo done by Marker and associates [134] again showed antigenicity in a high proportion (83 percent) of seronegative recipients and a trend toward less fever and leukopenia in the vaccinated group.

Prophylaxis has also been shown to be possible with the use of interferon-alpha [37,93]. In an initial six-week trial, which included both seropositive and seronegative transplant patients, Cheeseman and colleagues [37] reported that human leukocyte interferon given to kidney transplant recipients delayed cytomegalovirus excretion and decreased viremia with cytomegalovirus. In an additional evaluation of the effects of interferon-alpha given for 14 weeks to seropositive recipients of renal transplants, Hirsch and coworkers [93] found that 7 of 22 placebo-treated patients had clinical syndromes attributable to cytomegalovirus infection, whereas only one of 20 interferon-treated patients had a similar syndrome. On the basis of this encouraging information, a multicenter collaborative trial is now underway to test the role of interferon in the prevention of primary cytomegalovirus infection in this population.

*Bone marrow transplants.* The major impact of cytomegalovirus in the bone marrow transplant population appears to be in the pathogenesis of interstitial pneumonia. Interstitial pneumonitis is a syndrome that may complicate over 40 percent of allogeneic bone marrow transplants [151]. The clinical syndrome is not distinctive; patients develop fever, nonproductive or poorly productive cough, tachypnea, and sometimes, chest pains. The risk period is usually from one to four months posttransplantation [151], although in one recent series cases occurred up to six months after transplantation [245]. Diagnostic procedures short of open lung biopsy are not reliable, and most authors recommend open lung biopsy when possible to rule out other treatable causes of this syndrome [151,245].

Of the first 377 bone marrow transplant recipients reported by Meyers and Thomas [151] from the University of Washington, 60 (16 percent) patients had cytomegalovirus as the cause of interstitial pneumonitis. This represented 44 percent of all definable pneumonias in this series. In a series of 63 bone marrow transplant patients reported from U.C.L.A. [245], a total of 43 pneumonias were found, of which 10 (24 percent) were due to cytomegalovirus. This represented 37 percent of the 28 pneumonias in which a definable organism was found. The attack rate for cytomegalovirus-associated pneumonia in patients transplanted for acute leukemia has been reported to be twice that seen in patients transplanted for aplastic anemia [150]. Other risk factors for cytomegalovirus pneumonitis are positive cytomegalovirus serologic studies in the recipient before transplantation [167], seropositivity of the donor [150], and inability of the recipient to mount a fourfold or greater rise in complement fixation antibody titer after exposure to cytomegalovirus [167].

Prophylactic or therapeutic granulocyte transfusions have been reported to increase the risk of cytomegalovirus infection and disease as well [89]. In a study of 387 bone marrow transplant patients from the University of Washington, Hersman and coworkers [89] reported that acquisition of cytomegalovirus infection was higher in recipients of granulocyte transfusions but that this increase reached significance only in cytomegalovirus-negative patients. There did not appear to be any difference in incidence of interstitial pneumonias of all types between the treated and control group.

Because mortality from cytomegalovirus pneumonia in bone marrow transplant recipients has approached 90 percent in some series [151], treatment and prophylaxis of this disease have been attempted [148,149,234]. Treatment of seven cases with a combination of vidarabine and human leukocyte interferon resulted in little clinical evidence of efficacy and in hematologic toxicity in four of the cases [148]. A study of high-dose intravenous acyclovir in eight patients failed to show a significant beneficial effect [234].

In a trial of cytomegalovirus immune plasma for the prophylaxis of cytomegalovirus infection, Winston and associates [246] reported that the incidence of symptomatic cytomegalovirus infection and interstitial pneumonia were both significantly less in the plasma-treated group. Encouraging results were also obtained with prophylactic use of hyperimmune cytomegalovirus globulin by O'Reilly and colleagues [172]. The incidence of interstitial pneumonia and of cytomegalovirus infection was reduced in the hyperimmune globulin group. In another study with hyperimmune globulin, the incidence of cytomegalovirus infection was less only in seronegative patients who had not received granulocyte transfusions from seropositive donors [147]. It was not clear whether cytomegalovirus immune globulin decreased the severity of cytomegalovirus infection or the incidence of interstitial pneumonia in this group.

*Heart transplants.* As in renal and bone marrow transplant recipients, cytomegalovirus infection occurs with increased frequency in patients who are seropositive for cytomegalovirus before cardiac transplantation. Pollard and coworkers [181], in a prospective review of 36 cardiac transplant recipients,

reported that cytomegalovirus infection (defined as viral shedding) occurred in 100 percent of seropositive patients and 62 percent of seronegative patients. Primary infection was more frequently symptomatic in this study, and heart implantation from a seropositive donor to a seronegative recipient was significantly correlated with subsequent cytomegalovirus infection.

In a study to define the role of the donor heart and immunosuppressive therapy in herpes virus infections in cardiac transplant recipients, Preiksaitis and associates [185] reported that when cellular blood products from seronegative donors were used, all primary cytomegalovirus infections were due to transmission of cytomegalovirus from the donor heart. As in the study by Pollard's group, all patients who were seropositive before transplant and for whom the donor cytomegalovirus serologic status was known excreted cytomegalovirus within ten weeks of transplantation regardless of donor cytomegalovirus serologic results and/or use of screened or unscreened blood products. Patients with recurrent cytomegalovirus infection who received antithymocyte globulin had a longer period of cytomegalovirus shedding and more days of fever compared to the group who received cyclosporine as the primary immunosuppressive drug.

Although fever, atypical lymphocytosis, and pneumonia are the most common features of cytomegalovirus infection in the cardiac transplant recipient, cytomegalovirus hepatitis [181] and retinitis [157,182] have also been a problem. Pollard and colleagues [182] have reported 14 patients with cytomegalovirus retinitis, 7 of whom were cardiac transplant recipients. According to the authors, the ophthalmologic picture was characteristic and distinguishable from other forms of retinitis in immunocompromised patients. Several patients had minimal ophthalmologic changes and healed spontaneously. Several patients with more severe disease had a temporally related improvement in their chorioretinitis with adenine arabinoside (vidarabine) treatment.

Cytomegalovirus has also been implicated as a causal factor in the increased incidence of pulmonary superinfection observed in cardiac transplant patients [189]. Of 49 cardiac transplant recipients studied at Stanford University Medical Center from 1973 to 1977 [189], the incidence of bacterial and *Pneumocystis*-related disease (but not fungal) was significantly higher in patients with primary (but not reactivated) cytomegalovirus infection.

Little in the way of therapy for established cytomegalovirus infection in cardiac transplant recipients has been attempted. A single case of cytomegalovirus pneumonitis reported by Ashraf and coworkers [6] appeared to respond to a ten-day course of intravenous acyclovir. At the time of this writing, a prospective study is in progress to determine whether this agent will be efficacious in this setting.

HERPES SIMPLEX VIRUS  *Renal transplants.*  Almost all infections caused by herpes simplex virus in transplant recipients are due to reactivation of latent virus (see Chapter 35). One-half of those who are seropositive and two-thirds of those who excrete herpes simplex virus will develop mucocutaneous lesions [197]. In the renal transplant recipient, herpes labialis is most common in the first month posttransplant and is usually due to type I isolates [94]. These infections may be prolonged and result in extensive oral and esophageal disease. Primary pneumonia due to herpes simplex virus is felt to be rare. Viremia, hepatitis [59,236], keratitis [99], and central nervous system infection [94] have been reported but are also unusual. There is no known increased incidence of renal allograft rejection in patients with herpes simplex viral infection. A predisposition to oral *Candida* infection when mucocutaneous boundaries are involved by herpes simplex virus has led some centers to begin oral nystatin therapy at the onset of such lesions [197]. Very little has been reported in the way of treatment [41,85] or prophylaxis [37] of herpes simplex viral infections in renal transplant populations.

*Bone marrow transplants.*  Meyers and coworkers [146] studied infections with herpesviruses before and for the first four months after bone marrow transplantation in 441 patients. They report that 62 (82 percent) of 76 seropositive patients but only one of 65 seronegative patients developed herpes simplex viral infection. Virus was isolated from 15 patients before transplant and from an additional 40 patients within five weeks after transplant. Herpes simplex virus were not commonly cultured from the oropharynx or orofacial lesions. In the bone marrow transplant population, many patients begin to have active oral excretion or oral lesions with herpes simplex virus early after transplantation. Approximately 80 percent of seropositive patients excrete herpes simplex virus, most commonly from the oropharynx, in the first 50 days after transplantation [26]. Severe mucositis may occur as well as spread of lesion by autoinoculation or dissemination by bloodstream.

Recently, herpes simplex virus pneumonia in 20 patients, 16 of whom were bone marrow transplant recipients, was reported by Ramsey and associates [186]. Mucocutaneous herpesvirus infection preceded the onset of pneumonia in 17 patients. Of 12 patients with focal pneumonia, 10 had concomitant herpetic tracheitis, esophagitis, or both, suggesting contiguous spread. Eight patients had diffuse interstitial pneumonia of which six had dissemination of herpesvirus to other organs. In the majority of cases, herpesvirus pneumonia was felt to be due to reactivation of endogenous virus.

Prophylaxis with 5 mg/kg/day of adenine arabinoside did not reduce herpes simplex excretion in a study of bone marrow transplant recipients by Kraemer and colleagues [110]. Prophylaxis of 20 seropositive bone marrow transplant recipients with intravenous acyclovir was performed by Saral and coworkers, [204] at the Johns Hopkins University. At a dose of 250 mg/M$^2$ of acyclovir every eight hours continued for 18 days, none of ten treated patients, but seven of ten placebo-treated patients became culture-positive for herpes simplex virus. After the study drug was stopped, however, five of the ten treated patients developed mild culture-positive herpes simplex virus infection, and two had asymptomatic viral shedding. Acyclovir was a potent inhibitor of herpes simplex replication but did not eradicate latent virus.

Parenteral adenine arabinoside or acyclovir has been used for serious herpes simplex viral infections in this population, but the efficacy has not been substantiated [151]. In a trial of intravenous acyclovir to treat mucocutaneous herpes simplex viral infection after bone marrow tansplant, Wade and coworkers [235] reported that 13 of 17 patients given acyclovir had a beneficial response, compared to 2 of 17 given placebo. Recurrent infection with each herpes simplex virus was common in the treated group after therapy was stopped.

*Heart transplants.*  Pollard and associates [181] reported that 23 of 36 heart transplant patients had antibody to herpes simplex virus before transplantation. None of the 13 patients without antibody developed virologic or clinical evidence of primary herpetic involvement after transplant, whereas 95 percent of patients who were seropositive pretransplant shed virus or had clinical disease. Although 90 percent of the patients with positive cultures for herpes simplex virus had clinical lesions, none developed disseminated disease. Rand and associates [189] observed that when cyclosporine-treated patients were compared to patients receiving antithymocyte globulin, the cyclosporine-treated group had significantly less symptomatic illness due to herpes simplex virus in the first six postoperative months. This occurred despite the fact that there was no significant decrease in herpes simplex viral shedding between the two groups.

A controlled trial of intravenous acyclovir in cardiac transplant recipients was reported in 1981 by

Chou and colleagues [39]. Viral cultures of mucocutaneous herpes lesions became negative, and more rapid relief of pain and healing of lesions occurred in five patients given intravenous acyclovir compared to controls. As observed in other transplant groups, however, shedding of herpes simplex virus often occurred after therapy was stopped.

VARICELLA-ZOSTER VIRUS *Renal transplants.* Approximately 7 to 9 percent of renal transplant patients develop clinical varicella-zoster viral infection [165] (see Chapter 35). These infections have occurred from two months to three years posttransplantation. Herpes-zoster infection rarely disseminates in this group and is not associated with the mortality that may be noted in bone marrow transplant patients. Primary varicella infection such as occurs in children, however, may be quite virulent when it occurs in a renal transplant patient [61,101].

*Bone marrow transplants.* In nearly half of all bone marrow transplant patients, a varicella-zoster viral infection develops [8]. The median time to onset posttransplantation reported by the Seattle group was five months (compared to one month for herpes simplex viral infection) [151]. Most infections occurred in the first year posttransplant. Of the untreated cases, one-third had cutaneous dissemination. Twelve percent of those infected in the first four months after transplantation died. Graft-versus-host disease did not appear to predispose to varicella-zoster infection in this series.

*Heart transplants.* In the heart transplant group, Pollard and colleagues [181] found a 22 percent incidence of reactivation of varicella-zoster viral infection (8 of 28 patients). Disease occurred from four weeks to one year posttransplantation. One patient died from disseminated disease. The prolonged duration of skin lesions ($\geq$ 12 weeks) due to varicella-zoster infection sometimes seen in this group has been remarkable [72].

EPSTEIN-BARR VIRUS *Renal transplants.* Cheeseman and coworkers [36] have recently reported their experience with Epstein-Barr virus excretion and disease in renal transplant recipients (see Chapter 35). Of 38 patients, all had pretransplant antibodies to viral capsid antigen, 33 had antibody to Epstein-Barr virus nuclear antigen, and three excreted Epstein-Barr virus on entry to the study. By the fifth month posttransplantation, 40 to 50 percent had detectable excretion of Epstein-Barr virus. Nineteen of 31 cadaver kidney recipients excreted Epstein-Barr virus, as opposed to two of ten patients with living related donors. Increased immunosuppression by the addition of anti-thymocyte globulin also increased the likelihood of Epstein-Barr viral excretion. Fourfold or greater rises in titer of antibodies to viral capsid antigen and early antigen R (restricted) occurred exclusively among patients who received antithymocyte globulin. None of the patients with a rise in viral capsid antigen antibodies or Epstein-Barr virus nuclear antigen antibodies had clinical symptoms that could be attributed to the Epstein-Barr virus; six of the eight patients with a rise in early antigen-restricted antibodies, however, had severe leukopenia, four had fever, and one had pulmonary infiltrates. No correlation between Epstein-Barr viral infection and allograft rejection could be found.

Marker and associates [133] reported the antibody response and clinical illness in 88 renal transplant recipients. Thirty patients had at least a fourfold rise in Epstein-Barr virus antibody posttransplant, and in those with at least an eightfold rise (8 of 88), a high incidence of prolonged posttransplant fever was observed. One patient in the latter group died of a malignant Epstein-Barr viral infection, and lymphoproliferative disease developed in one. Additional evidence of the association of the Epstein-Barr virus with posttransplantation lymphoproliferative disease has recently been reported in renal [45,83,117] as well as cardiac [173,202] transplant patients.

Treatment of renal transplant recipients with Epstein-Barr viral infection has been reported rarely [36]. Cheeseman and colleagues [36] reported a decreased incidence of Epstein-Barr viral excretion in renal transplant recipients treated with human leukocyte interferon. This effect lasted only for the duration of treatment, however.

*Bone marrow transplants.* Lange and coworkers [115] studied 50 bone marrow transplant patients for serologic changes to Epstein-Barr virus. Epstein-Barr viral antibody appeared in patients who were seronegative pretransplant, even when they received marrow from a seronegative donor. This suggested to the authors that plasma transfusions were a source of antibody. Lange's group also showed that, just as in other immunodeficient patients, bone marrow transplant recipients may have abnormally high antibody titers to viral capsid antigen and early antigen. Persistent Epstein-Barr viral infection or reactivation can occur in the presence of preexisting antibody, but clinical disease in this population is uncommon.

*Heart transplants.* Ho and associates [96] and Dummer and colleagues [54] reported on 24 cardiac transplant recipients studied for IgG antibodies to capsid antigen of Epstein-Barr virus at the University of Pittsburgh. Each of the three patients who were seronegative for this antibody pretransplant seroconverted. Symptoms developed in two—one had fever, pulmonary infiltrates, and thrombocytopenia, and one had fever and the development of a histiocytic lymphoma. Of 21 seropositive patients pretransplant, 8 showed a fourfold or greater rise in Epstein-Barr viral antibody; 5 also had clinical symptoms consistent with Epstein-Barr viral infection.

The major concern regarding Epstein-Barr viral infection in cardiac transplant recipients, however, is its association with posttransplant lymphoproliferative disorders [54,173]. Such disorders have occurred in 6 of the 66 cyclosporine-treated transplant recipients studied by Oyer and associates [173] who were transplanted between December 1980 and May 1983 and followed up for a maximum of two and a half years at Stanford University Medical Center. All cases occurred within six months of transplantation. Four of five cases studied had a fourfold or greater rise in Epstein-Barr virus on posttransplantation serologic studies. The genome of Epstein-Barr was incorporated into the tumor-cell DNA of all four patients in whom this assay was performed.

HEPATITIS VIRUSES  *Renal transplants.*  Hepatitis remains a common problem in the renal transplant patient (see Chapter 35). Although the causes of liver test abnormalities in these patients are diverse, including infections (particularly hepatitis B virus, cytomegalovirus, and non-A, non-B hepatitis), drugs (particularly azathioprine), and toxic reactions [56], it is the hepatitis B virus that has been best studied and that remains the most controversial agent for its role in chronic liver disease [224], hepatocellular carcinoma [207], allograft dysfunction [231], and death [92] in these patients. Hepatitis B is common among the staff and patients at most hemodialysis centers [74] (see Chapter 17). Because of this, most renal transplant patients who develop hepatitis B infection do so while still on hemodialysis before transplantation [197,232]. Most posttransplant hepatitis B viral infections, therefore, are due to reactivation of the virus (i.e., an increase in viral shedding to a measurable level) [160]. It appears possible to transmit hepatitis B virus to the few patients who have not been exposed to hepatitis B virus pretransplant by transplantation with a kidney from a hepatitis B surface antigen-positive donor [248]. This occurrence must be rare, however, since only 1.5 percent (3 of 208) of donors tested in one series were hepatitis B surface antigen-positive [233].

The role of active hepatitis B surface antigenemia in either prolonging [190,231] or decreasing [180] renal allograft survival has been controversial. It has been suggested that the ability of the patient with chronic renal failure to form hepatitis B surface antibody may mark the patient as an "immunologic responder" who is more likely to develop graft rejection [126]. Several other prognostic factors that may affect renal allograft function, such as number of pretransplant blood transfusions [171], sex of the donor [125], or HLA phenotype [92], need to be considered in reviewing these series. It would appear, at least in the first one to two years posttransplantation, that the chronic hepatitis B surface antigen excreter is not at undue risk of increased morbidity or mortality in this respect [63]. However, there may be an increased late risk of significant morbidity and mortality (mainly related to liver disease) in patients who are chronically antigenemic with hepatitis B surface antigen.

Another major area of concern related to the hepatitis B surface antigen carrier in renal transplant patients has been the persistent risk these patients pose to others (particularly dialysis staff and patients) because of their prolonged shedding of antigen [33,104,142].

It appears that a significant proportion of liver function test abnormalities in the renal transplant population are due to non-A, non-B hepatitis, although this is still a diagnosis of exclusion [109]. The clinical characteristics are similar to those found in patients with liver abnormalities due to the hepatitis B agent, but it is not clear what role, if any, this agent plays in allograft dysfunction. Cytomegalovirus and occasionally other herpes-group viruses also can cause hepatitis in the renal transplant group. The risk of acquisition of hepatitis A infection has not generally been noted to be increased in renal transplant recipients.

*Other transplants.*  An outbreak of hepatitis considered to be due to the non-A, non-B hepatitis agent or agents has been reported in nine bone marrow transplant patients at the University of Washington [48]. Winston and colleagues [245] make reference to only 3 cases of viral hepatitis among 213 infectious episodes in 63 bone marrow transplant patients, and Atkinson and coworkers [7], in an analysis of infections that occurred six months or longer after bone marrow transplantation, mentioned no cases of viral hepatitis.

It is not clear whether heart or liver transplant patients are at significantly increased risk of hepatitis B infection after transplantation.

PAPOVAVIRUSES  *Renal transplants.*  The human BK virus was first isolated in 1971 from the urine of a renal transplant patient [73]. Since that time other reports have shown urinary excretion of this virus in from 7 to 20 percent of renal transplant patients [97,197], often for prolonged periods of time. In a recent study of 61 renal transplant patients, Hogan and associates [97] demonstrated papovavirus excretion in the urine of 20 percent and seroconversion in 41 percent. Half of these infections were considered to be due to BK virus on the basis of immunofluorescent studies. Infection with this virus occurs commonly in childhood, and most of these BK infections were considered to be secondary to reactivation of virus. The urinary excretion of BK virus was correlated with ureteral stricture, arterial occlusive disease, development of drug-requiring diabetes mellitus, and an increased incidence of allograft dysfunction.

The other half of papovavirus infections noted in the study by Hogan's group were due to the JK virus. This virus is now thought to be the probable agent of progressive multifocal leukoencephalopathy, and several cases of this disease have been reported in renal transplant patients [94,251].

A significant proportion of renal transplant recipients experience clinical infection with the papilloma virus. This virus may produce severe, extensive lesions after transplantation and may be associated with considerable morbidity. Adenovirus infections, particularly of the lung or bladder, have also been documented in renal patients posttransplant [91,106]; (see Chapter 35); disseminated disease may occur, and death has been reported [158,216].

*Infection Due to Fungi*
The incidence of invasive fungal disease in renal transplant series varies widely [96,179,188]. Disease may be due to reactivation of previous fungal disease because of immunosuppression, or to primary infection; these infections usually are of the lungs or brain and occur in the postoperative setting; often, they are nosocomial in origin. Ramsey and associates [188] noted invasive pulmonary infection due to fungi in 5 of 54 renal transplant patients treated with azathioprine and corticosteroids. Ho and colleagues [96], however, reported that only one of 64 renal transplant patients treated with cyclosporine and none of 17 treated with azathioprine and corticosteroids had invasive fungal disease of any type.

Fungal infection is common in bone marrow transplant recipients. Martin and coworkers [139] reviewed the postmortem records of 160 cases and found 55 histologically proven invasive fungal episodes in 48 patients. Thirty-five episodes were disseminated, and *Candida* infections were most common. The major risk factors appeared to be a hypoplastic marrow and prolonged duration of granulocytopenia. A positive correlation was also found between invasive fun-

gal disease and colonization of three or four body sites with fungus. Winston and associates [245] reported that 22 (37 percent) of 60 bone marrow transplant patients had invasive fungal disease. The majority of infections occurred within the first 30 days posttransplant. Sixteen episodes of fungemia occurred. In patients with disseminated candidiasis, risk factors included older age and significantly more surveillance cultures positive for fungi.

Infection due to fungi, especially *Aspergillus,* has been a major problem in cardiac transplant patients, particularly before the advent of cyclosporine [12]. Gurwith and colleagues [81] concluded that this was likely due to the antilymphocyte globulin that these patients received. Although this correlation has not always been substantiated in other transplant populations [153], it appears that the incidence of invasive fungal disease has decreased in cardiac transplantation since the institution of cyclosporine [223]. In the series mentioned previously by Dummer and coworkers [54], only one of 33 cardiac transplant recipients receiving cyclosporine had invasive fungal disease. Oyer and associates [173] reported that 5 of 57 cardiac transplant patients treated with cyclosporine between December 1980 and March 1983 had invasive fungal disease, with death due to fungus in 2 patients.

In a study of 100 consecutive recipients of liver homografts, Schröter [205] reported 29 instances of invasive fungal disease, 12 of which were disseminated to multiple sites. The problem of invasive fungal disease in liver transplant recipients was reconfirmed by Dummer [55], who reported that 11 (42 percent) of 24 liver transplant patients had documented invasive fungal disease.

ASPERGILLUS *Renal transplants.* Infection with *Aspergillus* in the transplant population is most often nosocomial in origin and most often appears either during an episode of neutropenia or after a viral or bacterial pneumonia in a patient treated with broad-spectrum antibiotics. The most common portal of entry and site of infection is the lungs. Ramsey and associates [188] studied 54 renal transplant patients with pulmonary disease and found 5 cases of aspergillosis, 4 of which were invasive. These cases appeared most commonly one to four months posttransplantation, but were also seen later (greater than nine months after) as well. The patients often presented with fever, sweats, nonproductive cough, and dyspnea. Survival was related to duration of infection before diagnosis.

Of the 518 renal transplant patients at the University of Minnesota followed from October 1977 to

September 1981 [179] (average follow-up, 22 months), invasive pulmonary aspergillosis occurred in 14 (2.6 percent). Five patients had only fungal infection—four with *A. fumigatus* and one with *A. flavus*. Of the nine patients in whom aspergillosis occurred as part of a polymicrobial infection, seven instances occurred in association with cytomegalovirus infection and two in association with bacterial pneumonia. Central nervous system involvement occurred in two of these nine patients. *A. fumigatus* was responsible for all six infections in which an antemortem identification of fungus was obtained.

In addition to causing pulmonary disease, *Aspergillus* is an important cause of central nervous system infection. In a study of 20 episodes of central nervous system infection in 300 renal transplant patients, Hooper and associates [98] found *A. fumigatus* to be the second most common cause of central nervous system infection overall, and the most common cause when infection occurred one to four months posttransplantation. *Aspergillus* brain abscess was the most common infectious cause of focal neurologic findings and an altered state of consciousness. In only two of seven patients was *Aspergillus* central nervous system infection diagnosed antemortem, and both patients died in spite of systemic amphotericin B therapy. *Aspergillus* infections in the transplant population should also be considered at sites other than the lung and central nervous system. Infection with this organism often disseminates, and *Aspergillus* has been reported as a cause of wound infections [245], cutaneous lesions [116], and epidural abscess [31].

*Bone marrow transplants.* In a study of 63 bone marrow transplant patients, Winston and colleagues [245] reported six cases of invasive pulmonary aspergillosis, three of which were disseminated. Of interest is that five of these cases occurred within 30 days of the bone marrow transplant, a point that the authors relate to the early onset of profound neutropenia and the early use of broad-spectrum antibiotics. The symptoms were similar to those mentioned previously in renal transplant patients, and three of the six patients died of their fungal infection.

*Heart transplants.* *Aspergillus* infection has also been a major problem of diagnosis and management in the cardiac transplant population. Of a total of 263 heart transplants performed at Stanford University Medical Center through May 1983, *Aspergillus* infection was documented in 56 (21 percent) patients; 32 of these were associated with a fatal outcome [223]. Among the 78 cyclosporine-treated cardiac transplant recipients followed from December 1980 to August 1983 at Stanford University Medical Center, eight cases of invasive pulmonary aspergillosis have been seen [223].

Of the six cases diagnosed antemortem, all were due to *A. fumigatus;* three involved only the lung, and three were disseminated. In the two patients diagnosed only at autopsy, disseminated disease was found. Thus the advent of cyclosporine as primary immunosuppressive therapy in this patient group appears to have decreased invasive disease with this pathogen. Additional evidence comes from the group of 33 cyclosporine-treated cardiac transplant patients from the University of Pittsburgh reported by Dummer and coworkers [54], in which no evidence of invasive aspergillosis was reported.

*Liver transplants.* Invasive aspergillosis has been a significant cause of morbidity and mortality in liver transplant patients. Schröter and associates [205], in a study of 100 consecutive orthotopic liver transplants, documented nine cases of aspergillosis, eight of which involved the lungs. Although *Aspergillus* was disseminated in three of the nine cases, it was felt to be the primary cause of death in only one case.

CANDIDA   *Renal transplants.* *Candida* infection in renal transplant patients has been reported by several authors [179, 188, 200]. Renal transplant patients in whom infection with *Candida* occurs are generally seriously ill or have other viral or bacterial infections simultaneously [179]. In a study of renal transplant patients with fever and pulmonary infiltrates, Ramsey and colleagues [188] did not observe any cases of primary *Candida* infection of the lung. Of 23 patients, however, 5 had pulmonary superinfection with *C. albicans*. All five had been on antibiotics in the week before recognition of pulmonary superinfection, and four of the five had oral candidiasis. In 518 renal transplant recipients reported by Peterson and coworkers [179], no cases of primary systemic *Candida* infection were observed. Eight patients with cytomegalovirus infection developed deep-seated *Candida* infection, however, and systemic candidiasis was diagnosed in an additional four patients with other types of polymicrobial infections. All 12 isolates were considered to be of nosocomial origin. *C. albicans* and *glabrata* (also referred to as *Torulopsis glabrata*) were the most common isolates.

*Bone marrow transplants.* *Candida* species are the most common cause of fungemia in the bone marrow transplant population. Meyers and Thomas [151] reported that 12 percent of all positive blood cultures taken before day 50 post–bone marrow transplantation were due to *Candida* species. After day 50, this percentage increased to 28 percent, which suggested to the authors that the frequency of *Candida* infections increased in patients with prolonged granulocytopenia. Winston and associates [245], however, found an earlier peak in the time of appearance of candidemia in their series. *Candida* species were responsible for 12 of 14 episodes of fungemia that occurred within the first 30 days posttransplantation. Only two additional cases of fungemia occurred more than 30 days posttransplantation, one of which was due to *Candida*. In patients with disseminated *Candida* infection, a significantly greater number of surveillance cultures were positive for *Candida* before the initiation of conditioning therapy, a large number of urine and stool cultures revealed *Candida* at the time of infection, and oral candidiasis was more common. An increased risk of invasive fungal infection was not associated with sex, corticosteroid therapy, trimethoprim-sulfamethoxazole use, leukopenia, or duration of disease. Mortality was 85 percent in patients with candidemia. Other sites of invasive candidiasis were lung (three cases), esophagus (three cases), and peritoneum (one case).

*Heart transplants.* At Stanford University Medical Center, 17 cardiac transplant patients with *Candida* infection were observed through May 1983 [223]. In eight of the cases, the fungal infection was associated with a fatal outcome. The majority of these infections occurred before the standard use of cyclosporine. Since 1980 only two cyclosporine-treated patients with *Candida* infection have been observed; one had pulmonary and the other had mediastinal involvement.

*Liver transplants.* *Candida* also poses a major problem in patients with liver transplants. Schröter and colleagues [205] described 18 patients with disease due to *Candida;* eight had disseminated and ten had local infection. Of the eight patients with disseminated infection, the most common sites of invasion were lung (seven cases), heart (six cases), esophagus (six cases), and peritoneum (five cases). Five of these patients also had positive blood cultures. Although all eight patients with disseminated infection died, the infection could only be implicated as the primary cause of death in one patient. Localized disease was found most commonly in the kidney or peritoneal cavity. In all 18 patients, damage to the gastrointestinal tract or a surgical complication was felt to be present before infection. Of 44 liver transplant patients studied by Ho and coworkers [96], serious fungal infections were found in 44 percent. Seventy percent were due to *Candida* species; three had disseminated infection, six had fungemia, seven had abdominal infection, and three had lung involvement. In the same publication the authors reported that only one of 64 renal transplant patients and only one of 33 cardiac transplant patients taking cyclosporine had documented fungal infection.

CRYPTOCOCCUS *Renal transplants.* *C. neoformans* represents the most common cause of fungal central nervous system infection in renal transplant patients. Except for *L. monocytogenes,* it is the most common cause of central nervous system infection in this patient group [98,227]. It most typically causes a subacute to chronic meningitis and may present with few clinical signs or symptoms. It appears most often in the late posttransplant period. In the 678 renal transplant patients observed over a 20-year period (March 1961 to January 1980) and reviewed by Tilney and associates [227], six cases of cerebral cryptococcosis were observed. One of these six patients died of cryptococcal central nervous system infection. In a review of 300 renal transplant patients from 1969 to 1979, Hooper and colleagues [98] reported 20 patients with central nervous system infections. *Cryptococcus* accounted for six infections, all of which occurred more than four months posttransplantation. Clinical symptoms such as fever and headache could not differentiate cryptococcal from *Listeria* meningitis; *Listeria,* however, occurred most often in the early posttransplant period and was associated with a higher rate of leukopenia and the use of high-dose corticosteroids. Cough or changes on the chest x-ray, in addition to the findings of fever or headache, suggested to the authors the possibility of cryptococcal disease, since a respiratory route of infection was common. Therapy with both amphotericin and 5-fluorocytosine has been recommended, although therapy with amphotericin alone may be curative [98]. *C. neoformans* may also cause widespread disseminated disease in the transplant patient. This is especially true in the renal transplant patient, in whom skin [103,114], soft tissue [118], bone, and urinary tract infections [86] are not uncommonly seen. A diagnosis of cryptococcal infection in any of these sites should alert the physician to the strong possibility of concurrent central nervous system infection.

*Other transplants.* *C. neoformans* has not been a common pathogen in recent series of bone marrow [245], cardiac [84,223], or liver [84,206] transplant recipients. Two of 78 cyclosporine-treated cardiac transplant recipients followed since December 1980 at Stanford University Medical Center have had cryptococcal lung infection [223] and one of 24 liver transplant patients reported by Dummer and coworkers [55] from the University of Pittsburgh had cryptococcal meningitis.

COCCIDIOIDES *Renal transplants.* Although most areas of the country have little if any problem with this infection, areas in the southwestern United States, where this disease is endemic, have reported significant morbidity and mortality due to *Coccidioides immitis*. At the Univeristy of Arizona, Cohen and associates [40] reported 18 cases (6.9 percent) of coccidioidomycosis among 260 renal transplant patients followed over a ten-year period (1970 to 1979). The annual incidence was highest in the first year after transplantation. Five patients had disease within two months of their transplantation. Infection occurred most often by reactivation. Thirteen patients had extrapulmonary dissemination; arthritis and meningitis were the most common sites. Diagnosis was most often substantiated by positive cultures from bronchoscopy; routine sputum cultures yielded the fungus on culture in only one case. Urine culture was positive for *Coccidioides* in eight of ten individuals with disseminated disease. In most cases, serologic testing was useful only for confirmation of the diagnosis and for prognosis. Mortality was 63 percent overall and was 72 percent when disseminated disease was present—even when patients were treated with systemic antifungal therapy. Male sex and the presence of blood type B were risk factors found to be associated with an increased incidence of dissemination. The authors concluded that renal transplantation may be performed in areas endemic for coccidioidomycosis with a reasonably low risk of this disease. At present, however, when feasible, they advise against transplanting patients with a known past symptomatic infection with *Coccidioides;* they also advise patients transplanted outside an endemic area not to move to or visit endemic areas. Treatment must be prolonged since relapse is common in survivors. Other authors have suggested the discontinuation of immunosuppressive therapy because of the high mortality with this disease [105].

*Other transplants.* Although capable of causing disease in other transplant populations, coccidioidomycosis has not been observed in recent series of bone [245], heart [223], or liver transplants [205,206].

PHYCOMYCETES Mucormycosis accounts for only a small portion of fungal infections reported in transplant patients. At Stanford University Medical Center, only one patient with *Mucor* and two with *Rhizopus* infections have been seen among 263 heart transplant patients through May of 1983 [223]. Peterson and associates [179] reported one case of rhinocerebral mucormycosis among 518 renal transplant patients at the University of Minnesota, and Dummer and colleagues [55] at the University of Pittsburgh reported one case of invasive *Mucor* infection in a liver transplant patient who also had *Candida* peritonitis.

OTHER FUNGI Like coccidioidomycosis, infection of transplant patients with *Histoplasma capsulatum* occurs most often in outbreaks of this disease in endemic areas [46,240]. Wheat and associates [240], at the Indiana University Medical Center in Indianapolis, reported ten episodes of histoplasmosis in eight renal allograft recipients. These cases occurred during an outbreak of histoplasmosis in Indianapolis. This represented a risk for acquisition of histoplasmosis of 2.1 percent among the 379 allograft recipients followed during the outbreak, compared with a baseline risk of acquisition of 0.5 percent in allograft patients during the two years preceding the outbreak. The disease was most often primary. Fever and respiratory symptoms were common. Dissemination was documented in seven of the nine patients. Of interest is the fact that central nervous system involvement, a rare clinical manifestation of histoplasmosis in normal populations, was observed in three of the nine patients. Two of the five cases of histoplasmosis in renal allograft recipients reported by Davies and coworkers [46] also had central nervous system involvement. In the Indiana series, azathioprine was discontinued in seven patients, and all were treated with systemic amphotericin B for two to three months. This resulted in clinical cure in seven cases with a follow-up of at least six months.

To our knowledge, only one case of blastomycosis (causing pneumonia only) has been reported in transplant patients. Young and coworkers [250] described an infection due to *Phoma* species that occurred in a patient with a transplanted kidney who had been maintained on prolonged immunosuppressive therapy before the clinical appearance of the infection. *Pencillium* species caused pulmonary lesions in one heart transplant patient at Stanford University Medical Center.

### Infection Due to Nocardia

*Renal transplants.* Opportunistic infection due to *Nocardia* has caused serious morbidity and death in renal transplant patients. Nosocomial *Nocardia* infection of renal transplant patients appeared to occur by person-to-person transmission in an outbreak of nocardiosis in eight patients on a urology ward at St. Peters Group of Hospitals in London, England [127]. Low-grade fever, pleuritic chest pain, and nonproductive cough were the most common symptoms; pulmonary nodules or cavities were the most common chest x-ray abnormalities. Only one patient had cerebral involvement in this series. Diagnosis was made in all cases by culture of the organism, and all strains were identical by biochemical, physical, and immunologic testing [222]. The authors also found serologic testing helpful but stressed the importance of the retention of clinical specimens for at least seven days in the hope of isolating *Nocardia* by culture.

*Heart transplants.*   A retrospective study of 160 cardiac transplant patients at Stanford University Medical Center between January 1968 and December 1978 revealed 21 (13 percent) with nocardiosis [212]. The lung was the primary and only detectable site of infection in 17 (81 percent). There were three cases of disseminated disease, all to soft tissue, and none had central nervous system involvement. The time of onset of infection following transplantation ranged from 43 to 982 days, with no specific peak. No deaths were attributable to nocardial infection. Among the 78 cardiac transplant recipients treated with cyclosporine since December 1980 at Stanford University Medical Center, three (3.8 percent) cases of nocardiosis occurred [223]. Two cases had lung involvement only, and one case had dissemination to soft tissue.

*Other transplants.*   *Nocardia* infections have not been a problem in recent series of bone marrow [245] or liver [55,207] transplant patients.

### Infection Due to Protozoa

TOXOPLASMA GONDII   *Heart transplants.*   Infection with *T. gondii* in transplant patients has been best studied in recipients of cardiac allografts. The trans-

planted heart was considered to be the source of *Toxoplasma* infection in two cardiac transplant recipients reported by Ryning and associates [201] in 1979. Both recipients were seronegative for past exposure to *Toxoplasma* and received hearts from donors that had serologic evidence of recent *Toxoplasma* infection. Another seronegative cardiac transplant patient who received a heart from a seropositive donor and acquired *Toxoplasma* infection was reported by Rose and colleagues [196]. In this febrile patient, *T. gondii* was demonstrated by endomyocardial biopsy.

In a study of 50 heart or heart-lung transplant patients at Stanford University Medical Center between 1976 and 1982, Luft and coworkers [130] reported three cases of primary *Toxoplasma* infection and ten cases most likely due to reactivation of the latent infection (Table 37-6). Of 31 patients who were seronegative before transplantation, four received a heart from a seropositive donor. Three of these four patients had clinical disease: one had encephalopathy and abnormal liver function tests, one had fever and endomyocardial involvement, and one had chorioretinitis initially, which later progressed to brain abscesses. None of the 27 patients who were seronegative before transplantation and who received a heart from a seronegative donor had clinical disease or seroconversion, but 10 of the 19 patients who had pretransplant antibodies against *T. gondii* developed

TABLE 37-6. Toxoplasmosis after cardiac transplantation

| Transplant number | Recipient Titer Before Transplant | | Donor Titer | | Peak Recipient Titer after Transplant | | Symptoms due to *Toxoplasma* infection |
|---|---|---|---|---|---|---|---|
| | Dye test | DS-IgM-ELISA [210] | Dye test | DS-IgM-ELISA | Dye test | DS-IgM-ELISA | |
| 115 | Neg | Neg | 256 | NA | 16,384 | 4096 | Chorioretinitis brain abscesses |
| 123 | Neg | Neg | 512 | NA | 256 | 1024 | Fever endomyocarditis |
| 189 | Neg | Neg | 32 | Neg | 128 | 64 | LFT abnormalities encephalopathy |
| 75 | 32 | Neg | Neg | Neg | 256 | 4096 | None |
| 95 | 16 | Neg | NA | NA | 512 | 256 | None |
| 128 | 8 | Neg | NA | NA | 128 | NC | None |
| 130 | 16 | Neg | NA | NA | 512 | NC | None |
| 152 | 256 | Neg | NA | NA | 4096 | NC | None |
| 155 | 128 | Neg | NA | NA | 512 | NC | None |
| 194 | 16 | Neg | Neg | Neg | 2048 | 256 | None |
| 195 | 32 | Neg | Neg | Neg | 512 | 256 | None |
| 198 | 64 | Neg | Neg | Neg | 512 | NC | None |
| 233 | 32 | Neg | Neg | Neg | 1024 | NC | None |

NA = not available; NC = no change; LFT =
*Source:* Luft, B. J., et al. *Ann. Intern. Med.* 99:27, 1983.

a significant, (fourfold or greater) rise in antibodies, including 4 who developed significant IgM antibodies. The peak antibody titers occurred most often around the sixth week posttransplantation and were seen more commonly in patients who received antithymocyte globulin, azathioprine, and corticosteroids than in those receiving cyclosporine and corticosteroids. None of these ten patients had clinically manifest disease, and none required treatment for toxoplasmosis.

The experience reported with cardiac transplant recipients at Papworth Hospital in England [161] appears to provide additional evidence for the occurrence of primary *Toxoplasma* infection in this transplant group, presumably due to transfer of viable parasites within the donor heart muscle. *Toxoplasma* antibody was detectable in 18 (35 percent) of 51 cardiac transplant recipients and 10 (26 percent) of 39 donors pretransplant. Of the four seronegative recipients who received a heart from a seropositive donor and in whom follow-up serum was available, three were considered to have acute *Toxoplasma* infection, and two of these died as a result of their infection. As was true for the Stanford experience, no clinical *Toxoplasma* infections occurred in patients initially seropositive to *Toxoplasma* or in those who were seronegative and transplanted with a heart from a seronegative donor.

*Other transplants.* *Toxoplasma* infection in renal transplant patients has been reviewed by Herb and coworkers [88]. All seven patients reported in this series had a systemic illness characterized by central nervous system and respiratory abnormalities. In each of the seven, *Toxoplasma* was demonstrated in sections of brain. Transmission of *T. gondii* by renal transplantation has been reported by Meija and associates [145]. Two renal allograft recipients who had no serologic evidence of previous exposure to *Toxoplasma* and who received their organs from the same seropositive cadaver donor developed acute *Toxoplasma* infection shortly after transplantation.

PNEUMOCYSTIS CARINII    *Renal transplants.* Historically, the incidence of *P. carinii* pneumonia in renal transplant populations has averaged 10 percent [51,58]. The incidence has decreased, however, in most recent series [179,188]. In a study of 518 renal transplant recipients at the University of Minnesota from 1977 to 1981, Peterson and colleagues [179] reported only one case of *P. carinii* pneumonia. This low incidence may reflect the routine use of prophylactic trimethoprim-sulfamethoxazole in this series. Ramsey and associates [188] from the Massachusetts General Hos-

pital reported only two patients with *P. carinii* infection among 227 patients who were followed from 1966 to 1978. In this study, trimethoprim-sulfamethoxazole was used either prophylactically in patients with symptomatic cytomegalovirus infection (because of the recognized close association between the occurrence of cytomegalovirus and the development of *Pneumocystis* infection) [35] or as long-term treatment of pyelonephritis. Of note is the fact that the incidence of *Pneumocystis* infection was also reported to be low in transplant patients who did not receive prophylaxis with trimethoprim-sulfamethoxazole. In the patients included in this report, primary immunosuppressive therapy was with azathioprine and corticosteroids. In a study from the University of Pittsburgh [96], 3.4 percent of renal allograft recipients on azathioprine and 9 percent on cyclosporine had *P. carinii* pneumonia. Prophylactic trimethoprim-sulfamethoxazole was not used during the period of this study.

*Bone marrow transplants.* Next to cytomegalovirus infection, *P. carinii* represents the most common identifiable cause of interstitial pneumonitis in bone marrow transplant recipients. Of the first 377 allogeneic bone marrow transplant patients at the University of Washington in Seattle, 30 patients (8 percent) had *Pneumocystis* infection of the lung documented by biopsy or autopsy [151]. An additional study by the same group showed a significant lower incidence (1 percent) in syngeneic bone marrow transplant patients [2]. The median time to onset in allogeneic transplants was nine weeks, with a range that overlaps that of other known causes of interstitial pneumonia. This fact, plus the observation that clinical symptoms and x-ray changes are often indistinguishable from other causes of nonbacterial pneumonia, made diagnosis difficult. Most experts recommend open lung biopsy for diagnosis in this setting [151]. Simultaneous infection with other organisms, especially cytomegalovirus, was common and markedly increased mortality.

Prophylaxis with oral trimethoprim-sulfamethoxazole has resulted in a marked reduction of *Pneumocystis* infections in bone marrow transplant patients [151,245]. At the University of Washington [151], only three cases of *P. carinii* pneumonia were reported among over 200 bone marrow transplant patients who were receiving trimethoprim-sulfamethoxazole prophylaxis. A total daily dose of 150 mg/M$^2$ (trimethoprim component) was given orally, starting when the patient had 500 circulating neutrophils and continuing through day 120 posttransplantation. In a separate study, Winston and associates [245] reported that none of 30 allogeneic bone marrow transplant patients treated with trimethoprim-sulfamethoxazole, three tablets three times a day for two consecutive days each week, developed *P. carinii* pneumonia, compared to three (38 percent) of eight patients who took no prophylaxis.

*Heart transplants.* The incidence of *Pneumocystis* infection among cardiac transplant recipients has markedly decreased since the advent of routine use of cyclosporine. At the Stanford University Medical Center, 32 episodes of *Pneumocystis* pneumonia occurred in 30 of the first 263 patients [223]. Most of these patients were receiving azathioprine and prednisone, and many also received antithymocyte globulin. Among the 78 patients treated with cyclosporine since December 1980 and followed through August 1983, no cases of *Pneumocystis* pneumonia have been observed. None of these patients have received prophylactic trimethoprim-sulfamethoxazole. At the University of Pittsburgh, only one case of pneumocystosis has occurred in 33 cardiac transplant patients receiving cyclosporine [54].

*Other transplants.* Among 93 orthotopic liver transplants performed at the University of Colorado, 10 cases (11 percent) of *Pneumocystis* pneumonia were seen [206]. The majority of these cases received azathioprine, prednisone, and antilymphocyte globulin.

### Infection Due to Parasites

*Strongyloides stercoralis* usually infects only the mucosa of the small intestine. Hyperinfection, or invasion of other organs by filariform larvae, usually occurs only in the compromised host [209]. Several recent case reports have demonstrated the ability of this parasite to cause systemic infection or death in renal allograft recipients [100,209,239]. Weller and associates [239] reported two cases of overwhelming infection in renal transplant patients who had previously visited endemic tropical areas, and commented on the relation of these infections to the use of high-dose corticosteroids. One patient died of this disease even after conventional doses of thiabendazole were used, which led the authors to suggest long-term therapy monitored by frequent examination of concentrated stool samples in this immunosuppressed group.

Hoy and coworkers [100] reported two cases of strongyloidiasis in patients who had received allografts from the same donor. One patient who received a standard course of thiabendazole died; the second patient, who received multiple courses of this drug, survived. It appears that this parasite should be added to the growing list of bacterial [52,132], viral [18],

fungal [170], and protozoal [201] pathogens that may be transmitted with the transplanted organ.

## REFERENCES

1. Andrus, C. H., Betts, R. F., May, A. G., and Freeman, R. B. Cytomegalovirus infection blocks the beneficial effect of pretransplant blood transfusion on renal allograft survival. *Transplantation* 28:451, 1979.
2. Applebaum, F. R., Meyers, J. D., Fefer, A., Fluornoy, N., Cheever, M. A., Greenberg, P. D., Hackman, R., and Thomas, E. D. Nonbacterial nonfungal pneumonia following marrow transplantation in 100 identical twins. *Transplantation* 33:265, 1982.
3. Armstrong, J. A., Evans, A. S., Rao, N., and Ho, M. Viral infections in renal transplant recipients. *Infect. Immun.* 14:970, 1976.
4. Armstrong, J. A., Tarr, G. C., Youngblood, L. A., Dowling, J. N., Saslow, A. R., Lucas, J. P., and Ho, M. Cytomegalovirus infection in children undergoing open heart surgery. *Yale J. Biol. Med.* 49:83, 1976.
5. Ascher, N. L., Simmons, R. L., Marker, S., Klugman, J., and Najarian, J. S. Tuberculosis joint disease in transplant patients. *Am. J. Surg.* 135:853, 1978.
6. Ashraf, M. H., Campalani, G. C., Qureshi, S. A., Froud, D. J., and Yacoub, M. H. Acyclovir in treatment of cytomegalovirus pneumonia after cardiac transplantation (letter). *Lancet* 1:173, 1982.
7. Atkinson, K., Farewell, V., Storb, R., Tsoi, M. S., Sullivan, K. M., Witherspoon, R. P., Fefer, A., Clift, R., Goodell, B., and Thomas, E. D. Analysis of late infections after human bone marrow transplantation: Role of genotypic nonidentity between marrow donor and recipient and of nonspecific suppressor cells in patients with chronic graft-versus-host disease. *Blood* 60:714, 1982.
8. Atkinson, K., Meyers, J. D., Storb, R., Prentice, R. L., and Thomas, E. D. Varicella-zoster virus infection after marrow transplantation for aplastic anemia or leukemia. *Transplantation* 29:47, 1980.
9. Balfour, H. H., Jr. Cytomegalovirus: The troll of transplantation (editorial). *Arch. Intern. Med.* 139:279, 1979.
10. Balfour, H. H., Jr., Slade, M. S., Kalis, J. M., Howard, R. J., Simmons, R. L., and Najarian,

J. S. Viral infections in renal transplant donors and their recipients: A prospective study. *Surgery* 81:487, 1977.

11. Batata, M. A. Pulmonary tuberculosis in a renal transplant recipient. *J.A.M.A.* 237:1465, 1977.

12. Baumgartner, W. A., Reitz, B. A., Oyer, P. E., Stinson, E. B., and Shumway, N. E. Cardiac homotransplantation. *Curr. Probl. Surg.* 16:39, 1979.

13. Bayer, W. L., and Tegtmeier, G. E. The blood donor: Detection and magnitude of cytomegalovirus carrier states and the prevalence of cytomegalovirus antibody. *Yale J. Biol. Med.* 49:5, 1976.

14. Bell, T. J., and Williams, G. B. Successful treatment of tuberculosis in renal transplant recipients. *J. R. Soc. Med.* 71:265, 1978.

15. Bennett, W. M., Beck, C. H., Jr., and Young, H. H. Bacteriuria in the first month following renal transplantation. *Arch. Surg.* 101:453, 1970.

16. Betts, R. F. Cytomegalovirus infection in transplant patients. *Prog. Med. Virol.* 28:44, 1982.

17. Betts, R. F., Freeman, R. B., Douglas, R. G., Jr., and Talley, T. E. Clinical manifestations of renal allograft-derived primary cytomegalovirus infection. *Am. J. Dis. Child.* 131:759, 1977.

18. Betts, R. F., Freeman, R. B., Douglas, R. G., Jr., Talley, T. E., and Rundell, B. Transmission of cytomegalovirus infection with renal allograft. *Kidney Int.* 8:385, 1975.

19. Bolivar, R., Satterwhite, T. K., and Floyd, M. Cutaneous lesions due to *Mycobacterium kansasii*. *Arch. Dermatol.* 116:207, 1980.

20. Bore, P. J., Sells, R. A., and Jameson, V. Transfusion-induced renal allograft protection. *Transplant. Proc.* 11:148, 1979.

21. Bottone, E. J., and Sierra, M. F. *Listeria monocytogenes:* Another look at the "Cinderella" among pathogenic bacteria. *Mt. Sinai J. Med.* (N.Y.) 44:42, 1977.

22. Bourgault, A. M., Van Scoy, R. E., Wilkowske, C. J., and Sterioff, S. Severe infection due to *Streptococcus pneumoniae* in asplenic renal transplant patients. *Mayo Clin. Proc.* 54:123, 1979.

23. Braun, W. E., and Nankervis, G. Cytomegalovirus viremia and bacteremia in renal-allograft recipients. *N. Engl. J. Med.* 299:1318, 1978.

24. Briggs, J. D., Canavan, J. S. F., Dick, H. M., Hamilton, D. N. H., Kyle, K. F., Macpherson, S. G., Paton, A. M., and Titterington, D. M. Influence of HLA match and blood transfusion on renal allograft survival. *Transplantation* 25:80, 1978.

25. Britt, R. H., Enzmann, D. R., and Remington, J. S. Intracranial infection in cardiac transplant recipients. *Ann. Neurol.* 9:107, 1981.

26. Buckner, C. D., Clift, R. A., Sanders, J. E., Meyers, J. D., Counts, G. W., Farewell, V. T., and Thomas, E. D. Protective environment for marrow transplant recipients: A prospective study. *Ann. Intern. Med.* 89:893, 1978.

27. Bunjes, D., Hardt, C., Rollinghoff, M., and Wagner, H. Cyclosporin A mediates immunosuppression of primary cytotoxic T cell responses by impairing the release of interleukin 1 and interleukin 2. *Eur. J. Immunol.* 11:657, 1981.

28. Burgos-Calderon, R., Pankey, G. A., and Figueroa, J. E. Infection in kidney transplantation. *Surgery* 70:334, 1971.

29. Butler, W. T., and Rossen, R. D. Effects of corticosteroids on immunity in man. *J. Clin. Invest.* 52:2629, 1973.

30. Byrd, L. H., Cheigh, J. S., Stenzel, K. H., Tapia, L., Aronian, J., and Rubin, A. L. Association between *Streptococcus faecalis* urinary infections and graft rejection in kidney transplantation. *Lancet* 2:1167, 1978.

31. Byrd, B. F., III, Weiner, M. H., and McGee, Z. A. *Aspergillus* spinal epidural abscess. *J.A.M.A.* 248:3138, 1982.

32. Calne, R. Y., Thiru, S., McMaster, P., Craddock, G. N., White, D. J. G., Evans, D. B., Dunn, D. C., Pentlow, B. D., and Rolles, K. Cyclosporin A in patients receiving renal allografts from cadaver donors. *Lancet* 2:1323, 1978.

33. Chan, M. K., and Moorhead, J. F. Hepatitis B and the dialysis and renal transplantation unit. *Nephron* 27:229, 1981.

34. Charpentier, B., Salmon, R., Arvis, G., and Fries, D. Tuberculous acute colitis in kidney-transplant patient (letter). *Lancet* 2:308, 1979.

35. Chatterjee, S. N., Fiala, M., Weiner, J., Stewart, J. A., Stacey, B., and Warner, N. Primary cytomegalovirus and opportunistic infections: Incidence in renal transplant recipients. *J.A.M.A.* 240:2446, 1978.

36. Cheeseman, S. H., Henle, W., Rubin, R. H., Tolkoff-Rubin, N. E., Cosimi, B., Cantell, K., Winkle, S., Herrin, J. T., Black, P. H., Russell, P. S., and Hirsch, M. S. Epstein-Barr virus infection in renal transplant recipients: Effects of antithymocyte globulin and interferon. *Ann. Intern. Med.* 93:39, 1980.

37. Cheeseman, S. H., Rubin, R. H., Stewart, J. A., Tolkoff-Rubin, N. E., Cosimi, A. B., Cantell, K., Gilbert, J., Winkle, S., Herrin, J. T.,

Black, P. H., Russell, P. S., and Hirsch, M. S. Controlled clinical trial of prophylactic human-leukocyte interferon in renal transplantation: Effects on cytomegalovirus and herpes simplex virus infection. *N. Engl. J. Med.* 300:1345, 1979.

38. Cheeseman, S. H., Stewart, J. A., Winkle, S., Cosimi, A. B., Tolkoff-Rubin, N. E., Russell, P. S., Baker, G. P., Herrin, J., and Rubin, R. H. Cytomegalovirus excretion 2–14 years after renal transplantation. *Transplant. Proc.* 11:71, 1979.

39. Chou, S., Gallagher, J. G., and Merigan, T. C. Controlled clinical trial of intravenous acyclovir in heart-transplant patients with mucocutaneous herpes simplex infections. *Lancet* 1:1392, 1981.

40. Cohen, I. M., Galgiani, J. N., Potter, D., and Ogden, D. A. Coccidioidomycosis in renal replacement therapy. *Arch. Intern. Med.* 142:489, 1982.

41. Condie, R. M., Hall, B. L., Howard, R. J., Fryd, D., Simmons, R. L., and Najarian, J. S. Treatment of life-threatening infections in renal transplant recipients with high-dose intravenous human IgG. *Transplant. Proc.* 11:66, 1979.

42. Copeland, J., Wieden, M., Feinberg, W., Salomon, N., Hager, D., and Galgiani, J. Legionnaires' disease following cardiac transplantation. *Chest* 79:669, 1981.

43. Cosimi, A. B., Wortis, H. H., Delmonico, F. L., and Russell, P. S. Randomized clinical trial of antithymocyte globulin in cadaver renal allograft recipients: Importance of T cell monitoring. *Surgery* 80:155, 1976.

44. Coutts, I. I., Jegarajah, S., and Stark, J. E. Tuberculosis in renal transplant recipients. *Br. J. Dis. Chest* 73:141, 1979.

45. Crawford, D. H., Thomas, J. A., Janossy, G., Sweny, P., Fernando, O. N., Moorhead, J. F., and Thompson, J. H. Epstein-Barr virus nuclear antigen positive lymphoma after cyclosporin A treatment in patient with renal allograft (letter). *Lancet* 1:1355, 1980.

46. Davies, S. F., Sarosi, G. A., Peterson, P. K., Khan, M., Howard, R. J., Simmons, R. L., and Najarian, J. S. Disseminated histoplasmosis in renal transplant recipients. *Am. J. Surg.* 137:686, 1979.

47. Davis, B. R., Brumbach, J., Sanders, W. J., and Wolinsky, E. Skin lesions caused by *Mycobacterium haemophilum*. *Ann. Intern. Med.* 97:723, 1982.

48. Dienstag, J. L. Non-A, non-B hepatitis. *Adv. Intern. Med.* 26:187, 1980.

49. Dijkmans, B. A., Versteeg, J., Kauffmann, R. H., van den Broek, P. J., Eernisse, J. G., van Zanten, J. J., Bakker, W., Kalff, M. W., and van Hooff, J. P. Treatment of cytomegalovirus pneumonitis with hyperimmune plasma (letter). *Lancet* 1:820, 1979.

50. Diosi, P., Moldovan, E., and Tomescu, N. Latent cytomegalovirus infection in blood donors. *Br. Med. J.* 4:660, 1969.

51. Doak, P., Becroft, D., Harris, E., Hitchcock, G., Laeming, B., North, J., Montgomerie, J., and Whitlock, R. *Pneumocystis carinii* pneumonia-transplant lung, *Q. J. Med.* 42:59, 1973.

52. Dong, R. L., Boyd, P. J. R., and Eykyn, S. *Staphylococcus aureus* transmitted in transplanted kidneys. *Lancet* 2:243, 1975.

53. Dowling, J. N., Saslow, A. R., Armstrong, J. A., and Ho, M. Cytomegalovirus infection in patients receiving immunosuppressive therapy for rheumatologic disorders. *J. Infect. Dis.* 133:399, 1976.

54. Dummer, J. S., Bahnson, H. T., Griffith, B. P., Hardesty, R. L., Thompson, M. E., and Ho, M. Infections in patients on cyclosporine and prednisone following cardiac transplantation. *Transplant. Proc.* (In press.)

55. Dummer, J. S., Hardy, A., Poorsattai, A., and Ho, M. Early infections in kidney, heart, and liver transplant recipients on cyclosporine. *Transplantation* 36:259, 1983.

56. Editorial. Immunosuppression and hepatitis after renal transplantation. *Br. Med. J.* 1:1102, 1979.

57. Egbert, P. R., Pollard, R. B., Gallagher, J. G., and Merigan, T. C. Cytomegalovirus retinitis in immunosuppressed hosts. II. Ocular manifestations. *Ann. Intern. Med.* 93:664, 1980.

58. Eickhoff, T. Infectious complications in renal transplant recipients. *Transplant. Proc.* 5:1233, 1973.

59. Elliott, W. C., Houghton, D. C., Bryant, R. E., Wicklund, R., Barry, J. M., and Bennett, W. M. Herpes simplex type 1 hepatitis in renal transplantation. *Arch. Intern. Med.* 140:1656, 1980.

60. European Multicenter Trial, Preliminary Results. Cyclosporin A as sole immunosuppressive agent in recipients of kidney allografts from cadaver donors. *Lancet* 2:57, 1982.

61. Feldhoff, C. M., Balfour, H. H., Jr., Simmons, R. L., Najarian, J. S., and Mauer, S. M. Varicella in children with renal transplants. *J. Pediatr.* 98:25, 1981.

62. Fiala, M., Payne, J., Berne, T. V., Moore, T.

C., Henle, W., Montgomerie, J. Z., Chatterjee, S. N., and Guze, L. B. Epidemiology of cytomegalovirus infection after transplantation and immunosuppression. *J. Infect. Dis.* 132:421, 1975.

63. Fine, R. N., Malekzadeh, M. H., Pennisi, A. J., Uittenbogaart, C. H., Ettenger, R. B., Landing, B. H., and Wright, H. T. HBs antigenemia in renal allograft recipients. *Ann. Surg.* 185:411, 1977.

64. Flight, R. J. Listeriosis in Auckland. *N. Z. Med. J.* 73:349, 1971.

65. Foster, R. S., Jr., Winn, W. C., Jr., Marshall, W., and Gump, D. W. Legionnaires' disease following renal transplantation. *Transplant Proc.* 11:93, 1979.

66. Foucar, E., Mukai, K., Foucar, K., Sutherland, D. E., and Van Buren, C. T. Colon ulceration in lethal cytomegalovirus infection. *Am. J. Clin. Pathol.* 76:788, 1981.

67. Franzin, G., Muolo, A., and Griminelli, T. Cytomegalovirus inclusions in the gastroduodenal mucosa of patients after renal transplantation. *Gut* 22:698, 1981.

68. Frenkel, J. K., Nelson, B. M., and Arias-Stella, T. Immunosuppression and toxoplasmic encephalitis: Clinical experimental aspects. *Hum. Pathol.* 6:97, 1975.

69. Friedman, H. M. Cytomegalovirus: Subclinical infection or disease? *Am. J. Med.* 70:215, 1981.

70. Fryd, D. S., Peterson, P. K., Ferguson, R. M., Simmons, R. L., Balfour, H. H., Jr., and Najarian, J. S. Cytomegalovirus as a risk factor in renal transplantation. *Transplantation* 30:436, 1980.

71. Gadler, H., Sundvist, V., Tillegard, A., and Wahren, B. Studies of cytomegalovirus infection in renal allograft recipients. *Scand. J. Infect. Dis.* 14:89, 1982.

72. Gallagher, J. G., and Merigan, T. C. Prolonged herpes-zoster infection associated with immunosuppressive therapy. *Ann. Intern. Med.* 91:842, 1979.

73. Gardner, S. D., Field, A. M., Coleman, D. V., and Hulme, B. New human papovavirus (B.K.) isolated from urine after renal transplantation. *Lancet* 1:1253, 1971.

74. Garibaldi, R. A., Forrest, J. N., Bryan, J. A., Hanson, B. F., and Dismukes, W. E. Hemodialysis-associated hepatitis. *J.A.M.A.* 225:384, 1973.

75. Glazer, J. P., Friedman, H. M., Grossman, R. A., Starr, S. E., Barker, C. F., Perloff, L. J., Huang, E. S., and Plotkin, S. A. Live cytomegalovirus vaccination of renal transplant candi-

dates: A preliminary trial. *Ann. Intern. Med.* 91:676, 1979.

76. Glenn, J. Cytomegalovirus infections following renal transplantation. *Rev. Infect. Dis.* 3:1151, 1981.

77. Goldstein, J. D., Keller, J. I., Winn, W. C., Jr., and Myerowitz, R. L. Sporadic Legionellaceae pneumonia in renal transplant recipients: A survey of 70 autopsies, 1964 to 1979. *Arch. Pathol. Lab. Med.* 106:108, 1982.

78. Gombert, M. R., Goldstein, E. J., Corrado, M. L., Stein, A. J., and Butt, K. M. Disseminated *Mycobacterium marinum* infection after renal transplantation. *Ann. Intern. Med.* 94:486, 1981.

79. Griffin, P. J., and Salaman, J. R. Urinary tract infections after renal transplantation: Do they matter? *Br. Med. J.* 1:710, 1979.

80. Gump, D. W., Frank, R. O., Winn, W. C., Jr., Foster, R. S., Jr., Broome, C. V., and Cherry, W. B. Legionnaires' disease in patients with associated serious disease. *Ann. Intern. Med.* 90:538, 1979.

81. Gurwith, M., Stinson, E., and Remington, J. S. *Aspergillus* infection complicating cardiac transplantation. *Arch. Intern. Med.* 128:541, 1971.

82. Haley, C. E., Cohen, M. L., Halter, J., and Meyer, R. D. Nosocomial legionnaires' disease: A continuing common-source epidemic at Wadsworth Medical Center. *Ann. Intern. Med.* 90:583, 1979.

83. Hanto, D. W., Sakamoto, K., Purtilo, D. T., Simmons, R. L., and Najarian, J. S. The Epstein-Barr virus in the pathogenesis of posttransplant lymphoproliferative disorders: Clinical, pathologic, and virologic correlation. *Surgery* 90:204, 1981.

84. Hardy, A. M., Wajszczuk, C. P., Hakala, T. R., Rosenthal, J. T., Starzl, T. E., and Ho, M. Infection in renal transplant recipients on cyclosporine: *Pneumocystis* pneumonia. *Transplant. Proc.* (In press.)

85. Heaton, A., Arze, R. S., and Ward, M. K. Acyclovir for life-threatening herpes simplex virus infection after renal transplantation (letter). *Lancet* 2:875, 1981.

86. Hellman, R. N., Hinrichs, J., Sicard, G., Hoover, R., Golden, P., and Hoffsten, P. Cryptococcal pyelonephritis and disseminated cryptococcosis in a renal transplant recipient. *Arch. Intern. Med.* 141:128, 1981.

87. Henle, W., Henle, G., Scriba, M., Joyner, C. R., Harrison, F. S., Jr., von Essen, R., Paloheimo, J., and Klemola, E. Antibody responses to the Epstein-Barr virus and cytomegalovirus

after open-heart and other surgery. *N. Engl. J. Med.* 282:1068, 1970.

88. Herb, H. M., Jontofsohn, R., Loeffler, H. D., and Heinze, V. Toxoplasmosis after renal transplantation. *Clin. Nephrol.* 8:529, 1977.

89. Hersman, J., Meyers, J. D., Thomas, E. D., Buckner, C. D., and Clift, R. The effect of granulocyte transfusions on the incidence of cytomegalovirus infection after allogenic marrow transplantation. *Ann. Intern. Med.* 96:149, 1982.

90. Hess, A. D., and Tutschka, P. J. Effect of cyclosporin A on human lymphocyte responses in vitro. I. CsA allows for the expression of alloantigenic-activated suppressor cells while preferentially inhibiting the induction of cytolytic effector lymphocytes in MLR. *J. Immunol.* 124:2601, 1980.

91. Hierholzer, J. C., Atuk, N. O., and Gwaltney, J. M., Jr. New human adenovirus isolated from a renal transplant recipient: Description and characterization of candidate adenovirus type 34. *J. Clin. Microbiol.* 1:366, 1975.

92. Hillis, W. D., Hillis, A., and Walker, W. G. Hepatitis B surface antigenemia in renal transplant recipients: Increased mortality risk. *J.A.M.A.* 242:329, 1979.

93. Hirsch, M. S., Schooley, R. T., Cosimi, A. B., Russell, P. S., Delmonico, F. L., Tolkoff-Rubin, N. E., Herrin, J. T., Cantell, K., Farrell, M. L., Rota, T. R., and Rubin, R. H. Effects of interferon-alpha on cytomegalovirus reactivation syndromes in renal-transplant recipients. *N. Engl. J. Med.* 308:1489, 1983.

94. Ho, M. Virus infections after transplantation in man: Brief review. *Arch. Virol.* 55:1, 1977.

95. Ho, M., Suwansirikul, S., Dowling, J. N., Youngblood, L. A., and Armstrong, J. A. The transplanted kidney as a source of cytomegalovirus infection. *N. Engl. J. Med.* 293:1109, 1975.

96. Ho, M., Wajszczuk, C. P., Hardy, A., Dummer, J. S., Starzl, T. E., Hakala, T. R., and Bahnson, H. T. Infections in kidney, heart, and liver transplant recipients on cyclosporine. *Transplant. Proc.* (In press.)

97. Hogan, T. F., Borden, E. C., McBain, J. A., Padgett, B. L., and Walker, D. L. Human polyomavirus infections with JC virus and BK virus in renal transplant patients. *Ann. Intern. Med.* 92:373, 1980.

98. Hooper, D. C., Pruitt, A. A., and Rubin, R. H. Central nervous system infection in the chronically immunosuppressed. *Medicine* (Baltimore) 61:166, 1982.

99. Howcroft, M. J., and Breslin, C. W. Herpes simplex keratitis in renal transplant recipients. *Can. Med. Assoc. J.* 124:292, 1981.

100. Hoy, W. E., Roberts, N. J., Jr., Bryson, M. F., Bowles, C., Lee, J. C., Rivero, A. J., and Ritterson, A. L. Transmission of strongyloidiasis by kidney transplant? Disseminated strongyloidiasis in both recipients of kidney allografts from a single cadaver donor. *J.A.M.A.* 246:1937, 1981.

101. Hurley, J. K., Greenslade, T., Lewy, P. R., Ahmadian, Y., and Firlit, C. Varicella-zoster infections in pediatric renal transplant recipients. *Arch. Surg.* 115:751, 1980.

102. Isiadinso, C. A. *Listeria* sepsis and meningitis: A complication of renal transplantation. *J.A.M.A.* 234:842, 1975.

103. Jennings, H. S., III, Bradsher, R. W., McGee, Z. A., Johnson, H. K., and Alford, R. H. Acute cryptococcal cellulitis in renal transplant recipients. *South. Med. J.* 74:1150, 1981.

104. Kaiser, L., Kelly, T. J., Patterson, M. J., Sanchez, T. V., Shapiro, R. S., and Mayer, G. H. Hepatitis B surface antigen in urine of renal transplant recipients. *Ann. Intern. Med.* 94:783, 1981.

105. Kaplan, J. E., Zoschke, D., and Kisch, A. L. Withdrawal of immunosuppressive agents in the treatment of disseminated coccidioidomycosis. *Am. J. Med.* 68:624, 1980.

106. Keller, E. W., Hierholzer, T. C., Rubin, R. H., Black, P. H., and Hirsch, M. S. Isolation of adenovirus type 34 from a renal transplant recipient with interstitial pneumonia. *Transplantation* 23:188, 1977.

107. Kirby, B. D., Snyder, K. M., Myer, R. D., and Feingold, S. M. Legionnaires' disease: Report of 65 nosocomially acquired cases and review of the literature. *Medicine* (Baltimore) 59:185, 1980.

108. Kissell, S. M., Hoy, W. E., Freeman, R. B., Byer, B., and Yarger, J. M. Renal transplant urinary tract infections: Effect of perioperative antibiotics and earlier catheter removal. *N.Y. State J. Med.* 82:1543, 1982.

109. Knodell, R. G., Conrad, M. E., and Ishak, K. G. Development of chronic liver disease after non-A, non-B post-transfusion hepatitis: Role of gamma globulin prophylaxis in its prevention. *Gastroenterology* 72:902, 1977.

110. Kraemer, K. G., Neiman, P. E., Reevers, W. C., and Thomas, E. D. Prophylactic adenine arabinoside following marrow transplantation. *Transplant. Proc.* 10:237, 1978.

111. Krieger, J. N., Brem, A. S., and Kaplan, M.

R. Urinary tract infection in pediatric renal transplantation. *Urology* 15:362, 1980.

112. Krieger, J. N., Tapia, L., Stubenbord, W. T., Stenzel, K. H., and Rubin, A. L. Urinary infection in kidney transplantation. *Urology* 9:130, 1977.

113. Kugler, J. W., Armitage, J. O., Helms, C. M., Klassen, L. W., Goeken, N. E., Ahmann, G. B., Gingrich, R. D., Johnson, W., and Gilchrist, M. J. R. Nosocomial legionnaires' disease: Occurrence in recipients of bone marrow transplants. *Am. J. Med.* 74:281, 1983.

114. Kyriakides, G. K., Simmons, R. L., and Najarian, J. S. Wound infections in renal transplant wounds: Pathogenetic and prognostic factors. *Ann. Surg.* 182:770, 1975.

115. Lange, B., Henle, W., Meyers, J. D., Yang, L. C., August, C., Koch, P., Arbeter, A., and Henle, G. Epstein-Barr virus-related serology in marrow transplant recipients. *Int. J. Cancer* 26:151, 1980.

116. Langlois, R. P., Flegel, K. M., Meakins, J. L., Morehouse, D. D., Robson, H. G., and Guttman, R. D. Cutaneous aspergillosis with fatal dissemination in a renal transplant recipient. *Can. Med. Assoc. J.* 122:673, 1980.

117. Leech, S. H., and Kumar, P. Epstein-Barr virus-induced B-cell lymphoma after renal transplantation (letter). *N. Engl. J. Med.* 307:896, 1982.

118. Leff, R. D., Smith, E. J., Aldo-Benson, M. A., and Aronoff, G. R. Cryptococcal arthritis after renal transplantation. *South. Med. J.* 74:1290, 1981.

119. Light, J. A., and Burke, D. S. Association of cytomegalovirus (CMV) infections with increased recipient mortality following transplantation. *Transplant. Proc.* 11:79, 1979.

120. Linnemann, C. C., Jr., and First, M. R. Risk of pneumococcal infections in renal transplant patients. *J.A.M.A.* 241:2619, 1979.

121. Linnemann, C. C., Jr., First, M. R., and Schiffman, G. Response to pneumococcal vaccine in renal transplant and hemodialysis patients. *Arch. Intern. Med.* 141:1637, 1981.

122. Linnemann, C. C., Jr., Kauffman, C. A., First, M. R., Schiff, G. M., and Phair, J. P. Cellular immune response to cytomegalovirus infection after renal transplantation. *Infect. Immun.* 22:176, 1978.

123. Lloveras, J., Peterson, P. K., Simmons, R. L., and Najarian, J. S. Mycobacterial infections in renal transplant recipients: Seven cases and a review of the literature. *Arch. Intern. Med.* 142:888, 1982.

124. Lobo, P. I., Rudolf, L. E., and Krieger, J. N. Wound infections in renal transplant recipients: A complication of urinary tract infections during allograft malfunction. *Surgery* 92:491, 1982.

125. London, W. T. Sex differences in response to hepatitis B virus. III. Responses to HBV and sex of donor and recipient in kidney and bone marrow transplantation. *Arthritis Rheum.* 22:1267, 1979.

126. London, W. T., Drew, J. S., Blumberg, B. S., Grossman, R. A., and Lyons, P. J. Association of graft survival with host response to hepatitis B infection in patients with kidney transplants. *N. Engl. J. Med.* 296:241, 1977.

127. Lovett, I. S., Houang, E. T., Burge, S., Turner-Warwick, M., Thompson, F. D., Harrison, A. R., Joekes, A. M., and Parkinson, M. C. An outbreak of *Nocardia asteroides* infection in a renal transplant unit. *Q. J. Med.* 50:123, 1981.

128. Lowder, J. N., Lazarus, H. M., and Herzig, R. H. Bacteremias and fungemias in oncologic patients with central venous catheters: Changing spectrum of infection. *Arch. Intern. Med.* 142:1456, 1982.

129. Luby, J. P., Ware, A. J., Hull, A. R., Helderman, J. H., Gailiunas, P., Butler, S., and Atkins, C. Disease due to cytomegalovirus and its long-term consequences in renal transplant recipients. *Arch. Intern. Med.* 143:1126, 1983.

130. Luft, B. J., Naot, Y., Araujo, F. G., Stinson, E. B., and Remington, J. S. Primary and reactivated *Toxoplasma* infection in patients with cardiac transplants: Clinical spectrum and problems in diagnosis in a defined population. *Ann. Intern. Med.* 99:27, 1983.

131. Luft, B. J., et al. Manuscript in preparation.

132. Majeski, J. A., Alexander, J. W., First, M. R., Munda, R., Fidler, J. P., and Craycraft, T. K. Transplantation of microbially contaminated cadaver kidneys. *Arch. Surg.* 117:221, 1982.

133. Marker, S. C., Ascher, N. L., Kalis, J. M., Simmons, R. L., Najarian, J. S., and Balfour, H. H., Jr. Epstein-Barr virus antibody responses and clinical illnesses in renal transplant recipients. *Surgery* 85:433, 1979.

134. Marker, S. C., Howard, R. J., Groth, K. E., Mastri, A. R., Simmons, R. L., and Balfour, H. H., Jr. A trial of vidarabine for cytomegalovirus infection in renal transplant patients. *Arch. Intern. Med.* 140:1441, 1980.

135. Marker, S. C., Howard, R. J., Simmons, R. L., Kalis, J. M., Connelly, D. P., Najarian, J. S., and Balfour, H. H., Jr. Cytomegalovirus infection: A quantitative prospective study of three hundred twenty consecutive renal transplants. *Surgery* 89:660, 1981.

136. Marker, S. C., Simmons, R. L., and Balfour, H. H., Jr. Cytomegalovirus vaccine in renal allograft recipients. *Transplant. Proc.* 13:117, 1981.

137. Marks, J. S., Tsai, T. F., Martone, W. J., Baron, R. C., Kennicott, J., Holtzhauer, F. J., Baird, I., Fay, D., Feeley, J. C., Mallison, G. F., Fraser, D. W., and Halpin, T. J. Nosocomial legionnaires' disease in Columbus, Ohio. *Ann. Intern. Med.* 90:565, 1979.

138. Marshall, W., Foster, R. S., Jr., and Winn, W. Legionnaires' disease in renal transplant patients. *Am. J. Surg.* 141:423, 1981.

139. Martin, D. H., Counts, G. W., and Thomas, E. D. Fungal Infections in Human Bone Marrow Transplant Recipients. In the *Seventeenth Interscience Conference on Antimicrobial Agents and Chemotherapy.* New York: American Society for Microbiology, 1977, abstract 406.

140. Mason, J. W., Stinson, E. B., Hunt, S. A., Schroeder, J. S., and Rider, A. K. Infections after cardiac transplantation: Relation to rejection therapy. *Ann. Intern. Med.* 85:69, 1976.

141. Mayers, D. L., Martone, W. J., and Mandell, G. L. Cutaneous cryptococcosis mimicking gram-positive cellulitis in a renal transplant patient. *South. Med. J.* 74:1032, 1981.

142. Mayor, G. H., Kelly, T. J., Hourani, M. R., and Patterson, M. J. Intermittent hepatitis B surface antigenuria in a renal transplant recipient. *Am. J. Med.* 68:305, 1980.

143. McDonald, J. C., Ritchey, R. J., Fuselier, P. F., Lindsey, E. S., and McCracken, B. H. Sepsis in human renal transplantation. *Surgery* 69:189, 1971.

144. McHenry, M. C., Braun, W. E., Popowniak, K. L., Banowsky, L. H., and Deodhar, S. D. Septicemia in renal transplant recipients. *Urol. Clin. North Am.* 3:647, 1976.

145. Meija, G., Leiderman, E., Builes, M., Henao, J., Arbelaez, M., Arango, J. L., and Borrero, J. Transmission of toxoplasmosis by renal transplant. *Am. J. Kidney Dis.* 2:615, 1983.

146. Meyers, J. D., Flournoy, N., and Thomas, E. D. Infection with herpes simplex virus and cell-mediated immunity after marrow transplant. *J. Infect. Dis.* 142:338, 1980.

147. Meyers, J. D., Leszczynski, J., Zaia, J. A., Flournoy, N., Newton, B., Syndman, D. R., Wright, G. G., Levin, M. J., and Thomas, E. D. Prevention of cytomegalovirus infection by cytomegalovirus immune globulin after marrow transplantation. *Ann. Intern. Med.* 98:442, 1983.

148. Meyers, J. D., McGuffin, R. W., Bryson, Y. J., Cantell, K., and Thomas, E. D. Treatment of cytomegalovirus pneumonia after marrow transplant with combined vidarabine and human leukocyte interferon. *J. Infect. Dis.* 146, 80, 1982.

149. Meyers, J. D., McGuffin, R. W., Neiman, P. E., Singer, J. W., and Thomas, E. D. Toxicity and efficacy of human leukocyte interferon for treatment of cytomegalovirus pneumonia after marrow transplantation. *J. Infect. Dis.* 141:555, 1980.

150. Meyers, J. D., Spencer, H. C., Watts, J. C., Gregg, M. B., Stewart, J. A., Troupin, R. H., and Thomas, E. D. Cytomegalovirus pneumonia after human marrow transplantation. *Ann. Intern. Med.* 82:181, 1975.

151. Meyers, J. D., and Thomas, E. D. Infection Complicating Bone Marrow Transplantation. In Rubin, R. H., and Young, L. S. (Eds.), *Clinical Approach to Infection in the Compromised Host.* New York: Plenum, 1981, p. 507.

152. Mezo, A., Jennis, F., McCarthy, S. W., and Dawson, D. J. Unusual mycobacteria in 5 cases of opportunistic infections. *Pathology* 11:377, 1979.

153. Monaco, A. P. Kidney transplantation. *Behring Inst. Mitt.* 51:135, 1972.

154. Moore, T. C., and Hume, D. M. The period and nature of hazard in clinical renal transplantation: I. The hazard to patient survival. *Ann. Surg.* 183:266, 1976.

155. Moulsdale, M., Harper, J. M., and Thatcher, G. N. Unusual mycobacterium infection in a renal transplant recipient (letter). *Med. J. Aust.* 2:450, 1980.

156. Murphy, J. F., McDonald, F. D., Dawson, M., Reite, A., Turcotte, J., and Fekety, R. F. Factors affecting the frequency of infection in renal transplant recipients. *Arch. Intern. Med.* 136:670, 1976.

157. Myerowitz, R. L., Pasculle, A. W., Dowling, J. N., Pazin, G. J., Sr., Puerzer, M., Yee, R. B., Rinaldo, C. R., and Hakala, T. R. Opportunistic lung infection due to "Pittsburgh Pneumonia Agent." *N. Engl. J. Med.* 301:953, 1979.

158. Myerowitz, R. L., Stalder, H., Oxman, M. N., Levin, M. J., Moore, M., Leith, J. D., Gantz, N. M., Pellegrini, J., and Hierholzer, J. C. Fatal disseminated adenovirus infection in a renal transplant recipient. *Am. J. Med.* 59:591, 1975.

159. Nagington, J. Cytomegalovirus antibody production in renal transplant patients. *J. Hyg.* (Camb.) 69:645, 1971.

160. Nagington, J., Cossart, Y. E., and Cohen, B. J. Reactivation of hepatitis B after transplantation operations. *Lancet* 1:558, 1977.

161. Nagington, J., and Martin, A. L. Toxoplasmosis and heart transplantation. *Lancet* 2:679, 1983.

162. Nankervis, G. A. Cytomegalovirus infections in the blood recipient. *Yale J. Biol. Med.* 49:13, 1976.

163. Naot, Y., Brown, A., Elder, E. M., Shonnard, J., Luft, B. J., and Remington, J. S. IgM and IgG antibody response in two immunosuppressed patients with legionnaires' disease: Evidence of reactivation of latent infection. *Am. J. Med.* 73:791, 1982.

164. Naraqi, S., Jackson, G. G., Jonasson, O., and Yamashiroya, H. M. Prospective study of prevalence, incidence, and source of herpesvirus infections in patients with renal allografts. *J. Infect. Dis.* 136:531, 1977.

165. Naraqi, S., Jonassen, O., Jackson, G. G., and Yamashiroya, H. M. Clinical manifestations of infections with herpesviruses after kidney transplantation. A prospective study of various syndromes. *Ann. Surg.* 188:234, 1978.

166. Nathan, A. W., Turner, D. R., Aubrey, C., Cameron, J. S., Williams, D. G., Ogg, C. S., and Bewick, M. *Corynebacterium hofmannii* infection after renal transplantation. *Clin. Nephrol.* 17:315, 1982.

167. Neiman, P. E., Reeves, W., Ray, G., Flournay, N., Lerner, K. G., Sale, G. E., and Thomas, E. D. A prospective analysis of interstitial pneumonia and opportunistic viral infection among recipients of allogeneic bone marrow grafts. *J. Infect. Dis.* 136:754, 1977.

168. Nieman, R. E., and Lorber, B. Listeriosis in adults: A changing pattern. Report of eight cases and review of the literature, 1968–1978. *Rev. Infect. Dis.* 2:207, 1980.

169. Oliver, W. A. Tuberculosis in renal transplant patients. *Med. J. Aust.* 1:828, 1976.

170. Ooi, B. S., Chen, B. T. M., Lim, C. H., Khoo, O. T., and Chan, K. T. Survival of a patient transplanted with a kidney infected with *Cryptococcus neoformans*. *Transplantation* 11:428, 1971.

171. Opelz, G., and Terasaki, P. I. Dominant effect of transfusions on kidney graft survival. *Transplantation* 29:153, 1980.

172. O'Reilly, R. J., Reich, L., Gold, J., Kirkpatrick, D., Dinsmore, R., Kapoor, N., and Condie, R. A randomized trial of intravenous hyperimmune globulin for the prevention of cytomegalovirus (CMV) infections following marrow transplantation: Preliminary results. *Transplant. Proc.* 15:1405, 1983.

173. Oyer, P. E., Stinson, E. B., Jamieson, S. W., Hunt, S. A., Perlroth, M., Billingham, M., and Shumway, N. E. Cyclosporine in cardiac transplantation: A 2.5 year followup. *Transplantation* (In press.)

174. Pasculle, A. W., Myerowitz, R. L., and Rinaldo, C. R., Jr. New bacterial agent of pneumonia isolated from renal-transplant recipients. *Lancet* 2:58, 1979.

175. Pass, R. F., Long, W. K., Whitley, R. J., Soong, S., Diethelm, A. G., Reynolds, D. W., and Alford, C. A., Jr. Productive infection with cytomegalovirus and herpes simplex virus in renal transplant recipients: Role of source of kidney. *J. Infect. Dis.* 137:556, 1978.

176. Pearce, W. G., and Mielke, B. M. End-stage cytomegalic inclusion retinitis and disseminated intravascular coagulation. *Can. J. Ophthalmol.* 16:88, 1981.

177. Pearson, T. A., Braine, H. G., and Rathbun, H. K. *Corynebacterium* sepsis in oncology patients: Predisposing factors, diagnosis, and treatment. *J.A.M.A.* 238:1737, 1977.

178. Peterson, P. K., Balfour, H. H., Marker, S. C., Fryd, D. S., Howard, R. J., and Simmons, R. L. Cytomegalovirus disease in renal allograft recipients: A prospective study of the clinical features, risk factors, and impact on renal transplantation. *Medicine* 59:283, 1980.

179. Peterson, P. K., Ferguson, R., Fryd, D. S., Balfour, H. H., Jr., Rynasiewicz, J., and Simmons, R. L. Infectious diseases in hospitalized renal transplant recipients: A prospective study of a complex and evolving problem. *Medicine* (Baltimore) 61:360, 1982.

180. Pirson, Y., Alexandre, G. P. J., and van Ypersele de Strihou, C., Long-term effect on HB$_s$ antigenemia on patient survival after renal transplantation. *N. Engl. J. Med.* 296:194, 1977.

181. Pollard, R. B., Arvin, A. M., Gamberg, P.,

Rand, K. H., Gallagher, J. G., and Merigan, T. C. Specific cell-mediated immunity and infections with herpes viruses in cardiac transplant recipients. *Am. J. Med.* 73:679, 1982.

182. Pollard, R. B., Egbert, P. R., Gallagher, J. G., and Merigan, T. C. Cytomegalovirus retinitis in immunosuppressed hosts. I. Natural history and effects of treatment with adenine arabinoside. *Ann. Intern. Med.* 93:655, 1980.

183. Pope, T. L., Jr., Armstrong, P., Thompson, R., and Donowitz, G. R. Pittsburgh pneumonia agent: Chest film manifestations. *A.J.R.* 138:237, 1982.

184. Powles, R. L., Clink, H. M., Spence, D., Morgenstern, G., Watson, J. G., Selby, P. J., Woods, M., Barrett, A., Jameson, B., Sloane, J., Lawler, S. D., Kay, H. E., Lawson, D., McElwain, T. J., and Alexander, P. Cyclosporin A to prevent graft-versus-host disease in man after allogeneic bone-marrow transplantation. *Lancet* 1:327, 1980.

185. Preiksaitis, J. K., Rosno, S., Grumet, C., and Merigan, T. C. Infections due to herpesviruses in cardiac transplant recipients: Role of the donor heart and immunosuppressive therapy. *J. Infect. Dis.* 147:974, 1983.

186. Ramsey, P. G., Fife, K. H., Hackman, R. C., Meyers, J. D., and Corey, L. Herpes simplex virus pneumonia: Clinical, virologic, and pathologic features in 20 patients. *Ann. Intern. Med.* 97:813, 1982.

187. Ramsey, D. E., Finch, W. T., and Birtch, A. G. Urinary tract infections in kidney transplant recipients. *Arch. Surg.* 114:1022, 1979.

188. Ramsey, P. G., Rubin, R. H., Tolkoff-Rubin, N. E., Cosimi, A. B., Russell, P. S., and Greene, R. The renal transplant patient with fever and pulmonary infiltrates: Etiology, clinical manifestations, and management. *Medicine* (Baltimore) 59:206, 1980.

189. Rand, K. H., Pollard, R. B., and Merigan, T. C. Increased pulmonary superinfections in cardiac transplant patients undergoing primary cytomegalovirus infection. *N. Engl. J. Med.* 298:951, 1978.

190. Rashid, A., Sengar, D. P., Coutre, R. A., Jindal, S., and Posen, G. Hepatitis B antigen infection and graft survival in cadaveric renal transplantation. *Trans. Am. Soc. Artif. Intern. Organs* 23:433, 1977.

191. Renner, E. D., Helms, C. M., Hierholzer, W. J., Jr., Hall, N., Wong, Y. W., Viner, J. P., Johnson, W., and Hausler, W. J. Legionnaires'

disease in pneumonia patients in Iowa: A retrospective seroepidemiologic study, 1972–1977. *Ann. Intern. Med.* 90:603, 1979.

192. Richardson, W. P., Colvin, R. B., Cheeseman, S. H., Tolkoff-Rubin, N. E., Herrin, J. T., Cosimi, A. B., Collins, A. B., Hirsch, M. S., McCluskey, R. T., Russell, P. S., and Rubin, R. H. Glomerulopathy associated with cytomegalovirus viremia in renal allografts. *N. Engl. J. Med.* 305:57, 1981.

193. Riska, H., and Kuhlbäck, B. Tuberculosis and kidney transplantation. *Acta Med. Scand.* 205:637, 1979.

194. Rogers, B. H., Donowitz, G. R., Walker, G. K., Harding, S. A., and Sande, M. A. Opportunistic pneumonia: A clinicopathological study of five cases caused by an unidentified acid-fast bacterium. *N. Engl. J. Med.* 301:959, 1979.

195. Rogers, T. R., White, S., Pallet, A., Lucas, C., and Tabara, Z. An investigation into the relationship between *Staphylococcus epidermidis* bacteremia and the use of Hickman catheters during marrow transplantation. *Exp. Hematol.* 10:12, 1982.

196. Rose, A. G., Uys, C. J., Novitsky, D., Cooper, D. K. C., and Barnard, C. N. Toxoplasmosis of donor and recipient hearts after heterotopic cardiac transplantation. *Arch. Pathol. Lab. Med.* 107:368, 1983.

197. Rubin, R. H. Infection in the Renal Transplant Patient. In Rubin, R. H., and Young, L. S. (Eds.), *Clinical Approach to Infection in the Compromised Host.* New York: Plenum, 1981, p. 553.

198. Rubin, R. H., Fang, L. S., Cosimi, A. B., Herrin, J. T., Varga, P. A., Russell, P. S., and Tolkoff-Rubin, N. E. Usefulness of the antibody-coated bacteria assay in the management of urinary tract infection in the renal transplant patient. *Transplantation* 27:18, 1979.

199. Rubin, R. H., Russell, P. S., Levin, M., and Cohen, C. National Institutes of Health. Summary of a workshop on cytomegalovirus infections during organ transplantation. *J. Infect. Dis.* 139:728, 1979.

200. Rubin, R. H., Wolfson, J. S., Cosimi, A. B., and Tolkoff-Rubin, N. E. Infection in the renal transplant recipient. *Am. J. Med.* 70:405, 1981.

201. Ryning, F. W., McLeod, R., Maddox, J. C., Hunt, S., and Remington, J. S. Probable transmission of *Toxoplasma gondii* by organ transplantation. *Ann. Intern. Med.* 90:47, 1979.

202. Saemundsen, A. K., Klein, G., Cleary, M., and Warnke, R. Epstein-Barr-virus-carrying lymphoma in cardiac transplant recipient (letter). *Lancet* 2:158, 1982.

203. Sanders, K. L., Walker, D. H., and Lee, T. J. Relapse of legionnaires' disease in a renal transplant recipient. *Arch. Intern. Med.* 140:833, 1980.

204. Saral, R., Burns, W. H., Laskin, O. L., Santos, G. W., and Lietman, P. S. Acyclovir prophylaxis of herpes simplex virus infections. *N. Engl. J. Med.* 305:63, 1981.

205. Schröter, G. P. J., Hoelscher, M., Putnam, C. W., Kendrick, P. A., and Starzl, T. E. Fungus infections after liver transplantation. *Ann. Surg.* 186:115, 1977.

206. Schröter, G. P. J., Hoelscher, M., Putnam, C. W., Porter, K. A., Hansbrough, J. F., and Starzl, T. E. Infections complicating orthotopic liver transplantation: A study emphasizing graft-related septicemia. *Arch. Surg.* 111:1337, 1976.

207. Schröter, G. P. J., Weil, R., III, Penn, I., Speers, W. C., and Waddell, W. R. Hepatocellular carcinoma associated with chronic hepatitis B virus infection after kidney transplantation (letter). *Lancet* 2:381, 1982.

208. Schweizer, R. T., Kountz, S. L., and Belzer, F. O. Wound complications in recipients of renal transplants. *Ann. Surg.* 177:58, 1973.

209. Scowden, E. B., Schaffner, W., and Stone, W. J. Overwhelming strongyloidiasis: An unappreciated opportunistic infection. *Medicine* 57:527, 1978.

210. Siegal, J. P., and Remington, J. S. Comparison of methods for quantitating antigen-specific immunoglobulin M antibody with a reverse enzyme-linked immunosorbent assay. *J. Clin. Microbiol.* 18:63, 1983.

211. Simmons, R. L., Matas, A. J., Rattazzi, L. C., Balfour, H. H., Jr., Howard, R. J., and Najarian, J. S. Clinical characteristics of the lethal cytomegalovirus infection following renal transplantation. *Surgery* 82:537, 1977.

212. Simpson, G. L., Stinson, E. B., Egger, M. J., and Remington, J. S. Nocardial infections in the immunocompromised host: A detailed study in a defined population. *Rev. Infect. Dis.* 3:492, 1981.

213. Slade, M. O., Simmons, R. L., Yunis, E., and Greenberg, L. J. Immunodepression after major surgery in normal patients. *Surgery* 78:363, 1975.

214. Spence, R. K., Dafoe, D. C., Rabin, G., Grossman, R. A., Naji, A., Barker, C. F., and Per-loff, L. J. Mycobacterial infections in renal allograft recipients. *Arch. Surg.* 118:356, 1983.

215. Spencer, E. S. Clinical aspects of cytomegalovirus infection in kidney-graft recipients. *Scand. J. Infect. Dis.* 6:315, 1974.

216. Stalder, H., Hierholzer, J. C., and Oxman, M. N. New human adenovirus (candidate adenovirus type 35) causing fatal disseminated infection in a renal transplant recipient. *J. Clin. Microbiol.* 6:257, 1977.

217. Stamm, A. M., Dismukes, W. E., Simmons, B. P., Cobbs, C. G., Elliott, A., Budrich, P., and Harmon, J. Listeriosis in renal transplant recipients: Report of an outbreak and review of 102 cases. *Rev. Infect. Dis.* 4:655, 1982.

218. Stamm, W. E., Tompkins, L. S., Wagner, K. F., Counts, G. W., Thomas, E. D., and Meyers, J. D. Infection due to *Corynebacterium* species in marrow transplant patients. *Ann. Intern. Med.* 91:167, 1979.

219. Starzl, T. E., Klintmalm, G. B., Porter, K. A., Iwatsuki, S., and Schröter, G. P. Liver transplantation with use of cyclosporin A and prednisone. *N. Engl. J. Med.* 305:266, 1981.

220. Starzl, T. E., Koep, L. J., Halgrimson, C. G., Hood, J., Schröter, G. P., Porter, K. A., and Weil, R., III. Fifteen years of clinical liver transplantation. *Gastroenterologoy* 77:375, 1979.

221. Starzl, T., Porter, K. A., Putnam, C. W., Schröter, G. P. J., Halgrimson, C. G., Weil, R., III, Hoelscher, M., and Reid, H. A. S. Orthotopic liver transplantation in 93 patients. *Surg. Gynecol. Obstet.* 142:487, 1976.

222. Stevens, D. A., Pier, A. C., Beaman, B. L., Morozumi, P. A., Lovett, I. S., and Houang, E. T. Laboratory evaluation of an outbreak of nocardiosis in immunocompromised hosts. *Am. J. Med.* 71:928, 1981.

223. Stinson, E. B. Personal communication.

224. Strom, T. B. Editorial retrospective: Hepatitis B, transfusions, and renal transplantation—five years later. *N. Engl. J. Med.* 307:1141, 1982.

225. Suwansirikul, S., Rao, N., Dowling, J. N., and Ho, M. Primary and secondary cytomegalovirus infection: Clinical manifestations after renal transplantation. *Arch. Intern. Med.* 137:1026, 1977.

226. Taylor, R. J., Schwentker, F. N., and Hakala, T. R. Opportunistic lung infections in renal transplant patients: A comparison of Pittsburgh pneumonia agent and legionnaires' disease. *J. Urol.* 125:289, 1981.

227. Tilney, N. L., Kohler, T. R., and Strom, T. B. Cerebromeningitis in immunosuppressed recipients of renal allografts. *Ann. Surg.* 195:104, 1982.

228. Tobin, J. O., Beare, J., Dunnill, M. S., Fisher-Hoch, S., French, M., Mitchell, R. G., Morris, P. J., and Muers, M. F. Legionnaires' disease in a transplant unit: Isolation of the causative agent from shower baths. *Lancet* 2:118, 1980.

229. Tobin, J. O., Warrell, M. J., and Morris, P. J. Cytomegalovirus infection and renal transplantation (letter). *Lancet* 1:926, 1979.

230. Tolkoff-Rubin, N. E., Cosimi, A. B., Russell, P. S., and Rubin, R. H. A controlled study of trimethoprim-sulfamethoxazole prophylaxis of urinary tract infection in renal transplant recipients. *Rev. Infect. Dis.* 4:614, 1982.

231. Toussaint, C., Cappel, R., Vereerstraeten, P., Kinnaert, P., Dupont, E., and Van Geertruyden, J. Graft survival and response to hepatitis B virus in kidney recipients. *Transplant Proc.* 11:89, 1979.

232. Toussaint, C., Dupont, E., Vanherweghem, J. L., Cappel, R., DeRoy, G., Vereerstraeten, P., Kinnaert, P., Thiry, L., and Van Geertruyden, J. Liver disease in patients undergoing hemodialysis and kidney transplantation. *Adv. Nephrol.* 8:269, 1979.

233. Vaisrub, S. Hepatitis in renal transplant recipients (editorial). *J.A.M.A.* 243:551, 1980.

234. Wade, J. C., Hintz, M., McGuffin, R., Springmeyer, S. C., Connor, J. D., and Meyers, J. D. Treatment of cytomegalovirus pneumonia with high-dose acyclovir. *Am. J. Med.* 73:249, 1982.

235. Wade, J. C., Newton, B., McLaren, C., Flournoy, N., Keeney, R. E., and Meyers, J. D. Intravenous acyclovir to treat mucocutaneous herpes simplex virus infection after marrow transplantation: A double-blind trial. *Ann. Intern. Med.* 96:265, 1982.

236. Walker, D. P., Longson, M., Lawler, W., Mallick, N. P., Davies, J. S., and Johnson, R. W. Disseminated herpes simplex virus infection with hepatitis in an adult renal transplant recipient. *J. Clin. Pathol.* 34:1044, 1981.

237. Walker, D. P., Longson, M., Mallick, N. P., and Johnson, R. W. G. A prospective study of cytomegalovirus and herpes simplex virus disease in renal transplant recipients. *J. Clin. Pathol.* 35:1190, 1982.

238. Wang, D., Felig, S., Marso, E., Winston, D., and Gale, R. P. Increased incidence of pneu-mococcal infections in bone marrow transplant recipients. (Abstract, p. 351) *I.C.A.A.C.* 1978.

239. Weller, I. V., Copland, P., and Gabriel, R. *Strongyloides stercoralis* infection in renal transplant recipients. *Br. Med. J.* (Clin. Res.) 282:524, 1981.

240. Wheat, L. J., Smith, E. J., Sathapatayavongo, B., Battergei, B., Filo, R. S., Leapman, S. B., and French, M. V. Histoplasmosis in renal allograft recipients: Two large urban outbreaks. *Arch. Intern. Med.* 143:703, 1983.

241. Whelchel, J. D., Pass, R. F., Diethelm, A. Y., Whitley, R. J., and Alford, C. A., Jr. Effect of primary and recurrent cytomegalovirus infections upon graft and patient survival after renal transplantation. *Transplantation* 28:443, 1979.

242. White, D. J. Cyclosporin A: Clinical pharmacology and therapeutic potential. *Drugs* 24:322, 1982.

243. Williams, D. M., Krick, J. A., and Remington, J. S. State of the art: Pulmonary infection in the compromised host. Parts I and II. *Am. Rev. Respir. Dis.* 114:359, 593, 1976.

244. Winston, D. J., Dudnick, D. V., Chapin, M., Ho, W. G., Gale, R. P., and Martin, W. J. Coagulase-negative staphylococcal bacteremia in patients receiving immunosuppressive therapy. *Arch. Intern. Med.* 143:32, 1983.

245. Winston, D. J., Gale, R. P., Meyer, D. V., and Young, L. S. Infectious complications of human bone marrow transplantation. *Medicine* (Baltimore) 58:1, 1979.

246. Winston, D. J., Pollard, R. B., Ho, W. G., Gallagher, J. G., Rasmussen, C. E., Huang, N., Lin, C., Gossett, T. G., Merigan, T. C., and Gale, R. P. Cytomegalovirus immune plasma in bone marrow transplant recipients. *Ann. Intern. Med.* 97:11, 1982.

247. Winston, D. J., Schiffman, G., Wang, D. C., Feig, S. A., Lin, C. H., Marso, E. L., Ho, W. G., Young, L. S., and Gale, R. P. Pneumococcal infections after human bone-marrow transplantation. *Ann. Intern. Med.* 91:835, 1979.

248. Wolf, J. L., Perkins, H. A., Schreeder, M. T., and Vincenti, F. The transplanted kidney as a source of hepatitis B infection. *Ann. Intern. Med.* 91:412, 1979.

249. Young, L. S. Infectious Complications in Bone Marrow Transplant Recipients. In *Proceedings of the Second International Symposium on the Compromised Host.* London: Academic, 1983, p. 27.

250. Young, N., Kwong-Chung, K., and Freeman, J. Subcutaneous abscess caused by *Phoma* sp. resembling *Pyrenochaeta romeroi*. *Am. J. Clin. Pathol.* 59:810, 1973.

251. ZuRhein, G. M., and Varakis, J. Progressive multifocal leukoencephalopathy in a renal allograft recipient. *N. Engl. J. Med.* 291:798, 1974.

# 38 OTHER PROCEDURE-RELATED INFECTIONS

Robert A. Weinstein

With yards of entrails, miles of vascular network, dozens of extravascular spaces, and several organ systems, any patient is a candidate for a staggering array of diagnostic and therapeutic procedures. Although many of these procedures provide information that is essential for sophisticated patient care, supplant more traumatic intervention, or are critical for life support, most procedures also bypass natural host defenses and place patients at increased risk of nosocomial infection [71,88]. It is not surprising, then, that the introduction of any new procedure is often followed closely by case reports of procedure-associated infections. Occasionally, epidemiologic experiments of nature, in the form of nosocomial outbreaks, provide more detailed information on certain procedure-related hazards, and eventually such hazards may be subjected to prospective study. In this chapter, we discuss a variety of procedure-associated infections that have been highlighted by retrospective or prospective investigations and that have not been discussed elsewhere in this volume.

Because of the seemingly eclectic contents of this chapter, it is important to recognize from the outset that the procedures to be discussed have certain themes in common. First, all the procedures are exquisitely vulnerable to inexperienced operators, to breaks in aseptic technique, and to contaminated equipment or ineffective antiseptics. Second, various procedures involving many different sites have the bloodstream as a common site of infection, although, as will be seen, the risk of infection differs depending on whether the bloodstream contamination is transient or persistent as well as on host and organism-specific factors. Finally, many procedures bear the burden that the specific risks have not been defined sufficiently to justify certain preventive measures, such as the use of prophylactic antimicrobial therapy.

## INFECTIONS FROM DIAGNOSTIC PROCEDURES INVOLVING THE VASCULAR SYSTEM

### Phlebotomy

Phlebotomy is one of the oldest and certainly the commonest invasive procedure practiced in hospitals and clinics, and ever since the leech was replaced by the sterile hypodermic needle, blood-drawing has been regarded by most clinicians as totally safe and simple.In the 1940s, however, it became apparent that despite sterile needles, epidemic jaundice was being transmitted by the nonsterile syringes that were used commonly for phlebotomy. With a mock venous system and methylene blue as a marker, investigators showed that reflux occurred from the syringe into the test system when tourniquet pressure was released. By sterilizing syringes between uses, clinic workers abruptly halted the transmission of phlebotomy-associated hepatitis [/4].

Historically, the next major risk of phlebotomy to be recognized was staphylococcal septic arthritis of the hip in neonates [4]. In the early 1960s it was noted that this complication occasionally followed five to nine days after femoral venipuncture. Localized suppuration at the puncture site and thrombosis of the femoral vein, both unusual findings with isolated septic arthritis, suggested a causal relationship between pyoarthritis and a preceding femoral venipuncture. Since it is common to strike the femoral head during femoral venipuncture in neonates (which denotes that the joint capsule has been entered), femoral "sticks" demand the same aseptic conditions used for arthrocentesis, rather than the more lax conditions under which venipuncture is frequently performed. In light of the severe disability that may follow septic arthritis, many pediatricians now condemn the use of femoral venipuncture and recommend at least ten other sites for pediatric phlebotomy. When heel punctures are employed, the most medial or lateral portion of the heel's plantar surface should be used to avoid calcaneal puncture and osteochondritis [11].

The most recent innovation in blood-drawing—the popular and ingeniously simple evacuated collection tube—has streamlined blood collection, but unfortunately it has also reintroduced the reflux, or backflow, hazard that was first recognized in the 1940s. When commercial evacuated tubes are not sterilized routinely, they may be a source of hospital-acquired sepsis. One hospital traced an outbreak of five cases of "primary" Serratia bacteremia to contaminated commercial vacuum tubes used for blood collection. This outbreak prompted a detailed study of the backflow phenomenon, and it was shown that reflux may occur not only when the tourniquet is released (after active flow of blood into the tube has ceased), but also when the tube is tilted upward, when blood touches the stopper, when pressure on the end of the tube compresses the stopper, or when a "short draw" occurs due to insufficient vacuum [44]. While practices that might increase the risk of backflow are proscribed in the package insert that accompanies many commercial vacuum tubes, such inserts are not always seen by those responsible for blood-drawing, and many of the recommendations, particularly those concerning the positioning of patients for phlebotomy, are difficult to follow.

Even when a sterile syringe is used to draw blood, backflow during serial inoculation of vacuum tubes and blood culture bottles can result in cross-contamination and false-positive blood cultures. Although potentially avoidable, such serial inoculation is a convenient and common practice, particularly when blood is obtained from pediatric patients for hemogram and culture, and it has resulted in two reported "outbreaks" of pseudobacteremia [40]. Although none of the patients was affected directly, false-positive cultures put them at risk of unwarranted antibiotic therapy.

Over 500 million commercial evacuated blood-collection tubes are used annually in the United States and Canada. The problems cited previously, as well as culture surveys of evacuated blood-collection tubes [84], have led to the routine marketing and use of sterile tubes. The preservative and diagnostic reagents present in many tubes may still pose a risk—one that is probably minimal but not fully evaluated. It is hoped that the major problem of backflow has been returned to the shelf with the leeches. Nevertheless, health workers should be aware of the hazard, particularly when investigating the source of a "primary" bacteremia.

### Cardiac Catheterization

Serious local and systemic infections may result from cardiac catheterization procedures, particularly when contaminated instruments or ineffective antiseptics (e.g., dilute aqueous benzalkonium chloride) are used inadvertently or when breaks in technique occur in the cardiac catheterization laboratory. The major pathogens are staphylococci and gram-negative bacteria.

Up to 50 percent of patients undergoing cardiac catheterization develop an increase in temperature of more than $1°C$ ($1.8°F$) within 24 hours after catheterization. Their fever, however, has been attributed to the use of angiocardiographic contrast material, rather than to infection [69]. In fact, bacterial endocarditis has been reported very rarely in large series evaluating the complications of cardiac catheterization, and individual examples may have been due to concurrent infection that was initially undetected.

In some studies, the febrile reactions after a cardiac catheterization have been traced to pyrogenic endotoxin present in sterile catheters [65]. Reusable cardiac catheters (and disposable catheters, which many institutions now reuse in efforts to contain costs) may be exposed to contaminated distilled water during the initial phases of cleaning. Despite subsequent sterilization, usually by ethylene oxide, residual bacterial endotoxin may be present in the lumen or on the surface of the catheters and lead to sporadic as well as epidemic cases of fever and hypotension following cardiac catheterization. Single-use disposable catheters may prevent this complication. If catheters are reused, rinsing with sterile water before sterilization may lessen the problem.

Pyrogen has also been noted on sterile latex surgical gloves [47]. The incidence of febrile reactions following catheterization was reduced in one study from 11.6 to 0.6 percent when rinsing of latex gloves before catheterization was made routine [48]. One lot of surgical gloves was called to our attention recently because of an offensive odor left on wearers' hands. The manufacturer attributed this to "sour" talc used in preparing the gloves. The Food and Drug Administration found high levels of endotoxin on the glove surfaces. However, there are no regulations requiring testing of gloves for endotoxin, and the frequency with which commercially available surgical gloves are contaminated with endotoxin, and its side effects, are unknown.

Transient bacteremia during cardiac catheterization has been observed to occur in 4 to 18 percent of patients. In the studies reporting such an incidence, however, blood cultures were obtained from the intravascular catheter or from the vessel from which the catheter had been removed; it is therefore possible that some of the isolates represented contamination of the external part of the catheter or the site of insertion and that bacteremia was actually less frequent. In a study designed to assess this possibility, blood for culture was obtained by standard techniques from a vein distant from the site of catheter manipulation [69]. Venous blood cultures of 106 patients, the majority of whom had valvular heart disease, were obtained in this manner during cardiac catheterization, and all were sterile. Three of 38 samples that were drawn through the catheter that was placed in the heart or aorta during the procedure grew diphtheroids or microaerophilic streptococci. It was concluded that contamination of the "hub" end of the catheter with normal skin flora led to an overestimation of the incidence of bacteremia. Removal of organisms by lung "filtration" may also have accounted in part for the failure to isolate organisms from distal sites. In either case, it is clear that some contamination of the catheterization cutdown field has occurred. With rigorous application of strict aseptic technique and adoption of the working principle that cardiac catheterization is a surgical procedure, catheterization-associated infection should be very infrequent, and systemic antibiotic prophylaxis does not appear justified.

*Indwelling Arterial Catheters*

Indwelling arterial catheters are being used with increasing frequency in patients whose precarious cardiovascular status necessitates pressure monitoring or repeated blood-gas determination (see Chapter 36). Even though they provide information that is essential for sophisticated patient care and eliminate the need for potentially traumatic repeated arterial punctures, such catheters also provide a continuing portal of entry for microbial invasion of the bloodstream.

The infectious complications of the use of arterial catheters have been studied most extensively in neonates. In different centers, the incidence of colonization of indwelling umbilical artery catheters varies from 6 to 60 percent [1,6,46,64]. Unexpectedly, however, the incidence of colonization fails to increase with duration of catheterization, which suggests that catheters become contaminated initially or soon after insertion through the umbilical stump, an area that is heavily colonized and impossible to sterilize completely by local or systemic antibiotics. Indeed, the same organisms usually are isolated from both the cord and catheter in any individual patient. The most frequent contaminants are staphylococci, streptococci, and gram-negative bacilli, particularly *Pseudomonas, Proteus, Escherichia coli,* and *Klebsiella.*

The clinical significance of umbilical catheter colonization is difficult to assess, because the incidence of sepsis in most studies has been low. When serial prospective blood cultures have been obtained from catheterized neonates, however, transient catheter-related bacteremia has been noted. In a prospective study of temporary (two to four hours) umbilical catheterization for exchange transfusion, investigators showed a 60 percent incidence of catheter contamination and a 10 percent incidence of transient bacteremia due to *Staphylococcus epidermidis* (and, in one case, *Proteus*) that occurred four to six hours after transfusion; this study suggests that the risk from umbilical catheterization may be greatest during the insertion and removal of catheters [3]. In this study and others, prophylactic systemic antibiotics failed to reduce the incidence of catheter contamination or bacteremia. At present, antibiotic prophylaxis does not appear to be beneficial during umbilical catheterization; instead, attention should be focused on meticulous cord preparation and care.

In adults, the rate of bacterial colonization of indwelling arterial catheters and the risk of associated sepsis have not been studied as extensively. Gardner and coworkers [34] demonstrated positive arterial catheter-tip cultures in 4 percent of 200 patients exposed to radial artery catheterization (the preferred site in adults). The source of these organisms was not evaluated, and no direct relationship with patient disease was established, but the incidence of colonization of radial catheters (in contrast to umbilical catheters) did appear to be related to longer durations of catheterization.

More recent studies in adults have emphasized the risk of endemic infections caused by arterial catheters used for hemodynamic monitoring [5,59]. A prospective study of 95 patients (130 catheters) in a medical-surgical intensive care unit showed a 4 percent risk of arterial cannula-related septicemia; 12 percent of all sepsis in this unit was the result of intraarterial catheters [5]. These bacteremias were caused by gram-negative bacilli, enterococci, and *Candida*. Risk factors for the catheter-related infections included catheter placements exceeding four days, placement of catheter by cutdown or in the femoral artery, and the presence of local inflammation.

Breaks in aseptic technique may create a greatly increased risk of arterial catheter contamination and sepsis, as was highlighted by an outbreak of *Flavobacterium* bacteremia [77]. In the affected hospital, the sterile, heparinized glass syringes used for clearing arterial lines and for withdrawing arterial blood samples were submerged routinely in ice for a few minutes before use. The ice machine in the hospital's intensive care unit was contaminated with *Flavobacterium* (an organism that can survive and grow at temperatures as low as $-38°C$ [$-36°F$]), and contamination of in-use phlebotomy syringes with this ice resulted in 14 cases of *Flavobacterium* sepsis. Control of the outbreak depended on improved aseptic technique, that is, on discontinuing the practice of cooling syringes in ice before blood withdrawal and of reinjecting blood to clear the catheter system.

Guidelines for prevention of infections related to intravascular pressure monitoring have been formulated by the Centers for Disease Control (CDC) (Table 38-1).

*Transducers*
Pressure-monitoring devices (transducers or gauges connected to a closed space by a length of fluid-filled tubing) are being used with increasing frequency for monitoring cardiovascular and cerebrospinal fluid (CSF) pressures of critically ill patients. These devices can provide a portal of entry for microbial invasion of the blood or CSF. Although such devices frequently are used in the setting of arterial cannulation or cardiac catheterization, we feel that the threat posed by monitoring devices is so prominent and so frequently overlooked that a separate section on transducer-related infection is warranted.

Although many hospital personnel assume that a protective pressure gradient exists between patients and transducers, contaminated monitoring devices have been the source of nosocomial infection in outbreaks of gram-negative bacteremia, candidemia, and dialysis-associated hepatitis [86]. As electronic monitoring has been used increasingly to measure CSF and intrauterine pressure, there have been occasional reports of transducer-related infections in neurosurgical and obstetric patients. In one study, epidemiologic evidence and culture suggested that contaminated intrauterine pressure transducers used during labor were a nosocomial source of group-B streptococcal colonization [24].

As in infusion-related sepsis, any organism that can survive in the fluid used in the monitoring system is capable of causing monitoring-related infection. *Pseudomonas* species and members of the tribe Klebsielleae (*Klebsiella, Enterobacter,* and *Serratia*) have caused the reported bacteremias. The *Pseudomonas* species— *P. cepacia* and *P. acidovorans*—that were implicated in three outbreaks may reflect an emphasis toward unusual epidemics that are more readily recognized and evaluated. Pathogens such as *P. cepacia,* however, may have selective advantages in the hospital environment because of their ability to grow with minimal nutrients and to resist commonly used disinfectants, such as dilute aqueous benzalkonium chloride.

In the outbreaks that we investigated, pressure-monitoring devices were contaminated most frequently by an index patient. Just as organisms from a contaminated transducer may migrate (or be flushed) through fluid-filled monitoring lines to infect a patient, organisms in the bloodstream of a patient with preexisting bacteremia or viremia may migrate (or be refluxed) through the lines to contaminate a transducer. If the transducer is not sterilized after use, cross-infection can result.

Although we do not know how often personnel fail to sterilize transducers between uses, there are several reasons to believe that this is a relatively common error. First, many hospital personnel, failing to recognize that transducers may be a source of infection, are loath to subject such expensive and relatively delicate instruments to adequate cleaning efforts. Second, transducers cannot withstand autoclaving, and heavy patient loads frequently may not allow time for the more lengthy gas or chemical sterilization procedures that these devices require. Finally, even when an attempt at proper care is made, the many "nooks and crannies" in the traditional dome-and-diaphragm transducer may hamper cleaning and sterilizing efforts.

TABLE 38-1. Guidelines for preventing infections related to intravascular pressure-monitoring systems

Category I*
1. Use intravascular monitoring only when clinically necessary and discontinue as soon as possible
2. Arrange systems as simply as possible; do not assemble or fill systems with flush solution until needed
3. Do not use glucose-containing solutions as the interface liquid between transducer head and chamber-dome membrane or as flush solution (since they support growth of many microorganisms)
4. Wash hands before inserting cannulas or manipulating system; wear sterile gloves for inserting central catheters and for cutdowns
5. Guidelines for inserting and maintaining intravascular pressure-monitoring systems are similar to those for IV cannulas (see Chapter 36)
6. During calibration of the system, contact should not occur between sterile fluid in the system and nonsterile solutions or equipment
7. Any stopcocks should be covered; any specimens should be obtained aseptically with care to avoid contaminating any sampling ports
8. The flush solution should be changed every 24 hours; disposable components should not be resterilized and reused
9. After use, transducer heads (and reusable domes) should be cleaned, receive high-level disinfection or sterilization, and be stored to prevent contamination before next use

Category II*
1. Disposable components, preassembled and sterile-packaged by the manufacturer, should be used
2. Closed, rather than open (syringe and stopcock), flush systems should be used to maintain catheter patency
3. The chamber dome, tubing, and continuous-flow device (if used) should be replaced at 48-hour intervals. (It is not known whether the transducer needs periodic disinfection-sterilization during prolonged use for a single patient)
4. The site of peripheral arterial cannulas should be changed after four days if possible
5. Cannulas should not be changed over a guide wire if this is done solely for infection prophylaxis

*Ranking scheme for recommendations:
 Category I. Strongly recommended for adoption
  Measures in category I are strongly supported by well-designed and controlled clinical studies that show effectiveness in reducing the risk of nosocomial infections or are viewed as useful by the majority of experts in the field. Measures in this category are judged to be applicable to the majority of hospitals—regardless of size, patient population, or endemic nosocomial infection rate—and are considered practical to implement.
 Category II. Moderately recommended for adoption
  Measures in category II are supported by highly suggestive clinical studies or by definitive studies in institutions that might not be representative of other hospitals. Measures that have not been adequately studied, but have a strong theoretical rationale indicating that they might be very effective are included in this category. Category II measures are judged to be practical to implement. They are *not* to be considered a standard of practice for every hospital.
Source: Adapted from *Infect. Control* 3:61, 1982.

Once transducers are sterilized for use, the many manipulations involved in using a monitoring system make extrinsic contamination of the equipment possible. As anticipated [86], the frequent use of unsterile mercury manometers for calibrating sterile transducers makes contamination likely [33]. Other potential vehicles for transducer contamination include cleaning solutions and intravenous fluids and medications, particularly those in multidose vials [83]. Infusion bacteremia caused by extrinsically contaminated IV fluid is rare (see Chapter 36); however, the fluid column in pressure-monitoring systems is at much greater risk of contamination (and sepsis) because it may be stagnant and subjected to frequent manipulations. In one study of 56 ICU patients with 102 intraarterial infusions, prospective cultures of the monitoring systems showed 12 episodes of contaminated fluid in the chamber domes [55]. Eight of

these cases had concordant bacteremia. In all eight cases, the transducer "chamber dome" (Fig. 38-1) had been used for more than two days, suggesting that with prolonged use the monitoring circuit (Fig. 38-2) should be replaced every 48 hours.

For reasons outlined previously, we suspect that transducer contamination is relatively common and that monitoring-related infections have been occurring sporadically since transducers were introduced into clinical medicine. As increasing use of invasive procedures places a large population at risk of monitoring-related infection, and as awareness of this problem increases, such sporadic cases and the means for preventing them should receive more attention. In each hospital, guidelines need to be established for the care of transducers and for surveillance and management of monitoring-related infection (Table 38-1). Ongoing surveillance of transducer-related in-

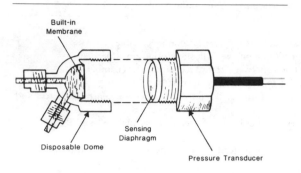

FIG. 38-1. Parts of disposable chamber dome and transducer.

fection in patients undergoing cardiovascular monitoring, as well as possibly obtaining periodic cultures from transducers and the fluid in monitoring lines, will help each hospital assess the adequacy of its monitoring practices and sterilization procedures.

Efforts are under way to improve the ease of transducer sterilization and to simplify the aseptic use of monitoring systems [85]. More recent innovations, not yet widely used, include miniature extravascular transducers that are built into the tips of standard Luer-Lok fittings and thus can be attached directly to monitoring lines (or designed for intravascular use), obviating the need for cumbersome domes; however, when sterilizing these miniature transducers, care must be taken to ensure that the area between the transducer and the Luer fitting is thoroughly cleaned and comes into full contact with the sterilizing medium. Inexpensive, disposable, pressure-monitor "isolating" devices are available also, but they allow only mean pressure readings, usually on a gauge-type manometer.

The traditional reusable transducer dome has been largely replaced by the disposable chamber dome (see Fig. 38-1), which has a thin membrane that abuts the transducer diaphragm and keeps the monitoring fluid within a sterile disposable circuit. The viability of this approach depends on the chamber dome not being reused and on the thin membrane reliably maintaining its integrity throughout a monitoring period [85]. Several outbreaks have documented the failure of disposable domes to prevent septicemia acquired from contaminated transducers [15,28]. The exact way that bacteria spread from contaminated transducers to the sterile circuit is not clear; however, hand transmission of organisms from transducer heads to dome fluid was shown experimentally during assembly, calibration, and manipulation of ports. Thus sterilization, or at least high-level disinfection, of

transducer heads appears necessary even when disposable chamber domes are used.

Finally, the most recently available advance in pressure monitoring is the totally disposable transducer system. At present, the relative costs and infection risks of disposable transducers compared to the chamber-dome system are not known. Moreover, it is not known to what extent current guidelines for intravascular monitoring, especially the frequency of changing systems, apply to the disposable transducers. In fact, since the publication of the CDC guidelines for preventing monitoring-related infections (Table 38-1), a prospective study of 117 patients has called into question the need to change routinely any component of the monitoring circuit [75]. In this study, no contamination of monitoring-system fluid was found despite prolonged (25 to 439 hours) use. The researchers felt that by placing the continuous-flow device just distal to the transducer (Fig. 38-2), they eliminated the static in-line fluid column, which in other studies [55] may have led to contamination. They also noted their meticulous care of stopcocks, a part of the transducer system most frequently manipulated and contaminated. Plugs were used for all stopcock sampling ports. The plugs were placed on a sterile sponge soaked with iodophor whenever the stopcock was manipulated, and the port was cleaned with iodophor before the plug was reinserted. Because studies of endemic contamination of transducer circuits are limited, the relative impact of eliminating the static fluid column, observing scrupulous asepsis during sampling, or changing transducer domes every 48 hours is not known.

## TRANSFUSION-ASSOCIATED INFECTIONS

This section will cover transfusion-associated infections [81] other than hepatitis and cytomegalovirus infections, which are discussed elsewhere (see Chapters 35 and 37).

### Blood Transfusion and Bacteremia

The first case reports of transfusion-related sepsis appeared in the 1940s and 1950s and involved shock syndromes produced by transfusion of cold-stored blood contaminated with psychrophilic organisms such as *Achromobacter* and some *Pseudomonas* species. Prospective microbiologic studies soon followed these reports and documented a contamination rate of 1 to 6 percent in banked blood [43]. The majority of contaminants were normal skin flora, presumably introduced with fragments of donor skin cored out during phlebotomy. Such contaminants were usually present in

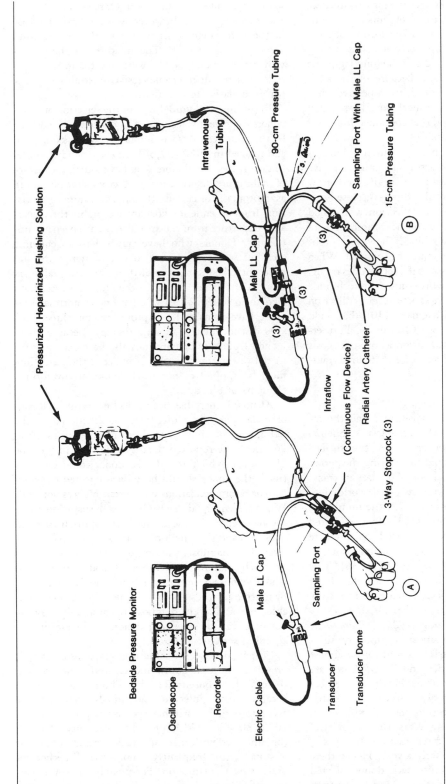

FIG. 38-2. Components of two arterial pressure-monitoring systems using continuous-flow devices. (System A from Maki, D. G., and Hassemer, C. A. *Am. J. Med.* 733:207, 1981. System B from Shinozaki, T., et al. *J.A.M.A.* 249:223, 1983, reproduced with permission.)

extremely low concentrations (several logarithmic factors below the level of $10^6$ to $10^8$ organisms per milliliter of blood associated with transfusion sepsis), and additional multiplication of organisms during storage seemed unlikely because of the long lag phase produced by refrigeration and because of the antibacterial action of blood. Indeed, retrospective studies failed to document any clinical illness associated with the transfusion of blood that contained low-level contamination with skin flora [12].

Today, as in 1940, the most common organisms associated with transfusion sepsis are gram-negative bacilli, particularly those able to survive and grow at 4°C (39°F). With the sterile, disposal, closed systems used at present for blood collection, with good collection technique, and with the prompt use of dated, refrigerated, banked blood, however, problems with blood transfusions should be minimal. When an episode of transfusion-associated sepsis does occur, it is important to search for breakdowns in technique or a contaminated common source (e.g., collection sets, disinfectants, and anticoagulants [10]) that could put other patients at risk (see Chapter 7). Furthermore, the possibility of transfusion-associated sepsis should be investigated in any case of febrile transfusion reaction [79].

*Blood Transfusion and Parasitemia*
The increased use of blood transfusions and the increased travel to countries where malaria is endemic have led to an increased occurrence of transfusion-related malaria. It is estimated that during the period between 1911 and 1950, about 350 cases of transfusion-associated malaria were reported worldwide, but during the period 1950 to 1972, the number of reported cases exceeded 2000 [113]. In the United States, 71 cases of transfusion-induced malaria were reported in the years 1958 to 1981 inclusive, of which 35 occurred between 1967 and 1972 [29,36]. This increase has been linked to imported cases of malaria: over 50 percent of the implicated donors had a history of recent military service in Southeast Asia [29].

Based on worldwide incidence data, *Plasmodium malariae* appears to be the most common cause of transfusion-associated malaria, accounting for almost 50 percent of cases. *P. vivax* and *P. falciparum* are second and third in worldwide incidence, respectively. This ordering probably reflects the fact that although *P. malariae* infection may persist in an asymptomatic donor for many years, the longevity of *P. vivax* malaria in humans rarely exceeds three years, and that of *P. falciparum,* rarely a year. Hence there is greater chance for an asymptomatic donor infected with *P. malariae* to escape detection and become the

source of an infected transfusion. Of note in the United States in the 1970s, however, was a relative increase in the percentage of cases due to the "malignant" species, *P. falciparum*. The majority of these cases were traced to donors who were infected in Southeast Asia, where antimicrobial-resistant strains of falciparum malaria are prevalent.

Recommended guidelines for the selection of blood donors to prevent transmission of malaria were adopted by the American Association of Blood Banks in 1970 and relaxed in 1974 [29,36]. In the amended guidelines, prospective donors who have a definite history of malaria are deferred for three years after becoming asymptomatic or ceasing therapy. Immigrants or visitors from an endemic area are acceptable three years after departure from the area if they have been asymptomatic. Donors who have traveled to an endemic area but who have remained free of symptoms and have not taken antimalarial drugs are acceptable six months after their return to the United States; travelers to an endemic area who have taken antimalarials must have remained symptom-free for three years after discontinuation of drug therapy. Because platelet and leukocyte preparations also have been incriminated in the transmission of malaria, the guidelines must be applied to potential donors of any formed elements of blood.

Although there has been a decline in the incidence of malaria in the United States, attributed to the termination of military involvement in Southeast Asia, 26 cases were reported during 1972–81. In 9 of the 18 cases in which an infected donor could be identified, the donor should have been rejected based on current recommendations but mistakenly was not [36]. When screening fails, a high index of suspicion about the recipient's disease is the best approach to rapid diagnosis and treatment of transfusion-associated malaria. The diagnosis should be considered in any patient who has received formed blood elements and who develops a fever for which no cause is determined by routine cultures. (Serologic methods are now available that accurately diagnose malaria, but they are not practical for screening donors or for rapidly diagnosing serious infection.)

Chagas' disease, or American trypanosomiasis, is prevalent through South and Central America, and there is a high potential for bloodborne transmission, because some infected individuals may become asymptomatic but still have persistent parasitemia for 10 to 30 years. Although the infectivity of blood contaminated with this parasite declines after ten days of storage, this frequently is not a useful method for preventing transmission. Fortunately, however, carriers of Chagas' disease can be detected by complement-fixation tests. In some areas of South America, 15 percent of potential blood donors are positive, and when blood from these donors has been used for transfusions, up to 25 percent of the recipients have developed clinical Chagas' disease. Thus serologic screening has become mandatory for the acceptance of blood donors in many South American countries.

Toxoplasmosis is a disease that is receiving increasing clinical attention, particularly as a cause of opportunistic infection in patients with impaired host defenses. A large portion of the general population, perhaps one-half of adults, have specific antibodies for *Toxoplasma gondii.* In one prospective survey of thalassemic patients who were frequently transfused, subclinical toxoplasmosis was detected at a rate comparable to that seen in a control group, and this was felt to be evidence against the transmission of toxoplasmosis by transfusion [45]. In another study, however, patients treated for acute leukemia developed toxoplasmosis following leukocyte transfusions from donors with chronic myelogenous leukemia; serologic data retrospectively obtained from donors revealed elevated anti-*Toxoplasma* antibody titers [75]. This inferential evidence for transfusion-associated toxoplasmosis is supported by the findings that the disease can be transmitted between animals by transfusion, that *Toxoplasma* organisms retain their viability in stored blood for up to 50 days, and that organisms can be recovered from the blood buffy-coat layers of patients with toxoplasmosis. Because it seems likely that toxoplasmosis can be transmitted if large concentrations of leukocytes are transfused, it has been recommended that blood from donors with high anti-*Toxoplasma* antibody titers not be used for leukocyte transfusion, particularly since the host defenses of recipients usually are severely compromised.

Transfusion-related babesiosis has also been documented recently [41,89].

### Blood Transfusion and Acquired Immunodeficiency Syndrome

Of the first 2157 patients with acquired immunodeficiency syndrome (AIDS), 3 percent did not fall into any recognized risk group; 18 patients without apparent risk shared the common factor of receipt of blood (or blood products) within five years before onset of AIDS [22]. In one case, a 14-month-old infant who had multiple transfusions at birth developed AIDS [2]. One of the baby's blood donors was a male homosexual who was well at the time of blood donation but died 17 months later of AIDS. Presumably he was incubating, and communicable for, AIDS at the time of donation. In several other cases of possible transfusion-associated AIDS, a male homo-

sexual with either fever and lymphadenopathy or a suppressed T helper–T suppressor lymphocyte ratio (findings either prodromal to or associated with AIDS) has been among the donors. No particular component of blood has been associated with these cases (see Chapter 35).

If AIDS can be transmitted by blood or blood products, the risk so far has been quite small; there is approximately one AIDS case per million transfusions. Despite the tentative nature of this association, several national groups have pushed for preventive measures including discouraging individuals in high-risk groups for AIDS from donating blood (promiscuous homosexual men, Haitians, IV drug addicts, hemophiliacs, and sexual partners or spouses of persons in high-risk groups) [16]. Other efforts include strict adherence to medical indications for transfusion, using cell savers during surgery, increased use of autologous transfusions, and most recently serologic screening of donated blood for antibody to the newly discovered AIDS virus, HTLV-III (Chapter 35).

### Platelet Transfusion

The incidence of bacterial contamination of platelet concentrates has been a source of controversy. While many investigators have reported no contamination, others have consistently found bacterial contaminants in 1 to 6 percent of concentrates [14]. Because it is now recommended that platelets be stored at room temperature (rather than 4°C [39°F]) to increase in vivo half-life, there is justifiable concern over the true incidence of "intrinsic" contamination and the possible proliferation of contaminants during storage. It seems reasonable to assume that platelet concentrates are as susceptible to contamination during collection as is blood, which is routinely found to have a 1 to 6 percent incidence of low-level contamination (see previous section). Moreover, platelet concentrates, unlike blood, have no protective antibacterial activity, and platelet transfusions are frequently obtained by pooling the contributions of several donors, which increases the risk of contamination additionally. Despite this seemingly grim picture, the majority of bacterial contaminants isolated from platelet concentrates have been normal skin flora, such as *Staphylococcus epidermidis* and diphtheroids, and they have been present in extremely low concentrations (less than 500 organisms per milliliter). Even in the highly susceptible patient populations that normally receive platelet transfusions, such contaminants have failed to produce any documented adverse reactions [21].

Although meticulous blood-banking techniques and the widespread use of closed collection systems have made platelet transfusion relatively safe, the occurrence of outbreaks emphasizes the possibility of sporadic, significant contamination of platelets. One outbreak involved seven cases of *Salmonella choleraesuis* sepsis that were traced to platelet transfusions from a blood donor with clinically inapparent salmonellal osteomyelitis and intermittent asymptomatic bacteremia [67]. (As an interesting aside, a long incubation period in this outbreak—that is, a mean interval of nine days between the transfusion with contaminated platelets and the signs of sepsis—was caused by coincidental administration of antibiotics at the time of platelet transfusion in several cases, and this initially delayed recognition of platelets as the vehicle of infection.) A second outbreak involved two cases of transfusion-induced *Enterobacter cloacae* sepsis [14]. An investigation prompted by the occurrence of these cases revealed that 20 percent of the platelet pools prepared in the affected hospital were contaminated. Although the majority of the contaminants were "nonpathogens" and present only in low concentrations, 6 of 258 platelet pools were shown to harbor *Enterobacter cloacae*. Despite extensive efforts, the source of these unusual contaminants was not discovered. A third outbreak with *Serratia,* was traced to contaminated evacuated tubes used following blood collection [10].

### Albumin Infusion

Because of faith in commercial manufacturing practices and the extremely low incidence of reactions to albumin infusion, most physicians consider commercial human serum albumin to be a completely safe product. A nationwide outbreak of albumin-related *Pseudomonas cepacia* sepsis, however, emphasized that any commercial product, particularly any blood component, is susceptible to contamination [78]. The outbreak involved four lots of commercial 25% normal human serum albumin. One of the lots had an estimated 1 percent contamination rate and resulted in at least seven cases of albumin-associated sepsis in one Maryland hospital; the other three lots caused isolated cases of albumin-related disease in patients in four other states. The organisms most likely gained access to the albumin vials during a hand-filling procedure.

In addition to emphasizing the risk of infection associated with the infusion of a nonformed blood component, it is worthwhile noting that the albumin outbreak points up several general problems in the detection and evaluation of low-frequency contamination of commercial products. First, nosocomial infections caused by low-frequency contaminants may be difficult to distinguish from endemic problems in

any one institution. In the Maryland hospital, the infusion-related infections became apparent only because of the enormous quantity of albumin that was used in the hospital. Second, since commercial products are usually prepared and sterilized in bulk lots, it is important to be able to trace the distribution of individual suspect lots. Although the Maryland hospital did not routinely record information on albumin distribution and use, an alert physician fortuitously noted the lot number and brand of albumin used in one case of suspected infusion-related sepsis. Third, sterility of an infusion product cannot be ascertained by visual inspection. Despite *P. cepacia* concentrations of $10^6$ to $10^8$ organisms per milliliter, the contaminated albumin was completely clear. Finally, when present in low frequency, some contaminants can be missed by the sampling schemes currently used for product quality control, and endotoxin may escape terminal filtration and be missed by currently used pyrogen tests. To facilitate the monitoring of albumin-related reactions, some hospitals now distribute this product through their blood banks.

Albumin-transmitted hepatitis is discussed elsewhere (see Chapter 35).

## INFECTION HAZARDS ASSOCIATED WITH ANESTHESIA

As noted in previous chapters, severe bacterial infections have been well documented in association with the use of contaminated equipment for local or spinal anesthesia or the use of contaminated anesthesia machines for delivery of general anesthesia. An additional well-recognized infectious complication of general anesthesia unrelated to the use of contaminated equipment is aspiration pneumonia attributable either to the passage of an endotracheal tube or to postoperative difficulties.

Aspiration of stomach contents into the lungs during or following obstetric anesthesia was first described by Mendelson [57], who found the incidence of this complication to be 0.15 percent during the preantibiotic era. In about two-thirds of these cases, aspiration was reported as having definitely occurred in the delivery room, but in the remainder, the complication went unrecognized until later. A common clinical pattern was that two to five hours after vomiting and aspiration, a dramatic onset of cyanosis, tachycardia, and shock was noted.

More recent investigations have shown a surprisingly high incidence of aspiration associated with general anesthesia. In one ingenious study, Evans blue dye was placed in the stomach preoperatively to be used as a "marker" for chemical aspiration; following anesthesia, the dye was sought by bronchoscopy [20]. Of 300 patients observed in this manner, 25 percent vomited, and aspiration was documented in 16 percent of the overall group. Interestingly, aspiration was "silent" and unnoticed by the entire operating team in one-half of those patients who did aspirate (an overall rate of 8 percent), and there were no obvious clues to the time of occurrence. No incidence of pneumonia was reported in this series, but it seems that in normal patients the aspirated inoculum is usually cleared without sequelae. Patients who have significant retention of gastric contents and preexisting pulmonary disease may be at much higher risk of developing a chemical aspiration pneumonitis and subsequent bacterial infection.

Despite these studies documenting intraoperative aspiration, it seems likely that postoperative aspiration accounts for the majority of aspiration pneumonias associated with general surgery. Surgical procedures involving the upper abdomen, thorax, or upper gastrointestinal tract have been the operations most commonly associated with aspiration pneumonia. The highest risk patients include those undergoing emergency procedures with a full stomach and those whose condition prevents the stomach from emptying well (e.g., full-term pregnancy, marked obesity, ileus, or massive ascites).

The upper respiratory and gastrointestinal passages are colonized by vast numbers of aerobic and anaerobic organisms, and a mixture of both types of organisms is usually found when specimens from a patient with aspiration pneumonia are cultured appropriately. Among the aerobic organisms, gram-negative bacilli are now encountered more frequently than staphylococci in hospitalized patients. Penicillin is commonly used in the initial therapy for aspiration pneumonia, but an added compound with activity against gram-negative organisms would seem preferable. Use of antimicrobial agents with broader coverage of anaerobic organisms has been advocated, but there is no convincing evidence of the clinical superiority of such agents over the penicillins in therapy of aspiration pneumonia. The prophylactic use of antibiotics and steroids is of unproven value. Therapeutically, the administration of corticosteroids may be of value, but it usually is carried out too late to minimize the chemical inflammatory reaction that is the hallmark of early aspiration.

Measures to prevent anesthesia-associated aspiration have included prolonged preoperative fasting, adequate sedation, attention to problems during anesthesia, insertion of a nasogastric tube before anesthesia, and careful monitoring of the patient in the early period postoperatively. Such principles can be readily applied to elective surgical intervention. Although the insertion of a nasogastric tube is felt to reduce the incidence of aspiration during anesthesia, more than half the cases of postoperative aspiration occur in patients whose nasogastric tubes have been left in place, and a quarter of cases of postoperative aspiration pneumonia have also been associated with tracheostomy. It is difficult to interpret these data, however, since the most seriously ill and aspiration-prone patients have tracheostomies or nasogastric tubes left in place.

In emergency procedures and for the high-risk patients cited previously, measures used to prevent aspiration or ameliorate its effect include attempts to empty the stomach (with metoclopramide or a large nasogastric tube); to decrease stomach acid (with anticholinergic drugs, $H_2$ blockers, or antacids—although some common antacids are suspensions of particulate matter that may themselves incite pulmonary inflammation if aspirated); to use cricoid pressure to occlude the esophagus during induction of anesthesia; or to pass an endotracheal tube with inflatable balloon under topical anesthesia with the patient awake (and empty the stomach after this).

### Endotracheal Intubation

Aside from aspiration, another potential hazard of anesthesia may be the occurrence of bacteremia secondary to the passage of an endotracheal tube. The organisms isolated from the blood usually are $\alpha$-hemolytic streptococci, both aerobic and anaerobic diphtheroids, and other anaerobic organisms that normally colonize the upper respiratory tract. There may, however, be a higher incidence of such bacteremia following the nasotracheal route of intubation (16 percent in one series) than following the less traumatic orotracheal route [8]. Prolonged nasotracheal (or nasogastric) intubation has also been associated with sinusitis, which may be quite occult.

## INFECTIONS OF THE CENTRAL NERVOUS SYSTEM: RESERVOIRS AND SHUNTS

Serious infection can complicate the insertion or prolonged use of two very important neurosurgical devices: the Ommaya-type subcutaneous reservoir, which is used for administering intrathecal therapy for fungal or neoplastic meningitis, and the ventricular shunt, which is used for decompression of hydrocephalus.

Complications have been observed frequently following the insertion or chronic use of subcutaneous intraventricular reservoirs [25,82]. In one series involving 21 reservoirs, nine patients developed CSF bacterial infections as a result of reservoir use or insertion, and complications associated with 17 reservoirs in 12 patients either necessitated reservoir removal or prevented their later use for intrathecal therapy [25] *Staphylococcus epidermidis*, *Corynebacterium acnes*, and α-hemolytic streptococci were the major causes of the reservoir infections, and this predominance of normal skin flora suggests that the bacteria gained access to the CSF during repeated percutaneous injections of antifungal or antineoplastic agents into the reservoir. Therapy of the bacterial superinfection usually is given systemically, because the efficacy of antimicrobials added to the reservoir, either for prophylaxis or for treatment of superinfection, has not been established. Furthermore, although in one study 80 percent of the patients who completed the treatment course were cured by systemic antimicrobial therapy alone [25], we still feel that infected spinal fluid devices should be removed.

The use of valved (Spitz-Holter type) catheters for the treatment of hydrocephalus (i.e., to shunt CSF from the lateral ventricle of the brain to the superior vena cava, the right atrium, or the peritoneum) has also been complicated by a high incidence of infections. In a number of series, the overall incidence of shunt infections has ranged from 6 to 23 percent, with a median of about 14 percent [54]. Most of these infections are caused by *S. aureus* or *S. epidermidis* and occur within two weeks to two months after surgery, which stresses the importance of intraoperative and perioperative shunt contamination in the pathogenesis of shunt infection. The equal risk of infection in patients with ventriculoatrial and ventriculoperitoneal shunts suggests that transient bacteremia is a less likely cause of such infections, since ventriculoperitoneal shunts are not exposed to the bloodstream [70].

Patients with infected ventricular shunts have several different clinical presentations. Some display a markedly toxic course with persistent pyrexia, progressive anemia, splenomegaly, and repeatedly positive blood cultures. More often there is a chronic, indolent course, and considerable clinical suspicion may be necessary before appropriate steps are undertaken. In certain cases, the clinical pattern may be related to the bacteriologic characteristics of the infection. Only about one-third of infected shunts, for example, exhibit visible wound infection and necrosis, but when these occur, they are important signs of underlying infection, usually with *S. aureus*. In contrast to cases with obvious local inflammation, *S. epidermidis* is found in the great majority of other cases, and this organism is most frequently associated with bacteremic infections.

The antimicrobial treatment of the shunt infections that complicate hydrocephalus is usually unsatisfactory unless the shunt is removed [42]. Although less than 10 percent of patients have their infection eradicated by systemic antimicrobial therapy alone, small numbers of patients have been treated with combinations of systemic and intraventricular antibiotics, and the addition of the latter appears to improve cure rates. Repeated administration of intraventricular antibiotics has its own complications, however, and when infection is widespread, the treatment of choice appears to be the administration of appropriate systemic antibiotics and the complete removal of the shunt to a new site. Preferably, some time should elapse between the removal of the infected shunt and the insertion of a new one. Despite this discouraging picture, it should be recognized that many of the antibiotics that were used to treat shunt infections in the past have been supplanted by newer agents that may prove to be more efficacious against this highly refractory infectious complication. In addition, the epidemiologic characteristics of shunt infections (e.g., perioperative acquisition of organisms) and the narrow spectrum of shunt pathogens suggest that the use of prophylactic antimicrobials at the time of shunt surgery may prove beneficial. Although one controlled study of relatively low-dose oxacillin prophylaxis failed to show that antibiotics had a significant protective effect [87], studies using larger doses of this or other drugs administered in such a way that high levels in the spinal fluid are attained at the time of surgery may be more successful.

## TRANSIENT BACTEREMIA FROM NONVASCULAR PROCEDURES

The occurrence of transient bacteremia associated with relatively noninvasive manipulation of colonized mucosa is well recognized [32]. Such bacteremia usually lasts no longer than 5 to 15 minutes, may shower at its peak 100 organisms per milliliter of blood (although the peak concentration is almost always much less), and is largely asymptomatic. Hundreds of studies have reported on bacteremia following oral treatments alone [19]. In this section, we discuss bacteremia following diagnostic gastrointestinal procedures, genitourinary instrumentation, and bronchoscopy; bacteremia following endotracheal intubation and invasive vascular procedures is covered earlier in this

TABLE 38-2. Characteristics of transient bacteremia associated with selected procedures

| Involved system | Maximum incidence of bacteremia (%) |
| --- | --- |
| Dental | 90 |
| Urologic | 80 |
| Airway | 30 |
| Gastrointestinal | 15 |
| Obstetric-gynecologic | 4 |

Concentration of bacteria per milliliter: < 20–130
Duration of bacteremia (minutes after procedure): 10–30
Predominant bacteria: anaerobes, enterococci, enteric gram-negative bacilli; occasionally, *Streptococcus pneumoniae*
Symptoms: usually none; fever more common with urologic-related bacteremia

chapter. Table 38-2 presents a summary of the characteristics of bacteremia associated with selected nonvascular procedures.

*Gastrointestinal Procedures*

Bacteremia has been reported as a sequel to a variety of gastrointestinal procedures, including sigmoidoscopy, colonoscopy, barium enema, esophagoscopy, biopsy of mucosal masses, injection sclerotherapy of esophageal varices, endoscopic retrograde cholangiopancreatography (ERCP), liver biopsy, esophageal dilatation, and rectal examination. In one prospective study of sigmoidoscopy, transient asymptomatic bacteremia was noted in 19 of 200 procedures [50]. The majority of organisms isolated were enterococci, and bacteremia was observed more frequently five minutes after than one minute after the termination of the procedure. Of note in this study, serial blood cultures were obtained through an indwelling venous needle. Although this convenient approach may have distorted or amplified culture results and is thus open to some criticism, the temporal profile and magnitude of bacteremia, as well as the types of organisms isolated, are consistent with bacteremia arising from the site of instrumentation. Other investigators using similar methods, however, have found bacteremia to be a rare complication of their sigmoidoscopic examinations, and they have concluded that other factors, particularly the experience of the sigmoidoscopist, need to be evaluated before routine antibiotic prophylaxis can be advocated for patients undergoing sigmoidoscopy [31].

In a study of colonoscopy, careful anaerobic cul-

turing and subsequent hourly temperature evaluation of patients showed a 27 percent incidence of transient bacteremia during the procedure and a 33 percent incidence of postprocedure fever in patients who had been bacteremic [62]. The greater trauma of colonoscopy compared to sigmoidoscopy may be responsible for the greater incidence of bacteremia and the more marked clinical response, although these are not consistently found [72]. Host factors may also influence the incidence and outcome of procedure-related bacteremia. In this regard, it is noteworthy that rare cases of symptomatic barium-enema septicemia have been reported in patients with impaired host defenses (acute leukemia) and in patients with active inflammatory bowel disease.

Although the role of antibiotic prophylaxis for endoscopy procedures is not certain, other preventive measures—particularly, careful disinfection of endoscopes and good aseptic technique—are of definite importance. The importance of such measures is highlighted by several anecdotal reports [27,30,34, 35,52]. In one report, two cases of *Pseudomonas* sepsis in leukemic patients undergoing esophagoscopy with mucosal biopsy were traced to exogenous bacteria introduced at the time of biopsy. Cultures of the esophagoscope and of the endoscopy room revealed widespread contamination with enteric organisms, including *P. aeruginosa*, and it was shown that in the routine handling of the instruments, aseptic technique was ignored [35]. In a second report, a case of cholangitis with polymicrobial sepsis followed ERCP in a patient without biliary tract obstruction. Inadequate disinfection of endoscopy equipment was implicated as the source of infection [30]. Large series of ERCP cases have also emphasized the better results obtained with experienced operators [9]. In a third report, several cases of infection with an uncommon, non-*typhosa*, *Salmonella* species were traced to an ineffectively cleaned endoscope [34]. Although endoscopy instruments pass through fields that are already grossly contaminated, the nosocomial organisms that may potentially be introduced by the equipment may be more invasive, more resistant, or more contagious than the patient's own flora. Clearly, any instrument that comes in contact with mucosal membranes during a procedure requires a high level of disinfection.

Percutaneous liver biopsy, although an invasive procedure, is not generally considered to be associated with infection risk. Two studies, however, have documented incidences of bacteremia of 6 and 14 percent following liver biopsy. In the first study, bacteremia was detectable in patients for several hours after biopsy, and it was associated in at least one patient with signs of gram-negative sepsis, but it may not have been attributable directly to the biopsy in all the cases [56]. In the second study, however, the bacteremias were transient, lasted for only 15 to 20 minutes after biopsy, and were asymptomatic [51]. In this study, cultures of liver biopsy specimens were positive in 7 percent of patients, and patients with positive specimens had a significantly higher incidence of bacteremia (83 percent) than did patients whose specimens were sterile (8.4 percent), which suggests a direct relationship between biopsy and bacteremia. One explanation of this relationship is that the hepatic reticuloendothelial cells that were in the process of "clearing" gut bacteria from the portal system were biopsied, resulting in a culture-positive biopsy specimen, a temporary defect in the bacterial clearance mechanisms of the biopsied area, and an associated transient bacteremia. The incidence and clinical significance of liver biopsy-associated bacteremia need additional evaluation, as does an association noted in the second study mentioned between liver biopsy and transient pneumococcal bacteremia in patients with cirrhosis. Antibiotic prophylaxis with liver biopsy is not warranted at present.

## Urologic Instrumentation

An association among urethral instrumentation, fever, and bacteremia has been recognized for many years. In various studies, the incidence of bacteremia associated with urologic procedures has been 2 to 80 percent, with the greatest risks of bacteremia occurring in patients with preexisting urinary tract infections, patients undergoing transurethral resection of the prostate, and patients with prostatitis that is evident on histologic section of biopsy specimens [80]. In 50 to 67 percent of patients in whom bacteremia develops after instrumentation, similar organisms are recovered from both preinstrumentation urine cultures and postinstrumentation blood cultures. The available evidence suggests that the sources of the other 33 to 50 percent of postinstrumentation bacteremias include occult prostatitis, the introduction of normal urethral flora (which perhaps explains the relatively large number of blood cultures that were positive for anaerobes in one study), and the contamination of equipment or irrigating fluids before or during instrumentation. It is apparent that careful evaluation for genitourinary tract infection before instrumentation, treatment of any infection, appropriate disinfection of equipment, and careful aseptic technique are mandatory. Moreover, because of the relatively frequent occurrence of enterococcal bacteremia after urologic instrumentation and because of the association of instrumentation with gram-nega-

tive sepsis as well as with infection at distal sites (e.g., joints), a brief pulse of systemic prophylactic antibiotics at the time of instrumentation may be warranted in high-risk patients, such as those with valvular heart disease, preexisting joint disease, or impaired host defenses [18].

## Bronchoscopy

Although fever and bacteremia have been documented in patients after rigid-tube bronchoscopy [18], bacteremia has not yet been documented prospectively in patients undergoing flexible fiberoptic bronchoscopy. There are, however, case reports of bacteremia related to fiberoptic bronchoscopy, including one report of fatal Pseudomonas bacteremia in a patient with preexisting Pseudomonas bronchitis. Furthermore, in one series of 100 patients who were followed carefully after fiberoptic bronchoscopy, 16 developed fever, 5 developed transient parenchymal infiltrates, and 1 developed rapidly fatal pneumonia. Older patients (more than 60 years old) and those with abnormalities on bronchoscopy were at greatest risk of complications. With the exception of the one fatal pneumonitis, however, all complicating infections resolved without antibiotic therapy, and prospective culturing failed to demonstrate bacteremia in any of the 100 patients [63].

## Conclusions

Two conclusions can be drawn from the studies of procedure-related bacteremia cited above: the equipment used for the procedures should be adequately disinfected or sterilized before every use, and proper aseptic technique should be employed by the operator (see Chapter 14). Beyond this, it is apparent that carefully planned, prospective multicenter studies would be needed to assess the incidence and clinical significance of procedure-related transient bacteremia, to determine which hosts are at risk of associated sepsis or infection at distal sites, to determine if specific risks for certain procedures can be sufficiently defined to justify preventive measures such as antibiotic prophylaxis, and to determine which prophylactic regimens would be most efficacious. Although such studies may not be available for some time (if ever), the procedures clearly will continue, and we have tried to note situations in which it seems reasonable to "cover" patients [18,32]. In this regard, it should be noted that for years dental patients with valvular heart disease have received endocarditis prophylaxis, largely on an empirical basis, although the specific regimens [61] and even the mechanisms by which prophylaxis may protect [39,53] have been called into question here too.

## OTHER PROCEDURES ASSOCIATED WITH INFECTIONS

### Cystoscopy

In addition to the risk of bacteremia associated with cystoscopy, a significant risk of urinary tract infection is associated with this procedure. Several remarkably similar outbreaks have been reported in which the use of dilute aqueous quaternary ammonium compounds as a cystoscope disinfectant was associated with procedure-related urinary tract infections with *Pseudomonas* species, particularly *P. cepacia* (also see Chapter 25). In these outbreaks, the quaternary ammonium compounds either were ineffective in decontaminating the equipment or were themselves actually harboring viable bacteria while in use as disinfectants [26].

Although the risk of infection associated with the use of dilute aqueous quaternary ammonium compounds has been known for at least 20 years, many hospital personnel persist in using these compounds as antiseptics and disinfectants. Such use has most likely resulted in many outbreaks of nosocomial urinary tract infection, as well as outbreaks of nosocomial bacteremia and occasional outbreaks of nosocomial respiratory tract and wound infection. To help decrease the risk of nosocomial urinary tract infection following cystoscopy, it is important that the equipment be thoroughly cleaned and properly disinfected between uses.

### Bronchoscopy

In addition to the risks of bronchoscopy cited, several outbreaks have highlighted the problems of pulmonary infection and false-positive culture results due to inadequately cleaned fiberoptic bronchoscopes. Especially worrisome is a report of the failure of povidone-iodine to kill *Mycobacterium tuberculosis* on bronchoscopes [60]. Preparations of this agent that are intended for skin degerming are often used inadvisably for decontaminating equipment. This experience has reemphasized the need for higher level disinfection (e.g., with glutaraldehyde) or sterilization of these scopes, especially after use on patients who may have tuberculosis.

### Arthrocentesis and Thoracocentesis

Although septic arthritis is caused most commonly by hematogenous spread of organisms, sporadic cases of staphylococcal arthritis and, at times, gram-negative bacillary arthritis have followed several days after invasive joint manipulations. During the mid-1960s, CDC epidemiologists investigated a cluster of cases of staphylococcal arthritis in which the infections occurred one to seven days after outpatient arthrocentesis or intraarticular injection of steroids. Epidemiologic evidence suggested that the physician who had performed these procedures was a disseminator of the epidemic strain, and microbiologic investigation showed that areas of chronic dermatitis on the physician's hands harbored the epidemic organism. A similar cluster of cases of staphylococcal arthritis, in which the infections occurred five to six days after arthrographic examination of the knee joint and three to four days after knee surgery, was traced epidemiologically to the surgeon who had performed these procedures, who was a nasal carrier of staphylococci.

Other diagnostic "taps," such as thoracocentesis [7], have also been associated with nosocomial infections, which emphasizes the fact that all invasive procedures should be performed only under strict aseptic conditions, with careful skin preparation, by an appropriately "scrubbed and gloved" operator, and using sterile equipment. While the relative rarity of centesis-associated infections may be considered testimony that good technique is generally employed in our hospitals and clinics, the lack of such infections also may be evidence of the capacity of the local tissue response to limit bacterial invasion in uncompromised hosts [23]. When procedures are performed in patients with compromised host defenses or on tissues that may have diminished ability to limit bacterial invasion (e.g., rheumatoid joints), the risk of procedure-associated infections may be considerable, which emphasizes the need for continued vigilance.

### Peritoneal Manipulation

Infectious complications of laparoscopy and amniocentesis are rare, presumably because of careful technique, sterile equipment, local host defense mechanisms, and the frequently healthy nature of the subjects. In fact, high-level disinfection of peritoneoscopes with glutaraldehyde instead of gas sterilization has appeared acceptable.

### Water Baths

Contaminated water baths have led to a large number of very similar outbreaks. Warm water baths used to thaw packs of cryoprecipitate for intravenous use by hemophiliacs, to warm peritoneal dialysate, or to warm radiopaque contrast material have led to outbreaks of *P. cepacia* bacteremia, *Acinetobacter* peritonitis, and endotoxemia, respectively [66,68,73]. Cold ice baths used to chill the cardioplegia solution for open heart surgery or to cool blood gas syringes have been implicated in outbreaks of mediastinitis and bacteremia [49].

The exact mechanism of bacterial transfer in these situations is often unknown but probably involves contamination of medication ports, splash onto operative fields, or hand transmission by staff. Possible preventive measures include using dry heat, using impermeable outer wraps and/or drying any immersed object before use, using sterile water or ice, and hand-washing after contact with water baths. The use of disinfectants in water baths has been suggested but not widely attempted.

### Ophthalmologic Examination

Manipulation of the conjunctiva and cornea occurs during tonometry, instillation of eye drops, and manual ophthalmologic examination, and it can result in transmission of conjunctivitis and other eye infections. The infection most commonly transmitted is epidemic keratoconjunctivitis, a highly contagious, frequently iatrogenic disease, which usually is caused by adenovirus type 8 [38] (see Chapter 35). Transmission of the virus occurs via fomites, such as inadequately disinfected tonometers and contaminated eye droppers, as well as by indirect person-to-person spread on the hands of health workers. Similar modes of transmission have been implicated in outbreaks of other viral and bacterial eye infection. Proper care of equipment and conscientious hand-washing between patient contacts is remarkably effective in halting the transmission of such diseases.

### Barium Enema

In addition to transient bacteremia, patients undergoing barium enema are at risk of two other infectious complications. First, infants may aspirate barium when faulty technique produces excessive retrograde flow of contrast material. Second, if the enema bag or tip is not replaced or is not adequately disinfected between uses, or if the barium is contaminated, the procedure may transmit enteric pathogens. This risk was highlighted by Meyers and Richards [58] when they demonstrated that attenuated poliovirus can be transferred via contaminated barium enema. At present, the use of disposable enema bags, tubing, and enema tips has largely put an end to such risks.

## REFERENCES

1. Adam, R. D., Edwards, L. D., Becker, C. C., and Schrom, H. M. Semiquantitative cultures and routine tip cultures on umbilical catheters. *J. Pediatr.* 100:123, 1982.
2. Ammann, A. J., Wara, D. W., Dritz, S., Cowan, M. J., Weintrub, P., Goldman, H., and Perkins, H. A. Acquired immunodeficiency in an infant: Possible transmission by means of blood products. *Lancet* 1:956, 1983.
3. Anagnostakis, D., Kamba, A., Petrochilon, V., Arsen, A., and Matsaniotis, N. Risk of infection associated with umbilical vein catheterization. *J. Pediatr.* 86:759, 1975.
4. Asnes, R. S., and Arendar, G. M. Septic arthritis of the hip. *Pediatrics* 38:837, 1966.
5. Band, J. D., and Maki, D. G. Infections caused by arterial catheters used for hemodynamic monitoring. *Am. J. Med.* 67:735, 1979.
6. Bard, H., Albert, G., Teasdale, F., Doray, B., and Martineau, B. Prophylactic antibiotics in chronic umbilical artery catheterization in respiratory distress syndrome. *Arch. Dis. Child.* 48:630, 1973.
7. Bayer, A. S., Nelson, S. C., Galpin, J. E., Chow, A. W., and Guze, L. B. Necrotizing pneumonia and empyema due to *Clostridium perfringens. Am. J. Med.* 59:851, 1975.
8. Berry, F. A., Blankenbaker, W. L., and Ball, C. G. A comparison of bacteremia occurring with nasotracheal and orotracheal intubation. *Anesth. Analg.* (Cleve.) 52:873, 1973.
9. Bilbao, M. K., Dotter, C. T., Lee, T. G., and Katon, R. M. Complications of endoscopic retrograde cholangiopancreatography (ERCP). *Gastroenterology* 70:314, 1976.
10. Blajchman, M. A., Thornley, J. H., Richardson, H., Elder, D., Spiak, C., and Racher, J. Platelet transfusion-induced *Serratia marcescens* sepsis due to vacuum tube contamination. *Transfusion* 19:39, 1979.
11. Blumenfeld, T. A., Turi, G. K., and Blanc, W. A. Recommended site and depth of newborn heel skin punctures based on anatomical measurements and histopathology. *Lancet* 1:230, 1979.
12. Braude, A. I., Sanford, J. P., Bartlett, J. E., and Mallery, O. T. Effects and clinical significance of bacterial contaminants in transfused blood. *J. Lab. Clin. Med.* 39:902, 1952.
13. Bruce-Chwatt, L. J. Blood transfusion and tropical disease. *Trop. Dis. Bull.* 69:825, 1972.
14. Buchholtz, D. H., Young, V. M., Friedman, N. R., Reilly, J. A., and Mardiney, M. R. Bacterial proliferation in platelets stored at room temperature. *N. Engl. J. Med.* 285:429, 1971.
15. Buxton, A. E., Anderson, R. L., Klimek, J., and Quintiliani, R. Failure of disposable domes to prevent septicemia acquired from contaminated pressure transducers. *Chest* 74:508, 1978.
16. Centers for Disease Control. Prevention of acquired immune deficiency syndrome (AIDS): Re-

port of inter-agency recommendations. *Morbid. Mortal. Weekly Rep.* 32:101, 1983.

17. Chmel, H., and Armstrong, D. *Salmonella oslo:* A focal outbreak in a hospital. *Am. J. Med.* 60:203, 1976.

18. Committee on the Prevention of Rheumatic Fever and Bacterial Endocarditis. Prevention of bacterial endocarditis. *Circulation* 70:1123A, 1984.

19. Crawford, J. J., Sconyers, J. R., Moriarty, J. D., King, R. C., and West, J. F. Bacteremia after tooth extractions studied with the aid of pre-reduced anaerobically sterilized culture media. *Appl. Microbiol.* 27:927, 1974.

20. Culver, G. A., Makel, H. P., and Beecher, H. K. Frequency of aspiration of gastric contents by the lungs during anesthesia and surgery. *Ann. Surg.* 133:289, 1951.

21. Cunningham, M., and Cash, J. D. Bacterial contamination of platelet concentrates stored at 20°C. *J. Clin. Pathol.* 26:401, 1973.

22. Curran, J. W., Lawrence, D. N., Jaffe, H., Kaplan, J. E., Zyla, L. D., Chamberland, M., Weinstein, R., Lui, K. J., Schonberger, L. B., Spira, T. J., Alexander, W. J., Swinger, G., Ammann, A., Solomon, S., Auerbach, D., Mildvan, D., Stoneburner, R., Jason, J. M., Haverkos, H. W., and Evatt, B. L. Acquired immunodeficiency syndrome (AIDS) associated with transfusions. *N. Engl. J. Med.* 310:69, 1984.

23. Dann, T. C. Routine skin preparation before injection: An unnecessary procedure. *Lancet* 2:96, 1969.

24. Davis, J. P., Gutman, L. T., Higgins, M. V., Katz, S. L., Welt, S. I., and Wilfert, C. M. Nasal colonization of infants with group B *Streptococcus* associated with intrauterine pressure transducers. *J. Infect. Dis.* 138:804, 1978.

25. Diamond, R. D., and Bennett, J. E. A subcutaneous reservoir for intrathecal therapy of fungal meningitis. *N. Engl. J. Med.* 288:186, 1974.

26. Dixon, R. E., Kaslow, R. A., Mackel, D. C., Fulkerson, C. C., and Mallison, G. F. Aqueous quaternary ammonium antiseptics and disinfectants: Use and mis-use. *J.A.M.A.* 236:2415, 1976.

27. Doherty, D. E., Flako, J. M., Lefkovitz, N., Rogers, J., and Fromkes, J. *Pseudomonas aeruginosa* sepsis following retrograde cholangiopancreatography (ERCP). *Dig. Dis. Sci.* 27:169, 1982.

28. Donowitz, L. G., Marsik, F. J., Hoyt, J. W., and Wenzel, R. P. *Serratia marcescens* bacteremia from contaminated pressure transducers. *J.A.M.A.* 242:1749, 1979.

29. Dover, A. S., and Schultz, M. G. Transfusion-induced malaria. *Transfusion* 11:353, 1971.

30. Elson, C. O., Hattori, K., and Blackstone, M. O. Polymicrobial sepsis following endoscopic retrograde cholangiopancreatography. *Gastroenterology* 69:507, 1975.

31. Engeling, E. R., Eng, B. F., Sullivan-Sigler, N., Bartlett, J. G., and Gorbach, S. L. Bacteremia after sigmoidoscopy: Another view. *Ann. Intern. Med.* 85:77, 1976.

32. Everett, E. D., and Hirschmann, J. V. Transient bacteremia and endocarditis prophylaxis: A review. *Medicine* 56:61, 1977.

33. Fisher, M. C., Long, S. S., Roberts, E. M., Dunn, J. M., and Balsara, R. K. *Pseudomonas maltophilia* bacteremia in children undergoing open heart surgery. *J.A.M.A.* 246:1571, 1981.

34. Gardner, R. M., Schwartz, R., Wong, H. C., and Burke, J. P. Percutaneous indwelling radial-artery catheters for monitoring cardiovascular function. *N. Engl. J. Med.* 290:1227, 1974.

35. Greene, W. H., Moody, M., Hartley, R., Effman, E., Aisner, J., Young, V. M., and Wienik, P. H. Esophagoscopy as a source of *P. aeruginosa* sepsis in patients with acute leukemia: The need for sterilization of endoscopes. *Gastroenterology* 67:912, 1974.

36. Guerrero, I. C., Weniger, B. C., and Schultz, M. G. Transfusion malaria in the United States, 1972–1981. *Ann. Intern. Med.* 99:221, 1983.

37. Guideline for prevention of infections related to intravascular pressure-monitoring systems. *Infect. Control* 3:61, 1982.

38. Hendley, J. O. Epidemic keratoconjunctivitis and hand washing. *N. Engl. J. Med.* 289:1368, 1973.

39. Hess, J., Holloway, Y., and Dankert, J. Incidence of postextraction bacteremia under penicillin cover in children with cardiac disease. *Pediatrics* 71:554, 1983.

40. Hoffman, P. C., Arnow, P. M., Goldmann, D. A., Parrott, P. L., Stamm, W. E., and McGowan, J. E. False-positive blood cultures: Association with nonsterile blood collection tubes. *J.A.M.A.* 236:2073, 1976.

41. Jacoby, G. A., Hunt, J. V., Kosinski, K. S., Demirjian, Z. N., Huggins, C., Etkind, P., Marcus, L. C., and Spielman, A. Treatment of transfusion-transmitted babesiosis by exchange transfusion. *N. Engl. J. Med.* 303:1098, 1980.

42. James, H. E., Walsh, J. W., Wilson, H. D., et al. Prospective randomized study of therapy in cerebrospinal fluid shunt infection. *Neurosurgery* 7:459, 1980.

43. James, J. D. Bacterial contamination of preserved blood. *Vox Sang.* 4:177, 1959.

44. Katz, L., Johnson, D. L., Neufeld, P. D., and Gupta, K. G. Evacuated blood-collection tubes: The backflow hazard. *Can. Med. Assoc. J.* 113:208, 1975.

45. Kimball, A. C., Kean, B. H., and Kellner, A. The risk of transmitting toxoplasmosis by blood transfusion. *Transfusion* 5:447, 1965.

46. Krauss, A. N., Albert, R. F., and Kannan, M. M. Contamination of umbilical catheters in the newborn infant. *J. Pediatr.* 77:965, 1970.

47. Kundsin, R. B., and Walter, C. W. Detection of endotoxin on sterile catheters used for cardiac catheterization. *J. Clin. Microbiol.* 11:209, 1980.

48. Kure, R., Grendahl, H., and Paulssen, J. Pyrogens from surgeons' sterile latex gloves. *Acta. Pathol. Microbiol. Immunol. Scand.* 90:85, 1982.

49. Kuritsky, J. N., Bullen, M. G., Broome, C. V., Silcox, V. A., Good, R. C., and Wallace, R. J. Sternal wound infections and endocarditis due to organisms of the *Mycobacterium fortuitum* complex. *Ann. Intern. Med.* 98:938, 1983.

50. LeFrock, J. L. Ellis, C.A., Turchik, J. B., and Weinstein, L. Transient bacteremia associated with sigmoidoscopy. *N. Engl. J. Med.* 289:467, 1973.

51. LeFrock, J. L., Ellis, C. A., Turchik, J. B., Zawacki, J. K., and Weinstein, L. Transient bacteremia associated with percutaneous liver biopsy. *J. Infect. Dis.* 131(Suppl.):104, 1975.

52. Low, D. E., Micflikier, A. B., Kennedy, J. K., and Stiver, H. G. Infectious complications of endoscopic retrograde cholangiopancreatography: A prospective assessment. *Arch. Intern. Med.* 140:1076, 1980.

53. Lowy, F. D., Chang, D. S., Neuhaus, E. G., Horne, D. S., Tomasz, A., and Steigbigel, N. H. Effect of penicillin on the adherence of *Streptococcus sanguis* in vitro and in the rabbit model of endocarditis. *J. Clin. Invest.* 71:668,1983.

54. Luthardt, T. Bacterial infections in ventriculo-auricular shunt systems. *Dev. Med. Child Neurol. (Suppl.)* 12:105, 1970.

55. Maki, D. G., and Hassemer, C. A. Endemic rate of fluid contamination and related septicemia in arterial pressure monitoring. *Am. J. Med.* 733:207, 1981.

56. McCloskey, R. V., Gold, M., and Weser, E. Bacteremia after liver biopsy. *Arch. Intern. Med.* 132:213, 1973.

57. Mendelson, C. L. The aspiration of stomach contents into the lungs during obstetric anesthesia. *Am. J. Obstet. Gynecol.* 52:191, 1946.

58. Meyers, P. H., and Richards, M. Transmission of polio virus vaccine by contaminated barium enema with resultant antibody rise. *Am. J. Roentgenol. Radium Ther. Nucl. Med.* 91:864, 1964.

59. Michel, L., Marsh, M., McMichan, J. C., Southorn, P. A., and Brewer, N. S. Infection of pulmonary artery catheters in critically ill patients. *J.A.M.A.* 245:1032, 1981.

60. Nelson, K. E., Larson, P. A., Schraufnagel, D. E., and Jackson, J. Transmission of tuberculosis by flexible fiberbronchoscopes. *Am. Rev. Respir. Dis.* 127:97, 1983.

61. Oakley, C., and Somerville, W. Prevention of infective endocarditis. *Br. Heart J.* 45:233, 1981.

62. Pelican, G., Hentges, D., and Butt, J. H. Bacteremia during colonoscopy. *Gastrointest. Endosc.* 22:233, 1976.

63. Pereira, W., Kovnat, D. M., Khan, M. A., Iacovino, J. R., Spivack, M. L., and Snider, G. L. Fever and pneumonia after flexible fiberoptic bronchoscopy. *Am. Rev. Respir. Dis.* 112:59, 1975.

64. Powers, W. F., and Tooley, W. H. Contamination of umbilical vessel catheters. *Pediatrics* 48:470, 1971.

65. Reyes, M. P., Ganguly, S., Fowler, M., Brown, W. J., Gatmaitan, B. G., Friedman, C., and Lerner, A. M. Pyrogenic reactions after inadvertent infusion of endotoxin during cardiac catheterizations. *Ann. Intern. Med.* 93:32, 1980.

66. Rhame, F. S., and McCullough, J. Follow-up on nosocomial *Pseudomonas cepacia* infection. *Morbid. Mortal. Weekly Rep.* 28:409, 1979.

67. Rhame, F. S., Root, R. K., MacLowry, J. D., Dadisman, T. A., and Bennett, J. V. *Salmonella* septicemia from platelet transfusions. *Ann. Intern. Med.* 78:633, 1973.

68. Rubin, J., Oreoponlos, D. G., Lio, T. T., Matthews, R., and deVeber, G. A. Management of peritonitis and bowel perforation during chronic peritoneal dialysis. *Nephron* 16:220, 1976.

69. Sande, M. A., Levinson, M. E., Lukas, D. S., and Kaye, D. Bacteremia associated with cardiac catheterization. *N. Engl. J. Med.* 281:1104, 1969.

70. Schoenbaum, S. C., Gardner, P., and Shillito, J. Infections of cerebrospinal fluid shunts. *J. Infect. Dis.* 131:543, 1975.

71. Schroeder, S. A., Marton, K. I., and Strom, B. L. Frequency and morbidity of invasive procedures: Report of a pilot study from two teaching hospitals. *Arch. Intern. Med.* 138:1809, 1978.

72. Schwesinger, W. H., Levine, B. A., and Ramos, R. Complications in colonoscopy. *Surg. Gynecol. Obstet.* 148:270, 1979.

73. Sharbaugh, R. J. Suspected outbreak of endo-

toxemia associated with computerized axial tomography. *Am. J. Infect. Control* 8:26, 1980.

74. Sherwood, P. M. An outbreak of syringe-transmitted hepatitis with jaundice in hospitalized diabetic patients. *Ann. Intern. Med.* 33:380, 1950.

75. Shinozaki, T., Deane, R. S., Mazuzan, J. E., Hamel, A. J., and Hazelton, D. Bacterial contamination of arterial lines: A prospective study. *J.A.M.A.* 249:223, 1983.

76. Siegel, S. E., Lunde, M. N., Gelderman, A., Halterman, R. H., Brown, J. A., Levine, A. S., and Graw, R. G., Jr. Transmission of toxoplasmosis by leukocyte transfusion. *Blood* 37:388, 1971.

77. Stamm, W. E., Colella, J. J., Anderson, R. L., and Dixon, R. E. Indwelling arterial catheters as a source of nosocomial bacteremia. *N. Engl. J. Med.* 292:1099, 1975.

78. Steere, A. C., Tenney, J. H., Mackel, D. C., Snyder, M. J., Polakavetz, S., Dunne, M. E., and Dixon, R. E. *Pseudomonas* species bacteremia caused by contaminated normal human serum albumin. *J. Infect. Dis.* 135:729, 1977.

79. Stenhouse, M. A. E., and Milner, L. V. *Yersinia enterocolitica:* A hazard in blood transfusion. *Transfusion* 22:396, 1982.

80. Sullivan, N. M., Sutter, V. L., Carter, W. T., Attebery, H. R., and Finegold, S. M. Bacteremia after genitourinary tract manipulation. *Appl. Microbiol.* 23:1101, 1972.

81. Tabor, E. *Infectious Complications of Blood Transfusions.* New York: Academic, 1982.

82. Trump, D. L., Grossman, S. A., Thompson, G., and Murray, K. CSF infections complicating the management of neoplastic meningitis. *Arch. Intern. Med.* 142:583, 1982.

83. Walton, J. R., Shapiro, B. A., and Harrison, R. A. *Serratia* bacteremia from mean arterial pressure monitors. *Anesthesiology* 43:113, 1975.

84. Washington, J. A. The microbiology of evacuated blood collection tubes. *Ann. Intern. Med.* 86:186, 1977.

85. Weinstein, R. A. The design of pressure monitoring devices. *Med. Instrum.* 10:287, 1976.

86. Weinstein, R. A., Stamm, W. E., Kramer, L., and Corey, L. Pressure monitoring devices: Overlooked source of nosocomial infection. *J.A.M.A.* 236:936, 1976.

87. Weiss, S. R., and Raskind, R. Further experience with the ventriculoperitoneal shunt. *Int. Surg.* 53:300, 1970.

88. Wenzel, R. P., Osterman, C. A., Donowitz, L. G., Hoyt, J. W., Sande, M. A., Martone, W. J., Peacock, J. E., Levine, J. I., and Miller, G. B. Identification of procedure-related nosocomial infections in high-risk patients. *Rev. Infect. Dis.* 3:701, 1981.

89. Wittner, M., Rowin, K. S., Tanowitz, H. B., Hobbs, J. F., Saltzman, S., Wenz, B., Hirsch, R., Chisholm, E., and Healy, G. R. Successful chemotherapy of transfusion babesiosis. *Ann. Intern. Med.* 96:601, 1982.

# INDEX

# INDEX